TAYLOR'S MANUAL OF FAMILY MEDICINE

Third Edition

TAYLOR'S MANUAL OF FAMILY MEDICINE
Third Edition

Editors

Paul M. Paulman, MD
Professor/ Predoctoral Director
Assistant Dean for Clinical Skills and Quality
Department of Family Medicine
University of Nebraska Medical Center
Omaha, Nebraska

Audrey A. Paulman, MD
Clinical Associate Professor
Department of Family Medicine
University of Nebraska Medical Center
Omaha, Nebraska

Jeffrey D. Harrison, MD
Associate Professor/Program Director
Department of Family Medicine
University of Nebraska Medical Center
Omaha, Nebraska

With 201 Contributors

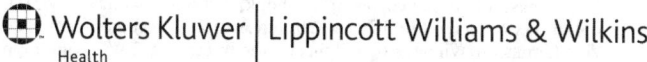

Wolters Kluwer | Lippincott Williams & Wilkins
Health
Philadelphia • Baltimore • New York • London
Buenos Aires • Hong Kong • Sydney • Tokyo

Acquisitions Editor: Sonya Siegafuse
Managing Editor: Dave Murphy
Marketing Manager: Kimberly Schonberger
Project Manager: Alicia Jackson
Manufacturing Coordinator: Kathleen Brown
Cover Designer: Becky Baxendell
Design Coordinator: Terry Mallon
Production Services: International Typesetting and Composition

3rd Edition
© 2008 by **Lippincott Williams & Wilkins, a Wolters Kluwer business**
530 Walnut Street
Philadelphia, PA 19106
LWW.com

Printed in the USA

Library of Congress Cataloging-in-Publication Data

Taylor's manual of family medicine / editors, Paul M. Paulman, Audrey A.
Paulman, Jeffrey D. Harrison ; with 195 contributors. —3rd ed.
    p. ; cm.
  Rev. ed. of: Manual of family practice / editor, Robert B. Taylor. 2nd
ed. c2002.
  Includes bibliographical references and index.
  ISBN-13: 978-0-7817-6654-8
  ISBN-10: 0-7817-6654-0
  1. Family medicine—Handbooks, manuals, etc.   I. Taylor, Robert B.   II.
Paulman, Paul M., 1953-   III. Paulman, Audrey A.   IV. Harrison, Jeffrey D.
V. Manual of family practice.   VI. Title: Manual of family medicine.
  [DNLM: 1. Family Practice—methods—Handbooks.   WB 39 T246 2008]
  RC55.M266 2008
  616—dc22
                                                            2007022191

Care has been taken to confirm the accuracy of the information presented and to describe generally accepted practices. However, the authors, editors, and publisher are not responsible for errors or omissions or for any consequences from application of the information in this book and make no warranty, expressed or implied, with respect to the currency, completeness, or accuracy of the contents of the publication. Application of this information in a particular situation remains the professional responsibility of the practitioner.

The authors, editors, and publisher have exerted every effort to ensure that drug selection and dosage set forth in this text are in accordance with current recommendations and practice at the time of publication. However, in view of ongoing research, changes in government regulations, and the constant flow of information relating to drug therapy and drug reactions, the reader is urged to check the package insert for each drug for any change in indications and dosage and for added warnings and precautions. This is particularly important when the recommended agent is a new or infrequently employed drug.

Some drugs and medical devices presented in this publication have Food and Drug Administration (FDA) clearance for limited use in restricted research settings. It is the responsibility of health care providers to ascertain the FDA status of each drug or device planned for use in their clinical practice.

The publishers have made every effort to trace copyright holders for borrowed material. If they have inadvertently overlooked any, they will be pleased to make the necessary arrangements at the first opportunity.

To purchase additional copies of this book, call our customer service department at (800) 638-3030 or fax orders to (301) 223-2320. International customers should call (301) 223-2300.

Visit Lippincott Williams & Wilkins on the Internet: at LWW.com. Lippincott Williams & Wilkins customer service representatives are available from 8:30 am to 6:00 pm, EST.

10 9 8 7 6 5 4 3 2 1

The editors would like to dedicate this book to Baby Boy Bryan, who grew along with the Manual, and who delayed his entry into the world long enough to allow his mother to help finish this book.

Alan M. Adelman, MD, MS
Jeanne L. and Thomas L. Professor
Department of Family and Community
Medicine
Pennsylvania State University
College of Medicine
Hershey, Pennsylvania

William A. Alto MD, MPH
Professor
Department of Community and Family
Medicine
Dartmouth Medical School
Hanover, New Hampshire

Navin M. Amin, MD, FAAFP
Associate Professor of Medicine
Department of Family Medicine
University of California Los Angeles
Los Angeles, California

Matthew R. Anderson, MD, MSc
Assistant Professor
Department of Family and Social Medicine
Albert Einstein College of Medicine
Bronx, New York

Kavitha K. Arabindoo, MD
Clinical Assistant Professor
Department of Family and Community
Medicine
University of Kansas Medical Center
School of Medicine
Wichita, Kansas

Elisabeth L. Backer
Clinical Associate Professor
Department of Family Medicine
University of Nebraska Medical Center
Omaha, Nebraska

Robert A. Baldor, MD
Professor and Vice-Chairman
Department of Family Medicine
and Community Health
University of Massachusetts Medical School
Worcester, Massachusetts

Denise D. Barnard, MD
Professor of Medicine
Department of Medicine/Cardiology
University of California San Diego
San Diego, California

Dennis J. Baumgardner, MD
Professor
Department of Family Medicine
University of Wisconsin School of Medicine
and Public Health
Milwaukee, Wisconsin

Keely J. Beam, Ed. S
Iowa Area Education Association
Red Oak, Iowa

Marvin Moe Bell, MD, MPH
Clinical Professor
Family and Community Medicine
University of Arizona
College of Medicine
Phoenix, Arizona

Michelle Anne Bholat, MD, MPH
Associate Professor
Department of Family Medicine
David Geffen School of Medicine
University of California Los Angeles
Los Angeles, California

Komalpreet Bhuller, MD
HOII, Second Year House Officer
Department of Family Medicine
University of Nebraska Medical
Center
Omaha, Nebraska

Shawn H. Blanchard, MD
Professor
Department of Family Medicine
Oregon Health and Science University
Portland, Oregon

Jennifer W. Boyden, MD
Assistant Professor of Family
Medicine
Department of Family Medicine
Mayo Clinic College of Medicine
Scottsdale, Arizona

Rachel Bramson, MD, MS
Associate Professor
Department of Family Medicine
Texas A & M University System Health
Science Center
College of Medicine
College Station, Texas

Dan Brewer, MD
Associate Professor
Department of Family Medicine
University of Tennessee
Knoxville, Tennessee

Dawn Brink-Cymerman, MD
Assistant Professor
Department of Family Medicine
SUNY Health Science Center
Syracuse, New York

Cory A. Brown, MD
School of Medicine
George Washington University
Washington, District of Columbia

Michael L. Brown, MD
Assistant Professor
Department of Psychiatry
Texas A & M University System Health
Science Center
College of Medicine
College Station, Texas

Bruce M. Bushwick, MD
Assistant Clinical Professor of Family
and Community Medicine
Department of Family Practice and
Community Medicine
Penn State College of Medicine
Milton S. Hershey Medical Center
Hershey, Pennsylvania

Laurie Carrier, MD
Resident
Family Medicine/Psychiatry
University of Cincinnati
Cincinnati, Ohio

Michael J. Cascio, MD

Jacintha S. Cauffield, Pharm.D., BCPS
Clinical Specialist-Ambulatory Care
Pharmacist Clinical Pharmacy Fellow in
Pharmacy Practice & Family Medicine
South West Washington Medical Center
Vancouver, Washington

S. Shekar Chakravarthi, MD
Medical Director
Senior Services
Hunterdon Medical Center
Flemington, New Jersey

Linda F. Chang, MD
Clinical Assistant Professor
Department of Family/Community Medicine
University of Illinois
College of Medicine
Rockford, Illinois

Jason Chao, MD, MS
Professor
Department of Family Medicine
Case Western Reserve University
Cleveland, Ohio

William E. Chavey, MD, MS
Assistant Professor
Department of Family Medicine
University of Michigan
Ann Arbor, Michigan

Joseph T. Cheatle
University of Nebraska College
of Medicine
Omaha, Nebraska

S. Lindsey Clarke, MD, FAAFP
Self Regional Healthcare
Ware Shoals Center for Family Medicine
Greenwood, South Carolina

Deborah S. Clements, MD
Associate Professor and Association Program
Director of Family Medicine
University of Kansas Medical Center
Ohio, Kansas

Brian Coleman, MD
Associate Professor
Department of Family Medicine
University of Oklahoma Health Science Center
Oklahoma City, Oklahoma

Maria R. Conroy, MD
OSU Family Practice at Gahanna
Gahanna, Ohio

Carol Cordy, MD
Clinical Associate Professor
Department of Family Medicine
University of Washington
Seattle, Washington

J. Steven Cramer, MD
Clinical Associate Professor of Family
Medicine
University at Buffalo
Buffalo, New York

Steven Crossman, MD
Clinical Assistant Professor
Department of Family Medicine
Virginia Commonwealth University
Richmond, Virginia

Peggy R. Cyr, MD
Associate Clinical Professor
Department of Family Medicine
University of Vermont
Burlington, Vermont

Mel P. Daly, MD, CMD, AGSF
Associate Professor of Medicine
Johns Hopkins University
School of Medicine
Baltimore, Maryland

Marilyn S. Darr, MD, PharmD
Associate Program Director
Family Medicine of Southwest Washington
Vancouver, Washington

Paul Dassow, MD, MSPH
Assistant Professor
Department of Family and Community
Medicine
University of Kentucky
Lexington, Kentucky

John E. Delzell, Jr., MD, MSPH
Associate Professor
Department of Family Medicine
Kansas University School of Medicine
Kansas City, Kansas

Lisa G. Dodson, MD
Assistant Professor
Department of Family Medicine
Oregon Health and Science University
Portland, Oregon

Patrick T. Dowling, MD, MPH
Professor and Chair
Department of Family Medicine
David Geffen School of Medicine
at UCLA
Los Angeles, California

Pamela Dull, MD
Associate Clinical Professor
Department of Family Medicine
Ohio State University
Columbus, Ohio

Kristy D. Edwards, MD
Assistant Professor
Department of Family Medicine
University of Nebraska College
of Medicine
Omaha, Nebraska

Nancy C. Elder, MD, MSPH
Associate Professor
Department of Family Medicine
University of Cincinnati
Cincinnati, Ohio

Ed Evans, MD
Program Director
Seneca Lakes Family Medicine Residency
Seneca, South Carolina

Paul Evans, DO
Vice Dean
Professor of Family Medicine
Georgia Campus
Philadelphia College of Osteopathic Medicine
Suwanee, Georgia

Ashley J. Falk, MD
Staff Family Physician
Urgent Care Clinic
Erling Bergquist Clinic
Offutt AFB, Nebraska

Nathan P. Falk, MD
Resident Family Physician
Department of Family Medicine
University of Nebraska Medical Center
Omaha, Nebraska

Jessica Farnsworth, MD
Fellow
Department of Family Medicine
The Nebraska Medical Center
Omaha, Nebraska

Brian J. Finley, MD
Assistant Professor
Department of Family Medicine
The Nebraska Medical Center,
Omaha, Nebraska

Carey Christiansen Ford, MD
Assistant Professor
Department of Family Medicine
University of Nebraska Medical Center
Omaha, Nebraska

Thomas Paul Forks, MD
Family Medicine
Brandon, Mississippi

Peter Forman, MD
Director Predoctoral Education
Family and Community Medicine
Albany Medical College
Albany, New York

Keith A. Frey, MD, MBA
Associate Professor
Department of Family Medicine
Mayo Clinic College of Medicine
Rochester, Minnesota

John D. Gazewood, MD, MSPH
Harrison Medical Teaching Associate
Professor
Department of Family Medicine
University of Virginia Health System
Charlottesville, Virginia

Dena L. George, MD
Resident
Family Medicine Residency Center
Carl R. Darnall Army Medical Center
Fort Hood, Texas

Aman Gill, MD
Assistant Professor
Interventional Radiology
University of Texas Medical Branch
Galveston, Texas

John R. Gimpel, DO, M Ed
Associate Professor
Department of Family Medicine
Georgetown University School
of Medicine
Washington, District of Columbia

Dwenda K. Gjerdingen, MD, MS
Professor
Department of Family Medicine &
Community Health
University of Minnesota
Minneapolis, Minnesota

Kristen H. Goodell, DM
Clinical Associate
Department of Public Health and Family
Medicine
Tufts University Family Medicine Residency
Walden, Massachusetts

Pepi Granat, MD
Voluntary Professor of Family Medicine
and Community Health
Department of Family Medicine
University of Miami
Miami, Florida

Joseph W. Gravel, Jr. MD
Residency Program Director
Tufts University Family Medicine Residency
Walden, Massachusetts

Lee A. Green, MD, MPH
Associate Professor
Department of Family Medicine
University of Michigan Medical School
Ann Arbor, Michigan

Michael A. Greene, MD
HOI
Department of Family Medicine
University of Nebraska Medical Center
Omaha, Nebraska

James L. Greenwald, MD
Associate Professor
Director, RMED
Department of Family Medicine
SUNY Upstate Medical University
Syracuse, New York

Samuel N. Grief, MD, FCFP
Assistant Professor in Clinical
Family Medicine
Department of Family Medicine
University of Illinois at Chicago
Chicago, Illinois

James K. Gude, MD
Clinical Professor, Departments of Medicine
and of Family & Community Medicine
University of California—San Francisco
School of Medicine,
San Francisco, California

Cecilia A. Gutierrez, MD
Associate Clinical Professor
Department of Family & Preventive Medicine
UCSD School of Medicine
San Diego, California

John G. Halvorsen, MD, MS
Thomas and Ellen Foster Chair and Professor
Department of Family and Community
Medicine
University of Illinois College of Medicine
Peoria, Illinois

Jimmy H. Hara, MD
Associate Clinical Professor
Family Medicine Department
David Gefffen School of Medicine
University of California Los Angeles
Los Angeles, California

Kathryn W. Hare, MD
Resident
Department of Family Medicine
Fairfax Family Practice
Fairfax, Virginia

Jefferey D. Harrison, MD
Associate Professor
Program Director
Department of Family Medicine
University of Nebraska Medical Center
Omaha, Nebraska

Russell Harrison, MD
Malmstrom, AFB, Montana

Meg Hayes, MD
Assistant Professor of Family Medicine
Medical Director, OHSU Family Medicine
at Marquam Hill
Portland, Oregon

John M. Heath MD, AGSF
Associate Professor
Department of Family Medicine Center
for Healthy Aging at Parker Stonegate
Robert Wood Johnson Medical School
New Brunswick, New Jersey

Fred E. Heidrich, MD, MPH
Clinical Professor
Department of Family Medicine
University of Washington
Seattle, Washington

James J. Helmer, MD
Assistant Clinical Professor
Department of Family and Community
Medicine
University of California
San Francisco, California

Michael J. Henehan, DO
Stanford University School of Medicine
Stanford, California

Charles E. Henley, DO, MPH
Professor and Vice Chair
Department of Family Medicine
University of Oklahoma College
of Medicine—Tulsa
Tulsa, Oklahoma

Joseph Hobbs, MD
Professor
Department of Family Medicine
Medical College of Georgia
Augusta, Georgia

William J. Hueston, MD
Professor and Chair
Department of Family Medicine
Medical University of South Carolina
Charleston, South Carolina

Scott W. Hughes, MD
HOII
Department of Family Medicine
University of Nebraska Medical Center
Omaha, Nebraska

Daniel G. Hunter-Smith, MD
Associate Professor
Department of Family Medicine
Rush Medical College
Chicago, Illinois

Douglas J. Inciarte, MD
HOIII
Department of Family Medicine
University of Nebraska Medical Center
Omaha, Nebraska

James W. Jarvis, MD, FAAFP
Associate Professor
Department of Family Medicine
Medical University of South Carolina
Greenwood, South Carolina

Kimberly J. Jarzynka, MD
Assistant Professor
Department of Family Medicine
University of Nebraska Medical Center
Omaha, Nebraska

Jeffrey G. Jones, MD, MPH, MSc
Medical Director
Travel Medicine
St. Francis Hospital
Indianapolis, Indiana

Sarah S. Jones, MD
Assistant Professor of Family Medicine
Department of Family Medicine
Uniformed Services
University of the Health Sciences
Bethesda, Maryland
Associate Program Director
Department of Family Medicine
David Grant Medical Center
Travis Air Force Base, California

Jennifer M. Joyce, MD
Associate Professor
Department of Family and Community
Medicine
University of Kentucky
Lexington, Kentucky

Daphne J. Karel, MD
Associate Professor
Department of Family Medicine
Medical University of South Carolina
Greenwood, South Carolina

Kenneth F. Kessel, MD
Professor
Department of Family Medicine
Rush Medical College
Chicago, Illinois

Mitchell S. King, MD
Associate Professor
Department of Family Medicine
University of Illinois
College of Medicine
Rockford, Illinois

Jeffrey T. Kirchner, DO
Clinical Associate Professor
Department of Family and Community
Medicine
Temple University School of Medicine
Philadelphia, Pennsylvania

George L. Kirkpatrick, MD
Emergency Department Physician
Mobile Infirmary Medical Center
Mobile, Alabama

Wendy Kohatsu, MD
Assistant Professor
Department of Family Medicine
Oregon Health and Sciences University
Portland, Oregon

Peter B. Kozisek, MD
Associate Program Director
Family Medicine Residency of Idaho
Boise, Idaho

Valerie B. Laing, MD
Affiliate Associate Professor
Department of Medicine/Dermatology
The Brody School of Medicine at East
Carolina University
Greenville, North Carolina

Walter L. Larimore, MD
Assistant Clinical Professor
Department of Family Medicine
University of Colorado Health Sciences Center
Denver, Colorado

Lars C. Larsen, MD
Professor
Department of Family Medicine
The Brody School of Medicine at East
Carolina University
Greenville, North Carolina

Kathryn E. Lazure
University of Nebraska College of Medicine,
Omaha, Nebraska

Kim E. LeBlanc, MD
Marie Lahansky Professor and Chairman
Department of Family Medicine
Louisiana State University Health
Sciences Center
New Orleans, Louisiana

Daniel T. Lee, MD
Associate Clinical Professor
Department of Family Medicine
David Geffen School of Medicine at UCLA
Los Angeles, California

William T. Leslie, MD
Assistant Professor
Division of Hematology/Oncology
Rush University Medical Center
Chicago, Illinois

Edward J. Lewis, MD

Jinn Liu, MD
Resident
Department of Family Medicine
Abington Memorial Hospital
Abington, Pennsylvania

Alison E. Lux, MD
Assistant Professor
Department of Family Medicine
University of Wisconsin
Milwaukee, Wisconsin

Paul E. Lyons, MD
Associate Chair
Department of Family and Community
Medicine
Temple University Hospital
Philadelphia, Pennsylvania

Megan R. Mahoney, MD
Assistant Clinical Professor
Department of Family and Community
Medicine
University of California at San Francisco
San Francisco, California

Russell G. Maier, MD
Residency Director
Central Washington Family Medicine
Yakima, Washington

Robert Mallin, MD
Associate Professor
Department of Family Medicine
Medical University of South Carolina
Charleston, South Carolina

Katherine L. Margo, MD
Predoctoral Director
Department of Family Medicine
and Community Health
University of Pennsylvania School of Medicine
Philadelphia, Pennsylvania

Thomas D. Masten, MD
Clinical Associate Professor of Physical
Medicine and Rehabilitation
Department of Family Medicine
and Orthopedics
Upstate Medical University
Syracuse, New York

Richard C. Mauer, MD
Ophthalmologist
Department of Surgery
Covenant Medical Center
Waterloo, Iowa

Todd A. May, MD
Associate Clinical Professor
Department of Family and Community
Medicine
University of California, San Francisco
San Francisco, California

Mary McDonald, MD
Assistant Professor
Department of Family Medicine
University of Kansas School of Medicine
Kansas City, Kansas

Donald B. Middleton, MD
Professor
Department of Family Medicine
University of Pittsburgh
Pittsburgh, Pennsylvania

Glenn D. Miller, MD
Associate Professor of Clinical Family
Department of Family and Community
Medicine
University of Illinois
College of Medicine at Peoria
Peoria, Illinois

Donald B. Milligan, MD, FAAFP, AAPM
Assistant Professor in Family Medicine
Chair, Committee on Pharmacy
and Therapeutics
University of Kansas Medical Center
Kansas City, Kansas

Stephen R. Mitchell, MD, FACP
Dean for Medical Education
Georgetown University School of Medicine
Washington, District of Columbia

Norman Montalto, MD
Professor
Department of Family Medicine
West Virginia University
Charleston Division
Charleston, West Virginia

Eric D. Morgan, MD, MPH
Commander
California Medical Department
Monterey, California

Karen E. Muchowski, MD
Family Physicians Group
Vancouver, Washington

Mary C. Murphy, MD
Assistant Clinical Professor
Department of Family and Community
Medicine
University of California, San Francisco
San Francisco, California

Jason L. Musser, DO
Family Medicine Resident
Department of Family Medicine
University of Nebraska Medical Center
Omaha, Nebraska

Randall H. Neal, MD, Col. USAF
Adjunct Associate Professor
Department of Family Medicine
University of Nebraska Medical Center
Omaha, Nebraska

Jon O. Neher, MD
Clinical Professor
Department of Family Medicine
University of Washington
Seattle, Washington

Gary R. Newkirk, MD
Clinical Professor of Family Medicine
Director, Family Medicine Spokane and Rural
Training Residencies
Spokane, Washington

Trang H. Nguyen, MD
Assistant Professor
Department of Family Practice and
Community Medicine,
UT Southwestern Medical Center
Dallas, Texas

Carole V. Nistler, MD
Olmsted Medical Center
Rochester, Minnesota

Michael L. O'Dell, MD, MSHA, FAAFP
Chair and Program Director
Department of Family Medicine
North Mississippi Medical Center
Tupelo, Mississippi

Sandra Christina Ogata, MD

Cynthia G. Olsen, MD
Professor & Executive Vice-Chair
Department of Family Medicine
Wright State University School of Medicine
Dayton, Ohio

Eugene Orientale, Jr., MD
Associate Professor
Department of Family Medicine
University of Connecticut Health Center
Farmington, Connecticut

Susan M. Ott, MD
Associate Professor
Department of Medicine
University of Washington
Seattle, Washington

Kalpana P. Padala, MD
Fellow in Geriatric Medicine
University of Nebraska Medical Center
Omaha, Nebraska

Prasad R. Padala, MD
Program Director
Geriatric Psychiatry Fellowship
Staff Psychiatrist
University of Nebraska Medical Center
The Veterans Affairs Medical Center
Omaha, Nebraska

Heather L. Paladine, MD
Visiting Assistant Professor of Clinical
Family Medicine
Department of Family Medicine
University of Southern California
Keck School of Medicine
Los Angeles, California

Pamela D. Parker, MD
Staff Physician
Department of Obstetrics and Gynecology
Memorial Hospital
Colorado Springs, Colorado

Douglas S. Parks, MD
Associate Professor
Family Practice Residency
University of Wyoming
Cheyenne, Wyoming

Sarah Parrott, DO
Assistant Professor
Department of Family Medicine
University of Kansas School of Medicine
Kansas City, Kansas

Nicole N. Paulman, MD
Resident Physician
Internal Medicine
University of Nebraska Medical Center
Omaha, Nebraska

Roger A. Paulman, MD
Resident Physician
Clarkson Family Medicine
The Nebraska Medical Center
Omaha, Nebraska

Kevin A. Pearce, MD, MPH
Professor
Department of Family and Community
Medicine
University of Kentucky
Lexington, Kentucky

Mhroos Peters, MD
Family Medicine Resident
University of Cincinnati
Cincinnati, Ohio

Michael B. Potter, MD
Associate Professor
Department of Family and Community
Medicine
University of California
San Francisco, California

Richard W. Pretorius, MD, MPH
Vice Chair for Medical Student Education
Department of Family Medicine
State University of New York at Buffalo
Buffalo, New York

Janey M. Purvis, MD
Adjunct Assistant Professor
Department of Family Medicine
Oregon Health and Sciences University
Portland, Oregon

Martin A. Quan, MD
Professor of Clinical Family Medicine
Department of Family Medicine
David Geffen School of Medicine at UCLA
Los Angeles, California

Kalyanakrishnan Ramakrishnan
Associate Professor
Department of Family Medicine
University of Oklahoma Health Science Center
Oklahoma City, Oklahoma

David C. Randolph

Joshua J. Raymond, MD
Assistant Professor
Robert Wood Johnson Medical
School/UMDNJ
Centrastate Healthcare Systems
Freehold, New Jersey

Carrie Riah

James P. Richardson, MD, MPH, AGSF
Clinical Professor
Department of Family Medicine
University of Maryland School of Medicine
Baltimore, Maryland

Mari A. Ricker, MD
Faculty Physician
Department of Family Medicine
Providence Milwaukie Hospital
Family Medicine Residency
Milwaukie, Oregon

Jonathan J. Rodnick, MD
Professor
Department of Family and Community
Medicine
University of California
San Francisco, California

Robert Ross, MD

Quinn Saigh

Shikar Saxena

Ted C. Schaffer, MD

Jeffery D. Schlaudecker, MD
Chief Resident
Department of Family Medicine
University of Cincinnati
Cincinnati, Ohio

L. Peter Schwiebert, MD
Professor
Family Medicine
University of Oklahoma Health Science
Center
Oklahama City, Oklahoma

Krupa Shah, MD
Resident Physician
Department of Family and Community
Medicine
Baylor College of Medicine
Houston, Texas

John P. Sheehan, MD
Assistant Clinical Professor
Department of Medicine
Case Western Reserve University
Cleveland, Ohio

Robert Sheeler, MD
Associate Professor
Department of Family Medicine
Mayo Clinic Graduate School
of Medicine
Rochester, Minnesota

Manel Silva

James W. Simmons, MD
Assistant Professor
Department of Family Medicine
University of Nebraska Medical Center
Omaha, Nebraska

William M. Simpson, Jr., MD
Professor of Family Medicine
Department of Family Medicine
Medical University of South
Carolina
Charleston, South Carolina

Ann K. Skelton, MD
Associate Clinical Professor
Department of Family Medicine
University of Vermont
Burlington, Vermont

Neil S. Skolnik, MD
Professor of Family and Community
Medicine
Temple University School of Medicine
Philadelphia, Pennsylvania

Charles Kent Smith, MD
Department of Family Medicine
Case Western Reserve University
Cleveland, Ohio

Christopher Smith, BS
College of Medicine
University of Nebraska Medical Center
Omaha, Nebraska

John L. Smith, MD
Assistant Professor
Department of Family Medicine
University of Nebraska Medical Center
Omaha, Nebraska

Ariel K. Smits, MD, MPH
Assistant Professor
Department of Family Medicine
Oregon Health and Science University
Portland, Oregon

Benjamin Soloman

Rhonda A. Sparks, MD
Associate Professor
Department of Family Medicine
University of Oklahoma Health Science Center
Oklahoma City, Oklahoma

Lois Starr

Elizabeth Steiner, MD
Research Assistant Professor
Department of Family Medicine
Oregon Health and Science University
Portland, Oregon

Curtis C. Stine, MD
Professor
Department of Family Medicine
and Rural Health
Florida State University
College of Medicine
Tallahassee, Florida

Denise K.C. Sur, MD
Vice Chair-Education, Associate Clinical
Professor
Department of Family Medicine
University of California
West Los Angeles, California

John E. Sutherland, MD
Clinical Professor
Department of Family Medicine
University of Iowa College of Medicine
Iowa City, Iowa

Angela W. Tang, MD
Associate Professor
Department of Medicine
David Geffen School of Medicine at UCLA
Los Angeles, California

Ruth E. Thatcher, MD
Assistant Professor
Department of Family Medicine
University of South Dakota
Sanford School of Medicine
Sioux Falls, South Dakota

William L. Toffler, MD
Professor
Department of Family Medicine
Oregon Health and Science University
Portland, Oregon

Michael L. Tuggy, MD
Clinical Associate Professor
Department of Family Medicine
University of Washington
Seattle, Washington

Marc Tunzi, MD
Assistant Clinical Professor
Department of Family and Community
Medicine
University of California
San Francisco, California

Amber M. Tyler, MD
Captain, United States Air Force Medical Corps
Family Medicine Resident
Department of Family Medicine
University of Nebraska Medical Center
Omaha, Nebraska

**Margaret M. Ulchaker, MSN, RN,
CDE, CNP, NP-C, BC-ADM**
Clinical Instructor
Department of Nursing
Case Western Reserve University
Cleveland, Ohio

Daniel J. Van Durme, MD, FAAFP
Professor and Chair
Department of Family Medicine
and Rural Health
Florida State University College of Medicine
Tallahassee, Florida

Edward C. Vincent, MD
Associate Clinical Professor, Department
of Family Medicine
University of Washington School
of Medicine
Seattle, Washington

Raymond R. Walker, MD, MBA
Associate Professor
Department of Family Medicine
University of Tennessee
Memphis, Tennessee

Anne D. Walling, MB, ChB
Professor
Department of Family and Community
Medicine
The University of Kansas School
of Medicine
Wichita, Kansas

Anne Walsh, PA-C, SCT (ASCP), MMSc
Clinical Instructor
Department of Family Medicine
University of Southern California
Los Angeles, California

Sally P. Weaver, MD, PhD
Research Director
Family Medicine Residency Program
McLennan County Medical Education
and Research Foundation
Waco, Texas

Stephanie L. Werner, MD
University of Nebraska Medical Center
Omaha, Nebraska

Joanne Williams

Pamela M. Williams, MD
Assistant Professor
Department of Family Medicine
Uniformed Services University of
the Health Sciences
Bethesda, Maryland

$\mathcal{T}$aylor's Manual of Family Medicine, third edition, is designed for the busy practitioner. The Manual is a point of care reference and will provide answers to the clinical questions most frequently encountered by the family physician and other generalists.

The editors and authors of the Manual have made every effort to preserve the practical style and format promulgated by Dr. Robert Taylor in the second edition of the Manual. New chapters "Bronchospasm," "Hematuria," and "Disability Determination" have been added, and some chapters have been removed, or their content assigned to other pertinent chapters. All chapters in this edition of the Manual have been updated with the latest clinical information and evidence, including electronic information resources.

The Manual's content emphasizes ambulatory care, with reference as appropriate to hospital, extended care facility, or home care, and emphasizes the family physician's approach to clinical problems. Throughout the Manual you will find information about the treatment, management, and prevention of commonly encountered clinical problems.

The Manual's chapter topics and information are also designed to assist the health profession student, resident, or practitioner prepare for certification or recertification examinations.

The hundreds of authors contributing to this work have done a tremendous job bringing practical, easy to understand, clinically useful information to their chapters. The editors are grateful. We could not have produced this volume without the able help, dedication, and organizational skills of Sarah Bryan; thank you, Sarah. We also thank the faculty and staff at the University of Nebraska College of Medicine, Department of Family Medicine, for their help and support during the production of this book. The production staff at Lippincott Williams & Wilkins, led by David Murphy, were incredible partners in this effort, and we thank them.

We hope you find this edition of the Taylor's Manual of Family Medicine useful and that it will become the book you reach for when you have a clinical question in your busy practice.

Paul M. Paulman, MD
Audrey A. Paulman, MD, MMM
Jeffrey D. Harrison, MD
Editors

CONTENTS

X: RESPIRATORY PROBLEMS

XI: GASTROINTESTINAL PROBLEMS

XII: RENAL AND UROLOGIC PROBLEMS

XIII: PROBLEMS RELATED TO THE FEMALE REPRODUCTIVE SYSTEM

XIV: FAMILY PLANNING AND MATERNITY CARE

XV: MUSCULOSKELETAL PROBLEMS AND ARTHRITIS

XVI: DERMATOLOGIC PROBLEMS

XVII: ENDOCRINE AND METABOLIC DISORDERS

XVIII: DISORDERS OF THE BLOOD

XIX: INFECTIOUS DISEASES

XX: INJURIES AND VIOLENCE

XXI: OCCUPATIONAL AND ENVIRONMENTAL PROBLEMS

XXII: THERAPEUTIC CHOICES

Disease Presentation
and Health Screening

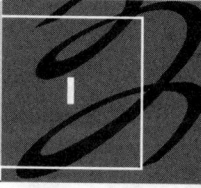

HEALTH MAINTENANCE FOR INFANTS AND CHILDREN
Russell Harrison

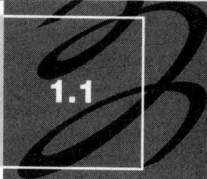

*H*ealth maintenance visits provide the physician with an excellent opportunity to practice preventative medicine and establish an ongoing relationship with the child and his or her family. At each visit, the child should be evaluated for early disease processes, and developmental and behavioral problems. In addition, the appropriate screening tests, immunizations, anticipatory guidance, and counseling must be provided. A good resource is the book Bright Futures: Guidelines for Health Supervision of Infants, Children, and Adolescents.

HISTORY AND PHYSICAL EXAMINATION

History

The initial history should address family history, social history, living environment, birth history, allergies, medications, and a complete medical history (including injuries, dietary history, growth, development, and behavioral problems). With each annual physical the history should be reviewed and updated for any changes.

Physical Examination

The physical examination should be complete, with particular attention to those aspects appropriate for the child's age.

Developmental Assessment

A child's developmental level should be assessed at each visit. The Denver Developmental Screening Test is a widely used assessment tool. Table 1.1-1 includes a listing of some developmental highlights that can be used for a rapid and informal developmental screening. Some questionnaires such as "Ages and Stages Questionnaires" can be purchased and may be used to help evaluate communication, gross motor, fine motor, problem-solving, and personal-social skills of children at different ages.

1

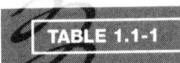

TABLE 1.1-1	Developmental Milestones[a]

Age	Developmental milestones
2 wk	Lifts head prone Follows to midline Responds to noise
2 mo	Smiles responsively Follows past midline Lifts head 45 degrees
4 mo	Grasps rattle Rolls over one way Laughs Squeals
6 mo	Sits briefly without support Reaches for objects Smiles spontaneously
9 mo	Transfers object from one hand to another Stands holding on Plays peek-a-boo Feeds self a cracker
1 yr	Stands momentarily Walks holding on to furniture Says mama, dada (now specific) Thumb-finger grasp
15 mo	Stands alone Walks alone Drinks from a cup Says three words other than mama, dada
18 mo	Mimics household chores (sweeping) Makes tower of two or three cubes Indicates wants
2 yr	Points to body parts Scribbles Handles a spoon well Says two-word sentences Kicks a ball

[a] These milestones should have been attained by 75% to 90% of children by the age indicated.

SCREENING

- Table 1.1-2 presents a summary of the screening recommendations outlined below.
- **Growth.** Measuring growth and following its progression over time can help identify significant childhood conditions. Height, weight, and head circumference should be measured at birth, at 2 to 4 weeks, and at 2, 4, 6, 9, 12, 15, 18, and 24 months of age. Height and weight should be measured at ages 3, 4, 5, 6, and every 2 years thereafter. Some disease-specific growth charts are available, for example, Down syndrome. See http://www.cdc.gov/growthcharts/.
- **Newborn screening.** Every state has its own regulations and, as such, clinicians should be familiar with their own state's guidelines and screen accordingly. Most states screen for at least phenylketonuria (PKU), congenital hypothyroidism, galactosemia, and sickle cell disease. Infants screened for PKU earlier than 24 hours after birth should be screened again before the second week of life. Primary care physicians must be aware

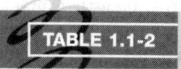

TABLE 1.1-2	Recommended Childhood Prevention Screening

Test/examination	Screening recommendation
Blood pressure	Age 3 and every 1–2 yr thereafter
Hearing	Newborn hearing screen, subjective assessment at all visits
Vision	Red reflex and corneal light reflex during first week of life and at 6 mo; visual acuity and cover–uncover at 3 yr and 5–6 yr
Anemia	Age 9 mo and consider repeat at 3–4 yr
Tuberculosis	No routine screening; annually in high-risk populations
Lead	Blood testing at 1 yr and again at 2 yr of age or screen based on high-risk exposure; screen with questionnaire at 6 mo to 6 yr
Cholesterol	No routine screening
Urinalysis	Consider screening urinalysis in preschool children; AAP recommends universal screen 4–5 yr

that the expanded newborn screen can have up to 3% false-positive results.[1] This can lead to increased parental stress and increased hospitalization rates. Other commonly screened diseases include congenital adrenal hyperplasia, maple syrup urine disease, homocysteinurea, biotinidase deficiency, and cystic fibrosis. Web sites with more information include:

- http://genes-r-us.uthscsa.edu/
- http://www.newbornscreening.com/
- http://www.hhs.state.ne.us/nsp/physicians.htm

- **Blood pressure.** Blood pressure should be measured beginning at 3 years of age and every 1 to 2 years thereafter during routine office visits. Hypertension in children is defined as persistent blood pressure elevation at or above the 95th percentile according to gender and age.[2]
- **Hearing.** A subjective assessment of hearing, including checking for a response to noise produced outside an infant's field of vision, noting an absence of babbling at 6 months of age, assessing speech development, and inquiring about parental concerns, should be performed repeatedly, especially during the first year of life. Even though more than 30 states require universal newborn hearing screening, the U.S. Preventive Services Task Force (USPSTF) has stated that there is insufficient evidence to recommend for or against routine universal screening of all newborns. In low-risk infants the false-positive rate can be around 90%. Screening patients who are high risk for sensorineural hearing loss is effective. The American Academy of Pediatrics (AAP) supports universal newborn hearing screening and also recommends "periodic hearing screening for every child through adolescence" but does not define what screening should be done or when that screening should occur. See www.ahrq.gov/clinic/3rduspstf/newbornscreen/newhearrr.htm#section2.
- **Vision.** All children should be screened for a red reflex (looking for malignancy of the retina) and a symmetrical corneal light reflex (looking for esotropia) during the first week of life and again at 6 months of age. In the first year of life children should also be screened with the cover–uncover test. At age 3 years, a photoscreen is recommended by some groups. The AAP recommends picture tests, such as LH test or Allen cards, at age 3 to 4 years old. AAP also states that children over 4 years old can be screened with Snellen letters, Snellen numbers, and Tumbling E charts.[3]
- **Anemia.** All children should be screened for anemia using either hemoglobin or hematocrit testing at approximately 9 to 12 months of age. Preterm infants and low-birth-weight infants who are fed with low-iron formulas should be screened by 6 months of age. Children with the following risk factors should have a repeat screening for anemia

6 months after their initial screen: preterm or low-birth-weight infants, breastfed infants who do not receive iron-supplemented foods after 6 months of age, children who consume more than 24 ounces of cows milk a day after age 12 months, and infants in low-income families. The cutoff point for a diagnosis of anemia at this age is a hemoglobin below 11 g/dL or a hematocrit below 33.0%.[4] Cutoff points should be adjusted upward for children who live at high altitudes. Clinicians may also consider repeat screening at age 3 to 4 years. The cutoff point for this age is a hemoglobin of 11. 5 g/dL or a hematocrit of 34.0%.

- **Urinalysis.** There is no consensus on either the necessity or timing of screening urinalysis to detect hematuria, proteinuria, glucosuria, or occult infection. However, it may be clinically prudent to perform a screening urinalysis in preschool children. The AAP recommends universal screening of all children 4 to 5 years old. Midstream clean-catch specimens are best, and the use of a plastic bag applied to the perineum should be avoided.
- **Tuberculosis.** Annual tuberculosis (TB) testing is recommended for children in high-risk populations. High-risk questionnaire:
  - Does your child have regular contact with adults who are at high risk for tuberculosis (such as homeless or incarcerated persons, persons with HIV, persons who use illicit drugs)?
  - Has your child had contact with someone infected with tuberculosis?
  - Is your child infected with HIV or other immunosuppressive disorders?
  - Was any household member, including your child, born in an area where TB is common (i.e., Africa, Asia, Latin America, Caribbean)? or Has anyone in your family traveled to one of these areas?

- Yes to any of these questions necessitates screening. The Mantoux test (0.1 mL of purified protein derivative containing 5 tuberculin units injected intradermally) should be used as the screening test. The test should be read in 48 to 72 hours by measuring the diameter of induration. A reaction is generally considered positive if any of the following is true:
  - The diameter of induration is 5 mm or greater and there is known or suspected HIV infection, close contact with an individual who has infectious TB, or a chest radiograph likely to represent old, healed TB.
  - The diameter of induration is 10 mm or greater in children younger than 4 years and those at high risk for TB.
  - The diameter of induration is 15 mm or greater in low-risk children. In general, bacille Calmette-Guérin–vaccinated individuals with positive Mantoux test results should be considered to have true infection.[5]

- **Lead.** All children aged 6 months to 6 years should be assessed for risk of lead exposure using a structured questionnaire (see questions below). Any child for whom an answer to any of the questions is yes should be considered high risk and should have whole-blood lead level testing. Those with blood levels less than 10 μg/dL should be retested once a year until age 6. Some groups advocate screening all children at 12 months of age. Following are recommended questions for assessing lead exposure risk (one yes or I don't know is considered positive):
  - Does your child live in or regularly visit a house that was built before 1950 and has peeling or chipping paint?
  - Does your child live in or regularly visit a house built before 1978 with recent, ongoing, or planned renovation or remodeling?
  - Does your child have a brother or sister, housemate, or playmate being followed or treated for lead poisoning (blood lead levels greater than 15 μg/dL)?
  - Does your child live with an adult whose job or hobby involves exposure to lead? (Examples include stained glass work, furniture refinishing, and ceramics.)
  - Does your child live near an active lead smelter, battery recycling plant, or other industry likely to release lead?

- **Cholesterol.** The American College of Physicians and USPSTF do not recommend cholesterol screening in pediatric patients. Patients who have familial hypercholesterolemia or risk factors for coronary artery disease should be screened at age 25 for males and age 35 for females with a fasting lipid panel. Long-term side effects of cholesterol medications are unknown, and there is concern that they may increase cancer risk. Children and adolescents should have their body mass index (BMI) calculated each annual physical.

If the BMI is elevated, behavioral counseling and dietary intervention should be initiated.[6] The AAP policy states that high-risk children over 2 years old should be screened. A high-risk child is one who has a parent or grandparent who had coronary artery disease diagnosed at <55 years old, parent who has a serum cholesterol >240 mg/dL, or if the child has risk factors such as obesity, hypertension, or diabetes. Screening includes a fasting lipid panel and stepwise approach to treatment can be followed.[7]

- **Depression and suicide.** There is insufficient evidence for or against routine screening for depression. It is part of the home/habits, education/employment/excercise, accidents/ambition/activities/abuse, drugs (alcohol, tobacco, others)/diet/depression, sex, suicide (HEADSS) exam for adolescents. Appropriate screening questions could include the following:

  - Over the past 2 weeks have you felt down, depressed, or hopeless?
  - Over the past 2 weeks have you felt little interest or pleasure in doing things?

Risk factors for depression in children include a history of verbal, physical, or sexual abuse; a history of parental depression; frequent separation from or loss of a loved one; and chronic illness.

- **Genetics.** Tracing the illnesses suffered by parents, grandparents, and other blood relatives can help the primary care physician predict the disorders to which a person may be at risk and take action to keep the patient and the patient's family healthy. Family history (preferably a three-generation medical history) is the single most important genetic tool currently available. Web-based genograms are available. See http://www.hhs.gov/familyhistory/, http://www.genetests.org/.

IMMUNIZATION

The Advisory Committee on Immunization Practices (ACIP), the Committee on Infectious Diseases of the American Academy of Pediatrics, and representatives from the American Academy of Family Physicians have worked together to develop the recommended childhood immunization schedule shown in Table 1.1-3 and http://www.cdc.gov/nip/recs/child-schedule.htm. It should be noted that vaccines are generally 90% to 95% effective. The Centers for Disease control (CDC) has "Guide to contraindications and precautions to commonly used vaccines" at http://www.cdc.gov/niP/recs/contraindications_vacc.htm and vaccine side effects at http://www.cdc.gov/NIP/menus/vaccines.htm.

- **Diphtheria, tetanus, and pertussis.** All children should be immunized against diphtheria, tetanus, and pertussis (DTP) at 2, 4, 6, and 15 to 18 months of age. The fourth vaccine can be given any time between 12 and 18 months, provided at least 6 months has passed since the third vaccination. The diphtheria, tetanus, and acellular pertussis (DTaP) vaccine is now recommended for the entire series. This vaccine contains an acellular pertussis preparation that has fewer side effects than whole-cell pertussis preparations. If a child younger than 7 years has a contraindication to pertussis vaccine, DT should be used. The recommended dosage of DTaP and DT is 0.5 mL, given intramuscularly. ACIP now recommends a booster (Tdap) during adolescence age 11 to 18 that contains tetanus and pertussis vaccine.

  - **Contraindications.** Prior anaphylactic reaction to vaccine or any vaccine component. Moderate or severe acute illness (do not postpone for mild illness). Encephalopathy within 7 days of administration of a previous DTP or DTaP.
  - **Precautions.** Fever exceeding 40.5°C (104.9°F), collapse or shocklike state within 48 hours of previous DTP or DTaP; seizures within 3 days of previous DTP or DTaP; persistent, inconsolable crying lasting 3 hours or more within 48 hours of previous DTP or DTaP; and history of Guillain–Barré syndrome.
  - **Adverse reactions.** Redness, swelling, or pain at injection site, fever greater than 38°C (100.4°F), and mild drowsiness, anorexia, and vomiting are common.

- **_Haemophilus influenzae_ type b.** All children should be immunized against _H. influenzae_ type b (Hib) at 2, 4, 6, and 12 to 15 months. There are currently three types of conjugate vaccine licensed for infant use. Ideally, the same type of vaccine should be given throughout the entire primary series, although current recommendations do allow for some interchangeability.[8] Hib vaccine is given intramuscularly.

TABLE 1.1-3 Recommended Childhood and Adolescent Immunization Schedule 2006*

Vaccine	birth	1 mo	2 mo	4 mo	6 mo	12 mo	15 mo	18 mo	24 mo	4–6 yr	11–12 yr	13–14 yr	15 yr	16–18 yr
Hepatitis B	HepB	HepB		HepB	HepB				HepB					
Diphtheria, tetanus, pertussis			DTaP	DTaP	DTaP		DTaP			DTaP	Tdap	Tdap		
Haemophilus influenza type B			Hib	Hib	Hib	Hib								
Inactivated polio virus			IPV	IPV	IPV									
Measles, mumps, rubella						MMR				MMR	MMR			
Varicella						Varicella			Varicella					
Meningococcal												MCV4		MCV4
Pneumococcal			PCV	PCV	PCV	PCV			PCV/PPV					
Influenza					Influenza Yearly									
Hepatitis A						Hepatitis A series								

*Note: Children/adolescents may not sequire all doses of some vaccines listed in this table. Schedules for some vaccinations vary and allow flexible timing of administeration of vaccines. For the latest recommended child/adolescent vaccination schedule go to: http://www.cdc.gov/nip/recs/childschedule.htm.

- **Contraindications.** Prior anaphylactic reaction to vaccine or any vaccine component. Moderate or severe acute illness (do not postpone for mild illness).
- **Adverse reactions.** Mild fever and pain, redness, or swelling at the injection site are possible side effects.

■ **Hepatitis B.** All children should be immunized against hepatitis B at 2, 4, and >6 months of life. Some groups advocate for a four-shot series, which would include one vaccine dose at birth prior to discharge from the hospital and then proceeding with the above schedule. Infants born to mothers positive for hepatitis B surface antigen (HBsAg) should receive hepatitis B vaccine and hepatitis B immune globulin within 12 hours of delivery. Infants born to mothers with unknown HBsAg status should receive hepatitis B vaccine, and mother's blood should be drawn; if positive for HBsAg, then immune globulin should be administered to infant within 1 week of delivery. All older children and adolescents at high risk for hepatitis B infections should receive a complete series of immunizations.

- **Contraindications.** Prior anaphylactic reaction to vaccine or any vaccine component (i.e., common baker's yeast). Moderate or severe acute illness (do not postpone for mild illness).
- **Adverse reactions.** Pain at the injection site (3% to 29%) and fever greater than 38°C (100.4°F) may occur in 1% to 6% of children.

■ **Measles, mumps, and rubella.** All children should be immunized against measles–mumps–rubella (MMR) at 12 to 15 months and 4 to 6 years old. Those who have not received the second dose should complete the schedule no later than age 11 to 12 years. It is a live attenuated viral vaccine. It is administered subcutaneously at a dose of 0.5 mL.

- **Contraindications.** Prior anaphylactic reaction to vaccine or any vaccine component (i.e., neomycin or gelatin). Most neomycin allergy is manifest as a contact dermatitis 48 to 96 hours after the vaccine is administered and is not a contraindication to the vaccine. Precaution must be used in patients who have had a prior anaphylactic reaction to eggs, although this is not an absolute contraindication to the vaccine. Algorithms published by several different groups can help in the decision-making process.[9] Moderate or severe acute illness (do not postpone for mild illness). Immunodeficient patients. Pregnancy or planned pregnancy within the next 3 months. Receipt of immune globulin or blood products within the preceding 11 months.
- **Adverse reactions.** Fever greater than 39.4°C (103°F) may develop 5 to 12 days after immunization and last up to 5 days (10% to 20% risk); 1% of children may develop mild joint pain and stiffness and even arthritis 1 to 2 weeks after receiving the vaccine. A transient rash may occur in 5% of vaccinees, and some children may experience swollen cervical and posterior auricular lymph nodes 1 to 2 weeks after immunization. Rare encephalopathy and thrombocytopenia (1/million).

■ **Poliovirus.** All children should be immunized against polio with the inactivated poliovirus vaccine (IPV) at 2 months, 4 months, 6 to 18 months, and 4 to 6 years of age. To eliminate the risk for vaccine-associated paralytic poliomyelitis, use of an all IPV schedule is now recommended. Administered subcutaneously or intramuscularly.

- **Contraindications.** Prior anaphylactic reaction to vaccine or any vaccine component (i.e., streptomycin, polymyxin B, or neomycin). Moderate or severe acute illness (do not postpone for mild illness).
- **Adverse reactions.** Mild fever and pain, redness, or swelling at the injection site are possible side effects.

■ **Varicella.** All children who have no history of varicella infection should be given the varicella zoster vaccine (VZV) at 12 to 18 months of age. Older children who have not been vaccinated and who lack a reliable history of chickenpox should receive one vaccine dose if <13 years old and two doses if >13 years old. It is a live attenuated viral vaccine. VZV is administered as a single 0.5-mL subcutaneous dose.

- **Contraindications.** Prior anaphylactic reaction to vaccine or any vaccine component (i.e., neomycin or gelatin). Moderate or severe acute illness (Do not postpone for mild illness). Immunodeficient children: Pregnancy or planned pregnancy within the next 3 months. Receipt of immune globulin or blood products within the preceding 5 months. VZV may be given to individuals who live in households with immunocompromised individuals. Vaccinees who develop a rash should avoid contact with immunocompromised individuals for the duration of the rash.

- **Adverse reactions.** Approximately 20% of children experience tenderness and erythema at the injection site. A generalized maculopapular or vesicular rash 1 month after immunization may occur in 3% to 4% of those receiving the vaccine. Transmission of the vaccine virus from healthy individuals who have been vaccinated to others is possible but has not been documented.

- **Hepatitis A.** As of October 2005, the ACIP put out updated guidelines that all children (irrelevant of high-risk status or not) should be immunized against hepatitis A with the first dose at >12 months old and the second dose >6 months after first dose. Administered intramuscularly.
  - **Contraindications.** Prior anaphylactic reaction to vaccine or any vaccine component. Moderate or severe acute illness (do not postpone for mild illness). Safety during pregnancy has not been determined.
  - **Adverse reactions.** Mild fever and pain, redness, or swelling at the injection site are possible side effects.[10]

- **Pneumococcal disease.** All children should be immunized with the 7-Valent pneumococcal conjugate vaccine (PCV7) at 2, 4, 6, and 12 to 15 months. Children age 24 to 59 months who are at increased risk for *Streptococcus pneumoniae* infections (e.g., those with sickle cell disease, cochlear implants, HIV infection, and other immunocompromised or chronic medical conditions) who did not receive PCV7 should be vaccinated according to the high-risk schedule (available online at www.cdc.gov/mmwr/PDF/rr/rr4909.pdf). The vaccine is administered intramuscularly as a 0.5-mL dose.
  - **Contraindications.** Prior anaphylactic reaction to vaccine or any vaccine component. Moderate or severe acute illness (do not postpone for mild illness).
  - **Adverse reactions.** Fever greater than 100.4°F (38°C) and local induration, tenderness, and erythema at the injection site are common. Fever is the most common reaction and occurs in 15% to 25% of recipients. The rate of fevers greater than 102.2°F (39°C) appears to increase after dose 2.

- **Meningococcal vaccine.** All children should be immunized with the meningococcal conjugate vaccine (MCV4) at age 11 to 12 years old or at entry into high school. College-age freshmen living in the dormitories should also be vaccinated. Any child >2 years old with terminal complement deficiencies, asplenia, and certain other high-risk groups should also be vaccinated. Meningococcal polysaccharide vaccine (MPSV4) is used for children age 2 to 10 years old. Administer 0.5 mL MPSV4 via the subcutaneous route (23 to 25 g, 5/8 needle) to patients ages 2 to 10 years in the anterolateral fat of the thigh in young children or in the posterolateral section of the upper arm for older children and teens. Administer 0.5 mL MCV4 via the intramuscular route (22 to 25 g, 1 to 1½″) in the deltoid muscle to patients ages 11 years and older.
  - **Contraindications,** prior anaphylactic reaction to vaccine or any vaccine component. Moderate or severe acute illness (do not postpone for mild illness).

- **Influenza vaccine.** Influenza vaccine is recommended annually for all children, especially those with the following risk factors: asthma, cardiac disease, sickle cell disease, HIV, diabetes, and children who are household members of health care workers. Children receiving the trivalent inactivated influenza vaccine (TIV) should be given an age-appropriate dose (0.25 mL if aged 6 to 35 months and 0.5 mL if >3 years). Healthy children >5 years old can receive the live attenuated influenza vaccine (LAIV) intranasally. Children <8 years old who are receiving the vaccination for the first time should receive two doses, separated by 4 weeks for TIV and 6 weeks for LAIV.
  - **Contraindications.** Prior anaphylactic reaction to vaccine or any vaccine component (i.e., egg protein). Moderate or severe acute illness (do not postpone for mild illness).

- **Rotavirus.** This vaccine is not a part of the routine vaccination schedule but is available as a live attenuated rotavirus with a recommended vaccination schedule at 2, 4, and 6 months old. The vaccination must be completed by 8 months of age. This is a liquid vaccine that is given by mouth. Although the prior rotavirus vaccine was removed from the market in 1999 because of increased risk of intussusception, the current vaccine has not been found to increase the risk of intussusception.

- **Contraindications.** Prior anaphylactic reaction to vaccine or any vaccine component.
- **Precautions.** Vaccine should not be administered to patients with acute, moderate to severe gastroenteritis until it resolves. Other precautions include pre-existing chronic gastrointestinal disease, prior intussusception, immunocompromised.[11] See http://www.cdc.gov/nip/vfc/acip_resolutions/0206rotavirus.pdf.

- **New and combination vaccines.** New combination vaccines are being tested such as the ProQuad (MMR + varicella) and a combination dTap-Hib-IPV. Combination vaccines represent one solution to the problem of increased numbers of injections during clinic visits. Package insert instructions and CDC recommendations regarding appropriate use should be followed.[8] Other disease for which vaccines are being developed include herpes simplex virus (HSV), cytomegalovirus/Epstein–Barr virus (CMV/EBV), respiratory syncytial virus (RSV), parainfluenza, group A and B streptococcus, human papillomavirus (HPV), and parvovirus.

ANTICIPATORY GUIDANCE AND COUNSELING

- **Anticipatory guidance.** Providing anticipatory guidance and health education surrounding issues likely to be encountered at specific ages is a cornerstone of the pediatric health maintenance visit. Clinicians should be familiar with common parental questions and be prepared to provide counseling and advice about child development, child behavior, discipline, nutrition, and safety.
- **Dental and oral health.** Dental and oral health counseling should be provided routinely, with referral for a dental visit occurring at 2 to 3 years of age. Parents should be instructed to wipe their infant's gums and teeth after each feeding with a moist washcloth. Once multiple teeth have appeared, parents should brush their infant's teeth daily using a pea-sized amount of toothpaste. To prevent tooth decay, infants should not be permitted to fall asleep with a bottle containing anything other than water. Infants should be encouraged to begin using a cup instead of a bottle at age 1 year. Fluoride supplementation should be administered according to the following guidelines:
  - Infants who are exclusively breastfed and those who live in an area without adequately fluoridated water should receive fluoride supplementation beginning at age 2 weeks and continuing until approximately age 16 years.
  - Children who live in an area where the local water supply contains less than 0.3 part per million (ppm) of fluoride should receive 0.25 mg fluoride daily until age 3 years, 0.5 mg fluoride daily from 3 years to 6 years, and 1.00 mg daily from 6 years to 16 years.
  - Children who live in an area where the local water supply contains 0.3 to 0.6 ppm of fluoride require no supplementation until age 3. From age 3 to 6 years, they should receive 0.25 mg fluoride daily, and from age 6 to 16 years, they should receive 0.50 mg daily.
  - No fluoride supplementation is required for children living in areas with more than 0.6 ppm of fluoride in the local water supply.

- **Safety.** Age-specific safety counseling should be provided routinely. Among the safety issues to be addressed are the following:
  - Sudden infant death syndrome: A sleeping infant should be positioned on his or her back and should not sleep prone.
  - Car seats/booster seats: Infants should be rear facing until 1 year old and weigh 20 lbs. A forward-facing car seat with a harness can the used until the child weighs 40 lbs. Booster seats can be used in children over 40 lbs until a seatbelt fits properly (usually children who are 58 inches tall and 81 lbs).
  - Use stair and window gates to prevent falls.
  - Keep objects that can cause suffocation and choking away from small children.
  - Avoid scald burns by reducing the water temperature of hot water heaters to below 120°F.
  - Keep medicines and other dangerous substances locked up and in child-resistant containers.

■ Always ensure that children wear safety helmets when riding bicycles.

■ Smoke alarms should be installed and maintained in the home.

■ Encourage parents not to keep a firearm in the home. If a gun is kept in the home, it should be stored unloaded and locked away, separately from ammunition.

References

1. McCandless S. A Primer on expanded newborn screening by tandem mass spectrometry. *Primary Care Clin Office Pract* 2004;3:583–604.
2. Rosner B, Prineas RJ, Loggie JM, et al. Blood pressure nomograms for children and adolescents, by height, sex, and age, in the United States. *J Pediatrics* 1993;123(6):871–886.
3. Eye examination and visual screening in infants, children and young adults. *Pediatrics* 1996;98:153–157. http://aappolicy.aappublications.org/cgi/reprint/pediatrics;98/1/153.pdf.
4. CDC criteria for anemia in children and childbearing aged women. *MMWR* 1989;38:400–404.
5. Potter B. Management of active tuberculosis. *Am Fam Physician* 2005;72(11). http://www.aafp.org/afp/20051201/2225.html.
6. Washington R. Interventions to reduce cardiovascular risk factors in children and adolescents. *Am Fam Phys* 1999;59(8). http://www.aafp.org/afp/990415ap/2211.html.
7. American Academy of Pediatrics. Cholesterol in childhood. *Pediatrics* 1998;101(1):141–147. http://aappolicy.aappublications.org/cgi/content/full/pediatrics;101/1/141.
8. Combination vaccines for childhood immunization. *MMWR* May 14, 1999;48:1–15.
9. Khakoo GA. Recommendations for using MMR vaccine in children allergic to eggs. *BMJ* 2000;320:929–932. http://bmj.bmjjournals.com/cgi/content/full/320/7239/929.
10. Prevention of hepatitis A through active or passive immunization: recommendations of the Advisory Committee on Immunization Practices. *MMWR* May 14, 2006;55 (RR07):1–23. http://www.cdc.gov/mmwr/preview/mmwrhtml/rr5507a1.htm.
11. Safety and efficacy of a pentavalent human-bovine reassortant rotavirus vaccine. *N Engl J Med* 2006;354:11–22. http://content.nejm.org/cgi/content/full/354/1/11.

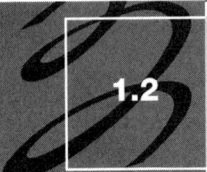

1.2 HEALTH MAINTENANCE FOR ADOLESCENTS
Norman Montalto

GENERAL PRINCIPLES

■ The 21st century has given us a **generation of complex teenagers from diverse backgrounds** who are being influenced by peers, society, and lifestyles of those around them. Many do not consider the impact their behaviors have on their present and future health as adults. **Our overall goal is to keep teens healthy, prevent accidental death, and help them reach adulthood with behaviors that will reduce premature death and disability as adults.**

■ This chapter **provides some tools and guidelines** to direct adolescents proactively to avoid injury, reduce risks of premature death, maintain health, and prevent the development of chronic disease as adults.

ADOLESCENT HEALTH MAINTENANCE

Injury and Disease Prevention, and Risk Management

■ **The adolescent years are a challenging period** for teens, their parents, and physicians. There are so many influences to be considered, choices to be made, and behaviors that will affect their futures.

■ **All adolescents (ages 11 to 21) should be evaluated** to determine current health status, assess risk factors, and be provided guidance for making choices that may have an impact on their health and well-being now and later as adults. Many teens engage in specific behaviors that are harmful or dangerous to themselves or their friends. In addition, some of these behaviors may have unhealthy consequences as the teens mature into adulthood. Some of these risky behaviors result in life-altering or fatal outcomes.

■ **More than 70% of deaths in adolescents are due to preventable causes** such as:
  • Motor vehicle accidents (31%)
  • Homicide (15%)
  • Unintentional injury (14%)
  • Suicide (13%)

■ **Family physician input is vital** to provide the teen with health care information, lifestyle guideposts, and direction that may influence their behaviors, health, and well-being for a lifetime.

  ■ The **complete care** of any patient, especially with adolescents, includes considering:
    • Emotional needs
    • Psychologic needs
    • Environmental needs
    • Social needs
    • Physical health needs

  ■ **Caring for teens is a complex task** because risk is everywhere, diversity abounds, habits are established, maturity levels vary, and clinical visits are sporadic. All teens, at every visit, should be provided the opportunity to obtain the health care guidance and services they need. Factors that influence access and utilization of healthcare services include:
    • Availability and use of insurance coverage
    • Single-parent families
    • Socioeconomic status
    • Educational status
    • Ethnicity
    • Sex of the adolescent
    • Health of the teen

■ In 2005, approximately two thirds of all adult mortality (age >25 years) in the United States was attributed to three conditions with similar risk factors: cardiovascular disease (39%), cancer (23%), and diabetes (3%). As teens mature into adulthood, the primary prevention of these conditions is desirable. Some believe the **health promoting behaviors that are developed in adolescence extend into adulthood.**

  ■ The lifestyle factors and behaviors that contribute to adult mortality and chronic disease (listed above) include, but are not limited to poor nutritional choices, lack of physical activity, and tobacco use. **Adolescence is a period of experimentation with behaviors** that can have immediate consequences, but also have an impact on their health as adults. The behaviors you suggest to prevent these chronic diseases are the same lifestyle and behavioral choices the teens may need to adopt as adults to treat these same conditions.
    • **Substance abuse** (tobacco, alcohol, marijuana, prescription drugs) increases the risk of addiction and unintentional injury and chronic disease.
    • Adoption of a sedentary lifestyle and unhealthy dietary **choices put their health at risk** as adults for developing obesity, diabetes, hypertension, cardiovascular disease, chronic lung disease, or cancer.

  ■ **Clinicians should identify these potential risk factors** for premature death and/or injury **and provide suggestions** to reduce risks that contribute to preventable causes of death.

  ■ To reduce the risk of chronic disease, several guidelines suggest that the minimum **frequency of contact with teens should be yearly.** This schedule may provide the adolescent and clinician opportunities to develop a trusting relationship over time. This also permits monitoring of the teen when not acutely ill, and possibly encourages openness to a discussion about topics that can have a lifelong impact on their health.

HEALTH MAINTENANCE GOALS, OBJECTIVES, AND RECOMMENDATIONS

Healthy People (HP2010)

The Centers for Disease Control and the National Center for Chronic Disease Prevention and Health Promotion **reviewed more than 100 objectives and identified 21 as critical,** because they represent most serious health and safety issues facing adolescents and young adults. The 21 critical health objectives (Table 1.2-1) are cited along with baseline and target goals for 2010.

Guidelines for Clinicians

- There are several **clinical practice guidelines** that clinicians may refer to for direction when providing health maintenance to adolescents.
- In general, these **guidelines are fairly similar** but do have **some subtle differences.** Some guidelines may be more helpful to some clinicians, and are listed for that reason.
  - The American Academy of Family Physicians (http://www.aafp.org/online/en/home/clinical/exam/age) and the American Academy of Pediatricians (http://www.aap.org/healthtopics/stages.cfm#) have provided **suggestions for the improvement of health care to adolescents.**
  - A review of three guidelines is listed in Table 1.2-2. These three organizations recommend specific **screening behaviors and counseling points** to educate teens and prevent injury.
  - For some clinicians who rely on evidence-based data to direct clinical care, they will find many of these **recommendations are based on expert opinion.** It is difficult to perform "outcomes-based research" on this very diverse population with a very heterogeneous background. The adolescent is a complex being influenced not by the health care professional alone, but by societal attitudes, parental behaviors and attitudes, peer groups, faith-based groups, media influences, and their own social and educational environment.
- Because a **significant amount of research has *not* been done on many of these recommendations,** some are suggested by experts based on the expected positive outcome. Research needs to validate cost-effectiveness and efficacy of these interventions, and the best methods to achieve them in various settings. The evidence to support health screening and immunizations is more soundly evidence based.

GAPS Health Service Record

- The use of the **GAPS Health Services Record (GAPS-HSR)** (Table 1.2-3) is one method to document and follow service delivery. The **GAPS Guidelines recommendations** (Table 1.2-4) are explained on the reverse side of the GAPS-HSR. The GAPS Guidelines will serve as a reference point for the remainder of this chapter, as the recommendations are concise and easy to follow.
- **Ensure confidentiality** with the adolescent patient **when you begin your visit.** It is important to make teens feel comfortable. As their physician, let them see that you are trustworthy and that you listen to them. Approach teens as unique, growing, developing beings with honesty, respect, fidelity, courtesy, and friendliness, and attempt to foster a relationship with them.
  - For teens to initiate or engage in discussion, the **clinician may consider a statement such as,** "*As you become older, my approach to your health care changes. We may talk about issues that you would not consider telling anybody else. I respect you as an individual and I will not share the information we discuss with your parents (guardian, caregiver) unless the information you discuss with me has the potential to cause harm to you or somebody else, or you give me permission to discuss it with them. Other than that, what we talk about now will be kept private between the two of us. Would that be okay with you?*"
    - The **intention of this statement** (or a similar one) is to **reduce communication barriers** between you and your adolescent patient, and encourage a more honest exchange of information while providing the patient with the respect and dignity of an adult patient. Messages like this, while not always immediately effective in building trust, may encourage trust and communication over time as you and your adolescent patient develop a clinical relationship.

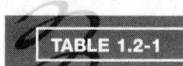

TABLE 1.2-1 | **Critical Health Objectives for Adolescents and Young Adults**

21 Critical Health Objectives for Adolescents and Young Adults

The 21 Critical Health Objectives represent the most serious health and safety issues facing adolescents and young adults (aged 10 to 24): mortality, unintentional injury, violence, substance use and mental health, reproductive health, and the prevention of chronic diseases during adulthood.

Obj. #	Objective	Baseline (year)	2010 Target
16-03 (a,b,c)	Reduce deaths of adolescents and young adults. 10- to 14-year-olds 15- to 19-year-olds 20- to 24-year-olds	21.5 per 100,000 (1998) 69.5 per 100,000 (1998) 92.7 per 100,000 (1998)	16.8 per 100,000 39.8 per 100,000 49.0 per 100,000
Unintentional injury			
15-15 (a)	Reduce deaths caused by motor vehicle crashes. 15- to 24-year-olds	25-6 per 100,000 (1999)	[1]
26-01 (a)	Reduce deaths and injuries caused by alcohol- and drug-related motor vehicle crashes. 15- to 24-year-olds	13.5 per 100,000 (1998)	[1]
15-19	Increase use of safety belts 9th-12th grade students	84% (1999)	92%
26-06	Reduce the proportion of adolescents with report that they rode, during the previous 30 days, with a driver who had bee drinking alcohol. 9th-12th grade students	33% (1999)	30%
Violence			
18-01	Reduce the suicide rate. 10- to 14-year-olds 15- to 19-year-olds	1.2 per 100,000 (1999) 8.0 per 100,000 (1999)	[1] [1]
18-02	Reduce the rate of suicide attempts by adolescents that required medical attention. 9th-12th grade students	2.6% (1999)	1.0%
15-32	Reduce homicides 10- to 14-year-olds 15- to 19-year-olds	1.2 per 100,000 (1999) 10.4 per 100,000 (1999)	[1] [1]
15-38	Reduce physical fighting among adolescents. 9th-12th grade students	36% (1999)	32%
15-39	Reduce weapon carrying by adolescents on school property. 9th-12th grade students	6.9% (1999)	4.9%
Substance Use and Mental Health			
26-11 (d)	Reduce the proportion of persons engaging in binge drinking of alcoholic beverages. 12- to 17-year-olds	7.7% (1998)	2.0%
26-10 (b)	Reduce past-month use of illicit substances (marijuana). 12- to 17-year-olds	8.3% (1998)	0.7%
06-02	Reduce the proportions of children and adolescents with disabilities who are reported to be sad, unhappy, or depressed. 4- to 17-year-olds	[2]	[2]
18-07	(Developmental) Increase the proportion of children with mental health problems who receive treatment.	[3]	[3]
Reproductive Health			
09-07	Reduce pregnancies among adolescent females. 15- to 17-year-olds	68 per 1,000 (1996)	43 per 1,000
13-05	(Developmental) Reduce the number of new HIV diagnoses among adolescents and adults. 13- to 24-year-olds	16,479 (1998) [4]	[3]
25-01 (a,b,c)	Reduce the proportion of adolescents and young adults with *Chlamydia trachomatis* infections. 15- to 24-year-olds		
	Females attending family planning clinics	5.0% (1997)	3.0%
	Females attending sexually transmitted disease clinics	12.2% (1997)	3.0%
	Males attending sexually transmitted disease clinics	15.7% (1997)	3.0%
25-11	Increase the proportion of adolescents who abstain from sexual intercourse or use condoms if currently sexually active. 9th-12th grade students	85% (1999)	95%

(continued)

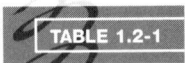

TABLE 1.2-1	Critical Health Objectives for Adolescents and Young Adults *(Continued)*		
Chronic Diseases			
27-02 (a)	Reduce tobacco use by adolescents. 9th-12th grade students	40% (1999)	21%
19-03 (b)	Reduce the proportion of children and adolescents who are overweight or obese. 12- to 19-year-olds	11% (1988-94)	5%
22-07	Increase the proportion of adolescents who engage in vigorous physical activity that promotes cardiorespiratory fitness 3 or more days per week for 20 or more minutes per occasion. 9th -12th grade students	65% (1999)	85%

Note: They are listed with the objective, baseline rates, and 2010 target goals. Critical health outcomes are underlined, and behaviors that substantially contribute to important health outcomes are in normal font.

[1] 2010 target not provided for adolescent/young adult age group.
[2] Baseline and target inclusive of age groups outside of adolescent/young adult age parameters.
[3] Developmental objective - baseline and 2010 target to be provided by 2004.
[4] Proposed baseline is shown but has not yet been approved by the Healthy People 2010 Steering Committee.

■ **When parents accompany teens into the examination room,** collect a history from each of them. This provides an opportunity to evaluate their relationship with the teen and the ways in which they communicate that may be helpful or harmful to their relationship. On occasion you may note dysfunctional patterns of communication that may assist you in understanding some of the frustrations of both the teen and the parents.

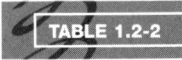

TABLE 1.2-2	Guideline Review		
	U.S. Preventive Services Task Force	**American Medical Association (AMA)**	**Maternal and Child Health Bureau**
Guidelines	USPSTF® 2005 Guideline to Clinical Preventative Services http://www.ahrq.gov/clinic/uspstfab.htm	Guidelines for Adolescent Preventive Services (GAPS) 2004 http://www.ama-assn.org/ama/pub/category/1980.html	Bright Futures 2002: For Health Supervision of Infants, Children, and Adolescents - 2nd Edition-Revised http://www.brightfutures.org/bf2/pdf/index.html
Scientific Rigor	Recommendations based on strength of evidence and effectiveness.	Recommendations based on strength of evidence and effectiveness.	
Target Population	11 to 24 yrs.	11 to 21 yrs.	0–21 yrs.
Clinical Scope	Eighty health conditions. Twenty-five interventions including screening, counseling, immunizations/chemoprophylaxis.	Twenty-four preventative service recommendations relating to health care delivery, health guidance, screening for biopsychosocial problems, and immunizations.	Detailed suggestions. Longitudinal approach, are given in the context of the community and family.
Comment	Unable to recommend for or against some interventions due to paucity of data to support it.	Yearly service visits.	Yearly visits.

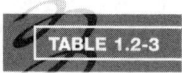

| TABLE 1.2-3 | **Health Service Record Guideline for Adolescent Service (GAPS)** |

Name _____   Date of Birth _____

| | Age of Adolescent | | | | | | | | | | |
| | Early | | | | Middle | | | Late | | | |
Procedure	11	12	13	14	15	16	17	18	19	20	21
Screening History											
(recommendation number)											
Eating disorders (13)											
Tobacco use (14)											
Alcohol/Drug use (15)											
Sexual activity (16)											
Depression (20)											
Risk for suicide (20)											
Physical, sexual, or emotional abuse (21)											
School performance (22)											
Physical Assessment											
Comprehensive examination (1)											
Blood pressure (11)											
Body mass index (13)											
Tests											
Cholesterol (12)											
Gonorrhea, Chlamydia, human papilloma-virus (17, 18)											
HIV, syphilis (17, 18)											
Pap smear (19)											
Tuberculosis (23)											
Immunizations											
Human papillomavirus (24)											
Measles, mumps, rubella (24)											
Tetanus-diphtheria (24)											
Hepatitis B virus (24)											
Varicella (24)											
Health Guidance											
Parenting (4)											
Development (5)											
Injury prevention (6)											
Diet and fitness (7, 8)											
Lifestyle (9, 10)											

This document is based on the GAPS recommendations. It may be copied and placed in the chart as a way to document and track what services have been provided or need to be performed during that visit or at a subsequent visit. Placing the date in the box when services are delivered is a rapid way to organize what needs to be done during a routine or acute visit. Each recommendation is numbered for an easy clinical reference by service and frequency, based on age. These guidelines are grouped under: Screening History, Physical Assessment, Tests, Immunizations, and Health Guidance. Boxes with interrupted lines are clinical decision points that the screening history and/or the physician's assessment of risk and especially the consequences may be individualized or tailored to each teen.

- **Excuse the parents** with a statement such as, "Well, (Mr. or Ms. Smith,) Joe is now at an age when I need to talk with him privately. Is this okay with you?" The usual response is "yes," but a **negative response may be cause for concern.**
- **Mental and physical abuse,** drug addiction, or relationship conflicts may result in a negative reply.
- To **collect a truthful history,** most teens will welcome meeting with you privately.
- Generally, female teens and some parents will feel more comfortable with a parent returning to the room **before the examination is performed.**

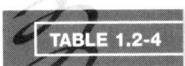

TABLE 1.2-4	Guidelines for Adolescent Preventive Services (GAPS)

These are brief summaries of the AMA GAPS Recommendations. Please see the Web Site for full explanation of each at http://www.ama-ssn.org/ama/upload/mm/39/gapsmono.pdf

Recommendation 1: From ages 11 to 21, all adolescents should have an annual preventive services visit.

Recommendation 2: Preventive services should be age and developmentally appropriate, and should be sensitive to individual and sociocultural differences.

Recommendation 3: Physicians should establish office policies regarding confidential care for adolescents and how parents will be involved in that care. These policies should be made clear to adolescents and their parents.

Recommendation 4: Parents or other adult caregivers should receive health guidance at least once during their child's early adolescence, once during middle adolescence and, preferably, once during late adolescence.

Recommendation 5: All adolescents should receive health guidance annually to promote a better understanding of their physical growth, psychosocial and psychosexual development, and the importance of becoming actively involved in decisions regarding their healthcare.

Recommendation 6: All adolescents should receive health guidance annually to promote the reduction of injuries.

Recommendation 7: All adolescents should receive health guidance annually about dietary habits, including the benefits of a healthy diet, and ways to achieve a healthy diet and safe weight management.

Recommendation 8: All adolescents should receive health guidance annually about the benefits of physical activity and should be encouraged to engage in safe physical activities on a regular basis.

Recommendation 9: All adolescents should receive health guidance annually regarding responsible sexual behaviors, including abstinence. Latex condoms to prevent STDs, including HIV infection, and appropriate methods of birth control should be made available, as should instructions on how to use them effectively.

Recommendation 10: All adolescents should receive health guidance annually to promote avoidance of tobacco, alcohol and other abusable substances, and anabolic steroids.

Recommendation 11: All adolescents should be screened annually for hypertension according to the protocol developed by the National Heart, Lung, and Blood Institute Second Task Force on Blood Pressure Control in Children.

Recommendation 12: Selected adolescents should be screened to determine their risk of developing hyperlipidemia and adult coronary heart disease, following the protocol developed by the Expert Panel on Blood Cholesterol Levels in Children and Adolescents.

Recommendation 13: All adolescents should be screened annually for eating disorders and obesity by determining weight and stature, and asking about body image and dieting patterns.

Recommendation 14: All adolescents should be asked annually about their use of tobacco products including cigarettes and smokeless tobacco.

Recommendation 15: All adolescents should be asked annually about their use of alcohol and other abusable substances, and about their use of over-the-counter or prescription drugs for non-medical purposes, including anabolic steroids.

Recommendation 16: All adolescents should be asked annually about involvement in sexual behaviors that may result in unintended pregnancy and STDs, including HIV infection.

Recommendation 17: Sexually active adolescents should be screened for STDs.

Recommendation 18: Adolescents at risk for HIV infection should be offered confidential HIV screening with the ELISA and confirmatory test.

Recommendation 19: Female adolescents who are sexually active or any female 18 or older should be screened annually for cervical cancer by use of a Pap test.

Recommendation 20: All adolescents should be asked annually about behaviors or emotions that indicate recurrent or severe depression or risk of suicide.

Recommendation 21: All adolescents should be asked annually about a history of emotional, physical, and sexual abuse.

Recommendation 22: All adolescents should be asked annually about learning or school problems.

Recommendation 23: Adolescents should receive a tuberculin skin test if they have been exposed to active tuberculosis, have lived in a homeless shelter, have been incarcerated, have lived in or come from an area with a high prevalence of tuberculosis, or currently work in a health care setting.

Recommendation 24: All adolescents should receive prophylactic immunizations according to the guidelines established by the federally convened Advisory Committee on Immunization Practices.

Screening History

■ **Detecting risks and making attempts to reduce them** should be a focus of care for adolescents at every visit. Age and maturity should be considered when guidance for parents and teens is offered.

   ■ The use of **mnemonic HEADS** (Table 1.2-5) is a method to **organize the clinician's thinking.** Address the topic areas listed to screen for opportunities to

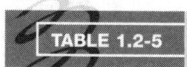

TABLE 1.2-5	Heads

HEADS—A mnemonic useful in the evaluation of adolescent patients.
H = Home, habits
E = Education, employment, exercise
A = Accidents, ambition, activities, abuse
D = Drugs (tobacco, alcohol, others), diet, depression
S = Sex, suicide

provide health guidance, perform a screening history to detect risky behaviors, educate about risk reduction, and promote healthy choices.

- Once these behaviors are identified, it is important to **document that the services have been provided;** making notations in the chart **on the GAPS-HSR** (see Table 1.2-3) of any history or findings relevant to the short- and long-term treatment plan.

■ Some important screening information is easier to obtain and manage than others. The **screening history following the HEADS format** (see Table 1.2-5) is a gentle way to break the ice, helps assess risk, and can be easily remembered. Some clinicians may prefer the **use of questionnaires** that have been developed by the American Medical Association (AMA) and other organizations (Table 1.2-6).

■ These **questionnaires completed by the parent/guardian and teen** are efficient ways to identify high-risk behaviors or topics of health concerns that need to be discussed.

■ The responses to these screening questions suggest **physical assessments or laboratory** tests **may be required.** Many components of the screening history are risk factors that can contribute to adult disease.

■ For many items identified in the screening history, or as a **resource for health guidance, web sites have been cited** to make the management of high-risk behaviors easier (see Weblinks).

■ Once information has been obtained, the clinician is encouraged to **use the format suggested by GAPS** (Figure 1.2-1) **to support a strategy** for encouraging healthy choices, promoting prevention, evaluating risk and identifying problems, and reaching solutions.

■ **Health Guidance (Recommendations 4 through 10).** Because nearly one third of adolescent mortality is due to unintentional injuries, the clinician should review these areas in depth.

■ **Talk with parents or caregivers** about their teens. **Give developmentally appropriate advice.**

■ Confirm and encourage consistent **seatbelt use.**

■ What **hobbies** does the teen participate in? What **sports?** Does the teen do them alone (i.e., swim)? Does the teen use sport- or work-appropriate **protective gear** (i.e., helmets, wrist protectors, eye or ear protectors, masks)?

■ Are there **guns within the home?** How are they kept? What does the teen do at work, around the home or farm, that may need **supervision for safety?** What **power tools** does the teen have access to that can cause harm? Are there **ATVs or other motorized vehicles** that can be used without permission?

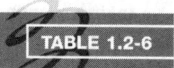

TABLE 1.2-6

Guidelines for Adolescent Preventive Services (GAPS) Implementation Materials
The following GAP questionnaires are available for download:

    Younger Adolescent Questionnaire
    Younger Adolescent Questionnaire Spanish
    Middle/Older Adolescent Questionnaire
    Middle/Older Adolescent Questionnaire Spanish
    Parent/Guardian Questionnaire
    Parent/Guardian Questionnaire Spanish
    http://www.ama-assn.org/ama/pub/category/1981.htm

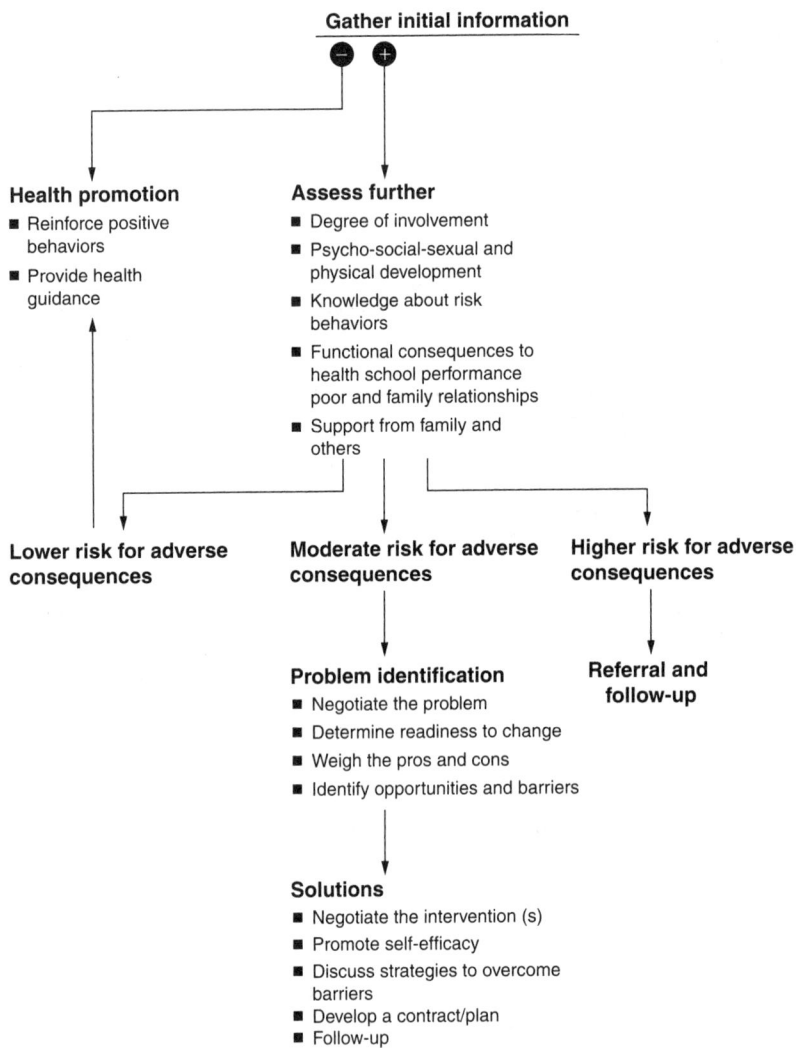

Figure 1.2-1. Steps for preventive screening and health promotion.

■ **Talking to teens about concerns with growth, maturation,** and **taking responsibility for all the choices they make,** including healthy ones, places teens in a position to take **control of their health and well-being.** Some teens are more willing and capable than others of accepting this responsibility.

■ **Parents can be involved in supporting healthy behaviors and modifying risky ones.** Teens can also support parents in their health goals when they are similar.

■ **Eating disorders (Recommendation 13), diet (Recommendation 7), and activity/ fitness (Recommendation 8)** are all related behaviors that *can* prevent or contribute *to* **development of adult chronic disease.**

■ Inquire about **body image and behaviors** that may suggest an eating disorder such as anorexia or bulimia. Be alert for **excessive weight loss or gain** as a sign of anxiety or depression.

- Explain the **value of diet and activity** in promoting health and preventing disease.
- Management of risks may require **extended visits or monitoring on a regular basis.**
- Review **dietary snack habits and beverage choices.** Ask about carbonated beverages, milk intake, fat content, and frequency of fast food.
- **Educate on how to make healthy food choices.** Teach them how to read food labels.
- **Encourage daily physical activity** to maintain both mental and physical health. Do they play sports for fun or competition daily? Do they have goals for their activities? Ask how much time is spent in front of the television, computer, or playing video games.

- **Tobacco (Recommendation 14) and alcohol (Recommendation 15).** The long-term effects of tobacco use are usually a result of **experimentation and subsequent addiction to nicotine as a teen.** Avoiding tobacco use during teen years reduces the likelihood of becoming an adult tobacco user.
    - **Evaluate their interest or experience(s)** with tobacco, alcohol, or other drugs of abuse. (See Recommendations 14,15.)
    - Try to **be honest and warn them how subtly addiction occurs** and how decision to use drugs and alcohol, especially tobacco, can affect their lives as teens and as adults.
    - **Minimizing experimentation, discouraging tobacco use,** and **promoting cessation** reduce the likelihood of adult tobacco-related illness.
    - **Family history of alcohol use and easy access to alcohol** are risk factors that should warrant intervention. It is estimated that nearly one half of U.S. high school students self-report current drinking in the past month; 60% of underage teens **binge drink** (five drinks or more for boys and four drinks or more for girls on a single occasion). Explore when or if this drinking occurs, how often, under what circumstances, and if other drugs or driving are involved.
    - **Drinking is** associated with **violence and injury,** and other high-risk behaviors.
    - **Marijuana** is the most commonly used illegal substance among teens (other than tobacco).
    - **Huffing** (inhalation of volatile substances) and the possibility of **prescription medication diversion and abuse** should be included in this discussion.

- **Sexual activity (Recommendation 16).** Approach the topic of sexuality **nonjudgmentally and openly.**
    - You might **ask teens to define the term** to see what their definition of "sex" is. (Some teens do not consider oral sex as sexual activity, and feel that it is safer.) The suggestions for health guidance (Recommendation 19) include recommending **abstinence and providing guidance about when to consider having sex.** When appropriate, encourage the use of **condoms and birth control,** which should be promoted to avoid pregnancy and sexually transmitted diseases (STDs). For those who are sexually active, screen for STDs.
    - Help teens with their understanding of **healthy relationships.**

- **Mental health (Recommendation 20).** Evaluate for **depression, anxiety, social phobia, posttraumatic stress disorder, anxiety, and attention-deficit disorder/ attention-deficit–hyperactivity disorder (ADD/ADHD),** which **may be uncovered by school performance changes (Recommendation 22),** changes in social groups, initiation or escalation of drug use, as well as subtle or acute and dramatic change in behaviors, such as eating, sleeping, self-care, hobbies, or activities.
    - **Teens with emotional stressors may turn to drugs of abuse,** especially tobacco, **if their treatment medications do not adequately control their symptoms.** Encourage and educate about behavioral coping strategies to reduce stress. Consider medication and referral when warranted.

- **Abuse (Recommendation 21). Invite teens to tell you** about the possibility of physical, sexual, or emotional abuse, and evaluate for potential **suicide risk (Recommendation 20).**
    - **Intervene directly** for these conditions if uncovered. Contact Child Protective Services **if you suspect that abuse may be occurring.** Document these findings carefully and ensure the teen is safe.

- **School performance (Recommendations 22).** Find out if teens **plan to finish school and what occupation, trade school, or college** they may be interested in. When school performance is evaluated, focus on what they like or what they enjoy doing (math, art, music, science, sports). Explore for any **learning problems or school difficulties** they may be facing or have faced in the past, and any other difficulties they may be experiencing at school.
    - Ask if they **feel safe at school.** Evaluate for fighting and bullying behaviors, and inquire about the presence of weapons at school.

PHYSICAL ASSESSMENTS/TESTS/IMMUNIZATIONS

- **Physical assessment** is recommended **on an annual basis,** and the focus should be on determining risk—for **obesity** (body mass index, BMI), **high blood pressure, cardiovascular disease, diabetes, or sexually transmitted diseases.** Obese teens are high risk and should be considered candidates to be screened for metabolic syndrome. Be alert for physical signs of injury (violence or abuse).
- Obtain appropriate **laboratory tests or imaging** based on each teen's individual risk, history, and physical examination findings.
- **Tests (Recommendations 12, 17 through 19, 23).** Some **laboratory evaluations are recommended** and should be considered based on the results of the history of physical assessment and on lifestyle. The family history, in some cases, may provide clues to the laboratory assessment of risk.
- **Immunizations (Recommendation 24).** The **most up-to-date information for adolescent immunizations** can be accessed online at http://www.cdc.gov/vaccines/specgrps/default.htm.
- **Scheduling follow-up visits** is beneficial to **evaluate progress and support behaviors intended to keep teens healthy.** These may include avoiding obesity or pregnancy, discouraging or treating tobacco use, treatment of hypertension, diabetes, or hypercholesterolemia.

SUMMARY

- This chapter is intended to **support a proactive, preventive focus to adolescent health care.** The delivery of health care to adolescents can be a significant challenge. One could cite poor reimbursement, poor utilization of time, or confusion about how to proceed with preventive service guidelines that may lack evidence-based clinical methods and outcomes for effectiveness. Similar issues arise for many health care conditions.
    - **Lack of training, physician perceptions, or confidence** about how to proceed with specific or multiple significant health risks may be overwhelming. **Developing a network of referrals is suggested.**
- **Guidelines have been overviewed, practical tips provided,** and **resources highlighted to facilitate the clinical care of teens.** Many believe that these types of services will reduce medical costs and improve the health of adolescents in the long term. All encounters with adolescents should be viewed as opportunities to provide individualized preventive services.
    - **Use the guidelines as a guide and focus on these six critical health behaviors:**
        - Alcohol and drug use
        - Injury
        - Violence (including suicide)
        - Tobacco use
        - Nutrition
        - Physical activity and sexual behaviors
    - **Provide the services and document their delivery.** Clinicians are encouraged to **adopt a systematic method** to gather information and **provide individual interventions,** and ensure appropriate services are offered and documented (see Figure 1.2-3).
    - **Do what makes sense.** Care for the child as if he or she were your child. **By providing comprehensive health care to adolescents, many opportunities will present themselves to encourage healthy decisions and choices as teens and prevent the development of chronic diseases as adults.**

Weblinks

1. AAFP News Now News Staff. 2006. Increased physical activity yields healthier kids, say experts [online]. Available from URL: http://www.aafp.org/online/en/home/publications/news/news-now/archive/.physicalactivity.html. Accessed September 7, 2006.

2. Agency for Healthcare Research and Quality (AHRQ). (n.d.) Up-to-date. Guide to clinical preventive services [online]. Available from URL: http://www.ahrq.gov/clinic/cps3dix.htm. Accessed September 7, 2006.

3. AACE, Stollings RD, Price W, et al. 2004. National summit on obesity: building a plan to reduce obesity in America [online]. Available from URL: http://www.ama-assn.org/ama/pub/category/12674.html. Accessed September 7, 2006.

4. American Medical Association. 1997. Guidelines for Adolescent Preventive Services (GAPS). Recommendations monograph [online]. Available from URL: http://www.ama-assn.org/ama/upload/mm/39/gapsmono.pdf. Accessed September 7, 2006.

5. National Center for Chronic Disease Prevention and Health Promotion (CDC). 2006. Healthy youth. Six critical health behaviors [online]. Available from URL: http://www.cdc.gov/HealthyYouth/healthtopics/index.htm. Accessed September 8, 2006.

6. National Center for Chronic Disease Prevention and Health Promotion (CDC). 2005. Healthy youth. Healthy people 2010 and the National Initiative to Improve Adolescent Health [online]. Available from URL: http://www.cdc.gov/HealthyYouth/Adolescent-Health/NationalInitiative/index.htm. Accessed September 8, 2006.

7. National Center for Chronic Disease Prevention and Health Promotion (CDC). 2006. Healthy youth. Publications and links [online]. Available from URL: http://www.cdc.gov/HealthyYouth/publications/index.htm. Accessed September 8, 2006.

8. National Center for Chronic Disease Prevention and Health Promotion (CDC). 2006. Healthy youth. Data & statistics. YRBSS: Youth Risk Behavior Surveillance System [online]. Available from URL: http://www.cdc.gov/HealthyYouth/yrbs/index.htm. Accessed September 8, 2006.

9. Grunbaum JA, Kann L, Kinchen S, et al. 2004. Youth risk behavior surveillance—United States, 2003. Available from URL: http://www.cdc.gov/mmwr/preview/mmwrhtml/ss5302a1.htm. Accessed September 8, 2006.

10. National Center for Chronic Disease Prevention and Health Promotion (CDC). 1999. Physical activity and health: a report of the surgeon general [online]. Available from URL: http://www.cdc.gov/nccdphp/sgr/sgr.htm. Accessed September 8, 2006.

11. Centers for Disease Control and Prevention, National Center for Health Statistics. 2006. America's children: key national indicators of well being 2005 [online]. Available from URL: http://www.childstats.gov/amchildren05/hea8.asp. Accessed September 8,2006.

12. Child Welfare Information Gateway. 2006. A new way to stay connected: (Formerly the National Clearinghouse of Child Abuse and Neglect Information and the National Adoption Information Clearinghouse) [online]. Available from URL: http://www.childwelfare.gov/. Accessed September 8, 2006.

13. Cohen E, Mackenzie RG, Yatis GL. et al. 1991. HEADS for adolescents [online]. Available from URL: http://chipts.ucla.edu/assessment/Assessment_Instruments/Assessment_files_new/assess_headss.htm. Accessed September 8, 2006.

14. National Institutes of Health Consensus Development Program. October 13–15, 2004. Preventing violence and related health-risking social behaviors in adolescents: an NIH State-of-Science Conference [online]. http://consensus.nih.gov/2004/2004YouthViolencePreventionSOS023html.htm. Accessed September 7, 2006.

15. U.S. Department of Health and Human Services, Health Resources and Services Administration, Maternal and Child Health Bureau. 2004. Child health USA: annual report on the health status and service needs of America's children [online]. Available from URL: http://www.mchb.hrsa.gov/mchirc/chus. Accessed September 8, 2006.

16. U.S. Department of Health and Human Services, Health Resources and Services Administration, Maternal and Child Health Bureau. 2004. Child health USA: adolescent mortality [online]. Available from URL: http://www.mchb.hrsa.gov/mchirc/chusa_04/pages/0473am.htm. Accessed September 8, 2006.

17. Reuters Health Information. 2006. Immunization Advisory Panel recommends HPV vaccine for all girls [online]. Available from URL: http://www.medscape.com/viewarticle/537674. Accessed September 8, 2006.

18. National Adolescent Health Information Center. 2006. The family environment & adolescent well-being: exposure to positive & negative family influences [online]. Available from URL: http://nahic.ucsf.edu/index.php/nahic/article/the_family_environment_adolescent_well_being/. Accessed September 8, 2006.
19. National Library of Medicine. 2000. Guide to clinical preventive services, 3rd ed. Recommendations [online]. Available from URL: http://www.ncbi.nlm.nih.gov/books/bv.fcgi?rid=hstat3. Accessed September 8, 2006.
20. National Institute of Diabetes and Digestive and Kidney Diseases (NIDDK). 2005. Talking with patients about weight loss: tips for primary care professionals [online]. Available from URL: http://win.niddk.nih.gov/publications/talking.htm. Accessed September 8, 2006.
21. U.S. Department of Agriculture 2005. My pyramid for kids [online]. Available from URL: http://teamnutrition.usda.gov/kids-pyramid.html. Accessed September 8, 2006.
22. Campaign for Tobacco-Free Kids. August 3, 2006. Special report: smoke-free laws protecting our right to breathe clean air [online]. Available from URL: http://tobaccofreekids.org/reports/shs/. Accessed September 8, 2006.

References

1. Eyre H, Kahn R, Robertson RM. Preventing cancer, cardiovascular disease, and diabetes; a common agenda for the American Cancer Society, the American Diabetes Association, and the American Heart Association. *CA Cancer J Clin* 2004;54:190–207.
2. Green M, Palfrey JS. *Bright futures: guidelines for health supervision of infants, children, and adolescents.* 2nd ed., rev. Arlington, VA: National Center for Education in Maternal and Child Health; 2002. Available from: URL: http://www.brightfutures.org/bf2/pdf/pdf/FrontMatter.pdf. Accessed September 7, 2006.
3. Montalto NJ. Implementing the guidelines for adolescent preventive services. Kansas City: American Academy of Family Physicians; 1998;57(9). Available from URL: http://www.aafp.org/afp/980501ap/montalto.html. Accessed September 7, 2006.
4. Confidential health care for adolescents [editorial]. *J Adolesc Health* 1997;21(6):408–415.
5. Healthy people 2010: with understanding and improving health objectives for improving health [editorial]. Washington, DC: U.S. Government Printing Office; 2000.

ACKNOWLEDGMENT

The author expresses his thanks and appreciation to Ms. Toni King for her technical assistance, editorial input, and support in the preparation of this manuscript.

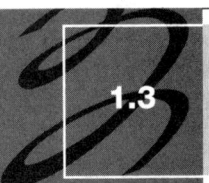

HEALTH MAINTENANCE FOR THE ADULT PATIENT
1.3
Paul E. Lyons

GENERAL PRINCIPLES

Family physicians and other primary care providers should follow guidelines and customize interventions based on the patient's personal profile (e.g., age, gender, family history, and other indicators of high-risk status).[1] They should also use efficient office systems to monitor and track the effectiveness of preventive interventions and to ensure compliance with recommendations. This chapter focuses on what to do and how to do it.

Definition

Primary prevention of adult morbidity and reduction of mortality through systematic, recurrent risk assessment and evidence-based intervention.

Classification

Adults represent a diverse population. Childhood is the age of congenital disease, adolescence the age of behavior-related morbidity. Adulthood represents the age of acquired illness.

Environment, genetics, activity (and inactivity), and advancing age contribute to a population that will increasingly manifest significant medical conditions. Because a uniform approach to this group of patients is not entirely possible, the U.S. Preventive Services Task Force (USPSTF) has divided this population into two age groups: 25 to 64 and 65 and older. Although these groupings are helpful, it may be useful to consider two additional subgroups, adults up to 40 and those over 80. The first group represents a generally healthy group of patients with relatively low risk for the most common causes of morbidity and mortality among adults (cardiac disease, cancer, renal disease, infectious disease such as pneumonia and influenza among others). This group will have considerably fewer screening tests. As the population ages, it seems apparent that those over the age of 65 are not a homogeneous group either. Recognize that the "young elderly" do not always fit the stereotypical profile of a geriatric patient and that the "older elderly" may have additional concerns that do not always apply to their younger peers.[2]

Adult patients should be viewed as a continuum rather than a series of distinct groups. Those age groups are useful for organizational purposes but must always be interpreted in the context of an individual patient and his or her personal medical story. The specific medical issues of each age group are influenced by the medical conditions of the previous age group and will, in turn, affect the health of patients as they age into the next age group. For this reason, comprehensive care of any given patient requires knowledge of current medical concerns as well as those that have gone before and those that will come and a willingness to help patients to help themselves achieve longer, healthier lives.

Etiology

- **Actual causes of death ranked by risk factor[3]**
  - Tobacco
  - Diet and activity patterns
  - Alcohol
  - Microbial agents
  - Toxic agents
  - Firearms
  - Sexual behavior
  - Motor vehicles
  - Illicit use of drugs

- **The 10 leading causes of death in adults.**[4] Table 1.3-1 presents the leading causes of death.

DIAGNOSIS

Clinical Presentation

Primary care physicians often see adults who present for a health maintenance visit, sometimes referred to by patients as a "check up" or "physical." Health maintenance is an integral component of the care and treatment of adult patients and one of the most important aspects of responsible health care by family physicians. Counseling and patient education activities, directed at asymptomatic healthy individuals, are as highly valued as the diagnosis and treatment of illnesses.[1] The leading causes of death and disability among adults are largely related to personal health and lifestyle behaviors and may, therefore, be preventable through routine health maintenance interventions in the form of counseling, screening, immunization, and chemoprophylaxis. These interventions are best delivered as an integral component of the provider–patient contact longitudinally—whatever the chief complaint—rather than as periodic, annual, or comprehensive physical examinations. As many provider–patient encounters occur only during times of illness or injury, the family physician must be prepared to be "opportunistic" and address health maintenance as a clinical issue whenever "teachable moments" arise, keeping in mind that, ultimately, patients must feel empowered to be responsible for their own health status. A few general guidelines will assist this process[2]:

- Form a therapeutic alliance with the patient. All meaningful change will come from the patient. It is the role of the physician to provide the necessary tools for all patients to be as healthy as possible. It is not the physician's role to make the patient change.

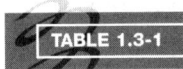

TABLE 1.3-1	Leading Causes of Death in Adults

Young adults (aged 19–39)	Middle adulthood (aged 40–64)
Motor vehicle crashes	Heart disease
Homicide	Lung cancer
Suicide	Cerebrovascular disease
Injuries (non–motor vehicle)	Breast cancer
Heart disease	Colorectal cancer
HIV infection (men)	Obstructive lung disease
	HIV infection (men)

Ten leading causes of death (all ages)

1. Heart disease	31.0%
2. Malignant neoplasms	23.2%
3. Cerebrovascular diseases	6.8%
4. Chronic obstructive pulmonary disease	4.8%
5. Accidents	4.2%
6. Pneumonia and influenza	3.9%
7. Diabetes mellitus	2.8%
8. Suicide	1.3%
9. Renal disease	1.1%
10. Cirrhosis	1.1%

- Listen fully, look carefully, test sparingly. The history will provide the overwhelming majority of the necessary information. The physical examination will add small but important additional pieces of information. Screening tests have an important but very limited role in adult care and should be ordered with careful consideration of their role in patient management.
- Counsel patiently. Behavior change is incremental and slow. Do not assume that the absence of change means the patient did not hear what you said. Repetition, understanding, encouragement, and patience will provide the best results. The family physician's adult patients (defined here as persons over the age of 19) are assumed to be motivated to protect and improve their health status and capable of being responsible for the maintenance of their health. Adults are motivated by economic issues related to work and family care responsibilities as well as the need for independence and security for their future as retirees.

Minimum Preventive Interventions
The recommendations in this chapter are based on the findings of two expert panels: the USPSTF[1] and the Commission on Public Health and Scientific Affairs of the American Academy of Family Physicians.[5] Recommendations listed in Table 1.3-2 cover minimal preventive interventions with widespread acceptability.

History
A systematic approach to these patients will allow for a structured, thorough, and focused visit that meets the current and future needs of your patients. Each of these visits will begin with a modified history. This history may be relatively comprehensive if the patient is new or may represent a review of important interval developments. The history will help direct the physical examination, limited screening tests directed toward prevalent, asymptomatic disease conditions, and patient counseling/education.[2]

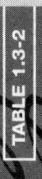

TABLE 1.3-2 Preventive Interventions for Patients Ages 19 to 64

Intervention	19	25	30	35	40	45	50	55	60	64
Screening										
Blood pressure					Every 2 yr					
Height and weight					Periodically					
Cholesterol					Every 5 yr					
Mammography							Every 1–2 yr (women)			
Pap smear				Every 1–3 yr (women)						
Prostate-specific antigen								Yearly (men)		
Sigmoidoscopy								Every 3–5 yr		
Stool occult blood								Yearly		
Urinalysis									Periodically	
Dental					Yearly					
Vision/glaucoma						Every 2–4 yr				
Breast		Every 1–4 yr					Yearly (women)			
Exams for cancer: thyroid, mouth, skin, lymph nodes, rectum (40+), prostate (men 50+)		Every 3 yr					Yearly			
Immunizations										
Tetanus–diphtheria					Every 10 yr					
Pneumococcal										Once
Influenza										
Counseling										
Smoking, alcohol and drugs, sexual behavior, HIV exposure, nutrition, physical activity, violence and guns, family planning, injuries, occupational health						Annual if indicated				
Chemoprophylaxis										
Folate (women 12–45)					Periodically					
Aspirin (men 40+)										
Estrogen (women 45+)										

History of Present Illness
- Although most patients will have no chief complaint, some will.
- Begin with open-ended questions ("tell me what brings you in today," "tell me what I can do for you today," "do you have any health concerns that I should be sure to address?").
- In the absence of specific concerns, the attention should turn to the other elements of the history.
- Should you uncover specific medical concerns these should be developed more fully.

Past History
- *Medical problems*—medical conditions now or in the past of which the patient is aware
- *Surgical problems*—including childhood surgeries such as tonsillectomy and any adult surgeries
- *Hospitalizations and emergency care*
- *Medications*—including prescription, over-the-counter, natural, herbal, and other complementary/alternative medicinal preparations
- *Allergies*—including which medications and the reaction that occurred
- *Toxic habits*—tobacco, alcohol, and illicit drug use (including quantity when present)
- *Obstetrical/gynecologic/sexual history*—including menstrual and pregnancy history for women and a sexual history for both men and women
- *Psychiatric history*—including psychologic concerns for which the patient may not have sought care
- *Health care maintenance*—including a review of age- and gender-appropriate health maintenance issues

Family History
A review of medical conditions that occur in the patient's family allows the physician to develop a broader understanding of health concerns that may arise in the future for this patient. A general family history should encompass three generations: up one generation (parents), down one generation (children, if any), and the index generation (siblings, if any). Basic information in the family history includes age, whether the person is alive or dead, and important medical conditions for each person. For persons who are dead, the age and cause of death should be noted as well as any additional medical conditions that may have been present.

Social History
The social history is a rich and varied component of the medical history. It may contribute to a broader understanding of the patient (e.g., hobbies, education, family status) and may also yield information with potentially important implication for the health of the patient (e.g., high-risk occupations, incarceration, travel to endemic disease areas, exercise and diet patterns).

Review of Systems
The well visit is often an excellent opportunity to review with patients "minor" complaints that they would not necessarily bring to the physician's attention. The review of systems allows for a broad, systematic but reasonably focused recapitulation of common complaints that may be indicative of broader medical issues.

TREATMENT

Counseling and Patient Education to Promote Healthy Lifestyles
- **Definition.** Adult health maintenance programs should promote lifestyle change by explaining the links between risk factors and health status. Risk factor assessment and counseling with adult patients should help them acquire information, motivation, and skills to adopt and maintain healthy behaviors. Recommended counseling strategies include the following:
  - Develop a therapeutic alliance.
  - Counsel all patients.
  - Ensure that patients understand the relationship between behavior and health.
  - Jointly assess barriers to change.
  - Gain patient commitment to change.

- Involve patients in selecting risk factors to change.
- Be creative, flexible, and practical, and use a combination of strategies.
- Design a behavior modification plan.
- Monitor progress through follow-up contact.
- Involve office staff (team approach).

Recommended Counseling Topics

- **Diet.** Nutritional assessment of intake of fat—saturated fats, polyunsaturated fatty acids (PUFAs), monounsaturated fatty acids (MUFAs)—cholesterol, complex carbohydrates, fiber, sodium, iron, and calcium (women) should be initiated. The Food Guide Pyramid and the Dietary Guidelines for Americans should be discussed: Eat a variety of foods; maintain a healthy weight; choose a diet low in saturated fat and cholesterol; choose a diet with plenty of vegetables, fruits, and grain products; use complex carbohydrates in moderation and limit intake of simple carbohydrates; use salt and sodium in moderation; and, if alcoholic beverages are used, use them in moderation.[6] Calcium is especially important for women beginning in their teen decade to reduce the risk of osteoporosis and bone fracture. Average daily intake should be 1,000 to 1,500 mg. The adverse effect of carbonated drinks with phosphorus on calcium and bone growth should also be discussed. Vitamin (especially antioxidants) and mineral supplementation should also be discussed with patients. Scientific evidence to date suggests that improving diet is more effective than supplementation alone.[7]
- **Exercise.** Patients should be given at least a brief exercise prescription, including selection of an exercise program to provide a source of regular physical activity. Such a program should be tailored to their health status and lifestyle, such as dynamic movement of large muscle groups for at least 20 minutes, 3 or more days per week, at an intensity of at least 60% of the maximum heart rate (220 beats per minute–age in years). Exercise at lower intensity and frequency levels can improve strength, flexibility, and cardiovascular fitness. Weight-bearing exercise is especially important for perimenopausal and postmenopausal women to avoid or decrease bone loss and osteoporosis.[1]
- **Substance use.** Include advice on cessation of tobacco use, limiting of alcohol consumption, health effects of other drugs, and not driving or doing other dangerous activities while under the influence of intoxicants (See Chapter 5.7). Smoking is the leading cause of preventable death in the United States. Studies have shown that multiple intervention strategies (one-to-one counseling, self-help materials, referral to community programs, prescription of nicotine substitutes) are most effective.[8] The basics of smoking cessation counseling should include providing a smoke-free office and hospital, designating an office smoking cessation coordinator, asking patients at every opportunity whether they smoke and assessing their readiness to stop if they do, using chart stickers if the patient smokes as a way of cueing office staff for ongoing interventions, providing multiple interventions to assist the smoker to stop, and following up to support patients who are motivated to stop.
- **Sexual practices.** Counseling efforts should focus on prevention of sexually transmitted diseases, including human immunodeficiency virus (HIV), and "safe-sex" recommendations: partner selection, condom use, and precautions regarding anal intercourse (See Chapter 19.4). Clinicians should take a complete sexual and drug history.[9] Sexually active adults should be advised that the most effective strategy to prevent infection is to abstain or maintain a mutually monogamous sexual relationship with an uninfected partner. Women of childbearing age need to be advised of the dangers of HIV and other sexually transmitted infections during pregnancy. Prevention of unintended pregnancy should also be discussed with individuals of childbearing age. Contraceptive options should be discussed with sexually active adults including information on efficacy limitations and proper use of available contraception techniques (See Chapter 14.1). Empathy and confidentiality are important aspects of this counseling.
- **Injury prevention.** Minimum counseling efforts in this area should include use of safety belts and helmets, prevention of violent behavior, safe use and storage of firearms, use of smoke and carbon monoxide detectors, not smoking near bedding or upholstery, and performing back conditioning exercises to prevent back pain and injuries. Intentional injuries include suicide and violence. Patients should be questioned regarding their risk of suicide and violence, with directed interventions when indicators are present. Injury to women as a result of domestic violence is one of the nation's most widespread and

least reported health problems. Unintentional injuries include motor vehicle–related injuries and environmental and household injuries. Advise patients never to drive while under the influence. To avoid other types of injuries, patients should be advised against alcohol, tobacco, or psychoactive drug use when participating in potentially dangerous activities; advised to check their smoke detectors regularly; and counseled to child-proof their homes and to prevent falls among elderly household members by securing loose throw rugs and electrical cords in pathways.

■ **Dental health.** Good personal oral hygiene, daily brushing and flossing, use of fluoride, and avoidance of sugary foods can control plaque and gingivitis. Individuals with current or history of use of tobacco or heavy use of alcohol are at risk for oral–pharyngeal cancers and should be advised to get a thorough checkup every 3 years up to age 40 and annually thereafter. Individuals engaged in sports potentially leading to dental trauma should be encouraged to use mouth guards.

■ **Preconception counseling.** Counseling and risk assessment, in addition to emphasizing general health promotion (abstinence from alcohol, drugs, and tobacco products and lowering risk of sexually transmitted disease), can reduce risk of congenital malformations and low birth weight, markedly improving outcomes by reducing infant morbidity and mortality. Health maintenance evaluations of a couple considering conception can include determining their emotional readiness to have children, the availability of sufficient financial resources, the risk of occupational toxin exposure for either person, and the need for genetic counseling and possible genetic diagnostic interventions. Counseling to reduce exposure to infections (rubella, cytomegalovirus, hepatitis B, toxoplasmosis, herpes simplex virus, chlamydia, human papillomavirus, and other sexually transmitted diseases) is very important. Exposure history should also be elicited to determine reproductive risk, for example, diethylstilbestrol (DES), other teratogens.[10,11]

Screening

■ **Definition.** Screening of asymptomatic adults is an important component in adult health maintenance and can often be accomplished at any patient visit. Scientific evidence strongly supports the screening of all adults for cardiovascular risk factors (tobacco use, hypertension, hyperlipidemia, sedentary lifestyle, family history), women older than 40 for breast cancer, and all adult women for cervical and ovarian cancer. Screening for colorectal cancer is recommended for adults older than 40 years.

■ **Criteria for screening.** Frame[12] developed criteria to consider when selecting a disease and test to use for screening:

■ The condition must have a significant effect on the quality and quantity of life.

■ Acceptable methods of treatment must be available.

■ The condition must have an asymptomatic period during which detection and treatment significantly reduce morbidity and mortality.

■ Treatment in the asymptomatic phase must yield a therapeutic result superior to that obtained by delaying treatment until symptoms appear.

■ Tests that are acceptable to patients must be available at a reasonable cost to detect the condition in the asymptomatic period.

■ The incidence of the condition must be sufficient to justify the cost of screening. Test sensitivity, specificity, and positive predictive value are important factors in the selection and evaluation of screening tests. Poor sensitivity or specificity can lead to a high rate of false-positive and false-negative results, both of which carry potentially serious consequences for patients.

■ **Selected screening interventions**
  ■ **Cancer screening[1,13]**
    • **Breast cancer.** There is universal consensus to offer mammography every 1 to 2 years for women aged 40 to 50, and annually thereafter. The American Cancer Society (ACS) recommends obtaining a baseline mammogram at age 35. There is no consensus at what age to stop screening. The USPSTF recommends routine screening until age 69, with continuing mammograms on an individual basis. Factors such as life expectancy, comorbidities, and general health are reasonable considerations for this and other screening tests. The ACS and the American

College of Obstetricians and Gynecologists recommend that clinical breast examinations be started prior to age 40. These examinations should be performed annually after age 40. There is insufficient evidence to recommend for or against teaching breast self-examination (See Chapter 13.8).

- **Colorectal cancer.** This is another important cause of cancer-related death in the United States (See Chapter 11.11). Colonoscopic screening should be directed to adults at higher than average risk. It is important to elicit family history to determine risk status. This should include history of colon cancer or adenomas and sporadic polyps in first-degree relatives, all now considered to be important predictors.[14] Persons with a positive family history should receive a colonoscopy by age 50. However, a recent study suggests that colonoscopic screening can detect advanced neoplasms in asymptomatic adults that were not detected with sigmoidoscopy.[15] Fecal occult blood tests (FOBTs) remain the most cost-effective screening tool in people older than age 50. If the test result is positive, follow-up examination with colonoscopy or flexible sigmoidoscopy plus air contrast barium enema (ACBE) should be undertaken. People older than 50 years may also benefit from screening with flexible sigmoidoscopy every 3 to 5 years. With a history of colon polyps, people should receive a colonoscopic screening every 5 to 10 years. The percentage of lesions detected by each method and the relative cost of the tests are estimated to be as shown in Table 1.3-3.
- **Prostate cancer.** Prostate-specific antigen (PSA) for prostate cancer is not recommended by the USPSTF but is recommended by the ACS and most other expert panels. The benefits of PSA screening remain controversial, whereas the risks resulting from screening are quantifiable and substantial. Digital rectal examination is not recommended as a screen for prostate cancer. If PSA tests are obtained, age-specific reference ranges should be used to eliminate unnecessary biopsies in patients older than 60 years with elevations due to the normal aging process[16] (See Chapter 12.5).
- **Cervical cancer screening.** Regular Pap testing is recommended for all women who are or have been sexually active and who have a cervix. Screening should begin with onset of sexual activity and be repeated at least every 3 years (See Chapter 13.4).
- **Melanoma and other skin cancers.** Patients with a history of skin cancer should have a complete skin exam annually. All adults with significant sun exposure and/or a prior history of sunburn should also receive a complete skin exam periodically.

■ **Screening for coronary artery disease and hypercholesterolemia**
- Blood pressure readings should be obtained at every office visit and at least once every 2 years. Total cholesterol should be measured periodically in men aged 35 to 65 and women aged 45 to 65; there is insufficient evidence to recommend for or against routine screening of younger men and women. Also, the appropriate frequency of and interval between screenings have not been established. However, after age 40, given the prevalence of cardiovascular disease, screening should occur at least every 5 years. Given the importance of lipid subfractions in therapeutic decisions, a fasting lipid profile should be obtained. All patients should be counseled about intake of dietary saturated fat and other measures to reduce coronary

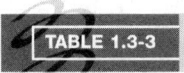

TABLE 1.3-3	Percentage of Colorectal Cancer Lesions Detected by Method and Relative Costs of Tests	

Method	Lesions detected (%)	Relative cost ($)
Fecal occult-blood testing	20–50	5
Flexible sigmoidoscopy	40	100–200
Air contrast barium enema	66–92	200
Colonoscopy	95	300–500

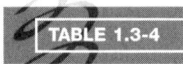

TABLE 1.3-4	Relative Risk for Coronary Artery Disease from Various Markers

Marker	Relative risk
Depression (men)	1.71
Depression (women)	1.73
Homocysteine	2.0
LDL-cholesterol	2.4
Apolipoprotein B	3.4
Total cholesterol/HDL ratio	3.4
High sensitivity C-reactive protein	4.4
Hostility	2.56

LDL, low-density lipoprotein; HDL, high-density lipoprotein.

heart disease (CAD) (See Chapter 17.4). The most important risk factors for CAD to screen for remain smoking, diabetes, and hypertension as well as hypercholesterolemia. Table 1.3-4 presents the relative risk of various markers for coronary artery disease.[17]
- It is important to have blood samples analyzed by an accredited laboratory. Abnormal results should be followed up by a second test, especially after 1–3 months of nonpharmacologic intervention (e.g., diet and exercise).

■ **Screening for osteoporosis.** Osteoporosis affects more than 25 million Americans, including 50% of women older than 45 years, and osteoporosis risk factors should be screened for in all women (See Chapter 17.6). Perimenopausal women at increased risk are white or Asian, have a history of bilateral oophorectomy before menopause, have a slender build, smoke or have smoked tobacco, have low calcium consumption patterns, a sedentary lifestyle, and a positive family history of the condition. There is insufficient evidence to recommend for or against routine bone density screening in asymptomatic men. After age 60, men also are at risk of osteoporosis; at least 20% of the 10 million Americans with osteoporosis are men. Only 3% of women older than 50 with an osteoporotic fracture ever received bone density evaluation. Screening by bone density measurement should be considered for high-risk individuals and all individuals older than 64 when the decision to use pharmacologic agents is to be based on bone mineral density measurements.

■ **Follow-up of screened patients is an important adult health maintenance strategy.** The single most important factor predicting whether cancer screening is obtained in the office setting may be the incorporation of a routine health maintenance visit in the practice regimen.[18] Screening results must be evaluated and incorporated into the patient record. This information is necessary to identify individuals for needed follow-up testing. Accuracy in testing and reporting of results is an important consideration. Laboratories used to analyze screening tests must adhere to national standards. Potential screening costs and morbidity may become issues for patients in the event of follow-up testing and treatment.

Immunizations
■ **Definition.** Vaccination against infectious diseases is an important and cost-effective component of adult health maintenance. Many adults have not received the vaccines and toxoids that are indicated to protect them against potentially life-threatening diseases.
■ **Recommended immunizations**
  ■ Tetanus–diphtheria (Td) booster every 10 years.
  ■ Hepatitis A vaccine for health care and lab workers, for injection or street drug users and their partners, for institutionalized persons and their caregivers, as well as for persons traveling abroad to endemic areas or wherever periodic outbreaks occur.

- Hepatitis B vaccine if high-risk status (health care workers, intravenous drug users, homosexual persons, dialysis recipients, blood product recipients).
- Pneumococcal vaccine if with medical condition or conditions that increase the risk of pneumococcal infection (chronic organ disease, HIV infection, sickle cell disease, asplenia, or older than age 55 and in an institution).
- Influenza vaccine annually if immune suppressed, a resident of a chronic care facility, or a health care provider; new evidence suggests that all adults should receive this vaccine to reduce days lost from work.
- Measles–mumps–rubella vaccine if born after 1956 and lacking evidence of immunity to measles.
- Varicella vaccine—consider for healthy persons without a history of chickenpox or prior immunization (consider serologic titer option).
- Occupational and environmental exposure-specific immunizations.[19]

- Office procedures to improve compliance with immunization recommendations are recommended and consistent with general office-based strategies to incorporate preventive services.
  - Have office staff routinely assess patient's immunization status, making sure that appropriately complete checklists are being used.
  - Generate reminders automatically.
  - Send reminder postcards.
  - Standing orders on outpatient and inpatient charts allow nurses to administer routine immunizations (e.g., annual influenza vaccine).
  - Provide patients with materials on vaccine-preventable diseases.
  - Provide chart audit feedback to clinicians on their patients' panel immunization rates.

Chemoprophylaxis

- **Definition.** This important component of adult health maintenance, often underprescribed, involves the use of medications or supplements prospectively to prevent potential future diseases. Indications (benefits), risks of use and nonuse, dosage, precautions, and possible side effects of chemoprophylactic agents are basic issues for the family physician in helping patients decide whether or not to adopt a specific intervention as a health maintenance strategy.
- **Recommended chemoprophylactic agents**
  - **Aspirin therapy.** Recent longitudinal trials indicate a benefit for women as well as men from daily or every-other-day use of aspirin after age 40 to prevent vascular disease, especially if the patient is at high risk or has a family history of coronary artery disease and no risk of stroke or bleeding. Other recent studies have suggested that regular aspirin at doses recommended for prevention of cardiovascular disease may also decrease the risk of and mortality from colorectal cancer for both men and women. There remains disagreement surrounding appropriate dosing and frequency of use.
  - **Skin protection from ultraviolet light.** Chronic overexposure to sunlight is responsible for 95% of all basal cell carcinomas. Individuals should be prescribed a sunscreen with a protection factor of at least 15 and encouraged to use it.
  - **Postexposure prophylaxis.** The USPSTF recommends prophylactic agents for people with exposure to *Haemophilus influenzae* type b disease and meningococcal infection (oral rifampin), hepatitis A (immune globulin), tuberculosis (isoniazid), hepatitis B (hepatitis B immune globulin and hepatitis B vaccine), and rabies (immune globulin) (See Chapters 6.3, 10.4, and 11.5).

Effective Physician and Office-based Strategies

The following strategies have been shown to enhance the quality and quantity of health maintenance interventions.[20]

- **Involve the office staff.** A team approach to the delivery of preventive services is highly effective. Nursing and other members of office or clinic staff are often able to communicate with patients very effectively. Examples of specific staff functions include reviewing records to prompt clinicians and patients regarding preventive care, updating patient care flow sheets or computerized records, issuing reminders to patients and clinicians, following up on test results, and helping patients gain access to community resources. All immunizations and many screening activities can be successfully provided by nurses or allied health professionals. The team approach resolves the major barrier physicians face in implementing preventive care and recommendations: lack of time.[21]

■ **Incorporate routine documentation tools into your practice.** The "Put Prevention into Practice" (PPIP) education and action kit of the U.S. Public Health Service targets the patient, the provider, and the office staff and system with easy-to-use materials and tools to foster a health maintenance approach. These include reminder postcards for patients to alert them of the need for specific prevention interventions, patient flow sheets for preventive care that may be added to the patient's chart (e.g., smoker, due for Td or mammogram), charts and posters that inform patients that health maintenance is a practice priority, and prevention prescription pads to allow the clinician to write brief risk-reduction behavioral prescriptions for patients. The *Clinician's Handbook of Clinical Preventive Services* is a user-friendly manual providing the basic steps of performing more than 60 preventive services. The kit also includes a Personal Health Guide as a portable health maintenance record for adults. (The PPIP kit can be obtained from the American Academy of Family Physicians Order Dept., 800-944-0000.)

■ **Facilitate patient compliance.** Make available patient education materials and information regarding community resources to help patients. Patient-held mini-records, such as the PPIP Personal Health Guide (see above), promote increased responsibility among patients for their own health maintenance activities and are available in Spanish and English. Patient education materials should also be appropriately directed in terms of the patient's literacy level and other pertinent factors (older than 60 years, requiring large print, etc.).

■ **Establish health maintenance guidelines (standards and objectives) for the practice and evaluate achievement through audits and continuous quality improvement approaches.** Practice systems to foster adult health maintenance activities can be most effectively evaluated through periodic reviews of charts and specifying other indicators of quality. To obtain or maintain National Commission on Quality Assurance (NCQA) accreditation, health care organizations are now required to conduct such audits, which usually include such indicators as immunization history, various cancer screening tests, and other health screening indicators such as hypertension, hypercholesterolemia, and domestic violence.

■ **Develop minicounseling topics.** Ten preventive topics, 3 to 10 minutes in duration and updated as necessary, can maximize the impact of "teachable moments." The list may include exercise, smoking cessation, stress reduction, injury prevention, discipline and parenting skills, and family health promotion.

■ **Reminder or prompting systems.** Generate compliance reminders, either manually or by computer, as a systemized approach to tracking patients in need of routine preventive care.[22]

References

1. U.S. Preventive Service Task Force. *Guide for clinical preventive services*, 2nd ed. Baltimore: Williams & Wilkins; 1995.
2. Lyons PE. Healthcare maintenance: children and adults. In: Paulman PM, ed. *Family medicine clerkship guide*, Amsterdam: Elsevier; 2005.
3. McGinnis JM, Foege WH. Actual causes of death in the United States. *JAMA* 1993;270:2207.
4. U.S. Centers for Disease Control and Prevention. *Natl Vital Stat Rep* 2000;48.
5. Commission on Public Health and Scientific Affairs, The American Academy of Family Physicians. Leawood, KS, 1995.
6. Thomson C, Ritenbaugh C, Kerwin J, et al. *Handbook of preventive and therapeutic nutrition handbook*. New York: Chapman and Hall, 1995.
7. Swain R, Kaplan B. Vitamins as therapy in the 1990s. *J Am Board Fam Pract* 1995;8:206.
8. U.S. Public Health Service. Smoking cessation in adults. *Am Fam Physician* 1995; 51:1914.
9. U.S. Department of Health and Human Services. *Clinician's handbook of preventive services*. Washington, DC: 1994.

10. Swan LL, Apgar BS. Preconceptual obstetric risk assessment and health promotion. *Am Fam Physician* 1995;51:1875.
11. Lyons PE. Preconception counseling. In: *Obstetrics in family medicine: a practical guide.* Humana Press; 2006.
12. Frame PS. Health maintenance in clinical practice: strategies and barriers. *Am Fam Physician* 1992;45:1192.
13. U.S. Public Health Service. Cancer detection in adults by physical examination. *Am Fam Physician* 1995;51:871.
14. Toribara NW, Sleisenger MH. Screening for colorectal cancer. *N Engl J Med* 1995; 332:861.
15. Lieberman DA, et al. Use of colonoscopy to screen asymptomatic adults for colorectal cancer. *N Engl J Med* 2000;343:162–168.
16. Ruckle HC, Klee GG, Oesterling JE. Prostate-specific antigen: concepts for staging prostate cancer and monitoring response to therapy. *Mayo Clin Proc* 1994;69:69.
17. Ridker PM, Hennekens CH, Buring JE, et al. C-reactive protein and other markers of inflammation in the prediction of cardiovascular disease. *N Engl J Med* 2000;342:836–843.
18. Ruffin MT, Gorenflo DQ, Woodman B. Predictors of screening for breast, cervical, colorectal, and prostatic cancer among community-based primary care practices. *J Am Board Fam Pract* 2000;13:1–10.
19. Zimmerman RK, Clover RD. Adult immunizations: a practical approach for clinicians, Part II. *Am Fam Physician* 1995;51:1139.
20. Yano EM, et al. Helping practices reach primary care goals. Lessons from the literature. *Arch Intern Med* 1995;155:1146.
21. Strange KC, et al. How do family physicians prioritize delivery of multiple preventive services? *J Fam Pract* 1994;38:231.
22. Frame PS. Computerized health maintenance tracking systems: a clinician's guide to necessary and optional features. A report from the American Cancer Society Advisory Group on Preventive Health Care Reminder Systems. *J Am Board Fam Pract* 1995;8:221.

HEALTH MAINTENANCE FOR OLDER ADULTS

James P. Richardson

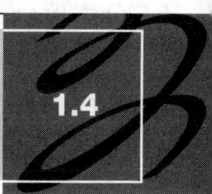

1.4

$\mathcal{T}$he proportion of the population that is elderly continues to grow. Because of the large influx of "baby boomers" into this group beginning in 2010, this demographic group will increase in size dramatically, guaranteeing that geriatric medicine will be a large part of every family physician's practice. Today's 65-year-old will live for an average of 13 to 17 years more. Thus, health promotion is not an activity that patients "outgrow."

As noted in previous chapters, many health promotion activities recommended in the past have not been supported by evidence of their effectiveness. Additionally, physicians cannot simply extrapolate recommendations for younger age groups because older adults often suffer from multiple comorbidities and reduced function. Physicians are often confused by the plethora of recommendations from government agencies, professional groups, and experts. A good source for the practitioner is the web site of the U.S. Preventive Services Task Force (USPSTF) www.preventiveservices.ahrq.gov.[1] This web site concisely reviews the evidence for more than 60 health promotion activities, ranking recommendations by the strength of the evidence. Besides making its own recommendations, this resource also includes the recommendations of organizations such as the American Cancer Society and evaluates whether these recommendations are supported by evidence from reliable studies. The task force now[3] evaluates prevention topics on a continuing basis, and the task force's web site should be monitored for future recommendations and revisions.

The following recommendations are largely consistent with the USPSTF guidelines but are the author's own. These recommendations apply only to asymptomatic people without risk factors.

INCORPORATING HEALTH MAINTENANCE INTO PRACTICE

Older patients are less likely than younger ones to request health promotion activities and are less tolerant of long appointments. A useful approach, therefore, is to attempt to include some elements of health maintenance activities with every visit. For example, a visit for hypertension follow-up in the fall is an opportune time to inquire about influenza, pneumococcal, and tetanus–diphtheria (Td) immunizations.

Many studies show that physicians believe they recommend health maintenance to their patients more often than can actually be demonstrated. Reminder systems and aids have been found effective in increasing health promotion use. The most effective are those that remove the physician from the decision loop.[2] In other words, physicians can provide health promotion activities by involving their nurses and other staff, or by using questionnaires to initiate discussions of health promotion. Office protocols and prompts from electronic medical record systems also are effective (e.g., immunizations, making a return appointment for cervical cancer screening). For a more detailed discussion of implementation strategies, (See Chapter 1.3).

As with all health care for older adults, health promotion activities should take into account quality-of-life concerns and patient preferences. Shared decision making is paramount.

PRIMARY PREVENTION

- **Definition.** Interventions that are primary types of prevention seek to prevent a given disease from ever beginning. A good example is immunizations to prevent infectious diseases.
- **Infectious diseases.** Prevention of infectious diseases is often neglected by patients and providers.[2] Together, influenza and pneumonia are the fifth leading cause of death in elderly individuals.
  - **Influenza.** Influenza vaccine should be administered in October or November in the United States to all elderly persons who consent and are not allergic to eggs. The vaccine is effective in reducing the incidence of influenza and pneumonia, as well as hospitalizations for these diseases.
  - **Pneumococcal vaccine.** This vaccine should be given at least once to all elderly individuals, as well as to younger patients with chronic diseases, such as pulmonary disease, chronic liver disease, and diabetes mellitus. High-risk individuals, defined as those older than 75 years or with severe chronic disease, should receive another booster after 5 years.
  - **Tetanus–diphtheria.** In the United States, tetanus is now a disease of the elderly population. Immunity to tetanus and diphtheria can be maintained by giving Td boosters every 10 years to patients who have had the primary series of three immunizations over 6 months. However, careful inquiry should be undertaken of all elderly people receiving Td boosters because many seniors, especially women, have never received primary immunization, and these individuals will not be protected with one booster.[3] Administration of tetanus immune globulin is necessary to elderly people with tetanus-prone (i.e., "dirty") wounds who have never completed a primary series.
  - **Tuberculosis.** Routine purified protein derivative (PPD) testing is not necessary for community-dwelling elderly individuals who are not HIV-positive but should be administered on admission to nursing homes or assisted living facilities. Two-stage testing (repeating the PPD 1 to 2 weeks after the first in those with an initial negative result) is necessary because of the booster phenomenon.
  - **Herpes zoster.** A vaccine to reduce the incidence of shingles, or herpes zoster, is now available. It is recommended for adults age 60 and older, but efficacy declines with increasing age.

- ■ **Prevention of sexually transmitted disease.** As with younger age groups, sexually active elderly individuals should be counseled to avoid high-risk sexual behavior and to use condoms with new partners.
- ■ **Routine dental care** remains important in the elderly population.
- ■ **Injury prevention.** Injuries are a frequent cause of death in elderly individuals.
  - ■ Elderly patients should be counseled regarding the dangers of falls and the benefits of exercise. Avoidable causes of falls include environmental hazards, such as poor lighting or throw rugs, visual deficits, and debilitation. Physicians should counsel older adults to gradually increase their exercise capacity by walking, gardening, or doing household chores. In addition to reduced fall risk, benefits demonstrated in population studies include lower incidence of cardiovascular disease, dementia, osteoporosis, and improved mood.
  - ■ Everyone should be counseled to wear safety belts (and bicycle or motorcycle helmets if applicable), to maintain working smoke detectors, to store firearms safely, and to keep hot water temperatures below 120°F.
  - ■ Although screening of all older drivers is not advocated, all providers should know the local laws governing driving restrictions should they become aware that a patient is no longer a safe driver. Many hospitals now offer testing by occupational therapists that might help with this determination.
- ■ **Osteoporosis.** Screening for osteoporosis in women by dual-energy x-ray absorptiometry (DXA) is recommended after age 65.
- ■ **Smoking cessation.** Benefits accrue to those who stop smoking at any age. Patients' smoking history should be obtained, and smokers should be encouraged to quit. Counseling patients to stop smoking is an effective intervention.
- ■ **Alcohol.** As alcoholism develops in some older people late in life due at least in part to slower metabolism, screening with the Cut down, Annoyed, Guilty, and Eye opener (CAGE) questions (See Chapter 5.3) is recommended.
- ■ **Lipid disorders.** Whereas secondary prevention of cardiovascular diseases with lipid-lowering drug therapy is well established, primary prevention for older adults remains controversial. There are scarce data regarding primary prevention in older adults, although the Cardiovascular Health Study found that statin therapy reduced the risk of both cardiovascular events and all-cause mortality in adults 65 and older with elevated cholesterol levels.[4] The National Cholesterol Education Program advocates screening elderly persons with a good life expectancy by measuring high-density lipoprotein and total cholesterol.[5] The decision must therefore be individualized, based on the senior's quality of life, life expectancy, other risk factors, cost, and patient preference.

SECONDARY PREVENTION: CANCER SCREENING

- ■ **Definition.** Interventions that seek to detect disease before individuals become symptomatic are secondary preventive measures. Examples include blood pressure measurement to detect hypertension and prevent cardiovascular diseases and cervical smears to detect cervical cancer.
- ■ **Breast cancer.** Almost half of all breast cancers in women occur in those aged 65 years and older. Breast self-examination has never been shown to be an effective tool in reducing mortality but is recommended by the American Cancer Society along with a yearly clinical breast examination. Mammography screening is more controversial because studies of mammography have included few women older than 75 years, and there is no evidence that mammography is effective after this age. Mammography combined with clinical breast examination has been proved to reduce mortality from breast cancer in women aged 50 through 69 years. The USPSTF guidelines recommend cessation of breast cancer screening at age 70. Nevertheless, because the aging breast has an increased proportion of fat, which makes it easier to examine radiologically (and therefore mammography has a higher positive predictive value in elderly individuals), clinical breast examination and mammography performed every 2 years can be recommended to women older than 70 with a good life expectancy who would have surgery should a suspicious lesion be found.[6]

- **Cervical cancer.** A significant proportion of elderly women have never had cervical (Pap) smears. Women with cervixes who are or have been sexually active should have smears at least every 3 years. Women who have had three or more technically satisfactory negative smears can stop undergoing screening after age 65 (See Chapter 13.4).
- **Colorectal cancer.** Rectal examination is not a useful screen in the asymptomatic patient. Fecal occult blood testing done yearly has been shown to reduce mortality from colon cancer by 33%,[7,8]) although the utility of this test may be less in the elderly individual due to a higher false-positive rate (and therefore lower positive predictive value) in elderly people. Rigid sigmoidoscopy has also been demonstrated to be effective in reducing mortality from cancer in the distal colon, but the optimal frequency of this screening is not clear.[9] There is insufficient evidence to recommend one test over the other.
- **Prostate cancer.** A digital rectal examination for prostate cancer has a very low yield. The prostate-specific antigen (PSA) test is elevated in older men, not only in those with prostate cancer, but also in men with benign prostatic hypertrophy as well. Although PSA testing identifies significant numbers of men with prostate cancer confined to the gland, it does not appear that mortality is reduced in those in whom early prostate cancer is found. Men older than 65 to 70 years most likely will die of a comorbid condition other than prostate cancer.[10] Therefore, with the possible exception of patients who request testing and have been informed of its drawbacks, PSA screening is not recommended for elderly men.
- **Skin.** A yearly examination of all skin for patients with significant sunlight exposure or with a history of skin cancer is recommended.

SECONDARY PREVENTION: OTHER DISEASES

- **Glaucoma.** Routine screening by primary care physicians is not recommended. High-risk populations (blacks older than 40, whites older than 65, and those with a positive family history, diabetes, or severe myopia) may be referred to eye specialists for screening. The optimal interval for screening is not known.
- **Hypertension.** Blood pressure should be measured at least yearly.
- **Hypothyroidism.** Routine screening is not recommended, but clinicians should have a low threshold for ordering thyroid function tests—for example, serum thyroid-stimulating hormone level (TSH and free T_4) because of its subtle presentation.
- **Abdominal aortic aneurysm.** A new recommendation of the USPSTF is that men between the ages of 65 and 75 who are current or former smokers should have at least one ultrasound of the abdominal aorta.

Geriatric Assessment

Although not as strongly supported by evidence as the above recommendations, most experts recommend some or all of the following activities for elderly individuals.[11]

- **Special senses.** Visual and hearing loss contributes to functional decline and cognitive impairment. Vision may be tested with the Snellen chart, and hearing loss may be screened by history.
- **Polypharmacy.** Simplifying drug regimens improves compliance, reduces the incidence of adverse drug reactions, and saves money. Common offending drugs are those whose indications were never clear or the indications for which have disappeared (e.g., digoxin). Anticholinergic drugs (e.g., antispasmodics, antihistamines) and sedatives are particularly problematic for older adults.
- **Cognitive impairment and depression.** Both of these are common in elderly individuals. The Folstein Mini-Mental State Examination[12] is specific but not very sensitive for dementia, especially in well-educated or intelligent older adults. Many simple depression-screening instruments (e.g., Geriatric Depression Scale) are available.[13]
- **Advance directives.** Although all elderly individuals should be encouraged to record their desires in formal advance directive instruments, simply recording the patient's desires in the medical record is often very helpful to other providers and family members

should the patient become unable to make his or her own decisions (See Chapter 22.5). More importantly, older adults should be encouraged to grant a power-of-attorney to someone to make decisions for them, should they become unable to communicate or lose decision-making capacity.

Chemoprophylaxis

- **Aspirin.** Although the value of aspirin is well established for secondary prevention of stroke and myocardial infarction, its role in primary prevention is less clear (for further discussion, See Chapter 1.3). The task force recommends that physicians discuss the use of aspirin with patients at high risk for cardiovascular disease (5-year risk >3%), although it also found that aspirin use increases the risk of gastrointestinal bleeding, and to a smaller extent, the risk of hemorrhagic stroke, particularly in older adults. Recently, aspirin at a dose of 100 mg every other day has been demonstrated to reduce the risk of ischemic stroke, myocardial infarction, and major cardiovascular events in women older than 65.[14] The optimal dose of aspirin for prophylaxis is not known.
- **Multivitamins.** Vitamin supplementation does not prevent cardiovascular disease, but diet supplementation with one multivitamin a day is safe and may benefit those older adults with poor diets.

References

1. Richardson JP. Considerations for health promotion and disease prevention in older adults. *Medscape* 2006. Available online at http://www.medscape.com/viewarticle/ 531942.
2. Richardson JP, Michocki RM. Removing barriers to vaccination use by older adults. *Drugs Aging* 1994;4:357.
3. Richardson JP, Knight AL. The prevention of tetanus in the elderly. *Arch Intern Med* 1991;151:1712 [Erratum *Arch Intern Med* 1991;151:2451].
4. Lemaitre RN, Psaty BM, Heckbert SR, et al. Therapy with hydroxymethylglutaryl coenzyme A reductase inhibitors (statins) and associated risk of incident cardiovascular events in older adults: evidence from the cardiovascular health study. *Arch Intern Med* 2002;162:1395.
5. Expert Panel on Detection, Evaluation, and Treatment of High Blood Cholesterol in Adults. Summary of the second report of the National Cholesterol Education Program (NCEP) Expert Panel on Detection, Evaluation, and Treatment of High Blood Cholesterol in Adults (Adult Treatment Panel II). *JAMA* 1993;269:3015.
6. Costanza ME, ed. Screening recommendations of the forum panel. *J Gerontol* 1992;47(special issue):5.
7. Mandel JS, et al. Reducing mortality from colorectal cancer by screening for fecal occult blood. *N Engl J Med* 1993;328:1365.
8. Winawer SJ, Fletcher RH, Miller L, et al. Colorectal cancer screening: clinical guidelines and rationale. *Gastroenterology* 1997;112:594–642 [Published errata in *Gastroenterology* 1997;112:1060 and 1998;114:635].
9. Selby JV, et al. A case-control study of screening sigmoidoscopy and mortality from colorectal cancer. *N Engl J Med* 1992;326:653.
10. Johansson J-E, et al. High 10-year survival rate in patients with early, untreated prostatic cancer. *JAMA* 1992;267:2191.
11. Gallo JJ, Bogner HR, Fulmer T, Paveza GJ, eds. *Handbook of geriatric assessment.* 4th ed. Gaithersburg, MD: Aspen Publishers; 2006
12. Folstein MF, Folstein SE, McHugh PR. Mini-Mental State: a practical method for grading the cognitive state of patients for the clinician. *J Psychiatr Res* 1975;12:189.
13. Gallo JJ, Wittnik MN. In: Gallo JJ, Bogner HR, Fulmer T, Paveza GJ, eds. *Handbook of geriatric assessment.* 4th ed. Gaithersburg, MD: Aspen Publishers; 2006:153.
14. Ridker PM, Cook NR, Lee I-M, et al. A randomized trial of low-dose aspirin in the primary prevention of cardiovascular disease in women. *N Engl J Med* 2005; 352:1293.

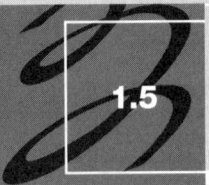

HEALTH CARE FOR THE INTERNATIONAL TRAVELER
Nancy D. Elder, Jeffery D. Schlaudecker, Mhroos Peters, Laurie Carrier

GENERAL PRINCIPLES
More Americans than ever are traveling to developing countries. Excess **mortality abroad is mainly due to accidents,** and **morbidity is primarily from traveler's diarrhea.** Serious infectious diseases, however, do threaten travelers' health, but many can be prevented or decreased with appropriate pretravel care. Unfortunately, less than half the travelers to developing countries seek travel medical advice.

APPROACH TO THE PATIENT
- **History** should include information about previous travel (including problems encountered), current itinerary (destinations, length of visit, type of accommodations, planned activities), and personal history (age, chronic diseases or problems, disabilities, habits, occupation, avocations). In addition, an up-to-date medication list, including over-the-counter and herbal preparations should be obtained, and an immunization history taken.
- The **physical examination** for young healthy patients needs nothing additional to that performed for health care maintenance. Patients with chronic illness will need special attention to maximize their current health prior to departure.

INTERVENTIONS AND RECOMMENDATIONS
Traveler's Diarrhea
- **Epidemiology. 20% to 50% of travelers** to developing countries have diarrhea in first 2 weeks. Symptoms last 4 days without treatment, 1/5 are bedridden for 1 day, 1/3 forced to alter activities.
- **Etiology. 50% to 80% bacterial etiology.** Primarily *Escherichia coli* in Latin America, Caribbean, Africa and *E. coli* and *Campylobacter* in Asia. Protozoa are uncommon; suspect if symptoms last more than 2 weeks.
- **Contaminated food and water** with fecal material is the primary cause including salads, unpeeled fruits, poorly cooked meats, unpasteurized dairy, and tap water. Food from street vendors especially risky. **Freezing does not kill;** thus, ice can be contaminated; even liquor with a high alcohol content does not sterilize contaminated ice. Rare person-to-person spread.
- **Definition**
  - Three or more unformed stools in 24 hours and at least one of the following: fever, nausea, vomiting, abdominal cramps, tenesmus, bloody stools. Dysentery is defined as diarrhea with fever and bloody, mucoid stools.
  - In children, it is defined as a twofold increase in number of stools.
  - Host factors that increase the likelihood include immunocompromise, extremes of age, adventurous travel (camping, staying with locals) and lowered gastric acidity (including using H2 blockers, proton pump inhibitors).
- **Behavioral counseling. "Boil it, cook it, peel it, or forget it."** Access to waterless hand cleaners could help reduce the risk. Bottled water safest; all water should be boiled >10 minutes. Traveler should avoid swimming in unclean waters. All foods need to be heated >65°C (not just warmed).
- **Medications:**
  - Antibiotic prophylaxis
    - Not recommended by the Centers for Disease Control and Prevention even for high-risk travelers, but some experts believe can be **appropriate for highest-risk**

travelers, including those with cardiac, renal, immunodeficiency, bowel disease, insulin-dependent diabetes.

- **Ciprofloxacin** 250 mg daily from day of arrival until 2 days after return, no longer than 3 weeks; 90% protective with side effects of skin rash, vaginal candidiasis, mild phototoxicity, gastrointestinal sensitivity, and rarely anaphylaxis. Not for children or in pregnancy.
- **Rifaximin** (Xifaxan), a nonabsorbed antibiotic, is well tolerated but limited data on effectiveness.

■ Probiotic prophylaxis
  - Protection up to 47% with *Lactobacillus* GG (Culturelle) in one study; other studies show limited or no benefit and optimal dosing is unknown.
  - Bismuth subsalicylate. 65% protective, but QID dosing limits utility. Not for patients on anticoagulation, other salicylates. Can interfere with doxycycline absorption. Stools and tongue temporarily discolored black.

■ **Treatment**
  ■ Antimicrobials
    - Debate exists regarding the use of empiric self-treatment of traveler's diarrhea. Successful use depends largely on pretravel education, but short-course therapy is unlikely to significantly contribute to worldwide resistance patterns.
    - Drug of choice for **empiric self-treatment is Ciprofloxacin** 500 mg bid for 3 days at first onset of gastrointestinal symptoms.
    - Alternatives include **levofloxacin** 500 mg once. **Zithromax** is recommended in places with high rates of quinolone-resistant *Campylobacter* (Thailand) and is dosed 1 g once; it is also recommended for children with traveler's diarrhea at 5 to 10 mg per kg once and is the drug of choice in pregnancy.

  ■ Antidiarrheals
    - **Loperamide** 4 mg at initial loose stool and then 2 mg after each loose stool up to 16 mg per day.
    - Limited clinical evidence suggests antimotility medications should not be used in cases of dysentery but are likely safe when used with an antibiotic.
    - Codeine should be avoided due to potential for central side effects and toxicity.

  ■ **Rehydration** is the most important treatment.
    - Oral Rehydration Solution (ORS) packets should be made available to travelers at high risk, or can make homemade ORS: 1 L of clean water, 1 teaspoon of table salt, 8 teaspoons of sugar; mix until dissolved and give after each emesis or loose stool. Bottled or treated water is acceptable in healthy adults.

Malaria

■ **Epidemiology.** Four species of *Plasmodium (P. malariae, P. vivax, P. falciparum,* and *P. ovale)* are passed from infected female anopheles mosquitoes to humans and cause disease. Only *P. falciparum* is life-threatening. There are more than 350 million cases and 1 million deaths from malaria each year, in Central and South America, Africa, the Middle East, the India subcontinent, and Oceania.

■ **Clinical presentation.** Flulike symptoms (fever, chills, muscle aches, headache) predominate. Severe *P. falciparum* may lead to liver and kidney failure; *P. vivax* and *P. ovale* may remain dormant in the liver for years and reappear months to years later.

■ **Behavioral counseling. Prevent mosquito bites** by avoiding outdoors at dusk and dawn; using **insect repellent** with high concentrations of diethyltoluamide (DEET) (>35%, although effectiveness plateaus at 50%, DEET is safe for children over 2 months old and pregnant women); spraying mosquito nets and clothing with permethrin; sleeping indoors or under a mosquito net. A second-line insect repellant, Picardin 7%, may be effective, but for only 1 to 4 hours per application. Educate patients about malarial symptoms, and the need for urgent medical evaluation and treatment.

■ **Medications:**
  ■ Prophylaxis
    - Resistance is constantly changing. Check up-to-date recommendations at web sites such as www.cdc.gov.

- Chloroquine (Aralen) is for adults, children, and pregnant women. Side effects are rare and minor (nausea, headache, dizziness). Adult dose is one 500 mg tablet (8.3 mg/kg salt for children) per week, starting 2 weeks prior to travel and continuing 4 weeks after leaving malaria area.
- Mefloquine (Lariam) is for adults and children over 9 kg only. Significant side effects, especially in those with seizure disorder, psychiatric history, or cardiac conduct abnormalities include neuropsychiatric disturbances. Adult dose is one 250 mg tablet (5 mg/kg salt for children) per week, starting 2 weeks prior to travel and continuing 4 weeks after leaving malaria area.
- Doxyclcline (Vibramycin) is for adults and children over age 8 only. Side effects include a photosensitivity reaction. Adult dose is one 100 mg tablet (2 mg/kg for children) per day, starting 2 days prior to travel and continuing 4 weeks after leaving malaria area.
- Atovaquone plus proguanil (Malarone) is for adults and children over 11 kg only. Side effects include abdominal pain, nausea, and headache. Adult dose is one 250 mg atoqaquone/100 mg proguanil tablet (pediatric tablet is 62.5 atovaquone/25 proguanil, number of tablets depends on weight) per day, starting 2 days prior to travel and continuing 7 days after leaving malaria area.

- Presumptive self-treatment
  - For travelers **unable to access medical care** within 24 hours. Atovaquone plus proguanil (Malarone) 4 tablets as a single dose daily for 3 days. Not for travelers who used Malarone for prophylaxis.

- **Treatment**
  - **Depends on region where malaria was acquired, as well as species of Plasmodium.** Details can be found at www.cdc.gov. In addition to medications above, medications include quinine (650 mg three times a day for 3 to 7 days); clindamycin (20 mg base/kg/day divided three times a day for 7 days); primaquine (30 mg base daily for 14 days). Internationally, the World Health Organization recommends Artemisinin Combination Therapy (ACT). Details of its recommendations are at http://www.who.int/malaria/docs/TreatmentGuidelines2006.pdf.

Vaccine-Preventable Infectious Diseases

- Diphtheria and Tetanus
  - Still **highly endemic** in the developing world
  - Immunization.
    - **Td** recommended booster **every 10 years for adults;** 5 years if prolonged trip planned with limited access to care and moderate or high risk of injury
    - **DTaP** for younger children, **Tdap** for older children or adults who have never received at least one previous dose of an acellular pertussis–containing vaccine
    - Side effects to Tdap, DT, and Td are rare, but may include soreness, redness, and swelling at the injection site

- Influenza
  - **Highly endemic** throughout the year in tropical climates
  - Immunization
    - Influenza vaccine contraindicated in those allergic to eggs

- Measles
  - Indicated for all travelers born in 1957 or later without history of disease or without two adequate doses of live vaccine at any point in life
  - Immunization
    - The live virus vaccine (mumps–measles–rubella, **MMR**) is generally well tolerated, but side effects can include fever and/or rash 7 to 12 days after vaccination
    - Not for immunosuppressed patients or in pregnancy

- Polio
  - All travelers should have the primary series of three doses. Those traveling to higher-risk areas should also have a one-time adult booster dose.

- Immunization
  - The injectable killed vaccine is used routinely in the United States and Canada.
  - Live attenuated oral vaccine not to be used in immunosuppressed, pregnancy.
  - Minor local reactions, like pain, redness, swelling may occur at the injection site, often within 6 to 12 hours.
- Hepatitis B
  - Vaccination series recommended for those travelers at high risk: **adventure travelers,** possibility of dental work or accessing health care, tattooing, or the possibility of a new sexual partner during the stay.
  - Immunization
    - **Three-dose series** (0, 1 to 2, 4 to 6 months).
    - Non-Food and Drug Administration (FDA)-approved **accelerated three-dose schedule** is available (given on days 0, 7, and 14), but requires fourth dose at 12 months for lifelong immunity.
    - Well tolerated, but minor local reactions, such as pain, redness, swelling, may occur at the injection site.
    - Safe, but less efficacious in pregnancy and immunosuppression.
- Hepatitis A
  - **Most frequent** vaccine-preventable travel-related illness. Risk is 300 per 100,000 per month of travel, five to seven times higher in high-risk areas and populations. **Indicated for most travelers** to the developing world.
  - Immunization
    - **Two dose series,** with second dose at least 6 months after the first. First dose provides **95% immunity** at 4 weeks; second dose provides **long-term** immunity.
    - Well tolerated, but minor local reactions, such as pain, redness, swelling, may occur at the injection site.
    - A combination hepatitis A/B vaccine is also available.
- Typhoid fever
  - Bacterial infection spread fecal–oral route, person to person, through contaminated food or water. Infection results in **high fevers, abdominal pain,** and frequently **diarrhea.** Especially high risk for pregnant travelers; causes preterm labor and/or spontaneous abortion. **Immunization recommended for most travel to the developing world,** or any travel that will include adventurous dietary habits, prolonged stays, or predominantly rural itineraries.
  - Immunizations: Two vaccines exist:
    - Oral Typhoid TY21a vaccine (Vivotif Berna)
      - Efficacy of 50% to 90% for this **live attenuated strain of *Salmonella typhi***
      - Duration of immunity is **5 to 6 years**
      - **Four doses** taken on days 0, 2, 4, and 6
      - Pills must be kept **refrigerated,** and not taken within 24 hours of mefloquin or antibiotics
      - Approved for ages 6 years and above, low risk of side effects, but should not be given to patients with congenital or acquired immunodeficiencies
    - **Injectable capsular polysaccharide vaccine** (Typhim Vi)
      - Efficacy of 60% to 80%
      - Duration of immunity is **2 to 3 years**
      - Well tolerated and low side effects
      - Safe for children aged 2 years and older and **for those with immunodeficiencies,** including HIV
- Yellow fever
  - Mosquito spread **viral illness** found in **South America** and **sub-Saharan Africa.** Mosquito precautions (see Malaria) are essential.
  - Immunization
    - Live virus vaccine with efficacy >95%.
    - Proof of immunization at approved site can be required for travel to or from endemic countries.

- Single dose becomes effective in 10 days, and protection lasts at least 10 years.
- Up to 5% of persons can experience flulike symptoms 5 to 14 days after immunization, and rarely encephalitis can occur.
- Not for patients with egg allergies, or in pregnant or immunosuppressed patients.
- Approved for patients 9 months or older.

- Meningococcal meningitis
  - Epidemics common in **sub-Saharan Africa,** but **uncommon** in travelers from the United States. Travelers to endemic areas of the world should be offered vaccination. **Legally required** for pilgrims making the **Hajj pilgrimage to Mecca, Saudi Arabia.**
  - Immunization
    - Meningococcal conjugate vaccine (MCV4, *Menactra*)
      - For persons older than 11 years of age
      - Increased effectiveness compared to MPSV4, see below, low risk of side effects, and may be used in pregnancy and immunosuppression
    - Meningococcal polysaccharide vaccine (MPSV4, *Menomune*)
      - For children aged 2 to 10 years, or acceptable alternative for older age groups
      - Similar side effect profile to MCV4

- Cholera
  - Epidemics of diarrhea in developing world. Best treated with prevention, oral rehydration.
  - Immunization: **Not recommended**

- Rabies
  - Endemic in most of the developed world. All animal bites or exposures in the developing world should be followed by vigorous washing and medical attention.
  - Vaccine **not indicated for most travelers,** but can be considered in high-risk persons, or those living >1 month in remote area with limited access to evacuation.
  - **Postexposure treatment still required** after pre-exposure vaccination.
  - Immunization
    - Inactivated viral preparation
    - Three-dose series on days 0, 7, 21, or 28
    - Chloroquine and mefloquin should not be taken until completion of vaccination series

- Japanese encephalitis
  - Arboviral infection transmitted by mosquitoes. Endemic or epidemic in some **Asian** countries, **India,** and parts of **Australia.** Low risk for short-term travelers and those staying in urban areas.
  - Immunization
    - **Inactivated vaccine** given subcutaneously on days 0, 7, and 30
    - Limited data in pregnancy or immunosuppression
    - Local and **allergic reactions common:** series should be completed 10 days prior to departure
    - Ensure access to emergency medical care

INJURIES AND ACCIDENTS
Definition and Epidemiology
- **Injuries** are among the leading causes of death and disability in the world, and they are the leading cause of preventable deaths in travelers.
- In **young adult travelers,** death rates due to injury are increased by a factor of 2 to 3 and most of these deaths are traffic or swimming related.
- **Unintentional injuries** include road traffic accidents, falls, fires, poisoning, and drowning, as well as injuries incurred during **extreme sporting events** and **recreational drug and alcohol use.**

Behavioral Counseling
- Travelers should be counseled on avoiding situations when traffic accidents frequently occur: at dusk, in poor weather conditions, at crossroads, while speeding, and while passing other drivers.

- **Seat belts** should be required as a condition of vehicle rental (as well as airbags if available), and those traveling with small children should bring appropriate **car seats.**
- Motorcycles, scooters, open trucks, and small, unscheduled aircrafts should be avoided.
- Travelers should ensure that companies specializing in extreme or recreational sports are credentialed and provide **proper supervision and safety equipment.**
- Travelers should select **lodging** that includes smoke detectors, sprinklers, and locks on the doors.
- **Health and evacuation insurance** is an option for travelers if their destinations include countries where there may not be access to good medical care.

SEXUALLY TRANSMITTED DISEASES

Definition and Epidemiology

- **Casual sexual encounters and increased sexual promiscuity** during travel play a major role in the transmission of sexually transmitted diseases (STDs). **Abstinence or mutual monogamy** is the most reliable way to avoid acquisition and transmission of STDs; correct and consistent use of the **latex condom** can reduce the risk of STD transmission.
- Many STDs, including HIV, have **high prevalence** in even the most obscure of travel destinations.
- **Some STDs are more prevalent in developing countries** (e.g., chancroid, lymphogranuloma venereum, and granuloma inguinale) and increased rates of infectious syphilis and quinolone-resistant gonorrhea have recently been reported among men who have sex with men.

Behavioral Counseling

- Travelers should be counseled to avoid sexual interactions with core groups of efficient STD transmitters (commercial sex workers) in endemic areas.
- Any traveler who may have been **exposed to an STD** and who develops a vaginal or urethral discharge, an unexplained rash or genital lesion, or genital or pelvic pain should seek medical care immediately.
- **Screening** for asymptomatic infection should be encouraged among travelers who have had casual sexual activity.

Medications

- **Knowledge of the clinical presentation, frequency of infection, and antimicrobial resistance patterns** (e.g., quinolone-resistant *Neisseria gonorrhoeae*) is important in the management of STDs that occur in travelers to specific destinations.
- **Treatment should be directed toward a specific pathogen** for most STDs in industrialized countries. Empiric treatment can be used in situations where laboratory testing is not available. A typical regimen in the United States includes ceftriaxone 125 mg IM once, azithromycin 1 g orally once, and metronidazole 2 g orally once.

ALTITUDE ILLNESS

Definition and Epidemiology

- A number of acute syndromes occur at high altitude. Some may occur at altitudes as low as 2500 m and all are more likely with increasing altitude.
- **Acute mountain sickness (AMS)** is defined as the presence of headache in an unacclimatized person who has recently arrived at an altitude above 2,500 m plus the presence of one or more of the following: gastrointestinal symptoms (anorexia, nausea, vomiting), insomnia, dizziness, and lassitude or fatigue. The symptoms typically develop within 6 to 10 hours after ascent, but can occur as early as 1 hour or as late as 96 hours.
- **High altitude cerebral edema (HACE)** is a clinical diagnosis, defined as the onset of ataxia and/or altered consciousness in someone with AMS, usually occurring within 48 to 72 hours upon arrival at a given altitude. Signs and symptoms include headache, confusion, loss of coordination, papilledema, loss of cerebellar control, decreased mental status, and coma.

- **High altitude pulmonary edema (HAPE)** accounts for the majority of deaths due to high altitude disease and usually begins 24 to 96 hours after arriving at altitude. HAPE often presents with an insidious cough, breathlessness out of proportion to work that does not respond to rest, and production of frothy, often rusty sputum. Physical signs include rapid respiration rate, cyanosis, elevated jugular venous pressure, and diffuse crackles on lung auscultation.
- **Risk factors** include a history of high altitude illness, rapid rate of ascent, residence at an altitude below 3,000 ft (900 m), physical exertion, obesity, age less than 50 years, and certain pre-existing cardiopulmonary conditions.

Behavioral Counseling

- **Altitude illness** can be prevented or modified by paying attention to the speed, height, and duration of ascent.
- **"Staging"** is the process of remaining at an intermediate altitude for a few days before attempting the ultimate altitude. The initial stage should be between 2,012 and 2,988 m. Then, depending on symptoms, ascent can continue at the rate of 305 m per day for 3,048 to 4,267 m and per 2 days over 4,267 m.
- If **symptoms of AMS** occur, further ascent should be delayed until symptoms resolve. If symptoms worsen, or if symptoms of HAPE or HACE occur, then descent should begin immediately.
- **Adequate hydration** can help decrease symptoms, as can good physical conditioning (but even athletes in excellent condition can experience altitude illness).

Medications

- **Acetazolamide** can help prevent or mitigate the symptoms of AMS. For prophylaxis, the dose is 125 to 250 mg orally twice a day 24 hours before ascent and for the first 2 days at high altitude. When treating symptoms, the dose is 250 mg twice a day until symptoms resolve.
- **Dexamethasone** can be administered in doses of 4 mg every 6 hours for the few days it takes an individual to acclimatize to high altitude.
- **Combining acetazolamide and dexamethasone** has been shown in some studies to have additive benefits in cases where there is a rapid progression of symptoms, particularly if descent will be delayed.
- **Oxygen therapy** can help alleviate many of the symptoms of AMS in the acute setting. It can be lifesaving in HAPE and improves the headache with AMS within minutes.
- **Theophylline** has been shown to have some efficacy in preventing or reducing the severity of AMS in several small studies.
- **Nifedipine** can be used to prevent HAPE in people with a previous history. The usual dose is 20 mg twice daily prior to ascent and then three times daily once climbers reach 3,400 m. Nifedipine 10 mg initially and then 20 to 30 mg every 12 hours can be used for the acute treatment of HAPE, while descent is being arranged.
- **Portable hyperbaric chambers,** which are becoming common equipment on mountaineering expeditions, may be a useful and lifesaving temporizing measure while descent is arranged in HACE and HAPE.

SPECIAL CONSIDERATIONS

- Prior to travel, maximize the health status of those with **chronic health problems,** such as diabetes, asthma, heart disease, arthritis, etc. Cardiovascular disease is the most common cause of death for Americans traveling abroad.
- Educate travelers using **life-sustaining medications** (asthma inhalers, antianginal medications, etc.) to bring twice as much as needed for the trip, in two separate containers in two separate locations (one always carried by the patient).
- Provide travelers with a **medication list** with generic names and doses, and include over-the-counter and herbal remedies. Travelers should also have **copies of important medical records,** including electrocardiograms, lists of diagnoses, and details on implantable devices (pacemakers, valves, defibrillators, etc.).

■ Consider the fetal impact of immunizations and prophylactic medications in **pregnant women,** and advise women about their own immunocompromised state. Adjust itineraries to avoid areas where teratogenic medications would be necessary for malaria prophylaxis. Discourage women with high-risk pregnancies from any international travel.

■ **Immigrants visiting friends and relatives** account for a disproportionately high volume of international travel. They are at increased risk of travel-related illness, as they have longer stays and spend time in high-risk areas. In addition, they rarely receive pretravel care, and often take inappropriate or no prophylaxis for malaria or other conditions. Physicians need to proactively query their immigrant patients about plans to visit friends and relatives abroad, and offer appropriate, culturally sensitive care.

References

1. Franco-Paredes C, Santos-Preciado JI. Problem pathogens: prevention of malaria in travellers. *Lancet Infect Dis* 2006;6:139–149.
2. Freedman D, Weld L, et al. Spectrum of disease and relation to place of exposure among ill returned travelers. *N Engl J Med* 2006;354:119–130.
3. Hackett PH, Roach RC. High altitude illness. *N Engl J Med* 2001;345:107–111.
4. Ryan E, Kain K. Health advice and immunizations for travelers. *N Engl J Med* 2000; 342:1716–1725.
5. Yates J. Traveler's diarrhea. *Am Fam Physician* 2005;71:2095–2100, 2107–2108.

Common Presenting Problems

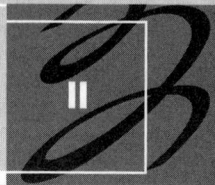

II

WEIGHT LOSS
Samuel N. Grief

2.1

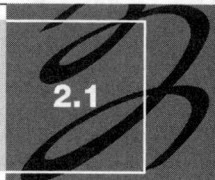

*I*nvoluntary or unintentional weight loss is a common complaint in primary care offices.[1,2] Weight loss is a challenging problem, often surrounded by fears on the part of both patient and physician of an occult malignancy. Recent studies and reports mitigate these fears.[3-5] Gastrointestinal and psychiatric disorders are usually the most prevalent causes of unintentional weight loss.[3,5] Although malignancy is a leading cause of weight loss, extensive and costly workups for occult cancers are rarely beneficial.[1,6] Evaluation of weight loss is not a simple task given the extensive potential list of causes (Table 2.1-1). In more than one study, 10% to 36% of weight loss remains undiagnosed.[3,5] Yet, basic principles of taking a comprehensive history, performing a pertinent and focused physical examination, and ordering appropriate laboratory testing will quickly uncover most causes of weight loss in the outpatient setting.

DIAGNOSTIC APPROACH

The key to the diagnosis of involuntary weight loss is a careful and complete history and age-appropriate physical examination. The approach begins broadly and then quickly focuses on specifics derived from the initial evaluation.

Quantify Loss

A loss of 5% or more from the baseline body weight (not ideal body weight) over 6 months is significant.[2-5] Serial measurements are the best method of verifying weight loss, but other considerations include family report and changes in clothing or belt size. For infants and young children, slowing or cessation of growth are red flags to initiate a diagnostic evaluation.

- **Categories of weight loss.** The causes of weight loss can be divided into four major categories: decreased intake; increased nutrient loss; increased metabolic demand; and impaired absorption (Table 2.1-1). A novel way of approaching typical causes of weight loss is by using the mnemonic device "Weight Loss MD" (Table 2.1-2).

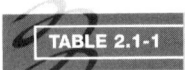

TABLE 2.1-1	Major Causes of Weight Loss

Decreased intake
    Malignancy, congestive heart failure, medications, dementia, depression, grief, electrolyte
        disturbances, poor dentition or taste, gastric or esophageal disease, electrolyte disorders,
        alcoholism, financial hardship, social isolation, HIV and AIDS
Increased nutrient loss
    Profuse vomiting or diarrhea, diabetes mellitus
Increased metabolic demand
    Fever, malignancy, tuberculosis, hyperthyroidism, chronic infection, drug abuse (cocaine,
        stimulants)
Impaired absorption
    Cholestasis, infection (parasitic, other), medications, pancreatic insufficiency, diabetic or HIV
        enteropathy, inflammatory bowel disease, celiac sprue, surgery

Special Considerations

A tailored approach in elderly people includes greater emphasis on social and environmental factors.[4,5,7] Unintentional weight loss in elderly people is often associated with increased morbidity and mortality.[4,5] The approach in human immunodeficiency virus (HIV) and acquired immune deficiency syndrome (AIDS) is more comprehensive, and special attention is given to disease-specific infections, nutritional changes, psychosocial issues, and neoplasia.[8–10] In the pediatric population, failure to thrive is still the most appropriate term for improper growth among infants and young children.[11] Anorexia nervosa and other psychiatric or behavioral disorders are the most common causes of weight loss in older children.[12]

History

■ **Initial data.** Begin with open-ended, general questioning followed by a complete review of systems. How do you feel about your weight? This open-ended question provides an opportunity for patients to disclose any concerns about their weight loss and help uncover undiagnosed eating disorders. More specific questions include: Is the loss intentional? Are you dieting, taking diuretics or laxatives, or suffering from any eating disorders? A yes to any of these questions would be classified as voluntary weight loss.

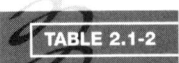

TABLE 2.1-2	Weight Loss MD: A Mnemonic for Common Causes of Unintentional Weight Loss in Adults

W	Wasting disease (e.g., cancer, AIDS)
E	Eating problems or disorders (anorexia nervosa, inability to feed self)
I	Income deprivation
G	Gastrointestinal problems (e.g., inflammatory bowel disease, parasitic infestation, chronic diarrhea)
H	Hyperthyroidism, hyperparathyroidism, hypoadrenalism
T	Toxic substances (e.g., alcohol, laxatives, illicit drugs)
L	Low-calorie diet (e.g., commercial weight loss programs, self-imposed diets)
O	Oral problems (e.g., sores, ulcers, caries, poor dentition or dentures)
S	Swallowing disorders (e.g., amyotrophic lateral sclerosis, Parkinson disease, progressive supranuclear palsy)
S	Social problems (e.g., isolation, stress)
M	Medication side effects or metabolic conditions (e.g., diabetes, thyroid disease)
D	Depression or other psychiatric disorders (e.g., schizophrenia, obsessive–compulsive disorder)

It is valuable to quantify the patient's average daily or weekly intake of food and drink and total calories. Food frequency questionnaires are useful tools for the above and are best administered by registered dietitians. The frequency of meals, appetite changes, and difficulty with food preparation can also be elicited. Quantify tobacco, alcohol, and drug usage as these substances often replace food intake and increase risk for nutritional deficiencies and subsequent weight loss. Focused and relevant past medical, surgical, psychiatric, and family histories will often provide clues to the underlying cause of weight loss. Ask about past bariatric or gastric bypass surgeries, previous or current mood disorders, and any history of endocrinopathies. Inquire about exercise habits—excessive exercise or forms of physical activity may hint at underlying body dysmorphic disorders. Medications (especially anorexiants) and herbal or vitamin supplements may also factor into weight considerations, and a detailed list of all pharmaceuticals should be obtained.[13] Social factors, including stress, isolation, and the cost and effort required to prepare and consume food, can have major impact on weight.

■ **Specific historical data.** The patient's symptoms and complaints should direct the clinician to greater detail. Focus your history using the mnemonic device Weight Loss MD (Table 2.1-2). Ask all patients about constitutional symptoms to evaluate their general state of health: Any nausea or vomiting? Change in bowel habits? Fever? How is their appetite? Energy level?

Physical Examination

The diagnostic utility of the physical examination in identifying the cause of weight loss has not been adequately evaluated.[5] However, some studies and reports demonstrate that physical findings are present in 66% of cases of involuntary weight loss.[1,14,15] First, quantify loss by serial weight measurements whenever possible. Measurement of vital signs, including body mass index, temperature, blood pressure, respiratory and heart rates, is always important. A focused examination based on clues from the history is appropriate. Physical findings such as a cachectic appearance, clubbing, generalized lymphadenopathy may also be relevant findings.[16]

Testing

■ **Basic laboratories.** Debate continues regarding the most useful and cost-effective laboratory testing for involuntary weight loss. A simple and structured approach is best[1,2,4–6] The first line of testing should include complete blood count, thyrotropin (thyroid-stimulating hormone; TSH) assay, urinalysis, and fecal occult blood testing. A comprehensive chemistry panel including transaminases, blood urea nitrogen, creatinine, and electrolytes (calcium, magnesium, phosphorus, sodium, and potassium) is essential. A chest radiograph is often useful but is not required.[1]

■ **Comprehensive analysis.** Careful observation and follow-up are superior management strategies to undirected diagnostic testing.[1,2,4–6] When indicated, upper gastrointestinal radiographs, endoscopy, and colonoscopy are the most useful second-line tests.[4,16] National Cancer Institute or U.S. Preventive Services Task Force age-specific screening guidelines should be evaluated and up-to-date for the patient. These can be accessed on the Internet at http://www.ahrq.gov/clinic/uspstfix.htm. Computed tomography and other expensive investigations are seldom beneficial in the absence of a specific indication.[1,4,5]

Differential Diagnosis

The integration of history, examination, and laboratory data will usually reveal the cause for involuntary weight loss. Cancer, including gastrointestinal malignancies, accounts for 24% of cases, whereas lung cancer represents 5% of cases. Gastrointestinal diseases account for another 25% to 31%.[3,4] If the initial steps in the evaluation are not conclusive, the best approach is careful observation. Follow-up examinations and testing should be done monthly for 6 months. If a physical cause exists, it will almost always be found within this period of time.[1] If an organic cause is present, this simple approach will expose it more than 75% of the time.[1,2,6] If an organic cause is not identified within the first 6 months, it is unlikely that one will be found.[3] However, these undifferentiated patients typically do well, and assuming they do not have continued and progressive weight loss, they have an excellent overall prognosis.[3] Malignancy is a significant cause of weight loss; however, a truly occult malignancy is rare, and an exhaustive search for one is neither cost-effective nor supported by the literature.[1–6]

TREATMENT

Nonpharmacologic and pharmacologic treatments are usually comingled in the treatment plan for unintentional weight loss.

■ **Nonpharmacologic treatment.** Involving ancillary health care providers, such as dietitians, social workers, home health care nurses, and immediate or extended family members is beneficial.[4,5] Increasing physical activity in patients with low energy may stimulate appetite and result in modest weight gain.[4,5] Nutritional supplements are a common modality in treating weight loss and often work best when used in conjunction with other treatment options.[4] Counseling patients to consume nutritional supplements in between, rather than instead of meals, is the best approach.[4,5] A broad-spectrum vitamin and mineral supplement should be considered in all patients with unintentional weight loss.[5]

■ **Pharmacologic treatment.** Several medications have been used in attempts to stave off continued weight loss and establish weight gain. Megestrol acetate is indicated for unexplained, significant weight loss in patients with AIDS.[17] Dronabinol is indicated for weight loss in patients with AIDS and in patients with cancer undergoing chemotherapy.[17] Other appetite stimulants or weight-gain-inducing medications include cyproheptadine, antidepressants, antipsychotics, and other mood-stabilizing drugs.[18] Treatment with any medication should initially be for a short period of time (<3 months); further treatment depends on response and condition of the patient.

References

1. Reife CM. Involuntary weight loss. *Med Clin North Am* 1995;79:299–313.
2. Thompson MP, Morris LK. Unexplained weight loss in the ambulatory elderly. *J Am Geriatr Soc* 1991;39:497–500.
3. Lankisch PG, et al. Unintentional weight loss: diagnosis and prognosis. The first prospective follow-up study from a secondary referral center. *J Intern Med* 2001;249:41–46.
4. Huffman GB. Evaluating and treating unintentional weight loss in the elderly. *Am Fam Physician* 2002;65(4).
5. Alibhai SMH, et al. An approach to the management of unintentional weight loss in elderly people. *CMAJ* 2005;172(6).
6. Wise GR, Craig D. Evaluation of involuntary weight loss. Where do you start? *Postgrad Med* 1994;95:143–146, 149–150.
7. Gazewood JD, Mehr DR. Diagnosis and management of weight loss in the elderly. *J Fam Pract* 1998;47:19–25.
8. Kotler DMD. Challenges to diagnosis of HIV-associated wasting. *JAIDS* 2004;37(S1):280–283.
9. Wanke CA. Algorithm for the management of HIV wasting. *JAIDS* 2004; 37(S1):284–288.
10. Tang AM, Jacobson DL, et al. Increasing risk of 5% or greater unintentional weight loss in a cohort of HIV-infected patients, 1995–2003. *JAIDS* 2005;40(1):70–76.
11. Olsen EM. Failure to thrive: still a problem of definition. *Clin. Pediatrics* 2006;45:1–6.
12. Behrman RE, Kliegman RM, Jenson HB. *Nelson textbook of pediatrics.* 17th ed. Amsterdam: Elsevier; 2004
13. Schiffman SS. Taste and smell losses in normal aging and disease. *JAMA* 1997;278:1357–1362.
14. Marton KI, Sox HC Jr, Krupp JR. Involuntary weight loss: diagnostic and prognostic significance. *Ann Intern Med* 1981;95:568–574.
15. Rabinovitz M, Pitlik SD, Leifer M, et al. Unintentional weight loss. A retrospective analysis of 154 cases. *Arch Intern Med* 1986;146:186–187.
16. Bilbao-Garay J, et al. Assessing clinical probability of organic disease in patients with involuntary weight loss: a simple score. *Eur J Intern Med* 2002;13:240–245.
17. *Physicians desk reference,* 60th ed. Thomson PDR; Birmingham: 2006.
18. Berkowitz RI, Fabricatore AN. Obesity, psychiatric status and psychiatric medications. *Psychiatr Clin North Am* 2005;39–54.

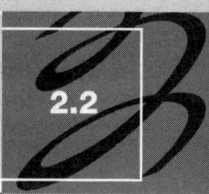

GENERAL PRINCIPLES

Definition

A state of increased discomfort and decreased efficiency resulting from prolonged or excessive exertion; loss of power or capacity to respond to stimulation.

Epidemiology

- Among the most common presenting complaints to family physicians
- Bimodal distribution by age: first peak in late teens/early 20s; second peak after 60
- Women present with fatigue more frequently than men (1.5 to 3.9 times)

Classification

- Acute fatigue: Fatigue of recent onset
  - Common as an incidental symptom
    - After stressful life experiences
    - Because of sleep deprivation
    - Because of common illnesses or conditions (pregnancy)
    - Because of medication side effects

  - Cause of acute fatigue usually apparent after history, physical exam, and basic labs.
  - If fatigue accompanies a self-limited process, it usually resolves spontaneously.

- Prolonged fatigue: Fatigue lasting at least 1 month
- Chronic fatigue: Unexplained fatigue lasting at least 6 months
  - Up to 50% of patients with chronic fatigue continue to have fatigue a year after their initial presentation to the physician.
  - In most cases, physician is unable to identify a specific cause of the chronic fatigue.

- Chronic fatigue syndrome (CFS): A clinical syndrome characterized by severe disabling fatigue of at least 6 months duration and a combination of symptoms that prominently include self-reported problems with concentration and short-term memory, sleep disturbances, and musculoskeletal pain. The Centers for Disease Control (CDC) web site is a good source of information about current information about CFS.

DIAGNOSIS

History

- Clarify and differentiate fatigue from weakness, shortness of breath, falling asleep during daytime activities, malaise, and related symptoms.
- Determine timing (onset/duration/progression) of fatigue
- Context of fatigue: What events were occurring around the time when the fatigue started?
- Associated symptoms:
  - Constitutional symptoms: fever, chills, night sweats, weight change, appetite change, obvious blood loss
  - System-specific symptoms: especially musculoskeletal, psychiatric (symptoms of depression), cardiovascular, respiratory, digestive, metabolic/endocrine, and neurologic

- Impact of fatigue on relationships, work, and leisure activities
- Environmental stress: personal, family, occupational, educational, financial
- Personal habits and behaviors: sleep, diet/nutrition, exercise, sexual activity/risk factors, alcohol use, recreational drug use

- Medications: prescribed and over the counter (OTC)
- Previous medical evaluations for fatigue, including location of those medical records
- Convening the patient's family may assist in particularly challenging patient presentations

Physical Examination

- Unlikely that the physical examination alone will establish a definitive diagnosis.
- General examination, to include:
  - Thorough general inspection: body habitus, skin color/texture, hair, sclera, nails/nail beds
  - Mental status
  - Neurologic
  - Musculoskeletal
  - Cardiovascular
  - Respiratory
  - Abdominal
  - Rectal
  - Endocrine (thyroid)
- More detailed exam of any additional body systems implicated in history

Laboratory Studies

- Helpful (confirmatory) in small percentage of cases.
- Review previous medical records to avoid unnecessary duplication of laboratory studies.
- General laboratory studies may include:
  - Complete blood count
  - Sedimentation rate
  - Liver function tests
  - Renal function tests
  - Urinalysis
  - Stool for occult blood
  - Thyroid-stimulating hormone
  - HIV
- More specific laboratory testing directed by findings in the history or physical examination.
- Probably not routinely indicated:
  - Other tests of immune function
  - Epstein–Barr virus (EBV) titers
  - Lymphocyte subpopulation analysis
  - Rheumatologic studies
  - Serologic studies

Differential Diagnosis

- Infectious diseases:
  - Viral syndromes (hepatitis, mononucleosis, influenza, HIV, etc.)
  - Bacterial infections (endocarditis, chronic genitourinary infection, tuberculosis, etc.)
- Toxin/drug effects:
  - Side effects of prescribed medication/OTC medication
  - Effects of alcohol or recreational drug use
  - Environmental or occupational exposures
- Metabolic/endocrine conditions:
  - Disorders of serum electrolytes, glucose, calcium, etc.
  - Malnutrition (starvation, dieting, or obesity)
  - Thyroid disorders
  - Diabetes mellitus
- Neoplastic disorders (leukemia, lymphoma, occult solid tissue malignancy)
- Vascular disorders (congestive heart failure, cardiomyopathies, valvular heart disease, etc.)
- Pulmonary conditions (chronic obstructive pulmonary disease, or COPD, restrictive lung diseases, etc.)

- Miscellaneous conditions:
  - Deconditioning
  - Anemia
  - Pregnancy
  - Connective tissue disease
  - Multiple sclerosis
  - Sleep disorders, including sleep apnea
- Psychosocial problems (depression, anxiety, adjustment reactions, situational life stress, sexual dysfunction, family violence, occupational stress, and professional burnout).

TREATMENT

General approaches to treatment: Treatment begins with meeting the patient for the first time, and gathering information about the patient's symptoms. Treatment continues at each visit throughout the evaluation and treatment process. Successful treatment of patients with fatigue is facilitated by physician sensitivity and empathy and aided by other activities that strengthen the doctor–patient relationship, like demonstrating interest in the impact of fatigue on the patient's life (relationships, work, and leisure activities). When treatable causes of fatigue are identified, treatment should be directed toward those specific causes.

Behavioral

- A symptom diary may be helpful for both, diagnosis and treatment.
- Assisting patients to develop health sleep habits may benefit the fatigued patient.
- A targeted exercise program may also benefit patients with chronic fatigue.

Medications

- Medications must be tailored to the specific disease/condition causing the fatigue.
- Antidepressants (tricyclics or selective serotonin-reuptake inhibitors) may help patients with disturbed sleep patterns.

Referrals

- Use consultants that will support and reinforce care plan.
- Avoid consultants who wish to run or repeat unnecessary diagnostic tests.
- Communicate clearly with all consultants about the purpose of referrals.

Counseling

- Referral for psychotherapy may be appropriate in selected patients. Common therapies utilized in the treatment of patients with fatigue may include:
  - Supportive psychotherapy
  - Cognitive–behavioral therapy
  - Brief dynamic psychotherapy

Patient Education

- Explain to the patient that the most common causes of fatigue in family practice are depression and other psychosocial disorders.
- For patients with a suspected psychosocial cause for their fatigue, reintroduce and probe these issues at each visit.
- Printed materials or articles on depression, CFS, and professional burnout may be helpful.
- Printed materials about starting an exercise program or maintaining good sleep habits may also assist selected patients.

References

1. Buchwald D, Komaroff AL. Review of laboratory findings for patients with chronic fatigue syndrome. *Rev Infect Dis* 1991;13[Suppl]:S12.0
2. Jones JF. Serologic and immunologic responses in chronic fatigue syndrome with emphasis on the Epstein–Barr virus. *Rev Infect Dis* 1991;13[Suppl]:506.
3. Kroenke K, Wood DR, Mangelsdorff D, et al. Chronic fatigue in primary care. *JAMA* 1988;260:929–934.

4. Morrison JD. Fatigue as a presenting complaint in family practice. *J Fam Pract* 1980;10:795–801.
5. O'Malley PG, Jackson JL, Santoro J, et al. Antidepressant therapy for unexplained symptoms and symptoms syndromes. *J Fam Pract* 1999;48:980–990.
6. Valdini AF, et al. One year follow-up of fatigued patients. *J Fam Pract* 1988;26:33. Available online at http://www.cdc.gov/cfs/cfs.

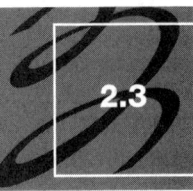

2.3   ## DIZZINESS
Donald B. Milligan

GENERAL PRINCIPLES

Definition

Dizziness is among the most common presentations in primary care, especially among elderly patients. It is the third most common reason for medical consultation, and is the most common reason for patients over 75 years of age. In some studies, as many as 42% of the population may complain of dizziness at some time. It may be a presentation of a number of physical problems, so must be approached systematically. Fortunately, the most common causes of dizziness are self-limited and not life-threatening.

- New-onset dizziness is usually diagnosed during the history. A focused physical examination and limited laboratory testing may be useful, but are usually confirmatory. Acute dizziness is usually due to a single diagnosis, and if life-threatening illness such as stroke is ruled out, symptomatic treatment and observation are usually sufficient.
- Chronic, persistent dizziness is more common in elderly patients, and more likely to be associated with multiple illnesses. Focusing on restoration of function rather than cure is the goal in this management.
- Laboratory testing is rarely the primary means of diagnosis. Multiple studies are available, but should be used to confirm the diagnoses established in the history and, to a lesser extent, in the physical examination.
- Initial differential diagnosis is very broad, but most patients are in a few common categories.

DIAGNOSIS

History

Dizziness is a subjective sensation of movement or disorientation in space. Many terms are used to describe this, but nearly all describe movement.

- **Avoid suggesting symptoms or etiology.** Most patients can be encouraged to describe their symptoms in a way that will fit one of the categories below.
- **Subtypes of dizziness.** Almost all causes will fall into four categories.
  - **Vertigo** —A sensation of movement, either in rotation or tilting. This is the classic description of dizziness most people visualize when they hear the term. It is a sensation most of us have experienced on a playground merry-go-round. It is normally associated with disorders of the vestibulocochlear system, although patients with psychologic disorders may describe it as well (e.g., panic disorder). Although acutely disabling, this is usually benign and self-limiting. Causes may include acute viral (or epidemic) labyrinthitis, benign positional vertigo, serous otitis media, vertebrobasilar vascular disease, Meniere disease, or atypical migraine.
  - **Presyncope**—This is commonly described as light-headedness or the feeling that one is about to faint. Most people recognize the symptom from times they stood up

suddenly. It is caused by inadequate cerebral circulation, and may result from postural hypotension, medication side effects, cardiovascular disease, hypovolemia, and vasovagal attacks.

- **Postural instability**—A sensation of unsteadiness, exacerbated by standing or walking, and often associated with a disturbance in gait. Often a secondary symptom, but presenting alone, it often represents neurologic disease, such as parkinsonism, cerebellar degeneration, axonal degeneration (multiple sclerosis), or peripheral neuropathy such as diabetes or B_{12} deficiency.
- **Other**—Vague, ill-defined, often associated with psychologic disorders, but may be associated other illnesses, such as with a change in refraction, either due to glasses or to an acute change in vision associated with other physical disorders.

- Younger patients will usually present with only one of the four categories above. Unfortunately, with increased age, it is common to have more than one of these, and the diagnosis is often more difficult.

Temporal Patterns of Illness

Continuous dizziness is most commonly found in psychologic disorders, but may also commonly be present in chronic physical illness.

- Episodic dizziness often has patterns that suggest specific diagnoses:
  - Benign positional vertigo—Episodes lasting less than 1 minute
  - Vasovagal episodes or cardiac arrhythmia—Presyncope lasting less than 1 minute
  - Transient ischemic attacks or migraine—Vertigo lasting 10 minutes to (in transient ischemic attacks) as long as 24 hours
  - Meniere disease—Episodic vertigo initially lasting 2 hours to 2 days, associated with tinnitus and gradual hearing loss
  - Recurrent vestibulopathy—Infrequent vertigo, usually lasting a day or less
- **Associated symptoms** often help establish the diagnosis:
  - Upper respiratory symptoms (rhinitis, sneezing, stuffiness, facial pain) may be associated with sinusitis or serous otitis media.
  - Dizziness brought on by exertion may indicate vascular disease (e.g., subclavian steal, carotid stenosis, aortic disease).
  - Numbness or tingling around the mouth or hands indicates hyperventilation, usually associated with anxiety disorders.
  - Loss of consciousness can indicate vasovagal episodes, arrhythmias, or seizures.
  - Neck pain on movement may indicate cervical osteoarthritis with vertebrobasilar insufficiency.
  - Hearing loss, especially unilateral, may indicate middle ear disease, Meniere disease, or acoustic neuroma.

Physical Examination

Physical examination follows the history. When history is unclear, vital signs and cardiovascular, otologic, and neurologic examinations should be carefully evaluated.

- **If benign positional vertigo is suspected,** perform Blake-Hallpike maneuver by rapidly moving the patient from sitting to head-hanging with the head rotated 30 degrees. A positive result involves reproduction of vertigo, rotary nystagmus, latency of onset (3 to 10 seconds), and fatigability with recurrent use of the movement.
- **Psychologic dizziness** can be sometimes provoked with hyperventilation.

Laboratory Tests

Usually confirmatory rather than diagnostic.

Imaging

- **Computed tomography**—Sometimes helpful for otoacoustic disease
- **Magnetic resonance imaging**—More useful for head imaging since most causes are in small areas of the posterior fossa

Clinical Laboratory
- Complete blood count for anemia
- Thyroid-stimulating hormone (TSH) or free T_4
- Testing for hypoglycemia (if indicated by history)
- BUN/Cr for uremia
- B_{12} for long-tract signs

Special Studies
- **Electronystagmometry**—Helpful in establishing vestibular diagnosis; may be more useful in elderly patients
- **Doppler vascular studies**—May be useful in cervical vertigo for subclavian steal or to distinguish vascular from arthritic causes in cervical vertigo
- **Holter monitoring**—Useful only if history suggests arrhythmia

TREATMENT
Management Principles
- **Treat specific diagnoses.** There is no specific treatment for unspecified "dizziness."
- **Avoid medication overuse:**
  - Drugs more common as causes of dizziness than as cures.
  - Meclizine—May be useful for acute labyrinthitis, Meniere disease, or recurrent vestibulopathy—but not otherwise.
  - Diazepam suppresses central responses to vestibular stimuli, so may be useful in some chronic dizziness problems.
  - Antidepressants may ameliorate psychologic illness.
  - Appropriately treat migraine, if present.

- Physical therapy is useful for many elderly patients. Deconditioning is common, and aggravates symptoms. In addition, physical therapy may be specifically useful for benign positional vertigo, vestibular loss, cervical vertigo due to arthritis (not circulatory), and cerebellar ataxias.

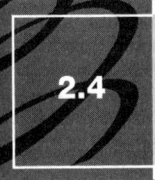

| 2.4 | **COUGH** |
| | *Jonathan J. Rodnick, James K. Gude* |

GENERAL PRINCIPLES
Definition
Cough is the chief complaint for 3.6% of office visits to U.S. physicians (about 30 million visits annually) and even comprises 40% of new patient visits to pulmonary specialists. Coughing is an involuntary visceral reflux that is regulated by vagal afferent nerves. However, there is some higher cortical control of this reflex. This chapter primarily addresses cough in adults. Conceptually, it is most important to know the division of cough to understand its etiology and treatment. Cough can be acute (<3 weeks duration), subacute (3 to 8 weeks duration), or (chronic >8 weeks duration) cough. The first question to ask a patient with cough is "how long have you had a cough?"[1]

DIAGNOSIS
Acute Cough
- Most acute cough is infectious and more than 200 viruses have been identified as causing the **common cold.** Rhinoviruses are the most common viral causes. A "cold" can

be an upper respiratory tract infection (URTI) or a lower respirator tract infection (LRTI), but the syndromes overlap.

■ Other causes of acute cough include exacerbation of pre-existing conditions, such as asthma, bronchiectasis, or chronic obstructive pulmonary disease (COPD) or an occupational or environmental exposure to an irritant (see chronic cough).

■ There are no recommended tests for the common cold. In the setting of an URTI, abnormalities seen on sinus films or computed tomography (CT) scans are often due to congestion from the infection and not diagnostic of a bacterial sinus infection. A diagnosis of bacterial sinusitis should not be made during the first week of symptoms.[2]

■ **Acute bronchitis** is defined as an acute LRTI with productive or nonproductive cough and no evidence of pneumonia or asthma. In patients with findings consistent with acute bronchitis, consider doing a chest x-ray to rule out acute pneumonia if the heart rate >100 per minute, the respirator rate >24 breaths per minute, the oral temperature is >38°C, or there are findings on chest exam (especially in the presence of pre-existing pulmonary disease, cardiac disease, or diabetes). Viral cultures, serologic assays, and spectrum analysis are not routinely performed.[2] The presence of purulent sputum is a poor predictor of bacterial infection.

■ **Influenza** usually presents with an abrupt onset of acute cough, fever, myalgias, pharyngitis, and/or headache. However, no one symptom rules influenza in or out, but an acute cough with fever and no history of flu vaccine make it more likely. There are a variety of rapid diagnostic tests for influenza A and B that use nasal scrubs, washes, and can give an answer (with greater than 70% sensitivity and 90% specificity) in less than 30 minutes. These tests do not add a lot to clinical judgment in outbreak settings.[3]

■ An underappreciated cause of severe respiratory infections in older adults, as in young children, is respiratory syncytical virus (RSV). One study found that in adults it is a more common cause of hospitalization than influenza.[4] Diagnostic testing should be done only on those with symptoms suggestive of influenza or hospitalized for viral pneumonia.

■ Although less likely, one needs to consider and exclude life-threatening diagnosis such as pneumonia, severe exacerbation of asthma or COPD, heart failure, or pulmonary embolism in those who appear quite sick.

Subacute Cough

■ The first question to ask in a patient with a cough lasting from 3 to 8 weeks is: "Is it related to a previous cold or bronchitis?" A **postinfectious** cough is the most common cause of subacute cough and can persist for 8 weeks (sometimes even longer) and is thought to be due to extensive inflammation of the respiratory mucus. If the cough has no relationship to a recent URTI or LRTI, proceed with working up as a chronic cough.

■ One should maintain a high index of suspicion for pertussis. One study found it in up to 20% of patients with a subacute cough. Think of pertussis if the cough gets worse when the runny nose dries up, is associated with posttussive vomiting, causes severe paroxysms, or has the characteristic inspiratory whooping sound. Diagnosis is by culture of nasopharyngeal secretions (from a wash or nasal swab).[5]

■ Lastly an **acute exacerbation of chronic bronchitis (AECB)** may last more than 3 weeks, especially in those with underlying COPD or bronchiectasis. A chest x-ray and/or spirometry should be considered if the chest exam is not normal or there is shortness of breath or other significant symptoms (such as hemoptysis, tachycardia, or wheezing).

Chronic Cough

■ In those with cough lasting longer than 8 weeks, first ask if the patient is taking angiotensin-converting enzyme (ACE) inhibitors. If so, have the patient stop. If the patient is a smoker, redouble your efforts to help the person quit. Third, order a chest x-ray. In patients with a clear chest x-ray, there are four common causes of chronic cough. They should be considered in the following order:

- **Upper airway cough syndrome (UACS).** Patients with this syndrome may need to frequently clear the throat and often have nasal congestion and/or hoarseness. There may be a history of allergic or nonallergic rhinitis or sinusitis symptoms. There is no definitive symptom or physical finding, and up to 20% of patients with UACS may have no upper respiratory symptoms.[6] The diagnosis is usually established by response to treatment (see below). If the patient suspected of UACS does not respond to treatment, sinus imaging may be indicated.
- **Asthma.** The history may be suggestive, but the patient with chronic cough and no history of asthma may still have "cough variant" asthma. In these patients, first do spirometry. If it is normal but you still suspect the diagnosis, the definitive test is a methacholine challenge test. If this test is not easily available, empiric treatment for asthma may be tried (see below).
- **Nonasthmatic eosinophilic bronchitis (NAEB).** This is a newly defined entity characterized by a chronic cough, no reversible airway obstruction, a negative methacholine challenge test, and a high eosinophil count in induced sputum. Patients often have an occupational or environmental allergy that triggers the cough.[7]
- **Gastroesophageal reflux disease (GERD).** In the nonsmoker with a normal chest x-ray, who is not taking an ACE inhibitor and has not responded to empirical treatments for UCAS or asthma, there is greater than 90% chance the cough is due to GERD. Patients with cough-generating GERD do not always have typical reflux symptoms (up to 75% do not have heartburn).[1] The "silent" GERD workup is expensive—a 24-hour esophageal pH test and/or endoscopy—and is usually done after empiric treatment is tried (see below).
- **Unexplained cough.** If the patient continues to have cough after the above workup and/or empiric treatments for UACS and silent GERD, referral to a pulmonary specialist is the final step. A diagnosis of habit or psychogenic should be made only after an extensive evaluation of other causes has been done.

TREATMENT

Most coughs are self-limiting. Investigations of the causes of chronic cough may not be easily accomplished, therefore empiric treatments are tried. Outlined below are some common therapies (listed in the order they are discussed above).

- **Common cold.** Try first-generation antihistamines (such as brompheniramine or chlorpheniramine) combined with a decongestant (pseudoephedrine). Nonsteroidal anti-inflammatory drugs (NSAIDs) (such as Naproxen) may also be used. Newer nonsedating antihistamines and other over-the-counter (OTC) products are ineffective. In those unable to take an antihistamine/decongestant, consider intranasal ipratropium if there are prominent rhinitis symptoms.[1]
- **Acute bronchitis.** No treatment is usually indicated. Short-term use of narcotic antitussives (such as codeine) or high-dose dextromethorphan (>30 mg or 3 tsp of many OTC products) may be considered.[8] If the patient is wheezing, consider inhaled beta-agonists. Other OTC expectorants, cough syrups, and drops, mucus-loosening agents, or antibiotics are not usually recommended. This is an opportune time to counsel smokers to stop.
- **Influenza.** Oseltamivir or zanamivir, if started within 48 hours of symptoms, will shorten the course by a few days and perhaps prevent spread.[9] Influenza vaccination is partially protective and should be given according to Advisory Committee on Immunization Practices (ACIP) guidelines.
- **Postinfectious cough.** If the cough interferes with the patient's quality of life, an inhaled anticholinergic (such as tiotropium or ipratropium) is the first step.[5] If the cough persists, try inhaled corticosteroids. If the patient has severe paroxysms, consider a 1-week course of oral prednisone (40 to 60 mg a day). Last, antitussives such as codeine or dextromethorphan can be used, especially for nocturnal cough.
- **Pertussis.** The effectiveness of antibiotic therapy wanes over time, and antibiotic treatment is not recommended if the cough has been present more than 3 weeks (most people present after this). Use a macrolide, such as a 5-day course of azithromycin, a 7-day

course of clarithromycin, or a 14-day course of erythromycin as treatment, or, more commonly, as postexposure prophylaxis.[10] Patients suspected of having acute pertussis should be isolated. Adolescents and adults age 64 or younger should be given a dTap vaccination in place of dT according to ACIP guidelines.

- **Acute exacerbation of chronic bronchitis.** A short course (1 to 2 weeks) of an antibiotic (such as doxcycline, TMP-SMX, amoxicillin/clavulante, or macrolide) may be tried. Use maximum doses of anticholinergic (ipratropium or tiotropium) bronchodilators. For severe exacerbations or for those with significant underlying disease, a short course of oral corticosteroids is sometimes used. Expectorants are not effective.
- **Upper airway cough syndrome.** First-generation antihistamine/decongestants (A/D) are the mainstay of treatment.[6] Continue at least 2 weeks, and if complete or partial resolution, for several weeks. With persistent nasal stuffiness, a trial of a nasal antihistamines, cromolyn, anticholinergics, or corticosteroids is warranted. If effective, continue for up to 3 months.
- **Cough variant asthma.** Treat with inhaled bronchodilators and corticosteroids for 8 weeks. If the cough is refractory, add an oral leukotriene receptor agonist. If that is not effective, a 5- to 10-day course of oral corticosteroids (40 to 60 mg of prednisone a day) may be necessary.[1]
- **Nonasthmatic eosinophilic bronchitis.** First, avoid the suspected allergen. Inhaled corticosteroids, as for asthma, are the key anti-inflammatory therapy. Other treatment protocols have not yet been established.[7]
- **GERD cough.** Twice-a-day proton pump inhibitors for 2 months should be tried. Lifestyle changes, including no smoking, no meals within 2 to 3 hours of retiring, weight loss, and head of the bed elevation should be initiated. Some foods, such as carbonated beverages, alcohol, citrus, spicy foods, and caffeine may aggravate reflux. Prokinetic agents (such as tegaserod or metoclopramide) should be reserved for those with definitive diagnosis. Antacids should not be used.

SUMMARY

- For patients with a chronic cough (>8 weeks duration) who are nonsmokers, are not taking ACE inhibitors, and have a normal chest film, the diagnosis is likely upper airway cough syndrome (UACS, formerly called postnasal drip), asthma, or GERD.
- The patient suspected of having UACS should be treated empirically with a first-generation A/D combination.
- The patient suspected of having cough variant asthma should have spirometry and, if suggestive, be treated with a standard antiasthma regimen of inhaled corticosteroids and bronchodilators.
- The patient with otherwise unexplained chronic cough may have reflux disease and should be treated with lifestyle modifications and acid suppression therapy.
- In summary for patients with chronic cough in whom the etiology is not clear, a series of empiric therapies may be tried. Usually start out with first generation A/D, followed by inhaled corticosteroids, with or without beta-agonists, then consider leukotriene inhibitors or oral corticosteroids and lastly try proton pump inhibitors.[11] Some patients will have more than one cause of their cough and need combination treatments.

References

1. Irwin RS, Dicpinigatis PV, Chang AB. Diagnosing and managing cough: clinical practice update. *Patient Care* May 2006:23–31.
2. Irwin RS, et al. Diagnosis and management of cough. Executive summary. *Chest* 2006;192:1S–23S (can be downloaded free at http://www.chestjournal.org).
3. Call SA, Volleunweider MA, Hornvng CA, et al. Does this patient have influenza? *JAMA* 1005;293:987–997.
4. Falsey AR, Hennessey PA, Formica MA, et al. Respiratory syncytial virus infection in elderly and high risk patients. *N Engl J Med* 2005;351:1749–1759.
5. Braman SS. Post infectious cough. ACCP evidence-based clinical guidelines. *Chest* 2006;129:138S–146S.

6. Pratter MR. Chronic upper airway cough syndrome secondary to rhinovirus disease (previously referred to as postnasal drip syndrome). ACCP evidence-based clinical practice guidelines. *Chest* 2006;129:63S–71S.
7. Brightling CE. Chronic cough due to nonasthmatic eosinophilic bronchitis. ACCP evidence-based clinical practice guidelines. *Chest* 2006;129:116S–121S.
8. Gonzales R. A 65-year-old woman with acute cough and an important engagement. *JAMA* 2003;289:2701–2708.
9. Jefferson T, Demicheli V, Rivetti D, et al. Antivirals for influenza in healthy adults: systematic review. *Lancet* 2005;367:303–313.
10. Centers for Disease Control and Prevention. Recommended antimicrobial agents for the treatment and postexposure prophylaxis of pertussis. 2005 CDC guidelines. *MMWR* 2005;54:1–15.
11. Pratter MR, Brightling CE, Boulet LP, et al. An empiric integrative approach to the management of cough. ACCP evidence-based clinical practice guidelines. *Chest* 2006;129:222S–223IS.

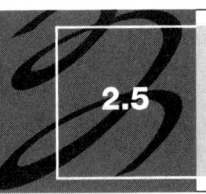

2.5 CHEST PAIN
Komalpreet Bhuller

GENERAL PRINCIPLES

Definition
Chest pain is the most common cardiovascular condition encountered in clinical practice. This presentation may be secondary to multiple causes, for example, any condition affecting the thorax, abdomen, cardiovascular system, muscular system, neurologic system can cause chest pain and finally it may be psychiatric.

DIAGNOSIS

Clinical Presentation
It is critical to delineate chest pain into emergent and nonemergent conditions. A careful history and physical examination can help the physician prioritize these two groups of patients. The first priority is to rule out life-threatening conditions such as myocardial infarction (MI), unstable angina, dissecting aneurysms, pulmonary embolism, pneumothorax, or the depressed patient with suicidal intent. Chest pain is a relatively common complaint.

History
The cardinal points of the history should include an accurate description of the chest pain noting the severity, frequency, location, radiation, quality, alleviating as well as aggravating features, and the duration of symptoms. Risk factors for cardiovascular disease should be elucidated from the history: Male gender, hypertension, diabetes, hyperlipidemia, smoking, personal, and family history of coronary artery disease (CAD), obesity, and substance abuse, as cocaine may cause angina or MI. The presence of systemic diseases such as lupus erythematosus, polyarteritis nodosum, or rheumatoid arthritis are associated with coronary arthritis. From this information, a differential diagnosis can be established and the physical examination will help clarify the relative probability of each cause.

Differential Diagnosis
■ **Angina:** May present with symptoms of heaviness, pressure, or squeezing substernally or in the anterior chest. This pain or discomfort may radiate to the upper back, neck, teeth, shoulder, or arm. Other accompanying symptoms may be nausea, diaphoresis, and/or lightheadedness secondary to hypotension. Symptoms vary from mild to severe

and onset can be gradual with resolution with rest within a few seconds. These episodes can last for minutes. Triggers can be exercise, emotional stress, hypoglycemia, or cocaine.

■ **Variant angina or Printzmetal angina:** Has similar history to angina; however, this pain can occur at rest or upon awakening. Patients may have an additional history of migraines or Raynaud disorder.

■ **Myocardial infarction:** Generally has similar but more severe symptoms as compared to angina. Symptoms may exceed 20 to 30 minutes and is not relieved by rest or nitroglycerine.

■ **Pericarditis:** Can resemble angina by presenting as substernal discomfort, can radiate to neck. However this pain is classically described to be felt at the top of the shoulder secondary to diaphragmatic irritation, in lateral chest and back in a dermatomal distribution. This pain lasts longer than angina. If patient is placed in a sitting position it will relieve pain whereas the pain increases upon lying down or swallowing. There can also be an association with connective tissue disease, following an MI, or viral illness.

■ **Aortic dissection:** A true pain not as vague as with angina. The regional of distribution is center of the chest radiating to the back with abrupt onset. The pain rapidly increases over hours and does not diminish or change with position.

■ **Pulmonary infarction from a pulmonary embolus:** Can range from deep, crushing pain similar to an MI to pleuritic pain. This can also be accompanied by weakness, nausea, vomiting, and dyspnea. Onset is usually sudden; however, 50% of the population will have symptoms of deep vein thrombus peripherally.

■ **Pneumothorax:** Often a sudden, unilateral sharp stabbing pain over the chest wall. Additional history of trauma or sports may be elicited.

■ **Pleural pain:** Can be sharp and knifelike or a dull ache felt superficially in the chest wall. The pain is associated with deep breathing, coughing, and positional changes.

■ **Tracheobronchitis:** Presents as a burning or aching after prolonged coughing. This accompanies or follows a respiratory tract infection.

■ **Esophagitis and gastroesophageal reflux:** Presents with a deep burning pain, which may be indistinguishable from an MI or angina felt in the epigastrium or substernally similar to angina. Onset is generally gradual with a chronic, fluctuating course. Alcohol, nonsteroidal anti-inflammatory drugs (NSAIDs), fatty foods, and large meals can aggravate symptoms.

■ **Gastric or peptic ulcer:** A deep burning or dull ache felt in the epigastrium or substernally approximately minutes after eating. Symptoms are made worse by anything that increases gastric or duodenal acidity, whereas milk or antacids relieve pain.

■ **Cholecystitis:** A cramping pain or ache in the epigastrium, right upper quadrant, or substernally felt minutes to hours after fatty meals.

■ **Costochondritis:** Ranges from a sharp to dull pain, which can last from seconds to weeks. Pain is worse with exercise or motion, and is reproducible on examination.

Physical Examination

First, it is critical to assess the general appearance of the patient. This is nonspecific; however, it may give insight to the severity of the underlying cause. Cyanosis indicates hypoxemia or low cardiac output. Diaphoresis is often associated with MI; also seen in high anxiety levels. Respiration rate may be increased in any cause of chest pain; however, use of accessory muscles may be a clue to a respiratory etiology.

The vital signs will determine whether the patient is stable or unstable. Tachycardia is often associated with anxiety, MI, pulmonary embolism (PE), and pneumothorax. Bradycardia may be associated with MI; however, it can be normal in a young athletic patient. Hypotension is more suggestive of an MI but may also be seen in patients with PE or other life-threatening conditions. A difference between blood pressures in either arm is suggestive of aortic dissection.

Auscultations will reveal absent breath sounds consistent with pneumothorax or tension pneumothorax. Pulmonary friction rubs may indicate plural inflammation; if heard overlying the heart can be suggestive of pericarditis. Ischemia may cause mitral insufficiency murmur or an S4 or S3 gallop. The cardiac examination may be entirely normal in a patient having an acute MI; however, a third heart sound is predictive. Pain on palpation of chest wall is suggestive of musculoskeletal disease. Hyperesthesia when associated with a rash is often due to herpes zoster. Localized tenderness in the right upper quadrant is suggestive of a biliary process. Extremity examination may reveal signs of a deep vein thrombosis (DVT), which can occur in up to 50% of those patients with a PE.

On the basis of the history and physical, chest pain can be characterized as emergent versus nonemergent or cardiac versus noncardiac. The Duke University database formula can be used for the pretest likelihood of CAD, considers the patients age, sex, cardiovascular risk profile, description of chest pain, and information from the resting electrocardiogram (ECG).

Laboratory Studies

Cardiac Studies

Troponin T and I, creatinine kinase CK-MB, and myoglobin are essential for confirming the diagnosis of infarction. The troponins are the most sensitive and specific cardiac markers. However, sensitivity of the tests is low until 4 to 6 hours after symptoms begin. A complete metabolic profile will give an indication of liver and renal function. A complete blood profile is an indication to an inflammatory process.

Ancillary Tests and Imaging

The **ECG** is a noninvasive and inexpensive test for identifying cardiac disease; however, the diagnostic yield may be low. Nonetheless, ECG abnormalities are an early sign of MI and can be identified within 90 minutes of symptom onset. Signs suggestive of an acute MI may include ST segment elevation, new Q wave, dysrhythmia, and T wave inversion. Clinically significant ST segment elevation is considered present if it is greater than 1 mm in two anatomically contiguous leads or 2 mm in two contiguous precordial leads. If possible, compare with an old ECG because Q waves may be consistent with a prior MI. Left ventricle hypertrophy which may be due to aortic stenosis or long-standing hypertension. ST depression may be associated with ischemia. Non-ST MI is represented by an ST depression or T wave inversion without Q waves. Noninfarction subendocardial ischemia is manifested by transient ST segment depression. Noninfarction transmural ischemia is represented by a transient ST segment elevation or paradoxical T wave normalization.

S1 Q3 T3, right bundle branch hyperacute P waves, or right access change may suggest PE or pneumothorax due to right ventricular strain. Diffuse ST elevation with PR depression and U waves may be suggestive of pericarditis.

A normal resting ECG predicts normal left ventricular function with a high degree of certainty; however, 20% of patients have a normal ECG. Left bundle branch block and pacing can interfere with an ECG diagnosis of coronary ischemia. The initial ECG is often not diagnostic in patients with acute coronary syndromes. An ECG should be repeated at 5- to 10-minute intervals if the patient remains symptomatic and there is a high clinical suspicion for an MI.

Chest x-ray may assist in the diagnosis of chest pain if cardiac, pulmonary, or neoplastic etiology is suspected. For example, it may reveal plural effusion, pneumonia, consolidation or pneumothorax, cardiomegaly, pulmonary edema, and aortic dissection. In the intermediate-risk patient there are a number of noninvasive tests; the decision of which test to perform is based on body size, associated medical conditions, the ability to exercise, and institutional experience with testing methods. These methods are stress test, echocardiogram, technetium-99 or thallium-201 perfusion scintigraphy. Women have a higher incident of false-positive results. Therefore, many physicians recommend that exercise be combined with imaging methods.

Cardiac echo is valuable in the evaluation of patients who have persistent chest pain suggestive of acute coronary syndrome (ACS), a nondiagnostic ECG, and serially negative cardiac enzymes. An echo can visualize regional wall abnormality within seconds of a coronary artery occlusion. In addition to detecting myocardial dysfunction or ischemia, it can also diagnose pericardial effusion of pericarditis, a dilated right ventricle (pulmonary embolism), and calcification and impaired excursion of the aortic valve leaflets (aortic stenosis). The sensitivity of an echo is very high, but the specificity is limited—the value of this test is to help exclude rather than diagnose an MI. Noninvasive stress testing influences clinical decision making when the pretest probability of CAD is intermediate. In a patient who is symptom free with normal or indeterminant test results, a stress test may provoke ischemia. An exercise electrocardiographic stress test is used to assess the functional capacity, or efficacy of current medical therapy in patients with known CAD. For patients who are unable to exercise due to physical limitations or severe pulmonary disease or general disability, pharmacologic stress agents such as dobutamine or persantine can be used. False positives occur with left ventricular hypertrophy, bundle branch block, pre-excitation syndromes, electrolyte abnormalities, and digoxin use. Patients with a low risk of CAD should not undergo noninvasive cardiac stress testing because an abnormal result would more likely be a false-positive result and a negative test result would confirm the low probability of CAD.

Nuclear imaging: Thallium-201 and technetium-99 sestamibi accumulate in myocardial tissue, which correlates to myocardial blood flow. Areas of ischemia demonstrate reduced radioactive counts. However, limitations are that a positive test is not diagnostic in patients with a prior MI and the test may be negative if chest pain has resolved for more than 3 hours. ECG-gated single photon emission computed tomography (SPECT) allows the calculation of left ventricular ejection fraction and evaluation of wall motion. This test is used when excessive body weight precludes thallium imaging.

Coronary angiography is considered the gold standard for the diagnosis and or intervention of CAD. It is reserved for:

- Patients with markedly positive noninvasive tests (i.e., hypotension and significant ST segment depression on ECG stress testing on a treadmill)
- Patients at high risk for CAD in whom empirical therapy has failed
- Patients with unstable or post infarction angina
- Patients with contraindication to exercise or pharmacologic stress testing.

Coronary angiography has certain limitations. Intravascular ultrasound studies have shown that coronary angiography may occasionally underestimate the severity of an area of narrowing.

Once illnesses requiring acute attention are excluded, it is important to differentiate the other causes of chest pain. Distinguishing cardiac and gastrointestinal causes may be difficult: cardiac causes, that is, angina, pericarditis, mitral valve prolapse, versus gastrointestinal causes, that is, gastroesophageal reflux disease (GERD), gastritis, ulcer, hiatal hernia, esophageal spasm. Patients should undergo a trial of acid suppression. One must consider a respiratory condition as well as not forget dermatologic disorders such as herpes zoster or cellulitis. If symptoms suggest a psychogenic cause, for example, depression, anxiety, somatoform disorders, evaluate the patient for a psychosocial source. A physical exam may indicate a musculoskeletal cause; if pain persists consider rib films, a bone scan, or CT of the chest. Always evaluate for overall atherosclerotic risk factors.

ABDOMINAL PAIN
Peter B. Kozisek

2.6

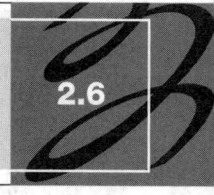

A bdominal pain is consistently ranked as one of the 10 most common undifferentiated problems presenting to the family physician. Despite the recent advances in diagnostic imaging and laboratory testing, the diagnosis and management of abdominal pain continues to require astute clinical judgment on the part of the physician. When the cause of abdominal pain constitutes a medical emergency, prompt diagnosis and treatment are mandatory. In nonemergent cases, the physician is called on to be efficient and cost effective in the use of laboratory and diagnostic imaging studies and to render an accurate diagnosis in a timely fashion.

DIAGNOSTIC APPROACH

History

A detailed history is critical in determining the cause of abdominal pain. Patients should be asked about the severity and quality of their pain as well as its location and the presence or absence of radiation. The setting and the time of origin of the pain should also be ascertained, as should any remissions or exacerbations. Factors that produce or worsen the pain and those that ease the pain require delineation. Associated symptoms such as nausea, vomiting, diarrhea, hematemesis, hematochezia or melena, and lightheadedness are often helpful in determining the etiology of the pain.

Physical Examination

A thorough and systematic physical examination, including inspection, auscultation, percussion, and palpation, is critical to an accurate and timely diagnosis of the cause of abdominal pain. Pelvic and rectal examinations are almost always indicated in the evaluation of abdominal pain. Visceral afferent pathways from the internal organs of the abdomen produce a pain that is typically dull, aching, or colicky in quality. Such pain may be difficult for the patient to accurately describe or localize. In contrast, somatic pain, resulting from the direct contact of the parietal peritoneum with blood, purulent discharge, or an inflamed organ, tends to be sharp and well localized. Guarding and rebound tenderness are important findings indicating potentially significant peritoneal irritation. Their presence should raise the index of suspicion for a potentially serious disorder, such as appendicitis, perforated diverticulum, ruptured ectopic pregnancy, perforated gastric or duodenal ulcer, ruptured abdominal aortic aneurysm, or bacterial peritonitis.

Diagnostic Studies

- **Laboratory tests**
  - **Urinalysis**
    - **Hematuria.** >5 red blood cells (RBC)/high-powered field (hpf) is suggestive of nephrolithiasis.
    - **Pyuria.** >5 white blood cells (WBC)/hpf is suggestive of pyelonephritis.
  - **Complete blood count (CBC).** The WBC count is frequently elevated in appendicitis, diverticulitis, cholelithiasis, mesenteric lymphadenitis, inflammatory bowel disease, pyelonephritis, pancreatitis, pelvic inflammatory disease (PID), gastroenteritis, and perforated viscus.
  - **Human chorionic gonadotropin (hCG).** A positive pregnancy test should alert the examiner to the possibility of an ectopic pregnancy.
  - **Amylase.** A significant elevation suggests pancreatitis. Serum amylase is sometimes elevated in inflammatory processes of the bowel mucosa, such as gastroenteritis.
  - **Liver function tests (LFTs).** Elevations commonly occur in cholelithiasis, hepatitis, and pancreatitis.

- **Diagnostic imaging**
  - **Abdominal radiographs.** Air-fluid levels suggest obstruction or adynamic ileus. A sentinel loop of dilated bowel may sometimes be present adjacent to an inflamed structure in the abdomen, such as the appendix, gallbladder, or pancreas. Free air beneath the diaphragm in upright films is suggestive of perforated viscus.
  - **Abdominal ultrasonography** is frequently helpful in the diagnosis of cholelithiasis, nephrolithiasis, pancreatitis, abdominal aortic aneurysm, ectopic pregnancy, pid, and ovarian cysts.
  - **Computed tomography (CT).** CT scanning is helpful in the diagnosis of pancreatitis, diverticulitis, ischemic bowel disease, abdominal aortic aneurysm, intra-abdominal abscess, and carcinoma.

THE ACUTE ABDOMEN

This refers to an acute and potentially life-threatening abdominal illness that requires immediate intervention. Differentiation of the acute abdomen from other, less serious causes of abdominal pain is the first challenge at the initial visit for abdominal pain. Signs and symptoms indicative of an acute abdomen include rebound tenderness, fever, an elevated WBC count with a left shift, severe or progressively worsening abdominal pain, abdominal distention, hypotension, shock, hematemesis, and rectal bleeding. The following illnesses may commonly present with an acute abdomen:

- **Acute appendicitis.** Acute appendicitis is frequently accompanied by anorexia, nausea, vomiting, and pain, which is initially periumbilical and later localizes in the right lower quadrant over the McBurney point. Patients often have low-grade fevers, and the CBC shows a leukocytosis with a left shift in typical cases. Immediate surgical referral is indicated when appendicitis is suspected.

- **Perforated viscus.** Perforation of the gallbladder or pancreas, peptic ulcer, or infected diverticulum may cause peritonitis, accompanied by the signs and symptoms of an acute abdomen. The chemical irritation of the peritoneum from bile, gastric secretions, and the contents of the pancreas typically causes abrupt and severe pain at the time of rupture. However, perforation of a diverticulum usually results in a more progressive evolution of peritonitis.

  - History, physical examination, laboratory studies, and appropriate imaging studies all contribute to the diagnosis of a perforated viscus. Immediate surgical referral is indicated if a ruptured viscus is suspected.

- **Intestinal obstruction.** Mechanical obstruction of the large or small bowel from tumor, volvulus, strangulated hernia, inflammatory bowel disease, impaction, adhesions, or a mass extrinsic to the bowel represents an acute abdominal emergency. Intestinal obstruction is initially manifested by nausea, vomiting, abdominal pain, and the absence of flatus. As the obstruction continues, abdominal distention becomes more prominent.

  - Auscultation of the abdomen may reveal "tinkles" or "high-pitched rushes" as the peristaltic action of the bowel encounters the obstruction. Abdominal radiographs in the supine and upright positions, along with a posteroanterior film of the chest, are the most important initial diagnostic tools in the diagnosis of obstruction. The presence of air-fluid levels on abdominal films indicates obstruction, although such findings can also be present with an adynamic ileus.

- **Mesenteric vascular occlusion.** Thrombotic or embolic occlusion of the mesenteric arteries or veins may result in intestinal infarction and gangrene of the affected bowel segment. Anorexia and steady, severe, slowly progressive abdominal pain followed by bloody diarrhea are the hallmarks of intestinal infarction. Pain out of proportion to the findings on physical examination is also characteristic of the disease. CT, arteriography, or direct visualization of the affected bowel segment may be necessary to make the diagnosis. Prompt surgical intervention is necessary to preserve both bowel function and life.

- **Ruptured abdominal aortic aneurysm.** The rupture of an abdominal aortic aneurysm constitutes an acute medical emergency and necessitates immediate surgical intervention. The onset of rupture is manifested by shock and vascular collapse accompanied by abdominal or flank pain. The diagnosis is usually made clinically on the basis of the presentation and the finding on examination of a pulsating abdominal mass. However, a ruptured aneurysm may not always pulsate, and in some cases ultrasonography, arteriography, or CT may be necessary to make the diagnosis. If surgery is performed within 2 hours of rupture, survival is more likely. Delay in diagnosis and surgical intervention is associated with high mortality secondary to vascular collapse and renal failure.

- **Ectopic pregnancy** (See Chapter 14.5). Ectopic pregnancy should be included in the differential diagnosis of abdominal pain in women of reproductive age. History, physical examination, quantitative hCG analysis, and ultrasonography aid in the diagnosis. A history of prior tubal sterilization should not deter the physician from considering ectopic pregnancy in the differential diagnosis.

SUBACUTE AND CHRONIC ABDOMINAL PAIN

Abdominal pain that is subacute or chronic may indicate a range of problems, from a potentially serious evolving illness to a self-limited illness requiring no further evaluation or treatment. Examples of such problems include the following:

- **Mesenteric lymphadenitis.** Mesenteric lymph nodes occasionally become inflamed and painful, presumably in response to viral infection. Symptoms may mimic those of acute appendicitis, and the diagnosis is sometimes made at the time of surgery. This illness is otherwise self-limited and requires no special treatment or intervention.
- **Gastritis or duodenitis** (See Chapter 11.1). Inflammation of the mucosal lining of the stomach and duodenum typically produces a dull, burning pain in the epigastrium or right upper quadrant. Symptomatic treatment is indicated as long as care is taken not to miss a bleeding or perforating ulcer.
- **Irritable bowel syndrome** (See Chapter 11.8). Irritable bowel syndrome is a self-limited illness that presents as a symptom complex of lower quadrant abdominal pain typically relieved by defecation, a mucus-like component of the stools, and periods of diarrhea alternating with constipation. Symptomatic treatment, with patient education, stress management, bulk laxatives, and antispasmodic medications, is the foundation of treatment.
- **Diverticulitis** (See Chapter 11.7). Inflammation and infection of a colonic diverticulum may produce a symptom complex of abdominal pain, fever, and anorexia. Typically occurring in older adults, diverticulitis is a potentially serious condition that can lead to intra-abdominal sepsis if rupture occurs.
  - Antibiotics are the treatment of choice with surgical consultation recommended in the more serious cases.
- **Cholelithiasis** (See Chapter 11.4). Right upper quadrant pain, particularly after a fatty meal, is a common presentation for cholelithiasis. Diagnosis is confirmed with ultrasonographic scanning of the gallbladder.
- **Inflammatory bowel disease** (See Chapter 11.9). Crohn disease and ulcerative colitis often present with abdominal pain and diarrhea. The clinical diagnosis is confirmed by tissue biopsy via flexible sigmoidoscopy or colonoscopy.
- **Gastroenteritis** (See Chapter 19.2). Crampy abdominal pain with diffuse diarrhea is the hallmark of gastroenteritis. Although most cases are self-limiting; more persistent or severe cases may require stool studies or flexible sigmoidoscopy, or both, for diagnosis.
- **Pancreatitis** (See Chapter 11.6). Pancreatitis may present as an acute or chronic illness. Approximately 80% of cases are secondary to either cholelithiasis or alcohol use. The diagnosis can usually be made by history and physical examination, in conjunction with serum amylase and lipase determinations. CT of the abdomen is important in determining the presence or absence of pancreatic pseudocysts.
- **Gynecologic causes of abdominal pain.** Common pelvic sources of abdominal pain include recurrent urinary tract infection, ovarian cyst, ovarian torsion, pid, endometriosis, and mittelschmertz.
- **Less common causes of abdominal pain.** Clinically important, but less common, causes of abdominal pain include chronic hepatitis, intra-abdominal abscess, somatization, nephrolithiasis, porphyria, Henoch-Schonlein purpura, diabetic ketoacidosis, drug ingestion, and food hypersensitivity.

References

1. Brunicardi FC, ed. *Schwart's principles of surgery.* 8th ed. New York: McGraw-Hill; 2005.
2. Silen W. *Cope's early diagnosis of the acute abdomen.* 19th ed. New York: Oxford University Press; 1996.
3. Townsend CM, Beauchamp RD, Evers BM, et al., eds. *Sabiston textbook of surgery.* 17th ed. Philadelphia: Elsevier Saunders; 2004.
4. Rakel RE, ed. *Textbook of family practice.* 6th ed. Philadelphia: Saunders; 2002.

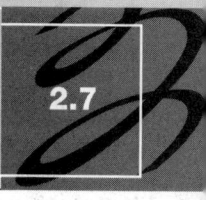

GENERAL PRINCIPLES

Definition

Jaundice is a yellowish discoloration of the skin, sclerae, and mucous membranes caused by an accumulation of bilirubin. Other causes of yellowish pigmentation, unrelated to hyperbilirubinemia, are excessive ingestion of foods rich in carotene (carrots) or lycopene (tomatoes) or certain drugs (quinacrine or busulfan).

Pathophysiology

Jaundice is not clinically evident until serum bilirubin levels exceed 2.5 mg/dL. Bile metabolism may be altered at four major points: overproduction (hemolysis), failure of uptake or excretion by the hepatocyte (transport defect), failure of conjugation (hepatocellular), or obstruction (extra- or intrahepatic).

DIAGNOSIS

Clinical Presentation

Signs and symptoms vary with the underlying etiology. Patients may be asymptomatic or have specific clinical manifestations that will help differentiate the cause.

History

- Nonspecific symptoms of liver disease include anorexia, nausea, vomiting, weight loss, fatigue, and malaise.
- Generalized pruritus is associated with cholestasis.
- Fever and chills are associated with biliary obstruction and cholangitis.
- Chronic weight loss especially preceding the jaundice suggests malignancy.
- Inquire about exposure to drugs, alcohol, or toxins. Agents known to cause jaundice are acetaminophen, certain antibiotics, chemotherapeutic agents, psychotropic medications, cholesterol-lowering agents, anticonvulsants, sex hormones, nonsteroidal anti-inflammatory drugs, inhalation anesthetics, thiazide diuretics, oral hypoglycemics, certain antihypertensives, certain antiarrhythmics, salicylates, cimetidine, warfarin (Coumadin), colchicine, allopurinol, penicillamine, gold, sulfa derivatives, and solvents.
- Blood transfusions, intravenous drug use, sexual contact, travel to endemic areas, ingestion of contaminated foods, and contact with jaundiced persons are associated with viral hepatitis.
- History of gallstones, biliary surgery, previous episodes of jaundice or inflammatory bowel disease, acholic stools, sudden-onset jaundice, and right upper quadrant pain suggest extrahepatic cholestasis.
- Family history of jaundice suggests an inherited defect in conjugation or bilirubin transport, hemolytic disorder, Wilson disease, α_1-antitrypsin deficiency, hemochromatosis, or benign idiopathic cholestasis.
- Abdominal pain suggests hepatic inflammation or congestion, obstruction, abscess, or tumor. Colicky right-upper quadrant pain is more often associated with common bile duct obstruction.

Physical Examination

- Palmar erythema, spider angiomas, gynecomastia, testicular atrophy, or ascites suggests of chronic liver disease or cirrhosis.

67

- Kayser–Fleischer rings are seen in Wilson disease.
- Xanthelasma is seen with chronic cholestatic liver disease, especially primary biliary cirrhosis.
- Signs of congestive heart failure suggest passive congestion.
- Hepatosplenomegaly, abdominal tenderness, mass lesions, and cachexia are suggestive of inflammatory or neoplastic disease.
- Courvoisier gallbladder (a nontender, palpable gallbladder) is a sign of pancreatic cancer.
- Large liver nodules suggest metastatic disease.

Laboratory Studies

- Initial laboratory tests should include transaminases—aspartate aminotransferase (AST) and alanine aminotransferase (ALT)—total and direct bilirubin, and alkaline phosphatase.
- A prothrombin time and albumin should be obtained if severe liver dysfunction is suspected.
- Specific tests include viral hepatitis serology, antimitochondrial antibody (primary biliary cirrhosis), iron studies (hemochromatosis), ceruloplasmin and urine copper levels (Wilson disease), and antinuclear and smooth muscle antibodies (autoimmune hepatitis).
- Gamma-glutamyl transpeptidase (GGTP), leucine aminopeptidase, and 5′-nucleotidase are used to confirm hepatic origin of alkaline phosphatase.
- **Liver biopsy may be necessary to completely determine the etiology.**

Imaging

- Ultrasonography can be used to identify extrahepatic obstruction and larger intrahepatic and extrahepatic masses (>1 cm).
- Computed tomographic (CT) scan has higher resolution than ultrasound and can detect smaller lesions (>5 mm) but is more costly and exposes the patient to contrast media.
- Magnetic resonance cholangiopancreatography (MRCP) provides images of the biliary tree without contrast media.
- Endoscopic retrograde cholangiopancreatography (ERCP) allows direct visualization of the biliary tree, but is more invasive than ultrasound or CT scan. Biopsy and therapeutic intervention is possible with this modality.
- Percutaneous transhepatic cholangiography is similar to ERCP but requires passing a needle through the liver parenchyma into a peripheral bile duct.

Differential Diagnosis

Evaluating the clinical presentation and pattern of initial laboratory tests delineates specific causes of jaundice.

- **Normal transaminases, alkaline phosphatase, and albumin suggest hemolysis or a defect of bilirubin conjugation or transport.**
  - Elevated unconjugated bilirubin (>80% to 85% of total) is seen with hemolysis or hereditary conjugating defects.
    - Obtain a complete blood count (CBC), blood smear, reticulocyte count, and lactate dehydrogenase (LDH).
    - If hemolysis is suggested, See Chapters 18.1 through 18.3.
    - If laboratory results are not consistent with hemolysis, suspect a defect in conjugation, especially if the total bilirubin is less than 6 mg/dL and conjugated bilirubin is normal.
    - Gilbert syndrome is the most common conjugating defect (7% of population): bilirubin is usually less than 3 mg/dL but increases with fever, fasting, or stress; patients are asymptomatic and have normal liver histology.
    - Crigler–Najjar syndrome is rare. In Type I bilirubin levels rise to 50 mg/dL and death occurs in infancy. In Type II bilirubin values may reach 20 mg/dL but no severe sequelae result except jaundice.
  - Elevated conjugated bilirubin (>50% of total) suggests a congenital defect in conjugated bilirubin transport. These conditions appear in childhood or adolescence with bilirubin levels up to 25 mg/dL, but cause no clinical sequelae. They follow an autosomal recessive inheritance pattern.

- Patients with rotor syndrome demonstrate visualization of the gallbladder on oral cholecystogram (OCG).
- In Dubin–Johnson syndrome the gallbladder is not seen on OCG; pathognomonic black pigment is found on liver biopsy.

■ **Predominant elevation of transaminases suggests hepatocellular injury**
  ▪ Acute or chronic viral hepatitis can be diagnosed by viral hepatitis serology.
  ▪ Alcoholic hepatitis clinically resembles viral or toxic hepatitis, but AST is usually greater than ALT (a reversal of the usual ratio); diagnosis is based on a history of heavy alcohol intake, absence of other causes of hepatitis, and liver biopsy.
  ▪ Hereditary liver disease
    - Wilson disease is confirmed by low ceruloplasmin levels and Kayser–Fleischer rings or liver biopsy.
    - Hemochromatosis is suspected in patients with a history of hepatomegaly, idiopathic cardiomyopathy, skin pigmentation, loss of libido, diabetes mellitus, or arthritis; elevated transferritin saturation and ferritin levels suggest the diagnosis, which is confirmed by genetic testing or liver biopsy.
    - α_1-Antitrypsin deficiency is associated with pulmonary disease and confirmed by decreased α_1-antitrypsin levels.
  ▪ Congestive and ischemic diseases including right-sided congestive heart failure, constrictive pericarditis, Budd–Chiari syndrome (hepatic vein or inferior vena cava obstruction), portal vein thrombosis, veno-occlusive disease, and hypotension are causes of jaundice and hepatocellular injury; diagnosis is based on other physical findings.
  ▪ Liver diseases in pregnancy that cause hepatocellular injury are acute fatty liver of pregnancy and toxemia.
  ▪ Drug-induced hepatitis can be confirmed by drug levels (e.g., acetaminophen), agent-specific patterns of hepatotoxicity, and, occasionally, liver biopsy.
  ▪ Autoimmune hepatitis is suspected when antinuclear antibodies, smooth muscle antibodies, or antimitochondrial antibodies are present; liver biopsy is helpful.

■ **Predominant elevation of alkaline phosphatase suggests cholestasis**
  ▪ Transaminases may also be elevated. 5′-nucleotidase and GGTP are usually elevated; if not, consider a bone source.
  ▪ If extrahepatic cholestasis is suspected based on history and physical examination, possible causes include choledocholithiasis, malignancies (pancreatic, bile duct, lymphoma, metastases), biliary stricture, sclerosing cholangitis, chronic pancreatitis, biliary atresia, and other rare conditions (Asian cholangiohepatitis, ascariasis, hemobilia).
    - Extrahepatic biliary obstruction requires prompt removal of the obstruction.
    - Obtain imaging of the biliary tree. Ultrasound is usually preferred due to lower cost, better detection of gallbladder stones, and avoidance of radiation exposure. CT gives better visualization of the pancreas and should be chosen if pancreatic pathology is suspected. Because ultrasound or CT scan can fail to detect up to 40% of intraductal stones, perform ERCP or percutaneous transhepatic cholangiography if suspicion is high.
  ▪ If intrahepatic cholestasis is suspected based on history and physical examination, order specific laboratory tests.
    - Consider ultrasound to rule out extrahepatic obstruction.
    - Acute and chronic hepatitis (viral, alcohol, and drug-induced) can be diagnosed by viral hepatitis serology and by withdrawal of toxins.
    - Cirrhosis is most commonly caused by long-term alcohol use and viral infections, especially hepatitis C. Rarer causes include genetic and metabolic diseases (Wilson disease, hemochromatosis, and α_1-antitrypsin deficiency) and autoimmune diseases (primary biliary cirrhosis, primary sclerosing cholangitis, and lupoid hepatitis). Liver biopsy may be helpful if the diagnosis or cause is unclear.
    - Chronic cholestatic syndromes include primary biliary cirrhosis and primary sclerosing cholangitis. Primary biliary cirrhosis is usually seen in middle-aged women; antimitochondrial antibodies are elevated in more than 90% of patients; liver biopsy confirms the diagnosis.

- Primary sclerosing cholangitis may be seen as an isolated finding or in association with inflammatory bowel disease, other fibrosclerosing syndromes, or AIDS; diagnosis is confirmed by ERCP or magnetic resonance cholangiogram.
- Benign recurrent intrahepatic cholestasis is diagnosed by recurrent episodes, family history, and absence of obstruction on cholangiography.
- Cholestasis of pregnancy is usually seen in the third trimester and often recurs in subsequent pregnancies or in association with estrogen use.
- Cholestasis can also be seen with sepsis, parenteral nutrition, postoperative state, or neoplasm.

■ **Neonatal jaundice**
  ▪ Evaluation of the newborn with jaundice is influenced by gestational age (preterm infants are at greater risk of sequelae), age of onset (clinical jaundice <24 hours of age is always abnormal), maternal illness (i.e., sepsis), and neonate signs and symptoms. Initial testing for significant jaundice include total and direct bilirubin, CBC, reticulocyte count, examination of the peripheral blood smear, blood typing (mother and baby), and Coombs test.
  ▪ Elevated unconjugated bilirubin
    • Physiologic jaundice
      ◦ Onset between day 2 and 4 of life, total bilirubin <15 mg/dL, predominantly unconjugated bilirubin (direct <1.5 mg/dL).
      ◦ Occurs in 50% of newborns.
      ◦ Resolution in 1 week (term) or 2 weeks (preterm).
    • Hemolysis
      ◦ Consider Rh and ABO incompatibility, spherocytosis, enzyme deficiency, and hemoglobinopathy.
    • Breast milk jaundice
      ◦ Onset between day 4 and 7 of life, peaking during the third week of life, elevated unconjugated bilirubin.
      ◦ Resolution between 3 and 10 weeks of age.
    • Other causes include polycythemia and cephalohematoma.
  ▪ Elevated conjugated bilirubin
    • Causes include sepsis, hepatitis, TORCH (toxoplasmosis, others such as syphilis, rubella, cytomegalovirus, and herpesvirus), biliary atresia, galactosemia.

References
1. Frymoyer CL. Jaundice. In: Taylor RB, ed. *Manual of family practice*. 2nd ed. Philadelphia: Lippincott, Williams & Wilkins; 2002:59–61.
2. Lidofsky SD. Jaundice. In: Feldman M, Friedman LS, Sleisenger MH, eds., *Sleisenger & Fordtran's gastrointestinal and liver disease*. 7th ed. Philadelphia: Saunders; 2002:256–259.
3. Schwiebert LP, Steiner GA. Jaundice. In: Mengel MB, Schwiebert LP, eds. *Ambulatory medicine: the primary care of families*. 3rd ed. New York: McGraw-Hill; 2001:213–221.

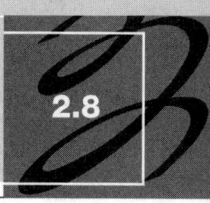

GENERAL PRINCIPLES

Definition
Clinically apparent interstitial fluid accumulation.

Anatomy
Edema can present in any tissue supplied by lymphatics, but is usually seen in the dependent-most parts of the body (e.g., legs, sacrum).

Pathophysiology
Imbalance of one of the **Starling forces** across the capillary endothelium leads to edematous tissue:

- Increased **hydrostatic pressure** in the capillary (πc) caused by obstruction downstream or an expansion of plasma volume. Arterial smooth muscle autoregulation protects against increases in systemic arterial pressure, and therefore patients with hypertension rarely develop edema.
- Changes in **oncotic pressure**—decrease in the capillary (πc) or increase in the interstitum (πi)—caused by a decreased rate of lymphatic clearance or by changes in plasma concentrations of protein or mucopolysaccarides.
- Increased **capillary permeability** also results in changes to oncotic pressure, but only indirectly through osmolarity. It is often secondary to local inflammation or trauma, and mediated by cytokines—tumor necrosis factor (TNF), interleukin-1 (INL-1), INL-10—and prostaglandins. Increased systemic histamine levels from seasonal allergies have similar effects.
- Edema often occurs in the context of an appropriate but destabilizing response to hemodynamic changes. For example, if effective circulating volume decreases, the kidneys respond by retaining sodium and water via activation of the renin–angiotensin–aldosterone (RAA) axis, which leads to edema. Although the excess sodium is checked by the release of natriuretics—atrial natriuretic peptide (ANP), brain-type natriuretic peptide (BNP)—the chronic RAA axis activation eventually overrides that equilibrium. However, because these controls on hemodynamics are fully functioning, the measured plasma volume and osmolality are most often normal.

Etiology
An intimidatingly diverse spectrum of disease states can lead to Starling disturbance, some insignificant, some life-threatening. Edema itself is relatively benign. However, it can indicate a serious underlying disease, and so finding its etiologic basis is crucial.

- Systemic causes:
  - *Drugs*: **Corticosteroids, antihypertensives** (calcium-channel blockers, or CCBs, vasodilators), hypoglycymics (glitazones), nonsteroidal anti-inflammatory drugs (NSAIDs), **hormones**
  - *Pregnancy-induced/menstrual*
  - *Cardiovascular*: Cardiomyopathies, **congestive heart failure** (CHF), pericarditis, large vessel obstruction
  - *Renal*: **Nephrosis, renal failure,** nephritis
  - *Liver*: **Cirrhosis, hepatitis,** hemochromatosis, Wilson disease

71

- *Hypoproteinemia*: Anorexia, malabsorption, protein deficiency, beriberi *Vasculitis*
- *Idiopathic edema* (also known as cyclic edema, periodic edema, fluid retention edema, orthostatic edema)
- Local causes:
  - *Venous*: **Deep vein thrombosis** (DVT), **venous insufficiency,** mass compression
  - *Lymphatic*: **Lymphedema,** lipedema, postsurgical trauma
  - *Musculoskeletal*: Trauma, overuse inflammation, bursitis compression
  - *Other*: Reflex sympathetic dystrophy, peripheral neuropathy, arteriovenous (AV) malformation, myxedema

DIAGNOSIS

Clinical Presentation

Edema is a relatively late stage presentation of interstitial fluid retention. Body water can increase by more than 15% before becoming clinically apparent. Besides **palpable swelling,** symptoms can include **restricted gait,** increased **abdominal width,** and **dyspnea** due to pressure on the diaphragm. Ascites and peripheral edema are two symptoms of overlapping disease pathways, and may present simultaneously.

History

- Onset
- Temporal **patterns**
- **Precipitating events:** trauma, recent surgery, menses
- **Ameliorating/aggravating factors:** elevation, position, diet
- **Associated symptoms:** pain, erythema, weight gain, tightening of shoes, rings, or waist bands
- **Past medical history** and comorbidities, especially related to cardiac, renal, hepatic, or malabsorptive diseases
- Current **medications**

Physical Examination

- **Pitting:** Press against a bony prominence for at least 5 seconds, then withdraw and note the degree of pitting. Nonpitting edema indicates lymphedema or organized edema.
- **Distribution:** Dependent, hand, facial/orbital, or full body (anasarca).
- **Symmetry**
- **Tenderness to palpation**
- **Vascular distension or cords**
- **Cardiac exam: Check for any new murmur, friction rubs, or rhythm disturbance.**
- **Abdominal exam: Check for ascites, organomegaly, or fluid waves.**
- **Skin exam: Check for erythema or signs of chronic liver disease. Hyperpigmentation of stasis dermatitis can indicate venous insufficiency.**
- **Lymphadenopathy**

Laboratory Studies

Lab testing is targeted at suspected etiology.

- **Liver function tests (LFTs), BUN/creatinine, UA, BNP,** and serum **albumin** comprise an appropriate initial panel to assess circulating fluid status and renal, cardiopulmonary, and hepatic condition.
- **24-hour urine collection** may be useful if renal etiology is suspected.
- Targeted **cultures and smears** can identify a suspected infection.
- **Stool studies** are helpful if malabsorption is suspected.
- **Thyroid studies** may reveal hypothyroidism and myxedema.
- Serum and urine **protein electropheresis** may help explain protein imbalances.

Imaging

Imaging studies should be considered if obstruction, cardiac, hepatic, or renal disease is suspected.

- **Chest x-ray (CXR), electrocardiography,** and **echocardiography** may be warranted to confirm cardiopulmonary causes.

- **Venous Doppler ultrasound** and **venography** can help reveal DVT, and should be ordered with unexplainable edema.
- **Ultrasound, computed tomography, and magnetic resonance imaging** may be useful in the workup of neoplastic, hepatic, or renal diseases.

Surgical Diagnostic Procedures

- **Cardiac catheterization** may be warranted to confirm cardiopulmonary causes.
- Vessel wall or cardiac muscle **biopsies** may warranted with adequate suspicion.

Monitoring

Serial evaluations are important to assess progression and monitor efficacy of underlying disease treatment.

Classification

- **Systemic** versus local
- **Symmetric** versus asymmetric
- **Pitting** versus nonpitting (brawny)

Staging

Edema grading is notoriously subjective, and rating systems differ widely among providers. A series of assessments by a single provider is much more useful clinically than any one single measurement.

- One system in common use is a 0 to 4 scale:
  - 0 = none
  - +1 = trace
  - +2 = mild, rebounds quickly
  - +3 = moderate
  - +4 = severe, indent remains >30 seconds
- Alternatively, a quantitative system is sometimes used, assessing pitting depth from 1 to ≥4 cm.
- Additional measurements can be useful in assessing severity, when measured over time:
  - Daily **weights**
  - **Patient position** at time of exam
  - **Extent,** or height up the limb

Differential Diagnosis

Workup should always begin by ruling out major organ failure. Beyond that, if a clear etiology is suggested by history and physical, a conservative diagnostic workup may be appropriate. Clinical suspicion should dictate diagnostic testing.

TREATMENT

Treatment should always be directed at management of underlying conditions. Empiric treatment may mask disease severity without correcting the imbalance in Starling forces, and therefore lead to missing a potentially serious underlying disease. Edema in itself is not dangerous and can be left untreated while a workup is under way.

Behavioral

- **Elevation** of affected limbs in most dependent edema temporarily reduces symptoms.
- **Compression stockings** are useful, but may worsen the condition, unless properly fit, by acting as a tourniquet. Careful sizing or custom fitting is essential.
- **Sodium restriction** can help offset renal sodium retention.
- Weight loss, smoking cessation, and stress reduction should all be encouraged as part of maintaining a healthy cardiovascular system.

Medications

- **Diuretics** are the mainstay for correction of peripheral edema, as they are relatively safe and target the pathology of the most common edema causes. Diuresis has an inherent maximal threshold, above which fluid is drawn from intravascular volume. The goal of treatment is to reach this threshold without exceeding it. Combining different diuretic classes may improve dieresis while avoiding high dosages.

- For patients with **CHF or renal disease,** correction is rapid because the body's full capillary system can be employed. Loop diuretics are first line. For patients with compromised renal filtration, larger doses may be required due to the severe sodium retention.
- With cirrhosis, aldosterone receptor antagonists such as **spironolactone** are first line, because these patients often develop secondary hyperaldosteronism.
- In patients presenting primarily with **ascites,** avoid rapid diuresis. Because only the peritoneal capillaries are available to draw off interstitial fluid, the maximal threshold is quickly surpassed.
- When **venous insufficiency** or **lymphatic obstruction** is the cause, diuretics have no effect on edema and draw only from plasma volume.
- Rarely, diuretics can induce edema. Consider this in patients on chronic diuretic treatment with new-onset edema.

■ Periodic **paracenteses** are sometimes used to avoid high diuretic doses, although the fluid drawn off is eventually replaced by new fluid.

■ Medications used to treat CHF—ACE inhibitors, vasodilators, beta blockers, digitalis—all improve cardiovascular efficacy, which helps alleviate edema.

Patient Education
Patients are often the first to notice edema, and often concerned about its cosmetic consequences. Offering reassurance and focusing discussion on the underlying disease can greatly alleviate the patient's concerns. Several valuable informational handouts are available online:

■ NIH, http://www.nlm.nih.gov/medlineplus/edema.html
■ AAFP, http://familydoctor.org/840.xml

References
1. Cho S. Peripheral edema. *Am J Med* 2002;113(7):580–586.
2. Kirton C. Assessing edema. *Nursing* 1996;26(7):54.

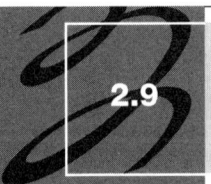

2.9 PELVIC PAIN
Steven Crossman

GENERAL PRINCIPLES
Pelvic pain is defined as pain in the pelvic region and can be acute or chronic in nature and can originate from a variety of causes. The true bony pelvis is that cavity bordered anteriorly by the pubic symphysis and superior rami, laterally by the ischium and ilium, and posteriorly by the sacrum and coccyx. This area contains the bladder, distal ureters, colon, rectum, pelvic neurovascular structures, and pelvic muscles. In women, it also contains the uterus, ovaries, and fallopian tubes, while in men it includes the prostate gland. Pelvic pain is much more common in women than men, and so this chapter focuses on female pelvic pain (see Special Considerations for a brief discussion of pelvic pain in men). Pelvic pain is a very common complaint in family medicine. The pathophysiology and management of pelvic pain depend on the nature of the underlying cause. A differential diagnosis of pelvic pain is listed in Table 2.9-1. Some of these problems are more often acute, others chronic, but many can present with acute exacerbations of an underlying chronic condition.

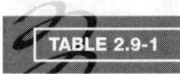

TABLE 2.9-1	Differential Diagnosis of Pelvic Pain

1) Skin
   a. Trauma[a]
   b. Shingles[a]
2) Musculoskeletal
   a. Trauma[a]
   b. Inflammatory arthritis[b]
   c. Piriformis syndrome[b]
3) Gastrointestinal
   a. Appendicitis[a]
   b. Gastroenteritis[a]
   c. Intestinal lymphadenitis[a]
   d. Constipation[c]
   e. Intestinal obstruction[a]
   f. Diverticulitis[a]
   g. Hernia[a]
   h. Irritable bowel syndrome[c]
   i. Inflammatory bowel disease[c]
4) Genitourinary
   a. Genital
      i. Pelvic inflammatory disease[a]
      ii. Sexually transmitted infections[b]
      iii. Pregnancy-related conditions
         1. Ectopic pregnancy[a]
         2. Miscarriage[a]
         3. Round ligament pain[a]
      iv. Ovarian cyst[b]
      v. Ovarian tumor[c]
      vi. Ovarian torsion[a]
      vii. Primary dysmenorrhea[c]
      viii. Vaginitis[a]
      ix. Fibroid uterus[c]
      x. Mittleschmirtz[c]
      xi. Endometriosis[c]
      xii. Adenomyosis[c]
   b. Urinary
      i. Urinary trace infection[a]
      ii. Renal stone[a]
      iii. Urethritis[a]
      iv. Interstitial cystitis[c]
5) Vascular
   a. Aneurysm[a]
   b. Ischemic colitis[b]
6) Psychologic
   a. Domestic violence[b]
   b. Sexual abuse[b]
   c. Vaginismus[c]

[a]Acute.
[b]Can be both acute and chronic.
[c]Chronic.

DIAGNOSIS (ACUTE)

Clinical Presentation

The clinical presentation of acute pelvic pain varies depending on the etiology. The patient complaining of pain may be mildly symptomatic to acutely ill and toxic appearing. Universal in the presentation is the report of pain, which may be reported in the lower abdomen, genital area, or lower back. Occasionally, the underlying pelvic pathology may lead to upper quadrant or generalized abdominal pain, with or without peritoneal signs.

History

As with any pain complaint, the history should begin with attempting to elucidate the PQRSTs of the pain: **p**alliative and **p**rovocative factors, the **q**uality of the pain, if there is any **r**adiation of the pain, the **s**everity of the pain, and the **t**iming of when the pain comes and goes. Second, the interviewer should ask about the presence of any associated symptoms. An organ system approach is helpful here, querying the patient on symptoms related to systems existing in the pelvic region, including the skin (rash, blisters, paresthesias), musculoskeletal (history of strain or trauma), genitourinary (vaginal discharge, dyspareunia, vaginal bleeding, urinary frequency or urgency, dysuria, hematuria), and gastrointestinal (nausea, vomiting, anorexia, hematochezia, constipation, diarrhea) systems. In women with pelvic pain, it is especially important to include an obstetrical, menstrual, and sexual history, asking about the last menstrual period, gravida/para status, past and current sexual partners, and history of sexually transmitted infections (STIs). It is helpful to know as well whether or not the patient has ever had any past abdominal or pelvic surgeries, especially appendectomy, hysterectomy, or oophorectomy. Eliciting the patient's own explanatory model for the symptoms is often extremely helpful, as it may reveal pertinent information (past history of similar pain, past medical evaluations) or important worries the patient may have ("I'm worried that I may have ovarian cancer").

Physical Examination

The physical examination should begin with review of the patient's vital signs, especially noting heart rate, blood pressure, and temperature. This should be followed by a general assessment of how ill the patient appears: for example, is the patient visibly uncomfortable (grimacing, grasping stomach, rocking back and forth), is she diaphoretic, etc.

Exam should then proceed to include the abdomen beginning with inspection looking for any skin lesions (rash or bruises) or any obvious distention or deformity. Auscultation follows to assess for presence or absence of normal bowel sounds. Palpation should uncover any tender areas as well as assess for peritoneal signs including rigidity, guarding, and rebound tenderness.

A pelvic exam is indicated as well and should begin with inspection of the external genitalia and urethral orifice looking especially for any skin lesions or discharge that might indicate an underlying infectious process, for signs of trauma, or for any anatomic abnormality. The speculum exam is then performed to allow direct visual inspection of the vaginal mucosa and the cervix, looking for signs of infection and also for any dilation of the cervix, or blood or tissue in the cervical os that could indicate an inevitable or threatened miscarriage. Samples can be obtained for STI screening and potentially for Pap smear testing (if patient is in need of this screening). Following visualization with the speculum the bimanual exam is completed to assess the cervix for cervical motion tenderness (also a peritoneal sign) and to assess for any uterine or adnexal masses or tenderness. The rectovaginal exam may be indicated based on clinical suspicion (need to rule out gastrointestinal bleed or fecal impaction, need to assess for possible retrocecal appendix, etc.).

Additional examination should be guided by the history and specific clinical situation.

Laboratory Studies

The most common testing ordered in the female patient with acute pelvic pain includes a complete blood count (CBC), urinalysis (UA), and pregnancy testing. Additional testing may include cervical cultures for *Neisseria gonorrhea* and *Chlamydia* and a vaginal wet prep and KOH slide. A high white count on the CBC may indicate an underlying infectious process. Anemia, if present and especially if associated with tachycardia or hypotension, could indicate a more serious process, such as a ruptured ectopic pregnancy or ovarian cyst. White blood cells, hematuria, and positive nitrite on the UA can suggest a diagnosis of urinary tract infection, while hematuria alone could indicate an underlying renal stone. The pregnancy test is crucial for any woman of childbearing age. An initial positive urine or blood test may need to be followed by a more specific serum quantitative test, which measures an exact amount of the human chorionic gonadotropin (HCG) hormone (this can be helpful in dating a pregnancy and in correlating with ultrasound findings). The vaginal wet prep can be diagnostic for bacterial vaginosis (if clue cells are seen) or *Trichomonas* vaginitis (if the flagellated trichomonads are seen). If the KOH slide is positive for yeast or fungal elements, then the diagnosis of *Candida* vaginitis is made.

Imaging

Although imaging is often not necessary in the evaluation of acute pelvic pain, there are situations where it will be helpful. If the patient is acutely ill and a reasonable diagnosis cannot be made based on the history, physical, and laboratory tests, then imaging may be needed to better define the problem.

Ultrasound imaging is readily available at most hospitals and even in some private offices. A pelvic ultrasound utilizing the transabdominal and transvaginal approaches can often identify many sources of pelvic pain including an ectopic pregnancy, ovarian pathology, uterine fibroids, pelvic inflammatory disease (PID), and even in some cases acute appendicitis. Ultrasound can also reveal the presence of uterine fibroids. Renal ultrasound can also be helpful in ruling out structural renal pathology and dilation of the ureters (hydronephrosis), which may result from an obstructing kidney stone.

Computed tomography (CT) imaging can also be helpful in assessing for signs of acute appendicitis and noncontrast spiral CT scan of the renal system has largely replaced intravenous pyelogram (IVP) testing to evaluate for the presence of nephrolithiasis. Some subtle changes may show up on the CT scan in cases of pid as well.

Magnetic resonance imaging (MRI) can also be used in the setting of acute pelvic pain; however, MRI is not always readily available and is more expensive.

Monitoring

Patients with acute pelvic pain should be monitored to ensure response to treatment. Depending on the diagnosis, patients may need to be admitted (acute abdomen) or re-examined within 48 to 72 hours (pid managed as an outpatient with oral antibiotics). Additionally, patients should be monitored until complete resolution of symptoms, as complications may arise and also as some acute pelvic pain may become chronic pelvic pain.

Surgical Diagnostic Procedures

In acute cases, surgical intervention for diagnosis (most often using laparoscopy) is generally reserved for those patients who are severely ill, where a diagnosis has not yet been made, or for patients who are failing to respond to treatment.

TREATMENT (ACUTE)

Specific treatments for a variety of common causes of acute pelvic pain are outlined below. Pain control will be an important feature for all patients with acute pelvic pain. For many diagnoses conservative treatment with ice or heat and rest, combined with over-the-counter acetaminophen or nonsteroidal anti-inflammatory drugs is sufficient. However, some patients may require narcotics to control their pain. Dietary modification may be useful in certain situations. Behavioral therapy in these cases is generally supportive as in some cases reassurance is all that is needed.

Medications

Many of the conditions that can cause acute pelvic pain are infectious and treatable with the correct antibiotic agent. Shingles can be ameliorated with the appropriate antiviral agent (acyclovir, valacyclovir, or famciclovir) especially if started early in the course.

Diverticulitis is usually managed with broad-spectrum antibiotic coverage to include Gram negative and anaerobic bacteria, usually trimethoprim-sulfa or a fluoroquinolone plus metronidazole. Most gastroenteritis though is viral in origin and requires only symptomatic care, though a bacterial pathogen may be more likely if the patient also has fevers, bloody diarrhea, and significant abdominal cramping.

Each sexually transmitted infection has its own specific management. When diagnosing an STI, it is important to remember to screen for additional infections, as when patients have one, they are at risk for others. Although the exact causative agent is often not identified in cases of pelvic inflammatory disease, it is often caused by *Chlamydia* or *N. gonorrhea* so empiric antibiotic coverage must be effective against both of these agents. Commonly, the combination of intramuscular ceftriaxone in one 250-mg dose plus oral doxycycline 100 mg twice daily for 2 weeks is used. Ofloxacin (400 mg twice daily) or levofloxacin (500 mg once daily) as a single oral agent for 2 weeks are alternative choices. Vaginitis is treated according to the causative agent: *Trichonomas* is treated with metronidazole 500 mg twice daily for 2 weeks, *Candida* infections are treated with topical (terconazole, clotrimazole, tioconazole, and nystatin) or oral (fluconazole) antifungals, and bacterial vaginosis is also treated with metronidazole, vaginally or orally, with clindamycin vaginally as the alternative. For urinary tract infection, there are many antibiotics that may be effective. These include the first-line agents of trimethoprim-sulfa, fluoroquinolones, macrodantin, and cephalexin.

Surgery

Surgery is the treatment of choice for acute appendicitis, ovarian torsion, and symptomatic hernias. Surgery is often indicated as well for bowel obstruction and for ectopic pregnancy (although in some instances ectopic pregnancy can also be managed medically) and may be indicated in diverticulitis or in cases of kidney stone (especially when there is concomitant obstruction).

Nonoperative

Many conditions may benefit from alternative therapies. Specifically, uterine artery embolization is now available in most communities and has provided an important non-surgical alternative to hysterectomy or myomectomy for the treatment of uterine fibroids.

Referrals

For pelvic pain with peritoneal findings, consultation with surgery (obstetrical, gynecologic, or general) is usually indicated.

Patient Education

Patient education should be provided to all patients to help them understand the etiology, treatment, and prognosis for their pelvic pain. Patients should also be educated to look for warning signs of disease progression. Follow-up should be encouraged when symptoms do not respond to therapy.

Complications

The potential complications from acute pelvic pain are wide-ranging. In most instances, the pain resolves and there are no long-term problems. However, many complications, including progression to chronic pain, are possible. pid can lead to chronic pain, infertility, and an increased incidence of ectopic pregnancies. Because of the increased risk of complications, hospitalization for patients with pid is indicated if the patient is pregnant, has severe illness, is unable to tolerate oral medication, has a tubo-ovarian abscess, or if there is failure to improve after 3 days on initial therapy.[1] Ectopic pregnancy can cause fallopian tube rupture, which can potentially lead to fatal blood loss. Fibroids (leiomyomata) of the uterus can lead to severe pain and anemia and may necessitate hysterectomy. Kidney stones, especially if recurrent or associated with obstruction, have the potential to lead to chronic kidney disease. Given the range of potential complications and the seriousness of many of the possible diagnoses, it is important for the health care provider to be careful and thorough in managing patients presenting with acute pelvic pain.

DIAGNOSIS (CHRONIC)

Clinical Presentation

The clinical presentation of chronic pelvic pain may be quite similar to that for acute. However, the time period will be in the range of 3 to 6 months or more, although the course may be intermittent.

History

With chronic pelvic pain, the history should be expanded to focus more in depth on the psychosocial situation of the patient as chronic pelvic pain may indicate a history of physical or sexual abuse. Furthermore, the physician should explore the impact of the pain on the patient's life at work, home, or school. Keeping a symptom calendar (sometimes referred to as pain diary) may be helpful in uncovering hidden patterns or associations.[2]

Physical Examination, Laboratory Studies, Imaging

The workup including physical examination, laboratory, and imaging studies should include the same items listed under acute pelvic pain.

Surgical Diagnostic Procedures

Diagnostic laparoscopy may be indicated in the workup of chronic pelvic when no obvious cause can be found on the initial workup.

TREATMENT (CHRONIC)

Medications

Medications for infectious etiologies are discussed above. For noninfectious gynecologic diagnoses there are often hormonal therapies that may be effective. The pain associated with endometriosis or adenomyosis can often be controlled by oral contraceptives or progestins, with or without over-the-counter analgesics. If unsuccessful, gonadotropin–releasing hormone analogues may be helpful.[3] These same medications are also often helpful in treating the pain from primary dysmenorrhea.[4]

Medications are also the mainstay of therapy in the treatment of inflammatory bowel disease and, along with lifestyle modification, may be helpful in treating irritable bowel syndrome. The most commonly used medications for inflammatory bowel disease are anti-inflammatories (like 5-acetylsalicylic acid compounds, such as sulfasalazine or mesalamine, and corticosteroids, such as prednisone and hydrocortisone) and immunosuppressant medications (like azathioprine, cyclosporine, and newer agents such as infliximab). In treating irritable bowel syndrome, it may be helpful to differentiate between constipation-predominant and diarrhea-predominant syndromes.

Referrals

If a gastrointestinal source is suspected, referral to a gastroenterologist for consideration of colonoscopy may be indicated. Additionally, when initial management fails to lead to significant improvement, additional surgical or gynecologic consultation may be required. When there is a significant psychosocial component, referral to a mental health specialist should be included. Finally, if a history of abuse is uncovered, the physician should make the patient aware of available legal and social supports in the community (including hotline numbers and names and numbers of local shelters).

SPECIAL CONSIDERATIONS (PELVIC PAIN IN MEN)

The differential diagnosis of pelvic pain in men includes the skin, musculoskeletal, gastrointestinal, urologic, and vascular possibilities listed in Table 2.9-1. For men, however, the prostate and scrotal contents must also be considered. Prostatis, which can be acute or chronic, is a common cause of pelvic pain in men as is referred pain from the scrotum.

Epididymitis, testicular torsion, torsion of the appendix testis, and a varicocele can all cause pain that is referred to the pelvis. Of these, epididymitis is usually infectious and is treated with appropriate antibiotics (in younger men less than 35 years old this is usually the same medications as used to treat pid in women, whereas for older men, fluoroquinolones are usually first-line agents). Testicular torsion is a surgical emergency, while torsion of the appendix testis (which only sometimes will have the classic "blue dot" sign) is almost always a benign, self-limited condition requiring only short-term analgesics. A varicocele is essentially a varicose vein in the scrotum and when symptomatic, or when there are concerns about fertility, urologic referral is indicated.

A patient with acute bacterial prostatitis is generally ill-appearing and often febrile. The patient will complain of pain, which may be anywhere from the lower back to the lower abdomen and pelvis. There will often be signs of urinary hesitancy or weakness of stream, and at times the patient may be unable to void altogether. Physical exam of an acutely infected prostate will reveal it to be enlarged, tender, and often boggy. The physician should avoid prostatic massage and vigorous prostate exam in this setting as there is concern this may increase bacteremia. The mainstay of treatment for acute bacterial prostatitis is antibiotic therapy targeting primarily Gram-negative pathogens using trimethoprim-sulfa or fluoroquinolones. However, in men younger than 35 there is again a higher likelihood of *N. gonorrhea* and *Chlamydia* infections so therapy should cover these agents as well. Therapy should continue for 10 to 14 days. However, bacterial prostatitis may be a chronic and less severe infection and in these cases may require antibiotic therapy for 1 to 3 months.

Some men may also suffer from chronic pelvic pain due to nonbacterial prostatitis (no bacteria on culture and no white cells seen in prostatic secretions). A variety of therapies have been tried including trials of antibiotics, anticholinergics, alpha blockers and non-steroidal anti-inflammatory medications.[5] Urologic consultation may be helpful for these patients.

References

1. Sexually transmitted diseases guidelines 2002. Centers for Disease Control and Prevention. *MMWR Recomm Rep* 2002;51(RR-6):1–78.
2. Williams R, Hern T. Pelvic pain. *Hosp Physician* 2002;6:1–12.
3. Mounsey AL, Wilgus A, Slawsone DC. Diagnosis and management of endometriosis. *Am Fam Physician* 2006;74:594–602.
4. French L. Dysmenorrhea. *Am Fam Physician* 2005;71:285–291.
5. Stevermer JJ, Easley SE. Treatment of prostatitis. *Am Fam Physician* 2000; 61:3015–3022.

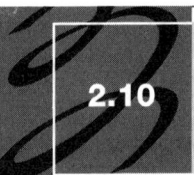

2.10   BACK PAIN

Katherine L. Margo, Thomas D. Masten

*B*ack pain, particularly low back pain (LBP), affects virtually everyone at some time. The etiology is often obscure, but once a serious medical problem has been eliminated the management is usually straightforward.

ACUTE LOW BACK PAIN

Definition

LBP refers to pain in the lumbar spine area.

Anatomy

Although LBP is most often related to the spine itself, other structures thought to contribute to LBP include paraspinal muscles, ligaments, facet joints, and intervertebral disks.

Etiology

Approximately 90% of all patients have nonspecific LBP, meaning no specific cause can be found. Potential causes include musculoligamentous injuries; disk herniation with nerve impingement; sacroiliac (SI) joint derangements; degenerative changes of the bone, disk, or facet joint; spinal stenosis; severe spondylolisthesis or scoliosis; underlying systemic diseases, such as cancer, infection, rheumatologic disease; and visceral diseases, such as aortic aneurysms or kidney disease. The first task for the clinician is to rule out a serious nonorthopaedic problem. Thereafter, defining a specific lesion is less important.

Diagnosis
Clinical Presentation
Patients can present either with insidious onset of LBP or abrupt onset. People with milder LBP often have ill-defined pain with a normal examination. People with a lumbar disk problem more typically have severe pain often with radiation down the leg ("sciatica"). There can be findings on physical examination but not always.

History
Serious conditions are found most frequently in patients older than 50 years. To rule out a potentially serious condition, ask about a history of trauma, cancer, unexplained weight loss or fever, failure of pain relief with bed rest, saddle anesthesia, bladder or bowel dysfunction, or a history that would indicate a risk of infection (e.g., HIV-positive status, intravenous drug use, and immune suppression).

Inquire about the onset of pain. Disk problems tend to occur suddenly, whereas other mechanical pain often comes on gradually. Information about the duration of the pain and previous episodes of back pain, as well as identification of precipitating situations at work or during exercise can be helpful. Pain below the knee, paresthesias, and weakness of the lower leg are consistent with nerve compression, usually due to a disk protrusion or herniation. Patients with unilateral low back and buttock pain that gets worse with standing in one position may be suffering from an SI joint derangement. A history in older patients of exacerbation of pain with walking that is relieved by leaning forward is suggestive of neural claudication due to spinal stenosis. It is important to assess current functional limitations, the employment history, and the psychosocial situation when planning a course of treatment. Chronic pain is defined as pain lasting longer than 12 weeks. The management for chronic LBP is different from that for acute LBP.

Physical Examination
Observation of the patient's posture and demeanor as you enter the room will assist you in assessing the severity of pain. Examine the spine for acute deviation, which is a sign of a disk derangement. Testing the range of motion of the spine looking for asymmetrical motion can also help identify disk problems. The walk test is performed by the examiner's positioning his or her thumbs over the patient's posterior superior iliac spines while the patient is standing and then watching to see if the thumbs move symmetrically when the patient's hips are flexed. Asymmetry of movement often indicates an SI problem.

Straight leg raising and extension of the knee while sitting (flip test) are tests for dural impingement usually from a disk; these tests are considered positive when sciatic type pain is produced in the leg as the leg is extended. Pain on the contralateral side is a strongly positive test result. Reproduction of pain to the back may also be significant, but is a less reliable finding.

Every back examination should include a neurologic examination that includes muscle testing, sensory examination, and testing of deep tendon reflexes, especially in the L4 to S1 distribution, because 95% of lumbar disk herniations occur at L4 to L5 or L5 to S1. Palpation for tenderness over the lumbar spinous processes and between L4 and the iliac crest over the ileolumbar ligament completes the examination.

Laboratory and Radiographic Studies
In the evaluation of nontraumatic LBP, laboratory or radiologic studies are not usually helpful during the first 4 weeks of the onset of back pain unless there are signs of a serious condition. Computed tomography (CT) and magnetic resonance imaging (MRI) can be misleading because of their high false-positive rate. In all 64% of asymptomatic people have either a bulge or a protrusion of a disk on MRI.[1] Even after 4 weeks, these tests should be reserved for the case in which surgery is contemplated. Blood tests are not indicated for the first 4 weeks unless there is a fever or other sign of systemic illness.

Treatment[2]

Patient Education

Because 90% of patients recover within 4 weeks despite method of treatment, patient education regarding the natural history of acute LBP is an important aspect of a successful outcome. Contemporary management of acute LBP, as expressed in the Agency for Health Care Policy and Research (AHCPR) Task Force report, moves beyond exclusively addressing pain control and bed rest to emphasis on improved activity tolerance and an early return to work. Taking time to discuss specific exercises and prevention by improving general fitness is also important. This also serves to avoid developing a disability mind-set.

Activity Level

Bed rest should be avoided except in the extreme cases, and even then patients should be put on bed rest for only 1 or 2 days. Usual activities should be instituted as soon as possible. However, all lifting and bending probably should be avoided temporarily. Exercise classes are useful for people with nonspecific LBP after 1 month.[3]

Medication

One well-designed study has shown that patients treated with fewer pain medications and less bed rest than other therapy have lower costs and equal functional improvement after 1 and 12 months.[4] Nonsteroidal anti-inflammatory drugs (NSAIDs) and acetaminophen should be used as first-line agents. Muscle relaxants including benzodiazepines are frequently used and are beneficial but are no more effective than NSAIDs, and no study has shown use of both NSAIDs and muscle relaxants to be better than either one alone. AHCPR guidelines suggest that opioids taken for longer than 2 weeks, oral steroids, and colchicine should be avoided altogether.

Physical Treatment Methods

Standard traction, biofeedback, and physical modalities (e.g., heat and cold packs, corsets) do not have good supporting research for their efficacy. Recently heat packs have been shown to give some benefit especially when paired with exercise. Specific back exercises may be beneficial if the correct type of exercise is chosen.[5]

Injections

Epidural injections can be helpful in radicular pain and in spinal stenosis. Trigger point injections are also used but have not been thoroughly investigated.

Surgery

Cauda equina syndrome requires immediate surgery; otherwise only 5% to 10% of symptomatic disk herniations require surgery. In fact, sciatica due to a herniated disk can resolve spontaneously in 9 to 12 months. Consider referral if a patient has persistent and severe sciatica and clinical evidence of nerve root compromise after 1 month of conservative care.

Behavioral

A poor social situation can alter a patient's reaction to pain, especially if there is job dissatisfaction. Other factors, such as pending litigation, can complicate or prolong the treatment. Assessment by a psychiatrist or other mental health professional may be helpful if the psychologic issues are complex.

Alternative Medicine

Manipulation by physical therapists, physicians, or chiropractors can be helpful during the first month of symptoms. There is no evidence that it is superior to other methods. It can also be used for the SI joint problems that are common in pregnancy.

Results

Recurrences of LBP are common, no matter what the treatment. It is important to recognize patients at risk for chronicity such as those with psychosocial risk factors such as depression or job dissatisfaction.

Chronic Low Back Pain

LBP lasting longer than 12 weeks is considered chronic and carries with it a worse prognosis. The longer the pain lasts, the less the likelihood of recovery. The goal of treatment should be to improve functional capacity despite the pain. Passive modality treatments should be avoided. An active exercise/reconditioning program with experienced therapists can be helpful. Ongoing psychosocial support is also crucial. Ligament injections are advocated by some physicians. Surgery should be avoided unless there is a proven source of pain. Many alternative therapies are available to these patients; unfortunately, few have been studied scientifically. Most do not cause harm and may be worth trying for selected patients.

CERVICAL PAIN

Diagnosis

History

A history of trauma, particularly that related to motor vehicle accidents, should be obtained. Pain down the arm with paresthesias in the distribution of C4 to C5 or below indicates nerve compression, often caused by disk protrusion. A story of waking up with a painful, deviated neck is consistent with an acute torticollis.

Physical Examination

Range-of-motion testing of the neck should be performed, including side flexion, rotation, forward flexion, and extension. A complete neurologic examination of both upper extremities should be performed, including motor, sensory, and reflex testing.

Laboratory and Radiographic Studies

Unless there is a reason to suspect a systemic illness causing the pain or there is a history of trauma, no radiographs or other radiologic studies are necessary on initial evaluation.

Management

When needed, immobilization with a soft or hard cervical collar should be limited to just a few days. The patient should start gentle range-of-motion exercises immediately. If the pain persists for more than 1 week, the patient should be referred for physical therapy. Medications should be limited to a mild analgesic, and a muscle relaxant should be added only if there is no response to the analgesic alone. Surgery is reserved for fractures or radiculopathy with disabling pain.

References

1. Jensen MC, et al. Magnetic resonance imaging of the lumbar spine in people without back pain. *N Engl J Med* 1994;331:115.
2. Koes BW, van Tulder MW, Thomas S. diagnosis and treatment of low back pain. *BMJ* 2006;332:1430–1434.
3. Moffett JK, et al. Randomized controlled trial of exercise for low back pain: clinical outcomes, costs, and preferences. *BMJ* 1999;319:279.
4. Von Korff M, et al. Effects of practice style in managing back pain. *Ann Intern Med* 1994;121:187.
5. Long A, Donelson R, Fung T. Does it matter which exercise? A randomized control trial of exercises for low back pain. *Spine* 2004;29(23):2593–2602.

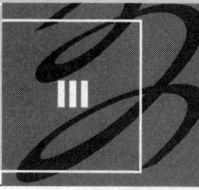

GENERAL PRINCIPLES

Definition

For the purpose of this chapter, the term *anaphylaxis* will refer to both anaphylaxis and anaphylactoid reactions.

- **Anaphylaxis** is a potentially fatal allergic, immunoglobulin E (IgE)-mediated, immediate hypersensitivity reaction affecting multiple organ systems in varying intensities.[1–3]
- **Anaphylactoid reactions** are clinically indistinguishable reactions that are non-IgE-mediated and are managed in the same manner as anaphylaxis.[1–3]

Epidemiology

True incidence is difficult to determine due to underdiagnosis, underreporting, and a lack of consensus on the definition. There has been an increase in the number of reported anaphylactic reactions in recent years, which may be due to an increase in therapeutic drug use, new food protein technologies, improved diagnosis, changes in diet, and increased latex exposure.[1,4–6]

- 1.25% to 16% of the general population is at risk for potentially experiencing an episode of anaphylaxis.[4,5]
- Incidence of severe anaphylaxis is 1 to 3 per 10,000 people and fatal anaphylaxis is 1 to 3 per 1 million people.[4,5]

Pathophysiology

Antigen-specific IgE on previously sensitized basophils and mast cells binds to the allergen causing release of multiple mediators including histamines, leukotrienes, prostaglandins, thromboxanes, and bradykinins. This release causes increased mucous membrane secretions, increased capillary permeability and leakage, reduced smooth muscle tone in blood vessels and bronchioles.[1,2,3,7]

Etiology

- Venoms: Aphids, honeybees, bumblebees, wasps, yellow jackets, hornets, fire ants, harvester ants, pit vipers, horseflies, deerflies

- Medications: Hormones, vitamins, succinate esters of hydrocortisone and methylprednisolone, nonsteroidal anti-inflammatory drugs, opiates, muscle depolarizers, antibiotics, allergen extracts
- Chemicals: Formaldehyde, ethylene oxide gas
- Foods: Nuts, milk, shellfish, legumes, citrus fruits, bananas, chocolate, fish, eggs, grains
- Foreign proteins: Vaccines (pertussis, typhoid, egg embryo), horse serum (antivenin), seminal plasma globulins (human, horse, rodent), antitoxins
- Latex
- Radiocontrast material
- Exercise
- Idiopathic[1–3,7]

DIAGNOSIS

Clinical Presentation

Symptom onset varies widely, usually within seconds to minutes of exposure, but may be delayed for several hours. Resolution of symptoms is usually within hours of treatment, but reactions may be protracted, lasting for up to 48 to 72 hours despite treatment. **Biphasic reactions** may occur with recurrence of symptoms 1 to 8 hours after recovery from initial presentation.[1,2,8]

- **Skin:** Pruritis, flushing, urticaria, angioedema, diaphoresis, erythema, maculopapular/mobilliform rash, pilor erecti
- **Eyes:** Conjunctival injection, lacrimation, periorbital edema, pruritis
- **Respiratory tract:** Pruritis of the lips, tongue, or palate; sneezing, rhinorrhea, nasal congestion, metallic taste, cough, wheeze, bronchospasm, tachypnea, dyspnea, accessory muscle use, hoarseness, choking sensation/tightness in the throat, laryngeal/oropharyngeal edema, stridor, cyanosis, respiratory arrest
- **Cardiovascular:** Chest pain, tachycardia, conduction disturbances, arrhythmias, myocardial ischemia/infarction, hypotension, bradycardia, cardiac arrest
- **Gastrointestinal:** Abdominal pain/cramping, bloating, nausea, vomiting, diarrhea
- **Neurologic:** Dizziness, weakness, syncope, seizure, sense of impending doom
- **Other:** Low back pain, uterine contractions[1–3,7,8]

History

- Onset and severity of symptoms
- Potential exposures or etiology (see above)
- Previous history of anaphylaxis, allergies, asthma, or atopy[1,3,8]

Physical Examination

- Frequent vital signs: Trendelenburg position if hypotensive. Application of a military antishock trousers (MAST) suit can buy time for other treatments to act.
- General appearance
- Respiratory and cardiovascular status: Stabilize airway. (May require endotracheal intubation or cricothyrotomy.)
- Identify any sting or injection site: Remove any remaining stinger and venom sac by scraping it off. (Do not pinch or squeeze the venom sac.) Consider applying a proximal tourniquet to decrease allergen absorption.[3,9]

Laboratory Studies

- **Arterial blood gas (ABG)** if respiratory symptoms present
    - PaO_2: May be normal or low depending on severity of respiratory symptoms.
    - $PaCO_2$: **Low** initially due to hyperventilation. **Normal** may suggest respiratory muscle fatigue. **Elevation** suggests impending respiratory failure.
- **Complete blood count (CBC) and electrolytes** if treatment is prolonged; or if patient has comorbid conditions or is hospitalized
- **Plasma histamine level, 24 hour urine N-methyl-histamine, or serum tryptase** to confirm diagnosis if uncertain[1,3,8,9]
- **Allergy testing:** Skin testing, radioallergosorbent test (RAST), serum antibody testing[1]

Imaging

- **Chest x-ray** if localized physical findings, poor response to treatment of bronchospasm, or uncertain diagnosis[3]

Monitoring

- **Continuous cardiac monitoring** with severe reactions, underlying cardiovascular disease, chest pain, hypotension, shock, concurrent β-blocker use, arrhythmias, and use of epinephrine or other vasopressors[3]
- **Continuous pulse oximetry** with respiratory symptoms[3]
- **Central venous pressure monitoring** with hypotension or shock[3]

Differential Diagnosis

- **Sudden loss of consciousness:** Vasovagal syncope, seizure, arrhythmia, hypoglycemia, cerebrovascular accident, drug overdose
- **Shock:** Hemorrhage, hypovolemia, sepsis, cardiogenic shock
- **Respiratory distress:** Status asthmaticus, chronic obstructive pulmonary disease (COPD) exacerbation, pulmonary embolism, epiglottitis, foreign body aspiration, pulmonary edema, respiratory infection, vocal cord dysfunction
- **Angioedema:** Hereditary angioedema, angiotensin-converting enzyme (ACE) inhibitor side effect
- **Skin symptoms:** Systemic mastocytosis, serum sickness, Chinese restaurant syndrome, scromboid toxin, medication side effects (red man syndrome, oral hypoglycemics with alcohol), peri/post menopausal hot flushes, autonomic epilepsy, idiopathic flushing, pheochromocytoma, carcinoid syndrome, medullary carcinoma of the thyroid, basophilic leukemia, acute promyelocytic leukemia, hydatid cyst, urticarial vasculitis, pseudoanaphylaxis, hyperimmunoglobulin E syndrome
- **Psychiatric symptoms:** Anxiety attack, globus hystericus, hyperventilation syndrome, Munchausen stridor, Munchausen by proxy, factitious anaphylaxis, malingering[1–3,7,9]

TREATMENT

The immediate goal of therapy is maintenance of the ABCs (airway, breathing, and circulation).

Medications for Routine Care

- **Epinephrine:** 0.3 to 0.5 mL of 1:1000 IM q 5 to 15 minutes. Peds: 0.01 mL/kg q 5 to 15 minutes to max of 0.3 mL per dose. Preferred in anterolateral thigh. 0.15 mL of 1:1000 can be injected at the site of a sting, vaccination, or medication injection with proximal tourniquet.
  - Indication: Moderate-to-severe reaction with respiratory distress, stridor, significant gastrointestinal symptoms, laryngeal edema, hypotension, syncope, dysrhythmia, rapidly progressing reaction
- **Oxygen:** High flow
- **Intravenous (IV) fluids:** 1 to 2 L bolus normal saline or colloid via two large-bore IV catheters; Peds: 20 mL/kg bolus continue as necessary
  - Indication: Orthostasis, hypotension, no response to one to two doses of epinephrine
- **Antihistamines:** Give H1 and H2 blockers together
  - **H1 blockers**
    - **Diphenhydramine:** 25 to 50 mg IV over 10 to 15 minutes, IM or PO with mild reactions q 4 to 6 hr; Peds: 1.25 mg/kg q 4 to 6 hr
    - **Chlorpheniramine:** 2 mg 4 tablets PO; Peds: Age <6 years 1 tablet PO, Age 6 to 12 years 2 tablets PO
    - **Hydroxyzine:** 25 mg PO; Peds: Age <6 years 50 mg PO qd divided tid-qid, Age >6 years 50 to 100 mg PO qd divided tid-qid
  - **H2 blockers**
    - **Ranitidine:** 1 to 2 mg/kg IV over 10 to 15 minutes or PO with mild reactions; Peds: 1.25 mg/kg IV or 2 mg/kg PO

- **Famotidine:** 20 mg IV or PO bid with mild reactions; Peds: 0.5 mg/kg/dose IV or PO bid
- **Cimetidine:** 300 mg IV, IM, or PO q 6 hr; Peds: 5 to 10 mg/kg IV, IM, or PO q 6 hr

■ **Bronchodilators:** Indication: bronchospasm, constant dry cough, respiratory distress
　▩ **Albuterol 0.5%:** 0.5 to 1 mL in 2.5 mL saline nebulized q 15 min or continuous; Peds: Age <2 years: 0.03 mL/kg, Age >2 years: 0.5 to 1.0 mL/kg
　▩ **Aminophylline:** 6 mg/kg over 30 min, then 0.5 to 0.7 mg/kg per hour; Peds: 5.6 mg/kg over 30 min, then 1 mg/kg per hour

■ **Corticosteroids:** Indication: to decrease incidence and severity of protracted, delayed, or biphasic reactions
　▩ **Methylprednisolone:** 40 to 250 mg IV or IM q 6 hr; Peds: 1 to 2 mg/kg IV or IM q 6 hr
　▩ **Prednisone:** 1 to 2 mg/kg PO q 8 hr[1–3,7–10]

Medications for Refractory Symptoms

■ **Epinephrine:** 0.5 to 1 mL of 1:10,000 IV or 3 to 5 mL per ET tube q 5 to 10 min; 5 to 15 μg/min continuous infusion, titrate to effect; Peds: 0.025 to 0.100 μg/kg/min
■ **Racemic epinephrine 2%:** 0.5 to 0.75 mL nebulized; Peds: 0.25 to 0.5 mL nebulized
　▩ Indication: Upper airway obstruction or persistent bronchospasm
　▩ **Ipratropium:** 3-mL vial mixed with albuterol and nebulized for refractory symptoms

■ **Glucagon:** 1 mg IV or IM q 1 min up to 5 mg or 1 mg IV bolus followed by continuous infusion of 1 to 5 mg IV/hr. Peds: 0.03 to 0.1 mg/kg up to 1 mg/dose repeat q 15 to 20 min
　▩ Indication: Concurrent β-blocker use

■ **Isoproterenol:** 0.1 mg/kg/min IV; Peds: 0.1 to 1.0 μg/kg/min IV
　▩ Indication: Concurrent β-blocker use and refractory to epinephrine, glucagons, IV fluids

■ **Atropine:** 0.3 to 0.5 mg IV, IM, or SQ q 10 min to max of 2 mg; Peds: 0.02 mg/kg to a max of 0.5 mg and 1 mg for adolescent; may repeat once
　▩ Indication: Bradycardia, concurrent β-blocker use

■ **Norepinephrine:** 0.5 to 30 μg/min IV; Peds: 0.1 to 1.0 μg/kg/min IV
■ **Dopamine:** 2 to 20 μg/kg/min IV infusion
■ **Phenylephrine:** 30 to 180 μg/min IV infusion
■ **Terbutaline:** 0.25 mg q 20 min SC; Peds: 0.01 mL/kg q 20 min
　▩ Indication: Refractory bronchospasm[1–3,7–10]

Referrals

Indication: Causative agent or diagnosis is unclear, patient education, recurrent reactions, consideration for allergy testing and desensitization.

■ **Immunotherapy** may be indicated to desensitize patients. Before consideration, sensitivity should be confirmed by a positive skin test result, RAST, or basophil histamine release test at least 2 to 4 weeks after the anaphylactic reaction.
　▩ **Hymenoptera.** All adults and children with a history of moderate to severe reactions should be considered. Treatment for adults with cutaneous symptoms only is controversial and for children is not recommended.
　▩ **Medications or vaccines.** Consider only if there is compelling indication for use of the drug.[9]

Risk Management

Potential pitfalls include failure to diagnose anaphylaxis in patients with unexplained syncope or shock, failure to counsel patients about avoidance and preventive measures, prescribing drugs to which the patient is allergic, failure to appreciate the potentially serious nature of symptoms, and complications of epinephrine use in patients without a clear indication.[3]

Patient Education

- **Avoidance techniques:** As much as possible, individual inciting agents should be avoided. Also avoid β-blockers, ACE inhibitors, angiotensin II receptor blockers, monoamine oxidase inhibitors, and some tricyclic antidepressants to avoid treatment medication interactions.
- **First aid (anaphylaxis action plan):** After appropriate instruction in use, epinephrine kits should be obtained and kept readily available to patient, schools, etc.
    - Epinephrine 1:1000 is available as Ana-kit two 0.3-mL doses plus four 2-mg chlorpheniramine tablets, EpiPen 0.3 mL/dose, and EpiPen Jr. 0.15 mL/dose, Twinject 0.15 mL or 0.3 mL/dose
    - Antihistamines. Diphenhydramine or chlorpheniramine should be taken.
    - Decrease absorption when appropriate with proximal tourniquet and epinephrine injection into site.
    - Seek medical attention.
- **Medical alert identification tags**
- **Pretreatment protocols for radiocontrast sensitivity**[1–3,8,10]

Follow-Up

- Hospital admission is recommended in many moderate and all severe reactions, incomplete response to treatment, recurrent reaction, secondary complication, comorbid illness, extremes of age, inadequate social support, poor access to emergency medical care.[1–3]
- Observation following recovery from mild to moderate reactions for at least 4 to 8 hours.[1,9]
- Continue oral antihistamines and prednisone for 3 to 5 days.[3]
- Symptoms may recur for up to 72 hours. Seek care immediately.
- Follow up closely with primary care provider.

Complications

Myocardial ischemia, arrhythmias, brain injury due to prolonged hypoxia, injury from fall due to syncope, death.[3]

References

1. O'Dowd LC. Anaphylaxis in adults. *Online UpToDate* (serial online). May 17, 2006; version 14.2.
2. Ellis AK, Day JH. Diagnosis and management of anaphylaxis. *Can Med Assoc J* 2003;169(4):307–311.
3. Krause RS. Anaphylaxis. *Online emedicine* (serial online). April 29, 2005.
4. Moneret-Vautrin DA, Morisset M, Flabbee J, et al. Epidemiology of life-threatening and lethal anaphylaxis: a review. *Allergy* 2005;60:443–451.
5. Sheikh A, Alves B. Hospital admissions for acute anaphylaxis: time trend study. *Br Med J* 2000;320(7247):1441.
6. Matasar MJ, Neugut AI. Epidemiology of anaphylaxis in the United States. *Curr Allergy Asthma Rep* 2003;3:30–35.
7. Becker LB, Billi JF, Eigel B, et al. Anaphylaxis. *Circulation* 2005;112:143–145.
8. Sampson HA. Anaphylaxis and emergency treatment. *Pediatrics* 2003;111:1601–1608.
9. Tang AW. A practical guide to anaphylaxis. *Am Fam Physician* 2003;68:1325–1332.
10. McLean-Tooke AP, Bethune CA, Fay AC, et al. Adrenaline in the treatment of anaphylaxis: what is the evidence. *Br Med J* 2003;327:1332–1335.

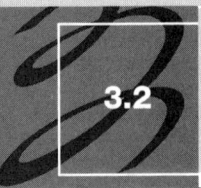

3.2 BRONCHOSPASM
Kimberly J. Jarzynka

GENERAL PRINCIPLES

Definition
Spasmodic contraction of the bronchial muscles causing narrowing of the bronchial lumen resulting in restricted airflow.[1]

Etiology
Asthma exacerbation, chronic obstructive pulmonary disease (COPD) exacerbation, anaphylaxis, infection (pneumonia, bronchitis, bronchiolitis, sinusitis), heart failure, aspiration, allergen exposure, irritant exposure (air pollutants, smoke, organic particles, chemicals, etc.), medication exposure, postnasal drip, foreign body aspiration, acid reflux, exercise, stress, weather changes, envenomation.[1,2]

DIAGNOSIS

Clinical Presentation
- Depends on severity and duration of bronchospasm
- Shortness of breath, cough, difficulty speaking, wheeze (may or may not be present), tachypnea, diaphoresis, accessory muscle use, anxiety, agitation, cyanosis, mental status changes, obtundation, respiratory or cardiac arrest[3,4]
- Pediatric patients may also present with weak cry, difficulty feeding, grunting, nasal flaring, irritability, inconsolability, and lethargy[3,4]

History
- Duration and severity of symptoms
- Precipitating factors
- Smoking/substance abuse history
- Current medication, compliance, and last use
- Drug or other allergies
- Prior hospitalizations and emergency department visits for bronchospasm, especially in the last year
- Prior episodes of respiratory failure, intensive care unit admission, intubation, or mechanical ventilation
- Other potentially complicating illnesses
  - Chronic pulmonary or cardiac disease
  - Diabetes, peptic ulcer disease, hypertension, psychosis, etc. (may be aggravated by systemic corticosteroids)[1,3]

Physical Examination
- Findings depend on severity and duration of symptoms (Table 3.2-1).
- Other signs: Diaphoresis, central cyanosis, nasal flaring and decreased capillary refill, etc.
- Look for signs of complicating condition: peripheral edema, stridor, subcutaneous emphysema, unequal breath sounds, fever, unilateral leg edema or tenderness, etc.[1,3–5,7]

Laboratory Studies
- **Complete blood count (CBC)** with fever, purulent sputum, or other signs of infection[1,3]
  - Leukocytosis is common with asthma exacerbations, significant stress, corticosteroid or catecholamine use
  - Eosinophilia

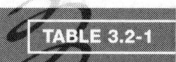

TABLE 3.2-1   Classifying Severity of Bronchospasm

	Mild	Moderate	Severe	Imminent respiratory arrest
Talks in	Sentences	Phrases	Words	Words or unable
Alertness	May be agitated	Usually agitated	Usually agitated	Drowsy or confused
Ability to lie flat	Able to lie flat	Sits	Tripod position	
Accessory muscle use, retractions	Usually not	Common	Usually	Paradoxical movement
Wheeze	Moderate, often only end expiratory	Loud, throughout exhalation	Usually loud, throughout inhalation and exhalation	Absent wheeze
Respiratory rate	Increased	Increased	Often >30/min	May be decreased
Heart rate	<100 bpm	100–120 bpm	>120 bpm	Bradycardia
Pulsus paradoxus	Absent <10 mmHg	May be present 10–25 mmHg	Often <25 mmHg adult, 20–40 mmHg child	Absence suggests respiratory muscle fatigue
PEFR (% predicted or personal best)	>80%	50–80% or response lasts <2 hr	<50%	<20–25% or unable to perform
SaO$_2$ (room air)	>95%	91–95%	<91%	

Adapted from Murphy S, Leneant C, Sheffer AL, et al. National Asthma Education and Prevention Program: Expert panel report II: Guidelines for the diagnosis and management of asthma. Bethesda, MD: National Heart, Lung, and Blood Institute, 1997. (NIH publication no. 97-4051.)

■ **Arterial blood gas (ABG)** with severe distress, peak expiratory flow (PEF) 30% predicted or less, or SaO$_2$ <90% after initial treatment[1,3,5]
  ■ **PO$_2$**
    • **Low** (<60 mmHg on oxygen) indicates impending respiratory arrest and increased risk of death[2,5,6]
  ■ **PaCO$_2$**
    • Initially **decreased** due to increased respiratory drive and hyperventilation.
    • **Normal** indicates severe airflow obstruction, respiratory muscle fatigue, and increased risk of respiratory failure.
    • **Elevated** (>42 mmHg) indicates inadequate ventilation and impending respiratory failure.[3,5,6]
■ **Serum electrolytes** with coexisting cardiovascular disease, diuretic or chronic steroid use[1,3]
  ■ Low potassium, magnesium, and/or phosphate may be secondary to frequent β$_2$-agonist or steroid use[1,3]
■ **Theophylline level** with current treatment[1]

Imaging

- **Chest x-ray (CXR)**
  - *Not* routinely recommended
  - Indication (suspected complicating cardiopulmonary process): fever, leukocytosis, unexplained chest pain, asymmetric breath sounds, hypoxemia, subcutaneous emphysema, peripheral edema, high-risk comorbidities (intravenous drug use, immunosuppression, granulomatous disease, recent seizures, cancer, chest surgery, congestive heart failure, etc.)[1,3-5]
  - Possible findings: Streaky infiltrates or hyperinflation[1,5]

Monitoring

- **Pulse oximetry**
  - SaO_2 90% or less in adults or 92% or less in children indicates severe airflow obstruction[1]
  - Oxygenation may decrease 4 to 10 mmHg with beta agonist inhalant therapy due to increases in v/q mismatch[1]

- **Spirometry/peak expiratory flow rate (PEFR)**
  - Serial measurements document response to therapy
  - Best method for assessment of the severity of an asthma attack[1,5]
  - Normal values differ with size and age, but 200 indicates severe obstruction in adults[1,5]

- **Electrocardiography (ECG)/Telemetry**
  - *Not* routinely obtained
  - Indication: Severely symptomatic, age 50, coexistent heart disease or COPD
  - Possible findings: Sinus tachycardia, right heart strain, supraventricular tachycardia (SVT) (consider theophylline toxicity), arrhythmias other than SVT are rare[1,3]

Differential Diagnosis

- Extrathoracic upper airway obstruction
  - Anaphylaxis, postnasal drip syndrome, vocal cord abnormalities or dysfunction, hypertrophied tonsils, epiglottitis, laryngeal edema, laryngostenosis, laryngocele, postextubation granulomas, retropharyngeal abscess, peritonsillar abscess, mobile supraglottic soft tissue, obesity, tumors, wegeners granulomatosis, cricoarytenoid arteritis, abnormal arytenoid movement, relapsing polychondritis, klebsiella rhinoscleroma[1,2,7,8]

- Intrathoracic upper airway obstruction
  - Tracheal stenosis, foreign body aspiration, airway tumors, intrathoracic goiter, tracheobronchomegaly, acquired tracheomalasia, herpetic tracheobronchitis, right-sided aortic arch[1,2,7,8]

- Lower airway obstruction
  - Asthma, COPD, emphysema, pulmonary edema, aspiration, pulmonary embolism, pneumonia, bronchiolitis, bronchitis, gastroesophageal reflux disease (GERD), cystic fibrosis, carcinoid syndrome, bronchiectasis, lymphangitic carcinomatosis, parasitic infections[1,2,7,8]

- Other
  - Panic disorder, hyperventilation syndrome, conversion disorder[1,7]

TREATMENT

Medications

- **Oxygen:** Maintain sats >90% to 92% and >95% with pregnancy and coexistent heart disease[1-3,6]
- **Short-acting β_2-agonist (albuterol)**
  - **Nebulized**
    - Intermittent: Adult 2.5 to 5 mg or peds 0.15 mg per kg (minimum 2.5 mg) q 20 to 30 min × 3 doses, then q 1 to 4 hour prn
    - Continuous: If severely ill or PEFR <200, adults 5 to 15 mg per hour or peds 0.3 to 0.5 mg/kg/hour

- **Metered-dose inhaler (MDI) with spacer/holding chamber** (four to eight puffs is equivalent to one nebulized treatment)
  - Four to eight puffs q 20 to 30 min × 1 to 4 hour prn, then q 1 to 4 hour prn
- **Parenteral:** If seriously ill with no improvement after two to three inhaled treatments; intravenous (IV) use is experimental.
  - **Epinephrine:** 1:1000 (1 mg/mL) adult 0.3 to 0.5 mg or peds 0.01 mg/kg sq q 20 min × 3 doses
  - **Terbutaline** (1 mg/mL) adult 0.25 mg or peds 0.01 mg/kg sq q 20 min × 3 doses, then q 2 to 6 hour prn[1,3,5,6]

- **Anticholinergics:** Add to albuterol if severe bronchospasm or slow response to initial β_2-agonist therapy; particular benefit with monoamine oxidase inhibitor (MAOI) use, COPD with asthmatic component, or asthma triggered by beta blockers.
  - **Ipratropium bromide (Atrovent)**
    - Nebulized: Adult 0.5 mg or peds 0.25 mg q 20 to 30 min × 3 doses, then q 2 to 4 hour prn
    - MDI: Four to eight puffs q 30 min × 3 doses, then q 2 to 4 hour prn[1,3,5,6]

- **Corticosteroids:** Start as soon as insufficient improvement with beta agonist is identified (<10% improvement in PEFR after first dose beta agonist, PEFR <70% after initial hour of treatment); start immediately in all patients currently taking oral corticosteroids; start early in pediatric population[1,3,5]
  - **Parenteral**
    - **Methylprednisolone (Solu-Medrol, Depo-Medrol)** adult 80 to 125 mg or peds load 2 mg per kg IV, maintenance 0.5 to 1 mg/kg/dose IV q 6 hour up to 5 days[1,3,6]
    - **Triamcinolone (Aristocort)** adult 60 mg IM × 1, followed by 20 to 100 mg IM when symptoms recur; peds <6 years: not recommended, 6 to 12 years: 0.03 to 0.2 mg per kg IM q 1 to 7 days[1]
  - **Oral:** In the absence of vomiting, efficacy is comparable to IV[1,5]
    - **Prednisone:** Adult 40 to 60 mg or peds 1 to 2 mg per kg po once, then adult 120 to 180 mg divided bid-qid × 48 hour, then 60 to 80 mg q day or peds 1 mg per kg q 6 hour × 48 hour, then 1 to 2 mg/kg/day divided bid (until PEF reaches 70% predicted)[1,3]
  - **Inhaled:** At discharge; do not wait until after taper (causes confusion and medication noncompliance)[5]

- **Methylxanthines:** Use is controversial, *not* generally recommended due to increased risk of toxicity, without added benefit[3,5]; may consider in refractory cases; check level with current treatment
  - **Theophylline (Aminophylline):** Adult 6 mg per kg lean body wt or peds 1 mg/kg/hour IV over 20 to 30 min followed by continuous infusion of 0.5 to 0.9 mg/kg/hour[1,6]

- **Magnesium sulfate:** Use is controversial, results of published trials are mixed[5]; may consider in refractory cases; 2 g over 30 min IV as high as 1 g per min up to 3 g IV[1]
- **Leukotriene receptor antagonist:** Use in acute setting is unclear; small studies indicate improvement in PEFR when given with acute bronchospasm[5,6]; may consider in refractory cases
  - **Montelukast:** 10 to 20 mg po[1]

- **Antibiotics:** *Not* recommended without signs of complicating bacterial infection (sinusitis, bronchitis, or pneumonia)[1–3,6]
- **Heliox:** Mixture of helium and oxygen; may improve oxygenation in refractory cases, but not proven consistently effective[6]; may consider in refractory cases
- **IV fluids:** Only to treat dehydration; young children and infants may become dehydrated due to tachypnea and decreased oral intake[1,3,6]
- **Sedatives:** *Not* recommended due to respiratory suppression unless intubated[3]
- **Mucolytics:** *Not* recommended; may worsen cough or bronchospasm[3]

Nonoperative

Endotracheal Intubation and Mechanical Ventilation

- **Indications:** Altered mental status, inability to speak, increasing or decreasing pulsus paradoxus, respiratory or cardiac arrest, diaphoresis in the recumbent position, acute barotrauma, severe lactic acidosis (especially in infants), silent chest despite respiratory effort, refractory hypoxemia ($PaO_2 < 60$ mmHg on max O_2), increasing $PaCO_2$ (50 mmHg and rising >5 mmHg/hour)[4]; see Table 3.2-1 above for findings associated with imminent respiratory arrest.
- **Risks:** High pressures causing hypotension (auto-PEEP), barotrauma, pneumothorax, pneumomediastinum[1]
- **Guidelines:**
  - Do not delay intubation once it is deemed necessary
  - Consult with or comanagement by physicians expert in ventilatory management
  - Best done semielectively, before the crisis of respiratory arrest
  - Perform in a controlled setting (intensive care unit or emergency room) by experienced physician
  - Maintain or replace intravascular volume to prevent hypotension caused by PPV
  - Permissive hypercapnia or controlled hypoventilation (adequate oxygenation and ventilation while minimizing high airway pressure and barotrauma)
    - Highest FiO_2 as necessary to maintain oxygenation
    - Accept hypercapnia
    - Treat respiratory acidosis with IV sodium bicarbonate
    - Adjust tidal volume, rate and I:E ratio to minimize airway pressures
    - Continue other therapy[3]

Referrals/Consultation

- Severe, refractory, or life-threatening symptoms with intensive care unit transfer or intubation with mechanical ventilation
- Recurrent emergency department visits or hospitalizations for bronchospasm
- Atypical signs and symptoms or difficult differential diagnosis
- Other complicating conditions
- Additional diagnostic testing indicated (allergy skin testing, rhinoscopy, pulmonary function tests (PFTs), bronchoscopy)
- Additional patient education is needed (problems with adherence or allergen avoidance)
- Confirmation of occupational or environmental exposure
- Pregnant patients with severe or recurrent symptoms
- Significant psychiatric, psychosocial, or family problems that interfere with care[1,3]

Risk Management

Failure to initiate steroid therapy or intubation, monitor electrolyte balance, admit a wheezing patient with normal PCO_2, treat expediently, educate patients upon discharge, identify other diagnoses (congestive heart failure, myocarditis, multiple pulmonary embolisms, surreptitious vocal cord dysfunction, panic disorder, hyperventilation, etc.)[1,6]

Patient Education

Monitoring PEFR at home with written action plan, importance of taking medication, proper medication use, proper use of inhalants and spacers, trigger avoidance, oral rinsing after inhaled corticosteroids, significance of nocturnal exacerbations, close follow-up[2–4]

Follow-Up

After initial treatment

- **PEFR ≥70% and minimal or absent symptoms:** Discharge with education and close follow-up
- **PEFR 50% to 70% and mild symptoms**
  - **Consider for discharge:** Improving lung function, low risk (good self-care skills and supportive home environment) and can obtain medications
  - **Hospitalize:** New-onset or labile asthma, multiple prior hospitalizations or emergency room visits, intensive care unit admission or intubation in the past year,

current use or recent withdrawal of oral corticosteroids at time of presentation with acute deterioration, severe symptoms that preclude self-care, other complicating conditions, psychiatric disease, drug use, or adverse socioeconomic conditions

- **PERF <50%:** Hospitalize[1,3–5]

Complications

Medication side effects, pneumothorax, pneumomediastinum, secondary infection, respiratory distress/arrest, death[1,6]

Special Considerations

- **Socioeconomic factors:** Inability to obtain medications can lower the threshold for admission. Consider discharging patient with medications in hand or IM steroid to avoid possible nonadherance.[1,5]
- **Pediatrics:** Treat as aggressively as adults in appropriate dosages, give corticosteroids early, more likely to become dehydrated due to increased work of respiration.[4]
- **Pregnancy:** Treat as aggressively as nonpregnant women to prevent maternal and fetal hypoxia. Hypoxia and respiratory acidosis can be detrimental to both the fetus and the mother. Continuous electronic fetal monitoring is recommended when fetus is potentially viable. Emergent delivery is usually unnecessary, fetus should recover with aggressive treatment of the mother. Obstetrical and pulmonary consultation with severe or refractory symptoms.[2,9]

References

1. Brenner B. Asthma. *emedicine* (On-line serial). Dec. 6, 2004.
2. Morris MJ, Perkins PJ. Asthma. *emedicine* (On-line serial). Dec. 6, 2005.
3. Murphy S, Lenfant C, Sheffer AL, et al. National Asthma Education and Prevention Program: Expert panel report II: guidelines for the diagnosis and management of asthma. Bethseda, MD: National Heart, Lung, and Blood Institute; 1997. (NIH publication no. 97–4051.)
4. Sawicki G, Dovey M. Acute severe asthma in children: assessment and prevention. *UpToDate* (On-line serial). Aug. 17, 2005; Version 14.1.
5. Fanta CH. Treatment of acute exacerbations of asthma. *UpToDate* (On-line serial). May 27, 2005; Version 14.1.
6. Saadeh C, Malacara J, Goldman M, et al. Status asthmaticus. *emedicine* (On-line serial). June 4, 2004.
7. Irwin RS. Diagnosis of wheezing illnesses other than asthma in adults. *UpToDate* (On-line serial). Mar. 3, 2005; Version 14.1.
8. Fakhoury K. Wheezing illnesses other than asthma in children. *UpToDate* (On-line serial). Aug. 13, 2004; Version 14.1.
9. Busse WW, Alving B, et al. National Asthma Education and Prevention Program: Working group report on managing asthma during pregnancy: recommendations for pharmacologic treatment. Bethseda, MD: National Heart, Lung, and Blood Institute, 2004. (NIH publication no. 05–5236.)

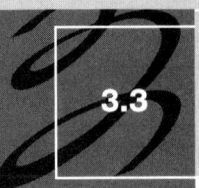

3.3 DRUG OVERDOSE
Jason L. Musser

GENERAL PRINCIPLES

- Rapid stabilization of any suspected overdose patient is the first priority.
- Quick determination of substance or substances used through interviews of the family and ambulance staff must be undertaken quickly to prevent delay of definitive therapy.
- Gastric lavage, emesis, whole bowel irrigation, activated charcoal, and use of cathartics should be considered to decrease gut absorption of toxic substances.
- Maintaining close contact with the poison control center (national toll free number 1-800-222-1222) or area toxicologists will likely be needed.
- Although not all overdoses are intentional, the care team should be alert to inconsistencies that indicate intentional overdose for self-harm or malicious intent and involve psychiatry and/or the appropriate authorities.

Suicide attempts, poisonings, pediatric accidental ingestion, and illicit drugs are the most commonly encountered drug overdoses. Ingestion of a toxic substance, either accidental or intentional, is the most prevalent route of exposure for human poisonings at 76% of cases presenting to a provider, thankfully only 3% of those cases require critical care. Analgesics (such as acetaminophen), alcohol, and antidepressants are the top three substances used in overdose situations. Today's era of drug parties, especially among teenage populations, is causing the number of accidental overdoses to increase. Continual experimentation with common substances and production of new illicit drugs to produce "altered perceptions" and "highs" will continue to confound clinicians.

There are a myriad of substances (both legal and illegal) that can and will be used by people to intentional harm themselves or be accidentally overdosed upon. As such, the text needed to include the pathophysiology of all these substances would take up a library in and of themselves. Health care providers should consult toxicologists, poison control centers, and the Internet for information on specific substances as well as up-to-date treatment options.

DIAGNOSIS

History and Physical Examination

Initially assess patients for the presence of life-threatening complications. Treatment should focus on the elimination of the drug and specific antidote and drug therapy. Question the patient, the patient's family or friends, and the paramedics about any drugs the patient is taking and whether any empty bottles or drug paraphernalia were found in the house. The approximate time and amount of ingestion along with the type and/or name of the drug taken helps determine whether to use agents to increase the elimination of the drug. A past medical history helps to determine whether the patient has other significant diseases that may complicate the overdose. A quick physical examination should focus on blood pressure, pulse, respirations, and pupils. Examine the skin for sweating, a cold or clammy feeling, and needle marks. Rales in the lungs point to pneumonia or pulmonary edema. Check the abdomen for an enlarged liver, and smell the breath for any distinctive odors (remember just because the person took a substance does not mean the person cannot have other processes going on such as a diabetic ketoacidosis). The neurologic examination should include level of consciousness, presence of nystagmus, the gag reflex, and deep tendon reflexes. Look for typical patterns or toxidromes of the suspected drug used, such as neuroleptic malignant syndrome, ocular changes, vital sign instability, etc.

Laboratory Tests and Imaging

The laboratory is of limited value in the initial evaluation of overdose patients. Standard blood tests common with the suspected agent can be obtained but waiting for the results of toxicology screens can be life-threatening. False-negative or false-positive drug screen results can be misleading. Baseline laboratory studies should include a complete blood count, electrolytes, urinalysis (including a check for hemoglobin to detect rhabdomyolysis), blood sugar, and blood urea nitrogen. Any patient with impaired respirations should have an arterial blood gas measurement, chest radiography, and electrocardiography.[2] A toxicology screen on the blood, urine, and any gastric contents is necessary as soon as possible as most substances metabolize quickly and some illegal drugs are not detectable within a few hours of ingestion even though their affects may be longer lasting.

The diagnosis of drug overdose is based on a good history and physical and lab results. As the physical findings vary based on the drug used, so too is the differential diagnosis wide. In general, however, the caring provider should include other causes for the patient's signs and symptoms such as infections and electrolyte disturbances. Further considerations are discussed in the treatment section below.

TREATMENT

Stabilization

In comatose or severely compromised drug overdose patients, establish an airway and ventilate the patient immediately. In lethargic or obtunded patients, check the gag reflex and, if it is not present, intubate the patient. If no blood pressure or pulse is present, begin cardiopulmonary resuscitation (CPR). Patients should be monitored for cardiac arrhythmias, and a large-diameter intravenous line should be placed. Decontamination should be considered as an additional "D" in the secondary ABCs of basic life support/advanced cardiac life support (BLS/ACLS) resuscitation. Gastric lavage can be attempted but is unhelpful if the ingestion was more than 60 minutes prior. Other methods to decrease the absorption of ingested substances include emesis, whole bowel irrigation, activated charcoal (1 g/kg), and use of cathartics to decrease bowel transit time. In cases of iron intoxication, lithium overdose, or a ruptured bag used in "body packing" (swallowing of small bags of illicit drugs to prevent detection during smuggling), whole bowel irrigation can decrease absorption. In these cases (i.e., body packing), whole bowel irrigation using various bowel prep solutions such as potassium chloride (Go-Lytely(r)), polyethylene glycol, or other electrolyte solutions can be used at a rate of 1 to 2 L per hour. Nasogastric administration of the solution may be required; patients should be lying at a 45-degree incline to help prevent aspiration. Airway protection and management is paramount in this procedure. It may take more than 5 hours to clear the contaminant; samples of the effluent from the rectum can be tested to ensure clearing of the drug.

Medication

During the initial treatment of drug overdose patients, empirically treat unconscious patients for possible hypoglycemia with 50 mL of 50% dextrose intravenous (IV). Before glucose is given, patients should receive 100 mg of IV thiamine to prevent an acute Wernicke syndrome in those with alcoholism. For potential narcotic overdoses, give naloxone (Narcan) to any patient with respiratory depression, 0.4 mg IV; if there is no response in 1 to 2 minutes, give 2 mg IV, and keep repeating the dose to a maximum of 10 to 20 mg IV. Flumazenil (Romazicon, formerly Mazicon), 0.2 mg IV over 30 seconds, and repeated if needed in 1 to 2 minutes, should be used in cases of suspected benzodiazepine intoxication. Further treatment is based on the drug use, and the most common are reviewed below.

Referrals/Counseling

Local poison control centers and toxicologists are good resources throughout the treatment process and especially helpful in uncommon overdoses. Psychiatrists and psychologists should be consulted in intentional overdoses for definitive therapy after the patient has been stabilized and cleared medically (depending on the drug and amount used, this may be several days). Close monitoring, usually from one-on-one supervision, may be needed during the time the patient has regained consciousness until he or she is well enough to go to an inpatient mental facility, if needed.

Prevention

Physicians play a critical role in preventing prescription drug overdoses. Evaluate all patients for their overdose potential. Give low-toxicity drugs to patients with a history of depression, substance abuse, previous suicide attempts, or overdoses and to those who may be more sensitive to drugs, such as elderly, young, or pregnant patients or patients on other drugs. Female patients are more likely to overdose than male patients. Give high-risk patients smaller amounts of the drug with more frequent refills. This is especially true in patients with seizure disorders requiring barbiturates. Barbiturates are 10 times more toxic than the benzodiazepines. In pain management, remember that propoxyphene is much more toxic in overdoses than other narcotics. For every written prescription, physicians should ask themselves:

■ What is the overdose potential of this patient?
■ Are there equally effective drugs that have less overdose toxicity?

SPECIFIC DRUG OVERDOSE TREATMENT

Cocaine and Amphetamines

Diagnosis

Patients with stimulant drug overdoses present with chest pain, cardiac arrhythmias, hypertension, stroke, paranoia, seizure, severe agitation, and triggering or worsening of asthma attacks. Severe cocaine intoxication may present as bradycardia and hypotension. Death is caused by cardiac arrhythmias, status epilepticus, cerebral hemorrhage, or hyperthermia. Suspect cocaine overdose in young patients presenting with chest pain and screen the urine and serum for benzoylecgonine (a metabolite of cocaine). Simultaneous ingestion of alcohol increases the production of cocaethylene, which causes prolonged drug toxicity. Smugglers may swallow large bags of cocaine to prevent detection, a practice known as body packing. Rupture of the bags causes severe cocaine intoxication. Whole-body irrigation (as noted above) is indicated in these circumstances.

Treatment

Treat hypertension with diazepam (Valium), 5 to 10 mg IV no faster than 5 mg per minute. If severe hypertension persists, start a sodium nitroprusside infusion, 0.5 to 10 µg/kg/minute. β-Blockers are contraindicated because they may cause a paradoxical increase in blood pressure and increase the mortality rate in cocaine overdose patients. Hyperthermia needs to be aggressively treated with rapid cooling to prevent rhabdomyolysis and subsequent renal failure. Treat myocardial ischemia with nitroglycerin and aspirin. Consider thrombolytic therapy and coronary catheterization in acute myocardial infarctions. Treat body packers with activated charcoal (50 to 100 g in adults) and a cathartic (if whole-body irrigation was not performed). Amphetamine psychosis, seen after "speed runs," can be managed with diazepam, 0.1 to 0.2 mg per kg IV or, in severe cases, haloperidol (Haldol), 5 to 20 mg IM or PO (but this may cause hyperthermia and a lowered seizure threshold).

Tricyclic Antidepressants

Diagnosis

Tricyclic antidepressants are frequently used in suicide attempts. Patients present with anticholinergic signs, including tachycardia, elevated temperature, confusion and delirium, decreased gastrointestinal motility, hyperreflexia, and dilated pupils. Patients presenting with arrhythmias, altered mental status, seizures, respiratory depression, or hypotension are at high risk, requiring close monitoring and usually admission to the hospital. Think of tricyclic antidepressant overdose if the patient has a QRS interval longer than 0.12 seconds with right axis deviation on the electrocardiogram.

Treatment

Because antidepressant overdoses decrease gastrointestinal motility, do gastric lavage and give activated charcoal every 4 hours. Treat cardiac toxicity and hypotension with sodium bicarbonate, 1 to 2 mEq per kg IV bolus, until the arterial pH is 7.45 to 7.55. If this does not control arrhythmias, give lidocaine. Glucagon (10 mg IV) has been used to treat severe hypotension in tricyclic overdoses. As a preventive measure, selective serotonin-reuptake inhibitors should be used in high-risk suicide patients.

Ethanol and Benzodiazepines
Diagnosis
Patients frequently use alcohol to "get the courage" to attempt suicide with other drugs. Adolescents may present with isolated alcohol intoxication due to experimental binge drinking. Symptoms include nystagmus, ataxia, hypoglycemia, vomiting, and coma. A blood level of 300 mg per dL causes coma in a "novice" drinker. In patients with severe coma and respiratory depression or arrest, consider the possibility of concomitant γ-hydroxybutyrate (GHB, one of the "date rape" drugs) ingestion.

Treatment
When managing ethanol overdoses, do a urine toxicology screen to determine which, if any, other drugs have been ingested. Time and supportive care (including intubation and blood pressure support as needed) are all that is needed for the majority of alcohol overdoses. Benzodiazepines should be used to control agitation and systemic affects (such as hypertension and tachycardia) in alcohol withdrawal. Flumazenil (Romazicon), 0.2 mg IV over 30 seconds, and repeated if needed in 1 to 2 minutes, can reverse the sedation and respiratory depressant effects in benzodiazepine overdoses, but it is rarely needed and can cause serious side effects (seizures if the patient is taking concomitant tricyclic antidepressants, and severe withdrawal effects and seizures if the patient is dependent on benzodiazepines). Temporary intubation and ventilatory support may be necessary in GHB overdoses or to prevent aspiration in sedative to hypnotic overdoses.

Opiates
Diagnosis
Opiate overdose is characterized by respiratory depression, pupil constriction, which may not be seen with meperidine (Demerol) or diphenoxylate (Lomotil) overdose, central nervous system depression, and low blood pressure and pulse. In severe overdose patients, apnea and pulmonary edema may occur. If alcohol has been ingested, opiate toxicity is increased. Fentanyl is not detected in standard urine toxicology screens.

Treatment
In propoxyphene (Darvon) overdoses, large doses of naloxone are needed. Treat cardiac arrhythmias caused by propoxyphene with IV sodium bicarbonate. Because the effect of naloxone is shorter than that of most opiates, treat patients with repeated doses every 2 hours.

Hallucinogens
Diagnosis
Lysergic acid diethylamide (LSD) is the most commonly abused hallucinogen. LSD causes sympathetic stimulation with tachycardia, hallucinations, paranoia, fear, dilated pupils, sweating, and fever. It can be difficult to differentiate hallucinogen intoxication from acute schizophrenic symptoms. Patients who have taken hallucinogens usually have no history of mental illness, know that the symptoms are drug related, and have visual instead of auditory hallucinations. Patients who have been at a "rave" dance club commonly ingest LSD, methylene dioxymethamphetamine (ecstasy or MDMA), or methylenedioxyamphetamine (Eve or MDA).

Treatment
Hallucinogens are rapidly absorbed into the bloodstream, and lavage and activated charcoal only increase agitation. Quiet reassurance helps patients to "come down." In severe cases, diazepam or lorazepam helps to quiet patients. MDMA can cause hyperthermia and muscle rigidity that can lead to rhabdomyolysis if untreated (cool the patient and use benzodiazepines for rigidity).

Phencyclidine
Diagnosis
Treatment of phencyclidine (PCP) overdose patients is dreaded by most health care professionals. Patients' behavior ranges widely, from quiet sedation to severe violence. PCP is frequently used as an adulterant in other illicit drugs, and patients may not know that they have ingested PCP. In mild intoxication, patients are lethargic, euphoric, and have hallucinations. In more severe intoxication, patients have hypertension, muscle rigidity, sweating, seizures, and coma. Suspect PCP intoxication in any patient with nystagmus and rapidly changing behavior.

Treatment
Because enterohepatic recirculation slows elimination, the effects of PCP last up to 24 hours. Decrease sensory input and administer activated charcoal to decrease reabsorption. Avoid the use of restraints, which can increase the risk of rhabdomyolysis. Treat violent behavior with benzodiazepines. Haloperidol may be used cautiously but it may increase muscle rigidity. Increased diuresis is advocated by some authors.

Acetaminophen
Diagnosis
This is based mostly on history but should be suspected in cases of elevated liver function tests in suspected drug overdose/intoxications. Acetaminophen is commonly available in most households and is frequently used by many for suicidal gestures. An acetaminophen level can be determined from serum samples. Nomograms are available to help determine total ingested dose and whether a toxic and/or lethal dose was consumed. Accidental chronic overdose is possible in situations where the children's formulation dosing is used for infant drops (which are more concentrated). Prompt recognition of the problem and instituting appropriate therapy is necessary to prevent significant morbidity and mortality.

Treatment
N-Acetylcystine is the antidote of choice for acute acetaminophen overdose where the serum level is in the toxic range on the nomogram. It should also be given to paracetamol and N-acetyl-p-aminophenol (APAP) overdose patients where the liver enzymes are elevated but the serum APAP level is undetectable as these patients are still in the toxic phase of APAP poisoning. Intravenous N-acetylcystine should be considered in severe overdose cases and considered in chronic overdose situations, especially when the AST and ALT are significantly elevated.

Referrals
Severe overdose, either acute or chronic, may require transfer to an intensive care unit. If this is the case, consultation with a liver transplant team should be done, as liver transplant may become necessary in severe cases.

Ethylene Glycol and Methanol
Diagnosis
Typical symptoms are nausea, vomiting, abdominal pain, pulmonary edema, hypotension, central nervous system depression, seizures, ataxia, and coma. Visual disturbances (blurred vision, blindness, optic disc hyperemia) are hallmarks of methanol toxicity. An anion gap metabolic acidosis with osmolar gap is present with both intoxications. Calcium oxalate crystals in the urine are suggestive of ethylene glycol intoxication.

Treatment
Aggressive supportive care is required for both substances. Stabilization and airway management must be closely monitored. Thiamine, folate, and multivitamin supplements should be used in both cases. Folinic acid (1 mg/kg up to 50 mg every 4 to 6 hour for 24 hours) should be used in methanol poisoning. Ethanol can be used, either orally or intravenously, to prevent metabolism of the substances to their toxic metabolites. Maintain a blood concentration of 100 to 150 mg per dL. Fomepizole (4-methylpyrazole), an inhibitor of alcohol dehydrogenase, can also be used. It has advantages over ethanol in that it does not exacerbate the intoxicated state. One protocol involves a loading dose of 15 mg per kg IV followed by 10 mg per kg IV bolus every 12 hours; after 48 hours the dose is increased to 15 mg per kg IV bolus every 12 hours. In either treatment, the therapy is continued until the concentration of methanol or ethylene glycol falls below 20 mg per dL. Hemodialysis can also be used. Indications for its use include significant or refractory acidosis, visual impairment, renal failure, and pulmonary edema. It is continued until the acidosis resolves.

References
1. Schulz JE. *Drug overdose. Manual of family practice.* 2nd ed. Philadelphia: Lippincott Williams & Wilkins; 2001.
2. Zimmerman JL. Poisoning and overdoses in the intensive care unit: general and specific management issues. *Crit Care Med* 2003;31(12).

3. Mokhlesi B. Adult toxicology in critical care: part I: general approach to the intoxicated patient. *Chest* 2003;123(2):577–592.
4. Rowden AK. Acetaminophen poisoning. *Clin Lab Med* 2006;26(1):49–65.
5. Mokhlesi B. Adult toxicology in critical care: part II: specific poisonings. *Chest* 2003; 123(3):897–922.

EPISTAXIS

Dena L. George, Pamela M. Williams

3.4

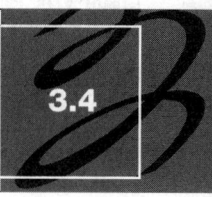

GENERAL PRINCIPLES

Definition

Epistaxis is simply defined as **bleeding from the nose.**

Anatomy

The vascular supply to the nose is through branches of both the internal and external carotid arteries. Epistaxis is described as **anterior** or **posterior** based on the location of bleeding. About 90% of cases occur in the region of the **Kiesselbach plexus** along the **anterior** septum. The usual location of posterior bleeding is the posterior septum.

Epidemiology

Epistaxis is the most common bleeding disorder of the head and neck region and is estimated to occur in about 60% of the population. Most cases require no medical intervention. The majority of cases occur in children <10 and adults >50 years old.

Etiology

Common causes for both anterior and posterior epistaxis are divided into **local** and **systemic** factors:

- Local:
  - Trauma/nose picking
  - Irritants/dry nasal mucosa
  - Tumors
  - Medications (nasal steroids)
  - Foreign body
  - Allergic rhinitis/sinusitis

- Systemic:
  - Coagulopathies
  - Hemophilia
  - Thrombocytopenia
  - Medications (anticoagulants/antihistamines/antihypertensives/anti-inflammatories)
  - Hypertension
  - Systemic infection
  - Recreational drugs
  - Alcohol

DIAGNOSIS

Clinical Presentation

Patients present with a **range of symptoms** from visible nasal bleeding to nausea, hemoptysis, and melena. **Assessment of hemodynamic stability** is a critical first step as some patients may require resuscitation prior to taking a history or performing a physical exam.

History

In the stable patient, key historical questions include: **duration** of current episode, **amount** of bleeding, **prior history** and treatment, **chronic medical conditions,** medications, recent illnesses, recreational drug use, prior surgeries, known bleeding disorders, nonprescription drugs and herbal medicines, and recent trauma.

Physical Examination

Unstable patients should have intravenous catheters and fluids started and cardiopulmonary monitor placed prior to the physical exam. Instruments necessary for adequate visualization include nasal speculum, light source, suction, and irrigator. The exam includes **inspection of the turbinates and septum** to identify the general condition of the mucosa and location of bleeding.

Laboratory Studies

Further evaluation and testing are **directed by the history and physical exam.** Patients with significant bleeding, known liver disease, or on anticoagulation therapy, should be evaluated with a complete blood count, and prothrombin/partial thromboplastin time. Patients with recurrent, unexplained epistaxis should be evaluated for a hereditary bleeding disorder. The most common one associated with epistaxis is von Willebrand factor (vWF).

Monitoring

The type and amount of monitoring for patient safety is **based on the resuscitation required,** extent or persistence of bleeding, and comorbid conditions. Patients may require hospital admission for ongoing monitoring and treatment.

TREATMENT

Behavioral

Sustained compression of the nose with the patient **leaning forward for 5 to 20 minutes** is the first step to control bleeding.

Medications

For bleeding unresponsive to compression, the next step is to achieve **vasoconstriction** using either **oxymetazoline** or **phenylephrine solution** applied directly to the mucosa or with soaked cotton/gauze. If no response, the next step is to apply **topical anesthetic** such as **lidocaine** or **4% cocaine. Chemical cautery** may also be performed on easily visualized bleeding vessels. **Silver nitrate** sticks should be applied to the area for no more than 5 seconds to prevent destruction of healthy tissue. This procedure has limited efficacy if bleeding is profuse, and can be associated with complications if applied aggressively, extensively, or on both sides of the septal wall.

Nonoperative

For persistent anterior bleeding, the next step is **nasal packing.** This may be accomplished with Bayonet forceps and nonadherent gauze or expandable nasal tampons. Packing material is directed in a posterior to anterior manner, and folded in layers until the superior aspect of the cavity is filled. All packing material should be coated with **topical antibiotic** to help reduce the risk of infections such as toxin producing Group A *Staphylococcus.* Other types of packing available include 3% bismuth tribromophenate (Xeroform), oxidized cellulose (Surgicell), and absorbable gelatin foam (Gelfoam). Packing may be left in **place for 3 to 5 days** for adequate clot formation, and moistened with normal saline prior to removal.

Referrals

All **persistent** or **posterior bleeding** unresponsive to the above interventions should be referred for specialty care. Further options include embolization, vessel ligation, and septoplasty.

Patient Education

Patients should be advised to return for care with any of the following: persistent bleeding, fever, hematemesis/vomiting, dizziness, dyspnea, or any concerns. Patients should also be educated on **steps to help prevent** future **occurrences** to include keeping the mucosa moist with petrolatum jelly or nasal saline.

Complications

Complications may occur as a result of any treatment intervention and include **infection** (localized or spread into surrounding tissues), **necrosis** of septum, **septal hematoma, abscess** formation, or **septal perforation.**

Follow-Up

Follow-up is based on the interventions performed. **Packing removal** should occur **3 to 5 days after placement.** Consideration should also be given to repeating any abnormal lab work and following anticoagulation status for patients on warfarin.

Special Considerations

Posterior bleeding: Posterior bleeding that does not respond to anterior nasal cavity packing is considered an **otolaryngologic emergency,** and patients are at risk for significant complications. Posterior packing requires special training, and is generally performed by an otolaryngologist. Foley bulb catheters or double balloon catheters are placed in combination with gauze packs to tamponade the posterior pharynx.

References

1. Frazee TA, Hauser MS. Nonsurgical management of epistaxis. *J Oral Maxillofac Surg* 2000;58:419–424.
2. Kucik CJ, Clenny T. Management of epistaxis. *Am Fam Physician* 2005;71:305–311.
3. Santos PM, Lepore ML. Epistaxis. In: Calhoun KH, Healy GB, et al., eds. *Head & neck surgery—otolaryngology.* 3rd ed. Philadelphia: Lippincott Williams & Wilkins; 2001:415–428.
4. Viducich RA, Blanda MP, Gerson LW. Posterior epistaxis: clinical features and acute complications. *Ann Emerg Med* 1995;25:592–596.

This chapter represents the views of the authors and does not represent the views of the Uniformed Services University, the U.S. Army, the U.S. Air Force or the Department of Defense.

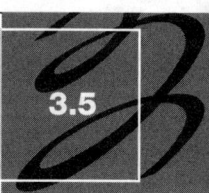

SYNCOPE
Carole V. Nistler

3.5

GENERAL PRINCIPLES

Syncope is the temporary cessation of cerebral blood flow causing loss of consciousness and postural tone followed by spontaneous recovery, not requiring resuscitation. Presyncope is the sensation of lightheadedness or faintness that may precede syncope or may represent an unrelated disorder.[1]

Syncope is a symptom of one or more underlying causes. Cardiac causes, related to mechanical obstruction or arrhythmic disruption of cardiac output, should be identified early in the workup of syncope because these factors are associated with double the risk of death from both cardiac and noncardiac causes.[1] Syncope should be distinguishable by history from other conditions that cause altered consciousness, such as seizure, vertigo, amnesia, concussion, migraine, hypoglycemia, drug or alcohol intoxication, narcolepsy, or coma. These conditions either are associated with other distinctive symptoms or do not cause an abrupt loss of consciousness followed by a spontaneous recovery.

Causes of Syncope (Table 3.5-1)

■ **Reflex or neurally mediated syncope** is due to abnormal cardiovascular reflexes that disrupt or reverse the normal compensatory autonomic response to standing or any other situation that reduces venous return to the heart.[2] Parasympathetic activity causes

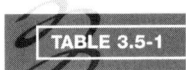

TABLE 3.5-1	Causes of Syncope

A. Reflex or neurally mediated
  1. Vasovagal attack (neurocardiogenic)
  2. Situational (micturition, defecation, cough, or sneeze)
  3. Carotid sinus hypersensitivity (tight collar, shaving, elderly)
B. Orthostatic causes
  1. Autonomic failure
    a. Primary (Shy–Drager syndrome)
    b. Secondary (diabetes, alcoholism, uremia, amyloidoses, pernicious anemia, Parkinson disease, cancer)
  2. Drugs (diurectics, tricyclic antidepressants, angiotensin-converting enzyme inhibitors, calcium channel blockers, phenothiazines, nitrates)
  3. Hypovolemic states (diarrhea, vomiting, gastrointestinal hemorrhage)
C. Cardiac
  1. Mechanical or obstructive (aortic or pulmonic stenosis, hypertrophic cardiomyopathy, pulmonary hypertension, pulmonary embolism, atrial myxoma, myocardial infarction, prosthetic valve malfunction)
  2. Arrhythmia (sick sinus syndrome, atrioventricular block, supraventricular or ventricular tachycardia, long QT syndrome, pacemaker malfunction)
D. Cerebrovascular
  1. Vertebrobasilar transient ischemic attack
  2. Subclavian steal syndrome
  3. Seizures?
E. Psychiatric (anxiety, panic, depression)
F. Unexplained

vasodilatation and bradycardia and overrides the normal increase in sympathetic output of the heart and blood vessels, resulting in peripheral blood pooling and right-sided heart underfilling.

- **Vasovagal attack** or neurocardiogenic syncope is the most common cause of syncope among people without heart disease.[1] Vasovagal attacks may be caused by stimuli such as emotional stress, the sight of blood, venipuncture, or prolonged standing. They may be preceded by symptoms of fatigue, weakness, diaphoresis, nausea, abdominal pain, or visual field changes.[2] They may be followed by mild confusion or disorientation.[3] Tilt-table testing can confirm a vasovagal cause for recurrent syncope.[4]
- **Situational syncope** is caused by vagal stimulation that accompanies decreased venous return due to the Valsalva maneuver associated with coughing, sneezing, micturition, and defecation.[4]
- **Carotid sinus hypersensitivity** is caused by maneuvers that increase vagal output via increased pressure to the carotid sinus such as head turning, shaving, or wearing a tight collar. It is more commonly seen in elderly individuals and can be diagnosed via carotid sinus massage[5] (see below).
- **Orthostatic causes** of syncope occur because of the failure of the autonomic nervous system to respond appropriately to a decrease in blood pressure or to volume depletion. Orthostatic hypotension is defined as a drop in systolic blood pressure of at least 20 mmHg or a drop in diastolic blood pressure of at least 10 mmHg within 3 minutes of standing. Syncope due to orthostasis is caused by autonomic failure (primary and secondary causes), medications, or hypovolemic states.[6]
- **Cardiac syncope** is due to decreased cardiac output from either mechanical obstruction or arrhythmia.[1] Obstructive causes are typically associated with exertion. Arrhythmias often cause abrupt unconsciousness, not related to exertion, and may be secondary to underlying structural heart disease, drugs, or electrolyte abnormalities.

Ventricular tachyarrhythmias associated with underlying heart disease may be life-threatening (See Chapter 9.6).

- **Cerebrovascular syncope** is an infrequent cause.[5] **Vertebrobasilar insufficiency** can cause loss of consciousness, but it is more likely to cause dizziness or drop attacks (falls without loss of consciousness). Severe disease should be associated with brain stem or focal neurologic deficits including vertigo, dysarthria, diplopia, or ataxia. **Atypical or unwitnessed seizures** may be confused with syncope and tonic-clonic movements can occur after a true syncopal episode. However, seizure disorders should be distinguishable from true syncope by the presence of warning auras, urinary or fecal incontinence, and postictal states (See Chapter 6.4) and the tonic-clonic movements that occur during a seizure are more likely to cause soft-tissue injuries.
- **Psychiatric syncope** may be associated with generalized anxiety disorder, panic disorder, or major depression. Its management consists of treatment of the psychiatric disorder[7] (See Chapters 5.1 and 5.2).
- **Unexplained** syncope may occur in 36% of patients undergoing evaluation.[1]

DIAGNOSIS

History

Should include a description of the syncopal event by the patient and, if possible, a witness; any preceding or residual symptoms (postictal state, neurologic deficit); any relationship to micturition, defecation, cough, swallowing, acute pain, postural change, exertion, shaving, or increased neck pressure. **Medications** that may cause syncope are nitrates, calcium channel blockers, β-blockers, angiotensin-converting enzyme inhibitors, phenothiazines, tricyclic antidepressants, monoamine oxidase inhibitors, barbiturates, diuretics, and drugs that cause prolonged QT syndrome, such as quinidine, trimethoprim–sulfamethoxazole, and the macrolides.

Physical Examination

Should focus on the detection of cardiovascular or neurologic disease with particular attention to blood pressure measurements, the cardiac exam, and evaluation of the carotid arteries.

- **Measurement of orthostatic changes** can be diagnostic, if they occur in conjunction with syncopal symptoms.
- Significant **differences in blood pressure or pulse between the right and left arms** may indicate subclavian steal syndrome or aortic dissection.
- **Cardiac auscultation** can identify the murmurs of aortic stenosis, mitral stenosis, or hypertrophic cardiomyopathy.
- **Carotid sinus massage** for 5 seconds in a supine patient may be attempted, with cardiac monitoring and intravenous access, to detect a cardiac pause of 3 seconds or a 50 mmHg decrease in systolic blood pressure and symptoms of presyncope or syncope. It should not be attempted in patients with a carotid bruit or ventricular arrhythmia, or in those who have had a myocardial infarction (MI), transient ischemic attack, or stroke within the preceding 3 months.[8]
- **Initial diagnostic tests** should include blood urea nitrogen, creatinine, electrolytes, glucose, calcium, hematocrit, and, if appropriate, a pregnancy test.[9,10] Cardiac enzymes, arterial blood gases, or drug screens may be indicated by the clinical picture. More importantly, an **electrocardiogram (ECG)** should be obtained to identify atrioventricular block, bifascicular block, Wolff–Parkinson–White syndrome, sinus node disease, prolonged Q-T interval, previous MI, or severe left ventricular hypertrophy, which could predispose to cardiac arrhythmia.
- **Additional cardiac testing** may be prompted by physical findings or an abnormal ECG.
- **Echocardiography** is indicated if obstructive causes are suspected. Evidence of coronary artery disease should prompt **stress testing.** The **continuous-loop ECG monitor,** which can be worn for several weeks and which records the immediate past 5 minutes of cardiac rhythm when the patient pushes a button, may provide a better method than Holter monitoring for detecting arrhythmic causes.[11] **Signal-averaged electrocardiography** is a noninvasive method of detecting the propensity for ventricular tachycardia.[12]
- **Electrophysiologic studies** are indicated for patients with evidence of underlying heart disease whose diagnosis has not yet been identified through noninvasive tests.

■ **Tilt-table testing** is indicated (a) in patients with recurrent syncope but without evidence of heart disease, (b) in patients with heart disease in whom cardiac causes have been ruled out, and (c) in patients who are at high risk for injury from recurrent syncope[4] (pilots, commercial drivers, etc.). Patients are placed on a table with electrocardiography and blood pressure monitors and are suddenly brought to an upright position of 40 to 90 degrees for 45 to 60 minutes. Syncopal symptoms represent a positive test result and provide 89% to 100% specificity for neurally mediated syncope.[4]

■ **Psychiatric evaluation** should be considered for patients with recurrent, noncardiac syncope.

TREATMENT

Treatment is not required for noncardiac, nonrecurrent syncope; otherwise, treatment is directed at the underlying disorder.

References

1. Soteriades ES, Evan JC, Larson MG, et al. Incidence and prognosis of syncope. *N Engl J Med* 2002;347:878–885.
2. Kapoor W. Syncope. *N Engl J Med* 2000;343:1856–1862.
3. Kenny RA. Neurally-mediated syncope. *Clin Geriatr Med* 2002;18:191–210, vi.
4. Kapoor W. Using a tilt-table to evaluate syncope. *Am J Med Sci* 1999;317:110–116.
5. Arthur W, Kaye GC. The pathophysiology of common causes of syncope. *Postgrad Med J* 2000;76:750–753.
6. Consensus Committee of the American Autonomic Society and the American Academy of Neurology. Consensus statement of the definition of orthostatic hypotension, pure autonomic failure, and multiple system atrophy. *Neurology* 1996;46:1470.
7. Linzer M, Yang EH, Estes NA III, et al. Diagnosing syncope. Part 2: unexplained syncope. *Ann Intern Med* 1997;127:76–86.
8. Puggioni E, Guiducci V, Brignote M, et al. Results and complications of the carotid sinus massage performed according to the method of symptoms. *Am J Cardiol* 2002;89:599–601.
9. Linzer M, Yang EH, Estes NA III, et al. Diagnosing syncope. Part 1: value of history, physical examination and electrocardiography. *Ann Intern Med* 1997;126:989.
10. Prodinger RJ, et al. Syncope in children. *Emerg Med Clin North Am* 1998;16:617.
11. Sivakumaran S, Krahn AD, Klein GJ, et al. A prospective randomized comparison of loop recorders versus Holter monitors in patients with syncope or presyncope. *Am J Med* 2003;115:1.
12. Kuchar DL, Thorburn CW, Sammel NL. Signal-averaged electrocardiogram for evaluation of recurrent syncope. *Am J Cardiol* 1986;58:949.

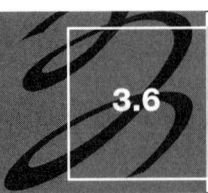

3.6

CEREBRAL CONCUSSION
Kim E. LeBlanc

GENERAL PRINCIPLES

■ Any physician may be called on to evaluate someone with a concussion.
  ■ The treating physician must maintain objectivity.
  ■ Several sets of guidelines have been proposed, but the use of these is no longer recommended.
  ■ The 2nd International Conference on Concussion in Sport in 2004 had specific recommendations that should be followed.

Definition

- Sports concussion is defined as a complex pathophysiologic process affecting the brain, induced by traumatic biomechanical forces.
- The terms *concussion* and *mild traumatic brain injury* are often used interchangeably.
- *Simple* concussion: Gradually resolves over 7 to 10 days without complication.
- *Complex* concussion: More than 1 minute of loss of consciousness (LOC), prolonged cognitive impairment after injury, specific sequelae, persistent symptoms.

Pathophysiology

- Caused by a direct blow to the head, face, neck, or elsewhere on the body with an impulsive force transmitted to the head.
- Typically results in rapid onset of short-lived neurologic impairment that resolves spontaneously.
- Clinical symptoms reflect a functional disturbance rather than a structural injury.
- Results in graded set of clinical syndromes that may involve loss of consciousness.
- Resolution of symptoms typically follows a sequential course.
- Grossly normal structural neuroimaging studies.

SYMPTOMS

- Posttraumatic amnesia poorly reflective of injury severity.
- LOC does not necessarily imply severity.
- Convulsive phenomena are generally benign and require no specific management.
- The most common manifestations of concussion are as follows:
  - Confusion
  - Disorientation
  - Amnesia

- Subtle manifestations may not be easily recognized. Examples include:
  - Slower responses to questions; difficulty following instructions
  - Disjointed speech patterns, vacant stares, deficits of memory
  - Emotional lability

- Symptoms usually seen in the first few minutes or hours:
  - Nausea and/or vomiting; dizziness and/or vertigo
  - Headache, inattentiveness, occasional problems with speech or vision

- Examples of late symptoms that may also occur (may not be apparent for days or weeks):
  - Lightheadedness, persistent mild headache, inability to concentrate
  - Lack of energy, frustration, intolerance to loud noises or bright light
  - Sleep disturbances; memory dysfunction

RECOGNITION

- The unconscious patient should be presumed to have a cervical injury until proven otherwise.
- Differential diagnosis include:
  - Subarachnoid hemorrhage
  - Hematomas: epidural, subdural, intracerebral
  - Intracerebral contusion
  - Second-impact syndrome

- Particular attention should be paid to signs of neurologic deterioration
  - Serial neurologic examinations should be performed at least every 5 minutes.
  - Once the patient's immediate needs are met, the physician may begin classifying the concussion: simple versus complex.

MANAGEMENT

- Neuroimaging adds little to concussion evaluation, as usually normal.
- Neuroimaging should be considered if intracerebral pathology suspected.

- Simple concussion: Limit activity while symptomatic
  - Most common form; must be evaluated by physician
  - No further intervention is required during period of recovery
  - No significant activity until all symptoms have resolved
  - Graded return to activity
- Complex concussion
  - Formal neuropsychologic testing and other testing should be considered.
  - Multidisciplinary approach to include those experienced in managing concussive injuries.
  - May have prolonged course.
- Stepwise return to previous activity level.
  - No activity until asymptomatic.
  - Once without symptoms, may begin light activities.
  - If no symptoms are induced, may begin more strenuous activity similar to work or play environment.
  - If symptoms are noted at any of the above stages, step back to previous asymptomatic stage and progress again after 24 hours.

References
1. McCroy P, Johnston K, Meeuwisse W, et al. Summary and agreement statement of the 2nd International Conference on Concussion in Sport, Prague 2004. *Br J Sports Med* 2005;39:196–204.
2. Cantu RC. Concussion severity should not be determined until all post concussion symptoms have abated. *Lancet* 2004;3:437–438.
3. Johnson K, Ptito A, Chankowsky J, et al. New frontiers in diagnostic imaging in concussive head injury. *Clin J Sports Med* 2001;11:166–176.

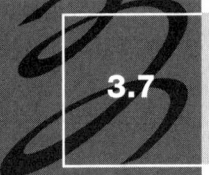

3.7 FRACTURES REQUIRING SPECIAL CONSIDERATION
Jessica Farnsworth

FRACTURE BASICS
Classification of Fractures
Complete fractures disrupt the entire cortex, whereas incomplete fractures involve only one side. Fracture location is usually related to anatomical landmarks or is described as involving the proximal, middle, or distal thirds of long bones. Closed (simple) fractures have no skin disruption that communicates with the bone, as compared with open (compound) fractures, which do disrupt the skin. Complicated fractures are those with associated soft-tissue injuries. Avulsion fractures occur when a tendon or ligament pulls away from the bone with an attached fragment. Alignment refers to the relationship of the longitudinal axis to the fracture fragments. Abnormal alignment is described by degrees of angulation. Position describes the relationship of the fragments to their normal location. Displacement describes the abnormal position of the fracture fragments. Impacted fracture fragments are pushed together, whereas distracted fracture fragments are pulled apart. Direction of fracture lines is indicated by the terms *transverse, oblique, comminuted,* and *spiral.* Transverse fracture lines are perpendicular to the axis of the bone, and oblique fracture lines cross the axis of the bone at an angle. Comminuted fractures have more than two fragments. Spiral fractures result from a torsional force.

Clinical Diagnosis of Fracture

The diagnosis of fracture should be considered any time there is a history of significant acute or chronic trauma to a bone resulting in the complaint of pain. Signs of fractures include localized pain, tenderness, ecchymosis, and edema. Gross deformity, decreased function, abnormal mobility, and crepitus may also be present. Do not dismiss the possibility of a fracture because it cannot be immediately visualized on a radiograph. A careful examination for associated injuries to viscera, tendons, nerves, and blood vessels should always be included.

Imaging Techniques

Most fractures are adequately visualized on plain radiographs, but some fractures require special imaging techniques for prompt diagnosis and optimal treatment. Radionuclide bone scanning is a very sensitive but nonspecific tool in the evaluation of fractures. It is most commonly employed to evaluate suspected occult or stress fractures that are not apparent on plain radiographs. Tomography is used to evaluate suspected fractures in bones that are frequently obscured by overlying structures. Computed tomography (CT) scanning is particularly helpful in confirming fractures of the pelvic and facial bones. Magnetic resonance imaging (MRI) is useful to diagnose occult fractures or injuries to cartilage, ligaments, and tendons.

Treatment Generalities
Stability

Stable fractures tend to maintain their position and alignment; unstable fractures tend to displace. Unstable fractures require early immobilization to prevent this result. If there is doubt about the stability of a particular fracture, it should be treated as unstable until consultation is obtained.

Associated injuries must be considered in the evaluation of any fracture. A detailed examination for damage to viscera, nerves, blood vessels, tendons, and overlying skin must be performed. The management of traumatized viscera usually takes precedence over fracture management. Neurovascular injuries should be recognized early and referred for repair. Most tendon ruptures also require surgical treatment. Open fractures require special consideration because even a small skin defect that communicates with the fracture greatly increases the patient's chances of developing osteomyelitis. These wounds should generally be debrided in the operating room and the patients given prophylactic antibiotics.

Reduction is the procedure that returns displaced fracture fragments to acceptable position and alignment. What constitutes acceptable position and alignment varies with the fracture location and type, patient age, and the functional demands placed on the bone. A neurovascular examination should always be repeated after reduction.

Immobilization of fractures is initially achieved by splinting to provide pain relief and to prevent further displacement, associated injuries, and the fat emboli syndrome. Definitive immobilization can be achieved through internal or external fixation. Internal fixation requires a surgical procedure. External fixation is provided by splinting or casting. Choosing the correct type and length of immobilization is critical for optimal healing. Inadequate immobilization can result in displacement, delayed union, or nonunion of fracture fragments. Prolonged or improper immobilization can result in stiffness and functional impairment. Consultation should be obtained if there is doubt about the appropriate type and length of immobilization.

SKULL FRACTURES

General Principles
Definition

Fracture to any of the eight cranial bones, including parietal, temporal, occipital, frontal, sphenoid, and ethmoid bones. Skull fractures are categorized by location (basilar vs. the skull convexity), pattern (linear, depressed, or comminuted), and whether they are open or closed. Complicated skull fractures are those that are open or depressed, those that involve a sinus, and those that cause intracranial air.

Diagnosis

Physical Examination

Basilar skull fractures are fractures of the base of the skull and may be manifested by a cerebrospinal otorrhea or rhinorrhea, mastoid ecchymosis (Battle sign), periorbital ecchymosis (raccoon eyes), hemotympanum, vertigo, hearing deficit, and seventh nerve palsy. Nasal discharge that is positive for glucose indicates a basilar skull fracture with cerebrospinal fluid (CSF) leak. Intracranial injury should always be suspected and a careful assessment of the patient's neurologic status should be performed, including the use of the Glascow Coma Scale.

Imaging

Skull radiographs should be obtained, but if they are negative and a fracture is strongly suspected, a CT scan should be obtained. CT scan should also be obtained if the patient exhibits altered mental status, focal neurologic deficits, signs of a basilar skull fracture, seizures, or a palpable depression of the skull.

Treatment

Scalp lacerations may hemorrhage and should be controlled as rapidly as possible, as the rich blood supply to the scalp can result in massive blood loss. Direct pressure can be used, as well as lidocaine with epinephrine infiltrated locally. Vessels can be clamped or ligated if still necessary. Open fractures should be carefully cleaned and repaired. Gentle wound exploration should be performed, with care taken not to drive bone fragments into the brain. Use of prophylactic antibiotics following an open skull fracture is controversial. In the case of a basilar skull fracture with a CSF leak, a third-generation cephalosporin such as ceftriaxone 1 to 2 g per day is a good initial choice. Fractures depressed beyond the thickness of the skull require operative repair. Closure of an open fracture should be undertaken only in consult with a neurosurgeon if a CT scan has not been obtained. Fractures that cross the middle meningeal artery or a major venous sinus may require neurosurgery expertise. Occipital fractures have a higher rate of subarachnoid hemorrhage and neurosurgery should be involved. Patients with a basilar skull fractures or altered mental status should be hospitalized. Periorbital and mastoid ecchymoses are often absent initially but may develop over the course of a few hours. Patients with a CSF leak have a higher risk of meningitis and antibiotics are indicated, but should be given only in consultation with a neurosurgeon. Most CSF leaks resolve within a week. Complications from skull fractures involve intracranial injury, infections, and seizures.

MAXILLOFACIAL FRACTURES

General Principles

- **Anatomy:** Facial bones consist of the zygoma, maxilla, lacrimal bone, nasal bone, mandible, sphenoid, frontal, ethmoid, and palatine. Cranial nerves II, III, VI, and branches of V course through the orbital foramina and may be compromised in orbit fractures.

Diagnosis

History and Physical Examination

Question the patient regarding whether he or she is experiencing abnormal vision, facial numbness, and abnormal alignment of teeth. Pain on eye movement suggests injury to the orbit or globe. Suspect domestic violence if the mechanism of injury does not seem plausible. Inspection should evaluate facial alignment and cranial nerve VII function. Palpate the face looking for tenderness or crepitus.

Imaging

Plain films or CT scan may be helpful, but should only be completed after management of head, chest, and abdominal trauma.

Treatment

- **Airway:** Always secure the airway first with maneuvers such as chin lift, jaw thrust, and oropharyngeal suctioning. With severe mandible fractures, the tongue may obstruct the airway and may need to be pulled forward. If the C spine has been cleared, the patient with tongue obstruction from a flail mandible may need to sit upright and lean forward to be able to breathe. Be careful not to get distracted from the routine trauma protocol by gross facial injuries. Avoid nasotracheal intubation as an injured cribiform plate may allow entry into the brain. Rapid sequence intubation in facial trauma is risky because bag-valve mask may be insufficient if intubation fails. Awake intubation may be necessary. Preparation for immediate backup cricothyroidotomy should be made in case intubation fails.

- **Nasal fractures:** In all cases involving nasal trauma, view the septum for a hematoma. If present, anesthetize with a topical anesthetic and incise the inferior portion of the hematoma and allow it to drain, then pack the nose with Vaseline gauze to prevent reaccumulation of blood. Nasal films are optional and may show a fracture, but referral to an ear, nose, and throat (ENT) specialist is needed only if there is obvious deformity or difficulty breathing through the nose. Consultation can be done on an outpatient basis in 5 to 7 days when edema has resolved.

- **Orbital fractures:** Blow-out fractures typically occur after blunt trauma to the eye or eyelids that is transferred to the weak floor of the orbit. This allows for the contents of the orbit to herniate through the floor, which may cause limitations in eye motion. The damage to the infraorbital nerve may cause anesthesia of the upper lip, nasal mucosa at the vestibule, lower eyelid, and maxillary teeth. If subcutaneous emphysema is found, suspect a sinus or facial fracture and consider starting antibiotics appropriate to sinus pathogens. Patients should avoid blowing their nose to prevent accumulation of subcutaneous air. A Waters view of the orbit or a CT evaluation is generally diagnostic for orbital fractures, and if positive, ENT referral should be made. Examine pupils for reactivity and whether the pupils line up in the horizontal plane. A teardrop-shaped pupil indicates a penetrated globe. Extraocular motions should be evaluated for restriction or pain. Visual acuity should be assessed using the Snellen chart, finger counting, and light perception. The swinging flashlight test may indicate optic nerve or retinal injury if the pupil initially dilates rather than constricts. If traumatic optic neuropathy is suspected, emergency ophthalmic consultation should be made in an effort to prevent blindness. Subconjunctival hemorrhage is often present with periorbital fractures. Widening of the distance between the medial canthi or pupils portends serious orbital injury.

- **Naso-ethmoidal-orbital fractures (NEO):** Suspect NEO injuries in those with trauma to the bridge of the nose or medial orbital wall. These fractures may involve lacrimal disruption and dural tears. A maxillofacial surgeon should be consulted if physical exam or CT scan suggests an NEO injury.

- **Zygomatic fractures:** Lateral subconjunctival hemorrhage often accompanies zygomatic fractures. Arch fractures are common and may be seen on arch view radiographs; these can be managed on an outpatient basis. Tripod fractures involve the infraorbital rim, diastasis of the zygomatic-frontal suture, and disruption of the zygomatic–temporal junction and are more serious. The eye may tilt when the fragment is displaced inferiorly. Tripod fractures can be seen on Waters view, and require admission for open reduction and internal fixation.

- **Mandibular fractures:** Fractures are often multiple because of the ring shape of the mandible. Malocclusion and pain on jaw movement indicate fracture. Lower lip and lower dental anesthesia occurs with mandibular fractures. Intraoral lacerations should be examined for to determine if the fracture is open or closed. Intravenous antibiotics should be started with open fractures, whereas closed fractures may be managed on an outpatient basis after consultation with an oral surgeon. If the patient has normal occlusion and a negative tongue-blade test, panoramic radiographs may be unnecessary. The tongue-blade test consists of having the patient bite down forcefully on a tongue blade. The physician then twists the tongue blade in an attempt to break the blade. Patients with an intact mandible will break the blade, whereas patients with a broken jaw will reflexively open their mouth.

- **Maxillary fractures:** Fractures of the maxilla require high impact and are usually associated with multisystem trauma. Facial stability can be assessed by rocking the maxillary arch and simultaneously feeling the central face for movement with the opposite hand. Fractures of the midface may require manual reduction of the face to stem bleeding; the hard palate can be grasped at the maxillary arch and fragments realigned.

Special Circumstances

- **Penetrating facial trauma:** Gunshot wounds to the face may injure the oral cavity and intravenous antibiotics should be given against oral flora.
- **Children:** Suspect nonaccidental trauma in cases of pediatric maxillofacial injury. Young children have a higher incidence of frontal bone injury due to its prominence, whereas adolescents have more midface fractures as their sinuses form. Cricothyroidotomy should be avoided in children younger than 12 as they are at higher risk for subglottic stenosis and tracheomalacia. Early fracture follow-up is important in all pediatric facial fractures as a child's facial skeleton heals quickly and can make delayed reduction difficult.

NECK FRACTURES

Cervical spine immobilization should always be performed when neck injury is suspected. Clinical exam of the cervical spine should involved palpation of the vertebrae and assessment of range of motion. It is generally safe *not* to obtain films if there is no midline cervical tenderness, no focal neurologic deficit, normal alertness, no intoxication, and no coexisting injury, which could distract the patient from feeling the pain caused by the neck injury. If films are needed, a lateral cervical radiograph that adequately demonstrates all seven cervical vertebrae is appropriate. To interpret films comfortably, remember the normal curves of the cervical spine (Figure 3.7-1): anterior and posterior vertebral body lines should form a smooth, continuous, lordotic curve, and the posterior cervical line should be a straight line connecting the bases of C1, C2, and C3. If the bases miss the line by more than 2 mm in either direction, suspect a pathologic process. Careful observation of these lines, along with the odontoid, can help the clinician rule out cervical fractures. If there is any doubt about the possibility of a significant cervical injury after viewing the cervical films, proceed with neurosurgical consultation while maintaining immobilization.

THORACOLUMBAR FRACTURES

Isolated, stable fractures that do not typically involve neurologic deficits include transverse process fractures, spinous process fractures, and pars interarticularis fractures. More serious fractures include wedge compression fractures, Chance fractures (involves the spinous process, lamina, transverse process, pedicles, and vertebral body), burst fractures, flexion distraction injuries (loss of height in the anterior portion of the vertebra with increased interspinous spaces posteriorly), and translational injuries (translation of vertebral segment on subsequent segments). Plain radiographs are generally adequate to make the diagnosis, although a CT scan may be required. Patients found to have acute spine fractures generally require hospital admission for further evaluation, treatment, and control of symptoms. They will benefit from bed rest (for at least 24 hours, longer in more significant fractures), analgesics (often liberal use of narcotics is necessary to control pain), and careful and serial neurologic reassessment. In the presence of neurologic deficit, emergent neurosurgic or orthopedic consultation is necessary.

THORACIC CAGE

- **Rib fractures:** Fractures of the first or second ribs generally result from serious trauma, and attention should be directed to injury to the great vessels, cervical spine, head, and brachial plexus. Other rib fractures, if at multiple levels, may result in a flail chest. This diagnosis is made by observing paradoxical inward movement of the chest during inspiration. Underlying pulmonary contusion will cause hypoxemia as fluid moves into the injured lung. Treatment is oxygen and adequate analgesia to allow adequate ventilation. If the patient cannot maintain adequate oxygenation, early ventilatory support is extremely important before the patient enters respiratory failure. Radiographic evaluation of the chest is necessary to confirm the injury as well as to rule out pneumothorax and hemothorax. Uncomplicated rib fractures are treated conservatively. Rib detail films are of questionable usefulness because approximately half of nondisplaced fractures cannot be seen in plain films, and treatment is the same for rib contusions and fracture. Other visceral injuries may be associated with rib trauma, and further evaluation of the liver, spleen, and kidneys may be indicated, depending on results of the physical examination. Chest wall supports should be used cautiously, if at all, because

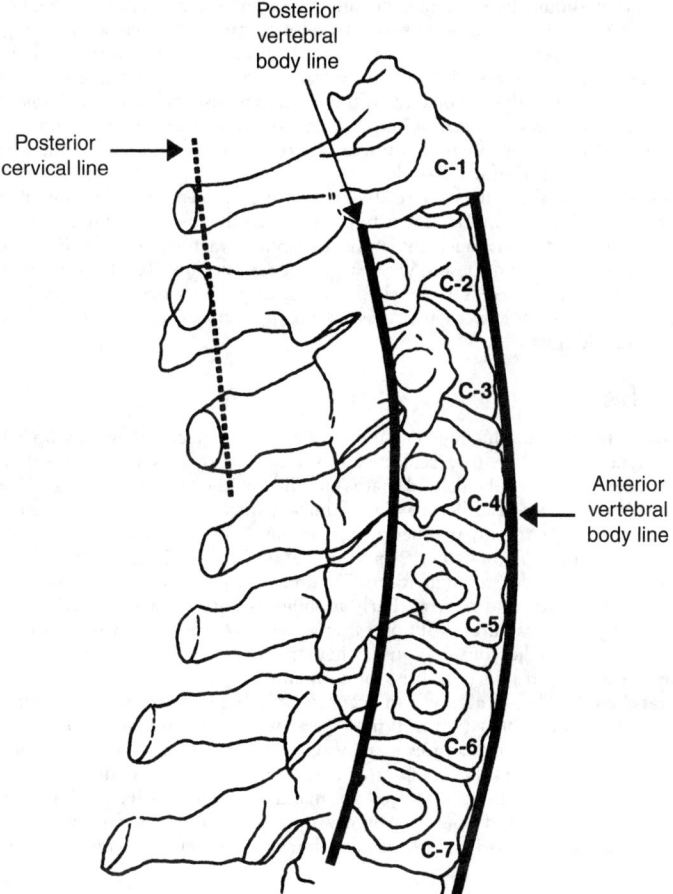

Figure 3.7-1. Normal landmarks of the cervical spine.

they impair the mechanics of ventilation and the clearance of pulmonary secretions, leading to atelectasis and pneumonitis. Visceral injury should be suspected in children because their rib cages are cartilaginous and flexible. Patients should be instructed on using a pillow for splinting and should deep-breathe and cough frequently. Healing usually takes 4 to 6 weeks.

- **Sternal fractures:** Sternal fractures can be associated with significant trauma and mortality and are commonly the result of steering wheel impact in motor vehicle accidents. Chest radiographs with lateral views of the sternum generally demonstrate the fracture. An electrocardiogram (ECG) should be obtained serially in these patients because myocardial contusion may be associated with this fracture.

SHOULDER GIRDLE

- **Clavicle:** Fractures of the clavicle are common, with fractures of the middle third the most common. Most patients have palpable swelling and tenderness at the fracture site and generally carry the affected arm in the adducted position, resisting motion of the arm. Because these fractures may be associated with neurovascular injury, a meticulous examination should be done and documented. Routine clavicle radiographs usually demonstrate the fracture. Nondisplaced fractures can be treated with a sling; if displacement is present, a figure-of-8 brace can be used. Fractures of the medial third of the clavicle may be associated with intrathoracic injuries or late-onset arthritis. Clavicular fractures that involve the distal third may disrupt the coracoclavicular ligament and nonunion may occur without operative repair. Consultation with a specialist is suggested for severely displaced fractures, complicated fractures, or fractures of the medial or distal third of the clavicle.

- **Scapula:** Scapular fractures are relatively rare and high energy is required to fracture this bone. One must consider coexisting injuries to the ipsilateral lung, thoracic cage, and shoulder girdle. Management of most scapular fractures includes immobilization with a sling, ice, and analgesics, with early range-of-motion (ROM) exercises. Surgical management may be necessary for significant or displaced articular fractures of the glenoid, angulated glenoid neck fractures, acromial fractures with rotator cuff tear, and some coracoid fractures.

HUMERUS

- **Proximal humerus:** This injury commonly occurs in elderly women who fall on an outstretched hand. A neurovascular exam should be performed with attention to sensation over the skin of the deltoid that is supplied by the axillary nerve. The Neer classification is used to describe proximal humerus fractures. A one-part fracture in the Neer system may have any number of fracture lines but no major segment (greater and lesser tuberosities, anatomic neck, and surgical neck) is significantly displaced (>1 cm separation or >45-degree angulation). Treatment of one-part fractures is immobilization, ice, anagelsics, and referral. Early mobility is critical for successful treatment of proximal humeral fractures. Multipart fractures (two or more segments) should prompt emergent orthopaedic consultation as they are more likely to involve neurovascular injuries, rotator cuff injury, and risk of nonunion.
- **Humeral shaft:** These fractures can occur in active young men or osteoporotic elderly women; metastatic breast cancer may present as a pathologic humerus fracture. Midhumeral transverse fractures usually result from a direct blow. A fall on an outstretched hand may result in a spiral fracture. Neurovascular injuries are a common complication. Most closed fractures are managed nonoperatively with immobilization, ice, analgesia, and referral. Surgery may be required for pathologic fractures, fractures associated with neurovascular injuries, or very proximal or very distal humerus fractures.

ELBOW AND FOREARM FRACTURES

- **Intercondylar fractures:** These fractures are more common in adults and any distal humerus fracture should be initially assumed to be intercondylar rather than supracondylar and a careful search should be made for a fracture line separating the condyles from each other and from the humerus. These fractures are associated with severe soft-tissue injuries. Joint reduction should be performed and the elbow immobilized and urgent orthopaedic referral made.
- **Supracondylar fractures:** These extra-articular fractures occur most commonly in children with posterior elbow dislocation. Patients with olecranon fractures have increased pain with elbow extension, whereas the pain of radial head fractures is usually aggravated by supination. Radiographs may reveal a fat-pad sign posteriorly or anteriorly. These signs may be the only radiologic abnormalities in nondisplaced radial head fractures. Suspected occult or nondisplaced radial head fractures can be treated with a posterior splint for 2 weeks followed by a sling and ROM exercises. Patients with displaced fractures of the radial head and fractures involving more than 30% of the joint surface should be referred to an orthopaedist, as should those with olecranon fractures. Undisplaced fractures are treated by casting whereas displaced fractures require surgical fixation. Neurovascular injuries are common, as well as other complications like nonunion, malunion, myositis ossificans, and loss of motion. Sensation and motor function should be

tested. The radial nerve provides wrist and finger extension and sensation to the dorsum of the hand. The median nerve controls wrist flexion, finger flexion, thumb abduction, and provides sensation to the palm of the hand. The anterior interosseus nerve arises from the median nerve and has no sensory component so specific muscles must be tested to discover injury. Testing consists of flexion at the index finger distal interphalangeal (DIP) and thumb interphalangeal joints (ask patient to make the "OK" sign). The ulnar nerve controls the intrinsic muscles and sensation to the ulnar side of the hand. Acute vascular injuries are possible and absence of a radial pulse is common in children, which is usually due to transient spasm. The most serious complication is Volkmann ischemic contracture, which can involve muscle and nerve necrosis and eventual severe fibrosis. Edema reduces venous outflow and arterial inflow, which induces ischemia, manifested by refusal to open the hand, pain with passive extension of the fingers and forearm tenderness. Supracondylar fractures with associated absent radial pulse should be reduced, immobilized, and emergent orthopaedic referral made.

- **Olecranon fractures:** The olecranon is commonly fractured and may involve ulnar nerve injury or radial head and neck fractures. Undisplaced fractures (<2 mm displacement) are immobilized with the elbow in 45 degrees of flexion with orthopaedic follow-up within a week. Displaced fractures are treated surgically.
- **Radial head fractures:** Radial head fractures are the most common elbow fracture and occur with a fall on a outstretched hand. A fat-pad sign in a patient with an appropriate mechanism of injury is sufficient to make a diagnosis of a radial head fracture. Undisplaced and minimally displaced fractures are treated with sling immobilization and early ROM, whereas all other fractures should be referred acutely to an orthopaedist.
- **Forearm fractures:** Mid-forearm fractures are usually the result of a direct blow. Associated radioulnar joint dislocations are common. The radiographic evaluation should include views of the elbow and wrist in addition to anteroposterior (AP) and lateral views of the forearm. Fractures that involve both the radius and ulna are rarely stable and usually require surgical fixation. A long arm cast can be used with minimally displaced or undisplaced fractures. Open fractures can involve nerve injuries. Complications can include compartment syndrome. Isolated undisplaced ulnar or radial fractures can be immobilized in a long-arm cast with close follow-up; displaced fractures require open reduction and internal fixation.
- **Distal radius and ulna fractures:** Colles fracture results from falls on the outstretched hand and consists of a distal radial metaphysis fracture that is dorsally angulated and displaced. Fractures should be reduced, using finger traps while the fracture fragment is pushed distal and palmar while the patient's forearm is firmly held. Immobilization should involve a long arm cast. Potentially unstable fractures have >20 degrees of angulation, intra-articular involvement, marked comminution, or more than 1 cm of shortening. Unstable fractures may require surgical intervention. The neurovascular examination is particularly important because of commonly associated median nerve and radial artery injuries. Smith fracture is a volar angulated fracture of the distal radius, or "reverse Colles fracture," and treatment is similar to that for Colles fracture.

WRIST FRACTURES

- **Scaphoid fracture:** Scaphoid fractures are the most common and complicated carpal fracture. They are usually caused by a fall on a hyperextended wrist. Patients have tenderness over the scaphoid in the anatomical snuffbox or with axial compression of the thumb. The radiographic evaluation should include AP, lateral, oblique, and scaphoid views. Nondisplaced scaphoid fractures frequently have negative acute radiographs. Suspected occult fractures should be immobilized in a short-arm thumb spica splint or cast and re-evaluated in 2 weeks. Displaced or unstable fractures should be placed in a long-arm thumb spica splint or cast. Healing of the scaphoid is hindered by its poor blood supply. Accordingly, avascular necrosis and nonunion are common complications. Persons with confirmed fractures should be referred to an orthopaedist because of the high incidence of complications.

HAND FRACTURES

■ **Distal phalanx:** These can be classified as tuft, shaft, or intra-articular. Fractures at the base may be associated with flexor or extensor tendon involvement. In general, these fractures can be treated as soft tissue injuries with protective splinting for 2 to 4 weeks. Small subungual hematomas (<25% of the nail bed area) should be drained. Larger hematomas are suggestive of a significant nail bed laceration and should be repaired for optimal cosmetic result. Extensor tendon avulsion fractures (mallet finger) may require splinting for 6 weeks.

■ **Proximal and middle phalanx:** The physical examination should focus on ruling out the presence of rotational deformity and tendon avulsions. If the hands are held palm up and the fingers flexed, they should point toward the scaphoid. Any overlap suggests a rotational deformity. Extensor tendon avulsion fractures of the proximal interphalangeal central slip result in a boutonniere deformity. Decreased active ROM accompanies tendon avulsions. Nondisplaced extra-articular fractures and volar plate fractures involving less than 15% of the joint surface can be splinted in flexion for 3 weeks followed by 3 more weeks of dynamic splinting. Most of these fractures are stable and can be treated with buddy taping. Midshaft transverse fractures, spiral fractures, and intra-articular fractures often require internal fixation. Other unstable fractures can be splinted after closed reduction. Splinting should be done from the elbow to the DIP with the elbow in 20-degree extension and the metacarpophalangeal joint in 90-degree flexion.

■ **Metacarpal fractures:** Metacarpal fractures are classified as head, neck, shaft, or base fractures. Metacarpal head fractures should be treated with ice, elevation, immobilization, and referral to a hand surgeon. Metacarpal neck fractures should be splinted with the wrist in 20-degree extension and the MP flexed at 90 degrees. Fracture of the fifth metacarpal neck is called a boxer's fracture and angulation of <40 degrees is acceptable. Angulation of <20 degrees is acceptable in the fourth metacarpal. In second and third metacarpal neck fractures, <15 degrees of angulation is acceptable. If the second and third metacarpal necks are significantly displaced or angulated, precise reduction and fixation is required. Nondisplaced shaft fractures can be treated with a gutter splint; otherwise, operative fixation is required. Metacarpal base fractures may be associated with carpal bone fractures; fourth and fifth metacarpal base fractures may result in paralysis of the motor branch of the ulnar nerve.

PELVIS AND HIP FRACTURES

■ **Pelvic fractures:** Pelvic fractures should be suspected in all victims of serious or motor vehicle trauma. Fractures may occur in a single pelvic bone, the pelvic ring, or the acetabulum. Because the pelvis is a ring, there is usually more than one fracture or ligamentous injury. Examination of the patient may reveal perineal and pelvic edema, ecchymoses, lacerations, and deformities. The pelvis should be compressed from lateral to medial and also anterior to posterior to appreciate pain or instability. The greater trochanters should be compressed and hip range of motion evaluated. Rectal examination should be done, with attention to tone, bone fragments, or rectal injury. Inability to void, hematuria, or a high-riding prostate suggests urethral injury. A standard AP view of the pelvis should be obtained in all victims of serious trauma. Serious pelvic fractures, namely, those that are unstable or that include displacement of the pelvic ring, are often associated with multisystem trauma and high mortality. Significant hemorrhage is common, and the patient may present in shock. In these patients, hospital admission with appropriate specialty consultation is advised. Temporary external fixation of the pelvis may be attempted with a tightly wrapped bed sheet. Single pubic or ischial ramus fractures are the most common fractures of the pelvis. Elderly fall victims often experience a single pubic or ischial ramus fracture and these can be treated conservatively with pain control and short-term bed rest with progression to ambulation with crutches. A cushion for sitting may help relieve pain. Iliac wing fractures usually result from acute trauma, and the treatment is similar to that listed for single pubic or ischial ramus fractures. Coccyx fractures result from falls in which the individual lands in the seated position. Localized pain to palpation and pain with sitting or defecation characterize such fractures. The diagnosis can usually be confirmed by rectal examination, and radiographic results are often negative. Treatment generally involves bed rest, sitz baths, laxatives, and cushions for sitting. Acetabular fractures are common in motor vehicle accidents and occur during hip dislocations. Treatment includes reduction of the dislocation, hospital admission, and early orthopaedic consultation.

■ **Hip fractures:** These fractures are classified as intracapsular (femoral head and neck) or extracapsular (trochanteric, intertrochanteric, subtrochanteric). Intracapsular fractures are at greater risk for avascular necrosis due to compromise of the femoral neck vessels. Radiographs should be obtained in all major trauma victims as well as elderly fall victims, even if the patient is ambulatory. Occult fracture should be suspected with negative films but significant pain with weight-bearing after trauma, and MRI may be helpful. Intertrochanteric fractures cause marked external rotation and shortening of the affected limb. Morbidity and mortality are relatively high in elderly patients with hip fractures due thromboembolic events and failure to regain normal function. Orthopaedic consultation should be made emergently with intracapsular fractures, whereas extracapsular fractures should be referred urgently.

LOWER EXTREMITY

■ **Distal and mid-femur fractures:** The mid-femur is a strong bone with excellent blood supply, a characteristic that predisposes patients with femoral shaft fractures to significant potential for hemorrhage. The muscles surrounding the femoral shaft frequently cause a deformity and displacement of any fracture. Patients generally present with severe pain, a shortened leg, and a swollen thigh. Routine films generally demonstrate the fracture. The extremity should be immobilized, and orthopaedic consultation should be urgently obtained as surgical fixation will be required. Open fractures should be irrigated and parenteral antibiotics started. Distal femoral fractures are uncommon and may be intra-articular or extra-articular. They are usually the result of direct trauma, and these patients present with pain, swelling, and deformity of the knee. Because of the close proximity of this area of the femur to the peroneal nerve (innervates space between the first and second toe) and the popliteal artery, it is essential that the neurovascular status of the leg be evaluated and documented early in the assessment of the patient. Initial treatment includes analgesics, immobilization, and emergent referral.

■ **Tibia and fibula:** Tibial fractures are the most common of long-bone fractures. They may be intra-articular or extra-articular. Fractures of the tibial plateau (medial and lateral tibial condyles) are easy to miss on standard radiographic films and are more readily seen on a tibial plateau view. Nondisplaced, single plateau fractures can be immobilized and outpatient orthopaedic referral made. Other plateau fractures should be referred quickly. Dislocations and fractures of the fibular head may appear innocuous but are often a marker for more significant knee injury. Displaced fractures of the tibia are often associated with displaced fractures of the fibula. Orthopaedic consultation is recommended for tibial and fibular fractures because of the frequently associated injuries (ligamental, meniscal, and vascular) and the frequently seen complications, which can result in chronic pain, knee dysfunction, and degenerative arthritis.

■ **Patella:** Patellar fractures most commonly result from direct trauma, but a violent contraction of the quadriceps may cause an avulsion fracture. Transverse fractures are most common, followed by stellate and comminuted types. Local tenderness and swelling are the most common presenting complaints. Active extension should be evaluated because the extensor mechanism can be disrupted. AP, lateral, and skyline views of the patella are usually sufficient to define any fractures. Because bipartite and tripartite patellae are relatively common and usually bilateral, comparison views may be helpful and smooth cortical margins should be seen. A nondisplaced patellar fracture with intact extensor mechanism should be treated with a knee immobilizer, ice, elevation, and analgesics followed by long leg casting. Aspiration of hemarthrosis may be helpful in lessening pain. Attention must be paid to maintaining quadriceps tone with exercises. Consideration should be given to specialist consultation because of the possibility of traumatic chondromalacia and avascular necrosis. In other types of patellar fractures, consultation is recommended.

■ **Ankle:** The ankle joint consists of three bones (tibia, fibula, and talus) and three main ligamentous structures (lateral ligament complex, medial deltoid ligament, and the syndesmosis, which joins the tibia and fibula). The Ottawa Ankle Rules should be used to determine whether films are needed when a patient presents with ankle pain. Radiographs are required if there is any pain in the malleolar zone and inability to bear weight both immediately and in the emergency room (ability to bear weight should be assessed by asking the patient to take four steps). The standard radiographs (AP, lateral, and mortise views) are usually adequate. Special attention should be paid to the malleolar–talar space. Ankle fractures and ligamental injuries often coexist. Disruption of the ankle at only one place generally results in a stable ankle injury that can be treated by conservative means (posterior splinting, nonweight bearing, and edema control). If two or more disruptions of the ankle are present, the ankle is not stable, and treatment is immobilization and emergent referral. Unilateral avulsion fractures of the distal tip of the malleolus are often treated like second-degree sprains. If there is any doubt about optimal management, discuss the case with an orthopaedic specialist. The risk for complications of ankle fractures (traumatic arthritis, chronic talar instability, chronic pain and swelling, and osteochondral fractures) is high.

- **Hindfoot fractures:** The hindfoot consists of the calcaneus and talus. Although standard films may demonstrate fractures here, CT scanning may be required for adequate visualization of injuries. Also, occult fractures are common in this area. For this reason, the clinical examination is critical in making decisions. Although full ankle motion may be present, heel pain with weight bearing after the appropriate trauma is common. Calcaneus fractures should prompt evaluation of the spine as they are usually caused by falls from a height. Compartment syndrome can occur with calcaneal fractures. Generally, the undisplaced fracture is treated with a well-padded posterior splint, nonweight bearing, elevation, and analgesics until swelling subsides, when a well-molded walking cast may be used. Partial weight bearing is generally needed for at least 8 weeks. Because of the high likelihood of posttraumatic arthritis and chronic pain and stiffness, patients bearing these fractures are often referred to an orthopaedic specialist. If any displacement is present, prompt referral is recommended.

- **Midfoot fractures:** The midfoot consists of the navicular, cuboid, and three cuneiforms. Isolated fractures of the cuboid and cuneiforms are rare and an injury to the Lisfranc joint should be sought, especially if there is point tenderness over the midfoot or when there is laxity between the first and second metatarsals in a dorsal–plantar direction. The Lisfranc joint consists of the tarsometatarsal complex and injuries here are often missed. A fracture of the base of the second metatarsal or gap >1 mm between the bases of the first and second metatarsals on radiograph is pathognomic of a ligamentous injury. Small, nondisplaced chip fractures of the navicular are usually treated with a compressive dressing for several weeks. Other nondisplaced navicular fractures can often be treated conservatively with a well-molded walking cast. Displaced navicular fractures and Lisfranc joint injuries with cuboid and cuneiform fractures should be referred for open reduction.

- **Forefoot fractures:** The metatarsals and phalanges comprise the forefoot; metatarsal fractures are divided into shaft and neck fractures. Metatarsal and phalangeal fractures usually result from direct crush injuries. Because of the large forces to the second and third metatarsals during the push-off phase of walking or running, this is also an area that is prone to stress fractures. Standard foot radiographic views are generally adequate to demonstrate fractures (with the exception of early stress fractures). A secondary ossification center in the base of the fifth metatarsal may sometimes be confused with a fracture, but this area generally has smooth, bilateral sclerotic margins. Early stress fractures may require a bone scan to visualize the problem. Nondisplaced shaft fractures are generally treated conservatively with a walking cast or orthopaedic shoe. However, the first metatarsal, if fractured, should be kept nonweight bearing. Displaced shaft fractures can be treated with closed reduction, casting, and nonweight bearing for 6 weeks. For neck fractures, open fixation is often required for displaced fractures. Fifth metatarsal fractures are the most common of the metatarsal fractures. The base of the fifth metatarsal is the most common metatarsal fracture, and an avulsion fracture and a transverse fracture (Jones fracture) of the base should be differentiated. The Jones fracture (transverse fracture 15 to 31 mm distal to the proximal part of the metatarsal) can be complicated by malunion or nonunion and thus orthopaedic referral should be made; 6 weeks of casting and nonweight bearing will be required. An avulsion fracture of the tuberosity of the base can appear similar to a Jones fracture but can be treated with only a cast shoe. Phalangeal fractures, if nondisplaced, can be treated with "buddy taping" and sometimes a cast shoe. Fractures of the first toe are not adequately immobilized by dynamic splinting, and a walking cast is usually necessary. Displaced fractures should be reduced if possible under digital nerve block; displaced fractures of the great toe may need surgical fixation.

PATHOLOGIC FRACTURES

Any fracture that results from insignificant trauma should be considered pathologic, meaning that the broken bone has pre-existing disease that has resulted in a loss of structural integrity. The patient may complain of pain that existed even before the fracture, and the actual fracture site may not be especially tender. The radiograph may have an altered appearance in that the trabecular patterns of the bone near the fracture can be disrupted. The most common causes of bone disease are osteoporosis, myelomas, and metastatic lesions (think of cancer of the thyroid, breast, prostate, bronchus, kidney, bladder, uterus, ovary, testicle, and adrenals). Less common—but more benign—causes include enchondromas (also called chondromas), solitary bone cysts, and giant cell tumors. Malignant primary bone tumors may also present with pathologic fractures, which generally require specialist evaluation and treatment.

FRACTURES UNIQUE TO CHILDREN

There are several unique factors about the diagnosis and treatment of fractures in children. These include the presence of the epiphyseal plate, the tendency to suffer incomplete fractures, and the evaluation for signs of child abuse (See Chapter 20.5).

Epiphyseal plate injuries are common because this site is the weakest portion of the immature skeleton. Injuries that would result in a ligamentous strain in adults frequently fracture the epiphyseal plate in children. The physical examination reveals tenderness and edema over the epiphysis. The radiographic evaluation may be difficult, and comparison views should be considered. Epiphyseal plate fractures are most commonly classified by the Salter–Harris system (Figure 3.7-2):

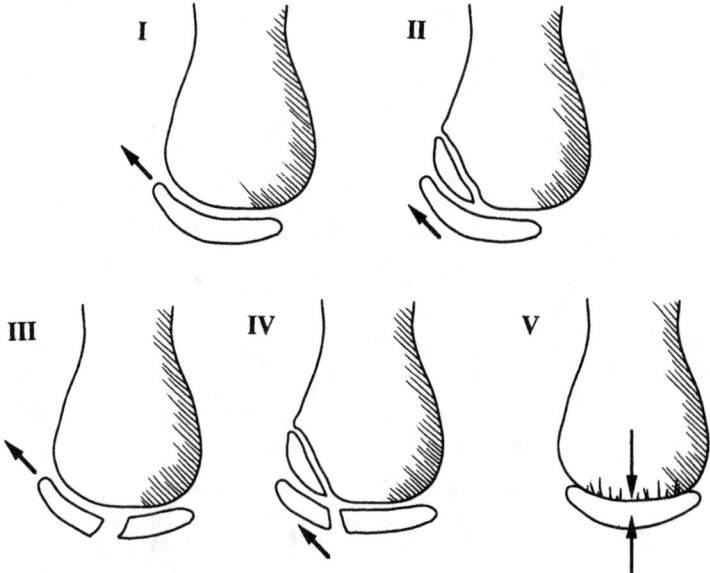

Figure 3.7-2. Salter–Harris system.

- Type I: Fracture through the epiphyseal plate
- Type II: Epiphyseal plate fracture with an associated metaphyseal fragment
- Type III: Fracture through the epiphysis onto the articular surface
- Type IV: Fracture through the distal metaphysis, epiphyseal plate, and epiphysis
- Type V: Impaction of the epiphyseal plate

Types I and II are treated with casting, often after closed reduction, and enjoy a good prognosis. Types III and IV have a higher risk of growth disturbance and should generally be referred. Type V is often diagnosed in retrospect, after a growth disturbance has occurred.

Incomplete fractures include torus fractures and greenstick fractures. Torus fractures occur when there is a buckling of one side of the cortex. They are usually caused by a compression force. Torus fractures occur commonly in the forearm after a fall on the outstretched hand. They are treated with a long arm cast for 4 to 6 weeks. Greenstick fractures occur when a long bone is bowed, resulting in a break in only the convex side of the cortex. These are generally stable fractures that most commonly occur in the forearm. Forearm greenstick fractures with less than 15 degrees of angulation should be placed in a cast for 4 to 6 weeks. Patients whose fractures show more than 15 degrees of angulation should be referred to an orthopaedist.

Physical abuse is a significant cause of early childhood fractures. Suspicion should be raised by an inconsistent or implausible explanation and by inappropriate parental behavior. The classic radiologic evidence of child abuse is multiple fractures in various stages of healing. Suspected victims should be evaluated with a skeletal survey, followed by the appropriate completion of forms and referrals to protective agencies.

Problems of Infants and Children

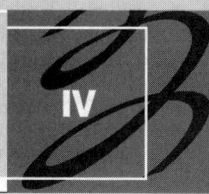

IV

DEVELOPMENTAL PROBLEMS IN CHILDREN

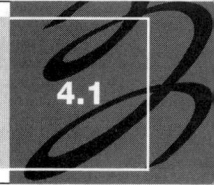

4.1

Dennis J. Baumgardner

GENERAL PRINCIPLES

Developmental problems of children include intellectual and special sensory deficits, motor dysfunction, and psychosocial disorders caused by nonprogressive central nervous system (CNS) dysfunction (behavioral problems are discussed in Chapter 4.9). Although up to 25% of children have developmental problems, diagnosis is often delayed due to overreliance on normal variation as explanations of subtle findings, inattention to specific milestone delays when the child is otherwise normal, reliance on strictly clinical impressions in deference to cumbersome screening devices, and the physician's or parents' reluctance to discuss their fears. This problem is best approached by ongoing surveillance in the context of a continuing relationship with the family.[1–4]

DIAGNOSIS

History

Should include open-ended questioning of the parents regarding their child's physical, cognitive, sensory, and social development, and any prior professional concern or workup. The medical history should document established developmental risk, such as known sensory deficit, chromosomal abnormality, myelomeningocele, and human immunodeficiency virus (HIV) infection. For example, children with conditions such as cleft lip or palate may be otherwise unaffected or may experience physical or psychological developmental problems resulting from the cleft, and perhaps additional problems if the cleft is part of a syndrome.

Risk Factor Assessment

Builds on prenatal care assessment. Biologic risk factors may be summarized as significant maternal disease, hazardous exposure, obstetric complication, congenital infection and malformation(s), and significant neonatal, infant, or childhood neurologic, cardiopulmonary, infectious, somatic, or metabolic disease. Family history may reveal risk factors, such as familial developmental or sensory deficits, history of autism, or chromosome abnormalities. Psychosocial risks include cognitive disability; serious emotional disturbance, substance abuse, or lack of parenting skills in caregivers; limited social or financial support; and stress, violence, or a history of abuse or neglect in the family.

Physical Examination

Physical examination is essential for detection of risk, or workup of developmental delay. Attention should be paid to growth abnormalities (including abnormal head circumference), congenital anomalies, skin findings (e.g., neurofibromatosis, tuberous sclerosis, Sturge–Weber syndrome), eye findings (e.g., retinal pigmentation of Tay-Sachs), organomegaly (neurodegenerative disorders), postural and transition movement disorders, as well as the neurologic examination. Key physical findings have been summarized by Levy and Hyman[3] and Bear.[4] Facies may be indicative of a specific syndrome (e.g., fetal alcohol) or may lead to erroneous conclusions. Many facially dysmorphic children have normal intelligence, whereas children deemed attractive may have any degree of cognitive impairment or autism.

Developmental Surveillance

Should be performed at each well-child visit by the use of milestones. This may be done "on the fly," along with immunizations, in children who are only presented for episodic care. The milestones in Table 4.1-1 were selected on the basis of objectivity, ease of parental

---

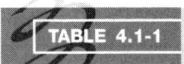 **TABLE 4.1-1**   **Developmental Milestones**

1 mo
    Raises head when lying prone (GM)
    Retains a ring or rattle (FM)
    Gives alerting response (1 wk) (A/L/C)
    Regards face in direct line of vision (Vis, FM)

2 mo
    Raises chest when lying prone (GM)
    Social smiling (6 wk) and cooing (A/L/C)
    Follows moving object across midline (Vis, FM)

3 mo
    Up on elbows when prone (GM)
    Hands unfisted more than half of time (FM)
    Blinks to visual threat (Vis)

4 mo
    Up on hands when prone (GM)
    No head lag when pulled to sitting (GM)
    Brings hands together (FM)
    Orients to voice (A/L/C)
    Symmetrical corneal light reflexes and normal eye cover testing (Vis)

5 mo
    Sits with support (GM)
    Transfers objects (FM)
    Laughs (A/L/C)

6 mo
    Sits with minimal support (GM)
    Has unilateral reach (FM)
    Babbles (A/L/C)

7 mo
    Sits without support (GM)
    Takes pellet (crude grasp) (FM)
    Searches for dropped object (A/L/C)

(continued)

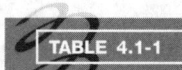 **TABLE 4.1-1** **Developmental Milestones** *(Continued)*

8 mo
 Comes to sitting position (GM)
 Has immature pincer grasp (FM)
 Says dada/mama (inappropriate) (A/L/C)
9 mo
 Stands holding on (GM)
 Bangs blocks together (FM)
 Plays peek-a-boo (A/L/C)
12 mo
 Walks with minimal assistance (GM)
 Has mature pincer grasp (10 mo) (FM)
 Releases voluntarily (FM)
 Says dada/mama (appropriate) and two other words (A/L/C)
 Searches for hidden object (A/L/C)
 Follows simple verbal commands (with gestures) (A/L/C)
 Drinks from cup (PS)
15 mo
 Walks alone well (GM)
 Puts in and takes out (pellets in a bottle) (FM)
 Follows simple verbal commands (without gestures) (A/L/C)
 Has three- to six-word vocabulary (A/L/C)
18 mo
 Climbs (GM)
 Stacks three or four blocks (FM)
 Knows three body parts (A/L/C)
 Imitates housework (A/L/C)
 Uses spoon (PS)
2 yr
 Runs (GM)
 Stacks four or five blocks (FM)
 Has 50-word vocabulary (A/L/C)
 Uses some two- to three-word sentences (A/L/C)
 Enjoys being read to, points to objects in book (A/L/C)
3 yr
 Walks up and down stairs, alternating feet (GM)
 Balances on one foot for 1 s (GM)
 Stacks nine blocks (FM)
 Copies a circle (FM)
 Knows own name and sex (A/L/C)
 Uses three- to four-word sentences (A/L/C)
 Dresses self except for buttons (PS)
4 yr
 Hops on one foot (GM)
 Throws a ball (GM)
 Copies a circle and a cross (FM)
 Counts to 4 (A/L/C)
 Recognizes three or four colors (A/L/C)
5 yr
 Walks heel-to-toe or skips (GM)
 Balances on one foot for 5–10 s (GM)
 Builds a stairway or building with blocks (FM)
 Copies a square (FM)
 Counts to 10 (A/L/C)
 Follows three commands (A/L/C)

A/L/C, auditory/linguistic/cognitive; FM, fine motor; GM, gross motor milestone; PS, personal/social; Vis, visual.

recall or demonstration in the office, and uniformity (e.g., crawling is omitted because some children never demonstrate this prior to walking). All four major streams of development (gross motor, fine motor, language, and personal–social) are represented. Developmental delay is defined as actual development that is 25% or more behind the expected rate in any or all of the four major streams.

Key points regarding milestones include the fact that development should occur in an orderly, predictable, intrinsically controlled fashion, although often in spurts. Parents and providers may focus on growth in the first 8 to 10 months, disregarding gross motor delay. Similarly, gross motor surveillance may overshadow that of fine motor development, the latter often being the earliest indicator of motor disability (hypertonia or primitive reflexes may mimic normal gross motor development in cerebral palsy). Warning flags are abnormal head size and failure to have hands unfisted at least 50% of the time by 3 months. The presence of handedness earlier than 18 months may represent an opposite-side hemiplegia. Gross motor achievement may be falsely reassuring because it does not indicate intelligence. Language development is the best predictor of intellectual potential and is therefore combined with cognitive development in Table 4.1-1. Fine motor skills combine visual maturation, hand function, and problem solving, and are the second best indicator of future intelligence.

Linguistic capacity develops in sequential, critically timed phases and depends on the adequacy of stored utterances (receptive vocabulary) in infancy. A common pitfall is to ignore a language milestone delay until age 2. A wide vocabulary by age 3 is predictive of reading level at Grade 2. Another cognitive warning flag is lack of appreciation of object permanence by the end of the first year. The average age of diagnosis of congenital deafness is 2 years; the pitfalls are parents' failure to seek the alerting response to sound in the nursery, and confusing the child's response to vibrations or to gestures as indicative of hearing. Expressive skills that are advanced in comparison with receptive skills may be a sign of a pervasive developmental disorder. Articulation problems are often not identified by the parents. Specific red flags for autism disorders include no babbling or pointing by 12 months, no sharing of interest in objects with another person; no single words by 16 months, or no two-word spontaneous phrases by 24 months; any loss of language or social skills at any age.[5,6] Follow-up of milestone delay should include formal developmental testing (by referral if necessary). Formal regular screening of all children for developmental delay, using one of a number of instruments, receives a C recommendation.[7] Autism-specific screening and diagnostic tools are available.[5]

Further Assessment

There is no routine laboratory workup. The results of state screening for certain inborn metabolic disorders must be known, and testing augmented if there is plateau or loss of milestone skills, vomiting and lethargy, movement or cutaneous disorders, failure to thrive, unusual body odor, or suggestive family history. Thyroid disorders must always be ruled out in developmental delay. Children with abnormal muscle tone should be screened with creatinine phosphokinase and aldolase. Neuroimaging is indicated for children with focal neurologic findings, significant prematurity, abnormal head growth (confirmed by magnetic resonance imaging), craniofacial anomalies, many genetic syndromes, seizures, sensory impairments, and other unexplained findings. Appropriate lead screening must be undertaken because relatively low-level toxicity can lead to impairment (See Chapter 1.1). Children with major or multiple anomalies suggestive of a syndrome should have chromosomal analysis (done best in consultation with a geneticist). Chromosomal mosaicism may present subtle findings and be missed by amniocentesis. DNA testing for fragile X and other genetic testing is done as indicated. Learning disabilities are confirmed by neuropsychometric testing.

SPECIFIC SYNDROMES AND MANAGEMENT

■ **Learning disabilities** (75 in 1,000 children) may be specific or global, and etiologic factors are often unknown. Learning disabilities are associated with increased comorbidities, including depression, anxiety, substance abuse, and sleep and eating disorders. Dyslexia is the most common disability, and it may affect written language and mathematical skills development. Sensory deficits must be ruled out. Preschool diagnosis is often difficult, and problems may not arise until adolescence and persist or even present in adulthood. Treatment should be individualized, with the focus on educational therapy. Retention is rarely useful and may negatively affect self-esteem and socialization.

- **Mental retardation** (25 in 1,000 children) is defined as a deficit resulting from disease, injury, or abnormality that existed prior to age 18, IQ of 70 to 75 or below, and deficits in at least 2 of the following 10 areas of adaptation: communication, self-care, home living, social skills, community use, self-direction, health and safety, functional academics, leisure, and work. Mild retardation may be isolated, but severe retardation is often accompanied by associated deficits, often as part of a syndrome, that also affect prognosis. Specific medical problems, such as gastroesophageal reflux or aspiration pneumonia, may also be present. Linguistic deficits are due to the cognitive deficits and contribute to the emotional and behavioral disorders that often occur.[2]

- **Cerebral palsy** (2.5 in 1,000 children) is a collection of disorders that variably manifest as abnormal motion and posture caused by early nonprogressive, CNS injury (most commonly during intrauterine development). The Swedish classification involves four types: spastic (abnormalities of the pyramidal tract including quadriplegia, diplegia, and hemiplegia), dyskinetic (choreoathetosis with variable tone or rigidity and dystonia), ataxic (broad-based gait, truncal titubation, and dysmetria), and mixed. Approximately half of affected children have associated mental retardation; most of those with normal intelligence have perceptual problems that may result in learning disabilities. Early neuroimaging is the most direct indication of pathogenesis, but a specific diagnosis often does not imply a specific prognosis. Treatment may include neurosurgery or orthopaedic surgery or devices; medical treatment for seizures, spasticity (potentially including intrathecal baclofen or botulism toxin injections), constipation, and gastroesophageal reflux; and appropriate therapies.[8]

- **Autism spectrum disorder** (6 in 1,000 children). This division includes a spectrum of neurodevelopmental disorders with multiple etiologic factors involving impaired reciprocal social interactions, verbal and nonverbal communication, and restricted interests and/or repetitive behaviors and resistance to change.[5] There are often associated global cognitive deficits and sensory abnormalities but not motor deficits (except for clumsiness). About 25% of patients manifest seizures. There is an apparent, but ill-defined genetic component. Children who demonstrate social interest and some degree of empathy and sustained interactions are considered to have pervasive development disorder rather than autism. Often, those with better socialization and no delay in language skills are diagnosed with Asperger syndrome. Early multidisciplinary medical, educational, language, behavioral and family therapy, and highly predictable daily routines and preparedness are treatment mainstays. Medications targeting specific behaviors may be useful.[6]

- **Hearing impairment** (6 in 1,000 children). Prompt recognition and habilitation, including early sign language instruction, can maximize language skill development and social and emotional growth. Risk factors for hearing loss include family history, congenital infections, craniofacial anomalies, birth weight less than 1,500 g, severe hyperbilirubinemia, bacterial meningitis, asphyxia, ototoxic medications, mechanical ventilation for 5 or more days, and suspected syndromes that may include hearing loss. One third of cases will be missed by these criteria, and the Joint Committee on Infant Hearing has endorsed universal hearing screening by age 3 months. The effect of recurrent or chronic otitis media on development is unclear as causality is difficult to prove. Delayed milestones should not be dismissed based on otitis media.

- **Visual impairment** (0.5 in 1,000 children) is present in many of those with developmental disorders. Conversely, an increased prevalence of developmental problems is seen in the visually impaired. Careful screening, prompt diagnosis, and referral to an ophthalmologist skilled in the care of children is essential.

- **Down syndrome** (1 in 1,000 children), or trisomy 21, is a common cause of mental retardation and may serve as a prototype for other chromosomal abnormalities with a wide range of medical, developmental, sensory, and emotional manifestations. Specific Down syndrome growth charts should be used along with screening for heart defects, hypothyroidism, atlantoaxial instability, and other associated conditions. Frequent office visits and provider education are required to anticipate and manage the various problems of children with any chromosomal abnormality or syndrome (See Chapter 14.3).

- **Other specific chromosomal disorders** such as Klinefelter syndrome (47,XXY) and trisomy X (47,XXX) may include various degrees of mental retardation or behavioral problems. Other examples include microdeletions such as Williams (7q23-), Prader–Willi (15q11-13 paternal), Angelman (15q11-13 maternal), velocardiofacial-DiGeorge (22q11-), chromosomal mosaicism, and other syndromes.
- **Fetal alcohol syndrome** (0.5 in 1,000 to 2 in 1,000 children) is diagnosed by documentation of (a) three specific facial abnormalities (smooth philtrum, thin vermillion border, small palpebral fissures); (b) growth deficit; (c) CNS abnormalities. Additional facial and hand abnormalities may be present in varying degrees. CNS impairment may not be apparent in the newborn; however, consequences are lifelong. Behavioral, learning, and adaptive difficulties are often greater than the degree of neurocognitive impairment.[9] Alcohol-related neurocognitive developmental disorder may be present without the typical facial features. Treatment includes referral to a multidisciplinary team, parent education, and individualized interventions to stabilize the home environment and improve parent–child interactions.
- **Fragile X syndrome** (0.25 in 1,000), the most common inherited cause of mental retardation, occurs in both males and females due to a mutation that causes expansion of a CGG-trinucleotide repeat unit found on the X chromosome. In affected families the mutation is inherited in an unstable fashion and undergoes intergenerational expansions. This syndrome can cause cognitive deficits ranging from subtle learning disabilities with a normal IQ to severe mental retardation with social avoidance, poor adaptation, and autistic behaviors. Females and those with fewer CGG repeats may be more mildly affected. Significant medical issues or malformations are rare, but may include the triad of prominent ears, a long, narrow face, and macro-orchidism (in boys). These and other variable findings may be subtle and less apparent in the younger child. Thus, this diagnosis should be considered in every child with delay in cognitive, adaptive, or communication milestones. DNA blood testing is diagnostic. Early intervention with appropriate therapies and family genetic counseling is beneficial.[10]
- **Failure to thrive** (inadequate physical growth) is particularly common in low-income families and may be caused by a variety of psychosocial, environmental, neurologic, and anatomical factors and their interactions. An excellent review is available.[11] There is evidence for a sensitive period for mental development that is mitigated by poor postnatal somatic growth, placing these infants at risk for cognitive delay. Prompt recognition and treatment are important.
- **Neurodevelopmental abnormalities due to HIV infection** are a spectrum of motor, cognitive, communication, social, and behavioral problems that may ultimately be seen in infected children. Appropriate antiviral and medical treatment and therapy and mainstream school settings are indicated (See Chapter 19.4).
- **Comprehensive primary care for children with developmental delay includes coordination and management of a team of medical and sometimes surgical and dental specialists, social workers, counselors (genetic, parental, family), habilitation or rehabilitation therapists, medical device services, and special educators.** Goals must be agreed on among physician, family, therapists, and educators and written progress reports shared. Knowledge of community and social services as well as advocacy for the child and family is essential.
- **Advice for the parents begins with frank, factual, unhurried, and compassionate discussions as soon as the diagnosis of delay is entertained.** Avoid speculation regarding intelligence and unnecessary pessimism. Expectations often affect outcomes: Low expectations may be a self-fulfilling prophecy. Helpful advice for rearing a child with special needs includes setting realistic goals, having routines, avoiding hours spent finding the "perfect educational toy," and acknowledging the baby's or child's own agenda (not feeling like one has to be teaching the child every minute to "catch up"). Maximizing communication in children with language disorders and helping parents foster special strengths of their child should help minimize the child's frustration and consequent additional emotional, behavioral, or social disturbances. Sports activities, including Special Olympics, are often helpful for weight management, fitness, development of physical coordination, and improvement of self-esteem.

Often activities involving gross motor skills are most appropriate, with attention to specific instances that increase the risk of injuries (e.g., atlantoaxial instability in Down syndrome). Consistent discipline, appropriate for the level of understanding, is important for the child, particularly in the context of his or her siblings (the child with special needs should not "get away with anything" at a given developmental age if the siblings did not). Parents should avoid allowing undesirable behaviors, such as chewing on a book, because this is "progress," only to have to work very hard later to extinguish the behavior.

PREVENTION

Involves optimization of preconceptual, prenatal (See Chapter 14.4), and postnatal care. The last includes not only avoidance of untoward exposure; early identification of toxic, metabolic, and medical disorders; appropriate therapy; and optimization of neurologic outcome; but also providing a nurturing environment. For the very premature, this should include careful application of appropriate stimuli and protected rest time. For the child in an at-risk home environment, a combination of social services, parental counseling and support groups, and an interested provider may improve outcome. Early diagnosis of visual or hearing loss should be made. Early exposure to books to encourage literacy and vocabulary building is recommended for all children. Finally, early identification of developmental delay or risk affords the best chance for affecting developmental change via a still malleable nervous system. It also empowers the family to be proactive in maximizing the child's abilities, perhaps avoiding secondary emotional and physical disability.

References

1. Johnson CP, Blasco PA. Infant growth and development. *Pediatr Rev* 1997;18: 224–242.
2. Daily DK, Ardinger HH, Holmes GE. Identification and evaluation of mental retardation. *Am Fam Physician* 2000;61:1059–1067.
3. Batshaw ML, ed. The child with development disabilities. *Pediatr Clin North Am* 1993;40 [entire volume].
4. Bear LM. Early identification of infants at risk for developmental disabilities. *Pediatr Clin North Am* 2004;51:685–701.
5. Spence SJ, Sharifi P, Wiznitzer M. Autism spectrum disorder: screening, diagnosis, and medical evaluation. *Semin Pediatr Neurol* 2004;11:186–195.
6. Wray J, Silove N, Knott H. Language disorders and autism. *Med J Aust* 2005;182:354–360.
7. Hamilton S. Screening for developmental delay: reliable, easy to use tools. *J Fam Pract* 2006;55:415–422.
8. Cerebral palsy in infants and young children: a synthesis. *J Pediatr* 2004;145:S1–S46 [entire supplement].
9. Wattendorf DJ, Muenke M. Fetal alcohol spectrum disorders. *Am Fam Physician* 2005;72:279–285.
10. Visootsak J, Warren ST, Anido A, et al. Fragile X syndrome: an update and review for the primary pediatrician. *Clin Pediatr* 2005;44:371–381.
11. Krugman SD, Dubowitz H. Failure to thrive. *Am Fam Physician* 2003;68:879–884.

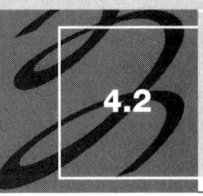

4.2 FEVER IN INFANCY AND CHILDHOOD
Peter Forman

GENERAL PRINCIPLES
Definition
Fever is the elevation of body temperature to 38°C (100.4°F) or higher. Rectal temperature most accurately reflects core temperature, especially in infants. Oral or tympanic temperatures are suitable for older children but can be inaccurate.

Epidemiology
Fever is a prominent symptom of many diseases in infants and children. Fever, as a presenting complaint, accounts for nearly one third of pediatric outpatient visits in the United States.[1]

Pathophysiology
Infectious agents, toxins, or mediators of inflammation stimulate monocytes, macrophages, and other cell types to release interleukin-1 (IL-1), tumor necrosis factor (TNF), IL-6, and interferons (IFNs) that act on the anterior hypothalamus (antipyretics act here). This elevates the thermoregulatory set point causing increased heat conservation and increased heat production. This results in fever.

DIAGNOSIS
History
- Duration, height, and pattern of fever
- Constitutional: Sleepy, cranky
- Respiratory: Rhinorrhea, sore throat, otalgia, and cough
- Gastrointestinal: Vomiting and diarrhea
- Urinary: Dysuria, frequency (often absent in infants)
- Pronounced lethargy and irritability are red flags for serious bacterial illness (SBI)
- Noninfectious: Collagen vascular disease, malignancy, or metabolic disorder, such as hyperthyroidism; salicylate or anticholinergic poisoning as well as excessive environmental temperature

Physical Examination
Observation of the older infant or child is very helpful in determining the index of suspicion for an SBI. A pink, alert, well-hydrated, smiling, or easily consoled infant is much less likely to have an SBI than a pale, lethargic, dehydrated, dull, or irritable child.[2]

- **Skin**
  - Petechial rash (meningococcemia)
  - Maculopapular rash followed by petechial rash (Rocky Mountain spotted fever)
  - Sandpaper papular rash (Strep A infection)
- **Head**
  - Bulging fontanelle or nuchal rigidity (meningitis)
- **Eyes**
  - Conjunctivitis (otitis media, or OM; Kawasaki disease; measles with cough; coryza)
- **Ears**
  - Red, dull, nonmobile tympanic membranes (OM)

- **Nose**
  - Purulent rhinorrhea (sinusitis)
  - Nasal flaring (pneumonia or respiratory distress)
- **Throat**
  - Stridor (laryngotracheobronchitis, i.e., croup)
  - Stridor with drooling, dysphagia, or aphonia (epiglottitis)
  - Petechia on soft palate and uvula (streptococcal pharyngitis)
  - Vesicles or ulcers on tongue, lips, and buccal mucosa (herpes stomatitis)
  - Strawberry tongue (streptococcal pharyngitis, Kawasaki disease)
- **Chest**
  - Tachypnea, retractions, decreased breath sounds, crackles (pneumonia)
  - Ronchi (bronchitis)
  - Wheezing (bronchiolitis, asthma, inhaled foreign body)
- **Cardiac**
  - Murmur (subacute bacterial endocarditis, rheumatic fever, may be normal due to increased cardiac output from the fever itself)
- **Abdomen**
  - Local tenderness worsening with movement (appendicitis, or peritonitis)
- **Musculoskeletal**
  - Refuses to bear weight or use the extremity (septic arthritis, osteomyelitis)

Laboratory Studies

- No test can detect every SBI in all febrile children, but the following values in infants older than 28 days deserve further investigation:
  - White blood cell (WBC) count of 15,000 per μL or more or WBC count of less than 5,000 per μL
  - Absolute band count of 1,500 per μL or higher
  - Presence of toxic granulation or vacuolization in neutrophils
- **Further investigative studies:**
  - *Urinalysis with culture* should be considered in male infants younger than 6 months of age, older uncircumcised male infants, and female infants younger than 2 years old when fever does not have a source.
  - *Blood culture* should be considered in the child younger than 36 months who is at high risk for SBI, as indicated by physical examination, fever of 39°C or higher, or WBC count of 15,000 per μL or greater.
  - *Lumbar puncture* should be performed in the presence of symptoms or signs suggestive of meningitis, such as excessive irritability or lethargy, seizures, or bulging fontanelle.
  - *Stool smear* of bloody or mucoid diarrhea demonstrating five or more WBCs per high-power field (hpf) suggests bacterial enteritis warranting stool culture for *Salmonella, Shigella, Campylobacter, Yersinia,* or pathogenic *Escherichia coli.*

Imaging

- Chest radiography is indicated in the presence of pulmonary symptoms, such as tachypnea. Rales are not always heard in young children with pneumonia. If any of the following are present there is a 33% chance of findings on chest x-ray: respiratory rate greater than 50, coryza, cough, nasal flaring, grunting, stridor, rales, rhonchi or wheezing, or WBC >20,000.
- *If none are present there is a less than 1% chance of finding on chest x-ray.*[3]

TREATMENT

Behavioral

Avoid fever phobia by educating parents that fever is a symptom of an underlying illness and is itself seldom dangerous.[4] The primary reason to treat fever is to make the child more comfortable.

Medications

Fever of 38.9°C (102°F) or higher may be treated with acetaminophen, 10 to 15 mg/kg/dose q4h up to maximum of 5 doses per day, or ibuprofen, 5 to 10 mg/kg/dose q6–8h in children 6 months or older. The child may subsequently be sponged with lukewarm water if the temperature exceeds 40°C (104°F). The child should be encouraged to drink liquids and may be covered with a light blanket.

Special Therapy

■ Management of the febrile child at risk for a serious bacterial infection. **Low-risk criteria** apply to those previously healthy term infants who appear generally well (nontoxic) and have no focal bacterial infection except OM. Laboratory studies include total WBC of 5,000 to 15,000 per µL, absolute bands less than 1,500 per µL, urinalysis less than 5 WBCs per hpf or negative Gram stain result, and stool with less than 5 WBCs per hpf. These criteria do not exclude all infants with SBI but have a negative predictive value of about 98% to 99%.[5]

   ■ **Infants younger than 28 days** should undergo a sepsis workup in the hospital and receive parenteral antibiotics pending culture results.

   ■ **Infants 28 to 90 days old** who are toxic or at high risk should be admitted for sepsis workup and treatment. Infants who are nontoxic and at low risk may be evaluated and treated as outpatients provided they have reliable caretakers and follow-up. Following cultures of the blood, urine, and cerebrospinal fluid (CSF), ceftriaxone (Rocephin), 50 mg per kg IM, up to 1 g maximum, should be administered. The child must be re-evaluated within 24 hours.[6]

   ■ **Nontoxic infants aged 3 to 36 months with a temperature less than 39°C** should have fever treated symptomatically. Focal symptoms should be addressed but the child re-examined if he or she appears worse or the fever lasts longer than 48 hours.

   ■ **Nontoxic infants aged 3 to 36 months** with a temperature of 39°C or higher should have screening WBC count and blood culture if there is no obvious focus for infection. Girls younger than 2 years and boys younger than 6 months (or older if uncircumcised) should have a urine culture. Chest radiography, lumbar puncture, or stool specimen should be obtained if clinically appropriate. Empirical antibiotic treatment with ceftriaxone or amoxicillin–clavulanate (Augmentin), 40 mg/kg/day of amoxicillin divided in three doses, may be considered,[7] especially if the WBC count is 15,000 per µL or greater. Oral cefixime (Suprax) 16 mg per kg on day 1 followed by 8 mg/kg/day for a total of 14 days may be used to manage urinary tract infection (UTI).[8]

■ Follow-up of infants and children with fever without source.

   ■ **Infants 28 to 90 days old** must be rechecked within 24 hours. A second dose of ceftriaxone may then be given. OM or UTIs may be treated on an outpatient basis in afebrile, nontoxic, and nonbacteremic children. The afebrile well-appearing child with *Streptococcus pneumoniae* bacteremia may also be treated with oral antibiotics. Children who are still febrile, appear ill, or have a positive CSF culture result, or bacteremia other than antibiotic-sensitive *S. pneumoniae* should be admitted for sepsis workup and treatment.

   ■ **Children 3 to 36 months old** should be rechecked in 24 to 48 hours. If the child is afebrile and nontoxic, antibiotics can be discontinued after 48 hours. Oral antibiotics should be given for OM, UTIs, or antibiotic-sensitive *S. pneumoniae* bacteremia. Children who are still febrile, appear ill, or have a positive CSF culture result require further evaluation or parenteral antibiotic treatment, or both.

   ■ **Structural evaluation of the urinary tract** should be performed on boys and young girls after their first documented UTI.

Complications

■ **Treatment of febrile seizures**

   ■ Febrile seizures occur in 2% to 5% of febrile children between the ages of 6 months and 5 years. Seizures that are complex, occur upon arrival in the emergency department, or are accompanied by abnormal neurologic findings are a red flag that causes such as meningitis should be investigated. Lumbar puncture should be strongly considered in infants younger than 12 months presenting with their first febrile seizure.[9]

- Simple seizures are generalized tonic-clonic events that last less than 15 minutes and do not recur within 24 hours.[9]
- Complex seizures last longer than 15 minutes, demonstrate focal signs, or recur within 24 hours or in a flurry.[9]

■ Ensuring adequate airway, breathing, and circulation is all that is usually required for a short febrile seizure. Intravenous lorazepam (0.05 to 0.1 mg/kg over 2 to 5 min) may be used for prolonged seizures or those compromising the child's cardiorespiratory status. If necessary, lorazepam may be repeated but the clinician should be prepared to assist the child's ventilation. Rarely, intravenous phenytoin (15 to 20 mg/kg) is given slowly (1 mg/kg/min) for persistent seizure. Rectal diazepam (0.5 mg/kg to maximum dose of 5 mg) is 80% effective in controlling febrile seizures.[10]

■ Recurrent febrile seizures may occur in 50% of children younger than 12 months and 30% of children older than 12 months at the time of their first simple seizure. Recurrent seizures are also more likely if seizures were complex, multiple, or occurred in children with underlying neurologic abnormalities or a history of afebrile seizures.[11] Epilepsy may develop in 1% to 2.4% of children with simple febrile seizures (See Chapter 6.4).

■ Prophylaxis of febrile seizures is rarely indicated for simple seizures but may be used for frequent or severe seizures. Phenobarbital at a blood level of 15 µg per mL is effective but causes behavioral side effects in 20% to 40% of children. Valproic acid is effective in children but can cause fatal liver failure in addition to thrombocytopenia, gastrointestinal disturbances, and pancreatitis in those younger than 3 years. Oral diazepam given at the time of fever reduces the risk of febrile seizures but can cause lethargy and ataxia that could mask a CNS infection.[11]

References

1. Finkelstien JA, Christiansen CL, Platt R. Fever in pediatric primary care: occurrence, management, and outcomes. *Pediatrics* 2000;105:260.
2. McCarthy PL. Observation scales to identify serious illness in febrile children. *Pediatrics* 1982;70:802–809.
3. Harper M. Update on the management of the febrile infant. *Clin Pediatr Emerg Med* 2004;5(1).
4. Schmitt BD. Fever phobia. *Am J Dis Child* 1980;134:176–181.
5. Jaskiewicz JA, et al. Febrile infants at low risk for serious bacterial infection: an appraisal of the Rochester criteria and implications for management. *Pediatrics* 1994;94:390–396.
6. Baraff LJ, et al. Practice guideline for the management of infants and children 0 to 36 months of age with fever without source. *Pediatrics* 1993;92:1–12.
7. Bass JW, et al. Antimicrobial treatment of occult bacteremia: a multicenter cooperative study. *Pediatr Infect Dis J* 1993;12:466–473.
8. Hoberman A, et al. Oral versus initial intravenous therapy for urinary tract infections in young febrile children. *Pediatrics* 1999;104:79–86.
9. Provisional Committee on Quality Improvement, Subcommittee on Febrile Seizures. Practice parameter: the neurodiagnostic evaluation of the child with a first simple febrile seizure. In: *Clinical practice guidelines of the American Academy of Pediatrics*. 2nd ed. Elk Grove Village, IL: American Academy of Pediatrics; 1999:73–85.
10. Fishman MA. Febrile seizures. In: McMillan JA, ed. *Oski's pediatrics: principles and practice*. 3rd ed. Philadelphia: Lippincott Williams & Wilkins; 1999:1949–1952.
11. Committee on Quality Improvement, Subcommittee on Febrile Seizures. Practice parameter: long-term treatment of the child with simple febrile seizures. In: *Clinical practice guidelines of the American Academy of Pediatrics*. 2nd ed. Elk Grove Village, IL: American Academy of Pediatrics; 1999:105–115.

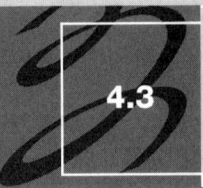

4.3 INSPIRATORY STRIDOR, CROUP, AND EPIGLOTTITIS

Neil S. Skolnik, Jinn Liu

GENERAL PRINCIPLES

Inspiratory stridor is a syndrome of upper airway obstruction, characterized by a harsh sound on inspiration. Etiologic factors include croup, epiglottitis, retropharyngeal abscess, peritonsillar abscess, foreign body, extrinsic laryngeal compression (tumor, cyst, hematoma), angioedema, laryngeal webs, vascular rings, bacterial tracheitis, acquired or congenital subglottic stenosis, and laryngomalacia.

Viral croup, often considered synonymous with laryngotracheobronchitis, is the most common form of upper airway obstruction in children aged 6 months to 6 years. It is caused by inflammation and edema of the subglottic region of the larynx. Parainfluenza viruses are the most frequent cause of croup, accounting for 75% of cases. Epiglottitis is a bacterial infection of the epiglottis that causes acute upper airway obstruction. It is usually caused by *Haemophilus influenzae* type b infection and has been nearly eradicated since the introduction of routine immunization with *H. influenzae* vaccine (See Chapter 1.1)

CROUP

Clinical Presentation

The mean age of children presenting with croup is 18 months, with age ranging from 3 months to 6 years. Croup is most common in early fall and winter, and usually, but not always, is preceded by a couple of days of upper respiratory symptoms followed by hoarseness, low-grade fever, and a "croupy" or barking cough.

Illness may progress no further or may go on to cause inspiratory stridor, flaring of the ala nasi, and suprasternal and intercostal retractions. The lungs are generally clear but about 5% of the time there is associated wheezing.

Diagnostic Studies

Usually no diagnostic studies are needed, and the diagnosis of croup can be made on clinical grounds. White blood cell (WBC) counts are usually normal or mildly elevated but are greater than 15,000 per mm^3 approximately 20% of the time. Lateral neck radiography shows widening of the hypopharynx. Posteroanterior radiographs may show a narrowed subglottic region known as a steeple sign. Classic signs of croup on radiography are seen only about half the time.

Treatment

The first decision in the treatment of croup is whether a child should be treated on an outpatient or inpatient basis. Indications for hospitalization include cyanosis or pallor, stridor at rest, respiratory distress, a toxic-appearing child, and hypoxemia. A helpful algorithm for treatment is shown in Figure 4.3-1.

- **Humidified air.** Provision of humidified air, either by having the parent hold the child in his or her arms in the bathroom at home with the shower turned on to generate steam or by using a croup tent in the hospital may be reasonable; however, studies have shown little efficacy for the use of humidified air in the acute care setting.
- **l-Epinephrine** (1:1000) at a dose of 0.5 mL/kg diluted in 3 mL normal saline (maximum doses: <4 years 2.5 mL/dose; >4 years 5 mL/dose) administered by nebulizer can be given to acutely decrease the upper airway obstruction seen in croup. l-Epinephrine has been shown to have equivalent potency and safety when compared to the much less available racemic epinephrine. Epinephrine works through α-adrenergic effects, which

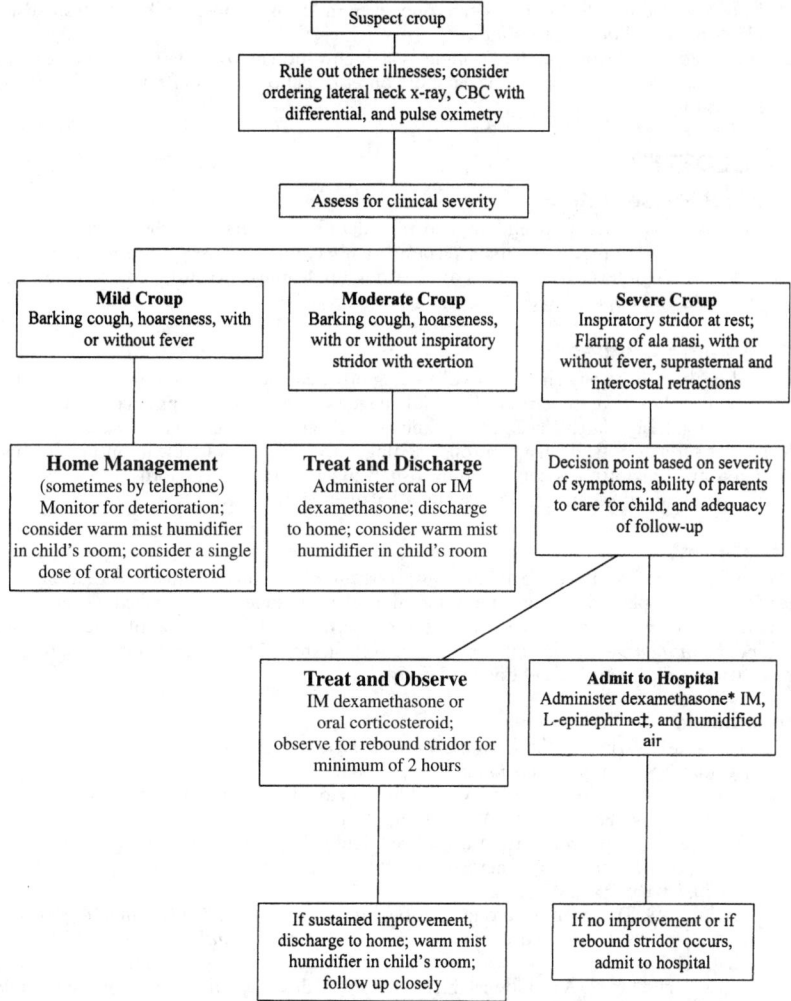

Figure 4.3-1. An algorithm for the treatment of croup. *, dosage 0.6 mg/kg; ‡, dosage l-epinephrine 1:1000, see text for dose. (From Skolnik NS. Croup. *J Fam Pract* 1993;37:168, with permission.)

lead to mucosal vasoconstriction that results in decreased edema in the subglottic region of the larynx. Time of onset of action is less than 10 minutes and duration of action is less than 2 hours. Treatment is very effective but transient; all children who receive racemic epinephrine must be observed for at least 2 hours because of the possibility of rebound stridor, and all such children should receive corticosteroid treatment.

■ **Adrenal corticosteroids.** Dexamethasone, 0.6 mg/kg IM or PO, is effective in decreasing airway obstruction, but it has a slow onset of action and often does not take effect for up to 6 hours. Oral and intramuscular dexamethasone appear to have equivalent efficacies and are more effective than nebulized corticosteroids. Prednisone, 3 mg/kg PO, is also probably effective but has not been studied as extensively. Adrenal corticosteroids should be considered for all children with croup; even mild cases appear to benefit from a single dose of oral dexamethasone.

- **Nebulized budesonide.** Budesonide is a highly potent topical steroid that can be administered by nebulizer. It has a short onset of action and is effective in decreasing inspiratory stridor.

EPIGLOTTITIS

Clinical Presentation

Epiglottitis tends to occur in children who are older (3 to 7 years) than the croup age group with no history of a preceding upper respiratory infection. The disease is of sudden onset, and there is a high fever. The child is often sitting up, leaning forward, and drooling without a cough, and appears toxic.

Diagnostic Studies

Lateral neck radiography shows a swollen epiglottis, classically referred to as the "thumb sign." If the clinical presentation of a child suggests epiglottitis, the physician should not waste time getting a lateral neck radiograph. Visualization of the epiglottis should be performed as soon as possible in a controlled setting with facilities available for intubation and tracheotomy. Epiglottitis is confirmed by visualizing a cherry-red epiglottis. Blood cultures should be obtained because this is usually a bacteremic disease.

Treatment

Treatment is twofold. First, the airway must be secured to ensure adequate ventilation. This is usually accomplished through endotracheal intubation done in a controlled setting where tracheostomy can be performed if necessary. Second, intravenous antibiotics effective against *H. influenzae* type b should be started (cefuroxime, 75 mg/kg/day divided into q8h, or ceftriaxone, 100 mg/kg/day divided into ql2h).

References

1. Knutson D, Aring A. Viral croup. *Am Fam Physician* 2004;69:3.
2. Skolnik NS. Croup. *J Fam Pract* 1993;37:165.
3. Scolnik D, et al. Controlled delivery of high vs low humidity vs mist therapy for croup in emergency departments. *JAMA* 2006;295:11.
4. Waisman Y, et al. Prospective randomized double-blind study comparing l-epinephrine and racemic epinephrine aerosols in the treatment of laryngotracheitis (croup). *Pediatrics* 1992;89:302.
5. Skolnik NS. Treatment of croup: a critical review. *Am J Dis Child* 1989;143:1045.
6. Russell K, et al. Glucocorticoids for croup. *Cochrane Database Syst Rev* 2004;(3): CD001955.
7. Bjornson CL, et al. A randomized trial of a single dose of oral dexamethasone for mild croup. *N Engl J Med* 2004;351;1306–1313.
8. Klassen TP, et al. Nebulized budesonide for children with mild to moderate croup. *N Engl J Med* 1994;331:285.
9. Klassen TP. Croup. An algorithm for the treatment of croup. *Pediatr Clin N Am* 1999;46:1167.
10. Mauro RD, Poole SR, Lockhart CH. Differentiation of epiglottitis from laryngotracheitis in the child with stridor. *Am J Dis Child* 1988;142:679.
11. Johnson DW, et al. A comparison of nebulized budesonide, intramuscular dexamethasone, and placebo for moderately severe croup. *N Engl J Med* 1998;339; 498–503.

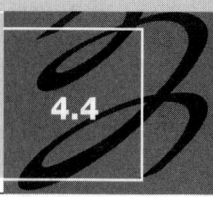

*A*irway hyperresponsiveness—the tendency of airways to constrict and cause obstruction due to inflammation—characterizes both asthma and wheezing respiratory illnesses in children.

DIAGNOSIS

History

- The most common symptoms include cough, wheezing, shortness of breath, and chest tightness. Determine if respiratory distress has occurred previously and associated phenomena (e.g., seasonally, with upper respiratory infections, or nocturnally).
- Associated diseases, including allergic rhinitis eczema or food allergies are common (See Chapters 8.6 and 16.5).
- Aggravating factors, such as smoke, animals, exercise, upper respiratory infections, and drugs, should be identified.
- A family history of allergies or asthma is common.

Physical Examination

- Obtain vital signs, including respiratory rate, temperature, pulse, and weight and oxygen saturation.
- Observe the child's color and degree of respiratory distress and anxiety. Fatigue and cyanosis signal a severe attack, and the clinician should be prepared for respiratory failure.
- Stridor indicates an upper airway problem, such as croup or foreign body (See Chapter 4.3).
- Check if the wheezing is bilateral and document retractions as well as the ratio of inspiration to expiration (I/E). In children without wheezing or who have normal respirations, check for a posttussive wheeze. Lack of wheezing and presence of a normal chest examination do not exclude asthma and in fact may indicate worsening of the clinical situation.
- Hydration status should be evaluated.
- A complete ear, nose, and throat examination should be performed with a focus on infections, nasal polyps (pathognomonic for cystic fibrosis), and signs of allergies.

Differential Diagnosis

The differential diagnosis is important as treatment for the various conditions is different: they include the following conditions:

- **Asthma** is characterized by recurrent episodes of cough, dyspnea, and diffuse wheezing and is difficult to diagnose in children younger than 3 years but usually begins before 3 years of age (See Chapter 10.1).
- **Bronchiolitis** is characterized by the insidious onset of wheezing, tachypnea, hypoxia, and chest wall retractions associated with a 2- to 3-day history of rhinorrhea, cough, and low-grade fever in a child younger than 3 years.[1] Respiratory syncytial virus (RSV) is the most common cause but bronchodilator therapy does not affect the course of the disease.
- Other conditions include **cystic fibrosis, bronchopulmonary dysplasia, gastroesophageal reflux and recurrent aspiration, congestive heart failure, pneumonia, sinusitis, croup, mediastinal mass, foreign body aspiration, congenital airway or heart anomalies, syndromes of ciliary dyskinesia.**
- **Large airway obstruction** can be caused by foreign bodies, vascular rings, tracheomalacia, tumors, and laryngeal webs.

Diagnostic Tests

- **Reversibility of airway obstruction** is diagnostic of asthma and can be evaluated with a trial of epinephrine or adrenergic aerosols.
- **Complete blood count and chest radiographs** are useful with fever to evaluate for pneumonia or if congestive heart failure is suspected. They are generally normal in reactive airway disease.
- **Pulmonary function tests** are usually reliable by age 5 to 6 years and are most useful for monitoring chronic asthma; they are not required for the diagnosis. If done to evaluate cough, provocation with methacholine might be needed.[1]
- **Sinus radiographs, pulmonary function tests, studies for reflux, and specific immunoglobulin E (IgE) antibodies or skin testing** (75% of people with asthma have environmental allergies) are indicated for patients whose asthma is resistant to the usual treatment or to evaluate for suspected inciting factors.
- **Oximetry** is useful for determining severity of respiratory compromise but is not helpful in the differential diagnosis.[2]

TREATMENT

Prevention

Warm-blooded animals should be removed from the home. Exposure to dust mites should be minimized by washing bedding and stuffed animals two times per week in water at least 130°F. Wipe off surface dust frequently using a damp cloth. Carpeting and upholstered furniture should be removed. The humidity level should be kept below 50%. Mattresses and box springs should be encased in airtight plastic covers with tape over the zipper. Regularly wash damp areas, such as shower stalls, basements, and window sills. Avoid environmental irritants. Do not allow smoking. Do not use woodstoves. Avoid strong odors or sprays. Do not clean when the patient is present. Reduce exposure to infections. Avoid daycare settings if possible, and vaccinate appropriately. If symptoms are severe or systemic and steroids are needed regularly, immunotherapy may be necessary.

Pharmacologic Therapy[3]

- **Cromolyn sodium (Intal aerosol spray) and nedocromil sodium (Tilade)** have few side effects. They are anti-inflammatory medicines and have no bronchodilator effect but inhibit mediator release from mast cells. The dosage is two puffs of multidose inhaler (MDI) three to four times per day or one unit dose via nebulizer mixed with a β-agonist. The treatment may be decreased to twice a day with adequate clinical response. They are a nonpreferred alternative monotherapy treatment for mild persistent asthma.
- **β-Adrenergic agonists** are bronchodilators effective in treating early asthmatic responses and exercise-induced asthma. They are the treatment of choice for acute episodes of bronchospasm and a rescue medication in all classes of asthma. Selective β-agonists are preferred due to fewer cardiac side effects. The β-agonists are available as MDIs, nebulizer solutions, oral preparations, and parental preparations.
- **Corticosteroids** are very potent anti-inflammatory medicines. Anti-inflammatory agents are the most important medicine in chronic recurrent asthma. They reduce inflammation, edema, and mucus secretions and restore β-adrenergic responses. According to the PEAK Trial, they are beneficial for treatment of symptoms at an early age but do not prevent the development of asthma. There is no evidence that children will have growth reduction secondary to use of inhaled glucocorticoids over the long term. The topical agents are quickly metabolized and rarely cause systemic symptoms. Inhaled steroids and cromolyn are best given 10 minutes after inhaled β-agonists. Oral doses are absorbed quickly and can be used for acute episodes.
- **Theophylline** is a bronchodilator whose use has markedly decreased in recent years due to side effects and lack of an anti-inflammatory component. It has a very narrow therapeutic window and serum levels must be monitored frequently.
- **Anticholinergics** function as bronchodilators in most patients with asthma and enhance the effect of the β-agonists. Ipratropium bromide (Atrovent) is poorly absorbed and has few systemic side effects. It is particularly useful in cold air–induced, irritant-induced, and emotionally induced asthma.

■ **Leukotriene modifiers:** Montelukast (Singulair), zafirlukast (Accolate), and zileuton (Zyflo). Montelukast is approved for age 2 and above, zafirlukast is approved for age 5 and above, and zileuton is approved for age 12 and above. Leukotriene antagonists work on the inflammatory cascade in asthma. They show some benefit for short-term symptom control and lower respiratory sequelae in infants with RSV.

■ **Long-acting beta agonists (LABA)** are not to be used as rescue medication or for acute bronchospasm. Salmeterol is approved for age 4 and above and formoterol is for ages 5 and above with neither being first-line treatment choice. Studies suggest that in children an increased dose of steroids may improve airway responsiveness to a greater degree than the addition of an LABA.

■ **Influenza vaccine** is useful in preventing virus-induced episodes of asthma or reactive airway wheezing secondary to inflammation. It is now recommended for children starting at age 6 months and repeated yearly.

Management

"Step-care" management strategy of asthma, in which the number of medications and frequency of use are increased as symptoms worsen, is recommended by the National Heart, Lung and Blood Institute.[3]

■ **Severe persistent**
  ▪ Long-term control—*Daily* anti-inflammatory: high-dose inhaled corticosteroid *and* long-acting bronchodilator. Oral corticosteroid tablets or syrup (2 mg/kg/day; do not exceed 60 mg/day) may be required intermittently.
  ▪ Quick relief—Short-acting bronchodilator; inhaled β-agonists as needed.

■ **Moderate persistent**
  ▪ Long-term control—*Daily* anti-inflammatory: inhaled corticosteroid, medium dose, *or* inhaled corticosteroid low-medium dose with long-acting bronchodilator, especially for nighttime symptoms. *If needed:* anti-inflammatory: medium-high dose inhaled corticosteroids *and* long-acting bronchodilator, especially for nighttime symptoms.
  ▪ Quick relief Short-acting bronchodilator; inhaled β-agonists as needed.

■ **Mild persistent**
  ▪ Long-term control—*Daily* anti-inflammatory: either low-dose inhaled corticosteroid. Cromolyn or nedocromil could be used as a second choice.
  ▪ Quick relief—Short-acting bronchodilator; inhaled β-agonists as needed.

■ **Mild intermittent**
  ▪ Long-term control—No daily medication needed.
  ▪ Quick relief—Short-acting bronchodilator; inhaled β-agonists as needed.

■ Leukotriene modifiers with a lower dose inhaled glucocorticoid as alternative to high-dose inhaled glucocorticoid therapy can be tried. Not all are responders to this drug class.

Flowmeters

Peak flowmeters, which measure peak expiratory flow rate (PEFR), are essential to manage asthma properly but not useful in very young children due to their inability to perform the exercise properly. The following are interpretations of flowmeter readings.

■ The green zone is defined as a PEFR of 80% to 100% of personal best: No symptoms are present; the patient can engage in full activity, and no change in medication is needed.

■ The yellow zone is defined as a PEFR of 50% to 80% of personal best: The patient is at increased risk of asthma attacks; treatment should be applied per the step-care management strategy (see above).

■ The red zone is defined as a PEFR of less than 50%. Call the physician; *emergency care is necessary.*

Indications for Admission

Continued wheezing an hour after administration of β-agonist in association with any sign of respiratory distress, persistent tachypnea, PCO greater than 40, PaO_2 less than 70, O_2 saturation less than 92%, and altered level of consciousness.

Indications for Consultation

Required if multiple hospital admissions, continuation of symptoms, PEFR less than 90% of predicted and never returning to baseline, and poor status following intubation.

Resources for Patient Education

- National Asthma Education Program, DHHS, Pub. No. 97-4051, 1997.
- American Lung Association, (800) 586-4872, www.lungusa.org.
- Asthma and Allergy Foundation of America, (800) 727-8462, www.aafa.org.
- Allergy and Asthma Network/Mothers of Asthmatics, Inc., (800) 878-4403, www.podi. com/health/aanma.
- National Asthma Education and Prevention Program, (301) 251-1222, www.nhlbi.nih. gov/nhlbi/nhlbi.htm.
- American Academy of Allergy, Asthma, and Immunology, (800) 822-2762, www. aaaai.org.

References

1. Barcy TL, Graber MA. Respiratory syncytial virus infection in infants and young children, *J Fam Pract* 1997;45:473–481.
2. Stemple DA, Redding GJ. Management of acute asthma. *Pediatr Clin North Am* 1992;39:1311.
3. Covar RA, Spahn JD. Practical guide for the diagnosis and management of asthma. National Asthma Education Program, DHHS Publ. No. 97-4051, 1997.
4. Covar, Spahn. Treating the wheezing infant. *Pediatr Clin North Am* 2003;631–654.

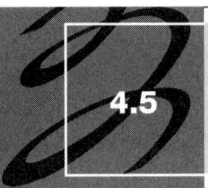

4.5   VIRAL EXANTHEMS OF CHILDREN
Jeffrey T. Kirchner

GENERAL PRINCIPLES

Viral exanthems of children are a common clinical problem encountered by the family physician. Numerous viral agents can produce a similar rash and other clinical symptoms, which makes the diagnosis challenging. A careful evaluation that includes age, immunization status, history of infectious diseases, exposures, medication use, type of prodromal period, features of the rash, fever, and the presence of pathognomonic signs is helpful in establishing a diagnosis. Laboratory testing may be available to confirm the diagnosis but often is not acutely useful due to the time delay in obtaining viral cultures or serologic antibody titers. The increasing availability of polymerase chain reaction (PCR) testing should improve the ability to diagnose many infectious illnesses. Treatment in most cases is supportive.

MEASLES

- **Causative agent.** Measles is caused by an RNA paramyxovirus that belongs to the genus *Morbillivirus*. Infected individuals are contagious up to 7 days after the onset of symptoms.
- **Clinical manifestations** may initially include fever, cough, conjunctivitis, and Koplik spots (an enanthem). Rash appears on the third or fourth day and begins as a purple–red maculopapular eruption along the hairline, forehead, and face. By the third day it spreads to the feet and it fades in the order of appearance. Acute encephalitis occurs in 1 to 2 per 1,000 reported cases and may be fatal.

- **Diagnosis.** This is usually made on clinical grounds, but viral cultures of body fluids or serologic testing is confirmatory. Specific immunoglobulin M (IgM) antibody is usually detectable by 72 hours after onset of the rash.[1]
- **Treatment** of uncomplicated infections is supportive. Vitamin A, 200,000 IU orally once daily for 2 days, is associated with lower mortality.[1]

RUBELLA (GERMAN MEASLES)

- **Causative agent.** Rubella is caused by a single-stranded RNA virus of the family Togaviridae. Infection is acquired through contact or droplet transmission.
- **Clinical manifestations** may include low-grade fever, postauricular adenopathy, headache, and myalgias. Rash consists of pink–red lesions that are discrete and do not coalesce. They appear first on the face and spread rapidly downward to the neck, arms, trunk, and lower extremities. The total duration is 3 to 4 days, with occasional brawny desquamation. Complications are rare but may include joint manifestations, thrombotic thrombocytopenia purpura, and encephalitis.
- **Diagnosis** is clinical but this can be unreliable. Diagnosis should be confirmed with serologic antibody testing for rubella IgM antibody or paired sera for IgG antibody titers.[2]
- **Treatment** is symptomatic and supportive.

ROSEOLA INFANTUM (EXANTHEM SUBITUM; SIXTH DISEASE)

- **Causative agent.** Roseola is caused by the human herpesvirus type 6 (HHV-6). It is the most common viral exanthem in children younger than 2 years.
- **Clinical manifestations** include abrupt onset of fever, commonly 40 to 40.6°C, which persists for 3 to 5 days with a rapid decline. Other symptoms include fussiness, rhinorrhea, and cough. Rash appears after defervescence. The lesions are pink macules or maculopapules 2 to 3 mm in diameter that blanch with pressure. They appear first on the trunk and then spread to the neck, face, and upper and lower extremities. The total duration is 1 to 2 days.
- **Diagnosis** is clinical. Serologic testing for HHV-6 IgM and IgG are available. The use of saliva specimens for HHV-6 DNA can be performed.[3]
- **Treatment** is symptomatic and supportive.

ERYTHEMA INFECTIOSUM (FIFTH DISEASE)

- **Causative agent.** Erythema infectiosum is caused by the human parvovirus B19. It is moderately contagious, with outbreaks occurring in families, daycare centers, and classrooms.
- **Clinical manifestations** include fever and myalgias. Potential complications include erythrocyte aplasia, arthropathy, and fetal hydrops. Rash has a sudden onset on the face, with marked erythema ("slapped cheek" appearance). This is followed by a generalized lace-like rash on the trunk and extremities that may persist for several weeks. Heat, bathing, sunlight, or local irritation may cause a flare up of the rash.
- **Diagnosis** is clinical but may be confirmed by serologic testing for parvovirus IgM antibody. IgG antibody may be helpful for determining past infection and immunity but substantial interindividual variation make it less useful. Direct B19 DNA hybridization methods are very reliable but more expensive.
- **Treatment** of uncomplicated cases is supportive. A 5- to 10-day course of immune globulin (0.4 mg/kg) has been curative in patients with congenital immune deficiency.[4]

ENTEROVIRAL INFECTIONS

- **Causative agent or agents.** The enteroviruses consist of numerous strains of echoviruses, Coxsackie viruses, and polioviruses. Incidence of these infections is greatest in the summer and fall.
- **Clinical manifestations** are varied and include fever, gastroenteritis, respiratory disease, meningitis, and myocarditis. Rash consists of exanthems that are often rubella-like in appearance. They tend to be generalized, maculopapular, and nonpruritic. Petechial lesions are sometimes seen with type 9 echovirus and Coxsackie virus type A. Hand,

foot, and mouth disease is characterized by vesicular stomatitis and cutaneous lesions of the distal extremities. Duration of enterovirus infections varies with age and viral type, lasting from a few days to 2 weeks.

- **Diagnosis** is clinical but may be difficult and often becomes one of exclusion. Serologic testing is available but is usually not acutely helpful. PCR testing of blood, cerebrospinal fluid (CSF), and feces is available but rarely indicated.
- **Treatment** of uncomplicated cases is symptomatic and supportive. Pleconaril and other compounds against enteroviruses are in various stages of development but not routinely available.

KAWASAKI DISEASE (MUCOCUTANEOUS LYMPH NODE SYNDROME)

- **Causative agent.** Kawasaki disease remains one of unknown cause; it predominantly affects infants and children under the age of 5 years.
- **Clinical manifestations** include fever ($\geq$5 days), nonpurulent conjunctivitis, erythema and fissuring of the lips, induration of the hands and feet, enlarged lymph node mass (>1.5 cm), and rash. The rash is deeply erythematous and polymorphic and most commonly manifests as pruritic plaques that vary from 2 to 10 mm. They may resemble urticaria or the target lesions of erythema multiforme. Distribution is variable and may be diffuse, truncal, or limited to the extremities. It slowly fades with resolution of clinical illness. Coronary artery aneurysms occur as sequelae of vasculitis in 20% to 25% of untreated children.[5]
- **Diagnosis** is clinical and must include five of the six clinical manifestations mentioned above. "Atypical Kawasaki disease," which is becoming increasingly recognized, is attributed to children who do not meet the case definition but have compatible laboratory findings and no other explanation for their illness. They are treated the same as patients with classic Kawasaki disease.
- **Treatment** includes intravenous γ-globulin (2 g/kg as a single 10- to 12-hour infusion) and aspirin (100 mg/kg/day until afebrile or 14 days into the illness; decrease to 5 to 10 mg/kg/day until erythrocyte sedimentation rate and platelet count normalize).

INFECTIOUS MONONUCLEOSIS IN CHILDREN

- **Causative agent.** Mononucleosis, which is caused by the Epstein–Barr virus (EBV), occurs in children but is most commonly seen in adolescents and young adults (See Chapter 19.3).
- **Clinical manifestations** usually include fever, tonsillopharyngitis, cervical lymphadenopathy, and splenomegaly. The rash with EBV infection occurs in 10% to 15% of patients and is usually on the trunk and arms. It is erythematous, macular and papular, or morbilliform. It appears during the first day or two of clinical illness and disappears by day 6 or 7. Inappropriate administration of amoxicillin or other antibiotic can result in a diffuse copper-colored rash.
- **Diagnosis** is made by serologic testing for EBV antibody, most commonly the Monospot test although more specific EBV antibody testing (VCA-IgG and IgM) is available.[6]
- **Treatment** is symptomatic and supportive for uncomplicated cases.

PRIMARY VARICELLA (CHICKENPOX)

- **Causative agent.** Varicella is caused by the varicella-zoster virus (VZV) and is one of the most contagious of childhood viral illnesses.
- **Clinical manifestations** include fever, headache, and malaise. Rash is characterized by the rapid evolution of macule to papule to vesicle. The vesicles, which resemble dewdrops, are 2 to 3 mm in diameter, pruritic, and rupture easily. The lesions appear in crops involving the face, extremities, and trunk. A unique feature of the rash is that the lesions in all stages may be found in the same anatomical area. They crust over by day 7 to 10.
- **Diagnosis** is clinical. Culture is the gold standard. Direct immunofluorescence (DFA) via monoclonal antibody can provide results in several hours. PCR is also available to differentiate between wild-type and vaccine VZV strains. Utility of serology (IgM and IgG) for rapid diagnosis has not been demonstrated.[7]

■ **Treatment** is usually symptomatic and may include antipyretics and antihistamines. Oral or intravenous acyclovir is sometimes used in complicated cases or for immuno-compromised children. The live-attenuated VZV vaccine is highly effective in preventing primary varicella although breakthrough cases do occur but are usually mild compared to primary infection.

References

1. Cochrane Library 2005; Issue 4:CD001479.
2. Weir E, Sider D. A refresher of rubella. *CMAJ* 2005;172(13):1680–1681.
3. Zerr DM, Meier AS, Selke SS. A population-based study of primary human herpesviurs 6 infection. *N Engl J Med* 2005;352:768–776.
4. Young NS, Brown KE. Parvovirus B19. *N Engl J Med* 2004;350:586–597.
5. Falcini F. Kawasaki disease. *Curr Opin Rheumatol* 2006;18:33–38.
6. Ebell MH. Epstein-Barr virus mononucleosis. *Am Fam Physician* 2004;70:1279–1290.
7. Hambleton S, Gershon AA. Preventing varicella-zoster disease. *Clin Micro Rev* 2005;18(1):70–80.

MUSCULOSKELETAL PROBLEMS OF CHILDREN AND ADOLESCENTS
John R. Gimpel, Stephen R. Mitchell

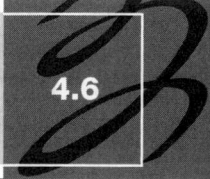

4.6

SCOLIOSIS

Scoliosis is a lateral and rotational spinal curvature. Curves greater than 10 degrees are present in 2% to 4% of adolescents at the end of their growth period. The majority of curves are due to idiopathic scoliosis and emerge in adolescence (age 10 to skeletal maturity), whereas infantile scoliosis (before age 3: less than 1% of cases) and juvenile scoliosis (age 3 to 10: 12% to 21% of cases) are much less common. Severe curves (greater than 100 degrees) are uncommon, are more likely to have an infantile or juvenile onset, and may lead to significant restrictive pulmonary disease and a shortened life expectancy. Secondary forms of scoliosis are caused by inherited disorders of connective tissue (e.g., Ehlers–Danlos syndrome, Marfan syndrome), neurologic disorders (e.g., syringomyelia, tethered cord syndrome, spinal tumors, neurofibromatosis, upper and lower motor neuron disease), and musculoskeletal conditions (e.g., herniated disc, osteogenesis imperfecta, spondylolysis, developmental dysplasia of the hip, leg length discrepancy).

Idiopathic Adolescent Scoliosis

This is the most common spinal deformity evaluated by primary care physicians, present in 2% to 4% of the general population, and is more common in females. The etiology is believed to be multifactorial, with a strong familial predisposition, although no single pattern of genetic predisposition has been accepted. Significant controversy surrounds the clinical recommendations for school-based screening as well as treatment of patients with scoliosis. The most common curve pattern is a right thoracic apex (90% of thoracic curves), followed by right thoracic–left lumbar, thoracolumbar, double thoracic, and left lumbar curves. Patients with other curve patterns or curves associated with pain or stiffness that are likely due to underlying pathology should undergo expedient evaluation.

■ **Clinical presentation.** Children generally present with cosmetic concerns or are referred through school screening programs. Significant pain may be suggestive of an underlying tumor or inflammatory process and is generally not part of idiopathic adolescent scoliosis. Neurologic symptoms should be elicited, which may be red flags for secondary causes.

- **Physical examination.** The physical examination reveals varying asymmetries in shoulder and iliac crest height, asymmetrical scapular prominence, and a flank crease. Curves are deemed as "right" or "left" based on their convexity, and named for the location of their apex vertebrae. The Adam forward bending test is the most sensitive and should reveal a right thoracic and possibly a left lumbar prominence. The neurologic examination and gait should be normal. Height measurements with the patient sitting and standing can be repeated every 3 to 4 months to monitor the growth spurt and gauge risk of progression. A scoliometer may be useful for follow-up and reassurance for the patient and family, but can be difficult to standardize and therefore somewhat unreliable.
- **Radiographs.** Patients with a scoliometer reading greater than 5 degrees or who are otherwise suspected of a significant curve can be screened with a single, standing, 36-inch posteroanterior (PA) film. The vertebral levels with the greatest tilt are identified and measured by the Cobb method (the angle between intersecting lines drawn perpendicular to the top of the most tilted vertebrae above the apex and the bottom of vertebrae below the apex is the Cobb angle). Magnetic resonance imaging (MRI) should be considered in patients with onset of scoliosis before age 8, an unusual curve pattern (e.g., left thoracic), rapid curve progression (more than 1 degree/month), neurologic symptoms or deficit, or significant pain.
- **Risk factors for progression**
  - Spinal growth correlates with ossification of the iliac apophysis from anteriolaterally to posteriomedially. Risser grades of 0 to 2 (Table 4.6-1) are associated with an increased risk, and patients closer to skeletal maturity (i.e., Risser grades 3 to 4) have a somewhat lower risk of progression. Assessing the epiphyseal status on wrist radiographs can also be used.
  - Girls, especially between the onset of the pubertal growth spurt (age 10 to 12) until cessation of spinal growth (Risser 4), are at risk for progression of scoliosis. On average, a girl with scoliosis generally has a relatively higher risk of progression before age 12, and a relatively lower risk after age 12.5. Girls generally have a tenfold higher risk of progression than boys.
  - Clinical markers of maturity, such as Tanner staging or age at menarche, are important in the evaluation. Peak curve progression occurs during Tanner stage 2 or 3. Delayed puberty and menarche are risk factors for progression. Hypoestrogen status delays maturation of osseous growth centers and allows an accentuated curve.
  - Thoracic curves or curves with their apex at a higher vertebral level are at greater risk.
  - Overall risk of progression: >10 degrees: 2% to 3%; >20 degrees: 0.3% to 0.5%; >30 degrees: 0.1% to 0.3%; >40 degrees, <0.1%.

- **Treatment**
  - **Curvature of 0 to 10 degrees is normal.**
  - For curvature of 10 to 15 degrees, follow up every 6 months for clinical recheck with forward bending test and scoliometer test to check for progression.
  - For curvature of 15 to 20 degrees, repeat radiographs every 3 to 4 months in a growing child with a larger curve. For smaller curves or near the end of growth, repeat radiographs in 6 to 8 months.

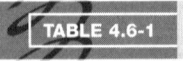

TABLE 4.6-1	The Risser Grading System for Spinal Maturity

Grade 0: No ossification
Grade 1: Ossification of 0% to 25%
Grade 2: 25% to 50%
Grade 3: 50% to 75%
Grade 4: 75% to 100%
Grade 5: Fusion to ilium

■ For curves greater than 20 degrees, refer to an orthopaedic subspecialist for consideration of close follow-up, bracing, and surgical options. Especially in light of the lack of evidence of progression to significant morbidity and mortality in most cases of scoliosis, the trend is currently away from bracing unless curves are 60 degrees or greater, or 40 degrees in patients lacking skeletal maturity. Surgical options (rod placement and bone grafting) for severe curves are generally used in only those patients with growth remaining.

SPONDYLOLYSIS AND SPONDYLOLISTHESIS

Spondylolysis is a bony defect of the vertebral pars interarticularis. It is generally considered to be a stress fracture due to repetitive lumbar hyperextension and is most common at L5 to S1. The pars defect may also be congenital, and is present in 5% to 6% of North Americans and more than 50% of Alaskan Native Americans or in those with a family history of spondylolysis. It is four times more common in gymnasts than in the general population, and should be considered in dancers, divers, cheerleaders, weightlifters, volleyball players, and football lineman, among other athletes, who present with back pain. Nonathletes may be genetically predisposed to pars breakdown with minimal stress, whereas athletes likely place undue stress on a normal pars. In 47% of athletes with back pain, spondylolysis is the cause. Spondylolisthesis is forward or anterior displacement of the cephalad vertebral body on the caudad one, and may be related to a history of spondylolysis, where bilateral defects allow the forward slippage. Grade I spondylolisthesis is displacement of 0% to 25%; grade II, 25% to 50%; grade III, 50% to 75%; grade IV, 75% to 100%; and grade V indicates slippage greater than 100%, which means no overlap of the two vertebral bodies.

Clinical Presentation

Low back pain develops in late childhood and early adolescence and is generally mild. Those with signs of inflammatory back pain, including prolonged morning stiffness, where pain is improved by exercise, and unrelieved by rest may in fact have anklylosing spondylitis (those who are HLA B27 positive have a 20% risk; See Chapter 15.2). In contrast, with spondylolisthesis or spondylolyis, back pain is aggravated with activities requiring lumbar hypertension, such as gymnastics, football (linemen), and ballet. The pain is midline or slightly lateral and may be referred to the buttocks or thighs. Radicular pain is unusual except in grade III slips or greater.

Physical Examination

Patients may have a stiff-legged gait due to tight hamstrings. Excessive lumbar lordosis is often present and there may be tenderness of the lumbar paraspinous muscles, or other evidence of somatic dysfunction (tissue texture abnormalities, asymmetry, decreased intersegmental range of motion, tenderness) at the affected level. Forward flexion does not aggravate the pain, whereas back hyperextension does. In the single-leg hyperextension ("stork" test) test, the patient stands, grasps one knee, and hyperextends the low back. Back pain on the weight-bearing side suggests an ipsilateral pars interarticularis defect.

Radiographs

The initial diagnostic workup for athletes with back pain of 3 or more weeks duration should include posteroanterior, lateral, and right and left oblique views of the lumbosacral spine. The most common site of involvement is between the fifth lumbar and first sacral segment. The pars interarticularis is best visualized on the oblique views, which show a lucent or sclerotic line known as the "collar of the Scottie dog." The lateral view demonstrates the amount of slippage in spondylolisthesis. If radiographs are normal and suspicion remains, a bone scan or single-photon emission computed tomography (SPECT) scan is indicated. SPECT is the most sensitive test and should be done if the plain bone scan is normal. MRI inadequately visualizes the pars in up to one third of cases and should not be relied on to rule out the diagnosis.

Treatment

- **Spondylolysis.** Any activity that causes pain should be restricted and the patient started on an antilordosis program of rehabilitation (abdominal and back strengthening, hamstring and hip flexor stretching). If pain persists in spite of conservative treatment, the patient should be placed in an antilordosis brace, such as a Boston overlap brace with 0 degree lordosis. The brace is worn during waking hours or up to 23 hours per day. For the first 2 to 3 weeks the patient performs only hamstring stretches. After 2 to 3 weeks or when pain subsides, lumbosacral stretches and abdominal strengthening out of the brace is added. Sporting activity while the brace is worn can be resumed when asymptomatic. Bracing can be weaned after 4 months if the individual is pain free with full sporting activity in the brace. The brace is tapered off by decreasing wear by 1 hour per day each week. Total bracing time is generally 6 to 9 months. Patients should be followed radiographically every 4 to 6 months for possible progression to spondylolisthesis. Patients with persistent pain should be referred.
- **Spondylolisthesis.** Patients with slippage up to 50% can be treated initially similarly to spondylolysis. Patients with slippage greater than 50% or with pain resistant to conservative treatment should be comanaged by an orthopaedic or spine surgeon.

JUVENILE KYPHOSIS (SCHEUERMANN DISEASE)

Scheuermann disease is an idiopathic condition resulting in anterior wedging of the thoracic vertebrae and a kyphotic deformity greater than 45 degrees. It occurs in approximately 4% to 8% of the population, is equally common in male and female adolescents, and affected individuals are likely genetically predisposed.

Diagnosis

Patients generally present at the onset of puberty (12 to 13 years) with a concern of a progressive "round back" deformity occasionally associated with pain. Pain is generally mild and activity related, but is not activity limiting or associated with easy back fatigability. The round-back deformity is accentuated by forward bending but does not fully correct with extension. Approximately one third of patients have associated scoliosis. Excess lumbar lordosis is common and predisposes to spondylolysis at L5 to S1. Severe kyphosis may be associated with cord compression, extradural cysts, thoracic disk herniation, or restrictive lung disease, but these manifestations are rare.

Radiographs

Complete evaluation requires full-length standing anteroposterior (AP) and lateral spine films. The lateral view shows irregularity of the involved vertebral end plates and anterior wedging of three or more contiguous vertebrae by 5 degrees or more. Kyphosis between T4 and T12 measured by the angle of Cobb is greater than 45 degrees. Only one or two vertebral bodies may be involved with thoracolumbar disease. The radiographs should also assess for associated scoliosis, lumbar hyperlordosis, and spondylolisthesis. Lateral hyperextension views are helpful in determining the flexibility of the deformity.

Treatment

- **General.** Treatment is based on the severity of deformity, presence of pain, and the patient's age. Curves of 45 to 60 degrees with no evidence of progression are treated with observation, an exercise program to correct lumbar lordosis (abdominal strengthening, increasing hip flexor, and hamstring flexibility), and thoracic spine hyperextension exercises. Recheck every 3 to 4 months.
- **Bracing** is indicated with significantly painful curves greater than 50 degrees, progressive deformity, or curves that are cosmetically unacceptable.[2] A modified Milwaukee brace is most commonly used in conjunction with exercises, is best if initiated before skeletal maturity, and generally requires 12 to 18 months of treatment. Comanagement with an orthopaedic or spine subspecialist is warranted.
- **Surgery** is indicated with severe deformities (generally >75 degrees) or persistent back pain unresponsive to conservative treatment.

BACK PAIN: MECHANICAL VERSUS INFLAMMATORY

Persistent back pain is generally uncommon in childhood—including the above topics. **Inflammatory back pain,** typified by onset of pain in adolescence or preadolescence, may reflect an underlying inflammatory condition (e.g., ankylosing spondylitis or Reiter syndrome; See Chapter 15.2). This pain is typically insidious in onset (over months), not associated with trauma or any visible abnormality described above, low back in origin, worse in the morning, associated with stiffness lasting an hour or longer, improving with exercise, and worsening after sitting.

Physical Examination

- Will sometimes reveal loss of normal lordotic curve (i.e., straightening), associated with decreased forward flexion of the lower 10 cm of the lumbosacral spine. The Schober maneuver measures 10 cm up from a line drawn between the sacroiliac "dimples" when standing fully upright and marks start and end of that distance. The child then bends forward and the distance between the two marked spots is remeasured. The normal lumbar spine expands from the baseline 10 cm out to 15 cm (expansion of 5 cm). Loss of normal lumbar expansion can indicate an early inflammatory spondyloarthropathy.
- In addition, when hip flexion, extension, internal and external rotation are normal—but crossing the leg, and pressing down on the knee and opposite pelvic brim (flexion, abduction, external rotation [Faber test]) causes pain in the sacroiliac joint, or the groin—there may be inflammation of the sacroiliac joint.

FLATFOOT (PES PLANUS)

Flatfoot is broadly categorized as either physiologic flexible flatfoot or pathologic flatfoot. Pathologic flatfoot in infants can be secondary to the common but benign calcaneovalgus foot or a more ominous congenital vertical talus. Older children may have a tarsal coalition, hypermobile flatfoot with tight heel cords, or neurogenic flatfoot.

Flexible Flatfoot

- **Etiology.** The normal arch is not present at birth and slowly develops around 4 to 5 years of age. Excessive laxity of the joint capsule and plantar ligaments allows the developing arch to flatten out while bearing weight. In young children, a fat pad may further obscure the arch.
- **Clinical presentation.** Children are generally brought to the family physician by the parents with a concern about potential problems related to the flatfoot. There is no complaint of pain by the child.
- **Physical examination.** The child's foot flattens with weight bearing but develops an arch while the child stands on tiptoe or actively dorsiflexes the great toe. Observed from behind, the calcaneus is in valgus position while the child is standing and inverts when the child stands on tiptoe. The child's ability to stand on the heels indicates adequate heel cord flexibility. The child should be able to stand both on the inner and outer borders of the feet indicating good muscular control and adequate subtalar motion.
- **Radiographs.** Radiographs are not needed unless other pathology is suspected.
- **Treatment.** Reassure parents that no treatment is necessary because there is gradual improvement with growth, generally by age 5 years. Arch supports do not generally make a difference in radiographic or clinical outcome. The occasional child who develops symptoms associated with the flatfoot (e.g., foot pain, patellofemoral pain) should be given medial longitudinal arch supports or a medial heel wedge, or both.

Pathologic Flatfoot

Pathologic flatfoot is characterized by limited ankle motion and, frequently, foot or ankle pain. Ankle motion may be limited in dorsiflexion by a tight heel cord and in inversion and eversion by subtalar pathology.

Hypermobile Flatfoot with Tight Heel Cord

- **Etiology.** A tight heel cord combined with a flexible flatfoot forces the calcaneus into a valgus position during ambulation. This compensatory hindfoot valgus allows for more ankle dorsiflexion. The resultant abnormal foot biomechanics lead to pain.
- Clinical presentation. Patients complain of foot or ankle pain.
- **Diagnosis.** The patient has a flattened arch and calcaneal valgus when standing. Observation from the side shows early heel lift-off during the gait and an arch that develops as the toes dorsiflex. Subtalar motion (calcaneal inversion and eversion) is normal but ankle dorsiflexion is limited to neutral or less.
- **Treatment.** Patients with mild symptoms can be initially treated with aggressive heel cord stretching and a medial longitudinal arch support with a medial heel wedge. Those with more severe symptoms can be treated with a short leg walking cast, with the ankle neutral for 4 weeks followed by heel cord stretching. Surgery for heel cord lengthening and correction of heel valgus may be necessary if conservative treatment fails.

Other Causes

Congenital vertical talus and a tarsal coalition are less common congenital causes of pathologic flatfoot, requiring referral to an orthopaedic or podiatric subspecialist.

HEEL PAIN

Severs Disease

- **Calcaneal apophysitis** is common in boys between the ages of 6 and 10, especially in obese children and athletes, secondary to repetitive microtrauma or overuse of the heel. Pain is usually on the posterior side of the calcaneus, and is more pronounced after activity. Acute treatment includes temporary avoidance of high-impact activities, heel lifts or heel cups, ice massage, and nonsteroidal anti-inflammatory drugs (NSAIDs). Once stretching is not painful, adding in stretching exercises and orthotic devices can be helpful. In refractory cases, cast immobilization may be needed.
- **Plantar fasciitis.** Plantar heel pain that is sharp and occurs with weight bearing on arising in the morning or after prolonged sitting is suspicious for plantar fasciitis. This is more common in adults, but can occur in overweight children and adolescents. Palpation of the medial calcaneal tubercle usually elicits tenderness, as compared to calcaneal stress fracture, where pain is elicited with medial to lateral compression of the calcaneus. Treatment is similar as for Severs disease, with orthotic devices that counteract pronation and disperse heel strike forces, and using local injections of corticosteroids in resistant chronic cases. Also remember that heel pain, stiffness in the morning, and inflammatory type back pain can be associated with inflammatory spondyoarthropathy.

BOWLEGS (GENU VARUS)

Varus angulation of the knee can be normal, secondary to metabolic disease, severe physiologic bowing, or osteochondrosis deformans tibiae (Blount disease).

- **Normal development.** Children are born with genu varum become maximally bowlegged by 6 months, and begin to straighten by 18 to 24 months. Genu valgum or "knock-knee" develops during the second to third year and peaks by the fourth year. Development then progresses back to the normal adult alignment of slight valgus by age 7 to 8 years. **Bowlegs should be fully evaluated if they have not corrected by age 2.**
- **Metabolic etiology.** Parents should be questioned regarding diet, and the child's growth curve should be reviewed. Rickets, abnormal calcium or phosphorus metabolism, and renal disease should be considered. If a generalized disorder is suspected, screening laboratory tests should be ordered, including serum calcium, phosphorus, alkaline phosphatase, creatinine, and hematocrit.

Severe Physiologic Bowing and Blount Disease

- **Clinical presentation.** The child has a painless bilateral genu varus that is of concern to the parents. Growth and development is otherwise normal.
- **Diagnosis.** Standing posteroanterior radiographs must be obtained while the child's feet are together or shoulder-width apart and patellae directly forward. A tibiofemoral angle of more than 20 degrees is abnormal.

- **Severe physiologic bowing.** This is characterized by medial metaphyseal beaking of the distal femur and proximal tibia, medial cortical thickening, and no pathologic changes of the proximal medial tibial epiphysis.
- **Blount disease.** This disorder is characterized by angulation under the posteromedial proximal tibial epiphysis, tibial metaphyseal irregularity, beaking of the proximal tibia, and wedging of the proximal epiphysis.
- **Treatment**
  - **Severe physiologic bowing.** Spontaneous correction generally occurs by age 7 to 8 years. Surgery may be indicated if the deformity persists past age 8.
  - **Blount disease.** Patients should be referred for consideration of surgery once the diagnosis is made or suspected.

INTOEING

General

Intoeing affects a large number of infants and children and is a major source of concern for parents, leading to consultation and questions. Understanding the primary cause of concern is helpful in counseling the parents of the child with intoeing. Knowledge of what is normal and what will self-correct with normal growth and development will prevent unnecessary treatment, identify the rare causes that need intervention, and reassure most parents that the condition will resolve over time with normal growth. The most common causes are metatarsus adductus, medial (internal) tibial torsion, and increased femoral anteversion, and vary in proportion to the age of the child.

Rotational Profile

The parents' attention focuses on the child's feet, but the source of intoeing can be anywhere in the lower extremities. Certain definitions are needed to facilitate evaluation of the gait and the lower extremities (Figure 4.6-1).

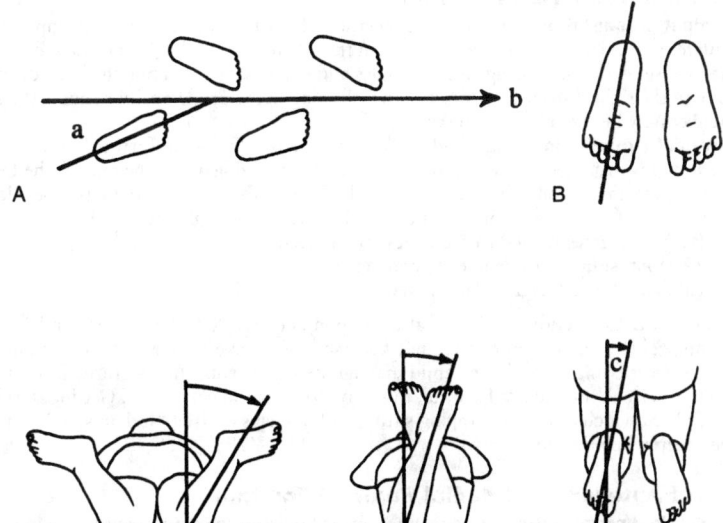

Figure 4.6-1. Rotational profile. **A:** The angle between the line of progression (b) and the foot axis is the foot progression angle (a). **B:** Foot axis. **C:** Internal (medial) femoral rotation. **D:** External (lateral) femoral rotation. **E:** Thigh–foot angle (c) is formed by the foot axis and the longitudinal axis of the femur.

- **Line of progression** is an imaginary line indicating the path of movement of the body while walking.
- **Foot axis** relates to metatarsus adductus. An imaginary line bisects the long axis of the foot from the mid-heel through the middle of the metatarsal heads.
- **Foot progression angle** is the angle of the intersection between the foot axis and the line of progression.
- **Internal and external femoral rotation** are indices of femoral version. The child lies prone with the knees flexed at 90 degrees. The pelvis is stabilized and the angle of gravity-assisted internal and external rotation of each leg is measured.
- **Thigh–foot angle** indicates tibial torsion. An imaginary line through the long axis of the foot is measured against the long axis of the femur, measured with the child in the prone position and the knees flexed at 90 degrees.

Metatarsus Adductus

- **Clinical presentation.** This is the most common cause of intoeing seen in the first year of life, either alone or combined with tibial torsion, and the most common congenital foot deformity (1 in 1,000 live births). Presentation may be unilateral or bilateral, and it is found more commonly in females, as well as more so on the left side. The most likely etiology is intrauterine positioning.
- **Physical examination.** The foot is convex laterally and concave medially, with possibly a prominence at the base of the fifth metatarsal. With the heel held in neutral position and pressure directed laterally at the first metatarsal head, a flexible deformity corrects to neutral but does not overcorrect (as do normal feet). Flexible deformities may self-correct if the lateral border of the foot is stroked. Rigid metatarsus adductus does not allow either active or passive correction of the deformity.
- **Treatment.** This condition resolves spontaneously by age 1 year in more than 90% of cases. Treatment of flexible metatarsus adductus involves having the parents passively correct the deformity with each diaper change. Referral for sequential casting is necessary for rigid metatarsus and is most effective if started early, preferably in the first month of life.

Medial (Internal) Tibial Torsion

- **Clinical presentation.** Parents are concerned about the appearance of asymptomatic unilateral or bilateral intoeing, generally in their 1- to 2-year-old. This is the most common cause of intoeing, being equal in males and females, but affecting the left side more so than the right. Intrauterine positioning, sleeping in the prone position, and sitting on the feet may be the primary causes.
- **Physical examination.** The child walks with the patella facing forward and the feet pointing inward. Determine the thigh–foot angle by gazing along the axis of the lower leg with the child prone and the knee flexed (Figure 4.6-1). Be sure there is no evidence of metatarsus adductus. Normal values of the thigh–foot angle are as follows:
  - Birth: 5 degrees medial to 5 degrees lateral version
  - 12 months: up to 10 degrees lateral version
  - Adults: 10 to 20 degrees lateral version
- **Treatment.** Correction is almost always spontaneous (90% by age 8), and braces, splints, cables, and orthotics have not been shown to be effective. The condition usually corrects by age 3 to 4. The child may habitually sit with the feet turned in toward the buttocks. Although not harmful, this may slow natural correction. Getting the child his or her own chair or encouraging sitting with the legs crossed "Indian style" in front may help while the child grows.

Femoral Anteversion (Medial Femoral Torsion)

- **Clinical presentation.** A congenital inward twist of the femur causes turning in of the knee, leg, and foot and commonly presents between 3 and 7 years of age. This is often familial, affecting girls more than boys.
- **Physical examination.** These children walk with their patellae and feet pointing inward. The gait appears very clumsy, with frequent tripping. With the child prone and the knees bent at a right angle, the degree of internal rotation of the thighs is

greater than that of external rotation. Medial rotation is normally less than 70 degrees for girls and 60 degrees for boys. Mild anteversion is 70 to 80 degrees, moderate is 80 to 90 degrees, and severe is greater than 90 degrees.

■ **Treatment.** Medial femoral torsion tends to correct spontaneously with growth (80%). Special braces are not necessary because it is impossible to "brace" the femur into external rotation. Rarely, patients may need surgical derotation in their teen years if there is a severe torsion resulting in significant cosmetic or functional problems. Discouragement of children from sitting in the "W" position (with their lower legs outside of their thighs) may help natural correction.

COMMON HIP PROBLEMS

Developmental Dysplasia of the Hip

Formerly referred to as congenital hip dysplasia of the hip, developmental dysplasia of the hip (DDH) includes several conditions associated with impaired development and growth of the hip. DDH in the infant represents a spectrum from subtle hip laxity to frank dislocation. The incidence is one to two cases per 1,000 children of European descent, and is rare is black Africans. It is four times more common in females and three times more common in the left hip than in the right. The most significant risk factor is a positive family history, and oligohydramnios. Newborn screening for this condition has greatly diminished the negative outcomes and is essential for early diagnosis and treatment, and a high index of suspicion is important to avoid missed or "late" diagnosis (beyond 3 months of age). Missing the diagnosis of DDH is the fourth most common cause of malpractice suits in pediatrics.

■ **Physical examination.** Serial physical examination remains the primary method for diagnosing DDH in infants, and should continue at well visits until the child is walking. Under optimal circumstances the infant will be relaxed during the examination and only one hip examined at a time.

■ **Barlow test.** One hand stabilizes the pelvis with the infant supine and the other hand holds the hip to be examined with the thumb in the groin and the forefinger over the greater trochanter. The hip is flexed to 90 degrees and gentle pressure is exerted posteriorly with the web space of the examiner's hand while lateral pressure is exerted with the thumb. With this maneuver the unstable hip can be felt to dislocate from the acetabulum ("dislocatable" and "positive" test).

■ **Ortolani test.** After Barlow's maneuver, the hip is abducted and gently lifted. Relocation of the dislocated femoral head is palpable (and sometimes audible) in a positive Ortolani reduction test. It is important to note that "clicks" or "pops" are not diagnostic of this condition but rather indicate a palpable femoral head leaving the acetabulum. Audible high pitched "clicks" without a sensation of instability usually have no particular significance.

■ **Older children** (>3 months) may be more difficult to examine, and are less likely to exhibit a positive Ortolani test. Signs to consider include tight or limited hip abduction; apparent shortening of the femur; uneven gluteal, groin, or thigh folds; telescoping of the affected hip; uneven knees when the child is supine with the hips flexed; or a limp or waddled gait.

■ **Imaging tests.** Plain radiographs are unreliable before 3 months of age. Radiographs may show proximal and lateral migration of the femoral head or poor acetabular development. Because of the dependence on positioning of the hips during examinations, there are many false-positive and false-negative results. Ultrasonography is the procedure of choice in the infant, and is best performed when the infant is 4 to 6 weeks old.

■ **Treatment.** The newborn who has a dislocated hip (positive Ortolani and irreducible) should be referred immediately to an orthopaedic specialist. In the 0- to 5 or 6-month age group, treatment is generally by Pavlik harness (a brace that places the hips in flexion and abduction) for the reducible hip and traction; closed reduction or spica cast is used for the unreducible hip or older child. As a dislocatable hip (positive Barlow) may stabilize within a few weeks, use of an abduction pillow and delayed referral and re-examination in 2 weeks may be an appropriate option. Avascular necrosis develops in 2.5 of 1,000 infants treated with the Pavlik harness prior to 6 months and 109 of 1,000 of those referred later. Surgical release of the adductor and iliopsoas muscles may be necessary in older infants than those who are walking, or even open reduction with femoral and/or pelvic osteotomy in children older than 2.

Legg—Calvé—Perthes Disease

Also known as avascular necrosis (osteonecrosis) of the femoral head, this is a mysterious disease with an unclear etiology. It is rare in toddlers but more common in children 4 to 9 years of age, has a male-to-female ratio of 5:1, and is bilateral 10% to 20% of the time.

- **Clinical presentation.** The patient usually presents with a limp, which is painless at first and then becomes painful only after activity. Pain becomes more constant and is frequently referred to the thigh or knee. Symptoms can be variable, and this entity must be considered in any child with a limp and/or groin, thigh, or knee pain. About 10% seem to be familial, and children with HIV seem to be at increased risk.
- **Physical examination.** The child may favor the hip and be unwilling to bear weight on it for any length of time. There may be slight limb shortening, and there is generally a decreased range of motion of the hip joint, especially in internal rotation and abduction. The most sensitive physical examination maneuver for intra-articular hip pathology is the prone internal rotation test.
- **Radiographs.** The diagnosis demands a high index of clinical suspicion, as radiographs are usually normal for the first 3 to 6 weeks of the disease. They may later show flattening or irregularity of the femoral head. Technetium bone scanning or MRI is useful to confirm early disease.
- **Treatment.** In younger children with early disease, treatment mainly consists of activity limitation and therapy to regain motion of the hip. The painful hip may require traction, crutches, Petrie cast, or abduction brace. Children identified before 6 to 8 years of age have a better prognosis. Recovery is more likely with disease diagnosed before age 5 to 6.[5] Orthopaedic specialist is recommended.

Slipped Capital Femoral Epiphysis

- **Clinical presentation.** Defined as a posterior and inferior slippage of the proximal femoral epiphysis on the metaphysis (femoral neck), slipped capital femoral epiphysis (SCFE) is the major hip disorder during the adolescent growth spurt, usually presenting in 11- to 14-year-old subjects and twice as often in boys as in girls. It occurs more commonly in obese children and in black or Polynesian children, and is bilateral in up to 40% of cases. The most common presentation is a chronic limp, although patients can present with acute hip pain and inability to walk, or more vague activity-related pain in the thigh, hip, groin, or knee. These symptoms warrant high suspicion and an immediate evaluation. Most cases are stable and have a good prognosis if diagnosed early.
- **Physical examination.** The child is generally overweight (80th to 100th percentile). Range of motion is limited in hip flexion, abduction, and internal rotation, and forced internal rotation causes groin or knee pain. Obligatory external rotation of the femur with passive hip flexion is a pathognomonic sign.
- **Radiographs.** Widening of the growth plate is an early visible sign on the supine AP view, but it may be more obvious on the frog-leg lateral view as the hip slips farther posteriorly than medially. Technetium bone scanning or MRI is useful in diagnosing preslips and questionable cases.
- **Treatment.** Once identified, this merits prompt orthopaedic referral. Treatment consists of avoiding any weight bearing and obtaining immediate orthopaedic evaluation. *In situ* fixation with a single central screw is the most widely used surgical treatment, and it is essential to recognize this condition early to avoid the complications of hip osteonecrosis and cartilage erosion.

Transient Synovitis

This relatively common disorder (0.2% annual incidence) typically occurs in children 3 to 8 years old, and is about two times more common in boys. It usually presents with unilateral pain and stiffness of the hip, but is bilateral in 5% to 10% of cases, and typically symptoms have been present for less than 1 week. Fever is typically absent or low grade, and children are nontoxic in appearance. Higher fevers and systemic symptoms, while they can occur, should prompt the urgent need to rule out septic arthritis. Of patients, 30% to 50% report having had a recent upper respiratory tract infection. Management is conservative, once septic arthritis has been excluded, and includes rest, NSAIDs, and return to full activity as tolerated. Radiographs, white blood count, and erythrocyte sedimentation rate can be followed by ultrasound-guided aspiration of the hip joint if necessary to exclude septic arthritis.

COMMON KNEE PROBLEMS

Osgood–Schlatter Disease

Commonly encountered in athletic children 10 to 15 years of age after a rapid growth spurt, especially in those who play jumping sports, such as soccer, gymnastics, basketball, and volleyball. This disorder is thought to be a traction apophysitis of the proximal tibial tuberosity at the insertion of the patellar tendon secondary to repetitive microtrauma.

- **Clinical presentation.** Anterior knee pain and swelling, which is bilateral in 30% of the cases. Swelling and tenderness of the tibial tuberosity. Hip examination should be performed to rule out referred pain (e.g., from slipped capital femoral epiphysis). Radiographs are generally not indicated unless symptoms are atypical or there are findings suggestive of osteomylelitis (e.g., warmth, erythema) or tumor.
- **Treatment.** Quadriceps stretching, ice, NSAIDs, and occasional resting periods are recommended, but complete avoidance of sports activities is generally not necessary or recommended. A protective pad over the tibial tuberosity may be helpful. The prognosis usually is excellent with conservative management.

Patellofemoral Pain Syndrome

Very common cause of retropatellar or peripatellar pain, particularly in adolescent female athletes. These patients typically have anterior knee pain that occurs with activity and worsens with steps or hills, and can also be triggered by prolonged sitting. It is likely due to overuse, overload, biomechanical factors, and muscular dysfunction. It is also found more commonly in patients with pes planus or pes cavus. Radiographs are appropriate in pain that persists for 4 to 6 weeks to exclude neoplasm or osteochondritis dessicans. Treatment includes ice, NSAIDs, relative rest, evaluation of footwear, and quadriceps strengthening. Taping, knees sleeves, and braces are somewhat controversial, and surgical approaches are considered a last resort (e.g., lateral release if excessive lateral tracking).

BENIGN ARTHRALGIAS OF CHILDHOOD

Growing Pains

Recurrent, self-limited pains in the extremities for which the child, parents, or physicians have no definitive explanation for are often labeled as "growing pains." These are benign, and usually resolve with 1 to 2 years of onset. Usually begin with ages 2 to 12, and may occur in 10% to 20% of school-aged children. Etiology unclear, but not actually caused by growth. Bilateral and symmetrical, usually hurt late in day or at night and usually do not interfere with daytime activities. Primarily in lower extremities, but may also occur in upper extremities, but usually in conjunction with lower extremity pain. Pain is deep, bilateral thighs or calf. Paroxysmal: quite severe at times, symptom free for days, and may interrupt sleep. Relieved by massage, heat, analgesics. Often the episodes may be associated with disruptive crying often within an hour of retiring and usually are better with parental massage. Accentuated by increased activity during the day, and may be related to overuse. Some have speculated that the pain originally starts with a mild increase in compartmental pressure that usually causes muscle pain more than joint pain. Physical exam normal. Often there may be significant psychologic overlay. It often responds to a period of nightly ibuprofen, especially on days with pain.

Benign Hypermobility

Some patients have hypermobility of joints and yet do not have another well-characterized connective tissue disease, such as Marfan syndrome or Ehlers–Danlos syndrome. Hypermobility may be present in 10% to 15% of girls, and somewhat less in boys. These patients can often extend the elbow more than 10 degrees beyond neutral, dorsiflex the fingers at the metacarpals to 90 degrees, retroflex the knee more than 10 degrees beyond vertical into recurvatum, oppose the thumb to the forearm, and place both palms on the floor without bending the knees. Most will have a passive flat foot. Some are asymptomatic, but others have joint pains and other recurrent somatic dysfunction and have been characterized as having benign hypermobile joint syndrome. Characteristically this can be daytime pain, and may disrupt walking and prolonged activities. Small joints in the hand may hurt with writing; this responds to using large pencils or padded pen holders to increase circumference. With growth, the adolescent usually has good athletic ability, but pain after prolonged activity. There is some increase in risk of ligamentous injury that will respond to preventive, periarticular muscular strengthening (e.g., quad strengthening). Some report brief episodes of joint swelling, as well as myalgias. There may be an association with fibromyalgia in some patients, and extra-articular manifestations may include anxiety, panic attacks, mitral valve prolapse syndrome, and cognitive disorders. Further study is needed.

ACKNOWLEDGMENT

The authors acknowledge Wade A. Lillegard and John P. Fogarty for their authorship of an earlier version of this chapter.

References

1. Tribus CB. Scheuermann's kyphosis in adolescents and adults: diagnosis and management. *J Am Acad Orthop Surg* 1988;6:36.
2. Bruce RW. Torsional and angular deformities. *Pediatr Clin North Am* 1996;43:867.
3. American Academy of Pediatrics. Clinical practice guideline: early detection of developmental dysplasia of the hip. *Pediatrics* 2000;105:896.
4. Biro F, Gewanter HL, Baum J. The hypermobility syndrome. *Pediatrics* 1983; 72(5):701.
5. Screening for developmental dysplasia of the hip. Evidence synthesis no. 42. Rockville, MD: Agency for Health care Research and Quality. Accessed March 29, 2006, at: hppt://www.ahrq.gov/downloads/pub/prevent/pdfser/hipdyssyn.pdf.
6. Shipman SA, Helfand M, Moyer VA, et al. Screening for developmental dysplasia of the hip: a systematic literature review for the U.S. Preventive Services Task Force. *Pediatrics* 2006;117:e557–576.
7. Frazer CH, Rappaport LA. Recurrent pains. In: Levine MD, Carey, WB, Crocker AC, eds., *Developmental behavioral pediatrics.* 3rd ed. Philadelphia: WB Saunders; 1999: 357.
8. The assessment and management of acute pain in infants, children, and adolescents. *Pediatrics* 2110;108:793.
9. Leet AI, Skaggs DL. Evaluation of the acutely limping child. *Am Fam Physician* 2000;61:4.
10. Cassas KJ, Cassettari-Wayhs A. Childhood and adolescent sports-related overuse injuries. *Am Fam Physician* 2006;73(6):1014–1022.
11. Sass P, Hassan G. Lower extremity abnormalities in children. *Am Fam Physician* 2003;68(3):461–468.
12. Screening for idiopathic scoliosis in adolescents; update of the evidence for the U.S. Preventive Services Task Force. Agency for Health care, Research and Quality. 2003. Accessed April 16, 2006 at www.preventiveservices.ahrq.gov.
13. Adib N, Davies K, Grahame R, et al. Joint hypermobility syndrome in childhood. A not so benign multisystem disorder? *Rheumatology* (Oxford) 2005;44:744.
14. Osgood-Schlatter disease. In: Greene WB, ed., *Essentials of musculoskeletal care.* 2nd ed. Rosemont, IL: American Academy of Orthopedic Surgeons; 2001:719.

ENURESIS 4.7

William L. Toffler, Shawn H. Blanchard

$\mathcal{E}$nuresis, or involuntary urination, is a common problem among children. Primary enuresis describes a pattern of never having achieved bladder control. Secondary enuresis occurs in an individual who had achieved control for at least 3 months but who has subsequently lost control. Each group can be subdivided further into nocturnal (night) or diurnal (daytime) enuresis.

Primary nocturnal enuresis (PNE), sometimes simply referred to as enuresis, is the most common group, responsible for 80% of cases.[1] PNE is more prevalent in boys. Age of diagnosis is of question as 20% of 5-year-old children are still wet at night, while only 7% of 7-year-olds will be.[1] Primary diurnal enuresis in older children and secondary enuresis are much less common and may represent more serious underlying etiologies.

Delayed bladder maturation, small functional bladder capacity, diminished vasopressin release, and poor sleep arousal alone or in combination may contribute to nocturnal enuresis in a given child. Posterior urethral valves, spinal dysraphism, diabetes are a few forms of complex enuresis requiring further evaluation and treatment.[2]

Enuresis can be disruptive to normal family life and can generate stress between parents and child. There may be anxiety about events like sleepovers and campouts, and there are significant costs in lost time, laundry, and bedding, as well as the potential for guilt and loss of self-esteem.[2] These concerns may well offset the inherent costs of treatment. The decision to intervene depends on weighing such factors and on consideration of the degree of frustration in either the child or parents.

DIAGNOSIS

The presentation varies by group:

- **Clinical presentation**
  - Whereas primary enuresis may or may not be perceived as a problem by either parent or child (or physician), secondary enuresis often proves problematic regardless of age. Infectious etiologies can be accompanied by dysuria, frequency, or urgency.
  - Urinalysis is a helpful screen for infection, but is usually normal.
- **Assessment**
  - **History.** Key questions should include periods of dryness, stress in the family, family history of enuresis (80% have a relative with enuresis[3]), bowel control (encopresis may signal stress or neurologic defect), peer interactions, and emotional changes. Never forget to ask about urinary infectious symptoms (frequency, volume, stream, retention, urgency, dysuria). Also inquire about age and results of previous efforts at bowel and bladder training, previous therapy, if any, and other health problems and medications, particularly any psychotropic or other drugs with sedative or autonomic effects. Voiding history questionnaires are useful and may be obtained from the National Kidney Foundation on the World Wide Web.[4]
  - **Physical examination.** The physical examination is often unrevealing but helps to exclude less common anatomic or neurologic defects. Genitalia should be examined for hypospadias, fistula, or other congenital anomalies. Gait, rectal tone, perianal sensation, and anal reflex are rarely abnormal but can be screened to avoid overlooking the possibility of neurologic etiologies.

- ■ **Laboratory studies.** Laboratory studies should be done selectively, depending on the history.
  - Urine dipstick and microscopic analysis are done to screen for infection, diabetes, and urinary tract abnormality.
  - Urine cultures may be obtained when indicated by urine microscopy.
  - Ultrasound of the kidneys, ureters, and bladder (prevoid and postvoid) may yield clues to anatomic or functional abnormalities.
  - Computed tomography (CT) urogram versus intravenous pyelogram (IVP) may be necessary when greater anatomic detail is desired, or if ultrasound fails to reveal adequate visualization.
  - Voiding cystourethrography can be considered when an anatomic defect or physiologic dysfunction is suspected, for example, when there is a history of daytime frequency, small stream caliber, or recurrent infection.

- ■ **Treatment**
  - ■ **Education.** Patient and parental education are paramount when choosing a treatment plan. Helpful information may be obtained from the National Kidney Foundation.[4]
  - ■ **Expectant management.** Enuresis spontaneously resolves in 15% of children with enuresis each year.[2] For some, the best treatment may be to monitor the child's progress. Either a parent or the child can record in a log the number of wet or dry nights per week. A review of the log at 6 months may indicate progress toward resolution.
  - ■ **Behavioral therapy.** Evidence suggests brief positive interventions prove constructive. Other techniques include arousal training, dry bed training, hypnotherapy, and alarm systems.[1] Enuresis alarms give improvement in dry nights provided that the parents and child are motivated. It is uncertain if this leads to long-term resolution. One parent often needs to wake the child and ensure that the child rises to void. The importance of parent compliance cannot be overemphasized.
    - Advantages of the alarm system include its relatively low cost and moderate success rate.
    - Disadvantages include the need for active parental participation to help wake the child (a major factor in failure), the potential inability of the alarm to awaken the child or parents, and the presence of external hardware.[1] Evidence suggests greater benefit from ultrasound bladder volume alarm than from wet alarms for long-term results.[5] The synergism between behavioral and pharmaceutical treatment is questionable.[6]
  - ■ **Desmopressin.** One to two sprays of desmopressin in each nostril at bedtime has a peak effect in 2 to 3 hours and may be effective the first night. The maximum dose is 40 μg (four sprays total). In tablet form, the initial dose is 0.2 mg orally 30 to 60 minutes prior to bedtime; 0.4 mg may be more effective and the dose may be titrated to a maximum of 0.6 mg as indicated.[2] Success occurs in approximately 50% of patients, but relapse rates can be as high as 50%. No long-term studies have been done to assess treatment longer than 12 months.[1] Advantages include the potential for immediate results, ease of administration, and some possible long-term improvement in decreased wetting frequency even if relapse occurs. Disadvantages are desmopressin's relatively high cost and high relapse rate. Side effects, such as hyponatremia and water intoxication, are rare when the drug is used in the recommended dosages and patients are advised to avoid excess water ingestion.[2]
  - ■ **Imipramine.** Less effective than desmopressin, imipramine is usually given in lower doses than those used in childhood depression, and its onset of action is rapid where its antidepressant effect is delayed. The initial dose is 10 to 25 mg at bedtime. Doses can be increased by 10 to 25 mg each 1 to 2 weeks, up to a maximum dosage of approximately 1 to 2 mg/kg/day. Although it may be helpful, the evidence suggests desmopressin is better and the relapse rate is high, up to 60%.[2] Advantages include low cost, ease of administration, and, as with desmopressin, possible long-term improvement in reduction in wetting frequency after relapse. The main disadvantages are the high relapse rate and the risk of overdose. An important issue is

informing parents about imipramine's potential toxicity and ensuring understanding of proper dosing.
- **Summary recommendation.** Success is 15% per year regardless of intervention. Some benefit is noted with brief interventions and added parental plan, the most successful of which appears to be using bladder volume alarms. Desmopressin works best for occasional nights when the child is traveling, visiting, or camping.[1]

References
1. Makari J, Rushton G. Clinical evidence concise: nocturnal enuresis. *Am Fam Physician* 2006;73(9).
2. www.uptodate.com, Nocturnal Enuresis.
3. Hogg RJ, Husmann D. The role of family history in predicting response to desmopressin in nocturnal enuresis. *J Urol* 1993;150:444.
4. National Kidney Foundation: www.kidney.org.
5. Pretlow RA. Treatmetn of nocturnal enuresis with an ultrasound bladder volume controlled alarm device. *J Urol* 1999;162(3pt2):1224–1228.
6. Gibb S, Nolan T, et al. Evidence against synergistic effect of Desmopressin with conditioning and treatment of nocturnal enuresis. *J Pediatr* 2004;144(3):351–357.
7. Gimpel GA, et al. Clinical perspectives in primary nocturnal enuresis. *Clin Pediatr* 1998;37:23.

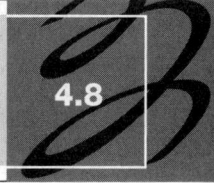

COMMON POISONING IN CHILDREN
Jason Chao

4.8

GENERAL PRINCIPLES

The ingestion of a potentially poisonous substance is a common medical emergency in children. U.S. poison control centers reported 2.4 million calls concerning potential poisonings in children in 2003 and 34 deaths. It is estimated that 85% of pediatric poisonings can be managed at home.

- Delayed effects of some poisons may not occur for hours to days. Remember to consider poisoning in the differential diagnosis of a child with serious unexplained symptoms or altered level of consciousness. Chronic poisoning may occur with few overt symptoms, especially with environmental toxins.
- More than 40% of ingestions involve household items such as cosmetics and personal care products. Cleaning products and plant ingestions are generally low-risk poisonings.
- Half of all poisoning deaths are due to medications, both prescription and over the counter. For ingestion of a substance of unknown toxicity, contact the local poison control center.

DIAGNOSIS

Common Toxidromes
- **Anticholinergic syndrome** (atropine, antihistamines, tricyclic antidepressants, etc.): Symptoms include mydriasis, dry skin, dry mouth, flushing, hyperthermia, urinary retention, ileus, tachycardia, hypertension, agitation, confusion, hallucinations, and seizures (See Chapter 3.3).
- **Cholinergic syndrome** (organophosphate and carbamate pesticides, certain mushrooms, etc.): Symptoms include salivation, lacrimation, bowel and bladder incontinence,

emesis, abdominal cramps, miosis, bronchospasm, diaphoresis, seizures, and bradycardia. (See Chapter 21.2).

■ **Sympathomimetic syndrome** (amphetamines, cocaine, etc.): Symptoms include mydriasis, sweating, fever, tachycardia, hypertension, agitation, confusion, hallucinations, seizures, nausea, vomiting, and diarrhea (See Chapter 3.3).

■ **Sedative syndrome** (opiates, barbiturates, clonidine, ethanol, benzodiazepines, etc.): Symptoms include sedation from lethargy to coma, hypotension, bradycardia, respiratory depression, miosis, hypothermia, and hyporeflexia. Opiates will produce additional miosis and decreased bowel sounds (See Chapter 3.3).

History

Attempt to determine the substance involved, quantity ingested, time of ingestion, and the cause of the exposure. For teens or adults, consider substance abuse and suicide attempt.

Physical Examination

Special attention should be paid to vital signs, mental status, pupil size, bowel and bladder function, mucous membranes, and skin moisture.

Laboratory Studies

■ There is debate on the utility of toxicology screens. Specific quantitative testing for a toxin or class of toxins can be helpful for certain drugs including acetaminophen, lithium, salicylate, carboxyhemoglobin, methemoglobin, theophylline, valproic acid, carbamazepine, digoxin, phenobarbital, iron, ethanol, methanol, and ethylene glycol.

■ Measurement of serum electrolytes and determination of an elevated anion or osmol gap may be helpful, but a normal osmol gap cannot rule out a significant ingestion such as a toxic alcohol.

Monitoring

■ Stabilization

■ **Establish the ABCs: airway, breathing, and circulation.** Perform a brief screening examination, including vital signs, mental status, and pupils, to identify the measures necessary in the first several minutes to prevent further deterioration of the patient.

■ Lethargic patients should have their blood glucose determined, or receive glucose if unable to do so (see below). Naloxone (Narcan) should be added for young children who may have ingested a narcotic. Use 0.1 mg per kg up to 2 mg IV. The dose may be doubled every 2 minutes if there is no response, to a total dose of 10 mg. The use of flumazenil in overdose management is controversial.

■ **Decontaminate skin and eyes with copious rinsing.** Eyes should be irrigated with lids open using normal saline. Avoid contamination of health care workers.

■ **Complete patient evaluation** is directed to identifying the type and amount of the toxic substance as well as the timing of the exposure, evaluating the severity of its clinical effects, and searching for associated complications and trauma. Begin general supportive care.

TREATMENT

■ **Activated charcoal**

■ Oral activated charcoal decreases systemic absorption of many drugs, including aspirin, acetaminophen, barbiturates, phenytoin, theophylline, and tricyclic antidepressants.

■ Activated charcoal may be readministered following gastric lavage. Protect the airway to prevent aspiration.

■ Dosage. Base dose on how much toxin must be adsorbed in a 10:1 activated charcoal/drug ratio, or give 1 g per kg to a maximum of 50 g. Can be mixed with chocolate or fruit syrup to increase palatability, or administered via gastric tube if not swallowed quickly.

■ Multiple-dose activated charcoal, given every 2 to 4 hours, may be used when large amounts or delayed-release drugs are ingested including carbamazepine, dapsone, phenobarbital, quinine, or theophylline.[1] Avoid dehydration if the activated charcoal is mixed with sorbitol.

- **Gastric lavage** has not been shown to improve clinical outcome.
  - Gastric lavage may be considered if (a) the quantity of substance ingested is potentially life-threatening and likely to pass through the lavage tube, and (b) a gag reflex is present. Lavage should be initiated within 60 minutes of ingestion.
  - Restrain the patient in a left lateral decubitus Trendelenburg position. Use a large-bore (24 to 32 French) single-lumen tube via the orogastric route. Instill aliquots of 10 to 15 mL per kg of saline and aspirate back until aspirated contents are clear.
  - Large volumes may be required. Protect the airway to prevent aspiration.

- **Syrup of ipecac** efficacy remains unproven. **Avoid** ipecac in patients with caustic ingestion, age younger than 6 months, a depressed mental status or expected to deteriorate rapidly, a need for rapid gastrointestinal (GI) evacuation, or who have ingested a substance with substantial morbidity if aspirated (hydrocarbons). It may have a limited role in home management of poisoning to provide early gastric evacuation, if rapid transport to the emergency department is not available. The American Academy of Pediatrics recommends that ipecac should no longer be a routine home treatment strategy.[2]

- **Improve elimination of the toxin**
  - Extracorporeal hemodialysis or hemoperfusion may be used in cases involving significant methanol, ethylene glycol or other toxic alcohol, lithium, salicylate, or theophylline ingestion.
  - Polyethylene glycol–electrolyte lavage solution (whole-bowel irrigation) may be considered for extended-release medications or substances not absorbed by activated charcoal such as iron or lithium. Dose: age 9 months to 5 years, 500 mL per hour; age 6 to 12 years, 1 L per hour.
  - Cathartics, such as sorbitol or magnesium citrate, are generally used only in conjunction with activated charcoal. Sorbitol is available premixed with activated charcoal. Stool output should be closely monitored if given.

INDIVIDUAL POISONS

Individual poisons have a specific effective antidote in less than 5% of poisonings.[3]
Provide general supportive care if no specific antidote is available.

Acetaminophen

- Emesis within 90 minutes of ingestion can decrease absorption by 50%.
- If time of ingestion is known, draw serum level at 4 hours after ingestion; otherwise draw serum level on admission.
- N-Acetylcysteine (Mucomyst) (NAC) is indicated if the history suggests an acute ingestion of more than 140 mg per kg or if plasma acetaminophen level falls on or above the line on a Rumack–Matthew nomogram (utoronto.ca/kids/aceta.htm). NAC is most effective if started within 8 hours of ingestion. The loading dose is 140 mg per kg either orally or by lavage tube after gastric lavage. After the loading dose, give 70 mg per kg every 4 hours for 17 doses. It may be diluted with a soft drink or juice to a 5% solution. NAC may be administered intravenously to patients with GI obstruction or inability to tolerate oral NAC.

Tricyclic Antidepressants

- Signs such as cardiac arrhythmia (QRS > 100 ms), hypotension, or seizures may occur soon after poisoning and without warning.
- Gastric emptying and activated charcoal decrease absorption. Avoid syrup of ipecac.
- Use norepinephrine for hypotension and benzodiazepines for seizures. Avoid quinidine-like drugs and dopamine, which may exacerbate dysrhythmias.

Antihistamines

- Cardiac monitoring, intravenous access, and lavage followed by activated charcoal are indicated for potentially significant ingestion.
- Acetaminophen and aspirin are frequently combined with antihistamine preparations, and levels for these drugs should be obtained.

- Physostigmine (Antilirium) is a specific antidote for significant anticholinergic toxicity including tachydysrhythmias with hemodynamic compromise, intractable seizures, severe agitation, or psychosis. It is given under close cardiac rhythm monitoring.

Insulin or Oral Hypoglycemic Overdose

- Hypoglycemia is the effect of overdose with these substances. Ethanol, aspirin, and β-blockers may also produce hypoglycemia. As little as one or two tablets of a sulfonylurea may be lethal to a small child.[4]
- Glucose as D10 is given for neonates at 5 mL per kg slow intravenous push. D25 is given for children up to 24 months, 1 g per kg slowly. Use D50, 1 to 2 mL per kg for children older than 24 months.
- Oral hypoglycemics may produce prolonged or recurrent hypoglycemia. Continuous glucose in fusion with glucose monitoring every 1 to 2 hours may be necessary. Octreotide is recommended for serious sulfonylurea toxicity or recalcitrant hypoglycemia; 4 to 5 μg/kg/day subcutaneous octreotide is given in divided doses every 6 hours to a maximum dose of 50 μg per dose.
- Glucagon may be administered if oral glucose is contraindicated and intravenous access for glucose is delayed. Use 0.025 to 0.1 mg per kg, intravenously, subcutaneously, or intramuscularly. The maximum amount per dose is 1 mg. Observe for emesis and aspiration because glucagon is an emetic.

Hydrocarbons

- Provide supportive therapy for hypoxia and respiratory failure. Coughing, gasping, or choking that persists is indicative of aspiration.
- Decontaminate skin with water, followed by soap or shampoo.
- Gastric emptying and/or charcoal is not indicated unless the hydrocarbon product is a substance known for its systemic toxicity, including camphor, halogenated hydrocarbon, aromatic hydrocarbon, metal, or pesticide.

Iron

- Induce emesis early with syrup of ipecac, or use whole-bowel irrigation because adult pills are too large for most lavage tubes, and activated charcoal is not effective.
- Deferoxamine (Desferal) is reserved for significant ingestions over 60 mg per kg elemental iron. Give intravenously at no more than 15 mg/kg/hour until the child is no longer ill or the urine is no longer colored. If given intramuscularly, the dose is 90 mg per kg to a maximum of 1 g.

Lead

- Succimer (DMSA) is given orally, 10 mg per kg every 8 hours for 5 days, followed by 10 mg per kg every 12 hours for an additional 2 weeks for moderately severe lead intoxication (50 to 69 μg/dL). The capsules can be mixed with juice, applesauce, or ice cream. Rebound increase in lead level is to be expected, and a repeat course of DMSA may be prescribed. Iron supplementation for iron deficiency anemia may be given concomitantly with DMSA.
- Symptomatic patients or severe lead poisoning should be admitted and treated with parenteral dimercaprol (British antilewisite, or BAL) and edetate calcium disodium (EDTA).

Salicylates

- Activated charcoal plus cathartic is effective in reducing absorption.
- Intravenous sodium bicarbonate 1 to 2 mEq per kg boluses every 3 to 4 hours to raise blood pH levels and enhance renal elimination.
- Hemodialysis should be considered early if a significant ingestion has occurred. Do not rely on the Done nomogram for predicting toxicity.[5]

Theophylline

- Avoid use of syrup of ipecac unless ingestion took place less than 1 hour before arrival because protracted vomiting may occur.
- Gastric lavage may be attempted, but tablets may be difficult to remove. In significant ingestions, repeated doses of activated charcoal should be administered, along with a cathartic.

■ Transfer to a facility with charcoal hemoperfusion or hemodialysis should be considered early, before the patient becomes too unstable for transfer.

Toxic Alcohols (Including Ethanol, Isopropanol, Methanol, and Ethylene Glycol)

■ Toxic alcohols are rapidly absorbed and many have toxic metabolites as well.
■ Fomepizole is a specific antidote for serious methanol or ethylene glycol ingestion. Give a 15 mg per kg loading dose, followed by 10 mg per kg every 12 hours for four doses, then 15 mg per kg every 12 hours until toxic alcohol level <20 mg per dL. If fomepizole is unavailable, an older alternative is ethanol 10% intravenous infusion to a serum concentration of 100 mg per dL, which competitively competes with toxic metabolites.
■ Hemodialysis should also be considered in significant toxic alcohol ingestions.

CONTINUING CARE AND PREVENTION

■ Consider child neglect or abuse in poisoning under the age of 12 months. After the age of 5 years, unintentional ingestion is unusual, and poisoning is due to stress, suicidal gesture or attempt, or drug-seeking behavior.
■ An adequate observation period should be established after diagnosis and initial treatment. Poison prevention education or social work assessment can be begun at this time. A referral source should be identified for follow-up treatment.

References

1. Gaudreault P. Activated charcoal revisited. *Clin Pediatr Emerg Med* 2005;6:76–80.
2. American Academy of Pediatrics Committee on Injury, Violence, and Poison Prevention. Poison treatment in the home. *Pediatrics* 2003;112:1182–1185.
3. Shannon M. Ingestion of toxic substances by children. *N Engl J Med* 2000;342:186.
4. Henry K, Harris CR. Deadly Ingestions. *Pediatr Clin North Am* 2006;53:293–315.
5. Eldridge DL, Dobson T, Brady W, et al. Utilizing diagnostic investigations in the poisoned patient. *Med Clin North Am* 2005;89:1079–1105.
6. McKay CA. Can the laboratory help me? Toxicology laboratory testing in the possibly poisoned pediatric patient. *Clin Pediatr Emerg Med* 2005;6:116–122.
7. Pharmaceutical drug overdose. Treatment guidelines. *Med Lett.* Sep 2006;4:61–66.

BEHAVIORAL PROBLEMS OF CHILDREN

Keely J. Beam

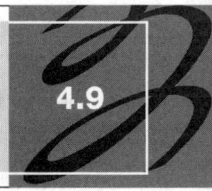

4.9

GENERAL PRINCIPLES

Appointments with the family physician (FP) provide important opportunities for screening and diagnosing behavioral problems in infants and children. FPs are often the first professionals to be consulted by parents when a behavior problem arises. Given that long-term outcomes are improved by early intervention it is important that FPs learn to screen, diagnose, and treat behavioral problems. Due to the limited time FPs have to spend with an individual patient, they must also know when to refer a child to a specialist for additional assessment and what community resources are available to assist both children with behavioral problems and their families.

■ **Prevention of behavioral problems.** Causation of behavioral problems are numerous and may include (but are not limited to) organic/genetic factors, physical factors, prenatal factors, early trauma, developmental delays, attachment disruptions, unrealistic parental expectations, poor parenting skills, poor parental mental health, parental substance abuse, physical/sexual/emotional abuse, and neglect. FPs should be aware of these factors and the impact they have on normal development. Providing anticipatory guidance is a focus of well-child care. FPs should also be aware of services in their community that will provide assistance to families in need at no or reduced financial cost. The Individuals with Disabilities Education Act (IDEA) guarantees services to children, from birth, with issues that will or do interfere with functioning in school. Under IDEA, public agencies have a duty to find children in need of assistance; FPs should know whom to contact, in their area, to initiate services. In cases of abuse and/or neglect, FPs should contact the appropriate authorities per their mandatory reporter requirement. Local human service departments provide many services as well as protection for children.

- **Stages of behavioral assessment.** The difference between behavioral problems and full-blown behavioral disorders is often situational. Behavioral problems may be a function of a given setting or interaction with a single person. Behavioral disorders manifest themselves across settings. In order to make an appropriate diagnosis and develop an effective treatment plan, FPs should work collaboratively with parents, psychologists (school, clinical, and developmental), school nurses, teachers, and social workers.
  - **Review records.** A review of records provides FPs with insight into the evolution of the presenting problem. In addition, it will provide clues to causation, which may provide direction for treatment.
  - **Interview.** Interview information, which may take the form of questionnaires or behavioral checklists, should be obtained from parents, teachers, and other significant caregivers, primarily to ascertain if the behavior is consistent over time and situation.
    - Behavior checklists should be normed, valid, and reliable for the behavior of concern. If the FP is unsure in regard to the validity and reliability of a given instrument, contact the school psychologist assigned to the patient's school. Statistics, assessment, and test development are core subjects in school psychology graduate programs.
  - **Observe.** Observations provide valuable data when making a behavioral diagnosis. In order to generate valid and reliable observations across settings FPs will have to collaborate with parents, school psychologists, school nurses, teachers, or social workers. Observations of events, such as tantrums or defiant behavior should follow the ABC model:
    - What was the **antecedent** of the event?
    - Describe the **behavior.** Do not include value judgments, but list measurable, nonjudgmental criteria.
    - What was the **consequence** of the behavior?
  - **Test.** Psychological testing of children with behavioral problems is time-consuming and fraught with issues that reduce the validity and reliability of the testing instrument. FPs should work collaboratively with psychologists in this endeavor.
- **Principles of behavioral intervention**
  - Children respond to respect from caregivers. Behavioral interventions will not be successful if parents treat the child disrespectfully.
  - Consistency of response is critical. Behavioral change only occurs in the context of consistent and predictable responses.
  - Positive reinforcement includes active education of the child about expected behavior and its beneficial consequences.
  - When negative reinforcement is necessary, it should be age and behavior appropriate.
  - Reassure parents that children need and want parents to exert consistent, reasonable controls on their behavior.
  - Tailor the plan to the child and the family. "One size fits all" does not apply to behavioral intervention, even in the same family. Plans must be specific—and communicated clearly to the child.
  - Review progress on a regular basis and adjust the plan as needed.
- **Overview of techniques for intervention**
  - Most parents learned their parenting techniques from their own upbringing and lack the skills to change what can often be a cycle of dysfunctional parenting. Although poverty can be an exacerbating factor, FPs should be aware that poor

parenting and the outcomes affect all socioeconomic groups. Parental training is a time-consuming process and generally outside the time allotment of an average office visit. FPs should be aware of community resources offered through schools, public mental health facilities, or churches, which offer free and/or reduced-cost parenting instruction.

■ **Classical and operant conditioning** principles can be effective at shaping behavior when used consistently. Positive and negative reinforcement and punishment, such as time-out, can be effective when used properly. Guidelines for implementing time-out suggest that 1 minute per year of the child's life is developmentally appropriate. Although rewards can also be effective, used in isolation, the expectations of the child will soon escalate. **Never ignore behavior!** Positive behavior should be reinforced and negative behavior should be dealt with. Children are attention-seeking beings, whether it is positive or negative attention. Ignoring a child, interrupting parental engagement and/or attachment, has been linked to serious mental disorders.

■ **Natural and logical consequences.** When safe, parents should let children learn about their environment through exploration and experimentation. In this model, parents prepare a child-friendly and child-oriented environment and utilize teaching moments—opportunities to model correct behavior and direct social instruction. Children experience the consequences, both good and bad, of their behavior. As a child grows in intellect, parents can discuss consequences, positive and negative and when necessary alternative behavior.

■ **Therapeutic model.** In cases where behavior problems are persistent or severe and are not responding to increased parental efficacy, the FP may consider referral to a mental health professional for testing and counseling. This approach is most successful when the FP collaborates with mental health professionals, parents, and patient (if appropriate). Children do not live in isolation, but in family and societal systems. Intervention is more successful when the system is treated instead of the patient in isolation.

■ **Mental health concerns in children.** Behavioral problems in children can be classified into three categories. First, there are problem behaviors that are normal for a child's age and development level, which will resolve with maturity and adequate parenting. Second, there are problem behaviors that were part of normal development, but that have persisted beyond what is age-appropriated and that will need intervention to resolve. Third, there are problem behaviors that indicate a serious underlying mental health problem. FPs should understand not only behavioral aberrations, but also normal behavioral development in order to differentiate. The American Psychological Association has compiled a classification system children with emotional/behavioral disorders in its *Diagnostic and Statistical Manual*, 4th ed. (DSM-IV). Although a complete listing accompanied by diagnostic criteria can be found in the DSM-IV chapter entitled, "Disorders of Infancy, Childhood or Adolescence," some common disorders that may cause behavior problems are listed here:

■ **Pervasive developmental disorders (PDD):** autism, Asberger syndrome. PDDs are characterized by social impairment and restricted behaviors. In addition, they may also be accompanied by language impairment, declining functioning, and mental retardation.

■ **Attention-deficient and disruptive emotional/behavioral disorders:** attention-deficient–hyperactivity disorder (ADHD), oppositional defiant disorder (ODD), conduct disorder (CD).
   • ADHD is characterized by inattention, hyperactivity, and impulsivity. These symptoms generally occur across settings, but are generally most noticeable during school and other times when seat work is required.
   • ODD is characterized by a continued pattern of defiant, disobedient, and hostile behavior.
   • CD is characterized bullying, threatening, and intimidating. In addition, rules of home, school, and society are often disregarded.

■ **Feeding and eating disorders:** pica, rumination, anorexia nervosa, and bulimia nervosa.

- **Tic disorders:** transient tic, chronic motor or vocal tic, Tourette disorder.
- **Elimination disorders:** enuresis, encopresis.
- **Internalizing disorders:** depression, anxiety.
  - Depression is characterized by depressed mood, irritability, loss of interest in activities and may also include physical symptoms. Pediatric bipolar is also a classification of depressive disorder in the DSM-IV. Research is currently being conducted on this disorder, which is difficult to differentiate from ADHD and depression. Depression can also lead to suicidal ideation, which is a national crisis. A 1998 study indicated that 20.5% of high school students had seriously considered suicide during a 12-month period, while 7.7% of students report making at least one suicide attempt.
  - Anxiety is characterized by constant and excessive worry. Anxiety disorders may also include separation anxiety (when not developmentally appropriate), social phobias, other specific phobias, panic attacks, obsessive–compulsive disorder, and posttraumatic stress disorder.

- There are other issues, not listed in the DSM-IV, because they are not considered disorders or because they are emerging through research conducted since the latest DSM-IV revision, which may also cause behavior problems.
  - **Learning disabilities** (which are listed in the DSM-IV, although behavior problems are not a diagnostic criteria) that are undiagnosed or unaided will often lead to anxiety, depression, and frustration.
  - **Oral habits** that persist beyond what is developmentally appropriate, such as nail-biting, digit-sucking, or refusal to relinquish a pacifier. These behaviors often act as self-soothing activities for children in times of stress and anxiety. By treating the underlying cause as well as the presenting problem these behaviors can often be extinguished.
  - **Sleep disturbances** such as night terrors are a normal developmental stage for toddlers. However, when these disturbances persist or intensify it may be an indication of anxiety or trauma. Other sleep disturbances may include sleepwalking and bedtime battles. Bedtime battles respond well to consistent bedtime routines and consistent expectations.
  - **Gay and lesbian issues** in adolescence have been linked to increased depression and anxiety. Due to continued social stigmatism, gay and lesbian teenagers may feel isolated and without social support. Gay and lesbian teenagers are 20 times more likely to attempt a suicide. Many communities and mental health providers have developed gay and lesbian support groups to help combat this sense of isolation.
  - **Early cigarette smoking and/or alcohol use** are considered problem behavior not only due to health/legal concerns, but because they are gateway drugs to more dangerous and harmful illegal drugs.

- **Working with other professionals.** In today's quickly changing society FPs need to become experts in collaboration. FPs deliver services much differently in today's managed health care system than they did even 10 to 15 years ago. Coordinating interventions from parenting advice/instruction to locating in-depth assessment and counseling for severe mental health disorders requires interdisciplinary partnerships among professionals.
  - Early intervention is the key to positive outcomes for children with behavior problems. Through well-child and other visits, the FP is usually the first professional to be alerted that development is not proceeding normally or that a family is struggling with a child's behavior. Every community has numerous mental health assets, however, as the primary health care providers FPs are usually the first professionals from whom parents seek advice. Of all the assets available in a community, a well-informed, collaborative-minded FP may be the most important.

References

1. Atkins MS, McKay MM, Talbot E, et al. DSM-IV diagnosis of conduct disorder and oppositional defiant disorder. *School Psychol Rev* 1996;25(3):274–283.
2. Callahan SA, Panichelli-Mindel SM, and Kendall PC. DSM-IV and internalizing disorders: modifications, limitations and utility. *School Psychol Rev* 1996;25(3):297–307.

3. Coleman MC. *Emotional and behavioral disorders: theory and practice.* 3rd ed. Needham Height, MA: Allyn & Bacon; 1996.
4. Eckert TL, Miller DN, DuPaul GJ, Riley-Tillman TC. Adolescent suicide prevention. *School Psychol Rev* 2003;32(1):57–76.
5. Kampaus RW, Frick PJ. *Clinical assessment of child and adolescent personality and behavior.* 2nd ed. Needham Heights, MA: Allyn & Bacon; 2005.
6. Power TJ. Promoting children's mental health. *School Psychol Rev* 2003;32(1):3–16.
7. Sattler JM. *Assessment of children.* 4th ed. San Diego: Jerome M. Sattler; 2001.
8. Steiner E. Behavioral problems of children. In: Taylor RB, ed. *Manual of family practice.* 2nd ed. Boston: Little, Brown; 1997:151–157.

ATTENTION-DEFICIT–HYPERACTIVITY DISORDER 4.10

Deborah S. Clements

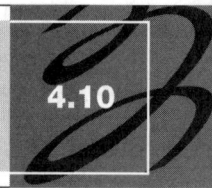

GENERAL PRINCIPLES

Attention-deficit–hyperactivity disorder (ADHD) is a condition that begins in early childhood and is characterized by symptoms of inattention, hyperactivity, and impulsivity. The symptoms broadly affect functioning in most areas of daily activity.[1] The prevalence of ADHD is estimated at between 8% and 10% of school-aged children. The condition occurs two to four times more commonly in boys than in girls and persists into adulthood in as many as 70% of cases.[2]

DIAGNOSIS

Clinical Presentation

Patients typically present as a result of concerns expressed by parents, teachers, or other caregivers during the primary grades of school. Although symptoms may not be apparent during the clinical visit, questions about school performance, behavior with friends and siblings, and completion of assignments and tasks both at home and at school are helpful in establishing a diagnosis.

- **Hyperactivity** presents as excessive talking or fidgeting, inability to remain seated during class, and difficulty playing quietly. Hyperactive features tend to predominate in the early years of childhood, peak at about 7 or 8 years of age and resolve during adolescence.
- **Impulsivity** is also observed in early childhood, although tends to persist into adulthood. Commonly, these children have difficulty waiting their turn, are disruptive in the classroom, often interrupting or intruding into others' activities. Occasionally, impulsivity results in peer rejection and can later manifest in substance abuse and difficulty managing finances.
- **Inattention** is manifested by forgetfulness, losing or misplacing homework or materials from school, disorganization, failure to complete assignments or tasks, poor attention to detail, and lack of concentration. These symptoms may appear later in childhood and also persist throughout life.

Because the differential diagnosis of ADHD includes hearing or visual impairment, diabetes, thyroid disorders, fetal alcohol syndrome, and seizure disorders, a complete physical and appropriate testing should be performed.

Diagnostic Criteria

The diagnostic criteria for ADHD were established by the American Psychiatric Association in the *Diagnostic and Statistical Manual of Mental Disorders*, 4th ed. (DSM-IV) and are summarized in Table 4.10-1.

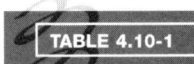

TABLE 4.10-1	**Diagnostic Criteria for ADHD**

A) One of the following two criteria must apply:
  1) Six or more of the following symptoms of inattention have persisted for at least 6 months to a degree that is maladaptive and inconsistent with level of development:
    a. Lack of attention to detail or careless mistakes in schoolwork
    b. Often has difficulty in sustaining attention during activities
    c. Often does not follow through on instructions or complete schoolwork or chores
    d. Often has difficulty organizing tasks and activities
    e. Often dislikes or avoids tasks that require sustained mental attentiveness
    f. Often loses things necessary for tasks or activities
    g. Often easily distracted by outside stimuli
    h. Often forgetful in daily activities

  2) Six or more of the following symptoms of hyperactivity-impulsivity have persisted for at least 7 months to a degree that is maladaptive or inconsistent with developmental level:
    a. Often fidgets with hands or feet or squirms in seat
    b. Often leaves seat in classroom or in other situations where remaining seated is expected
    c. Often runs or climbs in inappropriate settings
    d. Often has difficulty playing or engaging in quiet activities
    e. Often active or "on the go"
    f. Often talks excessively
    g. Often blurts out answer before question has been completed
    h. Often has difficulty waiting turn
    i. Often interrupts or intrudes on others

B) Some symptoms that caused impairment were present before age 7

C) Some impairment from the symptoms is present in two or more settings

D) There must be clear evidence of significant impairment in social, academic, or occupational functioning

E) The symptoms do not occur exclusively during the course of a pervasive development disorder, schizophrenia, or other psychotic disorder and are not better accounted for by another mental disorder (mood disorder, anxiety, personality disorder, dissociative disorder)

From American Psychiatric Association. *Diagnostic and statistical manual of mental disorders.* 4th ed. Washington, DC: American Psychiatric Association, 1994, with permission.

Assessment

- Office screening tests are available and relatively straightforward. These tools may be repeated following treatment to assess effectiveness.
- Standardized questionnaires completed by teachers, parents, and other caregivers are useful in both initial diagnosis and follow-up. These include the Conners Rating Scale, the AD/HD Rating Scale, BASC Monitor Rating Scale, and the Vanderbilt Assessment Scales (www.nichq.org/resources/toolkit), among others.
- Assessment may be done through progress reports submitted by teachers and caregivers.
- Safety and injury prevention should be discussed at each visit because children with ADHD are at increased risk for both intentional and unintentional injury.
- Because comorbidity is common, patients should be re-evaluated whenever new symptoms emerge or existing symptoms worsen.

Diagnosis of ADHD

- Children ages 6 to 12 years who present with symptoms of inattention, hyperactivity, impulsivity, poor academic performance, or behavioral problems should be evaluated

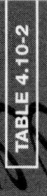

TABLE 4.10-2   **Medications Used in the Treatment of ADHD**

Agent	Dose schedule	Duration of action	Schedule
Stimulants			
Methylphenidate			
Ritalin, Metadata, Methylin	Two to three times daily	3–5 hours	5–20 mg bid to TID
Ritalin SR, Metadate ER, Methylin ER	Once or twice daily	3–8 hours	20–40 mg QD or 40 mg in morning and 20 mg in early afternoon
Concerta, Metadata CD, Ritalin LA	QD	8–12 hours	18–72 mg QD
Amphetamine			
Dexedrine, Dextrostat	bid to TID	4–6 hours	5–15 mg bid or 5–10 mg TID
Adderall, Dexedrine spansule	QD to bid	6–8 hours	5–30 mg QD or 5–15 mg bid
Adderall-XR	QD	8 hours	10–30 mg QD
Nonstimulants			
Atomoxetine			
Strattera	QD to bid	8 hours	1.2–1.4 mg/kg/day

Adapted from Smucker W, Hedayat M. Evaluation and treatment of ADHD, *Am Fam Physician* 2001;64;5:817–829.

for ADHD. For a diagnosis to be made, the child must meet the DSM-IV criteria as defined in Table 4.10-1 either in the context of the clinical visit or as observed by parents, teachers, or caregivers.[2]

- Pitfalls in accurate diagnosis:
  - Behavior may not be observed during the office visit.
  - Assessment questionnaires may convey a false sense of validity.
  - Discrepancies may exist in reports from teachers and parents or caregivers or history may be unavailable.
  - Other diagnostic tests such as laboratory studies, computed tomography, electroencephalogram are of little value in diagnosis of ADHD.
  - 20% to 35% of children have a comorbid psychiatric diagnosis or a learning disability.
  - Accurate diagnosis may require several office visits.

TREATMENT

Medications

- ADHD is a chronic condition that requires long-term treatment. Stimulants are first-line therapy for treatment of ADHD in children. With careful dose titration, up to 80% of children will respond to at least one stimulant without adverse effects.[3]
- Current medication choices include short-, intermediate-, and long-acting methylphenidate (Ritalin, Methylin, Metadate, Concerta) and dextroamphetamine (Adderall). Atomoxetine (Strattera), a nonstimulant medication, has also been approved for use in ADHD. A transdermal methylphenidate patch is also available (Daytrana) (Table 4.10-2).
- Adverse events associated with stimulant use include decreased appetite, headache, sleep disturbances, motor tics, and slowed growth velocity. Growth typically catches up during adolescence with discontinuation of medication use.

Behavioral Therapy

Although behavioral therapy alone is not proven to significantly reduce the core symptoms of ADHD, behavior problems can be improved. The goal of behavioral therapy is to focus on increasing the structure of the child's daily routine and to minimize distractions. A system of positive and negative reinforcements including praise and time-outs or loss of privileges can be useful.

Alternative Therapy

Dietary modification, nutritional supplements, homeopathy, and vision therapy have been suggested as treatments for ADHD in the lay press. Studies have indicated, however, that none of these alternatives has a response better than placebo.[4]

Referral

Evaluation by a pediatric subspecialist should be considered for children less than 6 years of age. Additionally, referral is appropriate for children with comorbid psychiatric diagnoses such as oppositional-defiant disorder, those with learning disabilities, speech or motor delay, a history of abuse, of severe aggression or emotional distress, or if response to treatment remains inadequate.

References

1. American Psychiatric Association. *Diagnostic and statistical manual of mental disorders.* 4th ed. Washington, DC: American Psychiatric Association; 1994.
2. Clinical practice guideline: diagnosis and evaluation of the child with attention-deficit/hyperactivity disorder. American Academy of Pediatrics. *Pediatrics* 2000;105:1158–1170.
3. Clinical practice guideline: treatment of the school-aged child with attention deficit/hyperactivity disorder. American Academy of Pediatrics. *Pediatrics* 2001;108: 1033–1044.
4. Baumgaertel A. Alternative and controversial treatments for attention-deficit/hyperactivity disorder. *Pediatr Clin North Am* 1999;46:977–992.

Human Behavior and Problems of Living

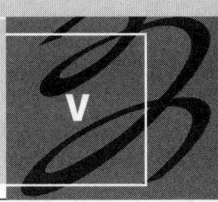

V

ANXIETY, PANIC DISORDERS, AND AGORAPHOBIA

Michael L. Brown, Rachel Bramson

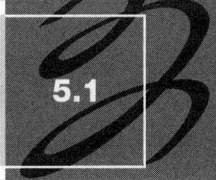

5.1

GENERAL PRINCIPLES

Anxiety disorders are the most common psychiatric illnesses.[1] Generalized anxiety disorder (GAD) and panic disorder (PD) are the most common anxiety disorders. Anxiety disorders have a high public health cost with markedly decreased role functioning, reduced health-related quality of life, and missed workdays.[2] Failure to recognize and treat anxiety disorders in primary care results in decreased quality of life for patients and inappropriate overutilization of health care services.[3,4] Only 50% of primary care patients with anxiety disorders are diagnosed by their physician.[5]

Definition

A diverse and heterogeneous group of mental health disorders including the following diagnoses: panic disorder with and without agoraphobia, agoraphobia without panic disorder, specific phobia, social phobia (social or performance anxiety often leading to avoidance), obsessive–compulsive disorder (OCD), posttraumatic stress disorder (re-experiencing an extremely traumatic event with arousal symptoms and avoidance of stimuli associated with event), acute stress disorder (immediate aftermath of extreme trauma), generalized anxiety disorder, anxiety disorder due to a medical condition, substance-induced anxiety disorder, and anxiety disorder not otherwise specified.[6]

Anatomy

Neuroimaging studies suggest anatomical brain differences in patients with anxiety disorders. This area warrants further investigation.[7]

Epidemiology

- More than one in four adults has at least one anxiety disorder in their lifetime.[8] Most anxiety disorders present in the mid-20s with prevalence about 1.5 times higher in women than in men. Although GAD has a 5% lifetime prevalence in the general population, 10% of women over 39 have GAD.[9]
- Many adults with anxiety disorders have experienced an anxious childhood or adolescence.[10] Lifetime prevalence of the anxiety disorders range from a low of 2% to 3% (OCD) to a high of 12% (social phobia).[8]

- Comorbidity with other mental health disorders is common. 80% of patients with social phobia and 50% of patients with GAD have other mental health disorders.[11]

Pathophysiology

- Diminished sensitivity to gamma-aminobutyric acid (GABA)/benzodiazepine complex (GABA is the main inhibitory brain neurotransmitter).
- Decreased alpha-2 adrenergic receptor sensitivity. This could be due to high levels of circulating catecholamines. This may be caused by an inappropriate/chronic activation of the fight or flight response.
- Studies are not uniform with regard to serotonin system but some show abnormalities in patients with GAD.
- Reduced autonomic responsiveness in GAD, possibly related to decreased vagal tone.[7]

Etiology

Not known but studies suggest familial patterns with a probable underlying genetic basis.[11]

Mechanisms of Injury

Early childhood stressors or emotional trauma may cause brain remodeling and neurochemical changes, which could increase the likelihood of anxiety disorders.

Presentation

Of patients with anxiety disorders, 83% present with somatic symptoms. The higher the number of symptoms, the higher the chance of an anxiety disorder. Unfortunately, physicians are less likely to recognize anxiety disorders when presented with physical symptoms alone.[10,12]

Diagnosis in the Primary Care Setting

Use of instruments can aid in primary care detection of anxiety disorders. The Zung Anxiety Scale is a brief screening instrument.[13] The Hamilton Anxiety Rating Scale and the Beck Anxiety Inventory can be used for confirmation of diagnosis and to document severity and improvement.[14,15] Short, two- and five-item screening questionnaires for PD have high sensitivity and adequate sensitivity to merit use.[16,17]

Special Therapy

Collaborative care interventions involving telephone contact with trained nonmental health professionals or behavioral heath specialists and psychiatrists have shown improvements in treatment outcomes, health-related quality of life, and employment patterns.[18,19]

Patient Education

- **Bibliotherapy**
  - *The Anxiety and Phobia Workbook*, by Edmund J. Bourne
  - *The Feeling Good Handbook*, by David R. Burns
  - *The Anxiety Disease*, by David V. Sheehan

- **Web sites**
  - **www.healthyminds.org**—Patient education site of the American Psychiatric Association (APA)
  - **www.nami.org**—National Alliance on Mental Illness (general information)
  - **www.ocfoundation.org**—The Obsessive Compulsive Foundation (for OCD)

COMMON DISORDERS

The most common anxiety disorders: GAD, PD, and agoraphobia are the focus of the rest of this chapter.

Generalized Anxiety Disorder

- **Clinical presentation.** GAD is characterized by worry that is pervasive, excessive, difficult for the patient to control, and that causes marked functional impairment or psychologic distress. The anxiety must be present for at least 6 months. Associated physical symptoms are characteristic, and include muscle tension, a feeling of being restless or "on edge," difficulty concentrating, irritability, insomnia, and fatigue.
- **Diagnosis.** Diagnosis of GAD is based on criteria enumerated in the *Diagnostic and Statistical Manual of Mental Disorders,* 4th ed. text revision (DSM-IV-TR).[6] The patient must experience excessive anxiety and an inability to control his or her sense of worry

for at least a 6-month period and have at least three physical symptoms related to motor tension, autonomic hyperactivity, and vigilance and scanning. Motor tension and hypervigilance better differentiate GAD from other anxiety states.

- **Differential diagnosis.** GAD is diagnosed when the anxiety is free floating and unrelated to the specific foci of other anxiety disorders, such as worry about panic attacks (PD) or worry that focuses exclusively on health concerns (such as somatization disorder or hypochondriasis). Generalized anxiety is a frequent finding in depressive disorders; in order to make a separate GAD diagnosis, the anxiety must be present in the absence of depression. Physiologic factors such as hyperthyroidism, medications, stimulant use or abuse (including over-the-counter or dietary stimulants) must not be responsible for provoking and maintaining the anxiety. Exacerbations of GAD may be provoked by clearly definable psychosocial stressors, but this differs from an adjustment disorder with anxious mood in that in adjustment disorder the duration of symptoms is less than 6 months.

- **Treatment**
  - **Medical therapy**
    - **Selective Serotonin-Reuptake Inhibitor (SSRI)** (Table 5.1-1) medications are generally considered to be first-line interventions for GAD. **Venlafaxine extended-release** (Effexor XR), **paroxetine** (Paxil), **escitalopram** (Lexapro), and **sertraline** (Zoloft) are Food and Drug Administration (FDA)-approved for treatment of GAD. **Citalopram** (Celexa) and **fluoxetine** (Prozac) are also effective. This class of medicines is generally well tolerated. The medications' tolerability, side-effect profile, and ease of dosing make them easy to use for the physician and easy to take for the patient. Nausea, flushing, headache, and tremor are common during the first week, and are dose related. Insomnia is a more common side effect than somnolence, so morning dosing is recommended to start with. GAD patients are frequently more sensitive to adverse effects of medications, so lower starting doses and smaller dose increments (compared to the treatment of depression, OCD, or PD) are recommended. While **increasing the dose at 2 to 4 week intervals,** patients may begin to experience improvement as early as 2 weeks, but typically 3 to 4 weeks at a therapeutic dose is required to determine efficacy. As with any other centrally acting medication, tapering the dose to change or discontinue it is always necessary.
    - **Buspirone** (Buspar). Buspirone is a novel medication unrelated to the SSRIs, tricyclic antidepressants (TCAs), or benzodiazepines. It is better tolerated than TCAs and can be used as a first- or second-line agent in GAD. Buspirone has been shown to be effective at total daily doses of 20 to 60 mg per day, usually divided bid or tid. Starting at 50% of the therapeutic dose (usually 7.5 mg bid) the dose is increased after a week. Dividing the dose into three, with the larger dose at night, may improve tolerability in patients who experience nausea or flushing. Like the SSRIs and TCAs, 3 to 4 weeks of treatment at a therapeutic dose are required for full response. Buspirone also plays a role in augmenting SSRIs or TCAs in patients who have a partial response to monotherapy with one of these agents. As with any other centrally acting medication, tapering the dose to change or discontinue it is always necessary.

TABLE 5.1-1   Common SSRIs in Anxiety Disorders

Drug	Starting dose	Target dose
Fluoxetine (Prozac)	10–20 mg QAM	20–60 mg
Sertraline (Zoloft)	25–50 mg QAM	50–200 mg
Paroxetine (Paxil)	10–20 mg QAM	20–60 mg
Citalopram (Celexa)	10–20 mg QAM	20–60 mg
Escitalopram (Lexapro)	5–10 mg QAM	10–20 mg
Venlafaxine XR (Effexor XR)	37.5 mg QAM	75–225 mg

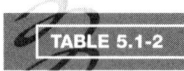

TABLE 5.1-2	Commonly Used Benzodiazepines			
Drug	Rate of onset	Usual daily dosage (mg)	Usual dose schedule	Active metabolites
Alprazolam (Xanax)	Rapid	1–6	0.5 mg TID-qid	No
Lorazepam (Ativan)	Intermediate	2–8	1 mg bid-TID	No
Clonazepam (Klonopin)	Intermediate	1–4	0.5 mg bid-TID	No
Diazepam (Valium)	Rapid	5–60	5–10 mg bid-TID	Yes
Chlordiazepoxide (Librium)	Intermediate	25–100	25 mg bid-TID	Yes
Clorazepate (Tranxene)	Rapid	7.5–60	7.5 mg bid-TID	Yes
Oxazepam (Serax)	Intermediate	30–120	10–20 mg bid-TID	No

- **Benzodiazepines.** Chronically anxious patients respond well to benzodiazepines, and all benzodiazepines are equally effective for the treatment of anxiety. The choice of one or another of these medicines is based on duration of action and pharmacokinetic factors, such as the accumulation of active metabolites, which can cause sedation or ataxia. Responders notice improvement within the first days of therapy. Benzodiazepines are appropriate in the treatment of chronic anxiety, although SSRIs are preferred as benzodiazepines may decrease alertness and psychomotor performance. Tolerance to these effects develops with consistent dosing. Absent a history of substance abuse, abuse of benzodiazepines by patients with GAD is very uncommon. However, physical dependence is to be expected. Initiating treatment with an SSRI or TCA for 1 to 2 months before attempting to taper benzodiazepines can reduce the chance of relapse. Benzodiazepines should be slowly tapered not faster than 10% to 20% of total dose per week. Many patients who are otherwise well controlled on other medications will benefit from using benzodiazepines on a prn basis for exacerbations of anxiety. Patients on benzodiazepines should not use any alcohol (Table 5.1-2).
- **Tricyclic antidepressants** are effective in GAD. **Imipramine** (Tofranil) has shown efficacy comparable to alprazolam. These have a greater side-effect burden, especially sedation and anticholinergic effects, compared to SSRIs or buspirone, and slower onset of action compared to benzodiazepines.
- **Monoamine oxidase inhibitors (MAOIs),** such as **phenelzine** (Nardil) and **tranylcypromine** (Parnate), are also effective, but their complexity of drug and food interactions make them unsuitable for general medical practice.
- **Other medications. Hydroxyzine** (Atarax or Vistaril), an antihistamine, is superior to placebo in GAD and has a rapid onset of effect. However, its utility is limited by its sedative properties and relatively low antianxiety properties compared to benzodiazepines. β**-Blockers** may be helpful for symptomatic relief of tremor, but do not have antianxiety properties.

■ **Psychotherapy.** Studies clearly demonstrate that various forms psychotherapy are helpful in treating GAD. **Cognitive behavioral therapy (CBT)** is superior to nondirective or supportive types of psychotherapy. **Biofeedback** and **progressive relaxation** can be helpful, especially in those patients with significant complaints of muscle tension, pain, or insomnia. Referral to a psychologist or licensed counselor with specific training in these forms of psychotherapy is appropriate when considering these treatments.

■ **Referral.** Referral to a psychiatrist should be considered in cases with comorbid psychiatric disorders or when the patient has not responded to several attempts at treatment by the primary care physician. Patients with substance abuse problems should be referred to a substance abuse counselor for treatment directed at the substance abuse disorder.

Panic Disorder and Agoraphobia

■ **Clinical presentation.** Panic attacks typically begin without warning. Pounding heart and dyspnea are common first symptoms, rapidly joined by dizziness or lightheadedness, diaphoresis, lightheadedness or faintness, chest pressure, and a sense of "impending doom"—a feeling of being about to die. The symptoms typically build to a peak over 10 to 30 minutes, and resolve over the next 30 to 60 minutes, on average. When their panic attacks begin, patients most commonly present to their family physician's office or to the emergency department. Patients will most commonly describe the physical sensations first, rather than fearfulness or anxiety. With the attacks comes an intense need to escape the immediate situation, whatever it is. Phobic avoidance develops from this, as patients gradually restrict their range of activities to exclude those settings in which attacks have occurred, where help might not be immediately available, or from which they might not be immediately able to escape in the event of an attack. Phobic avoidance that causes significant levels of distress or interference in the patient's life is diagnosed as agoraphobia. Up to two thirds of patients with PD have some degree of phobic avoidance.[10]

■ **Diagnosis (based on *DSM-IV-TR* criteria)**

■ **Panic disorder (PD).** Panic attacks are characterized by the abrupt onset of intense fear that peaks within 10 to 30 minutes of onset, and is associated with at least four autonomic symptoms, including palpitations, sweating, trembling, dyspnea, choking, chest pain, nausea, dizziness, depersonalization, paresthesias, hot or cold flashes, and fear of dying. Diagnosis requires recurrent panic attacks and either 1 month of behavior change in response to the attacks or persistent worry about additional attacks or their consequences. Panic attacks should not be due to a general medical problem or the direct effect of a substance (e.g., amphetamines). Routine laboratory screening for general medical problems at the time of initial presentation should include basic electrolytes, calcium (hypocalcemia due to hypoparathyroidism causes tetany and tremor; can be a complication of thyroid surgery), random glucose (hypoglycemia), thyroid-stimulating hormore (TSH) (hyper- and hypothyroidism), and urine drug screen. A 12-lead electrocardiogram (ECG) is usually obtained in the emergency department setting, and along with physical examination is sufficient to reassure the patient with PD about arrhythmia, although more extensive evaluation to rule out a cardiac event sometimes occurs. Patients not reassured by extensive evaluation may have comorbid hypochondriasis or other somatoform disorders. Sometimes PD and coronary artery disease coexist and long-term PD can cause coronary artery disease.[23] Isolated panic attacks can also occur in the context of other psychiatric conditions, most commonly other anxiety disorders and depressive disorders.

■ **Agoraphobia.** Agoraphobia is most commonly seen with PD. Diagnosis requires the presence of anxiety in situations where escape is difficult or help is unavailable. Such situations are either avoided, endured with marked distress, or require a companion to be tolerated. Avoidance must not be explainable by the existence of another mental disorder. Although panic attacks are the most subjectively distressing aspect of PD to patients, severe agoraphobia can be the most disabling and the most treatment-resistant part of their illness. Patients whose agoraphobia does not improve with successful medical treatment of their panic attacks should be referred for **cognitive–behavioral therapy** (CBT).

■ **Treatment.** In the emergency department or the office, offering patients a medical explanation and a diagnostic label for their experience can be very reassuring and therapeutic ("The workup is okay. What seems to have happened is you had a panic attack, sort of an 'adrenaline flood' in the brain"). It is not helpful to minimize or demean their experience ("it was just a panic attack")—after all, to patients, it felt like they really were about to die! If a medical cause for the panic attack is found, management begins with treatment directed at this condition. Dietary recommendations, such as the avoidance of nicotine, caffeine, and other stimulants, are helpful.[11]

■ **Medical therapy**

- The primary goal of treating PD is preventing recurrence of spontaneous panic attacks. Alprazolam, because of its rapid onset, can be effective in aborting a panic attack once it has begun, especially if taken sublingually. Patients with infrequent isolated panic attacks may only require prn doses of benzodiazepines, but PD typically requires daily medications to prevent recurrence. Effective treatment should be continued until patients are panic free for at least 6 to 12 months. Medication should be tapered slowly to avoid withdrawal symptoms or rebound panic attacks. Recurrence rates are greater than 50% after medication discontinuation, so ongoing maintenance therapy is commonly required. Buspirone and β-blockers are not effective in PD. Many patients with PD are sensitive to the side effects of antidepressant medications like SSRIs and TCAs, so treatment should be initiated with small doses and gradually titrated upward to therapeutic doses.

- **SSRIs** are first-line medications in PD, alone or in combination with benzodiazepines. **Fluoxetine** (Prozac), **sertraline** (Zoloft), and **paroxetine** (Paxil) are effective. Other SSRIs, including **venlafaxine extended-release** (Effexor XR) and **citalopram** (Celexa), can also be effective. Full antidepressant doses are required, beginning with half of the initial dose for the first week then increasing to the first target dose. Effective doses differ for each drug: fluoxetine, 20 to 60 mg per day; sertraline, 50 to 200 mg per day; paroxetine, 20 to 60 mg per day; citalopram 20 to 60 mg per day, and venlafaxine extended-release 75 to 225 mg per day (Table 5.1-1).

- **TCAs.** The efficacy of the TCAs is well established, and they are considered second-line if SSRIs fail or are not tolerated. **Imipramine** (Tofranil), **desipramine** (Norpramin), and **clomipramine** (Anafranil) are effective in PD. The initial starting dose should be 25 mg at bedtime and increased by 25 mg every 4 to 7 days as tolerated. Doses of 150 mg per day are usually required. The dosage may be slowly increased up to 300 mg per day if needed. **Nortriptyline** (Pamelor) is also very effective, and may be better tolerated; doses of 75 to 150 mg per day are used. An advantage of the TCAs is the ability to monitor blood levels within defined therapeutic ranges. Three weeks of treatment at an adequate dose is usually necessary before panic suppression is achieved.

- **Benzodiazepines.** High-potency benzodiazepines are highly effective in the treatment of PD, with efficacy similar to that of the SSRIs and TCAs. Compared to GAD, higher doses of benzodiazepines are required in PD: **alprazolam,** 2 to 8 mg per day divided tid-qid; **lorazepam,** 4 to 10 mg per day divided tid; or **clonazepam,** 2 to 6 mg per day divided bid-tid. Clonazepam is preferred for its longer duration of action, allowing less frequent doses and less risk for rebound panic between doses. As a rule, low doses should always be started, then gradually titrated upward to the lowest dose that provides the best clinical effect. For patients with severe symptoms, it may be indicated to initiate treatment with a benzodiazepine for rapid symptom relief at the same time that an SSRI or TCA is started, then gradually to reduce the benzodiazepine to prn use after a few weeks. Most patients who take benzodiazepines maintain their therapeutic benefit on a stable dose over time. Problems of misuse or abuse of benzodiazepines are probably limited to patients with histories of alcohol or drug abuse, or patients who increase their too-low medication doses on their own in an attempt to self-medicate ("pseudo-addiction"). Mood symptoms should be followed, as clonazepam can sometimes cause depressed mood and alprazolam can occasionally cause excitation or rarely mania.

- **MAOIs,** such as **phenelzine** (Nardil) or **tranylcypromine** (Parnate), may be even more effective than the tricyclics in resistant cases. Due to dietary restrictions and the potential for drug interactions, these drugs are not the first line of therapy and are not generally recommended in the primary care setting.

■ **Psychotherapy**

- **CBT** is effective in the treatment of PD and has been shown to increase the likelihood that patients can eventually reduce and even discontinue benzodiazepine treatment. The primary behavioral techniques include breathing retraining, relaxation training, and exposure to somatic cues, in which patients are taught to recognize and restructure their interpretations of their physical symptoms. This form of therapy is effective in both group and individual settings.

- Treatment involving gradual exposure of the patient with agoraphobia to feared situations is essential if agoraphobia is to be overcome. Focused CBT is more effective than nonspecific or purely supportive interventions in this regard. Supportive interventions and patient education are, however, helpful in encouraging the patient to undergo and work in therapy and confront these situations.

■ **Referral.** Referral to a psychiatrist should be considered in cases with comorbid psychiatric disorders or when the patient has not responded to several attempts at treatment by the primary care physician. Patients with substance abuse problems should be referred to a substance abuse counselor for treatment directed at the substance abuse disorder.

References

1. Hollander E, Simeon D. Anxiety disorders. In: *The American Psychiatric Association textbook of clinical psychiatry.* 4th ed. Washington, DC; American Psychiatric Press; 2003.
2. Stein M, Byrne P, Craske M, et al. Functional impact and health utility of anxiety disorders in primary care outpatients. *Med. Care* 2005;43(12):1164–1170.
3. Schmidt N, Kruse J. The relationship between mental disorders and medical service utilization in a representative community sample. *Soc Psychiatry Psychiatr Epidemiol* 2002;37(8):380–396.
4. Katon W. Panic disorder: relationship to high medical utilization, unexplained physical symptoms and medical costs. *J Clin Psychiatry* 1996;57(Suppl 10):1–8; discussion 19–22.
5. Ormel J, et al. Recognition, management, and course of anxiety and depression in general practice. *Arch Gen Psychiatry* 1991;48:700.
6. American Psychiatric Association. *Diagnostic and statistical manual of mental disorders: DSM-IV-TR.* 4th ed. text rev. Washington, DC: American Psychiatric Association; 2000:436–476.
7. Hidalgo R, Davidson J. Generalized anxiety disorder. *Dept Psychiatry Behav Sci* 2001;85(3):691–710.
8. Kessler R, Chiu W, Demler O, et al. Prevalence, severity and comorbidity of 12-month DSM-IV disorders in the National Comorbidity Survey Replication. *Arch Gen Psychiatry* 2005;62:617–627.
9. Wittchen H, Hoyer J. Generalized anxiety disorder: nature and course. *Clin Psychiatry* 2001;62(Suppl 11):15–19.
10. Culpepper L. Use of algorithms to treat anxiety in primary care. *J Clin Psychiatry* 2003;64(Suppl 2):30–33.
11. Griez E, Faravelli C, Nutt D, et al. *Anxiety disorders: an introduction to clinical management and research.* 2001,1–380.
12. Arikian S, Gorman J. A review of the diagnosis, pharmacologic treatment, and economic aspects of anxiety disorders. *Prim Care Companion J Clin Psychiatry* 2001;(3):110–117.
13. Zung W. A rating instrument for anxiety disorders. *Psychosomatics* 1971;12(6):371–379.
14. Shear M, Vander Bilt J, Rucci P, et al. Reliability and validity of a structured interview guide for the Hamilton Anxiety Rating Scale (SIGH-A). *Depress Anxiety* 2001;(12):266–178.
15. Beck T, Steer R. *Beck's anxiety inventory.* San Antonio: Psychological Corp.; 1990.
16. Stein M, Roy-Byrne P, McQuaid J, et al. Development of a brief diagnostic screen for panic disorder in primary care. *Psychosom Med* 1999;(61):359–364.
17. Means-Christensen A, Arnau R, Tonidandel A, et al. An efficient method of identifying major depression and panic disorder in primary care. *J Behav Med* 2005;28(6):565–572.
18. Rollman BL, Belnap BH, Mazumdar S, et al. A randomized trial to improve the quality of treatment for panic and generalized anxiety disorders in primary care. *Archives of General Psychiatry* 2005;62:1332–1341.
19. Craske MG, Roy-Byrne P, Stein MB et al. Treating panic disorder in primary care: a collaborative care intervention. *Gen Hosp Psych.* 2002;24:148–155.
20. Bourne EJ. The anxiety and phobia workbook 4th ed. Oakland, CA: New Harbinger Publications; 2005.
21. Burns DD. The feeling good handbook. New York: Plume/Penguin Books; 1999.
22. Sheehan DV. The anxiety disease. New York: Scribner; 1983.
23. Katerndahl D. Panic and plaques: Panic disorder and coronary artery disease in patients with chest pain. *J Am B Family Prac.* 2004;17(2):114–126.

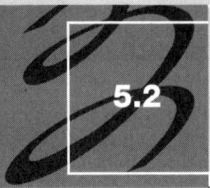

DEPRESSION
Prasad R. Padala, Kalpana P. Padala

GENERAL PRINCIPLES

Definition
Major depressive disorder (MDD) is characterized by persistent low mood and lack of interest and pleasure over at least 2 consecutive weeks.[1] The health care burden of MDD is comparable to that of cardiovascular diseases and is estimated, on a worldwide basis, to be among the top three in total expense. Family physicians treat more depression than any other professional.

Epidemiology
The lifetime population prevalence for MDD in the United States is 5% to 12% for men, and 10% to 25% for women.[2] The high variation can be explained by different settings such as in the community or in clinical population. Some variation is also due to differences in the methodology of the surveys. Irrespective of the methodology used, depression is twice as common in women as in men. Although the peak age of onset for depressive disorders is in the third decade, no age group is immune to the onset of depression. Late life depression with vascular etiology is being increasingly recognized.

Pathophysiology
The most replicated biologic finding in depression is elevated stress levels.[3] Bioamine hypothesis postulates decreased levels or activity of norepinephrine and/or serotonin responsible for development of depressive symptoms.[4] This has resulted in developing treatment strategies targeting these two neurochemical systems. Other, less specific findings include decreased latency to first rapid eye movement sleep phase and hypoperfusion of the frontal lobes in patients with MDD.

Cerebrovascular disease is increasingly recognized to have a significant relationship to mood disorders in elderly individuals. Deep white matter hyperintensities (DWMH) have been associated with chronicity of geriatric depression and its poor response to antidepressants.[5]

Etiology
Higher prevalence of depression in first-degree relatives of patients with major depression and higher concordance rates in monozygotic twins point to a genetic factor in the etiology of depression. Exposure to stressful life events such as death of a child and abuse can predispose patients to develop depression. Recently patients with short allele of serotonin transporter gene have been found to be more susceptible to adverse impact of stressful life events.[6] Thus, the etiology of depression has both genetic and environmental factors.

DIAGNOSIS

Clinical Presentation
Diagnosis of depression is mainly clinical. DSM-IV TR criteria for MDD are easily remembered using a mnemonic "SIGMECAPS" (Table 5.2-1). For the diagnosis of MDD, one has to suffer from five of the nine symptoms for at least 2 consecutive weeks. One of the symptoms has to be either depressed mood or markedly decreased interest in pleasurable activities. Several instruments can be used for detection of depression including the Beck Depression Inventory,[7] Zung Depression Self-Inventory,[8] Hamilton Depression Scale,[9] and more recently the Quick Inventory of Depressive Symptomatology[10] (QIDS), which not only assesses the severity of depression but also serves as a diagnostic tool based on the DSM-IV TR criteria.

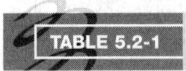

TABLE 5.2-1	Diagnostic Criteria for MDD Based on DSM-IV TR Criteria

Sleep disturbance, decreased or increased
Decreased **I**nterest or pleasure[a]
Feeling worthless or **G**uilt
Sustained low or depressed **M**ood[a]
Fatigue or loss of **E**nergy
Problems with memory and **C**oncentration
Appetite disturbance, weight loss or gain
Psychomotor agitation or retardation
Thoughts of death, **Suicidal ideation**

[a]Presence of one of these symptoms is a must to make diagnosis of MDD

Patients often present with somatic complaints to primary care providers and often deny mood symptoms. Corroborative history from family members and friends can be invaluable in making a diagnosis in poor historians. Denial of symptoms can have multiple reasons including stigma, negligence, and the fear of consequences of a diagnosis on their occupation and insurance status. Many older patients present with what otherwise looks like a depressive syndrome but steadfastly deny that they are depressed. This has been referred to as "masked depression" or "depression without sadness."[11]

Comorbidity is a rule rather than an exception. Anxiety disorders, substance use disorders, and other medical conditions complicate the course and treatment of depression and increase the risk for suicide.

Physical Examination

Physical examination is geared toward ruling out medical conditions such as hypothyroidism and parkinsonism that can manifest with depression.

Classification

Depression is a heterogeneous condition and is classified into MDD, dysthymia, depression secondary to general medical condition, substance-induced mood disorder, and depression not otherwise specified (NOS). Dysthymia is a low-grade depression that is present for more than 2 years. Substance-induced mood disorder usually has onset within a month of intoxication or withdrawal from substance use. MDD can often be complicated with psychotic symptoms. It is also further classified into primary and secondary depression and depression with or without melancholic symptoms. Yet another classification is based on presence or absence of atypical features such as hyperphagia, hypersomnolence, and hypersensitivity to rejection. This distinction is important as patients presenting with atypical features might respond better to monoamine oxidase inhibitors (MAOIs) such as phenelzine.

Differential Diagnosis

Bipolar disorder can manifest with depressive episodes. A history of mania in the past, family history of bipolar disorder, or past treatment with mood stabilizers alerts clinicians about the possibility of bipolar disorder. This distinction is essential to avoid the risk of switching to mania by initiating monotherapy with antidepressants in patients with bipolar disorder. Although the risk for manic switch is most robust with tricyclic antidepressants (TCAs), it is also seen with selective serotonin-reuptake inhibitors (SSRIs) and other agents such as venlafaxine and bupropion.

TREATMENT

Behavioral

The treatment of MDD includes both pharmacologic and psychologic interventions. Cognitive–behavioral therapy (CBT) and interpersonal therapy (IPT) are the most studied therapies for depression. Patients who respond to psychologic intervention are usually in the range of mild to moderate symptom severity. Combination of psychotherapy and pharmacotherapy has resulted in better results than either treatment alone.

Medications

Several classes of antidepressants are available, including MAOIs, TCAs, SSRIs, and mixed antidepressants. SSRIs are often considered the first-line treatment for depression due to their relatively better safety profile and ease of administration. The common doses of antidepressants are outlined in Table 5.2-2.

Most of the antidepressants have comparable efficacy at 50% to 60% response rate. The selection of an antidepressant is therefore dependent not on efficacy per se but on specific factors such as the side-effect profile, potential drug interactions, cost, ease of use, and formulation combined with patient-specific information such as comorbid medical conditions, and possibly the type of depressive symptomatology. TCAs should be used with caution in patients with cardiac disease. Similarly, TCAs should be avoided in people with dementia, narrow-angle glaucoma, urinary retention, and bowel obstruction because of their anticholinergic activity. The presence of a seizure disorder may preclude the use of bupropion.

Baseline symptoms often can help with selection of antidepressants. For example, "activating" antidepressants like fluoxetine and bupropion may be prescribed for patients with hypersomnia. Likewise, mirtazapine may be of value for patients with insomnia and anorexia. Drug interactions with concomitant medications may also inform which antidepressants to avoid (Table 5.2-3).

Special Therapy

■ Electroconvulsive therapy (ECT) has been employed successfully in the management of MDD. It is known to have 80% acute response but suffers from lack of persistent effects and often necessitates maintenance treatment. ECT is safe in elderly patients and often employed in patients with extreme anorexia, failure to thrive, and those with intractable suicidal thoughts.

TABLE 5.2-2   Doses of Common Antidepressants

Medication	Starting dose (mg/day)	Therapeutic dose (mg/day)
TCAs		
Amitryptyline	25–50	100–300
Nortriptyline	25	50–200
Imipramine	25–50	100–300
SSRIs		
Citalopram	10–20	20–60
Fluoxetine	10–20	20–80
Sertraline	25–50	100–200
Paroxetine	10–20	20–50
Escitalopram	10	20
MAOIs		
Phenelzine	45	180
Tranylcypromine	20	30–60
Mixed antidepressants		
Mirtazapine	7.5–15	15–45
Venlafaxine XR	37.5	75–225
Bupropion SR	100–150	300
Duloxetine	20–30	60

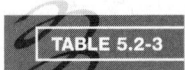

TABLE 5.2-3 **CYP-450 Enzyme Profiles of Commonly Used Antidepressants**

CYP-450 enzyme	Antidepressants	Major inhibitors	Major inducers
1A2	Fluvoxamine, mirtazapine	Ciprofloxacin, fluvoxamine, propafenone	Caffeine, carbamazepine, omeprazole
2C19	Citalopram, clomipramine	Fluvoxamine, omeprazole, ritonavir, ticlopidine	Phenytoin, valproic acid
2D6	Fluoxetine, mirtazapine, paroxetine, sertraline, venlafaxine	Fluoxetine, paroxetine, cimitidine, quinidine, ritonavir	
3A4	Citalopram, fluoxetine, mirtazapine, paroxetine, venlafaxine	Nefazodone, ciprofloxacin, ketoconazole, erythromycin, indinavir	Carbamazepine, phenobarbital, phenytoin, rifampin, ritonavir, St John's wort

■ **Augmentation of antidepressants:** Lithium, tri-iodothyronine, and methylphenidate have been used successfully in treating depression unresponsive to single antidepressants. Increasing use of atypical antipsychotics as augmentation agents is seen.

Risk Management

Major risk associated with depression is the high rate of suicide. About 15% patients suffering from depression lose life due to suicide.[11] The rates of suicide are highest among white men older than 60 years of age. Direct questioning and detailed past history can inform clinicians about potential suicide risk in a patient. SADPERSONS is a useful mnemonic for assessment of suicide risk in busy practices (Table 5.2-4).

Patient Education

Patients need to be educated about the common symptoms of depression and the need for treatment. It must be emphasized that depression is treatable and patients should be counseled not to stop antidepressants until they consult with their physicians. Several resources are available on the Internet about depression.[12,13]

TABLE 5.2-4 **Assessment Tool for Suicide Risk**

S	Male sex
A	Age (young/elderly)
D	Depression
P	Previous attempts
E	ETOH
R	Reality testing (impaired)
S	Social support (lack of)
O	Organized plan
N	No spouse
S	Sickness

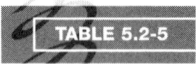

TABLE 5.2-5	**Geriatric Depression Scale**

Choose the best answer for how you have felt over the past week:
1. **Are you basically satisfied with your life?** YES / **NO**
2. Have you dropped many of your activities and interests? **YES** / NO
3. **Do you feel that your life is empty?** **YES** / NO
4. Do you often get bored? **YES** / NO
5. Are you in good spirits most of the time? YES / **NO**
6. **Are you afraid that something bad is going to happen to you?** **YES** / NO
7. **Do you feel happy most of the time?** YES / **NO**
8. Do you often feel helpless? **YES** / NO
9. Do you prefer to stay home, rather than going out, doing new things? **YES** / NO
10. Do you feel you have more problems with memory than most? **YES** / NO
11. Do you think it is wonderful to be alive now? YES / **NO**
12. Do you feel pretty worthless the way you are now? **YES** / NO
13. Do you feel full of energy? YES / **NO**
14. Do you feel that your situation is hopeless? **YES** / NO
15. Do you think that most people are better off than you are? **YES** / NO

Items in bold constitute the four-item scale.

Follow-Up

An increase in suicide rate is seen while recovering from an episode of depression, as the somatic symptoms of depression (sleep, appetite, and energy) are the first to improve and the cognitive symptoms (low self-esteem, guilt, and suicidal thoughts) are slower to improve. This increased risk for suicide during recovery necessitates continued monitoring while treating patients for depression.

SPECIAL CONSIDERATIONS

Late-life depression. There are several reasons depression in elderly individuals is difficult to diagnose. Older adults are less likely to endorse symptoms of depression than younger patients and often reject the diagnosis of depression. They are more likely to endorse low energy, anhedonia, and other somatic complaints, which are difficult to differentiate from general medical conditions. Likewise, there is a tendency to explain away depressive symptoms that are expressed as components of normal aging, grief, physical illness, or even dementia. Subsyndromal depression is much more common than major depressive disorder. To complicate matters further, suicide rates in elderly people are the highest of any age group. So a high degree of suspicion and specific inquiry is necessary for its detection and treatment. Specific rating scales such as geriatric depression scale are useful in screening for late-life depression (Table 5.2-5).[14] Even a four-item version of the geriatric depression scale (GDS) has high sensitivity for detection of depression and could be very helpful in busy practices.

References

1. American Psychiatric Association. *Diagnostic and statistical manual of mental disorders*. 4th ed., text rev. Washington, DC: American Psychiatric Association; 2000.
2. Eaton WW, Kramer M, Anthony JC, et al. The incidence of specific DIS/DSM-III mental disorders: data from the NIMH Epidemiologic Catchment Area Program. *Acta Psychiatr Scand* 1989;79:163–178.
3. Carroll BJ, Curtis GC, Mendels J. Cerebrospinal fluid and plasma free cortisol concentrations in depression. *Psychol Med* 1976;6:235–244.

4. Schildkraut JJ. The catecholamine hypothesis of affective disorders. A review of supporting evidence. *Int J Psychiatry* 1967;4:203–217.
5. Hickie I, Scott E, Mitchell P, et al. Subcortical hyperintensities on magnetic resonance imaging: clinical correlates and prognostic significance in patients with severe depression. *Biol Psychiatry* 1995;37(3):151–160.
6. Caspi A, Sugden K, Moffitt TE, et al. Influence of life stress on depression: moderation by a polymorphism in the 5-HTT gene. *Science* 2003;301(5631):386–389.
7. Beck AT, Ward CH, Mendelson M, et al. An inventory for measuring depression. *Arch Gen Psychiatry* 1961 Jun;4:561–571.
8. Zung WW. Development of a rating scale for primary depressive illness. *Arch Gen Psychiatry* 1965;13:508–515.
9. Hamilton M. A rating scale for depression. *J Neurol Neurosurg Psychiatry* 1960 Feb;23:56–62.
10. Rush AJ, Trivedi MH, Ibrahim HM, et al. The 16-Item Quick Inventory of Depressive Symptomatology (QIDS), clinician rating (QIDS-C), and self-report (QIDS-SR): a psychometric evaluation in patients with chronic major depression. *Biol Psychiatry* 2003;54(5):573–583.
11. Gallo JJ, Rabins PV. Depression without sadness: alternative presentations of depression in late life. *Am Fam Physician* 1999;60(3):820–826.
12. http://www.nami.org.
13. http://www.dbsalliance.org/info/depression.html.
14. Sheikh JI, Yesavage JA. Geriatric Depression Scale (GDS): recent evidence and development of a shorter version. In: *Clinical gerontology: a guide to assessment and intervention.* New York: Haworth Press, 1986:165–173.

ALCOHOLISM
Robert Mallin

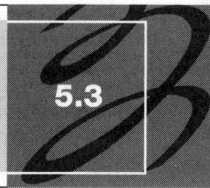

5.3

$\mathcal{T}$he prevalence of alcohol use disorders in primary care outpatients may be as high as 20%. The cost to society of these problems is staggering. Each year in the United States, alcoholism is responsible for 100,000 deaths and costs of $185 billion dollars.[1] Family physicians are in a unique position to identify and treat these problems.

GENERAL PRINCIPLES

Definition

- **Alcoholism is a primary, chronic neurobiologic disease** with genetic, psychosocial, and environmental factors influencing its development and manifestations. It is characterized by behaviors that include one or more of the following: impaired use of the drug alcohol, **compulsive use, continued use despite harm,** and **craving.**[2]
- Alcoholism or alcohol dependence is best defined by a **loss of control** over drinking.
- Because of the defense mechanism of **denial** patients are often not consciously aware of their loss of control, and tend to minimize the amount, frequency, and consequences of their alcohol consumption.
- **Alcohol abuse** refers to the harmful use of alcohol, usually meant for patients who are having consequences for their drinking but have not yet lost the ability to control their alcohol use.
- **Physical dependence** is a state of physiologic adaptation that is manifested by a drug class-specific withdrawal syndrome that can be produced by abrupt cessation or rapid

dose reduction of a drug or by administration of an antagonist.[2] In the case of alcoholism, physical dependence is sometimes but not always seen in the presence of alcoholism or alcohol dependence.

■ **Moderate drinking** is a term defined by not more than two drinks (a drink equals 1.5 oz liquor, or 12 oz beer, or 6 oz of wine) daily and no more than five in any given day for a male and no more than one drink daily for women with no more than three in any given day.

Epidemiology

■ Approximately two thirds of all American adults drink alcohol.
■ Each year 13.8 million Americans develop problems from drinking.
■ Lifetime prevalence for alcoholism is 20.1% for men and 8.2% for women.[3]
■ The prevalence of all alcohol use disorders is highest in young adults between the ages of 18 and 45.
■ For those who begin drinking before the age of 15 the rate of progression to alcoholism is 15 times that of those who begin drinking at age 21. In older adults the rates drop off precipitously.
■ Alcohol use disorders can be as high as 50% of patients admitted to a community hospital and are in the range of 25% to 27% in primary care practice visits.
■ Characteristics known to influence the epidemiology of alcoholism include gender, age, family history, marital status, employment status, and occupational/educational status.
■ The risk of alcoholism for the child of an alcoholic is approximately 50%. Single persons have a higher risk than married, and the unemployed and less educated have a higher risk.[4]

Pathophysiology

■ Alcoholism is a brain disease. A disorder in the reward system of the mesolimbic system of the brain results in dysregulated dopaminergic neurons.
■ This abnormality results in craving for alcohol and impairs individuals' ability to control their use of this drug. In addition to dopamine, multiple neurotransmitter systems are involved in this process including the gamma-aminobutyric acid (GABA) system, serotonin system, N-methyl-D-asparate (NMDA) system, glutamate. These systems modulate the effect of the drug and the reward system determines the craving for it.

Etiology

■ Family and twin studies show that there is a genetic component to a predisposition to alcoholism.
■ The development of alcohol dependence in patients who have no family history and the cases of strong family history that does not develop into alcoholism speak to environmental influences that must also play a part.

DIAGNOSIS

Screening

A primary screen for alcohol-related problems may be done as part of the review of systems or as part of a routine visit. Patients who drink at all, no matter how infrequently, should be asked questions from the "CAGE," a brief and practical primary screening tool for alcohol abuse. The term CAGE is an acronym for the key word in each of the four questions below. Any positive response justifies a more in-depth screen.

■ Have you ever felt you should *c*ut down on your drinking?
■ Have people *a*nnoyed you by criticizing your drinking?
■ Have you ever felt *g*uilty about your drinking?
■ Have you ever had a drink first thing in the morning to steady your nerves or to get rid of a hangover ("*e*ye opener")?

A slightly longer but more accurate alternative screening test is the Alcohol Use Disorders Identification Test (AUDIT) (Table 5.3-1). AUDIT questions are provided below along with the scoring values. Typically, a total of eight points or more on the AUDIT is suggestive of alcohol dependence.

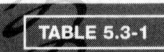

| TABLE 5.3-1 | The AUDIT Questionnaire |

1. How often do you have a drink containing alcohol?
   (0) Never
   (1) Monthly or less
   (2) Two to four times a month
   (3) Two to three times a week
   (4) Four or more times a week

2. How many drinks containing alcohol do you have on a typical day when you are drinking?
   (0) 1 or 2
   (1) 3 or 4
   (2) 5 or 6
   (3) 7 or 9
   (4) 10 or more

3. How often do you have six or more drinks on one occasion?
   (0) Never
   (1) Less than monthly
   (2) Monthly
   (3) Weekly
   (4) Daily or almost daily

4. How often during the last year have you found that you were not able to stop drinking once you had started?
   (0) Never
   (1) Less than monthly
   (2) Monthly
   (3) Weekly
   (4) Daily or almost daily

5. How often during the last year have you failed to do what was normally expected from you because of drinking?
   (0) Never
   (1) Less than monthly
   (2) Monthly
   (3) Weekly
   (4) Daily or almost daily

6. How often during the last year have you needed a first drink in the morning to get yourself going after a heavy drinking session?
   (0) Never
   (1) Less than monthly
   (2) Monthly
   (3) Weekly
   (4) Daily or almost daily

7. How often during the last year have you had a feeling of guilt or remorse after drinking?
   (0) Never
   (1) Less than monthly
   (2) Monthly
   (3) Weekly
   (4) Daily or almost daily

8. How often during the last year have you been unable to remember what happened the night before because you had been drinking?
   (0) Never
   (1) Less than monthly
   (2) Monthly
   (3) Weekly
   (4) Daily or almost daily

(continued)

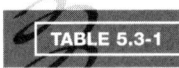

TABLE 5.3-1	The AUDIT Questionnaire *(Continued)*

9. Have you or someone else been injured as a result of your drinking?
   (0) No
   (2) Yes, but not in the last year
   (4) Yes, during the last year

10. Has a relative, friend, doctor, or other health worker been concerned about your drinking or suggested that you should cut down?
   (0) No
   (2) Yes, but not in the last year
   (4) Yes, during the last year

Clinical Presentation

■ **History**

  ■ Typically, because of denial, does not present straightforwardly.
  ■ Look for consequences from drinking in health, social, family, financial, legal areas (Table 5.3-2).
  ■ Diagnosis of alcohol dependence (Table 5.3-3).

■ **Physical Examination**

Although most patients with alcoholism will show no or only subtle physical findings, those with long-standing or severe disease will present with a variety of physical findings that are the result of alcohol-related health problems (Table 5.3-2).

Laboratory Studies

■ Because the hallmark of alcoholism is a loss of control over drinking, lab studies are useful in determining physiologic consequences from drinking, and can be markers of excessive drinking, but are not diagnostic.

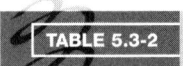

TABLE 5.3-2	Physical Signs of Alcohol Abuse

Acute or recent	**Chronic or prolonged**
Hypertension	Hypertension and/or cardiomyopathy
Sudden muscle necrosis	Chronic alcoholic myopathy
Nausea, vomiting, gastritis, reflux	Chronic atrophic gastritis
Delayed gastric emptying	Pancreatitis, pseudocyst formation
Alcoholic hepatitis	Cirrhosis, alcohol ketoacidosis
Increased sputum production	Decreased platelet function
Hypothermia	Megaloblastic anemia
Hypoglycemia, lactic acidosis	Decrease in polymorphonuclear leukocytes
Nystagmus, diplopia	Decreased cell-mediated immunity and T cells
Ataxia, stupor, coma	Peripheral neuropathy, dementia
Loss of magnesium, zinc, phosphorus, calcium, potassium, thiamine, and/or folate	Males: breast enlargement, gonadal atrophy Females: amenorrhea, anovulation
Holiday heart syndrome: atrial or ventricular dysrhythmia associated with heavy drinking	Wernicke–Korsakoff syndrome (triad of confusion, ocular disturbance, and ataxia)

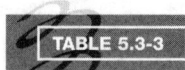

TABLE 5.3-3	Diagnosis of Alcohol Use Disorders

Alcohol abuse	Alcohol dependence
For a diagnosis of alcohol abuse the patient must show one or more of the following related to alcohol, on a *recurrent* basis: 1. Failure to fulfill major role obligations 2. Use in physically hazardous situations 3. Legal problems 4. Continued use despite having persistent or recurrent social or interpersonal problems related to the alcohol use	For a diagnosis of alcohol dependence at least three of seven criteria must be met: 1. Clinically significant tolerance 2. Clinically significant withdrawal 3. Recurrent failure of intent—drinks more or for longer duration than intended 4. Recurrent failure of control—persistent desire to stop or cut down usage 5. Preoccupation with alcohol 6. Predominance of alcohol-related activities 7. Continued alcohol use despite knowledge that the drinking contributes to a physical, social, psychologic, or other problem

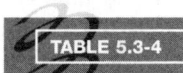

TABLE 5.3-4	Sample Detoxification Protocols

Basic orders
Multivitamin 1–2 qd
Quiet room with even lighting
Folate, 1 mg PO qd × 3 d
Thiamine, 100 mg ASAP and qd × 3 d
PO fluids as tolerated; IV usually not required
Magnesium supplement 1–2 tablets PO stat and qd; may give deep magnesium sulfate IM for severe withdrawal risk (2 g q8h)

Oxazepam
Over age 55 or hepatic dysfunction. 15–30 mg PO qh until symptoms remit or sedation occurs, then repeat total dose q6–8h for first day, reducing this dosage by 25% each day. Most patients will be off medication by day 5.

Diazepam loading
Under age 55 and healthy liver. 10–20 mg PO qh until sedated. Usually no further medication is required.

Phenobarbital taper
30 mg PO qid × 3 d, 15 mg qid × 2 d, and 15 mg bid × 1 d. Augment with sodium phenobarbital, 130–260 mg IM, early in treatment for severe withdrawal. Early use of IM phenobarbital for moderate to severe withdrawal is the key to success with this regimen. Use phenergan or hydroxyzine for nausea.

Severe agitation
Haloperidol, 5–10 mg, may be given PO, IM, or IV for severe agitation, in combination with any above withdrawal regimen; repeat as needed.

IM, intramuscular; IV, intravenous; PO, by mouth.
The above and other detoxification protocols may be modified for use in conjunction with instruments such as the Clinical Institute Withdrawal Assessment (CIWA-Ar) to better relate medication administration to actual withdrawal signs and symptoms.

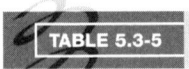

TABLE 5.3-5	Medications to Reduce Relapse in Alcohol Dependence	
Disulfram	Causes flushing and vomiting when drinking alcohol	250–500 mg daily (must be taken in observed setting to be effective)
Naltrexone	Reduces craving for alcohol	50 mg daily
Acamprosate	Reduces craving for alcohol	333 mg three times daily

- **gamma-Glutamyl transpeptidase (GGT)** is a liver enzyme that may be elevated by excessive alcohol consumption. It has poor sensitivity and specificity when used alone, but may be useful when used in conjunction with other markers such as:
  - **Mean corpuscular volume (MCV)** may be elevated from chronic excessive alcohol consumption.
  - **Carbohydrate deficient transferrin (%CDT)** when elevated suggests recent (7 to 14 days) heavy alcohol intake. CDT is useful for monitoring relapse to drinking.
  - **Ethyl glucuronide (EtG)** found in urine can detect even small amounts of alcohol up to 80 hours after ingestion.

TREATMENT

- Alcoholism can be treated successfully.
- **Brief interventions** have been shown to be successful. Often simply making the diagnosis of an alcohol problem and recommending a change in behavior may work.
- Once a diagnosis of alcohol dependence has been made, the appropriate recommendation is **abstinence** from alcohol and other addictive substances.
- More **formal interventions** can be designed for patients who do not respond to brief interventions, and are best handled by an addictions professional.
- **Detoxification,** treatment in an outpatient, inpatient, or residential setting is the appropriate recommendation for those who have a diagnosis of alcohol dependence (Table 5.3-4).
- For patients who have had symptoms of **withdrawal** in the past, medical detoxification is recommended (Table 5.3-4).
- Medications that are approved to treat alcoholism include disulfiram, naltrexone, and acamprosate (Table 5.3-5). These medications when used in the context of a comprehensive recovery program can help reduce relapse to drinking.
- Aftercare followed by involvement in Alcoholics Anonymous improves outcome in treatment for alcoholism.

References
1. Prescott CA, Kendler KS. Genetic and environmental contributions to alcohol dependence in a population based sample. *Am J Psychiatry* 1999;156(1):34–40.
2. Graham W, Schultz TK, et al., eds. *Principles of addiction medicine.* 3rd ed. Chevy Chase, MD: American Society of Addiction Medicine; 2003.
3. Grant BF. Prevalence and correlates of alcohol use and DSM IV alcohol dependence in the United States: results of the National Longitudinal Alcohol Epidemiological Survey. *J Stud Alcohol* 1997;58(5):464–473.
4. Harwood H. Updating estimates of the economic costs of alcohol abuse in the United States: estimates, update methods, and data. Report prepared by The Lewin Group for the National Institute on Alcohol Abuse and Alcoholism; 2000.

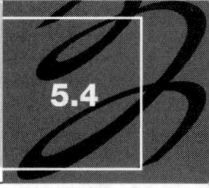

$\mathcal{S}$exual problems are common. They occur in almost half of all marriages, in at least 75% of couples who seek marital therapy, and in more than half of all adults who visit primary physicians' offices.

GENERAL PRINCIPLES

By definition, the sexual dysfunctions are disorders in sexual desire and in the psychophysiologic changes that occur during the sexual response cycle. The *Diagnostic and Statistical Manual of Mental Disorders* (4th ed). (DSM-IV) classifies them according to the following system:

- **Sexual desire disorders (SDDs)**
  - Hypoactive sexual desire disorder—deficient (or absent) sexual fantasies and desire for sexual activity.
  - Sexual aversion disorder—extreme aversion to, and avoidance of, genital contact with a sexual partner.

- **Sexual arousal disorders**
  - Female sexual arousal disorder—the inability to attain or maintain an adequate lubrication-swelling response of sexual excitement until sexual activity is completed.
  - Male erectile disorder (ED)—the inability to attain or maintain an adequate erection until sexual activity is completed.

- **Orgasmic disorders**
  - Female or male orgasmic disorder—delayed or absent orgasm following normal sexual excitement.
  - Premature ejaculation (PE)—ejaculation with minimal stimulation before it is wanted, before, during, or shortly after penetration.

- **Sexual pain disorder**
  - Dyspareunia—genital pain associated with sexual intercourse in either men or women.
  - Vaginismus—involuntary vaginal muscular spasm that interferes with sexual intercourse.

- **Sexual dysfunction due to a general medical condition**—sexual dysfunction that is fully explained by the physiologic effects of a medical condition.
- **Substance-induced sexual dysfunction**—sexual dysfunction that develops during or within a month of substance intoxication or when related to medication use.

DIAGNOSIS

Symptoms

Physicians should routinely ask about sexual relationships with open-ended questions, pursuing positive responses with queries directed to specific phases of the sexual response cycle. A more complete history incorporates the following categories.

- **Present history.** Pursue the presenting sexual concern with specific questioning, as one would further define any other problem.
- **Sexual history.** Explore all current and past sexual experiences (including sexual abuse), relationships, attitudes, emotional reactions, knowledge, sexual identity, and body image.

- **Developmental and family history.** Discuss family attitudes toward sexuality, parental modeling, religious influences, relationships with parents and siblings, family violence, and level of family function in the couple's families of origin.
- **Nature of current relationship.** Focus on the current relationship's development and stability, changes in feelings, unresolved conflict, loss of trust, and communication problems.
- **Current stressors.** Inquire about intrafamilial stresses (e.g., death, illness, problems with children, normative individual and family life cycle development transitions) and extrafamilial stresses (e.g., financial, occupational, legal).
- **Past medical history.** Identify any acute or chronic organic disease (diabetes mellitus is the most common organic cause), injury, or surgery that could affect sexual functioning. Inquire about psychologic problems (depression and anxiety are most associated with sexual dysfunction). Many commonly used drugs also affect sexual function, including anticholinergics, antidepressants, antihistamines, antipsychotics, anxiolytics, hormonal contraceptives, narcotics, sedative–hypnotics, and drugs of abuse (including alcohol and tobacco).
- **Self-report inventories.** The International Index of Erectile Function (IIEF) is a 15-item inventory that can help a busy clinician evaluate sexual functioning in men. The Female Sexual Function Index (FSFI) is a 19-question inventory that helps to evaluate sexual functioning in women.

Signs

A comprehensive physical examination further defines concurrent acute or chronic illness and associated physical conditions.

- **General.** Look for obesity, cachexia, and evidence of endocrine disease; determine vital signs.
- **Cardiovascular.** Search for bruits (especially femoral), peripheral pulses, evidence of venous stasis, arterial insufficiency (especially in the lower extremities), or a pulsatile epigastric mass.
- **Abdominal.** Look for pain, tenderness, mass, guarding, tympany, bowel activity, hernia, and evidence of prior surgery.
- **Neurologic.** Examine gait, coordination, deep tendon reflexes, pathologic reflexes, sensation, motor strength, integrity of the sacral reflex arc (S_2 to S_4) with perineal sensation, anal sphincter tone, and bulbocavernosus (S_2, S_3), bulbo-anal (S_3, S_4), and anal (S_4, S_5) reflexes.
- Observe the **male genitalia** for testicular size and consistency, penile size, malformations, and lesions. Examine the **prostate** for size, consistency, and tenderness. Obtain **penile blood pressure measurements** on any man with ED by inflating a 3-cm pediatric blood pressure cuff around the base of the penis and auscultating the central artery of the corpora cavernosa with a 9.5-MHz Doppler stethoscope as the cuff is deflated. The ratio between the penile systolic pressure and the brachial systolic pressure should exceed 0.75. Ratios less than 0.60 indicate penile vascular insufficiency.
- **Female pelvic examination.** Search for the following findings:
  - **External genitalia.** Search for dermatitis, atrophy, vulvar inflammation, warts, episiotomy or other scars, and clitoral inflammation, or adhesions.
  - **Introitus.** Look for hymeneal rigidity, tags, or fibrosis, urethral carbuncle, and Bartholin gland inflammation.
  - **Vagina.** Evaluate for spasm of the vaginal sphincter and adduction of the thighs with attempted vaginal examination, atrophy, discharge, inflammation, stenosis, relaxation of supporting ligaments, and tenderness along the vaginal urethra or posterior bladder wall.
  - **Bimanual examination.** Search for cul-de-sac masses or tenderness and adnexal mass or tenderness. Determine the presence, position, size, mobility, and tenderness of the uterus.
  - **Rectal examination.** Examine for hemorrhoids, fissures, constipation, and tenderness.

Laboratory Tests

- **Laboratory evaluation for systemic disease** includes a complete blood count, fasting blood sugar level, urinalysis, tests for sexually transmitted diseases, lipid profiles, and tests of thyroid, liver, and renal function.

- **Evaluation for SDD.** Obtain an early-morning serum bioavailable testosterone level in men. If levels are low or borderline, or if the low desire is associated with little or no sexual fantasy or masturbation history, then obtain a serum prolactin level.
- **Evaluation for female sexual arousal disorder.** Research techniques can now measure nocturnal clitoral and vaginal blood flow, and demonstrate vaginal engorgement cycles during rapid eye movement (REM) sleep, similar to erection cycles in men. Research techniques can also measure clitoral blood flow. These tools may become clinically useful to help differentiate organic from psychogenic sexual disorders in women and to determine the role of arterial factors in affecting sexual arousal and orgasm.
- **Evaluation for male erectile disorder**
  - Early morning **bioavailable serum testosterone levels** screen for hypogonadism. If the level is low, obtaining follicle-stimulating hormone (FSH), luteinizing hormone (LH), and prolactin levels can help to differentiate between primary testicular failure (high FSH and LH, normal prolactin) and secondary (pituitary-hypothalamic) failure (low FSH and LH, normal prolactin). If the FSH and LH are normal, but the prolactin is elevated, then a computed tomography (CT) scan or magnetic resonance imaging (MRI) can investigate the sella turcica for a pituitary adenoma.
  - **Nocturnal penile tumescence (NPT) evaluation** helps differentiate psychogenic interference (erections occur during sleep) from organic interference (erections do not occur). Several techniques evaluate and quantify NPT.
    - The **snap gauge** is a ring of opposing Velcro straps connected by three plastic strips. It is wrapped around the penis before sleep, and, by noting whether 0, 1, 2, or 3 bands break during sleep, one can estimate the maximum erectile response.
    - The **Rigiscan** is a small computer with two cables leading to rings that encircle the base and tip of the penis. The rings detect tumescence by passively expanding and detect rigidity by actively contracting. The Rigiscan records all erectile events and measures erection duration, tumescence, and rigidity.
    - The **NEVA system** uses electrode sets attached to the corona of the glans, to the base of the penis, and to the abdominal wall. These are attached to a monitor that records impedance data, which directly correlate to changes in penile volume.
    - **NPT monitoring** is performed in a sleep laboratory where electroencephalograph (EEG) tracings detect sleep cycles. Mercury strain gauges placed around the base and tip of the penis detect tumescence. Monitoring documents all erectile events; measures duration, tumescence, and rigidity (but not as well as the Rigiscan); and correlates erections with REM sleep.
  - When a **psychogenic etiology** is suspected the patient is evaluated for psychologic or psychiatric disorders.
  - When a **vascular etiology** is suspected, the following procedures can help to identify the cause.
    - **Intracavernous injection of vasodilators (papaverine or PGE$_1$)** helps to screen for a vascular etiology. Injections should cause an erection within 10 minutes that lasts at least 30 minutes. Delays longer than 15 to 20 minutes suggest arterial insufficiency, and a normal erection that is lost quickly suggests a cavernous leak.
    - The **Knoll/MIDUS System** is an office-based, bidirectional, continuous wave Doppler ultrasound system with spectral analysis that measures deep cavernous artery velocities. It can help to identify both arterial and venous insufficiency.
    - **Duplex ultrasound scanning** records blood flow in the cavernous arteries before and after a vasodilator (papaverine or prostaglandin E$_1$, or PGE$_1$) injection. Normal vessels should double in size, with an initial peak systolic flow velocity exceeding 30 cm per second.
    - When no arterial flow is demonstrated, then selective **internal pudendal angiograms** can determine if an arterial block exists that could be corrected by penile revascularization.
    - If persistent flow is present, then **cavernosometry and cavernosography** can be used to evaluate the veno-occlusive mechanisms of the corpus cavernosum. A vasoactive agent (20 μg PGE$_1$) is injected into a corpus cavernosum to cause

an erection; this is followed by a heparinized saline infusion to maintain it. Radiographic contrast is then infused, and radiographs are taken to identify leaks in specific veins and the glans-spongiosal system.

■ When a **neurogenic etiology** is suspected the first step is a trial of an oral phosphodiesterase-5 (PDE5) inhibiting agent such as sildenafil (Viagra). If the patient demonstrates no response, then the following tests may help to differentiate the problem.

  • **Bulbocavernosus reflex latency tests** measure the integrity of the sacral reflex arc (S_2 to S_4) by recording the time delay from stimulation of the glans by a pinch or squeeze to contraction of the bulbocavernosus muscle. Longer times suggest a neurologic cause for ED.

  • **Somatosensory evoked potentials** record waveforms over the sacrum and the cerebral cortex in response to dorsal penile nerve stimulation, and can help to localize neurologic lesions to peripheral, sacral, or suprasacral locations.

  • A handheld electromagnetic vibration device can be placed on the shaft of the penis to determine a threshold for **vibration perception.** Loss in perception suggests the presence of a peripheral neuropathy.

  • **Perineal electromyography** can help to detect disorders in the pudendal motor tracts that could be secondary to metabolic or toxic etiologies.

■ Evaluation for sexual pain disorders
  ■ **Office laboratory procedures** include saline and potassium hydroxide wet mounts of vaginal secretions to diagnose vaginitis or vaginosis; urinalysis, urine culture, and evaluation of prostatic secretions to diagnose associated genitourinary infections; and tests to diagnose chlamydial, herpes simplex, and gonococcal infections.
  ■ **Colposcopy** may diagnose specific vaginal or cervical pathology, such as human papillomavirus infections.
  ■ **Pelvic ultrasound** may diagnose adnexal, uterine, or cul-de-sac problems.
  ■ **Laparoscopy** may diagnose, and in some cases treat, adnexal or intraperitoneal pathology.
  ■ **Anoscopy or sigmoidoscopy** may identify associated colorectal problems.

TREATMENT

■ **Medical management**
  ■ **Testosterone** in the form of intramuscular (IM) testosterone enanthate (200 mg every 2 to 3 weeks) is effective treatment for hypogonadal men with testosterone values less than 100 ng/dL. Transdermal preparations (AndroGel, Androderm, Testoderm) applied daily will also raise testosterone levels to normal in 90% of men. Testosterone can also increase desire in women, but may produce androgenizing side effects.
  ■ **Bromocriptine mesylate (Parlodel)** treats hyperprolactinemia. Treatment begins with 1.25 mg daily, increasing by 1.25 mg every 3 to 7 days until the serum prolactin level is normal.
  ■ **Yohimbine (Aphrodyne)** theoretically enhances penile erections by restricting penile venous outflow and increasing libido through a central nervous system effect. Dosage is 6 mg PO tid.
  ■ The **PDE5 inhibitors** have become the drugs of choice for most men with ED. The recommended doses are as follows: sildenafil, 50 to 100 mg taken 1 hour prior to sexual activity; vardenafil (Levitra), 10 to 20 mg also taken 1 hour prior to intercourse; and tadalafil (Cialis), 10 to 20 mg taken 1 to 24 hours prior to intercourse. These drugs are contraindicated in patients taking organic nitrites because they potentiate their hypotensive effects.
  ■ **Oral phentolamine mesylate (Vasomax)** 20 to 80 mg taken 15 minutes prior to intercourse improves erectile function in men with mild-to-moderate ED. It is available in Mexico and Brazil, but not in the United States.
  ■ **Sublingual or transbuccal apomorphine (Uprima, Spontane)** is taken in 2 to 3 mg oral doses 20 minutes prior to sexual activity. It acts on the hypothalamic region to lower the threshold for erectile/ejaculatory reflexes. It is now available in England, but not in the United States.

■ **Intraurethrally inserted PGE₁ tablets (MUSE)** in strengths of 125, 250, 500, and 1,000 µg demonstrate effectiveness in 40% of men with ED from various causes.

■ **Topical nitroglycerin (Nitrol)** relaxes penile arterial smooth muscle, causing subsequent engorgement. Men with mild vascular, neurologic, or mixed arousal dysfunction may respond to 0.5 to 1.0 inches of 2% ointment applied to the penile shaft just prior to intercourse. The man must also wear a condom to avoid vaginal absorption by his partner. **Topical 2% minoxidil solution (Rogaine)** applied to the glans is reportedly as effective as nitroglycerin. Prophylactic analgesics help manage associated headache. **Topical PGE₁ (Topiglan, Alprox-TD)** is under study in men with ED. **Topical alpsrostadil (ALISTA)** may enhance clitoral arousal and vaginal lubrication in women. **Oral** and **vaginal phentolamine** are now being studied in women to determine whether they can enhance vaginal blood flow.

■ **Intracavernous injection of vasoactive drugs.** Patients may inject either papaverine or PGE₁(alprostadil) into a corpus cavernosum with a 27-gauge needle to induce an erection. Men with neurogenic disorders, mild vascular problems, combined neurogenic and vascular disorders, and psychogenic problems for which psychosexual treatment has failed may respond well. Injections also benefit men with PE because sexual activity can continue despite the premature orgasm. Therapy begins with a low dose of either drug (10 mg papaverine; 2.5 to 5.0 µg PGE₁) that is gradually increased to provide an adequate erection that lasts 1 to 2 hours. This usually requires 10 to 80 mg papaverine or 10 to 40 µg PGE₁. Injections are limited to 3 per week and 10 per month. In difficult cases these drugs may be mixed and used in combination. Bimix contains papaverine and phentolamine, and Trimix adds PGE₁. Injecting vasoactive intestinal polypeptide (VIP) 0.025 mg mixed with phentolamine 2.0 mg (Invicorp) reportedly demonstrates efficacy in men who have failed other injection therapies. It is not yet available in the United States.

■ **Tricyclic antidepressants** in antidepressant doses may help treat PE because they inhibit the cholinergic component of ejaculation.

■ **Thioridazine** at standard antidepressant doses may also benefit men with PE.

■ **Phenoxybenzamine (Dibenzaline)** is used by men with PE in daily doses of 20 to 30 mg. It should not be used by men who wish to procreate because phenoxybenzamine inhibits seminal emission.

■ **Clomipramine (Anafranil)** may benefit PE by increasing the sensory threshold for genital stimuli. Doses start with 25 to 50 mg 12 to 24 hours prior to sexual activity and increase until the man achieves ejaculatory control, experiences side effects, or reaches maximal recommended doses.

■ **Sertraline (Zoloft)** 50 to 100 mg, **paroxetine (Paxil)** 20 to 40 mg, and **fluoxetine (Prozac)** 20 to 60 mg taken 3 to 5 hours prior to sexual activity also delay ejaculation. Adding sildenafil 50 mg 1 hour prior to sexual activity increases the effectiveness of these drugs.

■ **Dapoxetine** may become the first Food and Drug Administration (FDA)-approved drug specifically indicated for PE. Studies indicate that 30 to 60 mg taken 1 to 3 hours before intercourse results in a three- to fourfold increase in ejaculatory latency time.

■ **A 2.5% lidocaine–2.5% prilocaine cream (EMLA cream)** applied to the glans and covered with a condom 30 minutes prior to intercourse also reportedly helps PE. It may also help women with introital dyspareunia and vaginismus.

■ **Water-based lubricating products (K-Y Jelly, Astroglide)** applied directly to the genital area prior to intercourse may reduce discomfort associated with intercourse without increasing infection or damaging condoms.

■ **Surgical management**
  ■ **Arterial revascularization.** Successful surgery for proximal artery occlusion can improve blood flow through the hypogastric vessels. Success depends on whether the distal vessels are patent and whether surgery damages the autonomic nerves that travel over the vessels.

- **Venous surgery.** Surgical procedures for venous incompetence have not demonstrated long-term success.
- **Penile prosthesis.** The penile prosthesis is the most reliable surgical option in the United States, with the inflatable prosthesis implanted most frequently. Prosthesis implantation is relatively uncomplicated, but most devices require replacement after 48 to 60 months.

■ **Mechanical management. Penile vacuum pumps (ErecAid)** can also aid erections. Air is withdrawn from a lubricated cylinder that the man places over his penis to create a vacuum that draws blood into the corpora cavernosum. An elastic band around the penile base maintains the erection when the cylinder is removed. A device that creates suction over the clitoris **(EROS-CTD)** is now approved by the FDA. It increases vaginal blood flow, as well as clitoral blood flow, erection, and sensitivity, and reportedly enhances sexual arousal and orgasm in women. Various **penile constriction rings (Soft Touch, Pressure Point, ACTIS Constriction Loop)** help to maintain erections in men with venous incompetence.

■ **Psychosexual therapy**
- **Standard principles** that undergird psychosexual therapy include the beliefs that people are responsible for their own sexuality; that growth in sexual attitudes, performance, and feelings results from behavioral change; that every person deserves sexual health; that physiologic relaxation is the foundation for sexual excitement; and that boundaries must be established with the nonsexual aspects of sexual dysfunction.
- **Cognitive—behavioral therapy** that incorporates behavioral therapy into other treatments is the treatment choice for managing most sexual dysfunctions. Behavior therapists assume that sexual dysfunction is learned maladaptive behavior that causes patients to fear sexual interaction. Therapy inhibits the learned anxious response.
- **Sensate focus exercises** heighten sensory awareness to touch, sight, sound, and smell. As patients focus on their own sensations they relax and overcome the barriers to their natural physiologic responses.
- **Hypnotherapy** helps remove symptoms and alter attitudes by teaching patients to use relaxation techniques before a sexual encounter and to learn alternative ways of dealing with anxiety-provoking sexual situations.
- **Group therapy** provides a strong support system to counteract sexual myths, correct misconceptions, and provide accurate information about sexual anatomy, physiology, and varieties of behavior.
- **Traditional marital therapy** is also important to manage the marital or relationship problems that generate stress, fatigue, and dysphoria.

■ **Specific sexual therapy techniques**
- **Directed self-stimulation** is the most effective treatment program to date for primary orgasmic dysfunction in women.
- **The stop-start technique of Semans** and the **squeeze technique** modification of Masters and Johnson help to manage PE.
- **Sexologic examination.** The vaginal sexologic examination helps treat women with arousal and orgasmic disorders by assisting them and their partners to identify specific erotically sensitive vaginal and genital foci. The examination is performed with the sexual partner, after the woman's signed consent.
- **Systematic desensitization** techniques successfully treat both dyspareunia and vaginismus.

References

1. American Psychiatric Association. *Diagnostic and statistical manual of mental disorders.* 4th ed. Washington, DC: American Psychiatric Association; 1994.
2. Halvorsen JG. The clinical evaluation of common sexual concerns. *CNS Spectrums* 2003;8(3):217–224.
3. Hellstrom WJG, ed. Treating erectile dysfunction: appropriate use of the PDE5 inhibitors. *J Fam Pract* 2005;Dec(S):2–46.

4. Laumann EO, Paik A, Rosen RC. Sexual dysfunction in the United States: prevalence and predictors. *JAMA* 1999;281(6):537–544.
5. Lue TF. Drug therapy: erectile dysfunction. *N Engl J Med* 2000;342(24):1802–1813.
6. Phillips NA. Female sexual dysfunction: evaluation and treatment. *Am Fam Physician* 2000;62(1):127–136, 141–142.

EATING DISORDERS
Cynthia G. Olsen

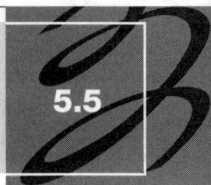

5.5

*E*ating disorders affect up to 7.5 million Americans or about 4% of the U.S. population, and involve a disturbed eating behavior and distorted body image. Bulimia nervosa is three times more common than anorexia nervosa. The male-to-female prevalence of eating disorders is approximately 1 to 10. The mortality rate for each is significant with that for anorexia nervosa 2% to 6%, mostly from starvation and suicide. The age of onset for anorexia begins at 13 years and that for bulimia is in later adolescence and young adulthood. Both are found predominantly in industrialized societies, where ideals about body size and the acceptance of dieting exist.

ANOREXIA NERVOSA

Diagnostic Criteria for Anorexia Nervosa (307.1)[1*]

- Refusal to maintain body weight at or above 85% normal weight for age and height.
- Intense fear of gaining weight or becoming fat.
- Disturbed perception of own body weight or shape, and denial of severity.
- Amenorrhea in postmenarchal female (at least three consecutive cycles).

Clinical Presentation

Anorexia nervosa presents often after a stressful life event, such as a school change, and may be episodic, relapsing, or chronic. The behavior of the anorexic includes impulse control problems and obsession with food. The two subtypes of anorexia nervosa include *restricting type* and *binge-eating/purging type*. Psychologic features include issues of loss and separation, indifference or vigorous denial, perfectionism, dichotomous thinking, alexithymia, conflicting self-denial and hedonism, and delayed psychosocial development. The stress of starvation causes the person to appear irritable, dysphoric, anxious, and angry.

Differential Diagnosis

Psychiatric disorders that may mimic anorexia nervosa include major depressive disorder, schizophrenia, body dysmorphic disorder, substance dependency, obsessive–compulsive disorder, and social phobia. Medical conditions include colitis, carcinomas such as brain tumor, pancreatic and bronchogenic carcinoma, acquired immunodeficiency syndrome, superior mesenteric artery syndrome, gastric outlet obstruction, and metabolic disorders such as Addison disorder, hyperthyroidism, or thiamine deficiency. The comorbidity of psychiatric and medical issues can make diagnosis and treatment challenging.

Symptoms and Physical Signs

The history is paramount in assessment and should include both the patient and family or friends. The clinician needs to verify body perception and weight loss behaviors. The anorexic patient may report aversion to meat, cold insensitivity, other compulsive behaviors,

*Adapted from DSM-IV.

exhaustion due to overactivity and exercise, sleep disturbance, paradoxical satiety, constipation, nausea, and abdominal pain and bloating. Measurement of height, weight, and body mass index is important to the assessment and monitoring of treatment. Findings include emaciation and decreased muscle mass, myopathy, lanugo of the trunk, peripheral edema, dry skin, petechiae, yellowed skin from hypercarotenemia, parotid gland hypertrophy, ketotic breath, bradycardia, hypothermia, and hypotension. Patients with anorexia who engage in binge-purge behavior may also have the findings of bulimia. Careful psychologic assessment should seek affective disorders, suicide risk, personality disorders, and substance abuse. In starving patients depression may be the result of metabolic disturbance and can resolve with weight gain and correction.

Laboratory studies may reveal normochromic normocytic anemia with leukopenia, electrolyte disturbance, hypothyroidism, low estrogen state with osteoporosis, diminished testosterone in males, increased liver functions due to fatty liver, hypercholesterolemia, increased growth hormone, renal insufficiency due to dehydration and hypokalemia, arrhythmias, and urine pH >7. Electrocardiogram is important in severely underweight patients (>25% of baseline weight) and those using chemical purgatives, especially syrup of ipecac (emetine) to rule out potentially life-threatening arrhythmia or disturbance. Magnetic resonance imaging usually reveals a decrease in brain size with ventricular dilatation.

BULIMIA NERVOSA

Diagnostic Criteria for Bulimia Nervosa (307.51)[1]*

- Recurrent binge eating, out of control, typically large amounts of food over a discrete time period (<2 hours).
- Recurrent compensatory acts to prevent weight gain (vomiting, laxatives, diuretics, enemas, fasting, diet pills, excessive exercise).
- Binge-purge cycle occur twice per month for 3 months.
- Preoccupation and criticism of body weight and shape.

Clinical Presentation

Bulimia can be further subtyped into *purging* (more common) and *nopurging types*. Bulimia is commonly found in families with a history of rigidity, substance abuse, sexual abuse, affective disorder, and obesity. Binge eating often begins after a period of dieting. The course may be chronic or intermittent with remissions, and long-term outcome is unknown. Patients with bulimia, unlike those with anorexia, have normal or slightly above normal body weight, admit more readily to their behaviors, have more somatic complaints despite being healthier, and are more outgoing and expressive. Psychologic features may include depressive disorders, emotional lability, low self-esteem, guilt and shame, negative self-criticism, dissociation during the binge-purge, substance abuse (one third), and personality disorders (one half). Behaviors include the consumption of sweets and high caloric foods, eating before and after parties, secrecy and attempts to hide behavior, manipulation of medications, and self-induced vomiting, the most common purge method (80% to 90%). Other common purge methods include regular use of laxatives, diuretics, diet pills, enemas, and syrup of ipecac. Unusual cases of medically ill patients withholding or abusing medical treatments for the purpose of weight loss have been reported.[2]

Differential Diagnosis

Psychiatric disorders that may mimic bulimia include anorexia nervosa (binge eating/purging type), major depression with atypical features, borderline personality disorder, and substance abuse. Mental illness comorbidity is high and can make diagnosis challenging. Neurologic conditions that have abnormal eating features include Kleine–Levin syndrome, Kluver–Bucy-like syndromes, Parkinson disease, migraine, temporal lobe epilepsy and other seizure disorders, brain tumors (posterior cranial fossa and pinealoma), postconcussive syndrome, and other conditions with increased intracranial pressure. Other medical entities include gastrointestinal carcinoma, pyloric obstruction, mesenteric artery syndrome, malignant hypertension, digitalis therapy, metabolic alkalosis, opiate withdrawal, and pilocarpine therapy.

---

*Adapted from DSM-IV.

Symptoms and Physical Signs

A careful history for binge eating and compensatory behaviors is necessary. Patients may report abdominal distention and discomfort, constipation, frequent pharyngitis, "heartburn," hematemesis, postbinge depression, and fluctuation of weight of 10 lb in a month. Self-induced vomiting frequently results in dental damage with posterior erosion from acidity, caries, and chips. The Russell sign is abrasions and scarring on the dorsum of the hand (typically unilateral and the dominant side) caused by scraping on the teeth. Other findings include bilateral, painless parotid and submandibular gland hypertrophy, abdominal striae, anal tears and fissures, dehydration, electrolyte disturbance, myopathy (especially proximal muscles), cardiomegaly, and arrhythmia. Unlike patients with anorexia who experience amenorrhea, patients with bulimia nervosa frequently have oligomenorrhea or irregular menses. Complications of purging can include gastric and esophageal rupture and tears, cathartic colon, aspiration and resulting pneumonitis, cardiac arrest, tonic-clonic seizures, carpopedal spasm, and hypokalemic nephropathy. Psychiatric assessment for comorbid conditions and suicide risk is necessary. Borderline personality disorder is a common comorbid condition, which makes treatment difficult and is characterized by self-destructive behavior, poor interpersonal relationships, and impulsive behavior.

Laboratory Findings

Abnormal laboratory findings may include occult blood in the stool, steatorrhea, hypocalcemia or hypomagnesemia, metabolic alkalosis, hypokalemia, impaired renal function, elevated serum amylase due to vomiting (30% of patients) and elevated liver enzymes particularly aspartate aminotransferase, lactate dehydrogenase, and alkaline phosphatase. Electrocardiographic abnormalities reflect electrolyte disturbance.

TREATMENT

Medical Treatment

The patient with an eating disorder is frustrating and requires the care of several providers that may include the family physician, psychologist, psychiatrist, social worker, and nutritionalist. Poorer outcome is associated with histories of sexual abuse, personality disorder, high pretreatment severity, and longer duration of illness. The first priority is to save the patient's life from complications; medical hospitalization is required for hemodynamic or metabolic disturbance, medication overdose, suicidal intent, and for the initiation of nutritional restoration. Psychiatric referral can help delineate the need for either outpatient or specialized inpatient care. Referral to a specialized program is prudent for patients with anorexia with >25% loss of their previous weight. A nutritionalist accesses lifetime dietary history and behavior and the patient's nutritional beliefs and values. Refeeding of the anorexic person begins by increasing the daily caloric intake by 300 calories and reducing activity by 50%. Refeeding syndrome, from overaggressive refeeding, results in fluid and electrolyte shifts, hypophosphatemia, congestive heart failure, hyper- and hypoglycemia, diarrhea myocardial dysfunction, and neurologic dysfunction including seizures. An energy intake of 1,200 kcal per day is appropriate for the first few days in severely starved, emaciated patients. Weekly weight gain expectations should be between 0.5 and 1.5 kg, depending on the program. Most adult females require 3,000 kcal of energy per day to achieve full weight restoration.[2] Total parental nutrition and tube feeding are invasive, remove responsibility from the patient, are often unsuccessful, and should only be used in dire situations. Learning appropriate eating behaviors include avoiding "dietary foods" aimed at weight loss, eating in company, and developing appropriate responses to both hunger and satiety. Patients with bulimia at normal weight need education on normal, relaxed eating behaviors, avoidance of restrictive practices, and tolerance of their body habitus.

Medical management of complications may necessitate hospitalization and referral. Cardiac monitoring of patients with electrolyte abnormalities, surgical consultation in the case of pneumothorax or Borhaave syndrome (25% mortality rate), or gastrointestinal specialist referral for cathartic colon, pancreatitis, or metabolic disturbance can be lifesaving. Pregnant patients have greater stress due to changes in body habitus, are at increased risk of hyperemesis gravidarium, and require close collaboration with an interested obstetrician. Pharmacotherapy has included prokinetic drugs for delayed gastric emptying, estrogens for osteoporosis, trace minerals and vitamins for nutritional depletion, topical fluoride and bicarbinate rinses for dental erosions, H_2 blockers for gastric reflux, and bulk fiber supplements in constipation. Cyproheptadine (Periactin) is a sedating, serotonergic antagonist, which may stimulate appetite but is usually not helpful.

Psychiatric Treatment

Psychiatric hospitalization is useful if the patient is depressed and suicidal, exhibits behavior unresponsive to outpatient therapy, displays psychosis, or a recalcitrant denial in need of confrontation and family therapy. Treatment goals include reduction of weight loss and binge-purge cycles and addressing unresolved psychologic conflicts. Behavioral "prescriptions" and contracts are useful. Professional psychologic testing is often performed. Psychotherapy (psychodynamic and cognitive–behavioral) in an individual or group setting is essential. Family involvement is almost always needed for assessment and resolution of interpersonal and family conflicts. Aftertreatment plans and relapse prevention plans should be prepared upon discharge. Psychopharmacotherapy for anorexia is disappointing. Distorted cognition does not respond to antipsychotic medications and they should be used only for psychotic features. Antidepressants, particularly selective serotonin-reuptake inhibitors (SSRI), are the primary drug treatment. Tricyclic antidepressants should be avoided in lower-weight patients at risk of cardiovascular complications. SSRIs with anxiolytic and antiobsessional properties are most useful.

In the absence of electrolyte disorders, patients with bulimia are usually managed in an outpatient setting. Patients with bulimia have a better response to drug treatment than do patients with anorexia. Antidepressants can be helpful in reducing binges, even in the absence of depression. The SSRIs (fluoxetine, paroxetine, and sertraline) have a low risk and side-effect profile are well suited for these patients.

References

1. American Psychiatric Association. *Diagnostic and statistical manual of mental disorders* (4th ed.) (DSM-IV). Washington, DC: American Psychiatric Association; 1994.
2. Garner DM, Garfinkle PE. *Handbook of treatment for eating disorders.* 2nd ed. 1997 New York: Guilford Press.

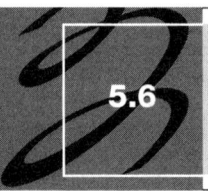

5.6 SLEEP DISORDERS
Carol Cordy

INSOMNIA

General Principles

Definition

Insomnia, primary or comorbid with medical, psychiatric, or neurologic disorders, is the inability to get adequate sleep even under ideal sleep conditions. This sleep disorder results in daytime fatigue, difficulty concentrating, irritability, and depression. Adequate sleep for adults ranges from 6 to 9 hours, averaging just over 8 hours.

Epidemiology

Approximately 50% of Americans complain of frequent insomnia, one in three experiences nightly insomnia, and up to 15% have chronic insomnia. Women and elderly people suffer from insomnia more often than men. Insomnia is associated with psychiatric and medical illness, poor quality of life, and poor memory, mood, and cognitive function; 6% of the population take over-the-counter sleep aids and 6% take prescription hypnotics.

Pathophysiology

The relationship between brain function and insomnia has not been well defined.

Etiology

Insomnia can be caused or exacerbated by other sleep disorders; psychiatric, medical, and neurologic disorders; disruption of the sleep–wake cycle; and medications. Caffeine, alcohol, nicotine, drugs of abuse, and poor sleep hygiene also cause insomnia.

Diagnosis

Clinical Presentation

Fatigue, impairment in daytime functioning, irritability, and depression may be a patient's presenting complaints. Patients who complain of insomnia report waking up feeling tired, waking up many times during the night, difficulty falling asleep, or waking up too early. Because the majority of patients with insomnia are not diagnosed, it is recommended that health care providers screen all patients with a brief sleep history.

History

A sleep history includes duration and frequency of symptoms of insomnia, number of hours of sleep per night, sleep conditions, medical illnesses, psychiatric illnesses, prescription and over-the-counter medications, and use of alcohol, tobacco, caffeine, and drugs of abuse. The patient's bed partner can help diagnose comorbid sleep disorders. Severe daytime drowsiness with frequent episodes of falling asleep during the day can help diagnose narcolepsy.

The diagnosis of primary insomnia is made if symptoms are not:

- Due to sleep deprivation. Patients with sleep deprivation are tired because they stay up too late or get up too early to get adequate sleep.
- Due to another sleep disorder such as obstructive sleep apnea (OSA), restless legs syndrome (RLS), periodic limb movement disorder (PLMD), narcolepsy, circadian rhythm sleep disorders (delayed or advanced sleep phase syndromes), nightmares, jet lag, or shift work.
- Comorbid with a psychiatric disorder, such as depression, bipolar disorder, generalized anxiety disorder, panic disorder, obsessive–compulsive disorder, posttraumatic stress disorder, a somatoform disorder, schizophrenia, acute stress, bereavement, trauma, or rejection. In all, 30% to 50% of insomnia is associated with a psychiatric disorder.
- Comorbid with a medical condition, such as asthma, allergies, hyperthyroidism, pain (arthritis, headaches), chronic obstructive pulmonary disease, congestive heart failure, frequent urination (benign prostatic hypertrophy, or BPH; stress/urge incontinence), menopausal symptoms, or gastroesophageal reflux.
- Caused by medications or drugs, such as steroids, antidepressants, antihypertensives, decongestants, bronchodilators, alcohol, nicotine, caffeine, or cocaine.
- Caused by a noisy or uncomfortable sleep environment or poor sleep hygiene. Up to 15% of insomnia is caused by poor sleep hygiene.

Physical Examination

A physical examination is indicated depending on the medical history.

Laboratory Studies

Ordered to rule out medical conditions based on the patient's medical history and physical examination.

Diagnostic Studies

Depression and anxiety questionnaires (Beck, Jung, Hamilton, PHQ) may be helpful in diagnosing psychiatric disorders. Sleep studies can be ordered if another sleep disorder is suspected.

Classification

Insomnia is classified as acute—lasting from 1 night to less than 1 month, or chronic—occurring at least three times a week for more than 4 weeks. Insomnia is also classified as primary or comorbid. The International Classification of Sleep Disorders lists 42 diagnoses associated with insomnia.

Treatment

If insomnia persists after successful treatment of another sleep disorder, psychiatric disorder, or medical condition, and medications and drugs that exacerbate insomnia have been stopped and proper sleep hygiene (see patient education) maintained, treatment with behavior therapy and/or medication is appropriate. Acute insomnia may be successfully treated with supportive counseling and a short course of hypnotic medication, which may help prevent chronic insomnia. Chronic insomnia is treated with behavioral therapy and a short course of hypnotic medications. Some patients may need a longer course of hypnotic or other sedating medications.

Behavioral

- **Stimulus control therapy** teaches patients to associate the bedroom only with sleep or sex. They are instructed to leave the bedroom if they are still awake after 15 to 30 minutes and return only when sleepy. This is repeated until they fall asleep.
- **Sleep restriction therapy** teaches patients to limit the time they spend in bed to their reported sleep time or a minimum of 4 hours. Daytime naps are not allowed. This state of sleep deprivation leads to more rapid sleep onset and efficient sleep.
- **Relaxation and cognitive therapies** may also be effective.
- **Bright light therapy** can help reset a disrupted sleep–wake cycle.
- **Daily exercise** may also improve sleep.

Medications

There is a risk of harm with the use of benzodiazepine and nonbenzodiazepine hypnotics as well as antidepressants and other medications for insomnia. These risks must be weighed against the benefits of adequate sleep.

Benzodiazepine and Nonbenzodiazepine Hypnotics. Approved indications for hypnotic medications are for brief and occasional treatment. Hypnotics have been shown to be of continued benefit for up to 6 months. Oversedation, poor coordination, and memory problems may occur early in treatment but usually resolve over time. The nonbenzodiazepine hypnotics act only on the type 1 benzodiazepine receptors in the brain and do not have muscle relaxant or antiseizure properties. Short-acting agents cause less daytime drowsiness. Intermediate- and long-acting agents cause less withdrawal and rebound insomnia. Triazolam (Halcion) has been associated with pronounced anterograde amnesia although all hypnotics have this potential side effect. These agents should not be used in patients with sleep apnea or active substance abuse. Half doses should be used in elderly individuals.

- **Short-acting nonbenzodiazepines—eszopiclone (Lunesta) 1 to 3 mg hs, zaleplon (Sonata) 5 to 20 mg hs, zolpidem (Ambien) 5 to 10 mg hs**
- **Short-acting benzodiazepines—triazolam (Halcion) 0.125 to 0.25 mg hs, oxazepam (Serax) 10 to 15 mg hs (off-label)**
- **Intermediate-acting benzodiazepines—temazepam (Restoril) 7.5 to 30 mg hs estazolam (Prosom) 1 to 2 mg hs, lorazepam (Ativan) 0.5 to 2 mg hs (off-label)**
- **Long-acting benzodiazepines—clonazepam (Klonopin) 0.25 to 1 mg hs (off label), flurazepam (Dalmane) 15 to 30 mg hs**

When patients stop taking hypnotics they may suffer from **rebound insomnia,** which can be treated with a few days of diphenhydramine 50 mg hs, trazodone 50 to 100 mg hs, or gabapentin 100 to 300 mg hs, or by restarting the hypnotic and tapering slowly.

Antidepressants. Antidepressants are not well studied or Food and Drug Administration (FDA) approved for the treatment of insomnia. They are recommended for patients with comorbid depression and anxiety or antidepressant-induced insomnia but may help patients with primary insomnia. Insomnia often responds to treatment of the underlying disorder, even with the more activating antidepressants. Trazodone can cause daytime drowsiness as well as orthostatic hypotension in elderly patients and, rarely, priapism. Tricyclic antidepressants are relatively contraindicated in elderly patients and in patients who abuse drugs and alcohol or are suicidal. Tricyclic antidepressants are the least safe in overdose. Selective serotonin-reuptake inhibitors and tricyclics may exacerbate RLS and PLMD.

- Trazodone (Desyrel) 25 to 200 mg hs
- Amitriptyline (Elavil) 10 to 25 mg hs, imipramine (Tofranil) 25 to 50, trimipramine (Surmontil) 25 to 50, nortriptyline (Pamelor) 10 to 25, doxepin (Sinequan) 25 to 50 mg hs
- Selective serotonin-reuptake inhibitors, mirtazapine, and venlafazine for comorbid depression.

Other Sleep Aids
- Gabapentin (Neurontin) 100 to 900 mg hs
- Diphenhydramine (Benadryl) or doxylamine (Unisom) in over-the-counter sleep preparations. Promethazine (Phenergan) 12.5 to 25 mg hs and hydroxyzine (Atarax) 10 to 100 mg hs have sedating effects.
- Melatonin 1 to 2 mg hs may help with jet lag, shift work, and delayed sleep phase syndrome, as well as chronic insomnia.
- Valerian and other herbals and L-tryptophan have little evidence to support their use.

Patient Education
- **Proper sleep hygiene** (not usually effective when used alone—poor sleep hygiene causes less than 20% of insomnia).
- Maintain a regular sleep–wake schedule, avoid daytime naps.
- Associate the bedroom with sleep, go to bed only when sleepy.
- Make the bedroom environment quiet, dark, and comfortable.
- Establish a regular bedtime ritual.
- Avoid caffeine, alcohol, and nicotine.
- Avoid heavy meals.
- Exercise regularly at least 3 hours before bedtime.

Referrals
Unless there is a history suggestive of OSA, RLS, PLMD, or narcolepsy, referral to a sleep disorder clinic for sleep studies/polysomnography is rarely necessary. Referral to a sleep disorder clinic may be appropriate for patients whose symptoms of primary or comorbid insomnia do not resolve with proper sleep hygiene, hypnotic medication, and adequate treatment of their comorbid disorder.

Counseling
Hypnotic medications should only be taken when a patient can get a full night's sleep. Possible side effects of medications should be discussed with all patients. Patients should not drive or operate machinery when they initiate treatment with sedative medications.

Follow-Up
Patients who require long-term use of medications for insomnia should be reassessed frequently and referred to a sleep clinic if they do not respond to treatment.

Complications
Daytime drowsiness can result in poor job performance, automobile accidents, decreased quality of life, and increased depression.

OBSTRUCTIVE SLEEP APNEA

General Principles
Definition
Obstructive sleep apnea is the occurrence of periodic abnormal and prolonged (greater than 10 seconds) pauses in breathing due to collapse or partial collapse and occlusion of the upper airway. Five or more episodes of apnea with hypopnea (decreased oxygen saturation) in 1 hour is diagnostic of sleep apnea.

Anatomy
Enlarged tonsils, uvula, or tongue, redundant tissue in the soft palate, small upper airways, nasal obstruction, or a loss of upper airway muscle tone may be present.

Epidemiology

OSA occurs twice as often in men (4% of middle-aged men) as in women. Obesity is a risk factor but OSA can also occur in normal-weight patients. There may be a genetic influence.

Pathophysiology

The arousal during sleep due to hypoxia and hypercapnea is thought to lead to adverse cardiovascular outcomes, insulin resistance, and metabolic syndrome.

Diagnosis

Clinical Presentation

Patients may present with a complaint of awakening suddenly gasping for air, morning headaches, nonrestful sleep, and daytime drowsiness. Also see Insomnia, above.

History

The patient's bed partner may notice loud snoring and episodes of choking or gasping. Also see Insomnia.

Physical Examination

A physical examination is indicated depending on the medical history. Physical abnormalities in the upper airways may not be obvious on physical exam.

Laboratory Studies

Complete blood count for polycythemia, thyroid-stimulating hormone (TSH) for hypothyroidism. Also see Insomnia.

Diagnostic Studies

Electrocardiogram to rule out cardiac abnormalities and a computed tomography or magnetic resonance imaging study if surgery is anticipated.

Diagnostic Procedures

Endoscopy if surgery is planned.

Classification

OSA can be differentiated from central sleep apnea, which is rare, with sleep studies.

Treatment

Comorbid conditions, including obesity, hypertension, and diabetes, should be treated. The effectiveness of surgery is controversial as is the use of oral devices.

Behavioral

Obese patients should lose weight. All patients should avoid the supine position during sleep, stop smoking, and avoid alcohol and sedating medications including hypnotics.

Medications

No medications have been particularly helpful although activating antidepressants may reduce daytime drowsiness.

Surgical

Some patients may respond to surgery to remove tissue that is obstructing the upper airways or craniofacial surgery to advance the mandible. Some patients may require tracheostomy.

Special Therapy

Referral to a sleep disorder clinic for nasal continuous positive airway pressure (CPAP) therapy is usually effective and reduces morbidity and mortality. The use of oral devices is controversial.

Referrals

Referral to a sleep clinic for diagnosis and treatment is always indicated.

Counseling

Patients need to understand the importance of using their CPAP device to avoid the morbidities and possible mortality of severe sleep apnea.

Complications
Untreated obstructive sleep apnea can lead to hypertension, heart attack, congestive heart failure, stroke, and even death, as well as car accidents and job-related accidents secondary to daytime fatigue.

RESTLESS LEGS SYNDROME

General Principles
Definition
RLS is an uncomfortable sensation of needing to move one's legs or arms when sitting or lying still.

Epidemiology
Approximately 2% to 15% of the population may have RLS. RLS is more common in women than men. There may be a genetic influence. RLS occurs more often in elderly individuals. As many as 20% of pregnant women complain of RLS. RLS is common in patients with end-stage renal failure. Of patients with RLS, 80% to 90% also have PLMD.

Etiology
RLS is usually idiopathic but may be secondary to anemia, uremia, neuropathy, varicose veins, pregnancy, or medications including tricyclic antidepressants, selective serotonin-reuptake inhibitors, lithium, and dopamine antagonists.

Pathophysiology
RLS may involve alterations in central dopamine mechanisms.

Diagnosis
Clinical Presentation
Patients complain of frequent uncomfortable sensations in their legs and occasionally their arms and the need to move to attempt to relieve this sensation. These symptoms are worse in the evening and at rest. If PMLD is present, patients may complain of symptoms of insomnia.

Diagnostic Workup
There is no test for RLS.

Physical Examination
A physical examination is indicated depending on the medical history. Check for varicose veins, neuropathy, and poor circulation.

Laboratory Studies
Complete blood count and ferritin for iron deficiency anemia, chemistry panel for uremia and diabetes, pregnancy test.

Treatment
Medications
Dopaminergic Agents
- Carbidopa—levodopa (Sinemet) 12.5/50 to 25/100 bid-tid

Dopamine Agonists
- Pergolide (Permax) 0.1 to 1.0 mg qd to bid, pramipexole (Mirapex) 0.125 to 1.5 mg tid, Ropinirole (Requip) 0.25 to 3.0 mg tid

Opioids (Particularly if Pain Is a Symptom)
- Codeine (Tylenol #3) 1 to 2 tablets hs-bid, hydrocodone (Vicodin 5/325) 1 to 2 tablets hs-bid, oxycodone (Percocet 5/325) 1 to 2 tablets hs-bid, propoxyphene (Darvon) 65 mg hs-bid, methadone 5 to 15 mg hs-bid, tramadol (Ultram) 50 to 100 mg hs-bid

Benzodiazepines (if Insomnia Is a Symptom)
- Clonazepam (Klonopin) 0.5 to 2.0 mg hs, triazolam (Restoril) 7.5 to 30 mg hs

Other Medications
- Gabapentin (Neurontin) 300 to 900 mg hs Clonodine (Catapres) 0.1 to 0.3 mg hs iron supplements for patients whose serum ferritin is below 50.

Referrals
Sleep studies if PLMD is suspected.

PERIODIC LIMB MOVEMENT DISORDER

General Principles
Definition
PLMD is the periodic and repetitive flexion of the legs and less frequently the arms that occurs every 20 to 90 seconds for minutes to hours during sleep.

Epidemiology
PLMD occurs in 5% of people age 30 to 50 and in 44% of people over the age of 65. Most patients with RLS have PLMD but most patients with PLMD do not have RLS; 12% of people with insomnia have PLMD.

Etiology
See RLS.

Diagnosis
Clinical Presentation
The patient may complain only of daytime drowsiness. The diagnosis is usually made by the patient's bed partner.

History
See Insomnia and RLS.

Physical Examination
Physical examination as indicated depending on medical history.

Treatment
Medications
If medical causes and RLS have been treated and offending medications have been stopped but symptoms persists, clonazepam (Klonopin) 0.5 to 2 mg hs or temazepam (Restoril) 15 to 30 mg hs may be helpful.

Referrals
The diagnostic workup may require referral to a sleep disorder clinic.

Complications
Complications of insomnia.

NARCOLEPSY

General Principles
Definition
Narcolepsy is a disturbance in rapid eye movement (REM) sleep causing periods of excessive daytime drowsiness and a tendency to fall asleep at inappropriate times. Narcolepsy can be associated with sleep paralysis, cataplexy, hypnagogic hallucinations, and disturbed sleep.

Epidemiology
Narcolepsy-cataplexy affects 1 in 2,000 people. Risk in first-degree relatives may be as high as 2%.

Etiology
Unknown.

Diagnosis
Clinical Presentation
The patient complains of sleep attacks lasting minutes to hours sometimes associated with cataplexy (loss of muscle tone), paralysis, or hypnagogic hallucinations.

History
See Insomnia.

Physical Examination
Physical examination as indicated depending on medical history.

Laboratory Studies
Laboratory and imaging studies may rule out comorbid insomnia based on the patient's medical history and physical examination. Depression and anxiety questionnaires (Beck, Jung, Hamilton, PHQ) can be used to rule out psychiatric disorders.

Treatment
Behavioral
Taking three or four short naps during the day may help reduce daytime drowsiness.

Medications
- **Daytime drowsiness**—modafinil (Provigil) 200 to 400 mg each morning, methylphenidate (Ritalin) 10 to 30 mg bid-tid 30 minutes before meals, dextroamphetamine (Dexedrine) 5 to 30 mg bid-tid
- **Cataplexy, sleep paralysis, and hallucinations**—fluoxetine (Prozac) 20 to 60 mg qd, paroxetine (Paxil) 20 to 60 mg qd, sertraline (Zoloft) 50 to 150 mg qd, clomipramine (Anafranil) 25 to 150 mg qd, imipramine (Tofranil) 25 to 100 mg qd, nortriptyline (Pamelor) 25 to 75 mg qd, or protriptyline (Vivactil) 10 to 60 mg qd, desipramine (Norpramin) 25 to 100 mg qd, venlafaxine (EffexorSR) 75 to 225 mg qd, atomoxetine (Straterra) 10 to 80 mg qd
- **Insomnia**—hypnotic medications

Referrals
Referral to a sleep clinic for diagnosis is indicated.

Patient Education
Patients with uncontrolled narcolepsy should not drive or handle dangerous machinery.

Complications
Dangers associated with daytime drowsiness while driving or handling machinery.

DELAYED SLEEP PHASE AND ADVANCED SLEEP PHASE DISORDERS
General Principles
- **Delayed sleep phase disorder (DSPD)** is common in teenagers and young adults who often feel more awake and productive late at night and compensate for late hours by sleeping in. When school and work obligations interfere, they become sleep deprived. DSPD generally resolves with age.
- **Advanced sleep phase disorder (ASPD)** is common in elderly individuals who fall asleep early and awaken very early. This early awakening can be particularly troublesome and potentially dangerous if the patient wanders or falls in the dark.
- Both of these **circadian rhythm disturbances** may respond to **bright light therapy** and **chronotherapy**—delaying or advancing bedtime over time until a normal schedule of sleep is achieved. **Good sleep hygiene** is also recommended.

References
1. www.nhlbi.nih.gov/health/prof/sleep
2. www.sleepfoundation.org
3. www.americaninsomniaassociation.org
4. www.ahrq.gov/clinic/epcsums/insomnsum.htm
5. http://consensus.nih.gov/2005/2005InsomniaSOS026html.htm
6. http://www.wemove.org/rls/
7. Schatzberg A, et al. *Manual of clinical psychology*. 5th ed. Washington, DC: American Psychiatric Publishing; 2005.

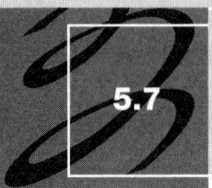

DRUG MISUSE DISORDERS

5.7

Lisa G. Dodson

$\mathcal{D}$rug misuse has long been recognized as a medical and societal problem. These disorders are common, accounting for billions of dollars in medical costs, lost productivity, and years of life lost.[1] Physicians are often in the position to first recognize the signs of drug abuse in patients presenting with other common problems. Patients suffering from drug use disorders may present with acute or chronic somatic complaint: psychiatric complaints; legal, occupational, or family problems; or drug-seeking behaviors. Physicians must maintain a high level of suspicion as well as a reasonable armamentarium of screening tools to recognize and treat these disorders. This chapter addresses both illicit and prescription drug use. Alcohol, tobacco, and drug abuse and overdose are addressed separately.

DEFINITIONS

Although any use of illicit substances and misuse of prescription or over-the-counter medications can be considered at-risk use, the *Diagnostic and Statistical Manual of Mental Disorders*, 4th edition (DSM-IV) identifies specific criteria for alcohol abuse and dependence outlined in Chapter 5.3. Substance abuse is a maladaptive pattern of substance use manifested by recurrent and significant adverse consequences related to the repeated use of substances.[2] Many substance uses do not meet the criteria for either abuse or dependence. It is important to recognize that such labels may be damaging to the patient if incorrectly applied and to be accurate and judicious in the use of these diagnoses.

RECOGNITION AND SCREENING

The most important screening tool for the practicing physician is maintaining a high level of suspicion for the presence of drug use and abuse. Substance abuse affects all social and economic groups and ages. Although there are a number of signs and symptoms characteristic of substance abuse, there is also wide variability in the manifestations of the disorder. In the earlier stages, the symptoms are primarily behavioral and psychologic, rather than physical. Complaints of depression, irritability, anxiety, paranoia, social withdrawal, poor memory, and poor concentration can be associated with drug use. Insomnia, loss of interest in activities, and marital, legal, or occupational difficulties can also signal substance use. Physical health problems may not manifest until late in the disease course. Early recognition and intervention is associated with improved health and social outcomes.[3]

Screening Tools

There are a variety of screening tools available for use in the office setting. The diagnostic standard for substance abuse is a careful diagnostic interview. The advantage of simple screening tools is ease of use and limited time commitment for the busy physician, but there are few data to suggest that these instruments offer advantage over other forms of history taking. One or more positive answers to CAGE or other drug screening questionnaires should prompt additional screening. There are a number of self-administered assessment tools, such as the Drug Abuse Screening Test (DAST), that have been validated for large populations and can be used for further screening. An adolescent-oriented version of DAST is also available. Alternatively, the patient can be referred to a specialist in substance abuse for more in-depth evaluation. Informing the patient of your level of concern about his or her drug use and offering advice regarding the consequences of drug use remains a powerful tool.

Laboratory Testing

Urinalysis remains the most commonly used and best validated method of laboratory testing for drugs of abuse. Advantages of urine testing include noninvasive collection of large sample volumes, well-established and cost-effective methodologies, and fairly standard excretion rates across populations. In addition, urine testing has been accepted for legal purposes. However, urine does not provide quantitative measures and is easily adulterated by addition of external substances or forced diuresis and dilution. Blood offers the advantage of quantitative and qualitative measurements but is limited by invasive collection procedures and the limited sample quantities available. Other body substances, including saliva, sweat, meconium, hair, breath, and breast milk, are potentially useful for identification of drug use, but each has advantages and disadvantages.[4] Meconium may be of use in determining intrauterine drug exposure in high-risk infants but is not recommended for routine use.

Prescription Drugs

Prescription drug abuse, misuse, and diversion is a significant medical and social problem. Street values for commonly prescribed narcotics and other controlled substances is increasing. Fear of being "scammed" or fear of regulatory actions against physicians has had a delirious impact on treatment of legitimate pain disorders and public confidence. Physicians should be concerned about their role in preventing misuse of prescription drugs. Prescribing practices that can help reduce the potential for misuse include:

- Maintaining high standards for charting, including flow sheets with prescription refills, next refill date, and diagnosis being treated
- Placing strict limits on after-hours prescribing
- Implementing prescription drug contracts with patients
- Exercising caution with brand name–only narcotic prescriptions (brand name drugs frequently have a higher street value and may offer little or no advantage in efficacy)
- Insisting on obtaining medical records from previous and concurrent providers
- Restricting controlled-substances prescription to one pharmacy per patient
- Being knowledgeable about pharmacology, abuse potential, and drug interactions
- Knowing federal and state statutes regarding controlled substances prescribing
- Carrying out appropriate diagnostic tests
- Consulting with pain or other specialists when appropriate

TREATMENT

- Treatment of substance disorders is difficult and costly. Although full treatment of severe substance abuse may be outside the scope of many primary care physicians, recent regulatory changes have created new options for physicians wishing to take on the primary treatment of patients with addiction and other drug misuse disorders.[5] Previously restricted to licensed centers, federal law now allows for the office-based treatment of opioid addiction with buprenorphine.[6] The waiver program authorizes qualified physicians who have attended a minimum of 8 hours of approved training to dispense and prescribe narcotics for the purpose of treating opioid addiction. Information on this program and training is available at http://buprenorphine.samhsa.gov.
- Primary care physicians play a crucial role in assisting the patient in recognizing problems associated with their use and the need for treatment. Brief intervention, a method of short counseling sessions focused on changing a specific behavior, has been shown to be effective in decreasing drug use.[3] The components of effective brief intervention include the following:
  - Feedback to patient about effects of substance use
  - Recommendations for behavioral change
  - List of options to achieve behavioral change
  - Discussion of patient reaction to feedback and recommendations
  - Follow-up to monitor and reinforce behavioral change
- The level of intervention and treatment required may exceed the limits of what is possible in the office setting. Referral to inpatient, outpatient, or residential care may be required in advanced cases. Familiarity with the principles of treatment, as well as local

resources available, allows the physician to remain involved in patient care and aids in transition, following treatment. Characteristics of effective treatment programs include the following:

- An individualized treatment approach
- Treatment of multiple problems, not just drug use
- Adequate duration of treatment
- Use of behavioral methods combined with medication when appropriate
- Identification and treatment of co-existing mental disorders
- Monitoring for potential drug use while in treatment
- Multiple episodes and types of treatment as needed

- Therapies include cognitive behavioral methods, such as relapse prevention therapy, individualized counseling, and motivational enhancement therapy. Twelve-step abstinence-based programs have been effectively adapted for a variety of substances and behaviors. The type of treatment that will be successful depends on a number of variables, including the motivation for entering treatment, social supports available, substance or substances of abuse, and age and gender. No one approach is universally successful. For example, adolescents, older adults, and pregnant women require substantially different approaches. Medications such as naltrexone, bupropion, and selective serotonin-reuptake inhibitors show some promise in reducing additive behaviors when combined with psychosocial and behavior therapies.

CONFIDENTIALITY

Federal statutes and regulations and many state laws require strict confidentiality surrounding medical records for drug abuse, screening, assessment, and treatment. Specific authorization for release of information is required; general medical consent is not sufficient.

References

1. Lewis DC. The role of the generalist in the care of the substance-abusing patient. *Med Clin North Am* 1997;81:831.
2. American Psychiatric Association. *Diagnostic and statistical manual of mental disorders*, 4th ed. Washington, DC: American Psychiatric Association; 1994.
3. Barnes HN, Sarnet JH. Brief interventions with substance-abusing patients. *Med Clin North Am* 1997;81:837.
4. Wolff K, et al. A review of biological indicators of illicit drug use, practical considerations and clinical usefulness. *Addition* 1999;94:1279.
5. Kuehn BM. Office-based treatment for opioid addiction achieving goals. *JAMA* 2005;294(7):784.
6. Lintzeris N, Ritter A, Dunlop A, et al. Training primary health care professionals to provide buprenorphine and LAAM treatment. *Substance Abuse* 2002;23(4):245.

Disorders of the Nervous System

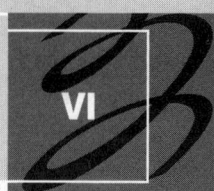

MIGRAINE HEADACHES
Anne D. Walling, Robert Sheeler

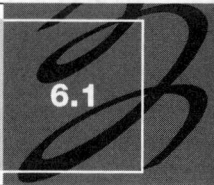

GENERAL PRINCIPLES

Definition

Migraine refers to a group of headaches syndromes characterized by episodes of pain lasting for up to 72 hours that is typically:

- Unilateral (predominantly temple/orbital but can extend to the occiput or neck)
- Moderate–severe intensity
- "Pulsating" "throbbing" "piercing" "splitting" in quality
- Exacerbated by exercise or activity and ameliorated by lying still or sleeping
- Accompanied by symptoms of photophobia (90%), phonophobia (74%), nausea (85%), vomiting (42%), or fatigue/somnolence

Epidemiology

Approximately 28 million Americans (18% of women and 7% of men) suffer from migraine. The condition usually begins in adolescents or young adults and rarely begins after age 40. In women, attacks may synchronize with menstruation and disappear during pregnancy. The number and severity of attacks tend to diminish with age. In children, migraine tends to be more common in boys and episodes may be dominated by vomiting and abdominal pain.

Classification

The International Classification of Headache Disorders recognizes several subtypes of migraine, based on the presence of aura before attacks or on predominant symptoms (e.g., ophthalmoplegic, basilar) but the same general management strategy is applicable to all migraine types.

Pathophysiology

- The pathophysiology of migraine is complex and incompletely understood. An inherited neurobiochemical predisposition to triggering the trigeminovascular system is certainly involved but the precise role of various factors and neuroreceptors (especially the serotonin $5HT_1$ group) remains to be clarified.

■ The U.S. Headache Consortium has produced evidence-based guidelines covering diagnosis, treatment, and prevention of migraine that are endorsed by AAFP and other leading medical specialty organizations.

DIAGNOSIS

History

The diagnosis is based on the history of typical episodes of unilateral headache plus the associated features (above). Age of onset and a family history are helpful in diagnosis. Aura (visual or neurologic symptoms prior to attacks) is pathognomonic but is only present in about 20% of cases. Many patients also describe sensitivity to certain foods (such as red wine, nitrates in smoked foods, or monosodium glutamate) or other factors (e.g., cigarette smoke, relief of stress, or menstruation) that can precipitate migraine attacks. The history may be complicated by the occurrence of more than one type of headache (e.g., tension or analgesic-rebound) in the patient with migraine. The individual features of each attack as well as the frequency, duration, severity, and impact on daily activities vary enormously between migraineurs. Migraine is reported to be underdiagnosed in primary care and questions about disabling headache, nausea, and light sensitivity are recommended to improve recognition of migraine.

Differential Diagnosis

The differential diagnosis includes:

■ Other recurrent headache syndromes (cluster, tension, rebound)
■ Other causes of unilateral headache (temporal arteritis, carotodynia, brain or scalp conditions, including trauma)

Physical Examination

Between attacks, physical examination is normal but a full neurologic examination is necessary to rule out alternative explanations for symptoms. During attacks, the patient looks fatigued, ill, and may be pale and vomiting. Characteristic behavior is to apply pressure and/or cold to the affected side of the head and to lie very still curled in a fetal position, in a dark, quiet room. No abnormalities are typically found on physical and neurologic examination during attacks.

Diagnostic Studies

The consortium concluded that neuroimaging is not warranted in patients with migraine who have no neurologic signs (Grade B recommendation). The estimated rate of finding clinically significant lesions in patients with migraine is estimated at 0.18% to 0.4%. Other laboratory tests are useful only to rule out alternative diagnoses suggested by the clinical presentation.

TREATMENT

Principles

As migraine is a recurring long-term condition, patients must be enabled to manage their attacks with support from the physician. Treatment goals are to:

■ Minimize the frequency, severity, and duration of attacks
■ Reduce migraine-related disability and improve quality of life
■ Prevent iatrogenesis or reliance on inappropriate medications
■ Avoid maladaptive behaviors by the patient and others.

The patient, physician, and others involved must have realistic expectations of treatment. Even with optimal, individualized treatment, migraine can only be managed, it cannot be eliminated. Treatment has to be individualized as patients respond differently to the available therapies. Tables 6.1-1 and 6.1-2 present appropriate therapies. No mechanism currently exists to predict which therapy will benefit an individual patient. Management also has to be adjusted over time as the migraine pattern evolves and the patient changes with age, health conditions, and lifestyle factors. Some experts recommend that the impact of migraine on the patient's life be documented using a standard assessment such as the Migraine Disability Scale (MIDAS) scale to help guide treatment strategy and monitor effectiveness. Patients should be encouraged to optimize their general health and to identify and minimize exposure to any migraine-precipitating factors.

TABLE 6.1-1   Most Effective Therapies for Acute Migraine

Medication class	Effective dose	Scientific/clinical effectiveness[a]	Adverse effects	Quality of evidence	Comments
Analgesics					
Aspirin	500–1,000 mg	+/+/+	GI upset	A	May be combined with antiemetics First-line therapy
Ibuprofen	400–2,400	+/+/+	GI upset	A	First-line therapy
Naproxen Na	750–1,750	+/+/+	GI upset	A	First-line therapy
Acetaminophen + aspirin + caffeine	500/500/130	+++/+/+	GI upset, insomnia	A	First-line therapy
Butorphanol spray	1 mg IN	+++/+++	Drowsiness, nausea, dizziness	A	Rescue medication; potential rebound/abuse
Acetaminophen + codeine	400–600 + 16–25 mg	++/++	Drowsiness, nausea, dizziness	A	Severe cases; potential rebound/abuse
Ergotamines					
DHE spray	0.5–4 mg I/N	+/+/+++	Nausea, nasal discomfort, vasoconstriction	A	Avoid in heart disease, claudication
DHE SC, IM, IV	1 mg	++/+++	Nausea, flushing, dysphoria, vasoconstriction	B	Use with antiemetics, moderate–severe cases, good in emergency room
Triptans					
Sumatriptan	25–50 mg (oral) 5–20 mg (nasal spray) 6 mg (SC)	+++/+++	Nausea, palpitations, hypertension	A	Moderate–severe cases; avoid in basilar, hemiplegic migraine, severe hypertension

(continued)

TABLE 6.1-1 Most Effective Therapies for Acute Migraine *(Continued)*

Medication class	Effective dose	Scientific/clinical effectiveness[a]	Adverse effects	Quality of evidence	Comments
Naratriptan	1–2.5 mg	++/+++	Nausea, palpitations, hypertension	A	Moderate–severe cases; avoid in basilar, hemiplegic migraine, severe hypertension
Rizatriptan	5–10 mg	+++/+++	Nausea, palpitations, hypertension	A	Moderate–severe cases; avoid in basilar, hemiplegic migraine, severe hypertension
Zolmitriptan	2.5–5 mg	+++/+++	Nausea, palpitations, hypertension	A	Moderate–severe cases; avoid in basilar, hemiplegic migraine, severe hypertension

[a]Scientific effectiveness: + less than minimal clinically significant benefit; ++ exceeds minimal clinically significant benefit; +++ far exceeds minimal clinically significant benefits. Clinical effectiveness: + few patients get clinically significant improvement; ++ some patients get clinically significant improvement; +++ most patients get clinically significant improvement.

GI, gastrointestinal; IM, intramuscular; IN, intranasal; IV, intravenous; SC, subcutaneous.

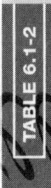

TABLE 6.1-2 Recommended Therapies for Migraine Prophylaxis

Medication class	Effective daily dose	Scientific/clinical effectiveness[a]	Adverse effects	Quality of evidence
beta-Blockers				
Propranolol	80–240 mg	++/+++	Fatigue; may exacerbate depression, asthma, Raynaud, bradycardia, hypotension	A
Atenolol	100 mg	++/++	As propranolol	B
Metoprolol	200 mg	+++/+++	As propranolol	B
Nadolol	80–240 mg	+/+++	As propranolol	B
Antiepileptics				
Divalproex Na	500–1,500	+++/+++	Nausea, asthenia, somnolence, weight gain, tremor, teratogenic	A
Sodium valproate	800–1,500	+++/+++	As above	A
Topiramate	50 mg	++/+++	Paresthesias, nausea, cognitive problems, weight loss	C
Antidepressants				
Amitriptyline	30–150 mg	+++/+++	Drowsiness, weight gain, anticholinergic effects	A
Nortriptyline	Not established	?/+++	As amitriptyline but may be better tolerated	C
Fluoxetine	20qod–40 mg	+/+	Insomnia, fatigue, tremor	B
Calcium channel blockers				
Verapamil	240 mg	+/+	Constipation, contraindicated in conduction block	B
Nimodipine	120 mg	+/+	Abdominal pain, expensive	B

[a]Scientific effectiveness: + less than minimal clinically significant benefit; ++ exceeds minimal clinically significant benefit; +++ far exceeds minimal clinically significant benefits. Clinical effectiveness: + few patients get clinically significant improvement; ++ some patients get clinically significant improvement; +++ most patients get clinically significant improvement.

209

Behavioral Therapies

Behavioral therapies are primarily used in migraine prophylaxis, either alone or as adjuncts to medication. Patients vary enormously in their response to such therapies. Based on a comprehensive review of behavioral and physical treatment modalities, the consortium recommended:

- Relaxation training with or without thermal biofeedback, electromyographic (EMG) biofeedback, and cognitive–behavioral therapy may be considered in preventing migraine (Grade A). No recommendations could be made about which modality is best suited to specific patients.
- Relaxation therapy and biofeedback may be combined with prophylactic medications to achieve additional clinical improvement (Grade B).
- No recommendations could be made concerning hypnosis, acupuncture, transcutaneous electrical nerve stimulation (TENS), cervical manipulation, occlusal adjustment, or hyperbaric oxygen (Grade C).[4,8]

Medications

Migraine Prophylaxis[4,8]

Preventive therapy aims to reduce migraine-associated disability by reducing the number, severity, and duration of migraine attacks and improving the patient's responsiveness to treatment of those attacks that occur despite prophylaxis. Prophylactic therapy should be considered when the patient perceives that the benefits of prophylaxis outweigh the disadvantages (e.g., adherence to daily medication, potential adverse effects, cost). Common circumstances for using prophylactic therapy include the following:

- Frequent, severe, prolonged, and disabling migraine attacks
- Poor response and/or adverse effects limiting use of acute migraine therapy
- Desire to reduce costs of acute therapy
- Rare migraine subtypes associated with potential neurologic damage (e.g., hemiplegic, basilar, prolonged aura)[4]

Although effective prophylactic therapy can halve the number of migraine attacks, fewer than 50% of migraineurs use this therapy.

Choice of a specific prophylactic medication depends on efficacy plus the potential for "added benefit" for an individual patient (e.g., antihypertensive or antidepressive effect) or adverse effect such as vasoconstriction or sedation. The selected medication should be started at a low dose and increased slowly until an effective dose is established. This requires several months of monitoring for effectiveness, compliance, and potential adverse effects.

Prophylactic Medications

- **Beta-blockers.** Agents without intrinsic sympathomimetic activity can reduce the number of migraine attacks in a significant proportion of patients but the effective dose varies enormously. The best evidence supports propranolol and timolol but atenolol, metoprolol, and nadolol are also effective. Patients should be initially screened then monitored for adverse effects to beta-blockers such as asthma, hypotension, bradycardia, Raynaud syndrome, or depression. If results are disappointing with the initial medication, another member of this class may prove successful.
- **Antiepileptics.** Divalproex sodium/sodium valproate was the antiepileptic agent with best evidence of clinical benefit in the consortium review. Modest effectiveness was reported for gabapentin and carbamazepine. The side effects of divalproex sodium, such as gastrointestinal upset, asthenia, and weight gain, as well as potential teratogenicity, hepatic and pancreatic damage, restrict its acceptability for many patients with migraine. Since the guidelines were published, clinical trials have suggested that topiramate may be comparable to divalproex or propranolol with a potential advantage of weight loss but disadvantages in fatigue, paresthesias, nausea, problems in memory and concentration, and significant expense.

■ The consortium concluded that propranolol, timolol, amitriptyline, and divalproex sodium had the best strength of evidence supporting efficacy with mild to moderate side effects.[4] Of the many other agents studied for migraine prophylaxis, the consortium also found limited evidence and lower efficacy for aspirin and certain nonsteroidal antiinflammatory drugs (NSAIDs), verapamil, feverfew, magnesium, and vitamin B_2.[4,8,9] Studies reported since the publication of the consortium guidelines also suggest a modest effect from angiotensin blockade (with lisinopril or candestartan) and Coenzyme Q10.[9] The NSAIDs such as naproxen and mefenamic acid are recommended for menstrually related migraine.

Treatment of the Acute Attack

General goals for the management of migraine attacks include:

■ Rapid and consistent relief of symptoms
■ Prompt return to normal functioning
■ Minimal risk of recurrence of symptoms
■ Limited/acceptable adverse effects
■ Minimize use of back-up medications
■ Cost-effective for patient and health systems[4]

Individualizing therapy is essential to obtaining the optimal relief of symptoms and enhancing adherence with therapy. Patients should be educated about migraine and encouraged to take significant responsibility for self-management. Factors in selecting therapy include the following:

■ The most troublesome symptoms (e.g., pain, vomiting, exhaustion)
■ Migraine pattern (e.g., speed of onset, time to peak symptoms, duration of symptoms, tendency to recur, time between attacks)
■ Comorbidities that limit medication choices (e.g., gastric bleeding, some forms of heart disease)
■ Patient confidence in medication and preference for route of administration
■ Cost and medication availability

From the many treatments studied, the consortium found pronounced statistical and clinical benefit for several analgesics, ergotamines, and triptans.[4]

Analgesics and Symptomatic Medications

Analgesics such as aspirin, ibuprofen, and naproxen can effectively control migraine symptoms (especially early in the attack) if absorbed in adequate doses. Several antiemetics also have some impact on migraine as well as addressing symptoms of nausea and vomiting. Analgesics and antiemetics are frequently given together (with due attention to potential side effects for an individual patient). Caffeine is a component of several nonprescription migraine medications as it has both a weak antimigraine effect and appears to enhance other medications. In appropriate doses, the combination of aspirin and metoclopramide is as effective as sumatriptan. The optimal symptomatic agent (or combination) and dose has to be developed for each patient but all should be counseled to treat early in the attack, control the dose and frequency of dosing to avoid rebound headache, and to report any adverse effects. The consortium found no role but significant potential dangers in the use of butalbital for migraine. Opiates can relieve pain but increase nausea and somnolence. The risk of abuse and availability of more effective agents lead most experts to recommend limiting opiate use to very specific circumstances such rescue medication for intractable attacks.

Ergotamines

These traditional migraine therapies are available for oral, injectable, nasal, or rectal use. The best evidence of efficacy is for dihydroergotamine (DHE) given nasally, intramuscularly, intravenously, or subcutaneously. The action is enhanced by combination with an antiemetic. The main adverse effects relate to vasoconstriction, nausea, and rebound headache. These medications must not be used during pregnancy or when vasoconstriction is contraindicated (e.g., peripheral vascular disease, coronary artery disease).

Triptans (Serotonin 5-HT$_{1B/1D}$ Agonists)

The seven currently available triptans differ mainly in bioavailability, speed of effect, and duration of action. Clinical efficacy appears similar within the group but a patient may respond well to one agent but not another. The choice of initial agent should be based on matching the pharmacologic properties of the drug (such as speed or duration of action) to the needs of individual patients. The form of administration can also be adapted to patient needs as some triptans are available in nasal or oral-dissolving forms and sumatriptan can be given subcutaneously. Triptans are contraindicated in basilar and hemiplegic migraine and in patients with heart disease or uncontrolled hypertension.[4] Nausea, flushing, and palpitations may occur. Triptans are significantly more expensive than most alternative treatments.

Surgery and Procedural Interventions

Small studies report significant improvement in the frequency and intensity of migraine following injection of botulinum toxin, removal of the corrugator supercilii muscles, and other procedures. Studies of patients treated for paradoxical cerebral embolism identified a high prevalence of migraine (especially with aura) that resolved or improved significantly after closure of patent foramen ovale.

SPECIAL CONSIDERATIONS

Migraine is a long-term condition that patients should be encouraged to manage with advice and support from their physicians. Depression and other stress-related conditions have traditionally had a high prevalence in patients with migraine. With positive coaching by physicians and individualized management utilizing the range of effective therapies, the impact of migraine on quality of life should be minimized.

References

1. Cady RK, Borchert LD, Spalding W, et al. Simple and efficient recognition of migraine with a 3-question headache screen. *Headache* 2003;44(4):323–327.
2. Lipton RB, Stewart WF, Diamond S, et al. Prevalence and burden of migraine in the United States: data from the American Migraine Study II. *Headache* 2001;41(7):783–791.
3. Headache Classification Subcommittee of the International Headache Society. The international classification of headache disorders. 2nd ed. *Cephalalgia* 2004;24:S9–160.
4. Silberstein SD. Practice parameter: evidence-based guidelines for migraine headache (an evidence-based review). *Neurology* 2000;55:745–762 (also available online at www.aan.com/professionals/practice/guideline/indes.efm).
5. Lipton RD, Dodick D, Sadovsky R, et al. A self-administered screener for migraine in primary care: the ID migraine validation study. *Neurology* 2003;61:375–382.
6. Morey SS. Practice guidelines: Headache Consortium releases guidelines for use of CT or MRI in migraine work-up. *Am Fam Physician* 2000;62:1699.
7. Stewart WF, Lipton RB, Kolodner KB, et al. Reliability of the migraine disability assessment score (MIDAS) in a population-based sample of headache sufferers. *Cephalalgia* 1999;19:107–114.
8. Morey SS. Practice guidelines: guidelines on migraine: Part 4. General principles of preventive therapy. *Am Fam Physician* 2000;62:2359.
9. Modi S, Lowder DM. Medications for migraine prophylaxis. *Am Fam Physician* 2006;73:72–78.
10. Huntington J, Yuan CL. Topramate for migraine prevention. *Am Fam Physician* 2005; 72:1563.
11. Tfelt-Hansen P. The effectiveness of combined oral lysine acetylsalicylate and metoclopramide in the treatment of migraine attacks. Comparison with placebo and oral sumatriptan. *Funct Neurol* 2000;15:196–201.
12. Ferrari MD, Goadsby PJ, Roon KI, et al. Triptans in migraine: detailed results and methods of a meta-analysis of 53 trials. *Cephalalgia* 2002;22:633–658.
13. Guyuron B, Kriegler JS, Davis J, et al. Comprehensive surgical treatment of migraine headaches. *Plast Reconstr Surg* 2005;115:1–9.
14. Reisman M, Christofferson RD, Jesurum J, et al. Migraine headache relief after transcatheter closure of patent ovale. *J Am Coll Cardiol* 2005;45:493–495.

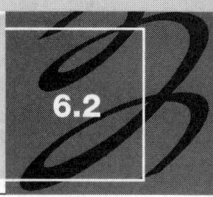

6.2

GENERAL APPROACH TO THE PATIENT WITH HEADACHE

Differentiating primary headache syndromes such as migraine, cluster, and tension from the potentially serious forms of secondary headaches caused by tumor, vascular problem, or infection is a critical task for the clinician when evaluating every patient with headache.

History

It is important to gather the patient's general medical history, neurologic history, and family history of headache. In particular one should inquire about patient's handedness, how many types of headaches the patient has, current age, and age of onset of different headaches. The frequency, duration, rapidity of onset intensity, location, and character of pain are all important, as is delineation of provoking and palliating factors including medicines (and frequency of use) that have or have not been effective. Associated nausea, vomiting, typical aura, focal neurologic and localized autonomic symptoms (such as lacrimation and rhinorrhea), and whether neck pain or stiffness has been noted should all be assessed. The presence or absence of fever and a history of any type of antecedent trauma can be important. Changes in mental status are of substantial concern. A previous history of cancer that could be metastatic is also important to assess. The patient's medications and any recent changes in regimen should be noted. Medication overuse can turn episodic into chronic headaches. A history of human immunodeficiency virus (HIV) changes the differential and workup substantially. New focal symptoms or a change or progression in a previously stable pattern of headaches is a concern, as is onset before age 5 or after age 50. A headache described as worst ever typically mandates an intensive evaluation.

Examination

Measure vital signs including temperature and blood pressure (BP). BP over 120 diastolic is believed to be a cause of headaches. Headaches with fever raise the possibility of infectious causes. Fundiscopic exam should be done to look for papilledema and the presence or absence of spontaneous venous pulsations (reassuring if present, not pathologic if absent). Cranial nerves, mental status, examination of the carotid arteries, cardiac exam, gait, reflexes, and motor and sensory exams should all be assessed. Neck exam for stiffness is critical in all febrile patients. The scalp should be palpated for tenderness as may occur in some tension pattern headache syndromes, and for defects of the skull in cases of trauma.

Laboratory and Imaging Studies

Most patients with typical migraine, tension headache, or other well-defined primary headache syndromes do not need further testing. Leukocyte patterns on complete blood count (CBC) can suggest viral or bacterial infection in a febrile patient. Sedimentation rate and/or C-reactive protein should be checked in patients older than 50 with new headaches or others suspected of having temporal arteritis or other vasculitis. Temporal artery biopsy is the definitive test for temporal arteritis. Antinuclear antibodies can be of value if vasculitis is suspected.

Neuroimaging

■ **Computed tomography (CT) or magnetic resonance imaging (MRI)** should be done in patients with new focal neurologic symptoms, worsening patterns of previously stable headaches, or for those with onset of new headaches before age 5 or after age 50 if another cause is not readily apparent, and in those who have a history of cancer that could be metastatic to brain. Neuroimaging is also appropriate in patients with headache after trauma or with any mental status changes.

- **Imaging the sinuses** (usually with CT) can find occult sinusitis, especially of the sphenoid sinuses. New headaches associated with cough, sex, or exertion should be evaluated by MRI to exclude underlying pathology. Unilateral headaches of acute onset and any focal symptoms should raise the concern of carotid artery dissection. Magnetic resonance angiography (MRA) imaging of the neck is helpful to exclude this as a cause.
- **Thunderclap** "worst-ever" headaches should be emergently evaluated with neuroimaging (usually CT). If on CT scanning herniation does not appear to be a risk, then lumbar puncture should be performed (looking for xanthochromia).
- **Lumbar puncture** should also be done with opening pressure measured if elevated intracranial pressure is suspected and whenever infectious causes beyond simple viral syndromes are thought to be possible causes.
- **HIV-positive** patients should be aggressively evaluated for possible central nervous system opportunistic infections.
- **Cerebrospinal fluid (CSF) Lyme disease tests** can occasionally be positive in the absence of positive peripheral titers. Urgent examination by an ophthalmologist is indicated if angle closure glaucoma or iritis/uveitis is suspected on the basis of a red painful eye. Sleep studies to exclude apnea are appropriate for headaches worse in the morning.
- Headache is a prominent component of carbon monoxide poisoning, which can be confirmed by carbomethoxyhemoglobin testing, but only when a high index of suspicion raises the question.

GROUP 1: CLUSTER AND OTHER TRIGEMINAL AUTONOMIC CEPHALALGIAS (TAC)

Key Points

- **Cluster and the related headaches**—Paroxysmal hemicrania and SUNCT (see definition below) are all severe unilateral headaches that involve activation of the trigeminal parasympathetic and/or sympathetic pathways. They are differentiated by their frequency, duration, and responsiveness to certain medications.

Definition/Diagnosis

Cluster is diagnosed when one to eight repeated, 15- to 180- minute attacks per day of moderately severe to severe unilateral orbital or temporal pain occur with at least one of the following associated: ipsilateral conjunctival injection and/or tearing, ipsilateral nasal congestion and/or rhinorrhea, ipsilateral eyelid edema, ipsilateral facial and/or forehead swelling, ipsilateral miosis, and/or ptosis or a sense of restlessness and agitation. Patients with cluster headache are usually pacing and restless as opposed to patients with migraine who are quiet and withdrawn. Attacks occur in spells, often nocturnal, often at the same time each day on the same side of the head. Clusters may be separated by months to years, and recurrent attacks may switch sides. About 10% to 15% of patients have chronic unremitting cluster-type headaches rather than groupings of headaches.

Pathophysiology/Epidemiology

Activation of the posterior hypothalamic gray matter, vasodilation, and activation of the trigeminal parasympathetic reflex with secondary sympathetic involvement are believed to occur. Men 20 to 40 years old are most commonly affected. The male-to-female ratio is about 3:1 (and appears to be decreasing as older studies showed ~5:1 ratios). Cluster and the other TAC headaches are all relatively rare affecting 1% of the population or less.

Workup

Detailed headache and neurologic history, family history, and complete neurologic exam are indicated. CT/MRI/MRA imaging or carotid ultrasound may be indicated if there are findings other than the usual associated trigeminal autonomic symptoms described above or if carotid artery dissection is suspected. Testing for glaucoma may be wise as intermittent angle closure can mimic some of these symptoms. Approximately 5% of cluster headaches are inherited in an autosomal dominant pattern.

Differential Diagnosis

The primary differential process is to determine if the patient has cluster (defined above), paroxysmal hemicrania, or short lasting unilateral neuralgiform headache with conjunctival injection and tearing (SUNCT). Paroxysmal hemicrania and SUNCT both require for diagnosis the presence of at least one of the ipsilateral autonomic symptoms described for cluster but in paroxysmal hemicrania the attacks last only 2 to 30 minutes, the patient must have at least five attacks per day, and by definition they are responsive to treatment with indomethacin. In SUNCT the attacks are similar in character but occur at a frequency of 3 to 200 per day and last only 5 to 240 seconds. The differential diagnosis when new onset also includes carotid dissection, angle closure glaucoma, and uveitis. Trigeminal neuralgia may mimic SUNCT but lacks the associated autonomic findings.

Treatment

- **Acute treatments** for cluster headache that have shown efficacy include triptans (most often given by injection), inhaled oxygen, and the somatostatin analogue octreotide. Most patients with cluster headache require prophylactic therapy.
- **Preventive therapies** that have been used with success include verapamil, prednisone, lithium, ergots, methysergide (use limited by side effects), cyproheptadine, and indomethacin; the last is also of special use in paroxysmal hemicrania. Table 6.2-1 presents a complete list of pharmacotherapies.
- **Surgery** on the trigeminal nerve and deep brain stimulators have also been used in patients with refractory cluster headache.
- **Complications:** Complications of cluster include the risk of suicide, violent behavior, secondary depression, loss of function due to the intensity of pain, and side effects from treatments.

Patient Education

Patients with cluster headache are a highly motivated group. They need to be educated about acute treatments that can be self-administered, adherence to preventive regimens, and avoidance of triggers such as alcohol and nitrates.

GROUP 2: TENSION TYPE HEADACHES (TTH) AND CHRONIC DAILY HEADACHES

Key Points

Tension headaches are extremely common, occurring in more than half the population. They exist in a spectrum from rare episodic to chronic daily tension pattern headaches; the latter can be extremely disabling.

Definition/Diagnosis

Tension headaches usually occur in the frontal and/or occipital areas in a bandlike pattern. They last 30 minutes to 7 days, are generally bilateral, of a nonpulsing quality (often described as pressing or tightening). They are of mild to moderate intensity and do not get worse with the activities of routine exertion. Unlike migraine, they do not have associated nausea or vomiting but either photophobia or phonophobia (but not both) may be present within the definition of TTH. Episodic tension headache is distinguished from chronic tension headache in frequency, the chronic form requiring headache to be present for more then 15 days per month for at least 3 months.

Pathophysiology/Epidemiology

Previously TTHs were thought to be psychogenic in origin. Further study suggests that at least the more severe and chronic forms are related to defects in central pain processing pathways. Approximately 90% of females and 70% of males experience some type of tension headaches, for a female-to-male ratio of about l.3 to 1. Chronic tension headaches are present in about 2% of the population. Episodic TTHs are so common that determining any genetic component is difficult.

Data suggest the more severe and chronic forms may be more common in patients with a family history of headaches.

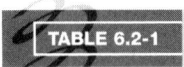 **TABLE 6.2-1**	Cluster and Trigeminal Autonomic Cephalalgias Pharmacotherapy	
Agent	**Headache type/ Rx class**
Abortive treatments	
Sumatriptan injection (Imitrex)[a]	Cluster: Triptan—
Sumatriptan (Imitrex), Zolmitriptan (Zomig) nasal	5HT(IB/ID) agonist
Sumatriptan (Imitrex), Zolmitriptan (Zomig), others oral	SUNCT headaches[b]
Oxygen by inhalation, high flow ~7–15 L/min	Cluster: Molecular agent— mechanism of action unknown
Ergotamine and Dihydroergotamine by various parenteral routes of administration (oral not generally effective for abortive treatment, but may be used as transitional agents to chronic prophylactic treatments)	Cluster: Vasoconstrictor, 5HT (1B/1D) agonist and suppresses neurogenic inflammation
Octreotide injectable (expensive, considered investigational)	Cluster: Somatostatin analogue
Indomethacin (Indocin)	Paroxysmal hemicrania: Response to this agent is uniform and diagnostic
Preventive treatments	
Verapamil	Cluster: Calcium-channel blocker
Prednisone/other steroids	Cluster: Corticosteroid
Lithium	Cluster: Ionic agent, class indeterminate
Methysergide (ergot derivative)—off U.S. market due to toxicity concerns	Cluster: Ergot derivative
Valproic acid (Depakote)	Cluster: Anticonvulsant
Topiramate (Topamax)	Cluster: Anticonvulsant
Indomethacin (Indocin)	Paroxysmal hemicrania: Highly effective
	Cluster: Possibly some degree of responsiveness

[a]Injectable triptan more effective than nasal or oral for cluster.
[b]SUNCT headaches are notably resistant to almost all treatments, some degree of response to triptans in a minority of patients has been seen.

Evaluation

Usual headache and neurologic history and physical plus palpation of the scalp for tenderness.

Laboratory Studies and Imaging

These are rarely indicated unless there are focal neurologic deficits, an accelerating pattern, or other worrisome features. An exception would be patients over age 50 with new headaches who should all have a sedimentation rate test to exclude temporal arteritis.

Differential Diagnosis

Tension type headaches that include either photo- or phonophobia can be mistaken for migraine. Similarly, transformed migraines can be mistaken for or overlap with chronic tension headaches. Medication-overuse headaches often complicate chronic tension headaches.

Withdrawal of frequently used abortive medication can lead to reversion of chronic headaches to episodic pattern tension headaches. Chronic subdural hematoma should be suspected in elderly persons with new headaches or in those who have suffered head trauma. Hemicrania continua is another primary headache type that is chronic. In hemicrania continua pain is unilateral, severe, indomethacin-responsive, and often associated with some degree of autonomic symptomatology.

Treatment

Aspirin, acetaminophen, and combinations containing one or both of these plus caffeine are often helpful for tension headaches. All nonsteroidal anti-inflammatory drugs (NSAIDs) seem to be effective. Combination medications such as isometheptene, dichloraiphenazone, and acetaminophen can be helpful. Butalbital containing combinations can be effective but have higher risk of rebound and abuse and may decrease the effectiveness of preventive medications. The muscle relaxant tinzidine can sometimes be useful. Occasional use of tramadol or mild narcotics such as acetaminophen with codeine can be considered for more intense pain. Preventive therapy for chronic headaches is often indicated. Tricyclic class medicines have the most literature support. Selective serotonin-reuptake inhibitors (SSRIs) may also be of use (Table 6.2-2). The application of heat, thermal biofeedback training, acupuncture, botox injections, and physical modalities such as massage may all be considered.

Complications

Anxiety and depression are both comorbid with chronic headaches. Whether the headaches have any causative role or not is unclear.

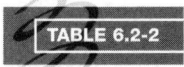

TABLE 6.2-2	Pharmacotherapy for Tension Headaches: Frequently Used Agents

Agent	Therapeutic class
Abortive treatments	
Aspirin	Salicylate
Acetaminophen	NSAID related
Ibuprofen, Naproxyn, others	NSAIDs
Toradol injectable	NSAID
Aspirin/acetaminophen/caffeine	Salicylate/NSAID related/combination
Acetaminophen/caffeine	NSAID related combination
Isometheptene; dichloraiphenazone, and acetaminophen (Midrin)	Vasoconstrictor, muscle relaxant, NSAID related/combination
Butalbital/aspirin/caffeine	Barbiturate/salicylate combination
Butalbital/acetaminophen/caffeine	Barbiturate/NSAID related combination
Tramadol (Ultram)	Atypical opioid
Acetaminophen with codeine (Tylenol #3, others)	Opioid derivative, NSAID related combination
Preventive treatments	
Amitriptyline (Elavil), nortriptyline (Pamelor), others	Tricyclic antidepressant
Prozac, others	SSRI—Selective serotonin-reuptake inhibitor
Tizanidine (Zanaflex)	Antispasmodic, central alpha-2 adrenergic agonist

Patient Education

For mild episodic headaches patients should be taught to use the safest effective medication on a prn basis. Education about the avoidance of medication overuse to minimize the risk of rebound headaches is warranted. Patients with chronic headaches should be taught the value of prophylactic medications. If chronic headaches persist, then patients should be given the opportunity to seek care at a specialized headache center.

GROUP 3: OTHER COMMON OR IMPORTANT HEADACHE SYNDROMES—SALIENT FEATURES

- **Hypnic headaches.** Moderate to severe, occur nightly, awaken patient from sleep, 2:1 female-to-male ratio. Last ~1 hour. Not associated with autonomic symptoms. Intracranial disorders should be excluded by neuroimaging such as MRI. Caffeine and lithium have been reported as effective treatments.
- **Cervicogenic headaches.** Head pain originating in cervical spine (usually Cl–3). Usually unilateral without side shifting, ablated by treating underlying pathology or temporarily by occipital and/or upper cervical nerve blocks.
- **Posttraumatic headaches.** Resemble tension headaches but within 7 days after head trauma and are often the most prominent symptom of a whole postconcussive syndrome that may include dizziness, memory and personality disturbances.
- **Exertional, cough-, and sex-associated headaches.** All associated with conditions that raise intra-abdominal pressure. More than 40% have some intracranial abnormality usually vascular (such as subarachnoid hemorrhage), or tumor, so complete workup and imaging such as MRI/MRA is indicated. Indomethacin is often helpful. There are some reports of beta-blockers being effective. Consider angina in differential of sex-associated headaches as anginal symptoms may be noted only in the head and neck in some patients.
- **Stabbing (ice-pick) headaches.** Stabbing pains lasting up to a few seconds one to many times/day. Felt in orbit, temple, and parietal areas in the distribution of the first division of the trigeminal nerve. No associated autonomic symptoms. Occur more commonly in patients with other headache types such as migraine or cluster. If strictly in one area, structural lesion should be excluded by imaging.
- **Idiopathic intracranial hypertension** (formerly called pseudotumor cerebri or benign intracranial hypertension). Progressive diffuse headache, usually daily, nonpulsating, and aggravated by straining or cough. Papilledema, sixth nerve palsy, visual and field defects are common. Elevated CSF pressure detected by lumbar puncture. Typical patient is a young obese woman. Oral contraceptives and tetracycline are risk factors.

References

1. Bigal ME, Lipton RB. Tension-type headache: classification and diagnosis. *Curr Headache Rep* 2005;9:423–429.
2. Castillo J, Munoz P, Guitera V, et al. Epidemiology of chronic daily headache in the general population. *Headache* 1999;39:190–196.
3. Diamond, S. Tension-type headache. *Clin Cornerstone* 1999;1(6):33–44.
4. Dodick DW. Chronic daily headache. *N Engl J Med* 2006;354:158–165.
5. Husid MS. Cluster headache: a case-based review of diagnostic and treatment approaches. *Curr Pain Headache Rep* 2006; 10(2):117–125.
6. Rasmussen BK, Olesen J. Epidemiology of headache. IASP Newsletter March/April 1996. Web reference: http://www.iasp-pain.org/TC96MarApr.htm.
7. Sandrini G, Tassorelli C, Ghiotto N, et al. Uncommon primary headaches. *Curr Opin Neurol* 2006;19(3):299–304.
8. Sjaastad O, Fredriksen TA. Cervicogenic headache: criteria, classification and epidemiology. *Clin Exp Rheumatol* 2000;18(Suppl 19):S3–6.
9. Smetana GW. The diagnostic value of historical features in primary headache syndromes. *Arch Intern Med* 2000;160:2729–2737.
10. International classification of headache disorders, 2nd ed. *Cephalalgia* 2004;24:1–160.

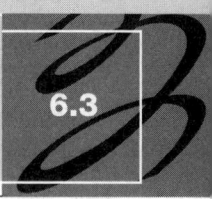

GENERAL PRINCIPLES

Definition

Meningitis is acute or subacute inflammation of meninges of the brain or the spinal cord. Acute meningitis (25% of cases) is an infection of less than 24-hour duration, whereas subacute meningitis (75%) evolves over a period of 24 hours to 7 days. Bacterial meningitis has a mortality of 30%; this mortality rate has remained unchanged in the last two and a half decades.

Etiology of Acute Meningitis

The most likely pathogens causing acute bacterial meningitis depend on several factors as follows:

- **Patient's age**
  - 0 to 5 weeks: Group B streptococci, *Listeria monocytogenes,* Enterobacteriaceae (predominantly *Escherichia coli*), *Enterococcus*
  - 5 weeks to 5 months: Group B streptococci, Enterobacteriaceae, *Haemophilus influenzae, Streptococcus pneumoniae, Neisseria meningitidis*
  - 5 months to 15 years: *S. pneumoniae, N. meningitidis, H. influenzae*
  - 15 to 55 years: *S. pneumoniae, N. meningitides*
  - Greater than 55 years: *S. pneumoniae, N. meningitidis, H. influenzae, L. monocytogenes,* Enterobacteriaceae, and other Gram-negative organisms

- **Immunocompromised or neutropenic status.** Causative organisms in this patient group are *Staphylococcus aureus*; Gram-negative pathogens, such as *E. coli, Pseudomonas, Serratia,* and fungi such as *Candida* and *Cryptococcus.*

- **With an intracranial shunt.** Patients with an intracranial shunt are likely to be infected with *Staphylococcus epidermidis, S. aureus,* and Gram-negative organisms.

Etiology of Subacute Meningitis

- **Mycobacterial causes** include *Mycobacterium tuberculosis* and *M. avium-intracellulare* complex (in HIV patients) (also see Chapter 19.4).
- **Spirochetal organisms** causing subacute meningitis are *Treponema pallidum* and *Borrelia burgdorferi.*
- **Fungal causes** include *Cryptococcus neoformans, Coccidioides immitis,* and *Histoplasma capsulatum.*
- **Viral organisms** causing meningitis include West Nile virus, herpesvirus types 1 and 2, echovirus, Coxsackie virus types A and B, *Enterovirus,* mumps, lymphocytic choriomeningitis, Epstein–Barr virus, cytomegalovirus, and arthropod-borne viruses.
- **Parasitic organisms** include *Naegleria* and *Angiostrongylus.*

DIAGNOSIS

Clinical Features

- The diagnosis of meningitis should be considered in every patient with fever and meningeal signs and symptoms. In bacterial meningitis, patients may have a precedent upper respiratory tract infection, otitis media, or pneumonia. Meningeal signs and symptoms include the following:

- Generalized headache (new-onset), nuchal rigidity, vomiting, photophobia, seizures, and changes in mental status, from mild confusion and obtundation to lethargy, drowsiness, and coma, are signs of meningeal infection.
- In the neonate, fever, decreased appetite, irritability, vomiting, or lassitude should alert the physician to consider meningitis. In elderly patients, there may be only fever and a change in mental status.

- Clinical examination in acute bacterial meningitis may reveal an ill-looking, toxic, febrile individual with neck rigidity and a positive Kernig or Brudzinski sign. There may be impairment of mental faculties or cranial nerve palsies (particularly involving nerves III, IV, VI, and VII). Focal neurologic signs include hemiparesis, monoparesis, or hemianopia with or without papilledema. In subacute meningitis, these classic signs may be absent, and the patient may have fever and altered mental status only. In infections due to *N. meningitidis*, a rapidly developing, purplish skin rash may be seen.

Laboratory Diagnosis
- **Cerebrospinal fluid (CSF) examination**
  - Elevated opening pressure is found in acute bacterial meningitis.
  - Purulent fluid with high polymorphonuclear cell count, increased protein, and low glucose indicates acute bacterial meningitis. Do counterimmunofluorescence/latex agglutination and Gram stain to identify the organism. Culture of CSF will specifically identify the offending pathogen.
  - Lymphocytic CSF with a normal glucose level is commonly seen in viral meningitis or partially treated pyogenic bacterial meningitis.
  - Lymphocytic CSF with a low glucose level is commonly seen in tuberculosis and fungal meningitis.

- **Other laboratory tests.** Two blood cultures, complete blood count (CBC), serum electrolytes, and radiologic studies of the chest or computed tomography (CT) scanning of the sinuses may be needed in some situations to rule out the primary focus of infection. CT scanning of the brain is essential if there is associated papilledema and before a lumbar puncture is done.

TREATMENT
It is of vital importance that empirical antimicrobial therapy is started immediately, preferably within 30 minutes of diagnosis.

Empirical Antibiotic Treatment
- Neonates (0 to 1 week) can be treated with ampicillin, 50 mg/kg IV q8h, and gentamicin, 2.5 mg/kg q8–12h, or cefotaxime (Claforan), 50 mg/kg IV q8h, or ceftriaxone (Rocephin), 100 mg/kg IV daily.
- Children, adolescents, and adults (5 weeks to 55 years) may be treated with one of the following regimens:
  - For children, cefotaxime: 150 mg per kilogram of body weight IV q6h or ceftriaxone 100 mg/kg body weight IV once or in two divided doses with vancomycin 60 mg/kg body weight/day IV in three divided doses.
  - For adults, cefotaxime: 2 g q6h IV or ceftriaxone 2 g q12h IV with vancomycin 1 g q12h IV.
- Patients older than 55 years can be treated with ampicillin, 2 g IV q4h, vancomycin 1 g q12h IV and cefotaxime or ceftriaxone. In patients allergic to penicillin, chloramphenicol, 25 mg per kg of body weight IV q6h, or trimethoprim–sulfamethoxazole (Bactrim), 10 to 15 mg/kg/day in four divided doses with gentamicin, 5 mg per kg IV per day in three divided doses.
- **Adjunctive therapy.** Corticosteroids, such as dexamethasone, 0.15 mg per kg of body weight q6h for 4 days, are recommended for infants and children.

■ **Specific therapy.** Once the specific pathogen is identified, specific cost-effective antibiotics should be substituted for empirical therapy.
  ■ *S. pneumoniae.* For infection in adults, give penicillin 4 million U IV q4h. Children should receive 30,000 U/kg of body weight in divided doses. Alternatives are chloramphenicol or a third-generation cephalosporin. For penicillin-resistant pneumococci, give cefotaxime or vancomycin, 1 g q12h IV.
  ■ *S. aureus.* For adults, give nafcillin, 2 g q4h IV. For children, give 100 to 300 mg per kg of body weight IV in divided doses. In case of methicillin-resistant *Staphylococcus aureus* (MRSA) infection give vancomycin.
  ■ *L. monocytogenes.* Give penicillin or ampicillin plus gentamicin. Alternative therapy is chloramphenicol or trimethoprim–sulfamethoxazole plus gentamicin.
  ■ *H. influenzae.* For β-lactamase-negative infections, give ampicillin; for β-lactamase-positive infections, give cefotaxime or ceftriaxone.
  ■ *N. meningitidis.* Give penicillin or ceftriaxone, cefotaxime, or chloramphenicol.
  ■ *E. coli or Enterobacteriaceae.* Give cefotaxime or ceftriaxone plus gentamicin.
  ■ **Tuberculosis.** Give a combination of isoniazid (INH), rifampin, pyrazinamide, and ethambutol, or streptomycin for 2 months, then INH and rifampin for an additional 7 to 10 months.
  ■ **Fungal etiology.** Give amphotericin B, 1 mg per kg of body weight IV or liposomal amphotericin, 5 mg per kg of body weight IV and 0.05 to 0.10 mg intrathecally of amphotericin B with or without flucytosine (5-FC, Ancobon), 150 mg per kg of body weight daily in divided doses. An alternative is fluconazole (Diflucan), 400 to 1,000 mg PO or IV, or voriconazole 200 mg PO or IV q12h, in *Cryptococcus* or *Coccidioides* meningitis.

■ **Duration of therapy.** Treatment of common bacterial meningitis continues for 7 days for *H. influenzae* and *N. meningitis*, 10 to 14 days for *S. pneumoniae*, 14 to 21 days for *Listeria* and group B streptococci, and 21 days for Gram-negative bacilli (other than *H. influenzae*).

Prevention

■ **Meningococcal meningitis.** Contacts should be given rifampin, 600 mg PO q12h for 2 days, or ciprofloxacin, 750 mg PO once. In pregnant patient 250 mg of ceftriaxone IM can be given. Meningococcal conjugate vaccine is now recommended by the Advisory Committee on Immunization Practices (ACIP) at ages 11 to 12 years or before high school entry or first-year college students living in dormitories and persons at increased risk like military recruits, travelers to countries with high incidence of meningoccocal disease, patients with anatomic or functional asplenia, and patients with terminal complement deficiency.
■ **H. influenzae meningitis.** Contacts younger than 12 months should receive rifampin 20 mg per kg of body weight for 4 days.

References

1. van de Beek D, de Gans J, Tunkel AR, et al. Community-acquired bacterial meningitis in adults. *N Engl J Med* 2006;354:44–53.
2. Tunkel AR, Hartmann BJ, Kaplan SL, et al. Practice guidelines for the management of bacterial meningitis. *Clin Infect Dis* 2004;39:1275.
3. van de Beek D, de Gans J, Spanjaard L, et al. Clinical features and prognostic factors in adults with bacterial meningitis. *N Engl J Med* 2004;351:1849–1859.
4. Feigin RD, McCracken GH Jr, Klein JO. Diagnosis and management of meningitis. *Pediatr Infect Dis J* 1992;11:785–814.

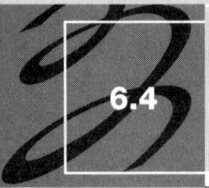

6.4 SEIZURES
Donald B. Middleton

GENERAL PRINCIPLES

A seizure is an involuntary, transient, electrical discharge from the brain. Recurrent seizures, usually stereotypic, define epilepsy. A seizure can produce motor (convulsive), sensory, autonomic, cognitive, or combined signs.

Clinical Presentation

Generalized seizures abruptly alter consciousness. Partial seizures begin with a localized symptom, often an aura, can remain localized (simple) or spread (generalize), or adversely affect consciousness (complex). An inciting event (e.g., hypoglycemia or strobe light exposure) or a noxious exposure (e.g., trauma or infection) helps to distinguish seizures from nonepileptic paroxysms (e.g., cardiovascular syncope or hysteria). Interictal apnea, micturition, defecation, tongue biting, or injury, especially a fracture or a broken tooth, or postictal headache, lethargy, confusion, or Todd paralysis is suggestive of seizure activity. Except for febrile seizures in childhood, the highest incidence of seizures is in elderly individuals.

GENERALIZED SEIZURES

- **Tonic-clonic, tonic, or clonic epilepsy (grand mal)** is recurrent sudden loss of consciousness with major motor activity, often heralded by a brief cry but without an aura. Postictal drowsiness or snoring is typical. Many of these common seizures are genetically determined or idiopathic, but secondary, reversible abnormalities, such as electrolyte imbalance, are often at fault.
- **Atonic seizures** cause sudden loss of muscle tone so often result in severe trauma.
- **Myoclonic seizures** are repetitive jerks of a single muscle group, often affecting the trunk or an extremity, usually with unimpaired consciousness. Examples are benign myoclonus of infancy and juvenile myoclonic epilepsy in adolescents. Myoclonic seizures frequently indicate underlying epileptic syndromes such as infantile spasms.
- **Absence seizures**
  - Typical spells **(petit mal)** usually last 5 to 10 seconds, produce minor facial twitches (e.g., eye blinking or lip smacking), occur dozens of times a day, and have no postictal state. Onset is after age 3 years and peak incidence is between ages 5 to 10 years. Most petit mal seizures resolve by early adulthood.
  - Atypical spells include postictal abnormalities and are common in the Lennox–Gastaut syndrome of childhood, associated with developmental delay.
- **Febrile seizures** affect infants or toddlers, may be generalized or focal, and reflect temperature change (see Chapter 4.2). These genetically linked seizures require no treatment unless multiple or recurrent.
- **Toxemia of pregnancy** can produce seizures related to hypertensive encephalopathy (see Chapter 14.8).
- **Drug-related seizures** can be due to lowering of the seizure threshold, as with antihistamines or phencyclidine, or withdrawal, as from alcohol or barbiturate (see Chapter 5.7).

PARTIAL SEIZURES

Partial seizures are always focal in onset but often spread to become generalized. Because of the possibility of an underlying central nervous system lesion, an effort to detect an aura or a sign of focal onset is required in all generalized seizure cases.

- **Simple spells** do not cause loss of consciousness.
- Motor seizures frequently occur with a jacksonian march, aphasia, chewing, or postural change. Localized Todd paralysis occurring postictally is suggestive of a partial seizure.
- Sensory spells can be visual, auditory, verbal, gustatory, somatic, or vertiginous.
- Autonomic attacks start with nausea, vomiting, pallor, diarrhea, or diaphoresis.
- Benign partial epilepsy of childhood (rolandic) occurs primarily during sleep in 4- to 13-year-old subjects and is self-limited. Consciousness is usually preserved.
- **Complex spells** alter consciousness or cognitive functioning. Patients may develop amnesia, déjà vu, abnormal behavior, or hallucinations. An aura and moderately prolonged postictal confusion distinguish temporal lobe (psychomotor) epilepsy from absence spells.

DIAGNOSIS

Diagnostic evaluation varies according to clinical presentation. In general the following tests are helpful:

- **Electroencephalography (EEG).** Although it is the most useful test, the EEG is not always diagnostic. Hyperventilation, sleep, photic stimulation, ambulatory recordings, videotaping, or repeat EEG improves diagnostic accuracy. A generalized three per second spike-and-wave pattern is diagnostic of absence spells. Partial complex seizures usually show a focal abnormality on the EEG.
- **Blood tests.** Serum electrolytes (especially sodium), calcium, magnesium, blood urea nitrogen, glucose, liver function tests—bilirubin, alkaline phosphatase, aspartate aminotransferase (serum glutamate oxaloacetate transaminase)—complete blood count, and, when indicated, toxin screens and alcohol level are sometimes diagnostic. An elevated prolactin or creatine phosphokinase level suggests recent seizure activity.
- **Imaging studies.** Magnetic resonance imaging (MRI) is the preferred study, but computed tomography (CT) can be done emergently to rule out intracranial hemorrhage or trauma (see Chapter 6.6). Patients older than 60 years or those with definite focal neurologic abnormalities should have an imaging study to investigate for a causal lesion (e.g., brain tumor or stroke).
- **Lumbar puncture** is indicated if infection or subarachnoid hemorrhage is suspected.
- **Anticonvulsant levels** are needed when control of seizures is poor, when drug toxicity is suspected, and within 2 weeks after drug dosage is changed or potentially cross-reacting drugs are added.

TREATMENT

Proper classification of the seizure is critical. Eyewitness accounts, history, neurologic assessment, and laboratory data point to the specific therapy most likely to succeed.

- Correction of blood chemistry abnormalities and combating inciting agents, such as drugs or infections, is essential.
  - **Hyponatremia.** Seizures or coma occur only if serum sodium is extremely low, usually less than 110 mEq per L. Hypertonic saline is best avoided. Slow correction at the rate of 12 mEq per day avoids central pontine myelinolysis.
  - **Hypocalcemia** requires one or two ampoules of calcium gluconate (90 mg/ampoule), IV over 5 to 10 minutes.
- Agents for epilepsy control are presented in Table 6.4-1; dosages are given below.[1,2] Drugs of choice are listed in Table 6.4-2.[1,3]
- Acetazolamide (Diamox), pyridoxine, adrenocorticotropic hormone (ACTH), biotin, or a ketogenic diet is useful under special circumstances.
- During pregnancy, the drug that has controlled the seizures should be continued. If the patient has been seizure free, an attempt to stop medication is warranted. Folic acid and vitamin D supplements may reduce birth defects (see Chapter 14.6) and vitamin K in the month prior to delivery can reduce neonatal hemorrhage.

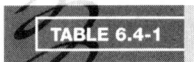

TABLE 6.4-1   Drugs for Seizures

Drug	Route	Adult (mg) SD	Adult (mg) UDD	Pediatric (mg/kg) SD	Pediatric (mg/kg) UDD	#DD	Therapeutic level (μg/mL)
Valproic acid (Depakene)	PO	500–1,000	1,000–2,000	10–15	15–60	1–3	50–120
Divalproex sodium (Depakote)	PO	Same as above		Same as above		1–3	SAME
Valproate sodium (Depacon)	IV	Same at ≤20 mg/min	—	Same at ≤20 mg/min		—	SAME
Carbamazepine (Tegretol, others)	PO	200–400	400–2,000	5–20	10–30	1–3	4–12
Phenytoin (Dilantin, others)	PO IV	300–400 15–20 mg/kg at ≤50 mg/min (up to 1,500 loading)	200–700	5 15–20 mg/kg at ≤50 mg/min (up to 1,500 loading)	4–15	1–3	10–20
Fosphenytoin (Cerebyx)	IV, IM IV	10–20 PE mg/kg at 150 mg/min	4–6 PE mg/kg	10–20 PE at 150 mg/min	4–6 PE	1–3	10–20
Phenobarbital (Luminal, others)	PO, IV	90–180	90–240	2–8 PO 10–20 IV	2–8	1–2	15–40
Primidone (Mysoline)	PO	100–125	250–1,500	10 (or 50 mg)	10–30	2–3	5–12 (primidone)
Gabapentin (Neurontin)	PO	300	900–6,400	10–15	10–30	3	2 and up
Lamotrigine (Lamictal)	PO	12.5–50	100–700	0.15–0.6	1–15	2	2–4
Ethosuximide (Zarontin)	PO	500	750–2,000	10–20	10–40	2	40–100
Clonazepam (Klonopin)	PO	1–1.5	1.5–20	0.01–0.03	0.05–0.2	2–3	20–80 ng/mL
Felbamate (Felbatol)	PO	600	1,200–4,800	15	15–60	3–4	30–130
Topiramate (Topamax)	PO	25–50	200–800	1–3	5–9	2	Not established
Tiagabine (Gabitril)	PO	4–8	8–56	0.1	0.4–0.7	2	Up to 550 ng/mL
Levetiracetam (Keppra)	PO	500	500–3,000	10–20	20–60	2	Not established
Oxcarbazepine (Triteptal)	PO	300	600–2,400	8–10	6–50	2	Not established
Zonisamide (Zonegran)	PO	100	100–600	1–2	6–8	1–3	20

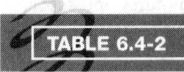

TABLE 6.4-2	Drugs of Choice for Seizures		
Type	**Seizure**	**First choice**	**Alternatives (adjuncts) in order of preference**
Generalized	Grand mal	Valproate Carbamazepine Phenytoin	Lamotrigine, topiramate, zonisamide, oxcarbazepine, levetiracetam, (gabapentin, pregabalin)
	Petit mal (absence)	Ethosuximide Valproate	Lamotrigine, clonazepam, zonisamide, levetiracetam; (acetazolamide)
	Myoclonic	Valproate Lamotrigine Carbamazepine	Topiramate, zonisamide, clonazepam, levetiracetam; rarely felbamate
Partial	Simple or complex	Phenytoin Lamotrigine Oxcarbazepine	Valproate, gabapentin, topiramate, tiagabine, zonisamide, levetiracetam, primidone, phenobarbital, pregabalin, rarely felbamate
Febrile seizures		Rectal diazepam	Valproate rectally

- Rectal diazepam or valproic acid are useful to achieve rapid seizure control, even in the home environment, especially for febrile convulsions.
- Vagal nerve stimulation can improve seizure control without drug side effects.
- Surgery offers some intractable seizure victims excellent outcomes.
- Withdrawal seizures as from alcohol are usually self-limited with low mortality so rarely require medication. Carbamazepine is contraindicated in this setting.

STATUS EPILEPTICUS

Status epilepticus is defined as continuous or repetitive convulsions lasting for 30 minutes or more and uninterrupted by consciousness even if seizure activity seemingly abates. The EEG confirms continued seizure activity.

- Evaluation is done as above, except that lumbar puncture is usually deferred unless bacterial meningitis is suspected.
- Treatment includes correction of abnormal findings and administration of the following drugs:
  - Thiamine, 100 mg IV, is given when alcoholism or malnutrition is possible.
  - Dextrose, 25 to 50 g IV, is given for adults; 2 to 4 mL per kg of 25% solution for children.
  - For adults, and as a second choice for children, phenytoin (Dilantin), 15 to 20 mg per kg IV infusion, is given at less than 50 mg per min, maximum 1 g in 20 minutes. A therapeutic level of 10 to 20 μg per mL is attainable within a few minutes.
  - Fosphenytoin (Cerebyx) is an alternative with fewer side effects given 20 mg per kg IV or IM at 150 mg per min (equivalent to 100 mg/min of phenytoin).
  - In children or if above recommendations are not effective in adults, one of the following two courses is taken:
    - Lorazepam (Ativan), 0.1 mg per kg IV, maximum 4 mg, given over 2 to 5 minutes, is the drug of choice in children and may be used in adults.
    - Diazepam (Valium), 0.3 mg per kg IV, maximum 20 mg, given over 2 to 5 minutes, is an alternative. A repeat dose may be administered. If the chosen drug fails, midazolam (Versed), 0.2 mg per kg IV, at 1 mg per minute, followed by a 0.2 mg/kg/hour infusion can be tried.

- Phenobarbital (Luminal), 10 mg per kg IV, given over 10 minutes and repeated once if needed can be tried. If this drug fails, pentobarbital (Nembutal), 2 to 8 mg per kg IV, at 25 mg per min, followed by a 0.5 to 5.0 mg/kg/hour infusion can still be effective.

- Propofol (Diprivan), 1 to 2 mg per kg IV over 5 minutes followed by 2 to 10 mg/kg/hour, can be added for continued seizures.

DRUG SIDE EFFECTS

Drug side effects are common but often controllable with serum levels. Periodic complete blood count and liver function tests are often required.

- Phenytoin (Dilantin) can produce stomach upset, rash, acne, gum hyperplasia (preventable with teeth cleaning), ataxia, nystagmus, folate deficiency, drowsiness, hirsutism, sedation, and osteomalacia.
- Carbamazepine (Tegretol) can produce rash, sedation, hepatitis, bone marrow suppression, and hyponatremia.
- Valproic acid (Depakene) can produce hepatitis, pancreatitis, sedation, hemorrhage, and hair loss.
- Benzodiazepines, including oxcarbazepine, can cause sedation and respiratory depression.
- Ethosuximide (Zarontin) can cause gastrointestinal upset, ataxia, sedation, hepatitis, and generalized seizures.
- Phenobarbital and primidone (Mysoline) can cause sedation, irritability, personality change, learning disability, rash, osteomalacia, and anemia.
- Gabapentin (Neurontin) and pregabalin (Lyrica) can cause sedation, ataxia, weight gain, and nystagmus.
- Lamotrigine (Lamictal) can cause rash, sedation, blurred vision, headache, ataxia, and vomiting.
- Topiramate (Topamax) can cause sleepiness, ataxia, psychomotor slowing, and kidney stones.
- Tiagabine (Gabitril) can produce dizziness and somnolence.
- Levetiracetam (Keppra) can cause dizziness and somnolence.
- Zonisamide (Zonegran) can produce ataxia, sleepiness, fatigue, and kidney stones.

PREVENTION

Prevention is aimed at avoidance of head trauma (e.g., with seat belts and bicycle helmets), infection (e.g., vaccines), drug abuse (e.g., drug education), stroke (e.g., blood pressure and cholesterol control), and cancer (e.g., smoking prevention). People with epilepsy should not swim alone or climb unassisted. Some states require that notification be made to driver's license authorities. Cardiopulmonary resuscitation (CPR) training can reassure some family members in their ability to deal with epilepsy.

References
1. Drugs for epilepsy. Treatment guidelines from the *Medical Letter* 2005;3:75–82.
2. LaRoche SM, Helmers SL. The new antiepileptic drugs; scientific review. *JAMA* 2004;291:605–614.
3. LaRoche SM, Helmers SL. The new antiepileptic drugs; clinical applications. *JAMA* 2004;291:615–620.

TRANSIENT ISCHEMIC ATTACKS
Sarah Parrott

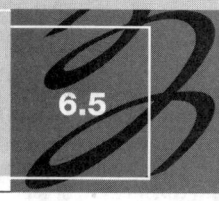

GENERAL PRINCIPLES

- Transient ischemic attack (TIA) is an ominous sign of brain ischemia and warns of the potential for future stroke.
- Rapid evaluation and treatment is important in the prevention of subsequent stroke.
- Most ischemic strokes occur within hours or days of a TIA.
- Antiplatelet or anticoagulation therapy is warranted for most causes of stroke.
- Tight control of diabetes, lipids, and hypertension can reduce the risk of subsequent stroke.
- Aggressive lifestyle modification can reduce the risk of subsequent stroke.
- TIA is often called **"mini stroke"** and is a warning that the patient is at increased risk for brain ischemia. The proposed new definition for a TIA is a "brief episode of neurologic dysfunction caused by a focal disturbance of brain ore retinal ischemia, with clinical symptoms lasting **less than 1 hour and without evidence of infarction."** An estimated 200,000 to 500,000 TIAs occur annually in the United States.

Pathophysiology

Large artery low-flow TIAs are considered "true TIAs." They are brief, recurrent, and with predictable symptoms. The causes include tightly stenotic atherosclerotic lesion in the internal carotid artery or the intracranial carotid artery when collateral circulation is not established. **Embolic TIAs** usually present with a single episode of focal neurologic symptoms lasting an hour or more. The embolus may be cardiogenic (atrial fibrillation, left ventricular thrombus or patent foramen ovale) or from a pathologic arterial process, usually extracranial. Hereditary clotting disorders may be involved.

DIAGNOSIS: HISTORY AND PHYSICAL EXAMINATION

Determining the **time of onset and duration of symptoms** is an essential piece of history. Further description of the **symptoms** may help the clinician determine the area of the transient ischemia. A **full neurologic examination** should follow, with specific attention to cranial nerve, motor, sensory, speech, language, coordination, and cognitive functions. The decision to proceed with **outpatient workup versus inpatient** depends on stability of the patient, resolution of all neurologic symptoms, and ability to proceed with testing in a timely manner as an outpatient. **Imaging:** If the symptoms have totally resolved by the time of evaluation, computed tomography (CT) imaging is not necessary. However, if symptoms continue, **CT without contrast** will rule out intracranial bleed. Magnetic resonance imaging (MRI) is more likely to identify areas of infarction, suggesting cerebrovascular accident (CVA), not TIA, should be the working diagnosis. **Carotid Doppler ultrasonography** can identify and quantify carotid atherosclerosis. Transesophageal echocardiogram with agitated saline to rule out atrial septal defect can be helpful. **Laboratory Data:** A **CBC and chem-12** will rule out hematologic and metabolic causes of neurologic symptoms. Further laboratory workup for clotting disorders should be considered, especially if there is a family history of thrombotic events. An electrocardiogram **(ECG)** to rule out atrial fibrillation and chest x-ray are standard.

    Symptoms of TIA include any of the following: visual disturbance in one or both eyes, unilateral or bilateral weakness of the face, arm, or leg. Decreased sensation or pain in the face, arm, leg, or trunk, slurring of words, difficulty pronouncing or "finding" words, clumsiness of arms or legs, loss of balance or falling to one side, apathy or inappropriate disorder, excessive somnolence, agitation, psychosis, confusion, memory changes, inattention to or denial of environment or body parts. The **differential diagnosis of TIA** includes seizures, migraine aura, syncope, distal nerve paresthesias, vestibulopathies, and hypoglycemia. Metabolic encephalopathis (hepatic, renal, or pulmonary) can cause alterations in behavior and movement.

TREATMENT

Risk Factor Moderation

Includes smoking cessation, weight loss for the obese patient, daily exercise, healthy diet including reduction/elimination of alcohol, achieving tight glycemic control, lowering lipids to acceptable range, and control of hypertension to meet Joint National Committee 7 (JNC-7) criteria (120/80).

Medications

Include anticoagulation (heparin or warfarin) if the cause is suspected to be atrial fibrillation, or antiplatelet therapy if the cause is vascular or unknown. Of the antiplatelet therapies available, the combination of long-acting dipyridamole and low-dose aspirin significantly reduced the incidence of stroke but not the incidence of death. Other considerations include clopidogrel, low-dose aspirin, or ticlopidine. Studies on the recommended antiplatelet regimen are ongoing. For lipid control, a statin or fibrate may be considered. Oral hypoglycemics or insulin should be used for tight control of blood glucose in patients with diabetes. Hormone replacement therapy should not be used in postmenopausal women with history of TIA.

Surgical Treatment

Includes carotid endarterectomy for stenosis >70%, carotid angioplasty and stenting for those with high risk for poor surgical outcome due to other medical illnesses, and intracranial stenting for tight, flow-limiting lesions identified by angiogram. These surgical interventions are preferably performed within 2 weeks of the TIA.

Complications

One study indicates that the cumulative risk for patients who seek care 1 week, 1 month, and 1 year after TIA is 7.2, 8.4, and 13.3, respectively. Therefore, a rapid response to the patient's complaint of symptoms is important. Office staff should be trained that "time is brain" and all neurologic changes should be evaluated immediately. Complications of anticoagulation and antiplatelet therapy are well documented and include bleeding. The clinician may consider a medication such as a proton pump inhibitor or H_2 blocker to protect the stomach from ulcer when prescribing daily aspirin.

Patient Education

The patient should be educated on the importance of lifestyle changes, the benefits of each medicine prescribed, and the importance of medication compliance to prevent stroke. Confirmation of smoking status might be considered on an intermittent basis if initial smoking cessation is achieved. The patient should be instructed to go to the emergency room immediately by ambulance if symptoms recur, as thrombolytic medications might be considered within the first 3 hours after symptom presentation in the case of stroke.

References

1. Sacco RL, Adams R, et al. Guidelines for prevention of stroke in patient with ischemic stroke or transient ischemic attack: a statement for healthcare professionals from the American Heart Association/American Stroke Association Council on Stroke; cosponsored by the Council on Cardiovascular Radiology and Intervention; the American Academy of Neurology affirms the value of this guideline. *Stroke* 2006;37:577–617. Available online at http://www./stroke.ahajournals.org/cgi/content /full/37/2/577.
2. Kistler JP, Furie KL, Ay H. Etiology and clinical manifestations of transient ischemic attack. Accessed 6/19/06 from UpToDate at http://wwwutol.com/utd/content/topic.do? topicKey+cva_dise/14351.
3. Kistler JP, Furie KL, Ay H. Treatment of transient ischemic attack and minor stroke. Accessed 6/19/06 from UpToDate at http://www.utdol.com/utd/content/topic.Do? topicKey=cva_dise/4620.
4. Solenski NJ. Transient ischemic attacks. Part I. Diagnosis and evaluation. *Am Fam Physician* 2004;69(7):1665–1674.

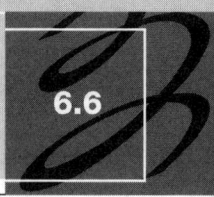

GENERAL PRINCIPLES

Definition

Stroke or cerebrovascular accident (CVA) is a syndrome characterized by acute onset of a focal neurologic deficit that persists for at least 24 hours and results from a disturbance in the cerebral circulation.

Epidemiology

In the United States, more than 157,000 people die of stroke annually and it is the third most common cause of death. Approximately 700,000 Americans experience a stroke each year, resulting in substantial disability among many stroke survivors.[1]

Classification

Strokes are classified into two main types: Hemorrhagic (20%) and ischemic (80%).

- Hemorrhagic strokes, or intracranial hemorrhages (ICH), occur when blood vessels rupture in the brain parenchyma or in the space around the brain.
- Ischemic strokes are caused by occlusion of blood vessels supplying the brain parenchyma, resulting in ischemia and infarction.

Mechanism of Injury

- Hemorrhagic strokes commonly are the result of head trauma, rupture of vascular malformations, and severe, uncontrolled hypertension. Other causes include coagulopathy, cocaine use, septic emboli, amyloid angiopathy, and bleeding into an area of ischemic infarct (hemorrhagic transformation).
- Ischemic strokes occur as the result of either embolism (60%) or thrombosis (40%). Emboli arise from the aortic arch, carotid arteries, and intracranial vessels. Cardioembolic sources include left atrial thrombus due to atrial fibrillation or atrial flutter, left ventricular thrombus, and paradoxical thromboembolism through a patent foramen ovale (PFO).
- Thrombotic strokes result from progressive atherosclerotic narrowing of vessels followed by acute thrombosis in the diseased artery. Large-vessel thrombosis occurs commonly in the carotid, middle cerebral, or basilar arteries. Thrombosis of smaller penetrating subcortical (e.g., internal capsule, thalamus) or brainstem arterioles are termed lacunar infarcts. Thrombotic disorders such as antiphospholipid syndrome and vasculitis also can cause ischemic strokes, and must be considered in patients less than 45 years of age and patients without risk factors.

DIAGNOSIS

Clinical Presentation

Patients experiencing a stroke can present with a wide variety and severity of symptoms. Depending on the location, mechanism, and size of the infarct, a patient may present with a classic, identifiable stroke syndrome (Table 6.6-1) or may report more subtle deficits, such as focal loss of sensation. Patients who have experienced embolic strokes often report sudden onset of the neurologic deficit that is maximal at onset, while thrombotic strokes typically evolve over minutes to hours. Patients with hemorrhagic events commonly experience severe headache, vomiting, and mental status changes.

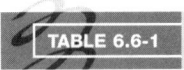

TABLE 6.6-1   Selected Acute Stroke Syndromes

Artery involved	Major symptoms
Anterior cerebral artery	Weakness of leg > arm, incontinence, personality change
Middle cerebral artery	Dominant hemisphere: Aphasia, weakness and sensory deficits in face, arm > leg; homonymous hemianopsia. Nondominant hemisphere: Neglect, weakness and sensory deficit (face, arm > leg)
Posterior cerebral artery	Isolated homonymous hemianopsia
Penetrating vessels/ lacunar infarcts	Weakness, unilateral (face = arm = leg) Weakness + sensory loss, unilateral Sensory loss, unilateral Dysarthria—clumsy hand syndrome
Basilar artery	Bilateral weakness, cranial nerve deficits, ataxia

History

Prompt diagnosis and treatment of stroke can improve the outcome. Note that if the patient is unable to communicate due to the neurologic deficit, other sources must be consulted. Ascertain:

- Subjective report of the neurologic symptoms
- The time of onset (when stroke symptoms are discovered on awakening, the time of onset is considered the time of the last known normal or baseline neurologic functioning)
- Presence of confounding or contributing factors such as alcohol or drug use, trauma, seizure activity, and risk for metabolic derangements
- History of atrial fibrillation, atherosclerotic disease, heart failure, prior venous thromboembolic event, diabetes, hyperlipidemia, and hypertension

Physical Examination

Physical examination of a patient with a possible stroke begins with assessment of vital signs and mental status. Ascertain the Glascow Coma Scale score and assess the patient's airway. Perform cardiovascular, pulmonary, and abdominal examinations. Once the patient is stable, a complete neurologic examination is required to assess and document the degree and localization of the deficit.

Laboratory Studies

Complete blood count, electrolytes, creatinine and BUN, hepatic enzymes, PT, PTT, and INR should be performed expeditiously. A stat finger stick blood glucose measurement is indicated to rule out hypoglycemia, which can present with focal neurologic deficits. An electrocardiogram should be performed on all patients to assess for arrhythmia, concurrent cardiac ischemia, or infarct. Perform serial measurements of troponin if there is suspicion for cardiac ischemia.

Imaging

Emergent noncontrast head computed tomography (CT) scan is required for all patients undergoing evaluation for stroke. The diagnostic yield of noncontrast head CT for detecting hemorrhage approaches 100%.[2] Providing the patient does not have significant renal dysfunction, a contrast head CT/cerebral angiogram can be ordered later to localize the vessels involved in an ischemic stroke. Patients presenting in the very early stages of a stroke may have a normal head CT. If there is a high clinical suspicion for cerebellar or brainstem infarction and the initial CT scan is negative, magnetic resonance imaging (MRI) is recommended owing to its superior sensitivity for posterior fossa processes.

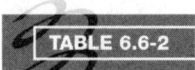

TABLE 6.6-2	Differential Diagnosis of Stroke
Hypoglycemia	Hypo-or hypernatremia
Seizure	Systemic infection (particularly in the elderly)
CNS tumors	CNS infection (abscess, meningitis, encephalitis)
Complicated migraine	Hypertensive encephalopathy
Todd's paralysis (postictal focal deficit that can persist up to 24 hours)	

Monitoring

Patients with stroke require close monitoring of multiple physiologic parameters. Level of alertness and ability to protect the airway must be followed closely. Initiate frequent neurologic checks to assess for progression of deficits. Continuous blood pressure monitoring is vital to prevent further brain injury. Perform frequent blood glucose measurements with a goal glycemic control of 110 to 180.

Differential Diagnosis

Numerous conditions can mimic a stroke. The most common mimickers of stroke are listed in Table 6.6-2.

TREATMENT

The treatment of acute stroke is dependent on the underlying physiology.

Operative Management

Hemorrhagic strokes require consultation with a neurologist and neurosurgeon to assess for ventriculostomy, intracranial pressure (ICP) monitoring, and possible surgical evacuation of hematoma. Surgical evacuation usually is reserved for posterior fossa (cerebellar) strokes, given the smaller anatomic space and higher risk for herniation.

Nonoperative Management

There is no role for operative management in an ischemic stroke with the rare exception of craniotomy for massive stroke with edema, severely increased ICP, and impending herniation. The goals of acute stroke management are to restore and maintain blood flow to the area surrounding the infarcted brain (the ischemic penumbra), prevent further injury to this vulnerable tissue, prevent secondary complications of stroke, and prevent subsequent strokes.

Restoring Blood Flow

- Thrombolytic therapy requires experienced stroke teams and strict adherence to protocols and exclusion criteria to achieve success rates equivalent to those reported in controlled trials.
- Alteplase (IV t-PA) is indicated for the thrombolytic treatment of ischemic stroke when therapy can be initiated *within 3 hours* of symptom onset and the neurologic deficit is serious enough to warrant the potentially fatal risks. Thrombolysis can improve the odds of complete or near-complete recovery from neurologic deficits at 3 to 6 months by about 11% (absolute difference, compared with placebo; number needed to treat, or NNT = 19). There is no mortality benefit. There is substantial risk for symptomatic intracranial hemorrhage (NNH = 17), including fatal hemorrhage (NNH = 40). The therapeutic index for thrombolysis is narrow and care must be taken to select patients in whom the benefits appear to outweigh the risks. Table 6.6-3 presents contraindications to thrombolysis.[3]

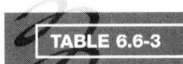

TABLE 6.6-3	Contraindications to Thrombolysis

Historical	Clinical
Stroke or head trauma within the prior 3 months	Rapidly improving stroke symptoms
Major surgery within 14 days	Seizure at onset of stroke
Lumbar puncture within 7 days	Pregnancy or lactation
Any prior intracranial hemorrhage	Active bleeding or acute trauma
Myocardial infarction within the prior 3 months	Minor or isolated neurologic signs
GI or GU bleeding within previous 21 days	Persistent SBP >185 or DBP >110
Laboratory:	
Platelets <100,000	
Elevated INR >1.7	

DBP, diastolic blood pressure; GI, gastrointestinal; GU, genitourinary; SBP, systolic blood pressure.

- Intra-arterial thrombolysis can be performed in select centers up to 6 hours after onset of symptoms. This is a non-Food and Drug Administration (FDA)-approved treatment and requires an experienced 24-hour neurointerventional service.
- More recently, mechanical thrombolysis of cerebral emboli has been studied. The MERCI Retriever system was approved by the FDA in 2005 and may be employed up to 8 hours after onset of symptoms.

Maintain Perfusion
- Early initiation of antiplatelet therapy is beneficial in patients who are not treated with thrombolytics. Aspirin 160 to 325 mg daily is recommended, with clopidogrel 75 mg daily as an alternative for aspirin-allergic patients. Immediate full-dose anticoagulation with IV heparin and SQ low-molecular-weight heparin (LMWH) is not associated with a significant reduction in death or dependency and is not recommended.[4]
- Blood pressure management is crucial in the treatment of acute ischemic stroke. The stroke-injured brain autoregulates systemic blood pressure to maintain cerebral perfusion pressure (CPP), which is equal to mean arterial pressure (MAP) minus ICP. The strategy of tolerating elevated blood pressures in the setting of acute ischemic stroke, sometimes termed "permissive hypertension," maximizes collateral blood flow to the ischemic penumbra.
- Numerous observational studies have demonstrated that blood pressure reduction in the first week after an acute ischemic stroke is associated with neurologic deterioration and worse outcomes.
- Treat elevated blood pressure when:
  - Systolic blood pressure >220
  - Diastolic blood pressure >120
  - Concurrent aortic dissection, congestive heart failure exacerbation, acute renal failure, hypertensive encephalopathy
  - Administering thrombolytics if needed to maintain SBP <185 and DBP <110

- When *acute* blood pressure reduction is indicated, labetolol is an efficacious and versatile drug, with a wide therapeutic index in intravenous and oral preparations. Enalapril is an alternative for those with contraindications to beta-blockers. Avoid use of hydralzine or intravenous calcium channel blockers (CCBs) due to risk of precipitous lowering of blood pressure and avoid nitrates and CCBs due to potential increases in ICP.
- In contrast to ischemic strokes, hemorrhagic strokes require aggressive blood pressure lowering to minimize the volume of hemorrhage.

Prevent Damage to Ischemic Penumbra

- Effective management of basic physiologic parameters can help preserve the viability of vulnerable brain cells in the ischemic penumbra.[5] Hyper- and hypoglycemia are deleterious to ischemic cells, so close attention to glycemic control is important (goal glucose 110 to 180). If intravenous fluid administration is required for resuscitation, isotonic fluids such as 0.9% saline are appropriate to avoid precipitating intracerebral fluid shifts that can occur with hypo- and hypertonic fluids.
- Aggressively control fever with anti-pyretics.
- Monitor SpO$_2$ and provide supplemental oxygen if needed.

Prevent Secondary Complications

- Aspiration is a substantial contributor to morbidity. All patients with cranial neuropathies or altered mental status should be nil per oral (NPO) with aspiration precautions until a speech and swallow evaluation is completed.
- Stroke patients have very high risk for venous thromboembolism (VTE). Pharmacologic prophylaxis with low-dose, low-molecular-weight heparin unfractionated heparin is strongly indicated in all patients unless there is specific contraindication. Mechanical VTE prophylaxis via intermittent pneumatic compression devices and graded compression stockings is recommended for patients with hemorrhagic strokes or other contraindication to low-dose heparin.
- It is prudent to order bed rest for the first 24 hours and until neurologic status has stabilized. Early mobilization, including passive range of motion exercises, with physical and occupational therapy helps improve function and decrease morbidity. Evaluation of skin integrity and use of air/circulating mattresses in bed-bound patients can help reduce the incidence of decubitus ulcers.
- Urinary retention, incontinence, constipation, and fecal impaction commonly occur after stroke and derangements of bowel and bladder function require prompt evaluation and treatment.
- Seizures occur in 5% to 10% of patients following stroke. Poststroke patients who develop seizures generally are treated with phenytoin. Prophylaxis is not warranted.

Risk Management
Prevent Subsequent Strokes

- One of the most important aspects of hospitalization for acute stroke is to identify the etiologic process to target prevention of recurrent strokes (Table 6.6-4).
- Anti thrombotic therapy is extremely important for secondary prevention after ischemic strokes. In patients who experience a noncardioembolic stroke, first-line therapy is aspirin at 75 to 150 mg daily. Patients who have experienced a stroke while taking aspirin are treated with aspirin/dipyridamole (25/200 mg BID) or clopidogrel 75 mg daily for secondary prevention. The combination of aspirin and clopidogrel is contraindicated for secondary stroke prevention. Chronic anticoagulation with warfarin is indicated when an embolic source (atrial fibrillation, ventricular thrombus) is identified.[4,6,7]
- Patients with high-grade ipsilateral carotid artery stenosis (70% to 99%) should be referred for evaluation for carotid endarterectomy (CEA). Carotid angioplasty and

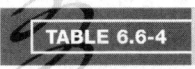

TABLE 6.6-4	Modalities to Work up Etiology for Stroke

A. Telemetry (atrial fibrillation and flutter)
B. Transthoracic echocardiogram with bubble study (intracardiac thrombus, PFO, and aortic arch)
C. Carotid artery imaging (CTA, MRA, or Doppler ultrasound)
D. CTA or MRA (intracranial vessels)

CTA, computed tomography angiography; MRA, magnetic resonance angiography; PFO, patent foramen ovale.

stenting is an alternative for patients with high-grade stenosis who are not candidates for CEA due to comorbid operative risk. Consider serial imaging every 6 to 12 months for patients with moderate carotid stenosis (50% to 69%).[6]

Risk Factor Modification

- All patients with ischemic strokes require aggressive long-term management of modifiable risk factors.
- Controlling blood pressure clearly is effective in reducing risk for subsequent strokes. Antihypertensive therapy should be initiated 10 to 14 days after stroke and must proceed slowly with a goal blood pressure of <135/80. The optimal drug regimen remains uncertain, but available data support the use of diuretics and combination therapy with diuretics and an angioten-converting enzyme (ACE) inhibitor or angiotensin receptor blocker (ARB).[6–8]
- Lipid management is important and the majority of patients likely would benefit from statin therapy. The current recommended low-density lipoprotein (LDL) goal is <100 and therapy with lipid-lowering agents such as statins will be required in many patients. Simvastatin 40 mg daily is FDA approved for secondary stroke prevention irrespective of LDL level.[7]
- Optimizing glycemic control results in more favorable outcomes for cardiovascular diseases, with a target HbA1C <7%.
- Counseling about lifestyle risk factor reduction should begin prior to discharge. Provide counseling and offer tobacco cessation assistance for all smokers.
- Recommend increasing regular physical exercise to reduce cardiovascular risk by lowering blood pressure, reducing obesity, and improving glycemic control.
- It is reasonable to recommend avoidance of heavy alcohol consumption, and a diet rich in fruits and vegetables and low in cholesterol and cholesterol-raising fatty acids.[6]

Referrals

- Because 40% of patients with stroke have moderate functional impairments and 15% to 30% have severe disability,[9] early evaluation for and referral to a multidisciplinary acute rehabilitation team is extremely important. Screening for admission to a rehabilitation program should occur as soon as the neurologic and medical conditions permit safe participation.
- Depression is very common after stroke, occurring in 30% to 60% of patients.[10] Screen all patients for depressive symptoms and counsel about the warning signs of depression that may emerge later.
- Patients who have profound disability after stroke or who had poor functional status prior to stroke may not be appropriate candidates for aggressive inpatient rehabilitation programs. These patients must continue to receive range of motion exercises, monitoring and treatment of contractures, and aggressive prevention of decubitus ulcers.

Patient Education

Counsel all patients with stroke about the warning signs of stroke and the importance of medication adherence. Family members play an important role in poststroke recovery and require education as to the nature of their loved one's neurologic deficit, prognosis for recovery, and plan for rehabilitation. All patients discharged on anticoagulation should receive intensive teaching about signs of bleeding, dietary issues, and activity modification.

Follow-Up

All patients who have experienced a stroke require follow-up care with primary care providers for long-term blood pressure management, lipid lowering, diabetes management, dietary and exercise counseling, smoking cessation, and management of anticoagulation if indicated. Clinicians also should monitor progress with rehabilitation therapy, changes in physical functional capacity, social functioning, and emergence of new cardiovascular symptoms or medication side-effects. Given the high prevalence, patients should be screened for depression at follow-up appointments.

References

1. American Heart Association. *Stroke facts 2006: All Americans.* Dallas, TX: American Heart Association; 2006.
2. Adams HP Jr, Brott TG, Crowell RM et al. Guidelines for the management of patients with acute ischemic stroke. A statement for healthcare professionals from a special writing group of the Stroke Council, American Heart Association. *Stroke* 1994;25:1901.
3. Lindbloom EJ. Thrombolytic therapy for acute ischemic stroke: risks and benefits. *J Fam Pract* 2003;52(10):757–761.
4. Albers GW, Amarenco P, Easton JD, et al. Antithrombotic and thrombolytic therapy for ischemic stroke: the seventh ACCP Conference on Antithrombotic and Thrombolytic Therapy. *Chest* 2004;126:483S–512S.
5. Fulgham JR, Ingall TJ, Stead LG, et al. Management of acute ischemic stroke. *Mayo Clin Proc* 2004;79(11):1459–1469.
6. Cohen SN. Preventing recurrent ischemic stroke: a 3-step plan. *J Fam Pract* 2005; 54(5):412–422.
7. Kirshner HS, Biller J, Callahan AS. Long term therapy to prevent stroke. *J Am Board Fam Pract* 2005;18(6):528–540.
8. AHA/ASA guidelines for prevention of stroke in patients with ischemic stroke or transient ischemic attack: a statement for healthcare professionals. *Stroke* 2006;37:577–617.
9. American Heart Association. *Heart and stroke statistical update 2005.* Dallas, TX: American Heart Association; 2004.
10. Sinyor D, Arnato P, Kaloupe K DG, et al. Post-stroke depression: relationships to functional impairment, coping strategies, and rehabilitation outcome. *Stroke* 1986;16: 1102–1107.

PARKINSON DISEASE

John D. Gazewood

6.7

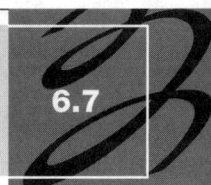

GENERAL PRINCIPLES

Definition

Parkinson disease (PD) is a progressive, degenerative neurologic disorder, characterized by tremor, rigidity, and bradykinesia.[1]

Anatomy/Pathology

PD is characterized by loss of dopaminergic neurons in the substantia nigra compacta in the midbrain that project to the striatal complex (putamen and caudate) in the forebrain. Lewy bodies (intracytoplasmic inclusion bodies) are present in affected neurons.[2]

Epidemiology

PD affects approximately 1% of the population over age 60. Currently 1 million Americans have PD and the prevalence will increase with the aging population. PD afflicts all ethnic groups, and occurs more often in men than woman.[1]

Pathophysiology

Possible causes include oxidative stress, apoptosis, and mitochondrial dysfunction; however, definitive proof that these mechanisms are involved in the pathway leading to degeneration is lacking. Accumulation of a toxic protein secondary to overproduction or to an abnormality in the ubiquitin-proteosomal system may be the underlying abnormality. Lewy bodies are composed of an abnormal protein (α-synuclein) that in normal form is found throughout normal brain tissues.[3]

Etiology

Combination of genetic and environmental factors. Approximately 10% to 15% of patients have a first-degree relative with PD. More than 10 different genes identified that play a role in PD have been identified.[4] It is unclear what environmental factors are involved in etiology.

DIAGNOSIS

Clinical Presentation

Patients with PD typically present with one of four symptom complexes[1]:

- Tremor
- Weak or clumsy limb
- Stiff or achy limb
- Gait disorder

History

The history is nonspecific in early disease, and includes insidious malaise, fatigability, and subtle personality changes (apathy). As disease progresses, motor symptoms predominate. Resting tremor is present in 75% of PD patients. Characteristics of the tremor include:

- Unilateral, typically involving upper extremity
- Worse with anxiety
- Better with sleep and motion of affected extremity

Stiffness and bradykinesia are also common and are manifest by such symptoms as trouble turning in bed, difficulty arising from a chair, loss of balance, trouble opening jars, and micrographia.[5]

Physical Examination

Diagnosis of Parkinsonism is suggested by the combination of bradykinesia with tremor and/or rigidity on physical exam:

- Tremor—Resting, coarse, four to six cycles per second, often referred to as "pill-rolling." Lessens with motion.
- Rigidity—Resistance to passive range of motion (ROM). While applying force across joint during ROM, cog-wheeling felt as a "jerky" or ratcheting type of resistance, with resistance followed by relaxation. Lead pipe rigidity is smooth resistance throughout ROM. Both types of resistance may be heightened with repeated ROM of limb.
- Rigidity must be distinguished from spasticity, which is characterized by resistance followed by giving away of strength (clasp-knife resistance).
- Bradykinesia—Difficulty in initiating and slowness of movement. Examples include masklike facies and gait abnormalities:
  - Difficulty initiating gait
  - Short, shuffling steps, with a normal base
  - Decreased arm swing
  - Bradykinesia can be elicited by having patients tap finger, "twiddle" their hands (roll them around each other), or tap their heels against the floor.[5]

Laboratory Studies

None typically needed.

Imaging

PD is a clinical diagnosis, and does not require imaging for diagnosis. Imaging can be useful in atypical presentations, and can help to differentiate PD from nonparkinsonian conditions, such as essential tremor. Imaging helps differentiate PD from progressive supranuclear palsy (PSP) or multisystem atrophy (MSA), conditions that can be mistaken for PD. For example:

- Conventional magnetic resonance imaging (MRI) usually normal in PD.[6]
- Novel MRI techniques (such as diffusion-weighted imaging) can differentiate PD from MSA and PSP.

■ Three-dimensional positron emission tomography (3-D PET) with 18F-Dopa shows asymmetric uptake and a greater decrease in uptake in caudal putamen than the caudate nucleus in PD.[2]

Differential Diagnosis

Other causes of parkinsonian symptoms include drug-induced parkinsonism, dementia with Lewy bodies, vascular parkinsonism, and the "Parkinson-plus" syndromes, which include PSP and MSA. PD may also be confused with essential tremor. These illnesses have important distinguishing features[7]:

■ Drug-induced parkinsonism: Use of antidopaminergic drug (e.g., metoclopromide, risperidol) with symptom improvement when medication withdrawn.
■ Vascular parkinsonism: Widespread deep bilateral lacunar infarcts associated with wide-based, shuffling, freezing gait, with a stepwise progression of illness.
■ Dementia with Lewy bodies: Dementia onset concomitant with onset of motor symptoms.
■ PSP: Supranuclear gaze palsy, gait instability with frequent falls early in course of illness, resting tremor uncommon.
■ MSA: Prominent dysautonomia (e.g., erectile dysfunction, orthostatic hypotension) early in course of illness, rapid course.
■ Essential tremor: Tremor bilateral and postural and can involve head. Is worse with motion, better with alcohol. Family history is common. No rigidity or bradykinesia.

TREATMENT

Goals of treatment are to minimize the disabling affects of PD. Starting treatment is not required at diagnosis, but is started when symptoms begin to impair function. Parkinson medications target the motor symptoms of the disease, and are more effective for treating the rigidity and bradykinesia than the tremor. There is no clear evidence that any PD medications have a neuroprotective effect.[8]

Medications (Table 6.7-1)

■ Monoamine oxidase-B (MAO-B) inhibitors (selegiline or rasigiline): Effective for mild symptoms.[9]
■ Levodopa/carbidopa: Most effective medication for PD. Its use is complicated by development of dyskinesias after 5 years. Long-acting dopamine preparations are no more effective than immediate-release dopamine and are more expensive.[9]
■ Dopaminergic agonist (bromocriptine, pramipexole, ropinorole, or carbegoline.) Effective, but are less effective than L-dopa. Their use is associated with a lower incidence of dyskinesias. However, they are more costly and have more central nervous system (CNS) side effects among elderly patients (hallucinations, drowsiness).[9]
■ Choice of levodopa/carbidopa or dopaminergic agonist as initial therapy: Dopaminergic agonists may be preferable for younger patients. For older patients, carbidopa/levodopa is preferred.[9]
■ Combination therapy: For patients who develop dyskinesias on levodopa/carbidopa, or when levodopa/carbidopa becomes less effective, addition of dopaminergic agent can be helpful. Catechol-O-methyltransferase (COMT) inhibitors (entacopone) increase duration of action of dopamine by inhibiting its degradation, and can be used to prolong its action. Anticholinergic agents may be useful for treating the tremor, although their use in elderly patients should be avoided because they are likely to cause delirium.[9–11] Amantadine is effective in treating dyskinesias.[3]

Surgery

Surgery is indicated for patients with advanced PD who have disabling symptoms despite optimal medical management.

■ PD tremor: Can be treated by ablation of the ventriculointermedius nucleus of the thalamus (thaladomotomy) or by electrical stimulation of this nucleus. The effectiveness of thaladomotomy diminishes over time, and thalamic stimulation was found to be better at 1 year than thaladomotomy in a randomized trial.[11,12]

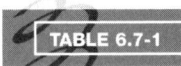

| TABLE 6.7-1 | Medications for Parkinson Disease |

Medication	Starting dose	Maximum dose	Price (starting, dose per month)[a]
MAO-B inhibitors			
Rasagiline	0.5 mg daily	1 mg daily	Brand only
Selegiline	5 mg daily	10 mg daily	Brand: $85.00 Generic: $30.00
Carbidopa/levodopa			
Carbidopa/levodopa	25 mg/100 mg TID	200 mg/2000 mg in divided doses	Brand: $79.00 Generic: $40.00
Carbidopa/levodopa sustained release	50 mg/200 mg BID	600 mg/2400 mg in divided doses	Brand: $111.00 Generic: $81.00
Dopamine agonists			
Amantadine	100 mg daily	400 mg in divided doses	Brand: $41.00 Generic: $34.00
Bromocriptine	1.25 mg BID	100 mg in divided doses (TID)	Brand : $112.00 Generic: $62.00
Cabergoline	Not approved for this indication		
Pramipexole	0.125 mg TID	1.5 mg TID	Brand: $110.00
Ropinirole	0.25 mg TID	3 mg TID	Brand: $165.87
COMT inhibitors			
Entacapone	200 mg/dose, given with carbidopa/ levodopa	1600 mg/day in divided doses	Brand: $69.00 (for 30)
Tolcapone (FDA Black Box warning for fatal hepatotoxicity)	100 mg TID	200 mg TID	Brand: $245.98
Anticholinergic agents			
Cogentin	0.5 mg/day	6 mg/day in divided doses	Generic: $7.99

[a]Prices from Epocrates Pro©, updated September 1, 2006.

■ Rigidity and bradykinesia: Can be treated by pallidotomy or stimulation of the subthalamic nucleus. Pallidotomy is also likely to be effective in reducing dyskinesias and on–off motor phenomenon. The effectiveness of subthalamic nucleus (STN) stimulation in reducing dyskinesias is uncertain.[11,12]

Special Therapy
There are insufficient data to conclude whether physical, occupational, and speech therapy are effective in PD. However, most clinicians will refer patients with more advanced PD for therapy, depending on the patients' specific needs. Therapy is typically not needed in early disease.

Referral
Consultation with a neurologist or geriatrician is appropriate when the diagnosis is uncertain, the patient responds poorly to medication, or when the physician is unable to adequately help the patient manage symptoms. The family physician needs to remain engaged with care after referral, as many neurologists do not address the disabling nonmotor symptoms of the

illness.[13] Referral to a neurosurgical center with expertise in PD is warranted for patients whose symptoms are disabling despite optimal medical therapy.

Patient Education

Patients require education about the course of the illness, how to use their medications, and side effects of therapy, which can be significant. Patients should be encouraged to develop an advanced directive. Patient support groups that include a large proportion of patients with advanced disease may be distressing for patients with mild PD. Some useful web sites for additional information are: www.michaeljfox.org; www.parkinson.org; www.apdaparkinson.org.

Complications

As the disease progresses, patients develop motor symptoms related to long-term therapy with L-dopa, including dyskinesias, as well as symptoms related to declining CNS dopamine levels, including wearing-off of L-dopa effectiveness early in dosing interval, on–off phenomenon, freezing, and gait abnormalities.[3] Additionally, the nonmotor symptoms of Parkinson disease are increasingly common with disease progression and 50% of patients rate their effect on daily living as significant.[13]

- Sleep disturbances: Include excessive daytime sleepiness and rapid eye movement (REM) sleep behavior disorder, where patients have vocalization and limb movement during REM sleep.
- Neuropsychiatric symptoms: The most common is depression, occurring in up to 45% of patients with PD. Hallucinations affect up to 40% of patients with advanced PD. About 15% will develop dementia.
- Autonomic symptoms: Include constipation, bladder dysfunction, orthostatic hypotension, erectile dysfunction, and hyperhydrosis.
- There are insufficient data to guide the therapy of these symptoms in patients with PD, so clinicians must extrapolate from therapy for other disorders.[13] A randomized controlled trial has shown that rivastigmine is effective for Parkinson dementia.[14]
- Prognosis: Population-based cohort studies indicate that median survival after diagnosis is 9.1 years. Patients with PD are more likely to be institutionalized and have a higher mortality rate than an age-matched population.[15,16]

References

1. Nutt JG, Wooten GF. Clinical practice. Diagnosis and initial management of Parkinson's disease. *N Engl J Med* 2005;353(10):1021–1027.
2. Piccini P, Whone A. Functional brain imaging in the differential diagnosis of Parkinson's disease. *Lancet Neurol* 2004;3(5):284–290.
3. Guttman M, Kish SJ, Furukawa Y. Current concepts in the diagnosis and management of Parkinson's disease. 2003;168(5):544. *CMAJ* 2003;168(3):293–301.
4. Scott WK, Nance MA, Watts RL, et al. Complete genomic screen in Parkinson disease: evidence for multiple genes. *JAMA* 2001;286(18):2239–2244.
5. Rao G, Fisch L, Srinivasan S, et al. Does this patient have Parkinson disease? *JAMA* 2003;289(3):347–353.
6. Seppi K, Schocke MFH. An update on conventional and advanced magnetic resonance imaging techniques in the differential diagnosis of neurodegenerative parkinsonism. *Curr Opin Neurol* 2005;18(4):370–375.
7. Tolosa E, Wenning G, Poewe W. The diagnosis of Parkinson's disease. *Lancet Neurol* 2006;5(1):75–86.
8. Schapira AHV, Olanow CW. Neuroprotection in Parkinson disease: mysteries, myths, and misconceptions. *JAMA* 2004;291(3):358–364.
9. Miyasaki JM, Martin W, Suchowersky O, et al. Practice parameter: initiation of treatment for Parkinson's disease: an evidence-based review: report of the Quality Standards Subcommittee of the American Academy of Neurology. *Neurology* 2002;58(1):11–17.
10. Rascol O, Goetz C, Koller W, et al. Treatment interventions for Parkinson's disease: an evidence based assessment. *Lancet* 2002;359(9317):1589–1598.
11. Goetz CG, Poewe W, Rascol O, et al. Evidence-based medical review update: pharmacological and surgical treatments of Parkinson's disease: 2001 to 2004. *Movement Disord* 2005;20(5):523–539.

12. Eskandar EN, Cosgrove GR, Shinobu LA. Surgical treatment of Parkinson disease. *JAMA* 2001;286(24):3056–3059.
13. Chaudhuri KR, Healy DG, Schapira AHV, National Institute for Clinical E. Nonmotor symptoms of Parkinson's disease: diagnosis and management. *Lancet Neurol* 2006; 5(3):235–245.
14. Maidment I, Fox C, Boustani M. Cholinesterase inhibitors for Parkinson's disease dementia. *Cochrane Database Syst Rev* 2006;1.
15. de Lau LML, Schipper CMA, Hofman A, et al. Prognosis of Parkinson disease: risk of dementia and mortality: the Rotterdam Study. *Arch Neurol* 2005;62(8):1265–1269.
16. Berger K, Breteler MM, Helmer C, et al. Prognosis with Parkinson's disease in Europe: a collaborative study of population-based cohorts. Neurologic Diseases in the Elderly Research Group. *Neurology* 2000;54(11 Suppl 5):S24–27.

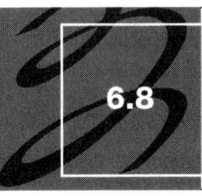

6.8   ALZHEIMER DISEASE
Kalpana P. Padala, Prasad R. Padala

GENERAL PRINCIPLES

Definition

Alzheimer disease (AD) is the leading cause of dementia in the elderly population. This progressive neurodegenerative disease presents with global cognitive decline, personality changes, behavioral complications, and functional impairments. This was first described in 1907 by Alois Alzheimer who found progressive loss of neurons and abnormal clumps and bundles of fibers in the brain of a woman who presented with disorientation, memory problems, paranoid delusions, and hallucinations.[1]

Epidemiology

Prevalence estimates of AD in the United States range from 5.7% to 10% among people aged 65 to 85 years and 25% to 45% in those 85 years of age or older. Currently there are 5.1 million Americans with AD in 2000. Conservative estimates project tripling of this number to 16 million by 2050.[2] The annual cost of caring for patients with AD in the United States is estimated to be around 148 billion dollars ranking third after heart disease and cancer.[3] This cost includes direct costs such as medications, physician visits, day care, hospitalization, and nursing home costs; and indirect costs such as the time caregivers spend with patients and associated loss of productivity in the workplace.

Pathophysiology

Intracellular deposition of neurofibrillary tangles and extracellular deposition of beta amyloid plaques are diagnostic of AD at autopsy.[4] Degree of cognitive impairment in AD is more closely related to the burden of the neurofibrillary tangles than the plaques. Hippocampus, basal forebrain, entorhinal, and temporal cortices, areas important in the processing of memory, have profound neuronal loss in AD.

Etiology

There is no single known etiology. Increasing age and positive family history are the two greatest risk factors for AD. Presence of ApoE4 allele increases the risk of AD. ApoE4 allele is present in 30% to 50% of patients with AD. Inheritance of one allele of ApoE4 increases the chances of developing AD twofold whereas inheriting both alleles raises the chances ten fold.[5]

DIAGNOSIS

Clinical Presentation

The diagnosis of AD is clinical and based on exclusion of common causes of memory dysfunction. The following criteria are outlined in the *Diagnostic and Statistical Manual of Mental Disorders*, 4th edition text revision (DSM-IV–TR)[6]:

- The development of memory impairment and at least one of the following cognitive disturbances: aphasia, apraxia, agnosia, and executive dysfunction.
- A significant decline from the previous level of functioning leading to significant impairment in social or occupational functioning.
- The cognitive decline is gradual in onset and progressive.
- The cognitive deficits are not due to any neurologic disease, systemic condition, substance use disorder, delirium, or other psychiatric disease.

The earliest symptom reported is impairment in recent memory. Other common deficits include learning deficits, language deficits, word-finding difficulty, repetitiousness, disorientation, and misplacing items (Table 6.8-1). Behavioral problems include depression, apathy, agitation, disinhibition, anxiety, hallucinations, paranoid delusions, and sleep disturbances. Functional decline manifested in difficulty cooking, handling finances, and driving often necessitate involvement of social services such as daycare programs and later institutionalization.

Physical Examination

A complete physical and neurologic examination is important to rule out systemic (such as hypothyroidism) and neurologic (such as cerebrovascular disease, Huntington disease, Parkinson disease) conditions. Frontal lobe release signs and anosmia are common neurologic findings in AD.

Laboratory Tests

Laboratory workup is necessary to rule out reversible and other causes of dementia. This includes a complete blood count, vitamin B_{12} and folic acid levels, comprehensive metabolic panel, thyroid-stimulating hormone, serologic tests for syphilis and human immunodeficiency virus. In some cases toxicology screen, cerebrospinal fluid exam, and chest x-ray may be necessary.

Imaging

A noncontrast computerized tomographic imaging of the brain is routinely done to rule out other causes of dementia such as normal pressure hydrocephalus. Other neuroimaging techniques, such as magnetic resonance imaging (MRI), are indicated with sudden deterioration of cognition, headaches, head injury, or abnormal neurologic exam.

Differential Diagnosis

- Vascular dementia: It is the second most common form of dementia comprising of 10% to 20% of all dementias. Cognitive decline is usually noted after a cerebrovascular event, followed by a plateauing of cognition until the next cerebrovascular event. This is often referred to as stepwise deterioration in cognition. Corresponding changes in MRI or computed tomography (CT) are usually seen.

TABLE 6.8-1	Ten Warning Signs of AD
Memory loss	Difficulty performing familiar tasks
Problems with language	Disorientation to time and place
Poor or decreased judgment	Problems with abstract thinking
Misplacing things	Changes in mood or behavior
Changes in personality	Loss of initiative

Source: Reference 7.

- Lewy body dementia: This neurodegenerative dementia is associated with parkinsonism, cognitive fluctuations, autonomic dysfunction, visual hallucinations, and neuroleptic sensitivity. It is characterized by presence of Lewy bodies in brainstem and cortex.
- Frontotemporal dementia: A heterogeneous group of rapidly progressive dementias, commonly seen in younger age group. Focal atrophy of frontal and temporal lobes is a characteristic finding. Inappropriate social behavior is an early clinical feature. Language dysfunction and behavioral abnormalities are the main clinical manifestations.
- Reversible causes of dementia include medication use, alcohol use, depression, thyroid disease, vitamin B_{12} deficiency, renal and hepatic dysfunction, hyponatremia, hypercalcemia, normal pressure hydrocephalus, subdural hematomas, chronic meningitis, and cerebral neoplasms.

TREATMENT

Medications

Although there is no cure for AD, two classes of medications are used to manage cognitive problems. Cholinesterase inhibitors increase the availability of acetylcholine, a neurochemical essential for memory. Three drugs are currently marketed in the United States and include donepezil, galantamine, and rivastigmine. Donepezil is administered once daily, usually started at 5 mg a day and titrated to 10 mg at 4 to 6 weeks. Galantamine is usually started at 4 mg twice daily and titrated to 8 mg twice daily at 4 to 6 weeks. Maximum approved dose is 12 mg twice daily, although clinical studies have shown no superiority of this dose over 8 mg twice daily dose. Rivastigmine is usually started at 1.5 mg daily and titrated up every 2 weeks in 1.5-mg increments to reach 6 to 12 mg daily dose. Although well tolerated some patients experience gastrointestinal side effects. Several strategies such as starting at a lower dose, slower titration, and taking the medications with food can be helpful.

The second class of drugs targets the glutamate receptors and prevents death of neurons by excessive influx of calcium (excitotoxicity). Memantine is an uncompetitive N-methyl-D-asparate (NMDA) receptor antagonist. It is started at 5 mg a day and titrated at increments of 5 mg weekly to reach the target dose of 10 mg twice daily. It can be used in combination with a cholinesterase inhibitor due to the different mechanisms of action.

Although mainly used for cognitive decline, cholinesterase inhibitors have been found to be helpful in the management of behavioral problems such as hallucinations and agitation. Specific treatments for behavioral problems such as selective serotonin-reuptake inhibitors for depression, atypical antipsychotics for hallucinations and delusions are often used (Table 6.8-2).

Behavioral Treatment

Nonpharmacologic interventions are crucial in the management of behavioral problems in AD and include several strategies such as structured activities, environmental interventions, sensory enhancement and relaxation techniques, social contact, and behavior therapy.

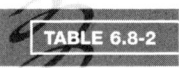 **TABLE 6.8-2**   **Medications for Behavioral Problems in AD**

Medication	Indication	Dose/day
Citalopram, Paroxetine, Fluoxetine	Depression, anxiety, and agitation	10–20 mg
Sertraline		
Risperidone	Psychosis,	25–100 mg
Olanzapine	agitation	0.25–2 mg
Quetiapine		2.5–10 mg
Aripiprazole		12.5–400 mg
		2.5–15 mg
Methylphenidate	Apathy	5–10 mg

Structured activities such as outdoor walks, physical activities, and recreational activities and environmental interventions such as having wandering areas and reduced stimulation go a long way in avoiding many behavioral problems.

Referrals/Counseling

A multidisciplinary team approach is necessary for the diagnosis and management of dementia. Referral to a geriatric evaluation clinic will often provide assessment from a geriatrician, geriatric psychiatrist, social worker, pharmacist, and nurse specialist. Several assessment tools can be used to monitor the progress of AD when such referrals are not available: Mini-Mental State Exam[8] and AD Assessment Scale-cognitive subscale[9] can be used for assessment of cognition. Activities of Daily Living scale and Instrumental Activities of Daily Living scale reliably assess the functional status of a patient. Neuropsychiatric inventory is a caregiver report of common behavioral problems seen in AD.[10]

Risk Management

Detailed evaluation of safety risks is essential at the intake and at each follow-up visit. Common safety concerns include cooking, driving, firearm safety, financial mismanagement, wandering in hazardous weather, and abuse. Involvement of family and social services can often help in management of these safety concerns. Small interventions such as involving meals on wheels, disabling the car, taking away the firearms or the ammunition, family involvement in fiscal management, wander guards can be life-saving. It is also crucial to establish advance directives and health care power of attorney.

Patient Education

Education about the disease, course of the illness, and the need for multiple interventions is essential. Family members need to be educated about various manifestations of dementia in different stages such as the cognitive problems, behavioral problems, and functional decline, all stemming from one disease process rather than multiple entities. It is also essential to educate about what to expect from medications used to treat dementia. Furthermore, educating about respite, accessing local support network such as the local chapter of Alzheimer association or office of aging can reduce caregiver burden. In the later stages of AD, families of patients need to be provided information on nursing homes in the local community and also about terminal care.

References

1. Fuller SC. Alzheimer's disease (senium praecox): the report of a case and review of published cases. *J Nerv Ment Dis* 1912;39:452–454. (Translated from Alzheimer's originally published notes.)
2. Hebert LE, Scherr PA, Bienias JL, et al. Alzheimer disease in the US: prevalence estimates using the 2000 census. *Arch Neurol* 2003;60(8):1119–1122.
3. http://www.alz.org/alzheimers_disease_alzheimer_statistics.asp.
4. Perl DP. Neuropathology of Alzheimer's disease and related disorders. *Neurol Clin* 2000;18:847.
5. Roses AD. Apolipoprotein E alleles as risk factors in Alzheimer's disease. *Annu Rev Med* 1996;47:387–400.
6. American Psychiatric Association. *Diagnostic and statistical manual of mental disorders.* 4th ed., text rev. Washington, DC: American Psychiatric Association; 2000.
7. http://www.alz.org/AboutAD/Warning.asp.
8. Folstein MF, Folstein SE, McHugh PR. Mini-Mental State: a practical method for grading the state of patients for the clinician, *J Psychiatr Res* 1975;12:189–198.
9. Mohs RC, Rosen WG, Davis KL. The Alzheimer's disease assessment scale: an instrument for assessing treatment efficacy. *Psychopharmacol Bull* 1983;19(3):448–450.
10. Cummings JL, Mega M, Gray K, et al. The Neuropsychiatric Inventory: comprehensive assessment of psychopathology in dementia. *Neurology* 1994;44(12):2308–2314.

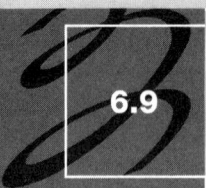

PERIPHERAL NEUROPATHY
6.9 *Krupa Shah*

GENERAL PRINCIPLES

Peripheral nerves contain motor, sensory, and autonomic fibers alone or in combination. Peripheral nerves may be damaged by various causes including hereditary, toxic, nutritional, ischemic, inflammatory, and paraneoplastic disorders. Peripheral neuropathies vary widely in their presentation, depending on the specific fibers involved, as well as on whether the axon itself or only the myelin sheath that is affected.

DIAGNOSIS

- **Signs and symptoms.** Patients with peripheral neuropathy may present with altered sensation, pain, weakness, or autonomic symptoms. In the early stages, patients may experience only pain or other subjective symptoms. Measurable sensory deficits are much less common. Motor dysfunction, if present, may range from mild weakness to complete paralysis, and usually more pronounced distally. Decreased tendon stretch reflexes are the earliest objective sign of motor dysfunction. Stumbling, tripping, or clumsiness of either hands or feet may also be reported, and often out of proportion to the degree of measurable weakness. Autonomic dysfunction is most often associated with diabetes (see Chapter 17.2).
- **Approach to the patient.** If particular symptoms are thought to represent a peripheral neuropathy, the identification of treatable causes or underlying medical conditions (particularly diabetes, alcoholism, and nutritional deficiencies) should be the first priority. History of recent viral illnesses or any new medications should be obtained. Work and hobbies should be reviewed for activities that cause repetitive nerve trauma as well as any potential toxic exposures. Hereditary neuropathies are common. A detailed family history is often helpful in previously unrecognized or long-standing distal neuropathies.

MONONEUROPATHIES

Mononeuropathies are usually due to entrapment, compression, or other physical injuries of peripheral nerves deep to fibrous bands (where they pass through bony openings or arch across bony prominences). Repetitive work or cumulative trauma may also be implicated. Electrodiagnostic studies are useful to confirm the diagnosis and quantify the injury. Treatment is generally conservative, including work or activity modification. Surgical exploration should be reserved for more chronic mononeuropathies that have begun to show evidence of weakness or atrophy. **Mononeuropathy multiplex** results from multifocal involvement of individual peripheral nerves; the clinical picture is highly variable and potentially confusing. Ischemic diabetic neuropathy, as well as vasculitides and chronic inflammatory demyelinating polyradiculoneuropathy (CIDP), accounts for most cases.

- **Trigeminal neuralgia** (tic douloureux) is relatively common and usually idiopathic. It is characterized as brief paroxysmal attacks of severe, lancinating facial pain in the maxillary or mandibular divisions of the trigeminal nerve (the ophthalmic division is rarely involved). Many patients report trigger points sensitive to even mild stimuli, such as chewing, tooth brushing, shaving, or talking. Carbamazepine (Tegretol) 200 to 300 mg tid is usually effective. Start with 100 mg at bedtime and increase by 100 mg every 1 to 3 days until symptoms are relieved. Some patients may require doses of up to 400 mg tid. Phenytoin (Dilantin), 300 to 600 mg daily, or baclofen (Lioresal), 5 to 20 mg tid, may be a useful alternative or an adjunct to carbamazepine.

- **Bell palsy** (idiopathic facial paralysis), an acute onset of isolated facial nerve paralysis, is common. It occurs at any age, and the etiology remains unclear. Although still somewhat controversial, evidence is accumulating that reactivated herpes viruses (simplex type 1 or zoster) in cranial nerve ganglia are the most common cause of Bell palsy. The prognosis, with or without specific treatment, is excellent, as almost all patients have spontaneous recovery in 1 to 3 weeks. However, 15% of patients (particularly those who are older or more severely affected) may show some residual weakness for several months or even permanently. Bilateral Bell palsy is rare and potentially more worrisome, with causes like Lyme disease, human immunodeficiency (HIV) infection, leukemia, syphilis, infectious mononucleosis, or sarcoidosis (see Chapters 19.3, 19.4, 19.5, and 19.10).
  - **Clinical presentation.** Symptoms typically develop overnight and the patient notices a facial droop on awakening. Many patients recall sitting in a draft or report a recent viral illness. The degree of impairment is widely variable, ranging from mild weakness and a delay in blinking to complete paralysis and inability to close the eye. Forehead muscles are involved in Bell palsy. Frontal sparing indicates a central nervous system (CNS) lesion. Corneal sensation is usually intact. Food may catch in the cheek on the affected side.
  - **Therapy.** Patient education about careful eye care is essential. The eye should be kept moist and lubricated with artificial tears or an ophthalmic ointment (Lacrilube). It may also be necessary to protect the eye with a shield or to tape it shut during sleep. If no contraindications to steroids exist, prednisone, 60 to 80 mg daily, tapered over 10 to 14 days, may be helpful, especially if started within the first 2 or 3 days. Adding an antiviral agent like acyclovir or valcyclovir to prednisone therapy may improve recovery rates compared with prednisone alone.
- **Brachial plexus neuropathies** are usually due to blunt or penetrating trauma. Any injury that is directed to the axilla or that forcibly stretches the head and shoulder may result in numbness and paresthesias of the arm and diffuse weakness of the arm and shoulder. Direct extension of apical lung tumors (Pancoast tumor) or metastatic brachial plexopathy, particularly from breast cancer, is common. Radiation therapy is also known to cause similar symptoms.
- **Carpal tunnel syndrome** (CTS) is the most common of all entrapment neuropathies. Any process that encroaches on the median nerve, either intrinsically or extrinsically, can cause a CTS (Chapter 15.5).
- **Ulnar nerve entrapment** in the ulnar groove or about the cubital tunnel is the most common ulnar neuropathy. Young athletes involved in overhand activities, particularly pitching, as well as patients who lean on their elbows at work or who have had prolonged elbow pressure after coma or general anesthesia, are susceptible. Patients experience intermittent paresthesias in the fourth and fifth fingers, as well as the dorsoulnar aspect of the hand and forearm. They may also experience generalized weakness of grasp and clumsiness of the hand and fingers, especially with fine manipulation. The ulnar nerve may also be compressed at the wrist (ulnar tunnel or Guyon canal syndrome) in individuals with certain occupations or in long-distance bicyclists. Motor symptoms are more pronounced with few, if any, sensory symptoms.
- **Radial nerve injuries** most commonly occur as a result of pressure in the axilla, such as occurrence after a drunken sleep with the arm draped over the back of a chair (Saturday night palsy) or from an ill-fitting crutch. Patients have a wrist-drop and paralysis of the finger extensors. There may also be weakness of extension at the elbow as well as of supination of the forearm. Entrapment of the posterior interosseus nerve (radial tunnel syndrome) at the level of the supinator muscle causes weakness of finger extensors without a wrist-drop.
- **Lumbosacral neuropathies**
  - **Meralgia paresthetica** is a compression neuropathy of the lateral femoral cutaneous nerve of the thigh. It is commonly seen in obese or diabetic individuals. Patients experience increasingly severe numbness, pain, paresthesias, and decreased sensation of the anterolateral thigh. There is no objective weakness.
  - **Femoral neuropathy** is most commonly due to a diabetic vascular mononeuropathy. It results in weakness of leg extension and paresthesias of the anteromedial thigh and the medial aspect of the lower leg and foot.

- **Peroneal neuropathy** may be caused by pressure at the level of the fibular head exerted by an ill-fitting cast, trauma, or improperly positioned delivery room stirrups. Diabetic, vasculitic, and hereditary neuropathies may also affect the peroneal nerve, leading to foot-drop and sensory changes of the dorsum of the foot and ankle.
- **Tibial neuropathy** (tarsal tunnel syndrome) most often is attributable to compression of the tibial nerve in the tarsal tunnel at the medial malleolus. This results in burning and paresthesias of the sole of the foot, and may be aggravated by walking or prolonged standing.

POLYNEUROPATHIES

Polyneuropathies are characterized by diffuse, bilateral, and symmetrical damage, producing a distal, stocking or glove pattern of paresthesias and sensory loss, later followed by decreased tendon reflexes and muscle weakness.

- **Diabetic neuropathy** is the most commonly encountered polyneuropathy. Some form of neuropathy develops in one half of all people with diabetes (also see Chapter 17.2). It usually develops after many years, although it may occasionally be the presenting feature of diabetes. Strict glycemic control and good daily foot care are key to preventing complications of diabetic neuropathy. Early recognition of diabetic neuropathy may decrease the incidence of lower extremity complications.
  - **Clinical presentation.** The primary types of diabetic neuropathy are sensorimotor and autonomic. A patient may have only one type of neuropathy or might develop different combinations of neuropathies. Most commonly, patients with diabetes experience a distal, symmetrical polyneuropathy with predominantly sensory involvement and mild motor signs. Initially, the patient may not perceive pain, thus initiating a cascade of events that may ultimately lead to the development of diabetic ulcers with potential for infection or amputation. Later, the patient may also experience severe burning discomfort or dysesthesias, particularly of the plantar surfaces of the feet. Involvement of large myelinated fibers may cause decreased joint position sense, leading to both sensory ataxia and secondary arthropathy (Charcot joints). Some patients with diabetes may have purely autonomic signs and symptoms. Postural hypotension is probably most common, but gastrointestinal (diabetic gastroparesis, intestinal hypomotility, and constipation or diarrhea) and genitourinary (impotence and atonic bladder) symptoms may also occur. Myocardial infarction is commonly silent in patients with diabetes because of loss of small pain fibers in the cardiac sympathetic system. Patients with diabetes frequently develop single as well as multiple mononeuropathies. These patients are more prone to both ischemic and entrapment neuropathies.
  - **Therapy.** Optimal glycemic control is most important for both prevention and treatment. Patient education about daily foot care is essential for preventing complications of diabetic neuropathy. The American Diabetes Association (ADA) recommends a thorough annual foot examination by a health care professional for all patients with diabetes. For pain control, the tricyclics, especially amitriptyline, 10 to 150 mg at bedtime, may be helpful. Either desipramine or nortriptyline, 75 to 150 mg, may be a useful alternative in patients unable to tolerate amitriptyline. Duloxetine, an antidepressant, in the doses of 60 to 120 mg was approved for the treatment of diabetic neuropathic pain. Pregabalin, an antiepileptic drug, was also approved for use. Oxycodone CR 10 to 60 mg twice a day, used judiciously, may be helpful. Gabapentin, 300 to 1,800 mg daily, carbamazepine, or phenytoin may also be used. Topical capsaicin 0.075% applied once daily may also help relieve diabetic neuropathy.
- **Inflammatory neuropathies**
  - **Herpes zoster** (shingles) is a painful rash that is caused by the reactivation of latent varicella virus in the distribution of the affected nerve (see Chapter 19.8). The characteristic vesicular eruption is unilateral and most often involves a thoracic dermatome. Risk factors for developing herpes zoster are increasing age, immunosuppression, intrauterine exposure to varicella (i.e., chickenpox), and outbreak of varicella at younger than 18 months.

- **Clinical presentation.** The prodrome of herpes zoster includes fever, malaise, and headache. These may precede the eruption by several days. Vesicles on the tip of the nose may indicate ophthalmic zoster. If there is eye pain, redness, or photophobia, refer the patient to an ophthalmologist. Involvement of the geniculate ganglion of the facial nerve may result in an acute facial nerve paralysis, accompanied by an eruption on the ear and within the ear canal (Ramsay Hunt syndrome). Weakness or paralysis, especially of the facial nerves, or disseminated zoster is more likely to occur in elderly individuals or in patients immunocompromised by HIV or malignancy.
- **Therapy.** High-dose acyclovir (Zovirax) 800 mg five times daily for 7 days, valacyclovir (Valtrex) 1,000 mg tid, or famciclovir (Famvir) 500 mg tid, also for 7 days have been shown to decrease both the duration and severity of acute symptoms if started early (within the first 72 hours of symptoms in all patients older than 50 years). There is evidence to support using antiviral therapy and possibly low-dose tricyclic antidepressants to prevent postherpetic neuralgia. The use of steroids has an unfavorable risk–benefit ratio. For established postherpetic neuralgia, there is good evidence to support treatment with gabapentin and tricyclic antidepressants.

■ **Lyme disease.** Bell palsy, which may be bilateral, or a polyradiculopathy may be seen in the early disseminated phase of Lyme disease (see Chapter 19.9).

■ **Leprosy.** Despite its low incidence in the United States, leprosy remains the most common cause of treatable peripheral neuropathy in the world. Leprosy must be included in the differential diagnosis whenever a patient from a high-risk group presents with a peripheral neuropathy. As leprosy and its attendant skin lesions progress, increasing anesthesia, with the potential for breakdown and injury, occurs in the lesions. Some degree of sensory loss is always present in leprosy. It is not unusual for symptoms of neuropathy to occur long before other manifestations of the disease.

■ **Acute inflammatory demyelinating polyradiculopathy** (AIDP) or **Guillain–Barré syndrome** (GBS). GBS is a syndrome of symmetrical, rapidly progressive, ascending muscle weakness with decreased or absent tendon stretch reflexes. Epidemiologic studies have linked it to infection with *Campylobacter jejuni* in addition to other viruses including cytomegalovirus and Epstein–Barr virus.
- *Campylobacter jejuni* gastroenteritis is the most frequent antecedent infection. All patients should be hospitalized to carefully monitor their cardiac and respiratory status, neurologic consultation and testing, and to initiate either plasmapheresis or immunoglobulin therapy. Most patients make a good recovery. Prognosis is worse in elderly patients and also in patients with more rapid progression of muscle weakness or evidence of axonal involvement.

■ **CIDP.** This disorder is a relatively common neuropathy that often goes unrecognized. Clinical and electrophysiologic diagnostic criteria have been established, allowing clinicians to distinguish CIDP from other acquired neuropathies. The usual clinical picture is a predominantly motor neuropathy with an elevated cerebrospinal fluid (CSF) protein value. Specifically, effective immunotherapies are available for CIDP.

■ **HIV** (see Chapter 19.4). The initial presentation of HIV infection may be as GBS or CIDP. HIV testing is indicated in these patients. In later stages, secondary opportunistic infections of the peripheral nervous system, primarily by herpes zoster or cytomegalovirus, or secondary malignancies may involve the peripheral nerves. Patients with late-stage HIV infection may have a particularly painful neuropathy.

■ **Nutritional neuropathies** are all related to B vitamin deficiencies. These generally occur in combination with one another, primarily in chronic alcoholics. Patients with anorexia or bulimia, malabsorption, and food faddists may also experience B vitamin deficiencies. A symmetrical distal polyneuropathy is common to all the nutritional neuropathies.

■ **Alcoholic neuropathy** is clinically indistinguishable from nutritional neuropathies due to vitamin deficiencies. In a few alcoholic patients, a neuropathy may occur despite an adequate diet. The prognosis for ultimate, but slow, recovery is good for patients who are able to stop drinking and resume a proper diet with multivitamin supplements (see Chapter 5.3).

■ **Vitamin B$_1$ (thiamine) deficiency,** or beriberi, most commonly occurs in chronic alcoholics. Although its primary form is a Wernicke–Korsakoff encephalopathy, a typical distal polyneuropathy may also occur. Both entities are treated with intramuscular injection of thiamine 100 mg every 12 hours the first day, followed by 100 mg daily PO.

■ **Vitamin B$_6$ (pyridoxine) deficiency** is caused by certain drugs that interfere with pyridoxine metabolism, notably isoniazid and dapsone. These drugs are used in the treatment of leprosy, which itself causes a sensory neuropathy—the clinical picture is potentially confusing. Pyridoxine supplements, 50 mg tid, may prevent this complication. However, excessive amounts of pyridoxine (>500 mg daily) may also cause a severe sensory neuropathy.

■ **Vitamin B$_{12}$ deficiency** may present initially with only vague paresthesias without objective signs. In older patients hematologic abnormalities may not be apparent until the neurologic complications have become irreversible. Diagnosis of vitamin B$_{12}$ deficiency is typically based on measurement of serum vitamin B$_{12}$ levels; however, about 50% of patients with subclinical disease have normal B$_{12}$ levels. A more sensitive method of screening for vitamin B$_{12}$ deficiency is measurement of serum methylmalonic acid and homocysteine levels, which are increased early in vitamin B$_{12}$ deficiency.

■ **Toxic neuropathies** develop over several weeks to months as a result of continued exposure to certain drugs, industrial toxins, or heavy metals. A progressive, symmetrical, ascending polyneuropathy is most frequently seen with occupational exposures. The most commonly implicated drugs include anticancer agents, particularly cisplatin and vinca alkaloids, as well as isoniazid, dapsone, nucleoside analogues, and amiodarone. Rare incidents of arsenic poisoning, either intentional or resulting from insecticide exposure, may cause a late-onset progressive polyneuropathy. Chronic lead exposure causes a predominantly motor neuropathy, typically beginning in the upper limbs, with an asymmetrical radial neuropathy and wrist-drop. Fluctuating symptoms may be due to intermittent exposures. Management is supportive care and avoidance from or removal of the offending toxin. The majority of toxic neuropathies are self-limited and improves gradually after toxin elimination.

■ **Hereditary neuropathies,** generally showing a slowly progressive and indolent course, are common. They are typically associated with high-arched feet (pes cavus) and hammertoe deformity, as well as slowly progressive weakness and wasting of peroneal muscle groups. Current therapy is limited to symptom relief. The ultimate prognosis is fairly good, with a manageable degree of disability.

■ **Miscellaneous.** Patients with peripheral neuropathies are occasionally found to have one of the dysproteinemias, most often monoclonal gammopathy of unknown significance. Multiple myeloma rarely causes a polyneuropathy. Monoclonal proteins may be detected by serum protein electrophoresis. Plasma exchange may be an effective therapy. Patients with distant, occult malignancy may present with a carcinomatous peripheral neuropathy. It is most commonly associated with small-cell lung carcinomas. Antineuronal nuclear antibodies may serve as serologic markers of these paraneoplastic syndromes, preceding detection of cancer by months or even years.

References

1. Poncelet AN. An algorithm for the evaluation of peripheral neuropathy. *Am Fam Physician* 1998;57:755–764.
2. Holland NJ, Weiner GM. Recent developments in Bell's palsy. *BMJ* 2004;329:553–557.
3. Aring AM, Jones DE, Falko JM. Evaluation and prevention of diabetic neuropathy. *Am Fam Physician* 2005;71(11):2123–2128.
4. Argoff CE, Backonja MM, Belgrade MJ, et al. Diabetic peripheral neuropathic pain: consensus guidelines for treatment. *J Fam Pract* 2006;55(6):1–20.
5. Mounsey AL, Matthew LG, Slawson DC. Herpes zoster and postherpetic neuralgia: prevention and management. *Am Fam Physician* 2005;72(6):1075–1080.
6. Hughes RA, Cornblath DR. Guillain-Barre syndrome. *Lancet* 2005;366(9497):1653–1666.
7. Oh R, Brown DL. Vitamin B$_{12}$ deficiency. *Am Fam Physician* 2003;67(5):979–986.
8. Grogan PM, Katz JS. Toxic neuropathies. *Neurol Clin* 2005;23(2):377–396.

Eye Problems   VII

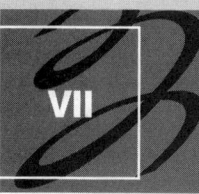

CONJUNCTIVITIS AND OTHER CAUSES OF A RED EYE   7.1
John E. Sutherland, Richard C. Mauer

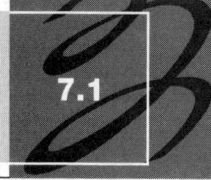

$\mathcal{T}$he most common causes of "red eye"—conjunctivitis, trauma, allergies, subconjunctival hemorrhage, and lid problems—are usually benign. However, some conditions presenting with a red eye require urgent evaluation and treatment. These include keratitis, episcleritis, scleritis, uveitis, orbital cellulitis, and acute angle closure glaucoma. Symptoms requiring immediate referral to an ophthalmologist are pain, proptosis, perilimbal injection, photophobia, tenderness, and decreased vision.[1]

INFECTIOUS CONJUNCTIVITIS (BACTERIAL OR VIRAL)
General Principles
- The most common cause of red eye: Outbreaks of conjunctivitis are not unusual in schools, childcare centers, military bases, and eye clinics.[2]

Diagnosis
Clinical Presentation
- **Bacterial conjunctivitis** presents with burning, irritation, glued eyes in the morning, and a purulent discharge that usually becomes bilateral within 2 days.
- **Viral conjunctivitis** discharge shows a more watery discharge and burning or gritty sensation and is often epidemic.
- **Chlamydial conjunctivitis,** more common in younger patients, shows a mucopurulent discharge, often is associated with urethritis or vaginitis, and tends to be subacute.

Laboratory Studies
Immunofluorescent tests on ocular scrapings for *Chlamydia trachomatis* and culture for *Neisseria gonorrhoeae* are required. Bacterial cultures should be obtained in neonates and patients who have severe inflammation or chronic or recurrent conjunctivitis. Results most commonly reveal *Staphylococcus epidermidis*, *S. aureus*, *Haemophilus influenzae*, and

Streptococcus pneumoniae. Viral studies are rarely performed. Urethral or cervical cultures may be indicated.

Physical Findings

Vision should be recorded and is normal unless the cornea is involved with keratitis. Hyperemia is highly diffuse involving both the bulbar and tarsal conjunctiva. Staining of the cornea with fluorescein should be performed, using topical anesthetic drops, cobalt blue filter, sterile irrigation fluid, and magnification with an ophthalmoscope or slit lamp. The cornea should be examined for a poor surface light reflex, infiltrate, ulcer, or ciliary or perilimbal injection. The presence of small papillae is common with viruses, and lid vesicles suggest herpesvirus infection. In herpes simplex, corneal involvement is usually dendritic.[1,3]

Treatment

Medications

- **Bacterial conjunctivitis (topical).** Even though this is mostly a self-limiting disorder, treatment results in earlier clinical remission. Antibiotic drops or ointment is given every 2 to 4 hours. It is best to choose an antibiotic with adequate Gram–positive coverage. All available ophthalmic antibiotics have strengths and weaknesses. Choices include bacitracin, sulfacetamide (Bleph–10), gentamicin (Garamycin, Genoptic), tobramycin (Tobrex), and erythromycin, or combinations, such as neomycin–polymyxin B–bacitracin (Neosporin ointment), gramicidin/neomycin/polymyxin B (Neosporin drops), trimethoprim–polymyxin B, (Polytrim), and polymyxin B–bacitracin (Polysporin). Neomycin preparations are more likely to invoke a hypersensitivity reaction. The topical fluoroquinolones ciprofloxacin (Ciloxan), levofloxacin (Quixin), gatifloxacin (Zymar), moxifloxacin (Vigamox), and ofloxacin (Ocuflox) are very effective, but because of increasing resistance should be reserved for severe or resistant infections.
- **Bacterial conjunctivitis (systemic)**
  - **H. influenzae.** Topical and systemic treatment is needed because of the risk of meningitis. Trimethoprim–polymyxin or quinolone eye drops are used for topical therapy. Systemic therapy choices are amoxicillin–clavulanate (Augmentin) or rifampin (Rifadin), or both.
  - **N. gonorrhoeae** in adults. Ceftriaxone (Rocephin), 1 g IM or IV is administered one time, augmented by topical antibiotics and frequent topical saline irrigation in endemic areas of penicillin-resistant gonorrhea.
  - **Chlamydial follicular inclusion and chronic bacterial conjunctivitis.** This is usually treated with oral tetracycline or erythromycin, 250 to 500 mg qid, or doxycycline, 100 mg bid, or clarithromycin, 250 to 500 mg bid for 3 weeks.[1–6]
- **Viral conjunctivitis (systemic and topical)**
  - **Adenoviral conjunctivitis.** This is extremely contagious for up to 14 days and may not resolve for up to 3 weeks. Because this is usually self-limited, treatment is supportive and includes ice-cold compresses, artificial tears, and naphazoline (Albalon, AK–Con, Vasocon, Naphcon) or naphazoline–pheniramine (Naphcon–A) qid if itching is severe. Ophthalmic antibiotics are often utilized because of patient expectations or to treat potential bacteria infection.
  - **Herpes zoster.** Referral is indicated for corneal involvement. If the trigeminal nerve is involved, treat with oral acyclovir (Zovirax), famciclovir (Famvir), or valacyclovir (Valtrex) for 7 days.
  - **Acute hemorrhagic.** This is caused by an enterovirus or coxsackievirus, both highly contagious and epidemic but self-limited. Treatment is supportive.
  - ***Molluscum contagiosum.*** Removal of the central core of the lesion present on the eyelid is sufficient to cure the conjunctivitis.
  - **Herpes simplex.** Referral is indicated for corneal involvement. Treatment is with trifluridine (1%) (Viroptic) for 7 days.
  - **Others.** Infectious mononucleosis, influenza, Lyme disease, cat-scratch fever, mumps, rubella, pharyngoconjunctival fever, and vaccinia viruses may be etiologic agents, and these are all treated supportively.[1,3]

NEONATAL CONJUNCTIVITIS

General Principles

It is imperative to make a specific etiologic diagnosis. Chemical irritation presents within 24 hours and most commonly is caused by prophylactic erythromycin, tetracycline, or silver nitrate. It is important to rule out sexually transmitted diseases such as gonorrhea and chlamydia. More commonly staphylococci or streptococci are the etiologic agent. Another common condition to differentiate is congenital nasolacrimal duct infection, which usually causes ocular discharge without redness. The presence of herpes simplex type 2 infection requires consultation.

Diagnosis

■ **Physical examination.** A detailed maternal history is important. Physical examination should assess for systemic illness.

■ **Laboratory studies.** Gram stain, Giemsa stain, immunofluorescent antigen detection, Papanicolaou stain, and specific cultures may be necessary.

Treatment

Medications

Topical therapy includes gentamicin for Gram-negative and erythromycin for Gram-positive organisms. Pseudomonal infection requires consultation. Systemic therapy for chlamydial infection is erythromycin syrup, 50 mg/kg/day qid for 14 days. For gonococcal infections, use ceftriaxone (Rocephin), 25 to 50 mg per kg qd IV or aqueous. Supportive treatment only is needed for chemical conjunctivitis. Most nasolacrimal duct blockage resolves spontaneously by the age of 6 months.

ALLERGIC CONJUNCTIVITIS

General Principles

Seasonal (SAC) and perennial (PAC) allergic conjunctivitis (AAC) are common immediate hypersensitivity reactions. Vernal (VKC) and atopic (AKC) keratoconjunctivitis are chronic, more severe, and may lead to sequelae.[5]

Diagnosis

History

AAC and PAC are characterized by pathognomonic bilateral itching, tearing, and mild eyelid swelling. VKC occurs in children and adolescents with more severe symptoms, including photophobia. This is most frequently seasonal, recurrent, and associated with other chronic allergy symptoms. AKC is associated with dermatitis and cataracts and typically reveals an atopic family or personal history.[4]

Physical Findings

A stringy discharge, mild redness, and edema occur in hay fever, whereas in atopic disease corneal involvement and blepharitis are common. Giant papillae are found on the conjunctiva in the vernal disorder and in contact lens–associated conjunctivitis.

Treatment

Medications

■ **Vasoconstrictors and antihistamines.** Vasoconstrictors, naphazoline 0.012% (AK-Con, Albalon, Naphcon) and Naphcon Forte 0.1% induce symptom relief quickly. The combination of naphazoline 0.025% and pheniramine 0.3% (Naphcon–A, Opcon-A) is more effective than either agent alone. New antihistamines levocabastine (Livostin), epinastine 0.05% (Elestat), emedastine 0.05% (Emadine) are all very effective. Oral antihistamines can also be of value.

■ **Mast cell stabilizers.** Pemirolast 0.1% (Alamast), Lodoxamide 0.1% (Alomide) qid, nedocromil 2% (Alocril) bid, or cromolyn 4% (Crolom) qid are effective in treatment during peak exposure. Olopatadine (Patanol), azelastine (Optivar), and Ketotifen 0.025% (Zaditor) are combination H_1 antagonist and mast cell stabilizers, which have the advantage of immediate and long-lasting benefit.

■ **Nonsteroidal anti-inflammatory drugs (NSAIDs).** Ketorolac 0.5% (Acular), Ketorolac 0.4% (Acular LS), nepafenac 0.1% (Nevanac), bromfenac 0.09% (Xibrom), flurbiprofen 0.03% (Ocufen), or diclofenac 0.1% (Voltaren) qid may also be effective treatment for allergic conjunctivitis.

- **Corticosteroids.** Prednisolone 0.1% (Inflamase Mild, AK Pred, Pred Mild), prednisolone 0.125% (Inflamase Forte, Pred Forte), dexamethasone 0.1% drops (Maxidex, Ak–Dex), fluorometholone 0.1% (FML or Flarex) or 25% (FML Forte), loteprednol 0.2% (Alrex) 0.5%, (Lotemax), or rimexolone (Vexol) two to four times per day are highly effective. Corticosteroids are used in severe cases but may cause cataracts or glaucoma with long-term use and should be administered under the direction of an ophthalmologist.
- **Nonpharmacologic treatment.** Cold compresses, saline irrigation, and ocular lubricants four to eight times daily may provide relief. Elimination or reduction of the allergen exposure should be attempted. In severe cases, desensitization or systemic steroids, or both, may be needed.[8,9]

KERATITIS
General Principles
Definition
Inflammation or infection of the cornea (the outermost portion of the eye).

Etiology
- **Bacterial** (Gram positive and negative)
- **Viral.**
  - Herpes simplex type I is the most common form. Varicella zoster, or shingles, is a post–chicken pox sequela seen in elderly and immunocompromised individuals. Adenovirus is an acute illness that produces corneal infiltration.
- **Fungal.** *Candida* occurs in debilitated patients. *Aspergillus* and *Fusarium* usually are the result of trauma.
- Contact lens overuse produces hypoxic damage.
- Foreign body retained in the cornea.
- Post-LASIK or other injury to the cornea.

Diagnosis
- Eye pain, photophobia, tearing, and blurred vision are prominent symptoms.
- **History.** Often contact lens usage is cited, but frequently appears without obvious causes.
- **Physical examination.** Perilimbal redness with slight focal whitening of the cornea.

Treatment
- If bacterial causes, the top choices are gatifloxacin or moxifloxacin.
- If viral, then topical trifluridine and/or oral valacyclovir is the treatment of choice.
- **Referral.** All cases should be referred to an ophthalmologist.
- **Complications.** Corneal scarring results in decreased vision.[10]

EPISCLERITIS
General Principles
Definition
Episcleritis is a superficial inflammation to the surface vessels of the eye. It affects the episcleral tissue that lies between the conjunctiva and sclera.

Pathophysiology
Poorly understood but inflammation is nongranulomatous with perivascular infiltration.

Etiology
- Most are idiopathic.
- Up to one third may have systemic collagen vascular condition, that is, rheumatoid arthritis, systemic lupus erythematosis (SLE), polyarteritis nodosa, inflammatory bowel disease, ankylosing spondylitis.
- Chemical injury.
- Atopy.
- Foreign body reaction.

Diagnosis
History
- Acute onset of painless to moderate discomfort
- Photophobia and watery discharge

Physical Examination
- Diffuse or localized injection of bulbar conjunctiva.
- Freely mobile nodule may be present.
- May have associated anterior uveitis.
- No exudate will be seen.

Laboratory Studies
- Not usually needed since condition is self-limited.
- A good review of systems often helpful.
- If recurrent and severe, consider uric acid, complete blood count (CBC) with differential, antinuclear antibody (ANA), rheumatoid factor (RF), erythrocyte sedimentation rate (ESR), VDRL, chest x-ray (CXR).

Differential Diagnosis
Viral conjunctivitis and scleritis

Treatment
Medications
- Since condition is self-limited, many will not need and may not respond to treatment.
- If pain is a factor, artificial tears and/or topical corticosteroids can be employed.
- Fluorometholone 0.1% or prednisolone acetate 1% are options.

Referrals
All cases should be referred to an ophthalmologist to determine if uveitis is involved.[11,12]

SCLERITIS
General Principles
Definition
- An acute, severe, vision-threatening inflammation of the sclera that may be diffuse (most benign) or nodular.
- Nodular form may progress to scleral thinning or perforation if untreated.

Pathophysiology
- Scleral inflammation is frequently part of a systemic immune-mediated collagen vascular disease.
- In rare cases this can progress to ischemic necrosis and loss of scleral tissue.

Etiology
- Rheumatoid arthritis in up to one third of patients.
- May also be seen in SLE, polyarteritis nodosa, ankylosing spondylitis, Wegener granulomatosis, relapsing polychondritis, sarcoidosis.

Diagnosis
History
- A severe, boring ocular pain of sudden onset.
- Photophobia and watering are prominent.
- No purulent discharge seen.
- Decreased vision may be seen.

Physical Examination
- A complete physical is mandatory, particularly of the skin, joints, heart, and lungs.
- Ocular injection is often bluish red.
- Globe is exquisitely tender.
- Globe inflammation may be segmental or diffuse.

Laboratory Testing
- Check CBC, lytes, ESR, fluorescent treponemal antibody absorbed (FTA-abs), uric acid, RF, ANA.
- Radiography of sacroiliac joint when ankylosing spondylitis is suspected.

Differential Diagnosis
Rule out episcleritis (more redness, less pain), conjunctivitis (discharge present), and uveitis (by slit-lamp exam).

Treatment
Medications
- Systemic corticosteroids are mandatory. Prednisone can be started at a 60 to 80 mg daily dose and gradually tapered over 6 to 12 weeks depending on patient response.
- Immunosuppressive agents are used in severe (necrotizing scleritis) disease often with rheumatologic consultation.

Referrals
An emergency condition mandating urgent ophthalmologic consultation.[11,13]

UVEITIS
General Principles
Definition
An acute, painful, vision-threatening inflammation of the uveal tract of the eye (iris ciliary body (retina or choroids).

Etiology
- Frequently idiopathic, but may have systemic collagen vascular disease associated.
- May be seen with rheumatoid arthritis, ulcerative colitis, syphilis, tuberculosis (TB), ankylosing spondylitis, Reiter syndrome, and Behçet syndrome.

Diagnosis
History
- Sudden, rapidly progressive, painful ocular injection with severe photophobia.
- Lacrimation is prominent without discharge.
- Decreased vision may be present.
- Occasionally a new onset of floaters is seen.

Physical Examination
- The pupil on the effected side is smaller.
- Perilimbal injection is diagnostic in anterior uveitis. If posterior involvement, injection will be more diffuse.
- Lack of purulent discharge is important.

Laboratory Studies
Same issues as in scleritis.

Differential Diagnosis
Conjunctivitis (discharge/nonpainful), episcleritis (lack of perilimbal involvement, minimal photophobia), scleritis (lack of perilimbal involvement)

Treatment
Medications
- Topical corticosteroids are required: 0.1% prednisolone acetate is the drug of choice.
- Occasionally periocular corticosteroid injection is used.
- For severe cases, oral prednisone starting at 60 to 80 mg is employed. Slow taper is important here over weeks to months based on response.

Referrals
- This is an ocular emergency and needs ophthalmologic consultation urgently.[14–16]

References

1. Leibowitz HM. Primary care: the red eye. *N Engl J Med* 2000;343(5):345–351.
2. Martin M, Turco JH, Zegans ME, et al. An outbreak of conjunctivitis due to atypical *Streptococcus pneumoniae. N Engl J Med* 2003;348(12):1112–1121.
3. Rietveld RP, ter Riet G, Bindels PJE, et al. Predicting bacterial cause in infectious conjunctivitis: cohort study on informativeness of combinations of signs and symptoms. *BMJ* 2004;doi:10.1136/bmj.38128.631319.AE.
4. Morden NE, Berke EM. Topical fluoroquinolones for eye and ear. *Am Fam Physician* 2000;62:1870–1876.
5. Marangon FB, Miller D, Muallem MS, et al. Ciprofloxacin and levofloxacin resistance among methicillin-sensitive *Staphylococcus aureus* isolates from keratitis and conjunctivitis. *Am J Ophthalmol* 2004;137:453–458.
6. Mah FS. New antibiotics for bacterial infections. *Ophthalmol Clin North Am* 2003;16:11–27.
7. Greenberg MF, Pollard ZF. The red eye in childhood. *Pediatr Clin North Am* 2003;50: 105–124.
8. Ono SJ, Abelson MB. Allergic conjunctivitis: update on pathophysiology and prospects for future treatment. *J Allergy Clin Immunol* 2005;115:118–122.
9. Bielory L, Kempuraj D, Theoharides T. Topical immunopharmacology of ocular allergies. *Curr Opin Allergy Clin Immunol* 2002;2:435–445.
10. Basic and Clinical Science Course. External Disease and Cornea. 2005-6; Section 8.
11. Jabs DA, Mudan A, Dunn JP, et al. Episcleritis and scleritis: clinical features and treatment results. *Am J Ophthalmol* 2000;BO(4):469–476.
12. Roy H. Episcleritis. E-medicine from Web M.D. 2006;1–12.
13. Naradzay J. Scleritis. E-medicine from Web M.D. 2006;1–22.
14. Smith JR. Management of uveitis. *Clin Exp Med* 2004;4(1):21–29.
15. Lustig MD, Cunningham ET Jr. Use of immunosuppressive agents in uveitis. *Curr Opin Ophthalmol* 2003;14(6):399–412.
16. Okhravi N, Lightman S. Cystoid macular edema in uveitis. *Ocular Immunol Inflammation* 2003;11(1):29–38.

AGE-ASSOCIATED EYE DISEASES: CATARACTS, GLAUCOMA, AND MACULAR DEGENERATION

7.2

Jon O. Neher

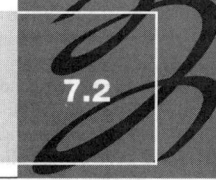

CATARACTS

General Principles

Definition

Cataracts are opacifications that form in the lens of the eye. Larger cataracts and those close to the visual axis may result in visual complaints.

Epidemiology

About **20 million people** in the United States over the age of 40 have an asymptomatic or symptomatic cataract in one or both eyes.

Etiology

Risk factors for cataracts include age, smoking, alcohol use, sunlight exposure, diabetes mellitus, ocular trauma, uveitis, the use of ocular corticosteroids or anticholinesterases.

Diagnosis

Clinical Presentation

- **Asymptomatic** cataracts are commonly noted in the family physician's office. Most cataracts are painless and develop slowly.

- **Trouble with driving** is the most common presenting complaint. Glare or halos around oncoming headlights and degradation of distance vision may make night driving especially difficult.
- **Trouble reading fine print** can also occur.

Physical Examination
- A **nondilated eye exam** with an ophthalmoscope will frequently confirm a suspected cataract.
  - A **milky discoloration** of the lens may be seen by illuminating the pupil with an ophthalmoscope held at 45 degrees to the examiner's eye.
  - **Changes in the red reflex** or difficulty clearly seeing the retina on direct ophthalmoscopy may also indicate the presence of a cataract.
- A **slit-lamp exam** may occasionally be required to confirm a cataract that is suspected by history.

Monitoring
No specific monitoring is required since a delay in therapy does not alter overall prognosis. Patients should be referred when lifestyle modifications (such as reducing night driving) become overly burdensome or are no longer sufficient to compensate for vision changes.

Treatment
Surgery
- **Removal of the lens** is the definitive therapy for cataracts. It is a low-risk procedure that is usually done under local anesthesia.
- In most cases, an **artificial lens is inserted** to replace the native lens. It is supported by the posterior lens capsule, which is left in place.

Results
- A postoperative **acuity of 20/40 is seen in about 90%** of patients.
- Pre-existing **ocular comorbidities reduce the effect** of lens replacement in a significant minority of patients.

Complications
- **Posterior capsule opacification** eventually occurs in about 20% of patients. It is treated relatively easily with laser capsulotomy.
- The **risk of macular degeneration** appears to be about fivefold higher in eyes that have had the native lens removed than in controls.[1] The association is confounded by the fact that cataracts and macular degeneration have several risk factors in common.
- **Rare complications** (<2%) include endophthalmitis, bullous keratopathy, lens malposition, cystoid macular edema, and retinal detachment.

AGE-RELATED MACULAR DEGENERATION
General Principles
Definition
Age-related macular degeneration (ARMD) is an **idiopathic process** that disrupts the normal microarchitecture of the central retina, resulting in central vision loss.

Epidemiology
- **More than 1.75 million people** in the United States are thought to have ARMD.
- **ARMD increases with age.** The rate of visual impairment due to ARMD rises from 6% between ages 65 and 74 to nearly 20% over age 75.

Classification
- Slowly progressive **dry macular degeneration** is the most common form. It consists of deposits of extracellular material known as drusen, chorioretinal atrophy, and alterations of the retinal pigment epithelium. It transforms into wet ARMD at a rate of 1% to 4% per year.

■ Rapidly progressive **wet macular degeneration** is characterized by abnormal neovascularization, retinal detachment, and retinal hemorrhages. Loss of central vision may occur over weeks to months.

Etiology
Risk factors include advancing age, hypertension, smoking, Caucasian ancestry, and family history.

Diagnosis
Clinical Presentation
■ **Gradual loss of vision** in one or both eyes generally accompanies dry ARMD. It may take place over months to years.
■ Patients often report resorting to **bright lights or magnifying lenses** to read fine print or perform other tasks that require fine visual acuity.
■ **Acute or rapidly progressive vision loss** suggests wet ARMD.
■ **Distortion of straight lines** also suggests wet ARMD.

Physical Examination
■ **Confirmation of retinal dysfunction** can be done in family physician's office using a Snellen chart at 20 feet and a standard pocket card. The patient should wear his or her usual corrective lenses. If acuity is poor, the tests should be repeated with the patient looking through a pinhole card, which will compensate for common refractive errors (but not for retinal disease).
■ **A retinal exam** may reveal the presence of drusen (which appear as yellow dots), edema, hemorrhage, or a grayish discoloration of the macular due to neovascularization.

Imaging
Fluorescein angiography is used by eye specialists to finely delineate the retinal vasculature in wet ARMD as an aid to plan therapy.

Monitoring
Amsler grids are used to monitor for retinal deformation or detachment. An Amsler grid looks like a sheet of graph paper with a dot in the middle. Patients are asked to look at the dot daily and report immediately if the grid lines appear curved.

Treatment
Medications
■ **Antioxidants** slow the progression of ARMD and reduce the chance of legal blindness in patients with moderate to advanced disease.[2] Shown to be effective is a daily combination of:
  ■ beta-Carotene 15 mg
  ■ Vitamin C 500 mg
  ■ Vitamin E 400 IU
  ■ Zinc 80 mg
  ■ Copper 2 mg

■ **Caution is advised recommending beta-carotene** since it is associated with an increased risk of lung cancer in smokers.

Special Therapy
■ **Conventional laser therapy,** which coagulates abnormal new blood vessels, is appropriate for about 15% of patients with wet ARMD. It can be performed with topical anesthesia. It delays the development of severe vision loss in well-selected patients by about 3 years.
■ **Photodynamic therapy** is appropriate for patients with abnormal vessels that overlie the fovea. A photo-activated dye is injected intravenously and the abnormal vascular bed exposed to a cool laser. The light activates the dye, which then scleroses the abnormal vessels.

■ **Angiogenesis inhibitors and macular translocation surgery** are still being studied and their roles are not well defined.

Referrals
Patients suspected of having wet ARMD (those with acute visual changes) should be immediately referred to an ophthalmologist. Patients with symptoms or findings of dry ARMD may be referred on a routine basis.

Patient Education
■ All patients need to be counseled about the need to **report acute changes** in vision and in the use of an Amsler grid.
■ **Reassure** patients that a high degree of independence and self-sufficiency is possible even though ARMD is not currently curable or reversible. Because the disease tends to spare peripheral vision, many people—even those with advanced central vision loss—retain the ability to move about safely in their environments.
■ **Low vision aides** (including large print books, print projectors, and large font computer screens) all work by allowing an image to fall on a larger area of retina.

Follow-Up
■ Patients with wet ARMD should be encouraged to obtain regular follow-up with their ophthalmologist.
■ Annual follow-up for dry ARMD with either an ophthalmologist or a family physician is reasonable.

PRIMARY OPEN ANGLE GLAUCOMA

General Principles

Definition
■ **Glaucoma** refers to a group of eye diseases characterized by damage to the optic nerve, commonly (although not universally) associated with an elevation of intraocular pressure (IOP).
■ **Primary open angle glaucoma** (POAG) is the most common type of glaucoma. POAG causes gradual, asymptomatic loss of peripheral vision in a characteristic pattern, followed by central vision loss if untreated.

Epidemiology
■ Over **2.5 million people** in the United States have POAG.
■ It is seen in **3%** of U.S. adults over the age of 55.

Etiology
Risk factors are elevated IOP, advanced age, severe myopia, diabetes, and family history.[3] It is also four to six times more common in black Americans than other ethnic groups.

Diagnosis

Clinical Presentation
Visual complaints are a late finding. If POAG is not diagnosed until it causes visual symptoms, significant irreversible retinal damage has already been done.

Physical Examination
■ **IOP measurement** will document a pressure above 21 mmHg in the affected eye in 80% of cases.
■ **Shiotz tonometers** may be used by some family physicians to measure IOP. The tonometer base is placed against the anesthetized eye to take a reading, so excellent cleaning between uses is critical.
■ **Ultrasound measurement** of IOP can also be achieved with a Tonopen. The Tonopen uses disposable rubber tips to prevent contact of the instrument with the eye.
■ **Air puff tonometers** are used in the ophthalmologist's office and measure resistance of corneal denting to a puff of air and do not touch the eye.

■ On **retinal exam** in the primary care office, glaucoma is suggested if the optic nerve cup-to-disk ratio is greater than 0.5.

■ **Confrontational visual field testing is not sensitive** enough to be of clinical use. However, rigorous visual field testing by an ophthalmologist is diagnostic.

Monitoring

■ **Screening for PAOG is controversial.**

▪ According to the American Academy of Ophthalmology, screening for glaucoma should be a part of every eye professional's comprehensive adult eye evaluation, starting at age 20, with a frequency that depends on the patient's risk factors.

▪ The U.S. Preventive Services Task Force found insufficient evidence to recommend for or against screening adults for glaucoma.[4]

Treatment

Medications

■ **Topical medications** may be given alone or in combination. Family physicians need to be aware of their potential side effects.

▪ Beta blockers are often a first choice, but may complicate heart failure management or increase airway resistance.

▪ Prostaglandins are also commonly a first choice and are generally well tolerated. Local effects include conjunctival injection, lengthening and color change of the lashes, and alteration in the color of the iris.

▪ Adrenergic agonists can contribute to hypertension, tachycardia, and dysrhythmias.

▪ Carbonic anhydrase inhibitors are sulfonamides and can produce hypersensitivity reactions.

▪ Cholinergic agonists may cause small, fixed pupils or headaches.

■ **Techniques to reduce systemic absorption** include refrigeration of the medications to increase viscosity and finger occlusion of the nasolacrimal duct for 5 minutes after instillation.

Surgery

■ **Surgery is indicated if medical therapy is ineffective** at lowering IOP or compliance is poor.

■ **Laser surgery** (trabeculoplasty) increases the aqueous outflow tract. Laser surgery is highly successful initially but frequently needs to be repeated after several years.

■ **Open trabeculotomy** or destruction of the ciliary body may be performed, but is obviously more invasive.

Results

Risk of visual field loss is reduced by about 45% in patients on therapy to normalize IOP.[5]

References

1. Wang JJ, Klein R, Smith W, et al. Cataract surgery and the 5-year incidence of late stage age-related maculopathy: pooled findings from the Beaver Dam and Blue Mountains eye studies. *Ophthalmology* 2003;110:1960–1967.
2. Age-Related Eye Disease Study Research Group. A randomized, placebo-controlled, clinical trial of high-dose supplementation vitamins C and E, beta carotene, and zinc for age-related macular degeneration and vision loss: AREDS report no. 8. *Arch Ophthalmol* 2001;119:1417–1436.
3. Distelhorst JS, Hughes GM. Open-angle glaucoma. *Am Fam Physician* 2003; 67:1937–1943.
4. U.S. Preventive Services Task Force. Screening for glaucoma: recommendation statement. *Ann Fam Med* 2005;3:171–172.
5. Maier PC, Funk J, Schwarzer G, et al. Treatment of ocular hypertension and open angle glaucoma: meta-analysis of randomized trials. *BMJ* 2005;331:134.

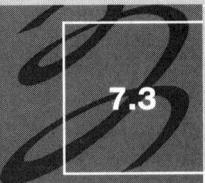

7.3

OCULAR INJURIES
Michael L. Tuggy, Douglas J. Inciarte

$\mathcal{T}$he incidence of ocular injuries in the United States is 3.15 per 1,000 population; rates are higher in males between 20 and 30 years of age. Most eye injuries are treated in the emergency department followed by private physicians' offices. Direct trauma, foreign body, and chemical injury are the most common causes of eye injuries. The significance of the injury varies greatly depending on the mechanism and extent of injury. Acute care of ocular injuries contributes on the maintenance on the visual acuity; the goal of the initial evaluation is to identify any injuries that could permanently affect vision and to relieve pain common to these injuries. Most patients are able to provide clear histories of the event, making the diagnosis simple and leaving the physician to rule out serious sequelae. Athletic facilities and industrial worksites are common places for eye injuries to occur. Physicians should emphasize the importance of protective eye equipment in patients who frequent such sites. The most important issue in the primary care setting consists in the identification of the eye injuries for early treatment and referral to the specialist.

GENERAL PRINCIPLES

- **Any ocular injury** requires a thorough history and examination to determine the nature of the injury, the effect of the injury on visual acuity, and the risk of possible penetration of the globe. All patients with eye injuries must have visual acuity testing with careful examination of the globe, cornea, fundus, pupillary responses, and extraocular movements. Each eye trauma is classified as an open or close globe injury, with different types or etiology, grade based on visual acuity, pupil examination and zone injured.
- **Slit-lamp examination.** If a slit lamp is available, a slit-lamp examination should be performed in cases of suspected abrasion, burn, or direct trauma.

Medications and Special Equipment

- Topical anesthetics (proparacaine or tetracaine) to facilitate removal of foreign bodies.
- Fluorescein dye with an ultraviolet light source.
- Antibiotic suspensions or ointments for prophylaxis.
- Sterile cotton-tipped swabs and 25-gauge needle to aid in removal of superficial foreign bodies.
- Mydriatics: Atropine, 1%, or homatropine, 5%, for relief of ciliary spasm.

SPECIFIC OCULAR INJURIES

Corneal Abrasion and Foreign Body
Presentation
Corneal abrasion is the most common urgent eye complaint seen in the primary care setting. The most common mechanism of this injury is wind-driven particulate matter entering and being trapped under the eyelid. These small particles are sensed acutely by the patient, who subsequently complains of constant pain in the eye. Marked tearing and injection of the eye usually accompany the pain of the abrasion.

Diagnosis
Corneal abrasions are best detected with fluorescein staining of the cornea. Use of topical anesthetics is not mandatory before staining of the eye. Fluorescein-tipped applicator paper is placed on the medial canthus of the eye and the patient is instructed to close the eye. Within 15 seconds, normal tearing will disseminate the stain across the cornea and scleral

conjunctiva. Under ultraviolet light, patches of fluorescein that adhere to the denuded epithelium identify abrasions.

The upper lid should be inverted to rule out the presence of a foreign body. If a superficial foreign body is present, then local anesthesia should be applied and the foreign body removed with a cotton-tipped applicator or 25-gauge needle.

Treatment

- Patching of the affected eye is no longer recommended because it may increase the risk of infection. Topical anesthetics should be avoided if no foreign body is present.[1]
- Atropine, 1%, or homatropine, 5%, two drops in the affected eye may be used to reduce pain symptoms from ciliary spasm. Oral nonnarcotic analgesics or topical nonsteroidal anti-inflammatory drugs (NSAIDs) can also be used for pain relief.[2]
- Application of topical antibiotic solution reduces the risk of secondary infection and is recommended for all abrasions. Corticosteroid suspensions are contraindicated.

Follow-Up

If symptoms resolve in 48 hours, no follow-up is necessary. If symptoms persist, re-examination is indicated to rule out retained foreign body or infection.

Hyphema
Presentation

Hyphema results from a direct blow to the eye or orbit, and is often related to sports activities. The patient has pain in the eye, decreased visual acuity, and injection of the globe.

Diagnosis

The finding of blood in the anterior chamber confirms the diagnosis. This finding may be delayed for hours to days following injury if bleeding is gradual.

Treatment

- Strict bed rest with head elevated at least 20 degrees.
- Bilateral eye patches to minimize eye movement.
- Instill atropine, 1%, two drops bid to reduce ciliary spasm.
- If an ophthalmologist is not readily available, intraocular pressure should be reduced by the use of oral acetazolamide or mannitol.
- Appropriate pain medications that are free of aspirin.

Follow-Up

Immediate ophthalmologic referral is indicated in all cases of hyphema.[3] Vitrectomy has been described as therapeutic for clotted hyphema.

Penetrating Injuries to the Globe
Presentation

Penetrating injuries to the eye are often caused by high-velocity missiles or severe blunt trauma to the orbit and globe. Vision is markedly decreased in the affected eye. Small projectile injuries may be very difficult to locate within the eye.

Diagnosis

Direct examination may reveal collapse of the anterior chamber or protrusion of the iris through the open cornea. Minute penetrations of the cornea may be made apparent by the seeping out of aqueous fluid through the cornea of a fluorescein-stained eye. Limit examinations of the eye to a minimum before an ophthalmologist is present. Penetrating injuries can be distinguished from perforated injuries by periorbital ecchymosis on presentation. Axial computed tomography (CT) scan can be considered to evaluate surrounding tissues and to identify penetrating intraocular injuries due to a foreign body.

Treatment

- Strict bed rest with head elevated at least 20 degrees.
- Apply bilateral eye patches to minimize eye movement. An eye shield should be placed over the injured eye.
- Do not put any medications into the eye.
- Give antiemetic such as chlorpromazine 25 mg IM every 4 to 6 hours to prevent emesis.
- Morphine 2 to 4 mg IV as needed for pain.

Follow-Up

Urgent ophthalmologic consultation is required for surgical repair with vitrectomy.

Orbital and Lid Injuries

Presentation

Orbital contusions or lacerations may have associated bony orbital injury. Many patients with orbital fracture complain of diplopia or increased pain with certain ocular movements due to entrapment of the extraocular muscles. Retro-ocular hematoma causes proptosis and requires urgent consultation for evacuation.[4]

Diagnosis

Careful palpation of the orbit reveals point tenderness and a palpable step-off if a displaced fracture is present. Restricted extraocular movements or proptosis should be ruled out. A Water view is the best radiographic study to identify orbital rim or orbital floor injuries in the office setting. Axial and/or coronal CT scan is now used more frequently to evaluate soft and hard tissues; also magnetic resonance imaging (MRI) can be considered an alternative.

Treatment

- The eye should be shielded but not patched after the examination is completed.
- Lid lacerations should be repaired by an ophthalmologist. It is important that the lacrimal ducts and cartilage of the lid be aligned properly at closure.
- Orbital fractures are treated with analgesics and local measures (ice) until the swelling is reduced. Even with some restriction of extraocular muscles, some patients will not require surgical intervention if the entrapment resolves within 2 weeks.

Follow-Up

Patients should be referred to an ophthalmologist within 12 hours.

Chemical and Thermal Burns

Presentation

Chemical burns are grouped by their relative pH values. Alkali burns are potentially the most serious as bases are more difficult to clear, although acid burns may cause more rapid destruction of tissue.[4] There are usually considerable pain and injection of the eyes with loss of visual acuity. The classification for thermal burns is similar to that for burns of the skin.

Diagnosis

History of chemical or thermal exposure followed by eye pain is adequate for the diagnosis of a burn injury. The cornea may appear eroded or hazy from edema.

Treatment

- Topical anesthetics should be applied for pain relief during irrigation or examination.
- All alkali and acid burns should be copiously irrigated with 2 L of normal saline. Do not attempt to neutralize the agent. Careful inspection after irrigation is important to prevent further injury with particulate matter.
- Alkali and thermal burns should have a mydriatic applied (atropine or homatropine).

Follow-Up

Patch the affected eye and refer the patient to an ophthalmologist.

References

1. Flynn CA. Should we patch corneal abrasions? A meta-analysis. *J Fam Pract* 1998;47:264.
2. Brown MD. Do ophthalmic nonsteroidal anti-inflammatory drugs reduce the pain associated with simple corneal abrasion without delaying healing? *Ann Emerg Med* 1999;34:526.
3. Hamill MB. Current concepts in the treatment of traumatic injury to the anterior segment. *Ophthalmol Clin North Am* 1999;12:457.
4. Baker SM. Management of orbital and ocular adnexal trauma. *Ophthalmol Clin North Am* 1999;12:435.
5. McGwin GM Jr. et al. Incidence of emergency department-treated eye injury in the United States. *Arch Ophthalmol* 2005;123(5):662–666.

6. McGwin et al. Rate of eye injury in the United States [miscellaneous article]. *Arch Ophthalmol* 2005;123(7):970–976.
7. Albert, Jakobiec. *Principles and practice of ophthalmology.* Clinical practice. Philadelphia: Saunders, 1994; Vol 5. 1994.
8. Ghazi-Nouri SG, et al. Periorbital ecchymosis as a sign of perforating injury of the globe. *Clin Exp Ophthalmol* 2005;33(2):194–196.
9. Kuhn/Pieramici DP. *Ocular trauma principles and practice.* New York: Thieme; 2002.
10. MacCumber MM. *Management of ocular injuries and emergencies.* Lippincott–Raven; 1998.

Ear, Nose, and Throat Problems

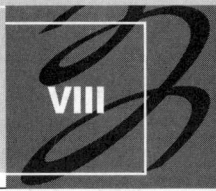

ACUTE OTITIS MEDIA
Carey Christiansen Ford

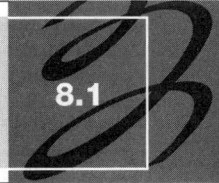

GENERAL PRINCIPLES
Definition
Acute otitis media (AOM) is an acute suppurative infection of the middle ear, often occurring in the setting of an upper respiratory infection. AOM may occur in adults, although more frequently develops in children. Generally short-lived, AOM in a healthy child has a self-limited course and only in some cases needs antibiotic therapy.[1]

Anatomy and Pathophysiology
The much higher propensity of children for AOM is in part due to the less steeply angled, shorter eustachian tube, which allows reflux of organisms and debris from the nasopharynx into the middle ear. With congestion of the tube from an upper respiratory infection, secretions can accumulate and bacterial pathogens can multiply, leading to inflammation and clinical symptoms.[1]

Epidemiology
AOM is the most common bacterial infection of children, with 5 million cases diagnosed per year. An estimated 30 million clinic visits for AOM are made each year.[1] It is also the most common reason for antibiotic use in children, and is the reason for 50% of antibiotics prescribed to preschool-age children.[2]

Risk may be reduced by breastfeeding for at least 6 months, ceasing pacifier use after 6 months of age, avoidance of "bottle-propping," and elimination of secondhand smoke exposure.[2] Other risk factors that are not modifiable include genetic predisposition, male gender, premature birth, Native American or Inuit ethnicity, family history, the presence of siblings in the home, and low socioeconomic status.[2]

Administration of influenza and pneumococcal vaccines may be of some benefit for reduction of the incidence of AOM.[2]

Etiology

Streptococcus pneumoniae, nontypable *Haemophilus influenzae,* and *Moraxella catarrhalis* are the most commonly found pathogens found on culture of middle ear fluid obtained by tympanocentesis.[2,3]

S. pneumoniae has been found in middle ear fluid in 25% to 50% of children with AOM, *H. influenzae* has been found in 15% to 30%, and *M. catarrhalis* has been found in 3% to 20%.[2]

The microbiology of AOM may be changing due to the administration of the pneumoccocal conjugate vaccine to infants, with an increase in *H. influenzae.*[2]

Viruses, including respiratory syncytial virus (RSV), rhinovirus, coronavirus, parainfluenza, adenovirus, and enterovirus, have been found in respiratory secretions and/or middle ear effusion in 40% to 75% of AOM cases and in 5% to 22% of middle ear effusion without bacteria.[4] Viruses may be the causative pathogen when antibiotic treatment is ineffective. However, viruses are the only pathogen in AOM in only 10% of cases.[2]

In 16% to 25% of cases of AOM, no organism can be found in middle ear fluid.[2]

DIAGNOSIS

AOM must be carefully distinguished from otitis media with effusion (OME) to avoid overdiagnosis and inappropriate antibiotic use.

A diagnosis of AOM requires (a) a history of acute onset of signs and symptoms, (b) the presence of middle ear effusion (MEE), and (c) signs and symptoms of middle ear inflammation.

Elements of the definition of AOM are all of the following: recent, usually abrupt, onset of signs and symptoms of middle ear inflammation and MEE.

1. The presence of MEE is indicated by any of the following:
   a. Bulging of the tympanic membrane
   b. Limited or absent mobility of the tympanic membrane
   c. Air-fluid level behind the tympanic membrane
   d. Otorrhea
2. Signs or symptoms of middle ear inflammation as indicated by either:
   a. Distinct erythema of the tympanic membrane or
   b. Distinct otalgia (discomfort clearly referable to the ear that results in interference with or precludes normal activity or sleep)[2]

Clinical Presentation

Signs and symptoms of AOM are nonspecific and may vary with age group. Cough, nasal discharge, and other upper respiratory symptoms are common and nonspecific. Fever, vomiting, otalgia, otorrhea, and hearing loss are variably present.[2]

Infants may present with irritability, fever, pulling on the ear, or anorexia. Clinical history alone is poorly predictive of the presence of AOM.[1]

Physical Examination

The position of the tympanic membrane (TM) is a key for differentiating AOM from OME; a red TM alone is inadequate for diagnosis.

■ **Pneumatic otoscopy.** Injection of the TM is found in 57% of AOM cases. The TM is bulging in 89% of cases and a bulging, opaque, immobile tympanic membrane had a 99% predictive value for AOM compared with the findings at tympanocentesis.[5]

■ Care must be taken to ensure an adequate exam. Important factors include adequate illumination, a functioning bulb, and obtaining a tight seal with the external auditory canal. A crying child's TM may appear pink or red, impairing the exam. Excess cerumen in the canal can also impair the exam and should be removed.[1]

■ **Tympanometry.** An adjunctive diagnostic technique to determine the pressure of the middle ear space. In one study, the sensitivity and specificity of a flat tympanogram for the presence of a middle ear effusion were 90% and 86%, respectively.[5] A seal must be made with the external canal for an accurate reading.

- **Acoustic reflectometry.** A seal does not need to be made, an advantage over tympa-nometery. Like tympanometry, acoustic reflectometry relies on measuring sound waves returning from the TM to measure the middle ear pressure.[5]
- **Tympanocentesis.** The gold standard for diagnosis of a MEE. Culture of fluid may be done to direct antibiotic use. Not routinely used, but an excellent diagnostic tool for refractory or recurrent AOM.[5]

Differential Diagnosis
- Otitis media with effusion
- Eustachian tube dysfunction
- Otitis externa
- Temporomandibular junction pain (TMJ)
- Dental pain
- Pharyngitis
- Upper respiratory infection

TREATMENT

Behavioral
Comfort measures for pain and fever relief (i.e., cool bath, relaxation, etc).

Medications
Antipyretics, including acetaminophen and ibuprofen. Topical agents such as benzocaine drops are beneficial, but short-acting.[2] There are no data supporting the use of deconges-tants and antihistamines for AOM; children treated with these medications have an increased risk of medication side effects.[6]

Observation Versus Antibiotic Use
The decision to observe a patient without prescribing antibiotics is directed by the patient's age and the severity of symptoms, as well as the certainty of the diagnosis. Additionally, observation should be reserved for those patients who can be observed by a caregiver with a reliable means of communication and follow-up. Initial treatment can consist of watchful waiting for 48 to 72 hours in children who are >2 years of age with either an uncertain diagnosis or with a certain diagnosis and nonsevere symptoms (mild otalgia and fever <39°C in the past 24 hours). Observation is acceptable in children aged 6 months to 2 years if diagnosis is uncertain and symptoms are nonsevere. Antibiotics are indicated in this age group and in children less than 6 months if the diagnosis of AOM is certain. A certain diag-nosis is one that meets all three criteria for AOM, as described above.[2] Symptomatic treat-ment with antipyretics is still indicated with the decision to observe. In the first 24 hours of observation the patient should experience a stabilization of symptoms, possibly after a period of worsening. By 72 hours if no improvement is noted, antibiotics are indicated.[2]

If antibiotic use is indicated, amoxicillin at high dose (80 to 90 mg/kg/day) is recom-mended for most children. In children with severe disease, amoxicillin–clavulanate (90 mg/kg/day of amoxicillin with 6.4 mg/kg/day of clavulanate) should be the first choice.[2] Duration of therapy is uncertain but typically 10 days of treatment is prescribed.[2]

- Amoxicillin allergy, not type I (i.e., no urticaria or anaphylaxis):
  - Cefdinir: 14 mg/kg/day in one to two doses
  - Cefpodoxime: 10 mg/kg/day in one dose
  - Cefuroxime: 30 mg/kg/day in two doses
- Amoxicillin allergy, type I:
  - Azithromycin: 10 mg/kg/day on first day, then 5 mg/kg/day on day 2 to 5
  - Clarithromycin: 15 mg/kg/day in two doses
- Other: Suspicion of resistant *S. pneumoniae*—Clindamycin 15 mg/kg/day in two doses
- Also acceptable, but have substantial resistance are erythromycin-sulfisoxazole (50 mg/kg/day of erythromycin) and sulfamethoxazole-trimethaprim (6 to 10 mg/kg/day of trimethaprim).
- If patient does not tolerate oral medication, a single dose of parenteral ceftriaxone (50 mg/kg) may be used, although a 3-day course is more effective.

- Failure of initial antibiotic therapy:
  - Amoxicillin–clavulanate: 90 mg/kg/day of amoxicillin, with 6.4 mg of clavulanate
  - Ceftriaxone: 50 mg per kg IM daily for 3 days

Referral

For refractory or recurrent AOM, a referral to an otolaryngologist may be warranted for tympanocentesis and placement of tympanostomy tubes.

Complications

Complications of AOM are rare, even without antibiotics or with delaying antibiotics, but include acute mastoiditis, intracranial abscess, bacterial meningitis, epidural abscess, brain abscess, lateral sinus thrombosis, cavernous sinus thrombosis, subdural empyema, and carotid artery thrombosis.[7] A more common complication is perforation of the tympanic membrane, resulting in purulent otorrhea. Infrequently, chronic suppurative otitis media may develop.[7] Complications of chronic or recurrent otitis may include school absenteeism, decreased hearing, and speech delay. MEE may persist for weeks after resolution of AOM, leading to transient hearing loss.[2]

Prognosis

Prognosis is excellent; most children with AOM recover without sequelae.

References

1. Rothman R, Owens T, Simel D. Does this child have acute otitis media? *JAMA* 2003;290:1633–1640.
2. American Academy of Pediatrics and American Academy of Family Physicians, Subcommittee on Management of Acute Otitis Media. Diagnosis and management of acute otitis media. *Pediatrics* 2004;113:1451–1465.
3. Berman S. Otitis media in children. *N Engl J Med* 1995;332:1560–1565.
4. Heikkinen T, Thint M, Chonmaitree T. Prevalence of various respiratory viruses in the middle ear during acute otitis media. *N Engl J Med* 1999;340:260–264.
5. Pichichero M. Acute otitis media: Part I. Improving diagnostic accuracy. *Am Fam Physician* 2000;61(7):2051–2056.
6. Flynn CA, Griffin GH, Schultz JK. Decongestants and antihistamines for acute otitis media in children. *Cochrane Database Syst Rev* 2004;3:CD001727.
7. Klein JO, Pelton S. Epidemiology, pathogenesis, clinical manifestations, and complications of acute otitis media (online). Available: http://www.uptodate.com.

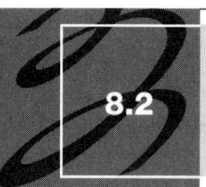

CHRONIC OTITIS MEDIA
Russell G. Maier

GENERAL PRINCIPLES

Chronic otitis media (COM) encompasses a broad area of ear disease that is discussed as three main clinical entities: otitis media with effusion (OME), chronic suppurative otitis media (CSOM), and COM. OME is defined as the presence of fluid in the middle ear without signs or symptoms of infection. Controversy exists regarding the diagnosis and treatment of OME. OME has been studied by evidence-based panels since 1994 that have developed objective treatment recommendations.[1] Much of the discussion on OME is based on the panel's recommendations for ages 2 to 12. CSOM is defined as chronic (6-week) otorrhea through a nonintact tympanic membrane. COM is defined as a perforation lasting longer than 1 month without drainage.

OTITIS MEDIA WITH EFFUSION

Clinical Presentation

In children and adults the presentation is similar; commonly there are no complaints. The diagnosis is made on a screening examination or follow-up for acute otitis media (AOM). If symptoms are present, they include behavioral changes, parental or patient complaints of diminished hearing, or a fullness or discomfort in one or both ears. Historically, the most common cause of OME is a prior ear infection.

Risk Factors

Risk factors for OME include recurrent AOM, group child care, passive smoke exposure, absence of breastfeeding as an infant, craniofacial abnormalities, and possibly allergies.

Clinical Examination

The diagnosis of OME is primarily clinical. There are few useful tests and no laboratory studies that aid in the diagnosis. It is important to document whether the effusion is unilateral or bilateral.

Physical Examination

By definition, there is no evidence for acute infection and a middle ear effusion is present. On examination, the external auditory canal should be normal. The drum may appear normal or thickened. A middle ear effusion may be noted as an air-fluid level, bubbles, or serous or serosanguinous fluid in the middle ear. If fever, a bulging erythematous eardrum, or drainage is present, the diagnosis of OME cannot be made.

Additional Tests

- **Pneumatic otoscopy.** Pneumatic otoscopy should be used as the primary diagnostic method.[1] A drum that appears normal may have fluid behind it. For pneumatic otoscopy to be accurate, a complete seal must be obtained in the ear canal. When slight positive and negative pressure is applied to the tympanum, it should move briskly back and forth. An effusion inhibits this movement.
- **Tympanometry.** If following clinical examination and pneumatic otoscopy the clinician is unsure about the diagnosis, tympanometry provides a useful adjunct and is accurate for infants 4 months and older. An effusion produces a flat, type B tympanogram.

Treatment

Treatment for adults and children is primarily medical but varies depending on the examination and underlying illnesses.

- **Children at risk.** Children at risk, those with sensory, physical, cognitive, or behavioral issues, should be considered for earlier evaluation. These children may be less tolerant of hearing loss. A hearing and, if necessary, speech and language assessment should be performed.
- **Normal child with OME for less than 3 months:**
  - **Watchful waiting.** In a variety of studies, the spontaneous resolution of OME ranges from 75% to 90% over 3 months. Given that approximately two thirds of all children improve without any treatment and with no risk to the child, watchful waiting is the recommended treatment course. Interval visits are optional after the initial diagnosis. At 3 months the child should be reassessed for resolution by pneumatic otoscopy and/or tympanometry.
  - **Antibiotics.** In the past, antibiotics have been an option for treatment during the first 3 months. Given the increasing difficulties and risks with resistant organisms, watchful waiting is now the preferred course.[2]
  - **Antihistamines and decongestants.** These are ineffective and have no role.[1]
  - **Steroids.** Steroids are not recommended because they show no benefit, especially in this early period.[3]
- **Risk factor reduction.** In all patients, there are several modifiable risk factors that contribute to OME. The child should not be exposed to any secondary smoke. Any smoking by family members or relatives should be done outside of the home or car, not in a different room. Group child care is a risk factor that rarely can be modified.

■ **Otitis Media with Effusion for 3 Months or More in Normal Children**
  ■ **Hearing evaluation.** At 3 months, all children with bilateral effusions should receive a hearing evaluation. If the hearing loss is 20 decibels (dB) or greater the patient should have language testing.
  ■ **Watchful `waiting.** Children at low risk who pass their hearing test may be reassessed at 3- to 6-month intervals. Asymptomatic OME tends to resolve spontaneously. If on reassessment the OME is present and the hearing evaluation is >39 dB, then surgery is recommended. From 21 to 39 dB of hearing loss a comprehensive audiologic evaluation is indicated. Treatment options depend upon the child's situation and parental preference. If the hearing loss is <21 dB a repeat test should be done in 3 to 6 months.
  ■ **Antibiotics.** Antibiotics have no benefit beyond 1 month. For parents adverse to surgery, a single course may be tried. A 10- to 14-day course of amoxicillin or trimethoprim–sulfamethoxazole would be first-line treatment, with amoxicillin doses at 40 to 80 mg/kg/day in three divided does. Repeat courses are not recommended.[1]
  ■ **Surgery.** Candidates for surgery have OME for 4 months or longer with persistent hearing loss, recurrent or persistent OME in children at risk (regardless of hearing status), or OME with structural damage to the tympanic membrane or middle ear. Tympanostomy tubes are recommended. If repeat tube placement is needed adenoidectomy is recommended. Myringotomy or tonsillectomy provides no benefit over watchful waiting. Myringotomy plus adenoidectomy is effective in children 4 years old or older.[4]
  ■ **Patient education.** Resources include patient handouts at http://familydoctor.org/330.xml, http://www.cdc.gov/drugresistance/community/files/GetSmart_OME.pdf, and for ear tubes http://www.entnet.org/healthinfo/ears/Ear-Tubes.cfm.

CHRONIC SUPPURATIVE OTITIS MEDIA AND CHRONIC OTITIS MEDIA

Clinical Presentation

CSOM often presents with drainage from an ear. Usually the individual feels fine or otherwise appears healthy. The patient may complain of otalgia, state that he or she is "out of sorts," or complain of hearing loss or difficulty hearing from the affected ear. COM is usually painless.

Risk Factors

Risk factors include recurrent AOM, immune impairment (e.g., from diabetes or chronic illness), allergies, craniofacial abnormalities, and an increased prevalence in certain subpopulations, including Eskimos and Native Americans. The use of tympanostomy tubes results in an approximately 1.6% to 3.0% incidence of chronic otorrhea.

Physical Examination

Clear otorrhea is unusual, and a cerebrospinal fluid leak should be considered. Especially in children, one needs to rule out a foreign body with secondary otitis externa as the cause of otorrhea. In adults as well, a careful examination and possibly a therapeutic trial must be done to rule out otitis externa as the cause of otorrhea. Once the external auditory canal has been cleaned, the tympanic membrane should be examined. Often a large central perforation is seen, with an abnormal middle ear noted. Marginal perforations are more often associated with cholesteatomas and other severe complications. If a cholesteatoma is noted, the patient should be referred to an ear, nose, and throat (ENT) physician. CSOM with cholesteatoma is primarily a surgical disease.

Laboratory Studies

If possible, cultures should be obtained. Material from the middle ear is most helpful. Drainage from the external auditory canal is acceptable, but the canal should be sterilized and the culture obtained from reaccumulated fluid. Culture should include both aerobes and anaerobes.

■ **Tympanometry.** If a perforation is suspected but not seen, a tympanogram will show a large canal volume but flat tracing or will fail to make a seal.
■ **Audiologic evaluation.** Because many patients complain of hearing abnormalities, it is helpful to document this finding so as to follow it during treatment. A conductive hearing loss of more than 30 dB is suggestive of disruption of the ossicular chain.
■ **Imaging studies.** The diagnosis of CSOM and COM is primarily clinical. If a cholesteatoma is suspected, if the diagnosis is uncertain, or if intracranial extension is suspected, computed tomography (CT) or magnetic resonance imaging (MRI) should be performed.[5]
■ **Immediate referral.** Patients with a facial palsy, labyrinthitis, or suspected intracranial suppuration should be referred immediately.

Treatment
Chronic Suppurative Otitis Media
Initial management is medical and involves removing the debris. If the practitioner does not have an operating microscope or suction, treatment may be better referred to an ENT physician. Following removal of debris, empiric antibiotic treatment with oral agents that cover *Streptococcus pneumoniae, Haemophilus influenzae, Moraxella catarrhalis, Streptococcus pyogenes, Staphylococcus aureus,* and *Pseudomonas aeruginosa* and anaerobes is recommended.[6] Amoxicillin clavulanate, 20 to 40 mg/kg/day in children or 850 mg bid to minimize diarrhea, may be prescribed. In conjunction with systemic therapy, topical otic suspension, such as neomycin, polymyxin B, and hydrocortisone (Cortisporin) or gentamicin otic drops, can be initiated. In adults, oral ciprofloxacin, 500 to 750 mg bid, may be added for pseudomonal coverage. The use of fluoroquinolones is contraindicated in children. If the combination of antibiotics and debridement does not stop the drainage, there are two other options.

■ **Aggressive medical management.** For CSOM refractory to conservative measures there are good data to support either inpatient or outpatient aggressive medical therapy: frequent suctioning and intravenous antibiotics for 6 weeks.[7,8] The primary care physician should refer the patient to an ENT physician for this care.
■ **Surgery.** If aggressive medical management fails (after 2 weeks of intravenous therapy there is no improvement), tympanomastoid surgery should be considered as the next step.

Chronic Otitis Media
A dry, uninfected middle ear does not require acute treatment other than being kept dry. Definitive repair is done electively in adults or at age 9 to 12 years in children.

Patient Education
For the acute draining ear, http://www.nlm.nih.gov/medlineplus/ency/article/003042.htm# Alternative%20Names.

References
1. http://www.pediatrics.org/cgi/content/full/113/5/1412. Accessed 6/30/06.
2. Dowell SF, et al. Otitis media: principles of judicious use of antimicrobial agents. *Pediatrics* 1998;101:165.
3. Mandel EM, Casselbrant ML, Rockette HE, et al. Systemic steroid for chronic otitis media with effusion in children. *Pediatrics* 2002;110:1071–1080.
4. Gates GA. Adenoidectomy for otitis media with effusion. *Ann Otol Rhinol Laryngol* 1994;103:54.
5. Kimmelman CP. Office management of the draining ear. *Otolaryngol Clin North Am* 1992;25:739.
6. Noble J, ed. *Textbook of primary care.* 3rd ed. St. Louis: Mosby; 2001.
7. Kenna MA, Rosane BA, Bluestone CD. Medical management of chronic suppurative otitis media without cholesteatoma in children: update 1992. *Am J Otol* 1993;14:469.
8. Dagan R, et al. Outpatient management of chronic suppurative otitis media without cholesteatoma in children. *Pediatr Infect Dis J* 1992;11:7.

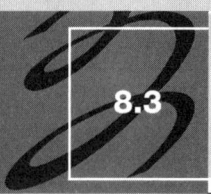

8.3   OTITIS EXTERNA
Paul Evans

GENERAL PRINCIPLES

Otitis externa is an inflammatory condition, usually self-limiting, of the external auditory canal (EAC). It is commonly seen in primary care because it affects all age groups. Otitis externa can be diffuse or circumscribed, acute or chronic, or can have eczematous features. Rarely, it can progress to necrotizing or "malignant" otitis externa in patients with diabetes or other immunocompromised patients, leading to serious illness, cranial nerve palsies, or death. Increases in summer are due to water exposure in swimming, increased humidity, and related activities that reduce cerumen protection. Other risk factors include trauma to the external auditory canal, swimming or moisture exposure, use of a hearing aid or other ear occlusive devices, and predisposing skin disorders, such as eczema, seborrhea, or psoriasis.

DIAGNOSIS
Clinical Presentation
- Symptoms. The most frequently described symptoms are itching, purulent discharge, otalgia, plugging of the ear, mild hearing loss, ear fullness, and tinnitus.
- Signs. On examination, there is pinnal tenderness, an erythematous and edematous external auditory canal, and a discharge. Pinnal eczema is often present.

Classification
- Acute otitis externa. This is usually infectious in origin, with *Staphylococcus aureus* or *Pseudomonas aeruginosa* the most common isolates. Fungi such as *Aspergillus, Candida,* and others have also been implicated. Anaerobes may also play a role. Cultures in acute otitis should be reserved for therapeutic failures because most patients respond to first-line therapy. Noninfectious causes, such as contact dermatitis, eczema, psoriasis, or trauma, should be sought.
- Chronic otitis externa. Chronic otitis is defined by symptoms lasting longer than 2 months. Causes similar to acute otitis externa are seen, but chronic otitis may be the result of failure to correctly diagnose and treat the pathogen initially. Predisposing factors remain important.
- Necrotizing or "malignant" external otitis. This is a rare but important infection seen most commonly in elderly patients with diabetes. Severe ear pain and systemic signs and symptoms may be present along with cranial nerve palsies. If not detected early and treated aggressively, this condition may progress to skull base osteomyelitis with possible erosion to the central nervous system. *Pseudomonas* is the most common pathogen.

TREATMENT
Acute Otitis Externa
- Clean out exudates and debris by gently suctioning or swabbing. Use of irrigation is controversial.
- Initial culture is not necessary.
- Topical drops that contain a mild acid (e.g., Domeboro Otic, 4 to 6 drops q2 to 3 hours) or antibiotics and a steroid, for example, neomycin, polymyxin B sulfates, and hydrocortisone (Cortisporin Otic suspension), 3 to 5 drops qid, are effective agents. Acidification lowers pH to inhibit *Pseudomonas* growth. Therapy should be used for about 7 to 10 days with sufficient quantity to contact all involved EAC tissues. If infection spreads to the concha or to the preauricular or infra-auricular area, systemic antibiotics should be

considered. If a fungal etiology is suspected, topical nystatin and clotrimazole have been successful first-line agents.

■ Cotton wicks for a severely swollen EAC assist in reducing swelling and more effectively getting topical therapy to targeted tissue. After 48 to 72 hours, the wick can usually be removed, with continuation of drops for the full 7 to 10 days.

■ Pain control with a topical anesthetic, for example, benzocaine, antipyrine, and dehydrated glycerin (Auralgan), 2 to 4 drops q1 to 2 hours as required, or with acetaminophen, or ibuprofen is usually successful. Occasionally, short-term narcotic analgesics may be necessary.

Chronic Otitis Externa

■ Maintain cleanliness of the EAC.

■ Because initial treatment has failed for 2 months or longer, bacterial and fungal cultures should now be done. A screening potassium hydroxide (KOH) preparation can rapidly detect fungal elements, which indicates otomycosis.

■ Re-examine for other conditions, such as chronic purulent otitis media with perforation, furunculosis, eczema, seborrhea, or psoriasis.

■ Carefully evaluate for contact dermatitis due to prior therapies. Common sensitivities to neomycin and other agents in topical preparations must be kept in mind.

■ If compliance has been ensured with an appropriate regimen for the cultured pathogen, a change to another antibiotic is indicated. Mixed bacterial and fungal infections may require multiple drug therapy. Addition of topical steroids reduces inflammation and the accompanying symptoms.

■ If all medical therapy fails, surgical consultation is appropriate for consideration for conchomeatoplasty or another procedure as a last resort.

Necrotizing or Malignant Otitis Externa

This rare condition requires early and aggressive therapy including consultation with an otolaryngologist. Hospitalization with antipseudomonal parenteral antibiotics (e.g., ceftazidime and gentamicin), careful debridement, and computed tomography (CT) or magnetic resonance imaging (MRI) to delineate the extent of bony or soft-tissue erosions are recommended. All elderly patients with diabetes with external otitis should be monitored for this serious complication.

SPECIAL CONSIDERATIONS—PREVENTION

■ **Infectious causes.** Because most of the bacterial and fungal organisms thrive on moist tissues, attention to drying the EAC and lowering the growth of pathogens with a mildly acidic environment is important. Over-the-counter preparations for preventing swimmer's ear that contain a drying agent and a mild acid are effective; similar home remedies can be made with a mixture of 50% isopropyl alcohol and 50% vinegar (5% acetic acid). When applied after moisture exposure, such a mixture is both efficacious and cost-effective.

■ **Noninfectious causes.** Maintaining good aural hygiene and getting early treatment of dermatologic problems lowers the incidence of otitis externa. Use of topical steroids for eczematous conditions as well as for allergic or contact dermatitis is helpful. Patients who use occlusive EAC devices, such as hearing aids, earpieces, or stethoscopes, must maintain a high level of attention to cleanliness to avoid bacterial or fungal contamination.

References

1. Kimmelman CP. Otitis externa. In: Rakel. *Conn's current therapy*. 57th ed. WB Saunders, Baltimore, MD: WB Saunders; 2005:221–223.
2. Eason JV. Otitis externa. In: *Ferri's clinical advisor: instant diagnosis and treatment*. St. Louis, MO: CV Mosby; 2006.
3. Roland PS, Stroman DW. Microbiology of acute otitis externa. *Laryngoscope* 2002;112:1166–1177.
4. Rubin Grandis J, Branstetter BR IV, Yu VL. The changing face of necrotizing otitis: clinical, radiological, and anatomic correlations. *Lancet Infect Dis* 2004;4:34–39.
5. Sander R. Otitis externa: a practical guide to treatment and prevention. *Am Fam Physician* 2001;63:927–936.
6. Beers SL, Abramo TJ. Otitis externa review. *Pediatr Emerg Care* 2004;20:250–256.

8.4 PHARYNGITIS
John L. Smith

GENERAL PRINCIPLES

Epidemiology
Acute pharyngitis is one of the more common illnesses seen by primary care physicians. Only about 10% of adults and 15% to 30% of children presenting with pharyngitis will have group A (beta)-hemolytic streptococcal (GABHS) infection.[1] Most pharyngitis, both viral and streptococcal, is transmitted by hand contact with nasal discharge and not oral contact.[2]

Etiology
Pharyngitis has both viral and bacterial causes, but GABHS is the only commonly occurring bacterial etiology.[1] Group C and G (beta)-hemolytic *Streptococcus, Neisseria, Chlamydia,* and *Mycoplasma* are much less likely bacterial causes.

DIAGNOSIS

Up to 70% of adults in the United States who present with a main complaint of sore throat are treated with antibiotics[3]; only about 10% have streptococcal pharyngitis. For this reason, various guidelines have been recommended using clinical and laboratory criteria to improve the accuracy of diagnosis and limit the inappropriate usage of antibiotics. The major problem in the diagnosis and treatment of adults with pharyngitis is not which of the multiple guidelines to follow, but that clinicians usually fail to follow any guideline at all.[4]

History
Although the symptoms of GABHS may be mild, frequent complaints are sudden onset of sore throat, headache, pain with swallowing, and fever. Abdominal pain, nausea, and vomiting may also be present.

Physical Examination
Frequent signs of GABHS are pharyngeal erythema, exudate, palatal petechiae, and anterior cervical lymphadenopathy. Sometimes a beefy red uvula is also present.[1] An associated sandpaper-like exanthem consisting of erythematous papules and located in the groin, neck, and axilla may be present and is referred to as scarletiniform (scarlet fever).

Laboratory Studies
The two tests most commonly used in the diagnosis of GABHS pharyngitis are a throat culture and one of a number of rapid antigen detection tests (RADT). The various RADTs have very good specificity at about 95%, but the sensitivities vary at about 80% to 90% depending on the specific tool. With that in mind, guidelines support a backup throat culture (gold standard) in children and adolescents with a negative RADT because of the small risk of acute rheumatic fever. Culture is not necessary in adults as the risk is substantially less.[5,6] Culture is also unnecessary with a positive RADT because of its high specificity.

274

Classification

Classifying pharyngitis as streptococcal and therefore warranting antibiotic therapy may be facilitated by utilizing clinical criteria established by Centor[4]: (a) subjective or objective fever, (b) absence of cough, (c) tender anterior cervical lymphadenopathy, and (d) tonsillar exudates. The American College of Physicians, American Academy of Family Physicians, and the Centers for Disease Control (CDC) recommend one of two approaches: (a) empirical treatment for three or four positive Centor criteria, or (b) empiric treatment only if four Centor criteria are present, but using an RADT in patients with two or three criteria and treating a positive test.[4] A recent study showed that these two approaches also overtreat, and that a strategy using RADT on all patients with two or more criteria and basing antibiotic usage only on a positive RADT is the most cost-effective approach.[7] These recommendations are for the adult population.

Differential Diagnosis

A sore throat can have other noninfectious etiologies such as gastroesophageal reflux disease, postnasal drainage, thyroiditis, seasonal allergies, a foreign body, and smoking.[2]

TREATMENT

The goals of therapy of GABHS are to prevent suppurative complications and rheumatic fever, decrease the length and severity of symptoms (may decrease symptoms by 1 to 2 days), and to limit the length of infectivity to allow earlier return to work or school.[1] Untreated GABHS may be infectious for up to 1 week after the acute illness,[2] and antibiotic treatment shortens that to 24 hours after the initiation of antibiotic treatment.[8]

Medications

The treatment of choice for GABHS continues to be penicillin because of its efficacy, narrow spectrum, and cost. Recommended regimens in adults are 250 TID–QID, 500 mg BID for 10 days, or 1.2 million units of benzathine penicillin G intramuscularly × 1. Children can be given 250 mg BID or TID for 10 days, or 600,000 units intramuscularly × 1 if less than 27 kg. Erythromycin and first-generation cephalosporins can be used in penicillin-allergic patients, although cephalosporins should not be used if the allergic response was an immediate-type hypersensitivity reaction.[5] Cephalosporins of varying generations have been shown to be twice as likely to give a bacteriologic cure for a GABHS infection in adults when compared to penicillin, but 19 patients would need to be treated for 1 additional cure.[9]

Azithromycin and a number of broader-spectrum cephalosporins have been effective in treating GABHS infections with a once-daily dosage; however, the expense and the broad spectrum make this option less desirable. Short courses of some of the same antibiotics may be effective, but also have the same disadvantages noted.[10] Once-daily amoxicillin is showing promise but awaits confirmatory studies.

If a patient has a recurrent episode shortly after treatment, noncompliance or re-exposure is more likely than treatment failure. Frequent, recurrent episodes of GABHS confirmed by culture or RADT in a symptomatic patient may be viral infections in a strep carrier (the *Streptococcus* is present in the pharynx with no immunologic response to it), or real GABHS infections. Amoxicillin/clavulanate or clindamycin have shown high rates of clearance of bacteria in this circumstance.

Other

Oral and intramuscular steroids have been shown to decrease duration and severity of pain in both children and adults with moderate to severe pharyngitis including GABHS infections. A single dose of 0.6 mg per kg of dexamethasone suspension to a maximum of 10 mg has been shown effective.[11]

Operative

Tonsillectomy is a reasonable option in patients with recurrent GABHS infections. A subsequent GABHS infection was three times less likely and two times less frequent in patients undergoing tonsillectomy.[12]

Risk Management

It is not necessary to test asymptomatic family contacts.[5] GABHS carriers are unlikely to infect close contacts, or develop secondary complications themselves. Up to 20% of school children in the winter/spring in temperate climates may be carriers.[5]

Follow-Up

It is not necessary to do a test of cure on asymptomatic patients.[5]

Complications

The suppurative complications are peritonsillar abscess, retropharyngeal abscess, mastoiditis, sinusitis, and otitis media. Nonsuppurative complications are rheumatic fever, which is rare in the United States and Europe, and poststreptococcal glomerulonephritis. There is no firm evidence that treating streptococcal pharyngitis will prevent glomerulonephritis.[1] Scarlet fever is a GABHS infection that produces an exotoxin, which induces the associated scarletiniform rash.[10]

References

1. Bisno AL. Acute pharyngitis. *N Engl J Med* 2001;344(3):205–211.
2. Vincent MT, Celestin N, Hussain A. Pharyngitis. *Am Fam Physician* 2004;69(6): 1465–1470.
3. Linder JA, Stafford RS. Antibiotic treatment of adults with sore throat by community primary care physicians: a national survey 1989–1999. *JAMA* 2001;286:1181–1186.
4. Linder JA, Chan JC, Bates DW. Evaluation and treatment of pharyngitis in primary care practice. The difference between guidelines is largely academic. *Arch Intern Med* 2006;166:1374–1379.
5. Bisno AL, Gerber MA, et al. Practice guidelines for the diagnosis and management of group A streptococcal pharyngitis. *Clin Infect Dis* 2002;35:113–125.
6. Merrill B, Kelsburg G, Jankowski TA. What is the most effective diagnostic evaluation of streptococcal pharyngitis? *J Fam Pract* 2004;53(9):734–740.
7. Humair J, Sylvie AR, et al. Management of acute pharyngitis in adults. Reliability of rapid streptococcal tests and clinical findings. *Arch Intern Med* 2006;166:640–644.
8. Snellman LW, Stang HJ, et al. Duration of positive throat cultures for group A streptococci after initiation of antibiotic therapy. *Pediatrics* 1993;91(6):1166–1170.
9. Casey JR, Pinichero ME. Meta-analysis of cephalosporins versus penicillin for treatment of group A streptococcal tonsillopharyngitis in adults. *Clin Infect Dis* 2004;38(11): 1526–1534.
10. Gerber MA. Diagnosis and treatment of pharyngitis in children. *Pediatr Clin North Am* 2005;52:729–747.
11. Olympia RP, Khine H, Avner JR. Effectiveness of oral dexamethasone in the treatment of moderate to severe pharyngitis in children. *Arch Pediatr Adolesc Med* 2005;159(3): 278–282.
12. Orvidas LJ, Stauver JL, Weaver AL. Efficacy of tonsillectomy in treatment of recurrent group A (beta)-hemolytic streptococcal pharyngitis. *Laryngoscope* 2006;116(11): 1946–1950.

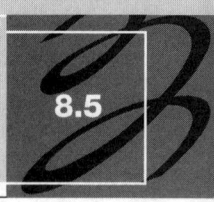
GENERAL PRINCIPLES

Definition
Rhinosinusitis is the term proposed by many authorities to replace the more commonly used term sinusitis.[1,2]

Anatomy
The frontal ethmoid and maxillary sinuses drain through the osteomeatal complex.

Classification
Acute bacterial rhinosinusitis (ABRS) by definition has less than a 4-week duration.[3] Chronic sinusitis is diagnosed with signs and symptoms lasting greater than 4 weeks.

Pathophysiology
The term rhinosinusitis more accurately reflects the pathophysiology of infection of the nasal and sinus cavities, because these cavities are contiguous. Impaired mucociliary clearance and osteomeatal obstruction contribute to the development of ABRS as well as chronic sinusitis.

Etiology
The majority of viral upper respiratory infections (URI) ("common cold") also affect the sinus cavities[4] and therefore could be termed a rhinosinusitis. Adults experience two to three colds per year and children from three to eight episodes.[5,6] Between 0.5% and 2% of upper respiratory infections in adults and 5% and 10% in children develop into ABRS. The majority of community-acquired rhinosinusitis in adults and children is caused by *Streptococcus pneumoniae, Haemophilus influenzae,* and *Moraxella catarrhalis.*[1] Chronic sinusitis, when cultures are performed, often reveal a mixture of anaerobic and aerobic bacteria to include *Prevotella, Fusobacterium,* anaerobic streptococci, staphylococci, as well as those bacteria usually responsible for ABRS.[3] Chronic sinusitis is often secondary to noninfectious causes such as allergy, non-eosinophilic rhinosinusitis, gastroesophageal reflux disease (GERD), cystic fibrosis, immunodeficiencies, and anatomic considerations such as nasal septal deformities, polyps, and malignancies.[3]

DIAGNOSIS

Clinical Presentation
One half to two thirds of patients with sinus symptoms who visit the family practice office are unlikely to have bacterial infection.

History
In the office, clinicians rely on patient history and physical examination to make the diagnosis. URI symptoms not improving after 10 to 14 days or worsening after 5 to 7 days have an increased likelihood of a bacterial infection.[1,3,7] The likelihood of bacterial disease also increases with a history of facial pain, purulent rhinorrhea, and postnasal drainage. Other frequent symptoms are congestion, facial and maxillary pain, headache, and cough. In children the symptoms of ABRS are less specific than in adults. Symptoms include persistent nasal congestion and cough lasting more than 10 days, high fever, and purulent nasal discharge. Children are less likely to present with facial pain or headache. Many have vomiting from the mucous drainage. A change in the color of the nasal discharge is not a

specific sign of bacterial infection, and may be due to the influx of neutrophils that may occur after a few days of viral infection.[1]

Physical Examination

Erythema of the nasal mucosa, sinus tenderness, and orbital swelling are indicative of bacterial disease, with purulent drainage at the middle meatus even more predictive.[2] Pain is often a less prominent symptom in chronic sinusitis.

Laboratory

Results of blood studies, such as elevated sedimentation rate and C-reactive protein, are nonspecific indications of sinusitis. Nasal cultures are of limited value because the mixed flora does not correlate with bacteria aspirated directly from the sinuses.

Imaging

Radiographic studies are usually reserved for confirmatory evidence when the patient's signs and symptoms are vague or uncertain, or when the response to treatment is poor.[3] Classically, standard radiography has been used to detect acute sinusitis with the Caldwell (anterior-posterior) view used for assessing the frontal sinuses and the Water (occipitomental) view for the maxillary sinuses, but they are not particularly sensitive. Computed tomography (CT) scanning is the imaging modality of choice for infectious and inflammatory involvement of the paranasal sinuses.[2,8] It is also the modality of choice for visualizing the osteomeatal complex and its possible obstruction, as well as the ethmoid sinuses. A limitation of CT scanning is that it cannot differentiate bacterial from viral disease.[7]

Differential Diagnosis

The differential diagnosis of acute bacterial rhinosinusitis includes protracted viral URI, dental disease, nasal foreign body, migraine or cluster headaches, temporal arteritis, tension headaches, and temporomandibular disorders.

TREATMENT

Medications

Antibiotic therapy for acute bacterial rhinosinusitis is associated with improved outcomes, and is therefore recommended and based on the most likely etiologic agents and their susceptibilities. Indiscriminate use of antibiotics for URIs has resulted in an increase in resistance to the point that almost 40% of *S. pneumoniae* have at least intermediate resistance.[1,9] Resistance of pneumococci to penicillin is usually based on alterations in the penicillin-binding proteins, which leads to decreased affinity[1] and therefore can often be overcome with an increased dose. *H. influenzae* and *M. catarrhalis* resistance to penicillins is primarily secondary to B-lactamase production.[1,5,9] Given the high rate of viral disease and also the spontaneous remission rate of ABRS that is 50% to 70%,[5] standard antibiotic regimens with amoxicillin are 83% to 88% efficacious, while high dose amoxicillin/clavulanate may reach 90% to 92%.[4,5] Specific recommendations for antibiotic choices[1,3,9]:

- Mild severity and no antibiotic treatment in last 4 to 6 weeks: Amoxicillin 500 to 1,000 BID or amoxicillin/clavulanate 875 BID (in children 45 mg/kg/day of the amoxicillin or amoxicillin component, and 6.4 mg/kg/day of clavulanate and divided BID–TID). In areas of increased resistance, the high-dose amoxicillin regimen may be used, with the amoxicillin component dosed at 90 mg/kg/day (maximum 4 g) and the clavulanate still at 6.4 mg/kg/day divided BID. Other first-line options are cefuroxime, cefpodoxime, and cefdinir. For patients who are allergic to beta-lactam antibiotics, trimethoprim/sulfamethoxazole has greater efficacy than the macrolides.
- Moderate severity, or mild severity and recent antibiotic use (within 4 to 6 weeks): High-dose amoxicillin/clavulanate, ceftriaxone, or, in adults, levofloxacin, moxifloxacin, or gatifloxacin are also recommended. Treatment with a macrolide after inadequate response to a cephalosporin may result in antibiotic failure 60% of the time.[4]
- The usual duration of treatment is 10 to 14 days; however, longer courses may be necessary in chronic sinusitis. If there is a lack of response after 3 to 5 days, re-evaluate the antibiotic regimen and consider other options.

- Topical and oral decongestants may help to decrease mucosal edema and improve drainage. Topical decongestants (oxymetazolone or phenylephrine) should not be used longer than 72 hours as rebound congestion (rhinitis medicamentosa) may occur.[3]
- Guaifenesin has not been shown to be useful in treating sinusitis. Nasal corticosteroids such as mometasone have been shown to be efficacious in improving the symptoms of rhinosinusitis.[6] Oral corticosteroids do not have proven efficacy, but may be helpful in patients who fail to respond to initial antibiotic therapy or have marked mucosal edema.

Special Therapy

Saline lavage or spray may help to liquefy secretions and improve drainage (1/4 tsp of salt in 8 oz of water).[3]

Surgery

Removing the adenoids has shown an improvement in rhinosinusitis in 70% to 80% of children.[2]

References

1. Anon JB, Jacobs MR, Poole MD, et al. Antimicrobial treatment guidelines for acute bacterial rhinosinusitis. *Otolaryngol Head Neck Surg* 2004;130(1 Suppl):1–45. Review.
2. Goldsmith A, Rosenfeld RM. Treatment of pediatric sinusitis. *Pediatr Clin North Am* 2003;50:413–426.
3. Slavin RG, Spector SL, Bernstein IL. The diagnosis and management of sinusitis: a practice parameter update. Joint Council of Allergy, Asthma, and Immunology. *J Allergy Clin Immunol* 2005;116:S13–47.
4. Poole MD, Portugal LG. Treatment of rhinosinusitis in the outpatient setting. *Am J Med* 2005;118(7A):45S–50S.
5. Poole MD. Acute bacterial rhinosinusitis: clinical impact of resistance and susceptibility. *Am J Med* 2004;117(3A):29S–38S.
6. Meltzer EO, Bachert C, Staudinger H. Treating acute rhinosinusitis: comparing efficacy and safety of mometasone furoate nasal spray, amoxicillin, and placebo. *J Allergy Clin Immunol* 2005;116(6):1289–1295.
7. Piccirillo JF. Acute bacterial sinusitis. *N Engl J Med* 2004;351:902–910.
8. Mafee MF, Tran BH, Chapa AR. Imaging of rhinosinusitis and its complications: plain film, CT, and MRI. *Clin Rev Allergy Immunol* 2006;30(3):165–186.
9. Anon JB. Treatment of acute bacterial rhinosinusitis caused by antimicrobial-resistant. *Streptococcus pneumoniae. Am J Med* 2004;117(3A):23S–28S.

ALLERGIC RHINITIS

Denise K.C. Sur

8.6

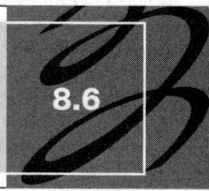

DEFINITION

Allergic rhinitis is a common condition affecting approximately 20% of the U.S. population and ranking as the sixth most prevalent chronic illness in the United States. Patients with this condition can be severely restricted in their daily activities and spend excessive time away from work and school.

DIAGNOSIS

History

- The history is the major diagnostic tool in recognizing allergy as a cause of rhinitis. The most common symptoms of allergic rhinitis are paroxysms of sneezing, rhinorrhea, nasal and palatal pruritus, ocular symptoms, and nasal obstruction. Allergic rhinitis can be either seasonal or perennial, with the seasonal type primarily related to pollen and the perennial type related to indoor allergens such as dust mites, cockroaches, and animal dander.

■ Other types of rhinitis include eosinophilic nonallergic rhinitis, vasomotor rhinitis, and rhinitis medicamentosa. Patients with eosinophilic nonallergic rhinitis or vasomotor rhinitis usually do not experience pruritus or paroxysms of sneezing. Patients with rhinitis medicamentosa usually have a history of repetitive topical decongestant use.

■ Nasal congestion associated with headache, purulent rhinorrhea, postnasal discharge, and halitosis suggests sinusitis (see also Chapter 8.5). Persistent unilateral obstruction suggests the presence of polyps or other structural obstructions.

■ Of note is that some studies have linked the early introduction of formula and foods to infants and the exposure of infants to cigarette smoke to the early development of allergic rhinitis.

Physical Examination

■ Patients with allergic rhinitis, whether seasonal or perennial, often have pale, bluish, boggy mucosa and clear secretions. Children may have darkening under the eyes and a nasal crease resulting from rubbing the nose. Conjunctivitis may or may not be present. The nonallergic patient, especially the patient with vasomotor rhinitis, is more apt to have erythematous mucosa with secretions of any color or consistency.

Laboratory Testing

■ Nasal smears for eosinophils are not diagnostic for allergic rhinitis but can be predictive of a favorable response to topical corticosteroids.

■ Skin testing or epicutaneous (prick) testing with appropriate antigens and positive and negative control substances is the most useful procedure for detection of allergic triggers in allergic rhinitis. Skin testing is specific and sensitive, and can assist in management by either avoidance or immunotherapy. It is important to note that food allergies need not be routinely tested because they rarely play a role in allergic rhinitis.

■ A specific serum immunoglobulin E (IgE) radioallergosorbent test (RAST) should be used in lieu of skin testing only when the patient has severe eczema or dermatographism. RAST testing is less sensitive and more expensive than skin testing.

MANAGEMENT

Three approaches may be used: avoidance, medication, and immunotherapy.

Avoidance

Avoidance of allergen exposure is always indicated, although it may be difficult to achieve. Measures that help control indoor allergen exposure include placement of dust-proof covers over pillows and mattresses, frequent dusting of surfaces and floors with a damp mop, maintenance of an indoor humidity below 50%, and avoidance or frequent bathing of indoor pets if the patient is sensitive to animals. Measures that help control outdoor allergens include closing of windows, running of air conditioners, and avoidance of lawn mowing and leaf raking.

Medications

■ **Antihistamines.** These medications relieve sneezing, itching, and rhinorrhea but not congestion. They are less efficacious than nasal steroids but equally or more effective than cromolyn[3,4]. Their most common adverse effects are sedation, performance/learning impairment, and anticholinergic effects (dry mouth, constipation, urinary retention, and abdominal pain). Compared with first-generation antihistamines, second-generation medications are equally or more effective, have fewer adverse effects, and are generally more expensive. Of the second-generation antihistamines, both loratadine and fexofenadine have Food and Drug Administration labeling as nonsedating, whereas cetirizine does not because it produces a higher incidence of somnolence and fatigue than placebo. Ceftirizine and desloratidine are appropriate for use in children >6 months

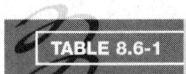

TABLE 8.6-1 | Commonly Used Antihistamines

Antihistamine	Usual dosage
Fexofenadine (Allegra)	60 mg PO bid
First-generation antihistamines	
Chlorpheniramine maleate (Chlor-Trimeton)	4 mg PO q4–6h
Clemastine fumarate (Tavist)	1.34–2.68 mg PO q12h
Diphenhydramine (Benadryl)	25–50 mg PO q4–6h
Promethazine (Phenergan)	12.5 mg PO q12h
Second-generation antihistamines	
Cetirizine (Zyrtec)	5–10 mg PO daily
Desloratadine (Clarinex)	5 mg PO daily
Loratadine	10 mg PO daily

of age[5]. Azelastine, an intranasal antihistamine preparation, offers acute symptomatic relief with minimal sedation. Its main drawback is that it leaves a bad taste in the mouth. Commonly used antihistamines are listed in Table 8.6-1.

■ **Decongestants.** Oral decongestants are α-adrenergic agonists. They have been shown to be effective but can cause side effects including nervousness, insomnia, irritability, headache, palpitations, and urinary obstruction. Their effects on blood pressure are still in dispute. They are contraindicated in glaucoma and during monoamine oxidase inhibitor therapy. Nasal decongestants should be used for only 2 to 3 days because prolonged use can lead to rebound congestion and rhinitis medicamentosa.

　■ The most commonly used decongestant is pseudoephedrine (Sudafed), 60 mg PO q4 to 6 hours.

■ **Inhaled steroids.** Topical nasal corticosteroids are the **most potent medical treatment** currently available for allergic rhinitis. They have been proved safe for long-term use but can occasionally cause nasal irritation, burning, and bloody nasal discharge. Rare reports of septal perforation have been made. Some nasal corticosteroids are approved for use in children older than 2 years. Commonly used inhaled steroids are listed in Table 8.6-2.

■ **Inhaled mast cell stabilizers.** Nasal cromolyn sodium (Nasalcrom) has been shown to be beneficial in treating allergic rhinitis and is approved for use in both adults and

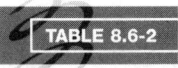

TABLE 8.6-2 | Commonly Used Inhaled Agents

Steroid	Dosage
Beclomethasone	1–2 sprays each nostril bid
Budesonide (Rhinocort)	2 sprays each nostril bid or 4 sprays each nostril qd
Flunisolide (Nasalide)	2 sprays each nostril bid
Fluticasone propionate (Flonase)	2 sprays each nostril qd or 1 spray each nostril bid
Triamcinolone acetonide (Nasacort)	2 sprays each nostril qd
Mometasone furoate	2 sprays each nostril qd
Dexamethasone sodium phosphate	2 sprays each nostril bid-tid
Antihistamine	
Azelastine	1–2 sprays each nostril bid
Mast cell stabilizers	
Cromolyn (Nasalcrom)	1 spray each nostril tid-qid

children. Its full effect may take up to 3 to 4 weeks, and adherence may be decreased secondary to need for use four to six times a day, but its use may eliminate the need for antihistamines and decongestants in the long term. Based on its human and animal safety profiles, cromolyn should be the first drug considered for the management of allergic rhinitis in pregnant women.

■ **Inhaled antihistamines.** One topical antihistamine, azelastine, is now available. It is shown effective in placebo-controlled studies and, like oral antihistamines, can cause sedation.

■ **Inhaled anticholinergics.** Ipratropium bromide relieves rhinorrhea only and is appropriate for patients 6 years of age or older with rhinorrhea not controlled with other medications.

Immunotherapy

■ Immunotherapy is the subcutaneous administration of increasing doses of allergens to which the patient is sensitive. It is indicated when severe symptoms are present that do not respond to avoidance or medication. Allergy injections given over a 3- to 5-year period may reduce symptoms in approximately 85% of cases.[1]

References

1. Noble SL, Forbes RC, Woodbridge HB. Allergic rhinitis. *Am Fam Physician* 1995;51:845.
2. Frew AJ. Advances in environmental and occupational diseases 2003. *J Allergy Clin Immunol* 2004;113:1161.
3. van Bavel, J, Findlay, SR, Hampel, FC Jr, et al. Intranasal fluticasone propionate is more effective than terfenadine tablets for seasonal allergic rhinitis. *Arch Intern Med* 1994;154:2699.
4. Welsch PW, Stickerk WE, Chu CP, et al. Efficacy of beclomethasone nasal solution, flunisolide, cromolyn in relieving symptoms of ragweed allergy. *Mayo Clin Proc* 1987; 62:125.
5. F-D-C Reports. Pharmaceutical Approvals Monthly 2002;7:15.

Cardiovascular Problems

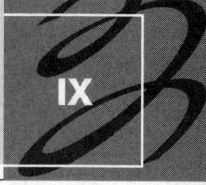

HYPERTENSION
Kevin A. Pearce, Paul Dassow

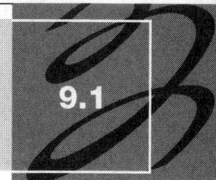

GENERAL PRINCIPLES

Systemic hypertension (HTN) in adults is defined as systolic blood pressure (SBP) of 140 mmHg or higher or diastolic blood pressure (DBP) of 90 mmHg or higher, based on the average of at least two readings taken with the patient comfortable and at rest. Prehypertension is defined as SBP 120 to 139 mmHg or DBP 80 to 89 mmHg.

The accuracy of the blood pressure (BP) determination rises with the number of BP readings averaged. Borderline readings should be averaged over at least three visits. Abnormal readings should be initially confirmed in the contralateral arm.

Hypertension is the most common diagnosis recorded during adult visits to primary care physicians. The prevalence of HTN rises with age, affecting 30% of American residents ages 40 to 59 years old and 65% of those 60 or older.

Risk factors for developing HTN include prehypertension, obesity, a family history of HTN, African American heritage, type 2 diabetes mellitus, and increasing age. Although common, it is not normal for BP to increase with age in adults, but the absolute health risks from HTN increase with age.

Hypertension is a powerful risk factor for myocardial infarction (MI), congestive heart failure (CHF), stroke, kidney failure, and premature death. The risk of developing cardiovascular disease doubles with each 20 mmHg increment of SBP or each 10 mmHg increment of DBP above 115/75 mmHg. In controlled clinical trials, treatment of HTN reduces the risk of CHF by 50%, stroke by 35% to 40%, and MI by 20% to 25%.

DIAGNOSIS

Clinical Presentation

Hypertension is usually asymptomatic until it produces morbid sequelae such as angina, MI, stroke, or CHF. Some patients get hypertension-related headaches, but it is often hard to determine whether the headache was a cause or an effect of elevated BP. Target organ damage (TOD) refers to symptomatic or asymptomatic hypertensive injury to the heart, brain, kidneys, eyes, or large arteries. TOD is common, but may be missed unless evidence for it is sought.

Hypertension is classified according to severity as Stage 1 (SBP 140 to 159 or DBP 90 to 99 mmHg) or Stage 2 (SBP >159 mmHg or DBP >99 mmHg). Classification is defined by either SBP or DBP, whichever falls into the higher stage.

History

The history should be obtained with three general aims in mind:

- Detection of exacerbating conditions or reversible causes of HTN
- Diagnosis of morbid sequelae from HTN
- Assessment of other risk factors for cardiovascular and renal disease

For each of these aims, history should be followed by careful physical examination and a few well-chosen tests.

The history should include assessment of lifestyle factors, comorbidities, and medications, which may cause or exacerbate HTN. The clinician should probe for alcohol or drug abuse, sleep apnea, pregnancy, renal artery stenosis (atherosclerotic if HTN began after age 50, congenital if onset was before age 30), hyperthyroidism or hypothyroidism, primary renal disease, panic disorder, primary hyperaldosteronism, and medication side effects (e.g., oral contraceptives, corticosteroids, stimulants). Although many patients may have one or more of these factors contributing to their HTN, only about 5% of patients have a solely reversible cause for their HTN.

The most common symptomatic morbid sequelae of hypertension are angina, MI, stroke, transient ischemic attack (TIA), and CHF. Hypertensive renal failure is relatively rare, as is visual loss. Hypertensive TOD underlies each of these sequelae. Asymptomatic TOD is even more common and must also be considered; including renal insufficiency, left ventricular hypertrophy, silent coronary artery disease, hypertensive retinopathy, and peripheral arterial disease (such as carotid stenosis or abdominal aortic aneurysm).

Risk stratification includes assessment of TOD and other major cardiovascular risk factors including family history, tobacco use, and history of diabetes, dyslipidemia, or renal insufficiency. Their presence and severity increase the clinical risk from HTN, and the importance of its control.

Physical Examination

The diagnosis of HTN depends on accurate BP readings that reflect the patient's usual BP. Readings taken when a patient is acutely ill or in pain should not be used to diagnose HTN. Routine BP measurements should be taken with the patient seated, after at least 5 minutes of rest, with the arm supported at the level of the heart (supine readings are acceptable). Note the index marks on the BP cuff to ensure proper placement and fit. SBP should be recorded at the onset of sounds, and DBP at their disappearance. At least two readings are recommended at each visit. Falsely elevated readings may occur if the BP cuff is too small or if severe atherosclerosis is present. If the radial artery is still palpable as a "cord" after inflating the cuff until the pulse is obliterated, then systolic readings are probably not reliable.

Home BP measurements are typically about 5 to 10 mmHg lower than those taken in the medical office, and average home BP levels above 135/85 mmHg should be considered hypertensive. Understanding this caveat, home BP readings can improve the accuracy of diagnosis and classification, and enhance patients' commitment to controlling their hypertension. A consistent and significant discrepancy between BP levels at home and in the medical office beyond 10 mmHg may warrant further investigation, including ambulatory BP monitoring.

Automatic ambulatory BP monitoring improves diagnostic and prognostic accuracy. But for reasons of practicality, it should be reserved for patients in whom a significant "white-coat" response is highly suspected, or for patients with symptoms of paroxysmal hypotension or paroxysmal hypertension.

The remainder of the physical examination should include height, weight, and assessments of cardiovascular and neurologic status. The latter include:

- Fundoscopic exam to look for signs of atherosclerosis and hypertensive retinopathy
- Auscultation of the heart and lungs to detect rales, heart murmurs, gallops, and arrhythmias
- Palpation and auscultation of the carotid arteries and major peripheral arteries to detect diminished pulses and bruits as signs of atherosclerosis

- Assessments for peripheral edema and jugular venous distension that may indicate CHF
- A neurologic survey exam to screen for signs of a past stroke

Laboratory Studies

Laboratory studies should be used to aid in assessments for TOD, to identify other cardiovascular risk factors, and to diagnose conditions that may exacerbate BP elevation or be reversible causes for HTN.

Unless the history and physical examination suggest otherwise, initial laboratory testing can be limited to:

- Serum electrolytes, BUN, and creatinine
- Complete blood count
- Fasting blood glucose level
- Fasting serum lipid profile
- Urinalysis and a spot urine albumin/creatinine ratio

A standard 12-lead resting electrocardiogram (ECG) should be performed as a baseline study and to assess for conduction abnormalities that may have implications for antihypertensive medication choices. ECG signs of left ventricular hypertrophy or ischemic heart disease should be given attention, but the resting ECG is not a good screening test for these problems.

TREATMENT

Behavioral

Beneficial lifestyle changes (diet, exercise, and alcohol restriction) should be included in the management of all hypertensive patients. These can suffice as the sole therapy for asymptomatic patients with Stage 1 HTN who have no evidence of TOD or diabetes, if BP can be kept lower than 140/90 mmHg. Those with chronic kidney disease or diabetes should have BP kept below 130/80 mmHg. If the lifestyle changes suggested below do not control BP after 6 months, drug therapy should be added for most patients. For patients with *no TOD and no other cardiovascular risk factor*, giving lifestyle changes up to 12 months is reasonable. Most patients with TOD or diabetes will require antihypertensive medication to achieve target BP. Nonpharmacologic treatment can be expected to lower BP on the order of 4 to 15/2 to 8 mmHg. The same lifestyle alterations are also recommended for the primary prevention of HTN.

The nonpharmacologic treatments for hypertension supported by evidence from controlled trials are as follows:

- **Weight loss:** Patients who are at least 10% above ideal body weight, or whose body mass index (BMI) exceeds 27, should be instructed on a regimen of diet and exercise that can be sustained indefinitely. Gradual and maintained weight loss is the goal.
- **Low-sodium diet:** The average American consumes 4 to 5 g of sodium (9.5 to 12 g of salt) daily, mostly in processed foods. Limiting dietary sodium to less than 2 g per day is recommended. Patients should be taught to use food labels and to make healthy choices in restaurants.
- **DASH diet:** A low-fat diet rich in fruits, vegetables, low-fat dairy, fish, poultry, whole grains and nuts, with little red meat, sweets, or sugary drinks is recommended. This diet also emphasizes potassium-rich foods such as bananas, citrus, tomatoes, broccoli, squash, and green leafy vegetables.
- **Moderation of alcohol** to less than two standard drinks per day: One drink equals 12 ounces of beer, 5 ounces of wine, or 2 ounces of liquor. Some patients (especially women) may be sensitive enough to alcohol that further restriction is necessary.
- **Regular aerobic activity:** Regular activities such as brisk walking, jogging, cycling, and tennis pursued on most days lower BP and overall cardiovascular risk independently of weight loss. Aerobic exercise also reduces overall cardiovascular risk by other mechanisms. A regular walking routine is a reasonable exercise regimen for most patients.

Adherence to treatment for a generally asymptomatic condition, whether behavior change or medication use, is often difficult for patients. The physician should set a schedule of regular follow-up and encourage open dialog with sensitivity to patient views, values, and culture.

Medications

There are more than 70 different drugs approved for use in the United States for treating hypertension. Grouping these drugs into pharmacologic classes aids in therapeutic decision making. The major classes and subclasses of antihypertensive drugs available in the United States, with one example of each, are shown in Table 9.1-1. Preparations containing two antihypertensive drugs are also available. Table 9.1-1 shows only starting doses; full prescribing information should be read be reviewed before prescribing.

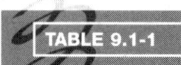 **TABLE 9.1-1**   **Antihypertensive Drug Classes with Example Drugs**

Class/subclass/drug name (trade name)	Starting dose[a]
Diuretics	
Thiazides	
Hydrochlorothiazide (HydroDIURIL, others)	25 mg qd
Potassium sparing	
Amiloride (Midamor)	5 mg qd
Loop	
Furosemide (Lasix)	20 mg bid
Beta-blockers	
Without ISA	
Atenolol (Tenormin)	50 mg qd
With ISA	
Acebutolol (Sectral)	200 mg bid
Alpha-beta-blocker	
Labetalol (Normodyne, Trandate)	100 mg bid
Angiotensin-converting enzyme inhibitors	
Lisinopril (Prinivil, Zestril)	10 mg qd
Calcium-channel blockers	
Dihydropyridines	
Amlodipine (Norvasc)	5 mg qd
Diltiazem (Cardizem, others)	120 mg qd (b)
Verapamil (Calan, others)	180 mg qd[b]
Angiotensin receptor blockers	
Losartan (Cozaar)	50 mg qd
Aldosterone antagonists	
Spironolactone (Aldactone)	25 mg qd
Alpha 1-blockers	
Doxazosin (Cardura)	1 mg qd
Central alpha 2-agonists	
Clonidine (Catapres)	0.1 mg bid
Peripheral antiadrenergics	
Reserpine (Serpasil)	0.1 mg qd
Direct vasodilators	
Hydralazine (Apresoline)	10–25 mg qid

ISA, intrinsic sympathomimetic activity.
[a]Review of full prescribing information is strongly advised.
[b]Sustained-release formulations recommended.

Medication regimens should be individualized for each patient based on the following:

- Evidence that the drug(s) will improve the patient's long-term health (not just lower BP)
- The patient's comorbidities and other cardiovascular risk factors
- The patient's past responses or reactions to medications
- Potential drug interactions
- Factors (such as cost and dosing convenience) that will affect the patient's ability to adhere to the prescribed treatment

African Americans and elderly patients tend to respond better to thiazide diuretics and calcium-channel blockers (CCBs) than they do to other classes of medications, but the other considerations above should take precedence over age and race.

High-quality evidence from controlled clinical trials has led to compelling indications for certain classes of antihypertensive drugs in the presence of certain types of TOD or comorbidity, as shown in Table 9.1-2. For all other patients, first-line medications are based on the strength of evidence that they reduce cardiovascular risk.

The first-line antihypertensive drugs classes are thiazide diuretics (TZD), beta-receptor blockers (BB), angiotensin-converting enzyme inhibitors (ACEI), calcium channel blockers (CCB), and angiotensin receptor blockers (ARB). Among these choices, a TZD should be included in most patients' regimens because of low cost of TZDs and consistent evidence for their high efficacy across multiple controlled trials. **Caution:** Thiazide diuretics can precipitate gout attacks, and should be avoided in patients with known gout.

For most patients, each medication should be started at the lowest recommended dosage and titrated upward, if necessary, at 2-week to 8-week intervals, depending on the severity of the HTN. Elderly patients may require even lower doses. Begin with a single-drug or a low-dose combination. More than one half of patients will require at least two medications to control their HTN. Dose titration and switching of medications are often both necessary. Patient education about this is important to engender trust and realistic expectations.

Follow-Up

Well patients with Stage 1 HTN should have follow-up visits every 1 to 2 months until the BP goal is reached without significant medication side effects (i.e., side effects that are unacceptable to the patient or the physician). Patients with Stage 2 HTN and/or complicating comorbidities should be seen every 2 to 4 weeks until the BP is clearly coming under control without unacceptable side effects. Once the BP goals are reached and stable on a given therapeutic regimen, follow-up can be stretched out to 6 months, unless other conditions dictate more frequent visits.

Goal BP levels should be SBP <140 mmHg and DBP <90 mmHg for most patients. For those with diabetes or chronic kidney disease, goal BP levels are lower: SBP <130 mmHg and DBP <80 mmHg. These patients usually require two or more antihypertensive medications to reach goal BP. Many clinicians choose to set target BP levels below these threshold because in population-based studies cardiovascular risk rises steadily with BP level; starting at SBP >115 mmHg or DBP >75 mmHg. However, care should be taken to avoid overly aggressive BP reduction in elderly patients, because they are at higher risk for orthostasis, tend to have stiffer arteries, and are at higher risk for stroke from episodic hypotension.

If treatment goals have not been met at the prescribed follow-up intervals, the medication dose should be changed, a different class of drug should be tried, or a second drug from another class should be added (see Table 9.1-1). Combining two first-line drugs from different classes at low to moderate doses is often effective, and including a diuretic is desirable. Avoid unwanted drug interactions, especially those that have cardiac and electrolyte effects. Central sympatholytics, alpha-1 blockers, and peripheral antiadrenergics are best reserved as second-line drugs (except in pregnancy, as discussed below). Direct vasodilators are useful for patients failing treatment with first- and second-line drugs, but they should be combined with a diuretic.

Laboratory tests at follow-up are determined by the type of therapy, comorbid conditions, and the baseline values.

TABLE 9.1-2 Guidelines for Choosing Initial Drugs for Hypertension Based on Comorbidities

Drug	Coexisting medical condition								
	Pregnancy	CAD	CHF	LVH	↓HR	DM	COPD	Gout	CKD
Diuretics									
Thiazide	—	—	Yes	—	—	Yes	—	No	No
Loop	—	—	Yes	—	—	—	—	No	Yes
Potassium-sparing	—	—	Yes	—	—	—	—	—	No
β-blockers									
Without ISA	—[b]	Best	Yes[c]	—	No	Yes[a]	No	—	Best[d]
With ISA	—	—	—	—	—	—[a]	No	—	—
Labetalol	Yes	—	No	—	No	—	No	—	—
ACE inhibitors	No	Yes	Yes	—	—	Best	—	—	Best[d]
Calcium blockers									
Diltiazem	—	—	No	—	No	—	—	—	Yes
Verapamil	—	—	No	—	No	—	—	—	Yes
Dihydropyridines	—	—	—	—	—	Yes	—	—	Yes
α₂-Agonist	—	—	—	—	—	—	—	—	—
Aldosterone antag	No	—	Yes	—	—	—	—	—	—
Angiotensin blocker	No	—	Yes	Yes	—	Yes	—	—	Best[d]
Methyldopa	Yes	—	—	—	—	—	No	—	No

Combined therapy with two drugs from different classes should be considered in most cases.
Best = first choice; Yes = drug is preferred; No = drug is relatively contraindicated; —, drug is acceptable but evidence is insufficient to rank treatment options.
ACE, angiotensin-converting enzyme; CAD, coronary artery disease; CHF, congestive heart failure; COPD, chronic obstructive pulmonary disease; CKD, chronic kidney disease; DM, diabetes mellitus; HR, bradycardia; ISA, intrinsic sympathomimetic activity; LVH, left ventricular hypertrophy.
[a]Caution in diabetes: Beta-blockers may blunt awareness of hypoglycemia
[b]Avoid atenolol in pregnancy
[c]Combine with diuretic and ACE inhibitor for systolic CHF.
[d]ACE inhibitors and angiotensin blockers are contraindicated in bilateral renal artery stenosis, or if serum creatinine is > 3.0 mg/dL.

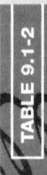

Special Therapy

Hypertensive crises are rare clinical emergencies in which high BP must be lowered immediately to prevent or limit a morbid complication. The situation, not the BP level alone, constitutes the emergency. Examples include:

- Acute pulmonary edema
- Acute MI
- Hypertensive encephalopathy
- Eclampsia
- Dissecting aortic aneurysm

In these situations, a controlled reduction of BP by 20% to 25% over a few minutes to a few hours is indicated.

Hypertensive urgencies are situations in which BP should be lowered to 160 to 170/100 to 110 mmHg within 24 hours to prevent complications. These include:

- Severe perioperative hypertension
- Accelerated malignant hypertension (BP > 220/120 mmHg and rising)

Precipitous decreases in BP should be avoided. The goal is clinical stabilization, not normalization of BP. Relatively short-acting parenteral (IV) antihypertensives, followed by oral therapy, usually work best. Suggested IV drugs and doses are listed in Table 9.1-3. If IV therapy is not an option, oral captopril (Capoten), 25 mg, clonidine (Catapres), 0.1 to 0.2 mg, or labetolol (Normodyne), 200 to 400 mg, can be used; each has a hypotensive effect within 1 hour. Sublingual administration is not more effective than oral.

In the setting of acute cerebrovascular attack (CVA), HTN should generally not be treated unless SBP is greater than 220 mmHg or unless there are signs of progressive intracranial bleeding. Quiet bed rest often results in a significant decrease in BP.

Complications

Antihypertensive medications have variable effects on cardiac conduction, cardiac contractility, arterial and venous tone, renal function, and electrolyte metabolism (especially potassium). The prescriber must be aware of these potential side effects when deciding on therapy and during follow-up examinations. Drug interactions may potentiate or ameliorate symptomatic or metabolic side-effects. New signs or symptoms of cardiac arrhythmia, dyspnea with exertion, edema, or fatigue should be thoroughly investigated. The serum electrolyte panel, BUN, and creatinine should be checked at least once per year; abnormalities should be addressed and followed up. Patients with existing cardiac disease, renal disease, or diabetes, and those on multiple medications, are at the highest risk for

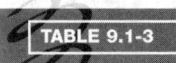

TABLE 9.1-3	Parenteral Drugs for Hypertensive Crisis

Drug name (trade name)	Dose for hypertensive crisis[a]
Labetolol (Normodyne)	20–40 mg IV q10 min
Methyldopa (Aldomet)	250–500 mg IV q6 hr
Hydralazine (Apresoline)	20–40 mg IV q1–2 hr nonpregnant 5–10 mg IV q20 min in pregnancy
Diazoxide (Hyperstat)	50–150 IV q15 min
Enalaprilat (Vasotec IV)	1.25 mg IV q6 hr
Nitroprusside (Nipride)	0.2–10 µg/kg/min IV (Use low dose in pregnancy)

[a]Review of full prescribing information is strongly advised.

complications. Such patients also are likely to gain more absolute benefit from control of HTN than are patients without diabetes or TOD.

SPECIAL CONSIDERATIONS

Hypertension in Pregnancy

Hypertension occurs in 12% to 22% of pregnancies in the United States. It is associated with significant maternal morbidity including seizure, stroke, encephalopathy, and hemorrhage. Additionally, HTN in pregnancy is a major contributor to uteroplacental insufficiency, placental abruption, prematurity, and fetal demise.

Hypertension in pregnancy is classified as either chronic or gestational. Criteria for diagnosis of either form are similar to the nonpregnant state:

- **Mild chronic or gestational HTN** is defined as SBP of 140 mmHg or greater or DBP of 90 mmHg or greater
- **Severe chronic HTN** is defined as SBP of 180 mmHg or greater or DBP of 110 mmHg or greater
- **Severe gestational HTN** is defined as SBP of 160 mmHg or greater or DBP of 110 mmHg or greater

Hypertension in pregnancy should be diagnosed only after an elevated blood pressure is documented on at least two readings taken 6 hours apart with the patient in the sitting position after a 10-minute rest. The HTN is considered chronic if the patient was diagnosed prior to conception or prior to the 20th week of gestation. Women with no recent blood pressure readings who present for prenatal care after the 20th week, and who meet the criteria for HTN, should be considered to have gestational HTN. If HTN persists beyond the usual postpartum period, a diagnosis of chronic HTN can be made in retrospect.

Pre-eclampsia is a pregnancy-induced, multisystem disease defined by gestational HTN with proteinuria. Given the increased risk of morbidity and mortality associated with pre-eclampsia, all women diagnosed with HTN during pregnancy should have a 24-hour quantitative urine protein measured. For those women with chronic HTN, a baseline measurement will document possible pre-existing renal disease that may influence subsequent diagnosis of pre-eclampsia. Chronic HTN is a known risk factor for the development of pre-eclampsia. The classification of pre-eclampsia as well as its treatment is covered in Chapter 14.8.

Treatment for chronic HTN in pregnancy and gestational HTN (without proteinuria) is dictated by the known effects of antihypertensive medications on uteroplacental blood flow and fetal outcome studies. Because numerous controlled trials have failed to demonstrate fetal or maternal benefit from treating *mild* HTN in pregnancy, the American College of Obstetrics and Gynecology (ACOG) recommends *not starting* antihypertensive medication for mild chronic or gestational HTN in pregnancy, unless there are comorbid conditions such as HTN-associated headaches, TOD, or rising BP levels.

For women already taking antihypertensive medication at the time of pregnancy diagnosis, current data support stopping therapy if HTN is mild, or switching treatment to the smallest effective dose of a first-line antihypertensive drug for use in pregnancy.

- **First-line antihypertensive drugs for HTN during pregnancy:**
  - Methyldopa 250 to 500 mg PO tid-qid
  - Labetolol 100 to 400 mg bid-tid

- **Acceptable second-line choices:**
  - Other beta-blockers (*excluding* atenolol which has been associated with growth restriction)
    - Metoprolol 50 to 200 mg bid
    - Pindolol 5 to 15 mg bid
  - Calcium-channel blockers
    - Nifedipine 10 to 30 mg tid
    - Nicardipine 20 to 40 mg tid

- Hydrochlorothiazide 25 to 50 mg qd
- Hydralazine 10 to 50 mg qid
- **Contraindicated in pregnancy:**
  - ACE inhibitors
  - Angiotensin-receptor blockers
  - Aldosterone antagonists

The use of ACE inhibitors during pregnancy is associated with a variety of renal and pulmonary toxicities in the fetus.

Treatment of acute, severe HTN in pregnancy should occur expeditiously to reduce the risk of maternal stroke and placental abruption.

Hydralazine has been the preferred agent in the United States due to its long history of safety and rapid onset of action; however, thrombocytopenia has been rarely reported in neonates born to women treated in the third trimester.

- **Recommended antihypertensive drugs for acute severe HTN in pregnancy:**
  - Hydralazine 5 to 10 mg IV every 15 to 20 minutes
  - Labetalol 20 mg IV bolus with 20 to 40 mg every 15 minutes as needed
  - Nifedipine* 10 mg PO q15 minutes, max 30 mg
  - Nicardipine* 5 mg per hour IV, increase at 2.5 mg per hour q5 to 15 minutes up to 15 mg per hour
  - Sodium nitroprusside 0.25 μg/kg/minute IV, increase 0.25 μg/kg/minute q5 minutes up to 5 μg/kg/minute

References

1. National High Blood Pressure Education Program. The seventh report of the Joint National Committee on Prevention, Detection, Evaluation and Treatment of High Blood Pressure (JNC 7). National Heart, Lung, and Blood Institute. Bethesda, MD: NIH; 2003: Pub. 03–5233.
2. ALLHAT Collaborative Research Group. Major outcomes in high-risk hypertensive patients randomized to angiotensin-converting enzyme inhibitor or calcium channel blocker vs diuretic: the Antihypertensive and Lipid-Lowering Treatment to Prevent Heart Attack Trial (ALLHAT). *JAMA* 2002;288(23):2981–2997.
3. Appel LJ, Champagne CM, Harsha DW, et al. Effects of comprehensive lifestyle modification on blood pressure control: main results of the PREMIER clinical trial. *JAMA* 2003;289(16):2083–2093.
4. Dahlof B, Devereux RB, Kjeldsen SE, et al. Cardiovascular morbidity and mortality in the Losartan Intervention for Endpoint reduction in hypertension study (LIFE): a randomised trial against atenolol. *Lancet* 2002;359(9311):995–1003.
5. Demers C, McMurray JJ, Swedberg K, et al. Impact of candesartan on nonfatal myocardial infarction and cardiovascular death in patients with heart failure. *JAMA* 2005;294(14):1794–1798.
6. Casaa P, Weiliang C, Stavros L, et al. Effect of inhibitors of the renin-angiotensin system and other antihypersensitive drugs on renal outcomes: systematic review and meta-analysis. *Lancet* 2005;2005;366;2026–2033.
7. Sibai BM. Diagnosis and management of gestational hypertension and preeclampsia. *Obstet Gynecol* 2003;102:181–192.
8. Chronic hypertension in pregnancy. *ACOG Pract Bull* July 2001;Number 29.

---

*Caution must be exercised with the concomitant use of calcium-channel blockers and magnesium as the combination has been reported to cause neuromuscular blockade and severe hypotension.

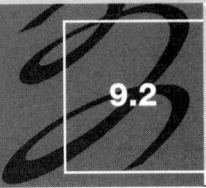

ISCHEMIC HEART DISEASE
William E. Chavey, Lee A. Green

GENERAL PRINCIPLES

Ischemic heart disease (IHD) is a chronic medical condition prone to acute exacerbations and affecting a sizable percentage of the adult population. The manifestations may be broad and have impact on inpatient and outpatient care. This chapter focuses on outpatient diagnosis and management.

Ischemic heart disease is a term interchangeable with coronary artery disease (CAD), coronary heart disease (CHD), and atherosclerotic heart disease (ASHD). Although in the most precise sense the terms are not identical, generally they all refer to a condition of obstructed blood flow in the coronary arteries that may result in ischemia or infarction of the myocardium. Clinically, patients with IHD may be asymptomatic, may have chronic stable angina, may present with an acute coronary syndrome (ACS; see below), or may present with sudden death as their initial symptoms.

Classification

The estimated prevalence of CHD is 13,200,000, and one in three American adults is estimated to have some type of cardiovascular disease (CVD).[1] Since 1900, CVD has been the number 1 cause of death every year except 1918.[1] It is also the most costly medical condition in the United States.[1]

Acute coronary syndromes are classified as unstable angina (UA), non-ST segment elevation myocardial infarction (NSTEMI) or ST segment elevation MI (STEMI) depending on serologic evidence of myocardial damage and on electrocardiographic (ECG) findings.

Several classification schemes exist for grading stable angina, although the most commonly utilized may be the Canadian Cardiovascular Society system commonly referred to as CCCS.

Canadian Cardiovascular Society[2] Class	Description
I	Ordinary physical activity does not cause angina
II	Slight limitation of ordinary physical activity
III	Marked limitation of ordinary physical activity
IV	Inability to perform any physical activity without discomfort

Most commonly in IHD, an obstruction develops due to atherosclerosis. Atheroslcerotic plaques may be stable and result in a pattern of chronic angina precipitated when myocardial oxygen demand exceeds the supply that is available across a coronary artery obstruction. ACS typically occurs when an unstable coronary artery plaque ruptures, promoting thrombus formation on the surface and acutely obstructing the vessel lumen.

The degree of coronary obstruction does not necessarily correlate with the likelihood of an acute coronary event; high-grade stenoses may never progress to infarction while less obstructive plaques may rupture and cause infarction. Some patients with angina have normal appearing coronary arteries. This situation can occur when the etiology of the symptoms is not cardiac, but it can also occur among patients who develop cardiac ischemia from coronary artery vasospasm (Prinzmetal angina). Those with Prinzmetal angina are typically younger and have fewer traditional IHD risk factors. The etiology is unclear and the prognosis (absent concomitant CAD) is favorable. Other patients may have microvascular disease or diffuse disease that is hard to detect on routine catheterization. These patients are more commonly women and may still have a substantial risk for progression to MI.

Atherosclerosis is a chronic inflammatory disease resulting from a complex interplay between cellular and chemical factors affecting the vascular endothelium. The atherosclerotic process occurs over years; is triggered by traditional IHD risk factors such as smoking, obesity, diabetes, hypertension, hyperlipidemia, and genetics; and results in the formation of obstructing plaques. Investigation into other contributor factors continues, but the most recent evidence shows that 80% to 90% of patients with IHD have traditional risk factors[3] and 87% to 100% of patients who suffer fatal IHD events have at least one traditional risk factor.[4]

A number of novel serum markers have been found to be associated with heart disease. Some are risk factors and others are only markers of disease. High-sensitivity C-reactive protein (hs-CRP) has derived the most attention and appears to be an independent risk factor for heart disease. Lipoprotein-a is a nonmodifiable risk factor that is genetically programmed and signifies risk for early-onset heart disease. In contrast, elevated homocysteine elevates risk for heart disease but lowering homocysteine levels does not reduce the risk of heart disease and is thus considered only a risk marker.

IHD is associated with obstructive sleep apnea and snoring, but the nature and direction of this association is not yet clear.

DIAGNOSIS

Clinical Presentation

An ACS may present with "typical" chest pain, atypical angina, sudden fatigue, congestive heart failure symptoms, or even nausea and vomiting. Diagnostic and management decisions must be made quickly and implemented immediately because the efficacy of many of the available treatments declines rapidly with time from onset of ischemia. Patients presenting with symptoms consistent with ACS should be classified very rapidly as having probable noncardiac pain, stable angina, unstable angina/NSTEMI, or STEMI meeting reperfusion criteria.

Stable angina commonly presents as exertional chest pain, tightness, shortness of breath, or fatigue. It has often been occurring for weeks or months before the patient consults a physician.

IHD presents in enough ways and across a broad enough spectrum of patients that it would be misleading to describe a "typical" patient or presentation. Rather, a high index of suspicion should be maintained for IHD among men over 40 and women over 50, with a rapidly increasing prior probability with advancing age.

Primary prevention of IHD is an important part of family practice. Baseline risk among asymptomatic adults should be estimated using the National Cholesterol Education Program (NCEP) framework,[5] either by counting risk factors or by calculating risk using the Framingham equation (accessible at http://hp2010.nhlbihin.net/atpiii/riskcalc.htm). The NCEP framework does overestimate risk among low-prevalence populations and can underestimate risk in some high-prevalence groups (e.g., Indian and other south Asian populations) by as much as 50%, so clinical judgment is required.

History

History is the most important information in the decision process for suspected IHD. It should address the following parameters:

- The location, character, and time course of the symptoms. Chest or left arm pressure or pain of a steady, dull nature is classic for cardiac ischemia. The feeling may be profound but vague and not even termed pain or pressure by the patient. Alternatively, some patients will insist that the sensation is one only of pressure, not pain. Occasionally pain may be present only in the jaw or scapular area. Sharp or pleuritic pain weighs against the diagnosis, as does pain that can be localized with one finger. Paresthesias (especially perioral tingling) suggest panic attack. Water brash has high specificity for gastroesophageal reflux. Reduced pain upon sitting up and leaning forward suggests pericarditis. Women may frequently present with vague symptoms that may be considered "atypical."

■ Prior history of IHD.

■ Classic epidemiologic risk factors: smoking, hyperlipidemia, hypertension, obesity, and family history. These have little or no diagnostic value for ACS,[6] but should be assessed in evaluating chronic angina. Those that are modifiable are key points in primary and secondary prevention.

■ Diabetes. Patients with long-standing diabetes often lack the characteristic pain of acute ischemia.

■ A complete listing of current medications including over-the-counter and alternative or herbal preparations and a list of any illicit drugs being used, especially cocaine.

A full cardiac and vascular review of systems should be included in the history for suspected chronic angina, but gathering this information should not be allowed to delay the rapid evaluation of ACS.

Physical Examination

Physical examination in cases of suspected ACS should be expeditiously conducted and directed to key findings, which include pulmonary edema, particularly sudden or "flash" edema; mitral valve murmur, particularly if of new onset; marked hypertension; hypotension or shock; confusion or other mental status changes; other neurologic deficits consistent with stroke; and hypoxia. These findings can be detected by a careful assessment of the ABCs (airway, breathing, and circulation), review of vital signs, as well as a heart, lung, and focused neurologic exam.

For patients with suspected chronic angina, a more complete directed physical examination emphasizing cardiovascular findings should be carried out. Carotid, abdominal, and renal bruits, pedal pulses (and ankle-brachial indices if pulses are diminished), and jugular venous waveform should be included. Chest tenderness to palpation that completely reproduces the presenting pain may make ACS less likely but does not exclude the possibility and this finding must be interpreted within the context of other clinical data.

Laboratory Studies

ECG is, with history, the foundation of diagnosis and risk stratification for suspected ACS. Certain crucial features are important:

■ ST segment elevation of at least 1 mm in two contiguous leads
■ New-onset left bundle branch block (LBBB)

Either of the above findings on an ECG in a patient with chest pain is diagnostic of STEMI and the patient should be triaged appropriately and emergently for reperfusion therapy via either thrombolytic therapy or emergent percutaneous coronary intervention (PCI). Patients with ST segment depression in the anterior leads in a pattern consistent with a posterior MI may also benefit from emergent reperfusion. Patients meeting these criteria must be identified immediately and emergently triaged from the outpatient setting to appropriate facilities to receive thrombolysis within 30 minutes or PCI within 90 minutes. Patients not meeting these criteria should not receive reperfusion therapy as it worsens outcomes.[7]

Other ECG findings such as Q waves of 1 mm or greater not known to be present previously, T-wave inversion, hyperacute T waves (greater than or equal to 50% of the maximal QRS amplitude), ST segment depression, and new conduction abnormalities or arrhythmias may also be important markers of ischemia.

Cardiac troponins T and I are more than 90% sensitive and similarly specific at 8 or more hours from the onset of pain.[8] Either or both may be assayed, generally for levels >0.1 ng per mL. Positive troponins with normal ECG can distinguish NSTEMI from UA and help identify patients who are at increased risk for infarction or sudden death.

All patients suspected of IHD should have a fasting lipid profile, glucose, complete blood count (CBC), estimated glomerular filtration rate (GFR), and electrolytes measured. Evaluation of ACS should not be delayed to obtain them; lipids may be measured fasting up to 24 hours after symptom onset.[7]

Imaging

Patients suspected of IHD should have a chest radiograph performed for pulmonary edema and cardiac enlargement. Evaluation of patients with ACS and initiation of reperfusion therapy, however, should not be delayed for radiography.

Stress testing is employed to assess cardiac structure and function. It is commonly used to assess the probability of significant coronary artery disease among those who have anginal symptoms or who are preparing for noncardiac surgery. A number of different stress and imaging modalities are available. The advantages and disadvantages of the most commonly utilized forms are displayed in Table 9.2-1. If stress testing is to be used for this purpose, pretest probability needs to be considered before ordering an exam. If the pretest probability is very low, the result of a stress test may not influence decision making. If the

TABLE 9.2-1   Comparison of Stress Test Options[9]

	Sensitivity	Specificity	Advantages	Disadvantages/cautions
Stress ECG	67	72	Cost effective Readily available Good measure of function	Not reliable with baseline ECG changes or for patients on digoxin High false-positive rate among women
Stress myocardial perfusion (thallium or sestamibi)	89	76	Very sensitive Good measure of function	Costly No assessment of structure
Stress echocardiogram	85	86	Good measure of function Very specific Good measure of cardiac structure More affordable than myocardial perfusion	Images may be compromised by obesity
Adenosine myocardial perfusion (thallium or sestamibi)	90	70	Very sensitive	Costly Caffeine ingestion may lead to false negatives Adenosine may cause bronchospasm No assessment of structure
Dobutamine echocardiogram	82	85	Very specific Good measure of cardiac structure More affordable than myocardial perfusion	Dobutamine may induce tachyarrhythmias Images may be compromised by obesity

risk is very high, then a negative test may not influence the decision whether a catheterization is necessary but may be helpful in targeting vessels for future revascularization.

Stress-testing may also be useful for assessing a patient's functional capacity, assessing myocardial viability post MI, and occasionally for guiding medical management of IHD.

Left heart catheterization is the gold standard for evaluating coronary artery anatomy. It is generally safe and is appropriate for identifying the location and extent of obstructive disease. If suspicion for Prinzmetal or vasospastic angina is high, a heart catheterization may also be used with ergonovine to assess for the presence of coronary artery spasm.

CT scan has evolved as an emerging technology that may have significant potential for heart disease. Multidetector computed tomography (CT) and CT angiography are both being utilized and investigated but the role that these emerging technologies will ultimately play in the diagnosis and management of heart disease is not yet clear.

Differential Diagnosis

Patients presenting with chest pain and related complaints have ACS in a minority of cases, approximately 30% in the emergency department setting[8] and less than 5% in the primary care physician's office setting.[10] Other high-probability diagnoses that should be considered are panic attack, gastroesophageal reflux disease, musculoskeletal pain, and pleurisy. Panic attack and gastroesophageal reflux disease are often close mimics of angina, and both are more common than angina in primary care settings. Both can result in morbidity, if misdiagnosed as angina, from inappropriate cardiac workups and from failure to treat the patient's real condition. Also consider other life-threatening diagnoses such as aortic dissection, pulmonary embolus, pneumothorax, or perforating ulcer, among others.

TREATMENT

Outpatient management of ACS focuses on rapid identification and risk stratification, immediate transport of reperfusion candidates to properly equipped facilities, and appropriate referral and transport of moderate- and high-risk patients. Patients without known true hypersensitivity or active bleeding should receive 325 mg of aspirin stat and be placed on 2 L per minute of oxygen by nasal cannula or mask while awaiting transport. If ECG monitoring is available it should be in place. Nitroglycerine can be administered sublingual every 5 minutes as tolerated by blood pressure for pain relief. A defibrillator should be ready, and personnel trained in its use should be with the patient continuously. Time is of the essence in ACS. American College of Cardiology/American Heart Association (ACC/AHA) standards are to keep total ischemic time to less than 120 minutes.[7] Patients with evidence of STEMI should be transported rapidly to a facility capable of providing appropriate reperfusion—thrombolysis or PCI.

Outpatient management of IHD consists of primary and secondary prevention. Inpatient management of ACS is outside the scope of this chapter. Common to both primary and secondary intervention is risk factor reduction—weight loss, smoking cessation, and good control of hypertension, hyperlipidemia, and diabetes (in order of absolute benefit) if present. Risk factor reduction occurs through both behavioral and medical interventions. Treatment of hypertension should be to a BP goal of <140/90 for all patients and to a BP <130/80 for those with renal disease or diabetes. Lipid lowering should be achieved with a statin, if tolerated, and in conjunction with the NCEP goals as described below.[5] National treatment goals for diabetes are for a HbA1C < 7.0, though available evidence does not clearly demonstrate reduced ACS risk for such tight diabetes control.

Population	Goal
<2 risk factors	Low-density lipoprotein (LDL) < 160 mg/dL
2 or more risk factors	LDL < 130 mg/dL
Known IHD or diabetes	LDL < 100 mg/dL
Very high-risk patients	Optional LDL target of 70 mg/dL (recent ACS, IHD plus diabetes; metabolic syndrome)

Operative interventions, for example, coronary artery bypass grafting (CABG) or percutaneous intervention (PCI) with stent placement, are available for treatment of disease in appropriate patients.

Behavioral

Smoking is the most powerful modifiable risk factor for IHD and smoking cessation is essential for both primary and secondary prevention. Physicians should ask about smoking habits at each visit, advise the patient to quit, assess the willingness to quit, and assist the patient in quitting smoking.

Depression is thought to be an independent risk factor for IHD and ACS and is associated with a worse prognosis. Treatment with selective serotonin-reuptake inhibitors (SSRIs) improves depression morbidity though not cardiac outcomes.[11] Current expert opinion is to use SSRIs among patients with IHD as needed in a manner consistent with how they would be used in the absence of heart disease.

Weight loss is an important component of reducing risk for MI. Body mass index (BMI) has traditionally been used as a measure of risk with the goal being <25, but waist to hip ratio has emerged as a more reliable measure of risk. Weight loss should target a waist circumference of <40 inches in men and <35 inches in women.[12]

Exercise both reduces risk directly and is an important component of weight loss. A written exercise prescription should be given for 30 to 60 minutes of activity, defined as brisk walking, 5 to 7 days per week,[12] and progress toward that goal should be monitored and reinforced at every visit. Patients may opt for more vigorous activity based on stress test results.

Medications

Medical management of IHD can involve a diverse array of medications. The most common are described in Table 9.2-2. The three medications in bold type are recommended to all patients unless contraindicated, with regular assessment of compliance. Intensive medical therapy is capable of achieving regression of coronary plaques and reducing ACS events.

Surgery

Emergent reperfusion therapy reduces mortality and morbidity, and is the standard of care for STEMI meeting the criteria above. PCI is preferred in high-volume centers if door-to-balloon times of 90 minutes or less can be achieved. Thrombolysis should be initiated (with a target door-to-needle time of 30 minutes) if suitably skilled PCI is not available in that time frame.[13] The primary care physicians must honestly assess the procedure volume and skills of their referral facility and the realistically likely time to initiation of therapy in making referral decisions.

Among stable angina patients, CABG improves survival for patients with left main disease, severe proximal left anterior descending (LAD) disease, or three-vessel disease with diminished left ventricular (LV) function. (A vessel is considered diseased if it has ≥50% obstruction on coronary angiography.) Recent improvements in angioplasty technology, particularly stenting, may make percutaneous revascularization an appropriate alternative for some such patients. Patients with diabetes do not fare as well with percutaneous revascularization as with CABG.

Anginal pain, ability to exercise, and daily role function are important patient-oriented outcomes. Consultation and evaluation for revascularization (either percutaneous or by CABG) to reduce pain and improve function is appropriate for many patients with stable IHD, even if mortality is unlikely to be reduced.

Special Therapy

Yearly influenza vaccine is indicated among patients with IHD. Also, patients with IHD should have a pneumovax once, which is to be repeated when the patient is older than 65 if the first pneumovax was administered before the patient was 65 years old.

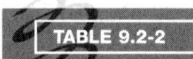

| TABLE 9.2-2 | Drugs Used Commonly in the Treatment of IHD |

Intervention	Dose	Primary prevention	Secondary prevention	Comments[a]
ACE inhibitors	Drug dependent	N/A	Only for high risk or for LVSD	Class effect May substitute ARB if intolerant of ACE Contraindicated if allergic, renal failure, hyperkalemia, hypotension, renal artery stenosis, pregnancy
Aspirin	75–162 mg daily	Moderate or high risk (e.g., Framingham 10 yr risk estimate >6%)	Standard of care; with-hold only for documented hypersensi-tivity or active bleeding	Higher doses associated with increased risk, but no benefit Contraindicated if allergic or if significant bleeding risk
Beta-blockers	Drug dependent	HTN	Standard of care; with-hold only for proven intolerance (asthma and patients with COPD should receive cau-tious trial)	Class effect except for LVSD Use only bisoprolol, carvedilol, or metoprolol succinate with LVSD Contraindicated in heart block, hypotension, severe reactive airway disease
Calcium-channel blockers	Drug dependent	N/A	Angina relief	Avoid short-acting nondihy-dropyridines (DHPs), e.g., verapamil, diltiazem Non-DHPs may cause heart block if combined with beta blockers Non-DHPs are not to be used with LVSD Contraindicated in hypotension, heart block
Eplerenone	25–50 mg daily	N/A	<14 days post MI if also with LVSD or diabetes	Aldactone in the same class but never tested for this indication Contraindicated with renal failure, hyperkalemia
Nitroglycerine	Drug dependent	N/A	Angina relief	Contraindicated in hypotension or within 24 hours after PDE inhibitor use (e.g., Viagra)
Clopidogrel	300 mg load 75 mg daily	Possible harm	if ASA intolerant + ASA post PCI or UA/NSTEMI[c]	Contraindicated if allergic or if significant bleeding risk

(continued)

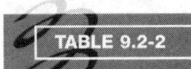

| TABLE 9.2-2 | | Drugs Used Commonly in the Treatment of IHD *(Continued)* | | |

Intervention	Dose	Primary prevention	Secondary prevention	Comments[a]
Statins	Drug dependent	Based on NCEP recommendations per risk profile	Standard of care; withhold only for documented intolerance	Class effect For secondary prevention, titrate to LDL <100 or optional, to LDL <70 in high-risk patients

[a]Assume contraindications considered before any medication given; the list of contraindications described here is not exhaustive; please consult a drug reference for a more comprehensive list.
[b]LVSD is left ventricular systolic dysfunction, i.e., EF <40%.
[c]Clopidogrel should be administered for 1-12 months post PCI with bare metal stent or post UA/NSTEMI without stenting. It should be administered for at least 12 months post drug eluting stent.

SPECIAL CONSIDERATIONS

The prevalence and the magnitude of impact of IHD have made appropriate management of this condition a high priority among groups following the quality of care for chronic diseases. Physicians should follow quality standards such as aspirin, statins, and beta-blockers for secondary prevention and should develop systems for identifying and tracking patients with IHD.

References

1. Heart disease and stroke statistics 2006 update. A Report from the American Heart Association Statistics Committee and Stroke Statistics Subcommittee. *Circulation* 2006;113:e85–e151.
2. Goldman L, Hashimoto B, Cook EF, et al. Comparative reproducibility and validity of systems for assessing cardiovascular functional class: advantages of a new specific activity scale. *Circulation* 1981;64:1227–1234.
3. Khot UN, Khot MB, Bajzer CT, et al. Prevalence of conventional risk factors in patients with coronary heart disease. *JAMA* 2003;290(7):898–904.
4. Greenland P, Knoll MD, Stamler J, et al. Major risk factors as antecedents of fatal and nonfatal coronary heart disease events. *JAMA* 2003;290(7):891–897.
5. National Cholesterol Education Program. National Heart, Lung, and Blood Institute. Available online at http://www.nhlbi.nih.gov/guidelines/cholesterol/atp_iii.htm. Accessed 30 June 2006.
6. Jayes RLJ, et al. Do patients' coronary risk factor reports predict acute cardiac ischemia in the emergency department? A multicenter study. *J Clin Epidemiol* 1992;45:621.
7. Antman EM, Anbe DT, Armstrong PW, et al. ACC/AHA guidelines for the management of patients with ST-elevation myocardial infarction; a report of the American College of Cardiology/American Heart Association Task Force on Practice Guidelines (Committee to Revise the 1999 Guidelines for the Management of Patients with Acute Myocardial Infarction). *J Am Coll Cardiol* 2004;44(3):E1–E211.
8. Ebell MH, Flewelling D, Flynn CA. A systematic review of troponin T and I for diagnosing acute myocardial infarction. *J Fam Pract* 2000;49:550.
9. Murthy TH, Bach DS. Comparative review of stress tests. *Clin Fam Pract* 2001;3(4):814.
10. Klinkman MS. Episodes of care for chest pain. *J Fam Pract* 1994;38:345.
11. Agency for Healthcare Research and Quality. Post-myocardial infarction depression (Evidence report/technology assessment report 123). AHRQ Publication 05-E018-02. Rockville, MD: U.S. Government Printing Office; May 2005.
12. Smith SC, Allen J, Blair SN, et al. AHA/ACC guidelines for secondary prevention for patients with coronary and other atherosclerotic vascular disease: 2006 update. *Circulation* 2006;113:2363–2372.
13. Van de Werf F, Gore JM, Avezum A, et al. for the GRACE Investigators. Access to catheterisation facilities in patients admitted with acute coronary syndrome: multinational registry study. *BMJ* 2005;330:441–444.

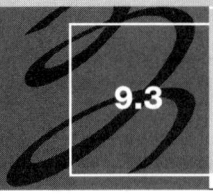

9.3

MURMURS AND VALVULAR HEART DISEASE
Kathryn E. Lazure

GENERAL PRINCIPLES

A heart murmur may have no pathologic significance—simply a representation of physiologic increases in blood flow. However, a murmur may be an important indicator of the presence of valvular abnormalities. The history and physical examination are valuable screening tools for all patients. In certain instances, further evaluation with electrocardiogram, chest x-ray, echocardiogram, and heart catheterization is required. Diagnosis is critical in valvular heart disease in order to achieve timely management prior to the onset of irreversible damage. Timing of surgical intervention correlates with good outcome. Generally, patients with stenotic valvular lesions can be monitored clinically until symptoms appear. On the other hand, patients with regurgitant valvular lesions require careful echocardiographic monitoring for left ventricular function and may require surgery even in the absence of symptoms. A brief discussion of some basic diagnostic tools is listed below. In addition, the most common valvular heart diseases as well as murmurs in pregnancy, murmurs in athletes, and murmurs in infants and children are reviewed in the following text.

DIAGNOSIS

History

History suggesting valvular heart disease is directed at symptoms potentially related to dysfunction of a valve. These symptoms can be thought of as relating to diminished forward flow (fatigue and decreased exercise tolerance) and symptoms relating to pulmonary congestion (paroxysmal nocturnal dyspnea and orthopnea).

Physical Examination

The physical examination focuses on the location, timing, duration, and quality of the murmur. In addition to these cardinal elements, various provocative maneuvers can cause changes in the murmur, changes that aid diagnosis. The Valsalva maneuver and standing decrease preload. Squatting or raising the legs increases preload. Handgrip increases afterload. There is no maneuver that decreases afterload. The beat after the long pause associated with a premature beat may also give clues to the etiology of a murmur by causing increased filling of the left ventricle.

Laboratory Studies

- **Electrocardiogram (ECG).** The ECG is not a specific tool for the diagnosis of valvular heart disease. Findings such as atrial enlargement or left ventricular hypertrophy (LVH) often occur late in the course of valvular heart disease.
- **Chest x-ray (CXR).** Like the ECG, the CXR does not offer early or specific diagnostic clues to valvular heart disease. Radiographic evidence of cardiomegaly or pulmonary congestion is a late finding.
- **Echocardiogram.** The echocardiogram is the definitive indicator that rules in or rules out the presence of valvular heart disease. It should be used when there is moderate clinical suspicion of valvular heart disease.

300

SPECIFIC DIAGNOSIS AND TREATMENT BASED ON VALVULAR DISEASE OR CONDITION

Aortic Stenosis (AS)

General Principles

Pathophysiology Left ventricular outflow obstruction leads to increased left ventricular pressure. In order to maintain normal wall stress, the left ventricle undergoes concentric hypertrophy. Subsequently, a decrease in contractile performance and in ejection fraction is noted.

Etiology of Valvular AS Senile AS (age-related degenerative calcific changes), congenitally bicuspid vale with superimposed calcification, rheumatic heart disease.

Diagnosis

Clinical Presentation Exertional dyspnea, angina pectoris, syncope, congestive heart failure, sudden death

Physical Examination

- **Murmur:** Harsh, diamond-shaped **systolic** murmur. AS murmur is heard best in second right intercostal space and radiates into neck vessels. It gets softer with maneuvers that increase afterload (handgrip).
- Diminished intensity (or absence) of aortic valve closure
- Weakened **(parvus)** and delayed **(tardus)** upstroke of carotid artery pulsation
- **Narrow** pulse pressure

Treatment

Management Asymptomatic AS management includes close clinical follow-up to monitor aortic valve area (normal is 3 to 4 cm^2). In addition, patients require endocarditis antibiotic prophylaxis and avoidance of medication that could result in hypotension. Symptoms occur late in the course of disease and are an ominous sign. Onset of symptoms triggers the need for surgical evaluation.

Surgery Aortic valve replacement is indicated if the patient becomes symptomatic, if there is evidence of left ventricular dysfunction, or if the patient has an expanding poststenotic aortic root. Percutaneous balloon aortic valvuloplasty is preferable in children and young adults with congenital, noncalcific AS.

Special Considerations: Subvalvular Aortic Stenosis

Hypertrophic Cardiomyopathy (with Outflow Obstruction) This is a familial disease characterized by marked hypertrophy of the left ventricle, most commonly the interventricular septum. The murmur is similar to valvular AS, but differs in that any maneuver that will make the left ventricle larger in diastole with make the subvalvular AS murmur softer. Conversely, any maneuver that will decrease the left ventricular size in diastole will make the murmur louder. This is the most common cardiac abnormality found in young athletes who die suddenly during vigorous physical activity.

- **Special therapy:** Beta-blockers are the standard of therapy while calcium-channel blockers are sometimes useful.
- The guidelines for surgical intervention (myomectomy) are not well defined.
- The incidence of sudden death is 2% to 4% per year in adults and 4% to 6% per year in children and adolescence.

Mitral Stenosis (MS)

General Principles

Pathophysiology Thickening and immobility of the mitral valve leaflets cause obstruction of blood flow from the left atrium to left ventricle and increased pressure within the left atrium, pulmonary vasculature, and right heart. A decreased mitral valve oriface (normal 4 to 6 cm^2) requires an abnormally elevated left atrioventricular pressure gradient to move blood from the left atrium to the left ventricle. The elevated pulmonary venous and pulmonary arterial (PA) wedge pressures reduce pulmonary compliance, contributing to clinical symptoms.

Etiology Mitral stenosis and mixed MS and mitral regurgitation (MR) are generally rheumatic in origin. Other etiologies include infective endocarditis and mitral annular calcifications. Rarely, congenital defects, endomyocardial fibroelastosis, malignant carcinoid syndrome, and systemic lupus erythematosis (SLE) cause MS.

Diagnosis

Clinical Presentation Many patients deny symptoms because patients gradually reduce activity with the slow progression of disease. Clinical presentation includes:

- Exertional dyspnea (most common and often only symptom)
- Hemoptysis
- Thromboembolism
- Chest pain
- Infective endocarditis
- Right-sided heart failure

Physical Examination

- Murmur: Low-pitched, rumbling, diastolic murmur, heard best at the apex with the patient in the left lateral decubitus position. (Duration of the murmur corresponds with the severity.)
- Accentuated S_1
- Opening snap (OS)
- Prominent "a" wave in jugular venous pulsations with normal sinus rhythm

Treatment

Management An annual history and physical examination, as well as a chest x-ray and ECG, are recommended in asymptomatic patients. Endocarditis prophylaxis in indicated in patients with MS; however, no further medical therapy is indicated. When mild symptoms develop, diuretics may be helpful in reducing left atrial pressure and decreasing symptoms. If symptoms are more than mild or if there is evidence of pulmonary hypertension, mechanical intervention is warranted and delaying intervention worsens prognosis.

Surgery

Mitral balloon valvotomy is indicated in symptomatic patients with isolated MS whose valve orifice is <1.7 cm². Balloon valvotomy is the procedure of choice in individuals with mobile, thin leaflets with no or little calcium. If balloon valvotomy is not possible, a surgical ("open") valvotomy can be performed. Mitral valve replacement is indicated in individuals with MS and significant associated MR.

Aortic Regurgitation (AR)

General Principles

Etiology

- Abnormalities of valve leaflets: Rheumatic heart disease, endocarditis, congenital
- Aortic root disease: Aortic dilation/dissection, syphilitic aortitis, Marfan syndrome, rheumatoid spondylitis

Pathophysiology In AS, an abnormal regurgitation of blood from the aorta to the left ventricle occurs during diastole. As a result, the left ventricle must pump the regurgitant volume in addition to the normal volume returning from the left atria. An increase in left ventricular end-diastolic volume is the main hemodynamic compensation. The left ventricle undergoes adaptive change, namely, dilation and eccentric hypertrophy.

Diagnosis

Clinical Presentation Symptoms of dyspnea on exertion, fatigue, and decreased exercise tolerance appear due to left ventricular failure. Also, patients with AR may experience an uncomfortable sensation associated with large pulse pressure.

Physical Examination
- Murmur: Blowing diastolic murmur which is best heard with the patient leaning forward, after exhaling. The murmur may get louder with increased afterload (handgrip).
- Bounding pulse
- Widened pulse pressure
- Displaced cardiac impulse (down and to patient's left)

Treatment
Management Asymptomatic patients require regular clinical evaluation, assessment of left ventricular function, and endocarditis antibiotic prophylaxis. The mainstays of medical management in symptomatic patients are afterload reduction (vasodilators), which reduces the amount of aortic regurgitations. Long-acting nifedipine has been shown to delay the need for valve surgery.

Surgery Compelling evidence supports surgical correction before the onset of permanent left ventricular damage, even in asymptomatic patients. AR should be corrected in patients who remain symptomatic despite optimal medical therapy. Aortic valve replacement should also be performed with progressive left ventricular dysfunction and a left ventricular ejection fraction <55% or left ventricular end-systolic volume >55%—"55/55 Rule" (even if asymptomatic).

Mitral Regurgitation (MR)
General Principles
Pathophysiology A portion of the left ventricular output is forced backward into the left atrium (LA) leaving the forward cardiac output into the aorta reduced. In acute MR, the LA is normal size and relatively noncompliant. LA pressure rises dramatically with subsequent pulmonary edema and right heart failure. In chronic MR, dilation and eccentric hypertrophy of the LA occurs making the LA more compliant; therefore, pulmonary edema is less likely to develop.

Etiology
- Acute MR: Endocarditis, ruptured chordae, papillary muscle dysfunction
- Chronic MR: Rheumatic heart disease, myxomatous degeneration, congenial anomaly, infective endocarditis, hypertrophic cardiomyopathy

Diagnosis
Clinical Presentation The most common symptoms with chronic, severe MR include fatigue, exertional dyspea, and orthopnea. Patients with pulmonary vascular disease can develop right-sided heart failure. In acute, severe MR, left ventricular failure with acute pulmonary edema is common.

Physical Examination
- Murmur: Apical, holosystolic murmur at apex with radiation to left axilla. The murmur of MR will become louder with increased afterload (handgrip).
- Presence of S_3, which indicates severe disease
- Laterally displaced cardiac impulse

Treatment
Management Asymptomatic patients require regular clinical evaluation, assessment of left ventricular function, and endocarditis antibiotic prophylaxis. In a normotensive patient with acute severe MR, nitroprusside can be utilized to diminish the amount of MR, in turn increasing forward output and reducing pulmonary congestion. For the asymptomatic patient with chronic MR, there is no generally accepted medical therapy. There are no large long-term studies to indicate that the use of vasodilators are beneficial in chronic MR. Heart rate should be controlled with digitalis, rate-lowering calcium-channel blockers, or beta-blockers if atrial fibrillation develops.

Surgery The optimal timing of surgery in patient with chronic MR can be a difficult decision. Routine echocardiographic evaluation should be performed in individuals with severe MR. Surgery is recommended when a patient is symptomatic despite optimum medical management. Surgery should also be considered when left ventricular dysfunction is progressive, with left ventricular ejection fraction declining below 60% (even if asymptomatic).

Special Considerations

Mitral Valve Prolapse (MVP) MVP is an exceedingly common condition and often asymptomatic. Patients may present with symptomatic arrhythmia, atypical chest pain, or exaggerated autonomic symptoms. Physical examination reveals a click (with or without a murmur), which move toward S_2 with increased preload and increased afterload. Some patients require endocarditis antibiotic prophylaxis. The degree of pathology is related to the degree of MR. Beta-blockers can be used for symptomatic treatment of chest pain.

Valvular Heart Disease in the Athlete

Preparticipation Physical

The preparticipation physical should focus on a family history of heart disease; sudden death; personal history suggesting syncope, near syncope, or arrhythmia; and evaluation of heart murmurs in supine, sitting, standing, squatting, and postsquatting positions.

High-Risk Murmurs

Most common causes of serious valvular heart disease in athletes causing sudden death are mitral prolapse and subaortic stenosis (caused by hypertrophic cardiomyopathy).

Risk Assessment

The main issue with mitral valve prolapse is the degree of ectopy present, especially with exercise. In hypertrophic cardiomyopathy, the most significant problem is the degree of outflow obstruction, which is usually related to the thickness of the septum.

Valvular Heart Disease in Pregnancy

Etiology

Most murmurs in pregnancy are physiologic as there is a 50% increase in circulating blood volume during pregnancy.

Pre-Existing Disease

Pre-existing valvular heart disease often is exacerbated by pregnancy. The increased blood volume and enhanced cardiac output associated with normal pregnancy can accentuate the murmurs associated with **stenotic** heart valve lesions (e.g., MS, AS) whereas murmurs of AR or MR may actually ease in the face of lowered systemic vascular resistance.

Valvular Lesions with Increased Maternal and Fetal Risk

- Severe AS with or without symptoms
- MR or AR with NYHA functional Class III to IV symptoms
- MS with NYHA functional Class II to IV symptoms
- Valve disease resulting in severe pulmonary hypertension (pulmonary pressure $> 75\%$ of systemic pressures)
- Valve disease with severe left ventricular dysfunction (EF < 0.40)
- Mechanical prosthetic valves requiring anticoagulation
- AR in Marfan syndrome

Valvular Heart Disease in Infants and Children

Etiology

The physician must consider valvular heart disease as a subset of congenital heart disease. In diagnosis of murmurs in infants and children, think of congenital problems and then rule in or out a valvular etiology.

- **Left to right** shunts, e.g., VSD or atrial septal defect (ASD)
- **Obstructive lesions,** such as aortic stenosis, pulmonic stenosis, coarctation of the aorta
- **Valvular insufficiency**

Relative frequency of pathologic murmurs in infants: Of murmurs in congenital heart disease, 63% are caused by the six most common congenital defects:

- Pulmonic Stenosis > PDA > ASD > Coarctation of the aorta > Aortic Stenosis

Diagnosis

Findings more common in infants and children than in adults include grunting, poor feeding, sweating, poor weight gain, wheezing, decreased exercise tolerance, cough, and squatting after exercise (to increase preload). Cyanosis and edema are very late findings.

Treatment

Referrals Pediatric cardiologists do not order echocardiograms in a large percentage of patients seen in referral for murmur. This makes the strategy of referring all questionable murmurs to a pediatric cardiologist more cost-effective than ordering echocardiograms and referring only the pediatric patients with positive findings on echo.

Surgery Children who have congenital heart disease that might require surgery should be treated with input from a pediatric cardiologist. Reasons not to operate include the fact that some structural problems, such as VSD and PDA, sometimes resolve on their own. Other reasons not to operate include the fact that younger children are poorer operative candidates and that artificial valves will need to be replaced as the child grows. Reasons not to wait too long include irreversible processes (such as pulmonary hypertension) and irreversible structural damage (such as dilatation or hypertrophy of the ventricles).

References

1. Bonow RO, Carabello B, de Leon AC, et al. Guidelines for the management of patients with valvular heart disease: executive summary. A report of the American College of Cardiology/American Heart Association Task Force on Practice Guidelines (Committee on Management of Patients with Valvular Heart Disease). *Circulation* 1998;98:1949–1984.
2. Boon NA, Bloomfield P. The medical management of valvular heart disease. *Heart* 2002;87:395–400.
3. Carabello BA, Crawford FA. Valvular heart disease. *N Engl J Med* 1997;337:32–41.
4. Davies MK, Gibbs CR, Lipp GYH. ABC of heart failure—investigation. *BMJ* 2000;2730:297–300.
5. Liberthson RR. Sudden death from cardiac causes in children and young adults. *N Engl J Med* 1996;334:1039–1044.
6. Rosenhek R, et al. Predictors of outcome in severe asymptomatic aortic stenosis. *N Engl J Med* 2000;343:611–617.
7. Scognamiglio R, Rahimtoola SH, Fasoli G, et al. Nifedipine in asymptomatic patients with severe aortic regurgitation and normal left ventricular function. *N Engl J Med* 1994;331:689–694.
8. Shipton B, Wahba H. Valvular heart disease: review and update. *Am Fam Physician* 2001;63.
9. Spirito P, Bellone P, Harris K, et al. Magnitude of left ventricular hypertrophy and risk of sudden death in hypertrophic cardiomyopathy. *N Engl J Med* 2000;342:1778–1785.
10. Stapleton JF. Natural history of chronic valvular heart disease. *Cardiovasc Clin North Am* 1986;16:105–149.

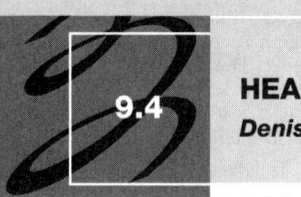

9.4

HEART FAILURE
Denise D. Barnard

GENERAL PRINCIPLES

Definition

Heart failure (HF) is a symptom complex deriving from cardiac dysfunction that may either be acute or chronic in its presentation. The "classic" presentation of acute, severe HF evokes an image of a patient with pink frothy pulmonary edema fluid and poor tissue perfusion. However, identical hemodynamic derangements are commonly found in the patient with chronic HF without extreme symptoms or dramatic physical examination signs, reflecting a slower, insidious onset. Therefore, while acute HF is readily diagnosed, signs and symptoms of chronic HF are frequently overlooked in clinical practice. This chapter focuses on the diagnosis, evaluation, and treatment of the patient with chronic HF due to left ventricular (LV) dysfunction.

HF results when the heart is unable to generate cardiac output sufficient to meet and maintain the metabolic requirements of the body without a marked elevation in filling pressure (either at rest, upon exertion, or under other physiologic demands). This working definition does not identify disease physiology in terms of the degree of systolic (ejection-related) or diastolic (relaxation-related) LV dysfunction, or consider disease etiology. HF may be associated with a wide spectrum of LV functional abnormalities, which may range from patients with normal LV size and preserved ejection fraction (EF) to those with severe LV dilatation and/or markedly reduced EF. In most patients, abnormalities of systolic and diastolic dysfunction coexist, regardless of EF.

Epidemiology

HF is a progressive syndrome affecting more than 5 million persons in the United States. It is the only cardiovascular disorder with increasing prevalence, especially among elderly individuals and in women. More than 550,000 new cases of HF are diagnosed annually. The incidence of HF approaches 10 per 1,000 population after age 65 and approximately 80% of patients hospitalized with HF are more than 65 years old. This common, yet *generally preventable,* syndrome is characterized by high mortality, frequent hospitalization, and reduced quality of life. HF is the most common Medicare diagnosis-related group and more Medicare dollars are spent for the diagnosis and treatment of HF than for any other diagnosis. It was estimated that the health care cost related to HF in the United States in 2005 was approximately $27.9 billion. Despite marked advances in medical therapy over the past two decades, the morbidity and mortality from HF remain unacceptably high, averaging 10% mortality at 1 year and 50% mortality at 5 years.

Classification

In 2001, the American College of Cardiology and the American Heart Association took an innovative approach to the classification of HF, one that emphasizes both the development and progression of the disease. This categorization identifies four stages involved in the development of the HF syndrome. The first two stages (A and B) are clearly not clinically overt HF, but are an attempt to help health care providers identify patients who are *at risk* for developing HF with the goal of prevention in mind. Stage C denotes the majority of patients diagnosed with clinical HF, and Stage D denotes patients who have developed refractory HF despite optimal therapy (Figure 9.4-1).

Within Stage C, the New York Heart Association (NYHA) classification system is traditionally used to categorize HF symptoms and estimate prognosis in clinical trials. To be useful in practice, one must be consider patients' baseline subjective symptoms in reference

	STAGE A	STAGE B	STAGE C	STAGE D
Stage descriptor	High risk for developing HF but does NOT have structural heart disease or symptoms of HF.	Has structural heart disease but does NOT have signs or symptoms of HF.	Has structural heart disease AND either prior or current symptoms of HF.	Has structural heart disease with refractory HF symptoms that requires special interventions.
Patient profile	Hypertension, diabetes, atherosclerotic disease, obesity or metabolic syndrome. Patients using cardiotoxins, with family history of cardiomyopathy.	Left ventricular hypertrophy, prior myocardial infarction, valvular or other heart disease but remains asymptomatic.	Any structural heart disease with symptoms or signs of HF. Even if symptoms resolve on medical therapy, patient remains Stage C.	Symptoms at rest despite maximal medical therapy, recurrent hospitalizations, or requiring special interventions such as cardiac transplantation or hospice care.
Key point	Heart failure is preventable at this stage.	Heart failure is still preventable at this stage.	Heart failure treatment slows disease progression and reduces morbidity and mortality at this stage.	End-stage HF has limited therapeutic options.

Figure 9.4-1. AHA/ACC classification system for chronic HF in the adult.

to a normal expected activity level for someone their age. NYHA Class I patients have no perceived symptoms or limitations in performing their regular daily physical activities. Class II patients have symptoms of HF with slight or moderate levels of activity. Class III patients have marked limitation of activity but are comfortable at rest. Class IV patients have symptoms of HF at rest.

Pathophysiology

HF is the clinical syndrome resulting from acute, chronic, or repetitive cardiac injury. Inciting factors include conditions as diverse as myocardial infarction (MI) and myocyte damage due to a viral infection or chemotherapeutic agent. This is explained by the observation that regardless of the initial injury, the adaptive systemic response to altered cardiac function as well as the resultant cardiac structural changes and cellular processes that develop within the heart itself are remarkably consistent. The characteristic pathophysiology of HF derives from systemic and local cardiac neurohormonal activation designed to be compensatory in nature, but results in deleterious changes in myocardial structure and cellular function in areas that were previously normal. This process is termed "*cardiac remodeling*," whose key features include the following:

- Remodeling is initiated by a threshold-reaching injury to the heart resulting in systemic and local neurohormonal activation—renin–angiotensin–aldosterone (RAAS) and sympathetic nervous systems.
- Neurohormonal activation results in additional myocardial damage that continues after resolution of the initiating event and tends to progress over time.
- Cardiac remodeling therefore results in increased cardiac chamber volumes and muscle mass (eccentric LV hypertrophy), increased extracellular matrix deposition, and myocardial fibrosis.

Etiology

The most frequent etiology of HF in the United States is coronary artery disease. Hypertensive or valvular heart disease and primary cardiomyopathy (familial or idiopathic) are also common entities. Myocardial dysfunction can also be secondary to infectious, metabolic, endocrine, nutritional, or toxic causes (notably alcohol and anthracyclines); connective tissue or pericardial diseases; neuromuscular or autoimmune disorders; as well as infiltrative diseases (amyloidosis, hemochromatosis, sarcoidosis) or undiagnosed congenital heart disease. This chapter does not address the category of high-output HF (due to thyrotoxicosis, sepsis, severe anemia, beriberi, Paget disease, myeloma, pregnancy, or significant arteriovenous shunting).

DIAGNOSIS

Clinical Presentation

The clinical presentation of a patient with HF can be quite subtle, and patients with significant degrees of LV dysfunction may be asymptomatic. Because early diagnosis and treatment reduce morbidity and mortality, successful therapy depends on clinical suspicion and screening for signs and/or symptoms of HF in all patients at risk for its development (Stages A and B). The clinical presentation of a patient with Stage C (overt) HF may be acute but often is more insidious and progressive. Acute or sudden-onset HF (minutes to hours) should prompt evaluation for myocardial ischemia/infarction, arrhythmia, abrupt valvular or LV structural deterioration, or hypertensive urgency producing an acute change in LV pressure or volume-loading conditions. Subacute-onset HF (days to weeks) is quite common, as mild symptoms of HF are often unrecognized or ignored by the patient until they become severe or persistent at rest.

History and Symptoms

- **Pertinent history** should include information regarding the risk factors for or extent of existing myocardial injury. These include hypertension, diabetes, dyslipidemia, coronary or peripheral vascular disease, myopathy, valvular heart disease, rheumatic fever, mediastinal irradiation, sleep-disordered breathing, exposure to cardiotoxic agents, current or past alcohol or amphetamine abuse, smoking, collagen vascular disease, HIV infection, thyroid disorder, pheochromocytoma, and morbid obesity. In addition, a family history of sudden cardiac death, cardiomyopathy, or tachyarrhythmias should be sought.
- **Symptoms** *strongly suggesting* a diagnosis of HF include dyspnea at rest or on exertion, orthopnea, paroxysmal nocturnal dyspnea (PND), nocturnal or recumbent cough or other sleep disturbance, pedal or scrotal edema, impaired exercise capacity or endurance. Less specific presentations of HF include early satiety, nausea and vomiting, abdominal discomfort or bloating, ascites, exertional wheezing, unexplained fatigue, weakness, or malaise, mental confusion or impaired concentrating ability, and daytime oliguria with recumbent nocturia. The spectrum of symptoms in a given patient reflects the relative extent of systemic and/or pulmonary venous congestion related to fluid overload versus reduced cardiac output (hypoperfusion).
- In a patient with known LV dysfunction and previously diagnosed HF, provocative and exacerbating factors should also be reviewed. Common precipitants are dietary sodium excess, medication noncompliance, interaction, or errors, substance abuse, uncontrolled diabetes or hypertension, infection, thyroid dysfunction, arrhythmia or silent myocardial ischemia, renal or hepatic insufficiency, over-the-counter medication use of nonsteroidal anti-inflammatory drugs (NSAIDs), pregnancy, and other physical or emotional stressors.

Physical Examination

- **Acute, decompensated HF.** The classic findings of acute, decompensated "congestive" HF include a resting tachycardia, tachypnea, diffuse pulmonary rales, and an abnormal apical impulse (enlarged, diffuse, displaced, dyskinetic, or sustained). In acute, decompensated "low output" HF, systemic hypoperfusion may be manifest as by hypotension, a reduced pulse pressure or pulsus alternans, diminished carotid upstroke volume,

Cheyne–Stokes respirations, cool extremities, and altered mentation. These patients will generally require acute hospitalization.

- **Chronic HF.** In chronic HF it is very common to find fairly clear lung fields with coarse breath sounds or reduced respiratory diaphragmatic excursion. Bibasilar or diffuse rales are observed typically when filling pressures are rapidly or markedly elevated. Pleural effusions, when present, are more right-sided than left, or bilateral. The greater the number of symptoms and signs observed in a given patient, the more reliable is the diagnosis of HF. The most specific physical findings are an elevated jugular venous pressure, an S_3, a laterally displaced apical impulse, pulmonary rales that do not clear with cough, and peripheral edema not due to venous insufficiency. Nonspecific physical findings include cardiomegaly or an abnormal apical impulse, an S_4, and tachypnea.

- Signs of biventricular or predominant "right-heart" failure include an elevated jugular venous pressure, right ventricular (RV) parasternal lift or subxiphoid tap, RV gallop, loud P_2 (pulmonary hypertension), abdominojugular reflux, pulsatile or tender hepatomegaly, ascites, and peripheral (dependent) edema. Signs of right-sided HF without signs of LV dysfunction may redirect your attention to primary or secondary pulmonary vascular diseases. Murmurs may reveal the cause of HF (valvular stenosis or regurgitation, hypertrophic cardiomyopathy with outflow tract obstruction) or in the case of mitral regurgitation, a possible consequence of LV remodeling and enlargement.

Diagnostic Testing

- **Electrocardiography.** The baseline electrocardiogram should be assessed for signs of infarction, arrhythmia, conduction delays, chamber enlargement or hypertrophy, which may provide clues suggesting the underlying etiology. Low QRS voltage may indicate an occult primary or secondary infiltrative myocardial disease such as amyloidosis. Nonspecific ST-T wave abnormalities are common. The QT interval may be prolonged, and implies electrolyte abnormalities, myocardial disease, drug effects, and/or risk for ventricular tachycardia.

- **Chest radiography.** It is important to note that a normal chest radiograph does not rule out the diagnosis of HF, but may afford a differential diagnosis. The chest x-ray can yield information on HF etiology and the degree of fluid overload or hemodynamic compensation. The cardiothoracic ratio and silhouette show that cardiac chambers are grossly enlarged. The amount of pulmonary vascular crowding, upper lobe redistribution, edema, Kerley B lines, or pleural effusions points more to volume status in the chronic setting and to the time course of hemodynamic alterations in the acute setting.

- **Blood tests.** Laboratory tests that should be obtained include thyroid-function tests (especially thyroid-stimulating hormone), because both hyperthyroidism and hypothyroidism can be a primary or contributory cause of HF. For guiding medical management, perform a complete blood count (CBC), serum electrolytes, creatinine, albumin, liver function tests, and urinalysis. Obtain other laboratory tests such as HIV or other viral serologies, serum transferrin and iron saturation, rheumatologic only if indicated by history and physical examination.

- When uncertainty exists about the diagnosis of HF, a low plasma brain natriuretic peptide (BNP) or pro-BNP level may be used to exclude HF as a cause of dyspnea with a high degree of certainty (high negative predictive value). Several natriuretic peptides are synthesized by and released from the heart in response to hemodynamic perturbations. The BNP concentration has *not* been shown to be effective in screening and identifying asymptomatic patients with ventricular dysfunction. Elevations in plasma BNP levels are seen in acute, decompensated and chronic HF, acute MI, myocardial ischemia and LV hypertrophy. Marked elevations in BNP levels correlate with symptoms and the degree of LV systolic dysfunction (EF). However, a modestly elevated BNP level can occur in other settings, such as pulmonary embolism and cor pulmonale. Likewise, the normal range of BNP is higher in women than men, and in both sexes increases with age and with declining renal function. Further, in the setting of morbid obesity, BNP levels may be disproportionately low.

- **Echocardiograpy.** The most valuable and cost-effective test in the diagnosis of HF is two-dimensional echocardiography with Doppler imaging, which facilitates the detection of abnormalities in myocardial, valvular, and pericardial structure and function.

One major determinant of the appropriate course of therapy for HF is determination of whether the LV EF is preserved or reduced. This information is quantified by echocardiography, along with cardiac chamber dimensions and/or volumes, LV wall thickness, and ventricular filling dynamics. Further, it provides an estimation of intracardiac hemodynamics, and an evaluation of chamber geometry and regional wall motion. Alternatively, LV or RV EF and filling dynamics can be determined by radionuclide imaging. An EF greater than 0.50 is considered normal by these techniques, while an LV EF of 0.40 or less reflects significant systolic dysfunction. Diastolic LV dysfunction can be present and contribute to HF symptoms in the setting of a low, normal, or increased EF. Population studies suggest that up to 40% of patients with significant HF have preserved EF and predominant diastolic LV dysfunction. Magnetic resonance imaging or computed tomography is useful in evaluating ventricular size, function, and mass, detecting right ventricular dysplasia or pericardial disease, and in some cases can distinguish viable myocardium vs. infarcted or fibrotic scar tissue. It is more expensive, however, and less widely available.

■ **Other diagnostic testing.** Once the clinical diagnosis of HF is confirmed with supportive data from echocardiography, the remainder of diagnostic testing is directed at determining the underlying etiology. Irrespective of LV EF, in all patients with HF, the etiology that is most important to consider and exclude is coronary artery disease. Strategies involving noninvasive evaluation or coronary angiography are best chosen based on symptoms, signs, and coronary heart disease risk factors.

Prognostic Assessment

An assessment of prognosis should be considered an integral part of the evaluation of a patient with HF at the time of diagnosis and periodically thereafter. Each of the following is an easy-to-measure variable that lends independent, additive prognostic information.

■ **Extent of LV dysfunction.** LV EF less than 0.35 with lower values worse, significant LV enlargement, dilation, or concomitant restrictive filling dynamics (significant diastolic dysfunction) denote an extremely high-risk patient. Concomitant RV enlargement or dysfunction worsens prognosis further.

■ **Symptom class.** Risk worsens with higher NYHA class, with NYHA IV having a 30% to 50% annual mortality risk. Persistent moderate to severe HF symptoms despite standard medical therapy warrants consideration of patient referral to an HF specialist.

■ **Hemodynamics.** Clinical, echocardiographically estimated or measured pulmonary hypertension in the setting of LV systolic dysfunction carries a worse prognosis and is an indication for more aggressive therapy.

■ **Exercise capacity.** Although age dependent, the inability to walk more than 300 meters in a 6-minute walk test (for any reason) infers substantially greater annual risk of death or morbidity compared with a patient who can walk 450 meters or more. Markedly impaired oxygen consumption with exercise, measured as a VO_2 max <15 mL/kg/min, or achieving less than 4 to 5 metabolic equivalents (METS) of work on bicycle or treadmill exercise test has a markedly adverse prognosis. Significant exercise impairment corresponds to a 1-year mortality rate of 20% or higher.

■ **Arrhythmia.** Atrial fibrillation, atrial or ventricular tachyarrhythmias, or evidence of other conduction system disease such as arteriovenous (AV) nodal block or left bundle branch block worsen prognosis. Any family history of sudden death. Approximately 50% to 70% of patients with low EF and symptomatic HF have episodes of nonsustained ventricular tachycardia on routine ambulatory electrocardiographic monitoring; this is generally not indicated for screening purposes in the absence of symptoms.

■ **Hyponatremia.** Serum sodium concentration of 135 mg per dL or less is generally related to intense renin–angiotensin system activation and denotes a higher-risk patient.

■ **Chronic kidney disease.** Significant renal insufficiency not due to expected (reversible) medication effects.

Assessment of Comorbidities

Patients and practitioners often underestimate the substantial influence of comorbid diagnoses or conditions on the clinical course and stability of patients with HF. These common conditions include atherosclerosis, hyperlipidemia, diabetes, hypertension, thyroid dysfunction, anemia, obstructive sleep apnea, and obesity. Treating them reduces ongoing or prevents additional cardiovascular injury. Intercurrent infections can trigger HF decompensation due to fever and physiologic stress and should be treated early and aggressively. Immunizations and general health care maintenance should be kept up to date.

Differential Diagnosis

The differential diagnosis of a patient with prominent *dyspnea* ± *edema* includes pulmonary parenchymal disease (obstructive vs. interstitial), pulmonary thromboembolic disease, cor pulmonale, pulmonary veno-occlusive disease, primary or secondary pulmonary arterial hypertension, exertional asthma, severe anemia, mitral stenosis, neuromuscular disease, constrictive pericarditis, or metabolic causes (i.e., acidosis). The differential diagnosis of a patient with predominant *edema* ± *dyspnea* includes severe venous insufficiency, nephrotic syndrome, cirrhosis, lymphedema, combined vascular insufficiency, and adverse medication effects (i.e., dihydropyridine calcium-channel blockers).

TREATMENT

Pharmacologic Management of Chronic HF and Systolic LV Dysfunction

The majority of clinical research trials that have established the foundation of traditional medical therapy have focused on HF with systolic LV dysfunction (LVD). The implicit goals of treating chronic HF are (a) improve patient symptoms and quality of life, (b) slow or reverse the progression of cardiac dysfunction, and (c) reduce HF mortality, morbidity, and therefore the cost burden of acute care. Since the pathophysiology of HF is complex, so follows the pharmacologic regimen. Angiotensin-converting enzyme inhibitors (ACE-Is) and beta (β)-blockers have become the cornerstone of therapy to delay, halt, or reverse cardiac remodeling and improve mortality. In addition, the roles of diuretic therapy, aldosterone inhibition, digoxin, and other vasodilator therapy are reviewed.

Angiotensin-Converting Enzyme Inhibitors

Contemporary treatment guidelines for systolic LVD mandate that an ACE-I be utilized as primary therapy unless contraindicated. ACE-Is improve hemodynamics by reducing afterload and attenuate the vasoconstrictor activity of angiotensin II (Ang II). Ang II also has thrombogenic, atherogenic, profibrotic, and other effects that contribute to progressive LV remodeling. ACE-Is improve HF symptoms and quality of life. The progression of HF is slowed by ACE-I therapy, as evidenced in clinical trials by a survival benefit and fewer hospitalizations. ACE-Is are indicated for use in the primary prevention of HF in patients at risk, post-MI patients regardless of EF, and in patients with documented LVD regardless of symptoms (AHA Stages A to D).

ACE-I are typically initiated at low dose and up-titrated over days to weeks until side effects are noted or the dose reaches the equivalent of those used in the HF trials (Table 9.4-1). In general, higher achieved doses result in greater reductions in morbidity and hospitalization for HF, but mortality reduction is seen at virtually all doses. Electrolytes and renal function should be checked before initiation, after every dose increase, and after addition of other medications. Hypotension is seen most frequently during the first few days of initiation or dose increase, particularly in patients with hypovolemia, a recent large diuresis, or severe hyponatremia (serum sodium under 130 mmol/L). ACE-Is lower blood pressure and alter intrarenal hemodynamics, inducing a predictable increase in serum creatinine. A modest elevation and plateau in blood urea nitrogen and serum creatinine concentration are expected with the use of diuretics and/or vasodilator therapy in HF. Progressively worsening renal function, however (i.e., serum creatinine increase of more than 0.3 mg/dL over a normal baseline, or a serum creatinine >2.5 to 3.0 mg/dL, may represent renal hypoperfusion due to a reduction in cardiac output or renal perfusion pressure.

In the absence of hyperkalemia, most HF experts will still initiate ACE-I therapy in a patient with a serum creatinine ≤3 mg per dL, employing an agent that is hepatically

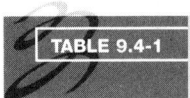

TABLE 9.4-1	Angiotensin-Converting Enzyme Inhibitors (ACE-Is) and Angiotensin Receptor Blockers (ARBs) Commonly Used for the Treatment of Chronic HF (Generic Names Listed)	

ACE-I	Starting dose	Maximum dose
Captopril	6.25 mg 3 times daily	50 mg 3 times daily
Enalapril	2.5 mg twice daily	10–20 mg twice daily
Fosinopril	5–10 mg daily	40 mg daily
Lisinopril	2.5–5 mg daily	20–40 mg daily
Perindopril	2 mg daily	8–16 mg daily
Quinapril	5 mg twice daily	20 mg twice daily
Ramipril	1.25–2.5 mg daily	10 mg daily
Trandolapril	1 mg daily	4 mg daily
ARBs	**Starting dose**	**Maximum dose**
Candesartan	4–8 mg daily	32 mg daily
Irbesartan	75 mg daily	150–300 mg
Eprosartan	300 mg daily	800 mg daily
Losartan	25–50 mg daily	50–100 mg daily
Olmesartan	10 mg daily	20–40 mg daily
Telmesartan	20 mg daily	40–80 mg daily
Valsartan	20–40 mg twice daily	160 mg twice daily

cleared to prevent drug or metabolite accumulation and profound hypotension. Other side effects of ACE-Is include orthostatic hypotension, dizziness, hyponatremia, cough, and angioedema. Cough develops in 5% to 10% of patients on an ACE-I but is much more common, up to 50%, in Asian/Chinese populations. Cough represents the most common reason for drug withdrawal. Note that cough may also represent worsening HF or other conditions, and if not resolved after a temporary discontinuation of the drug, the ACE-I should be restarted. Angioedema can be mild, or life-threatening in severe cases. Its prevalence is estimated at <1%, but is more common in black populations.

Angiotensin Receptor Blockers

This class of drugs has become an acceptable alternative to ACE-Is for both the prevention and treatment of HF. The most convincing data regarding the efficacy of angiotensin receptor blockers (ARBs) in HF therapy derives from the recent Candesartan in Heart Failure Assessment of Reduction in Mortality and Morbidity Trial (CHARM). The CHARM study had three placebo-controlled arms, one evaluating candesartan as an alternative to an ACE-I, the second as added therapy, and the third as therapy in patients with HF and preserved LV EF. In each arm, therapeutic benefit was observed.

Like ACE-Is, ARBs are also initiated at low dose and up-titrated over days to weeks (Table 9.4-1). An ARB is the best substitute for an ACE-I when the latter induces cough. The risk of angioedema is much lower with ARBs, but has been observed in approximately 8% of patients given an ARB *after* developing angioedema to the former drug. Other ARB side effects are quite similar to those of the ACE-I class of agents. Aside from the pathway of drug metabolism, little difference exists between the available ACE-Is and ARBs, the choice of agent becomes clinician or formulary preference.

β-Blockers

The pivotal trials that provided incontrovertible evidence of the efficacy of β-blocker therapy in patients with chronic HF were the U.S. Carvedilol Trials Program, Cardiac Insufficiency Bucindolol Study-2 (CIBIS-II), and the Metroprolol CR/XL Randomized Intervention Trial in Congestive Heart Failure (MERIT–HF) study. HF guidelines state

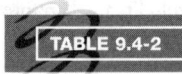

TABLE 9.4-2	**Beta (β-) Blocking Drugs Approved for the Treatment of Chronic HF with Systolic Left Ventricular Dysfunction**	
β-Blocker	Initial dose and typical increment during up-titration	Treatment dose goal in clinical trials
Bisoprolol	1.25 mg daily	10 mg daily
Carvedilol	3.125 mg twice daily	25 mg twice daily 50 mg twice daily if >85 kg
Metoprolol CR/XL	12.5–25 mg daily	200 mg daily

that only carvedilol, metoprolol, or bucindolol should be added to background ACE-I or ARB therapy (Table 9.4-2). The reason for this is that β-blockers are a very heterogeneous group of agents, exhibiting variable selectivity for β-receptors, marked differences in pharmacokinetics, and many have ancillary vasodilating or additional antioxidant properties. First, the patient should be carefully evaluated for clinical stability and should be considered euvolemic.

β-Blockers should be started at low dose and in general, up-titrated approximately every 2 weeks, with target doses reached in about 8 to 12 weeks. Patients should be followed carefully for signs of impending decompensation or side effects (fluid retention, hypotension, dyspnea, fatigue, bradycardia, or heart block). Patients who manifest worsening HF symptoms or fluid retention should have diuretic medications adjusted. A temporary dose reduction in ACE-I, ARB, or other vasoactive medications may be necessary when symptomatic hypotension is present. With careful observation the vast majority of patients can tolerate β-blocker therapy and achieve target doses. In general, patients on chronic β-blocker therapy experiencing an acute decompensation should remain on their β-blocker, or be given a reduced dose and up-titrated again following symptomatic resolution. Avoid abrupt discontinuation, especially in patients with underlying ischemic heart disease. If the initiation or up-titration of β-blockers to target doses proves difficult, consider referral to an HF specialist.

Other Vasodilators

For patients with HF and LV systolic dysfunction intolerant of ACE-I or ARB therapy (due to renal dysfunction or hyperkalemia), the combination of hydralazine (H) and isosorbide dinitrate (ISDN) is recommended. The mortality benefit with H-ISDN is not as great as that seen with ACE-Is or ARBs but is significantly better than those of placebo or vasodilatory α-blockers (prazosin). The H-ISDN combination is appealing in chronic kidney disease, as it tends to increase renal cortical blood flow. Side effects including headache, dizziness, diarrhea, tachycardia, and somnolence are significant with this regimen; up to 25% of patients will discontinue one or both. The benefit of nitrates is presumed to be related to enhanced nitric oxide bioavailability. Hydralazine is a direct-acting vasodilator, but also reduces nitrate tolerance. Nitrate therapy is useful in decreasing orthopnea and PND and tends to improve exercise tolerance in patients who have persistent limitations despite optimization of other therapies.

The African-American Heart Failure Trial (A-HeFT) enrolled 1,050 self-identified African American patients who had NYHA class III or IV HF with LV dilation and systolic dysfunction. A new fixed-dose combination of H-ISDN (or placebo) was utilized in addition to background therapy of an ACE-I or ARB, a β-blocker, and a loop diuretic. Many patients were also taking digoxin and an aldosterone antagonist. Patients receiving the H-ISDN combination demonstrated a 43% reduction in all-cause death and a 33% reduction in first HF hospitalizations and a significant improvement in quality of life. The fixed dose combination (BiDil) includes 37.5 mg H and 20 mg ISDN, and was titrated to 225/120 mg per day in three divided doses in this study.

The Prospective Randomized Amlodipine Survival Evaluation Trial-2 (PRAISE-2) added amlodipine or placebo to background HF therapy of an ACE-I, digoxin, and diuretics in nonischemic cardiomyopathy and symptomatic HF. There was no survival advantage (or disadvantage) attributable to amlodipine administration in this population, and very little data regarding patients also taking β-blockers. Amlodipine therefore becomes a third- or fourth-line choice, generally when another antihypertensive agent is necessary despite the medications discussed above.

Digitalis

Digoxin remains a useful drug in HF with systolic LVD two centuries after its initial use. Digoxin withdrawal from patients with stable chronic HF on an ACE-I contributes to decompensation requiring treatment or hospital admission, reduced exercise capacity, and lower quality-of-life scores. In the Digitalis Investigation Group (DIG) trial, the addition of digoxin to baseline therapy had a neutral effect on mortality but decreased hospitalizations for HF. Digoxin increases EF by 3% to 5% due to its positive inotropic effects mediated by sodium–potassium pump inhibition. More importantly, digoxin improves rest and exercise LV hemodynamics, and is sympathoinhibitory, attenuating the neurohormonal and baroreceptor abnormalities seen in chronic HF. This latter role as neurohormonal antagonist may be the more important mechanism of action, as all other agents with positive inotropic activity have increased HF mortality in clinical trials.

Digoxin therapy may be limited by renal insufficiency and conduction abnormalities (heart block, slow atrial fibrillation) but is generally well tolerated, with few side effects at recommended doses. Current guidelines state its use should be considered if HF symptoms remain after ACE-I and β-blocker titration when the EF remains less than 0.40. Loading doses are unnecessary and most patients should be prescribed a dose of 0.125 mg daily. Measurement of digoxin levels is now recommended, as data from the DIG trial data suggest adverse outcomes are related to a serum digoxin concentration greater than 0.8 to 1.0 ng per mL. Digoxin trough levels should also be obtained if there is clinical suspicion of toxicity due to signs or symptoms and to determine if dose (or dose frequency) reduction is indicated in the setting of worsening renal function, loss of lean body mass, or if additional medications are prescribed that have known or possible interactions that may elevate the serum digoxin concentration (verapamil, quinidine, amiodarone, spinolactone, and some antibiotics).

Diuretics

Diuretic therapy is indicated for symptoms or signs of systemic or pulmonary congestion due to volume overload. Diuretics relieve congestive symptoms by promoting excretion of excess sodium and therefore water (Table 9.4-3). There are no controlled clinical trial data prospectively evaluating the overall impact of diuretic therapy on mortality in patients with HF. Diuretics promote activation of the RAAS, potentiate the hypotensive effects of ACE-Is/ARBs, and may decrease cardiac output, especially in patients with diastolic LVD. Chronic diuretic therapy can be limited by the development of diuretic resistance or refractoriness. Diuretics also induce hypokalemia, hypomagnesemia, hyperuricemia and promote calciuria. Electrolytes magnesium, require close monitoring when diuretics are used.

Thiazide diuretics should be used if fluid retention is mild, but are effective only when the glomerular filtration rate is greater than 30 mL per minute. Loop diuretics are the

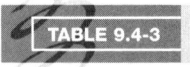

TABLE 9.4-3	Commonly Used Diuretic Drugs for the Treatment of Sodium and Fluid Retention in Chronic HF	
Thiazide class	**Initial oral dose**	**Recommended maximal oral dose**
Chlorothiazide	250 mg daily	500 mg daily
Hydrochlorothiazide	25 mg daily	50–100 mg daily
Metolazone	2.5 mg daily	10 mg daily
Loop diuretics	**Initial oral dose**	**Recommended maximal oral dose**
Furosemide	10–40 mg daily or twice daily	200 mg daily or twice daily
Bumetanide	0.5–1.0 daily or twice daily	4-5 mg daily or twice daily
Torsemide	10 mg daily	200 mg daily

mainstay of diuretic therapy in HF when congestion is moderate. When fluid retention is extreme or the patient has become refractory to loop diuretics, intravenous administration of a loop diuretic or the addition of the thiazide-like agent metolazone (1 to 5 mg 30 minutes to 1 hour prior to loop agent) can dramatically increase natriuresis. Potassium-sparing diuretics should be used with caution in patients on ACE-Is or ARBs and in patients with diabetes prone to type IV renal tubular acidosis.

Aldosterone Inhibitors

The Randomized Aldosterone Evaluation Study (RALES) demonstrated a beneficial effect on mortality due to progressive HF from low-dose spironolactone in patients with a recent hospitalization, and continued moderate to severe HF symptoms on ACE-I or ARB therapy. Only one third of the RALES population received β-blockers. Clinical guidelines recommend that normokalemic patients with serum creatinine less than 2.5 mg per dL and moderate to severe HF receive spironolactone 12.5 to 25 mg daily. Serum sodium and potassium should be checked at 1 week, frequently thereafter, and at any time there is a change in dosage of any medication that may influence potassium balance. Strong consideration should be given to lowering or eliminating supplemental potassium when spironolactone is added to the regimen, to lessen the risk of potentially fatal hyperkalemia.

Pharmacologic Management of Chronic HF and Preserved LV EF

Coronary artery disease and hypertension should be aggressively treated, if present. β-Blockers, ACE-Is, ARBs, and calcium-channel blockers have all been shown to be useful and may promote regression of LV hypertrophy and attenuate cardiac remodeling. Diuretics are typically necessary for congestive symptoms, but excessive preload reduction (nitrates, diuretics) can impair cardiac output and exacerbate hypotension and should be used cautiously. There is no apparent role for digoxin therapy in a patient with diastolic LVD. Patients with atrial fibrillation and rapid ventricular response intolerant of or refractory to β-blocker therapy, calcium-channel blocker therapy, or amiodarone therapy should be referred to an electrophysiologist for possible catheter ablation.

Evaluation of Exacerbating or Provocative Factors

Assess frequently for medication nonadherence or dietary noncompliance (sodium, alcohol, excess fluids), drug abuse, medication additions (calcium-channel blockers in systolic LVD, NSAIDs, glitazones, remicade, and other agents), uncontrolled hypertension or diabetes, decreasing renal or hepatic function, thyroid abnormalities, anemia, infection, ischemia or infarction, arrhythmias, pulmonary embolism, new valvular dysfunction, sleep apnea, and certain over-the-counter medication or supplement use. Because depression is common in HF and worsens clinical course, patients should be screened and treated.

Nonpharmacologic HF Therapies

Patient Education

Discuss with the patient *and family* the diagnosis and reason(s) for the development of HF, including prognosis and intended treatment plan. Symptoms referable to HF should be reviewed and patients instructed to call if symptoms are noted or increased, particularly rapid weight gain or loss. Emphasize sodium restriction to 3 or preferably 2 g per day, along with daily weight monitoring. Stress the importance of medication adherence, good nutrition, and physical activity. Fluid restriction is necessary only when excessive or when volume status is difficult to manage with diuretics and sodium restriction. Smoking cessation should be advocated. Guidelines recommend that patients' literacy, cognitive status, psychologic state, culture, and access to social and financial resources be taken into account for optimal education and counseling.

Written educational materials are quite useful and downloadable from the Heart Failure Society of America web site (www.hfsa.org or www.abouthf.org). Consider referral to a dietician or disease management program (home or clinic based, or via telemonitoring services) when patient understanding is an impairment to the success of your plan of care. These programs have been shown to significantly reduce HF hospitalizations, produce shorter lengths of stay, lower health care costs, and improve both quality of life and survival.

Exercise

Several controlled trials have shown that exercise training can lessen symptoms, increase exercise capacity, and improve the quality of life of patients with chronic HF. Exercise prescriptions (aerobic and light resistance training) are generally safe in compensated HF. Exercise testing may give patients more confidence in beginning a moderate exercise program or in resuming more of their normal activities, including sex. Cardiac rehabilitation programs may be an option, based on eligibility and insurance coverage.

Biventricular Pacemakers

Dyssynchronous contraction between the LV and RV can be improved by electrically activating the right and left ventricles in a synchronized manner with a biventricular pacemaker device. Cardiac resynchronization therapy (CRT) appears to improve LV EF, reduce secondary mitral regurgitation, and improve HF symptoms (when moderate to severe), as well as exercise capacity and quality of life. There is strong evidence to support the use of CRT to improve survival and to decrease hospitalizations in patients with persistently symptomatic HF receiving optimal medical therapy who have cardiac dyssynchrony (evidenced by a prolonged QRS duration) and an EF of 35% or less.

Automated Implanted Cardiac Defibrillators

Current guidelines recommend prophylactic automated implanted cardiac defibrillators (AICD) implantation in patients with EF less than 30% and mild to moderate HF symptoms when at least 1-year survival with good functional capacity is expected. Again, optimal medical therapy should be previously employed with a sustained reduction in EF. AICDs are generally not warranted in patients with refractory HF (Stage D) or in patients with concomitant diseases that shorten life expectancy independent of HF. The management of patients with an LV EF between 30% and 35% remains controversial. AICDs have bradycardia and antitachycardia pacing capabilities as well. Although highly effective in preventing sudden death, frequent shocks (appropriate or inappropriate) reduce quality of life and increase patient anxiety.

Mechanical Circulatory Assist Devices and Cardiac Transplantation

Cardiac transplantation is currently the only established surgical approach for refractory (Stage D) HF, but it is available to fewer than 2,500 patients in the United States each year. Nonetheless, patients with refractory HF despite standard therapy should be referred to a transplant center for evaluation. Cardiomyoplasty and left ventriculectomy (Batista procedure) have been abandoned as they had high mortality and survivors failed to show meaningful clinical improvement. Mechanical circulatory assist devices are utilized primarily as a "bridge to transplant," as high 1-year mortality and the cost of these devices have limited their application as "destination" therapy for patients ineligible for transplantation.

Advanced Directives

It is mandatory that discussions about advance directives occur in context with prognosis. These are best performed in the office setting following HF diagnosis, and after hospitalization or change in clinical status. Include the spouse, or a close family member. Consider referral to a Disease Management or Advanced Heart Failure Treatment Program. Utilization of end-of-life care services such as hospice care should occur after full and appropriate application of evidence-based pharmacologic and nonpharmacologic treatments.

References

1. American Heart Association. *Heart disease and stroke statistics: 2005 update.* Dallas, TX: American Heart Association; 2005.
2. Masoudi FA, Havranek EP, Krumholz HM. The burden of chronic congestive HF in older persons: magnitude and implications for policy and research. *Heart Fail Rev* 2002;7:9–16.
3. Cohn JN, Ferrari R, Sharpe N. Cardiac remodeling-concepts and clinical implications: a consensus paper from an international forum on cardiac remodeling. *J Am Coll Cardiol* 2000;35:569–582.
4. Greenberg B, Hermann D. *Contemporary diagnosis and management of heart failure.* 3rd ed. Newtown, PA: Handbooks in Healthcare; 2005.

5. Chatterjee K. Physical examination in heart failure. In: Hosenpud JD, Greenberg BH, eds. *Congestive heart failure, pathophysiology, diagnosis and comprehensive approach to management.* 3rd ed. Philadelphia, PA: Lippincott Williams & Wilkins; 2007:615–627.

6. Zile MR, Brutsaert DL. New concepts in diastolic dysfunction and diastolic heart failure: Part I. Diagnosis, prognosis and measurements of diastolic function. *Circulation* 2002;105:1387–1393.

7. Vitarelli A, Tiukinhoy S, Di LS, et al. The role of echocardiography in the diagnosis and management of heart failure. *Heart Fail Rev* 2003;8:181–189.

8. Hermann DD, Greenberg BH. Prognostic factors In: Poole-Wilson P, Colucci W, Massie B, et al., eds. *Heart failure: scientific principles & clinical practice.* Churchill Livingstone; New York 1997;439–454.

9. Mueller C, Scholer A, Laule-Kilian K, et al. Use of B-type natriuretic peptide in the evaluation and management of acute dyspnea. *N Engl J Med* 2004;350:647–654.

10. Heart Outcomes Prevention Evaluation Study Investigators. Effects of angiotensin-converting-enzyme inhibitor, ramipril, on cardiovascular events in high-risk patients. *N Engl J Med* 2000;342:145–153.

11. Hunt SA. ACC/AHA 2005 guideline update for the diagnosis and management of chronic heart failure in the adult: a report of the American College of Cardiology/American Heart Association Task Force on Practice Guidelines. *J Am Coll Cardiol* 2005;46(6):e1–82. Erratum in: *J Am Coll Cardiol* 2006;47(7):1503–1505.

12. HFSA 2006 comprehensive heart failure practice guideline. *J Cardiac Failure* 2006;12(1):1–86. Available at http://www.hfsa.org/hf_guidelines.asp, accessed 9/18/2006.

13. Garg R, Yusuf S. Overview of randomized trials of angiotensin-converting enzyme inhibitors on mortality and morbidity in patients with heart failure. Collaborative Group on ACE Inhibitor Trials. *JAMA* 1995;273(18):1450–1466.

14. Granger CB, McMurray JJ, Yusuf S, et al. Effects of Candesartan in patients with chronic heart failure and reduced left-ventricular systolic function intolerant to angiotensin-converting-enzyme inhibitors: the CHARM-Alternative Trial. *Lancet* 2003;362:772–776.

15. McMurray JJ, Ostergren J, Swedberg K, et al. Effects of Candesartan in patients with chronic heart failure and reduced left-ventricular systolic function taking angiotensin-converting-enzyme inhibitors: the CHARM-Added Trial. *Lancet* 2003;362:767–771.

16. MERIT-HF Study Group. Effect of metoprolol CR/XL in chronic heart failure: metoprolol CR/XL randomized intervention trial in congestive heart failure. *Lancet* 1999;353:2001–2007.

17. Packer M, Bristow MR, Cohn JN, et al. The effect of carvedilol on morbidity and mortality in patients with chronic heart failure. *N Engl J Med* 1996;334:1349–1355.

18. CIBIS Investigators and Committees. The Cardiac Insufficiency Bisoprolol Study II (CIBIS II): a randomized trial of beta-blockade in heart failure. *Lancet* 1999;353:9.

19. Cohn JN, Johnson G, Ziesche S, et al. A comparison of enalapril with hydralazine-isorbide dinitrate in the treatment of chronic congestive heart failure. *N Engl J Med* 1991;325:303–310.

20. Taylor AL, Ziesche S, Yancy C, et al. Combination of isosorbide dinitrate and hydralazine in blacks with heart failure. *N Engl J Med* 2004;351:2049–2057.

21. Packer M, O'Connor CM, Ghali JK, et al. Effect of amlodipine on morbidity and mortality in severe chronic heart failure. *New Engl J Med* 1996;335:1107–1114.

22. Packer M, et al. Withdrawal of digoxin from patients with chronic heart failure treated with angiotensin-converting enzyme inhibitors. *N Engl J Med* 1993;329:1.

23. The Digitalis Investigation Group. The effect of digoxin on mortality and morbidity in patients with heart failure. *N Engl J Med* 1997;336:525.

24. Pitt B, Zannad F, Remme WJ, et al. The effect of spironolactone on morbidity and mortality in patients with severe heart failure. *N Engl J Med* 1999;349:709.

25. Pitt B, Williams G, Remme W, et al. The EPHESUS trial: eplerenone in patients with heart failure due to systolic dysfunction complicating acute myocardial infarction: Eplerenone Post AMI Heart Failure Efficacy and Survival Study. *Cardiovasc Drugs Ther* 2001;15:79–87.

26. Brater DC. Diuretic therapy. *N Engl J Med* 1998;339:387–395.

27. Dormans TJ, Gerlad PG, Russell FM, et al. Combination diuretic therapy in severe congestive heart failure. *Drugs* 1998;55(2):165–172.

28. Leier CV, Cas LD, Metra M. Clinical relevance and management of the major electrolyte abnormalities in congestive heart failure: hyponatremia, hypokalemia and hypomagnesemia. *Am Heart J* 1994;128:564–574.

29. Philbin EF, Rocco TA Jr. Use of angiotensin-converting enzyme inhibitors in heart failure with preserved left ventricular systolic function. *Am Heart J* 1997;134(2Pt1):188–195.

30. Yusuf S, Pfeffer MA, Swedberg K, et al. Effects of Candesartan in patients with chronic heart failure and preserved left-ventricular ejection fraction: the CHARM-Preserved Trial. *Lancet* 2003;362:777–781.

31. Hermann D. Naturoceutical agents and cardiovascular medicine—the hope, hype and the harm. *ACC Curr J Rev*, 1999;Sept/Oct:53–57.

32. Bristow MR, Saxon LA, Boehmer J, et al. Cardiac-resynchronization therapy with or without an implantable defibrillator in advanced chronic heart failure. *N Engl J Med* 2004;350:2140–2150.

33. Cleland JG, Daubert JC, Erdmann E, et al. The effect of cardiac resynchronization on morbidity and mortality in heart failure. *N Engl J Med* 2005;352:1539–1549.

34. Fonarow GC, Stevenson LW, Walden JA, et al. Impact of a comprehensive heart failure management program on hospital readmissions and functional status of patients with advanced heart failure. *J Am Coll Cardiol* 1997;30:725–732.

35. Shah NB, Der E, Ruggerio C, et al. Prevention of hospitalizations for heart failure with an interactive home monitoring program. *Am Heart J* 1998;135:373–378.

36. Butler J, Khadim G, Paul KM, et al. Selection of patients for heart transplantation in the current era of heart failure therapy. *J Am Coll Cardiol* 2004;43:787–793.

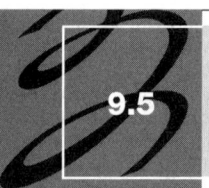

9.5 ATRIAL FIBRILLATION AND OTHER SUPRAVENTRICULAR TACHYCARDIAS
Kavitha K. Arabindoo

ATRIAL FIBRILLATION
General Principles
Epidemiology

Atrial fibrillation (AF) is one of the most common cardiac dysrrhythmias. There are about 2.5 million patients with this condition in the United States. The prevalence of AF is strikingly related to age, affecting as many as 10% of those older than 75 years. As the median age of the U.S. population continues to increase, so does the prevalence of AF. AF is a considerable health burden in that it increases total mortality twofold, heart failure threefold, and stroke rates fivefold. It is responsible for 10% to 15% of all strokes in the United States.

Classification

The following classification has been proposed by the 2001 American College of Cardiology/American Heart Association/European Society of Cardiology Board Task Force. Management of AF is dependent on recognition of the appropriate classification:

- **Paroxysmal AF** is self-terminating and lasts less than 7 days and usually less than 48 hours. It can further be subdivided into first-episode paroxysmal AF and recurrent paroxysmal AF. Therapy here should focus on prevention of recurrence.
- **Persistent AF** is not self-terminating and lasts longer than 7 days. This can again be first-episode or recurrent. Therapy should focus on modulation of heart rhythm or rate and preventing recurrence.
- **Permanent or chronic AF** has been present for more than 1 year and cardioversion has either not been attempted or has failed. Control of ventricular rate is the usually preferred therapeutic option.

Over a 5-year period, about 25% of patients with paroxysmal AF will progress to persistent AF; the likelihood is increased in patients with other risk factors that are discussed below.

Etiology
Besides age, other independent risk factors for AF include valvular heart disease, heart failure, coronary heart disease, obesity, obstructive sleep apnea, hypertension, and diabetes. Some other potentially **reversible causes** of AF include any cause of arterial hypoxemia, hypokalemia, hypomagnesemia, acute alcohol consumption, pericarditis, myocardial infarction (MI), and hyperadrenergic states such as postoperative period including postcardiac surgery, theophylline, or other stimulant toxicity and endocrinopathies (hypo/hyperthyroidism, pheochromocytoma). About 10% of patients with AF have none of the above identifiable risk factors; they are considered to have **"lone" AF.**

Pathophysiology
The pathogenic property common to all risk factors for AF is diastolic dysfunction of the left ventricle, which in turn leads to left atrial dilatation, stretch, and fibrosis and subsequent vulnerability to AF.

Diagnosis
Clinical Presentation
Symptoms can often be vague and include fatigue, lightheadedness, palpitations, breathlessness, and exercise intolerance. Younger and more active patients and those with paroxysmal AF are more likely to report symptoms. Acute presentations may include decompensated congestive heart failure and angina.

History and Physical Examination
Initial evaluation of the patient with AF includes a careful history and physical examination to assess for presence of symptoms, other comorbidities, and potentially reversible causes as noted above. An irregularly irregular pulse that is usually greater than 100 beats per minute (bpm) is characteristic of AF. **"Slow" AF** may indicate associated disease of the conduction pathway. It is important to assess if the patient is **hemodynamically stable** or **unstable** as this would dictate further course of management.

Laboratory Studies
- Basic laboratory workup including screening thyroid tests and metabolic panel are warranted, especially for a first episode of AF.
- All patients with AF should have an **electrocardiogram (ECG)** and a **transthoracic echocardiogram (TTE)** to help identify AF and quantify any underlying cardiovascular disease and guide subsequent management.
- The **ECG** demonstrates chaotic electrical activity with an irregularly irregular rate and rhythm. This is evidenced by constantly changing R-R intervals and no discernible P waves before the QRS complexes. The fibrillation waves are best seen in leads II, III, aVF, and V_1. The fibrillation pattern may be fine or coarse. A few patients have fine AF with little evidence on the ECG. The irregular ventricular pattern should allow determination of AF. Some patients have coarse fibrillation waves, making it difficult to distinguish from atrial flutter. This can again be distinguished by the erratic ventricular response. The QRS complexes are narrow unless there is aberrant ventricular conduction. The ECG may also reveal evidence of acute myocardial ischemia, pre-excitation, sinus node or conduction system disease, or QT prolongation (Figure 9.5-1).
- The **TTE** determines left atrial size (a predictor for AF recurrence), presence of any valvular and/or pericardial heart disease, and can also detect left ventricular hypertrophy and ventricular dysfunction that will influence management decisions. **Transesophageal echocardiogram (TEE)** is more sensitive for identifying atrial thrombi.
- Intracardiac **electrophysiologic studies** may be useful in young patients with idiopathic lone AF to detect underlying pre-excitation or conduction pathway disease.
- **Stress testing** is indicated only if the initial evaluation suggests the presence of ischemic heart disease.

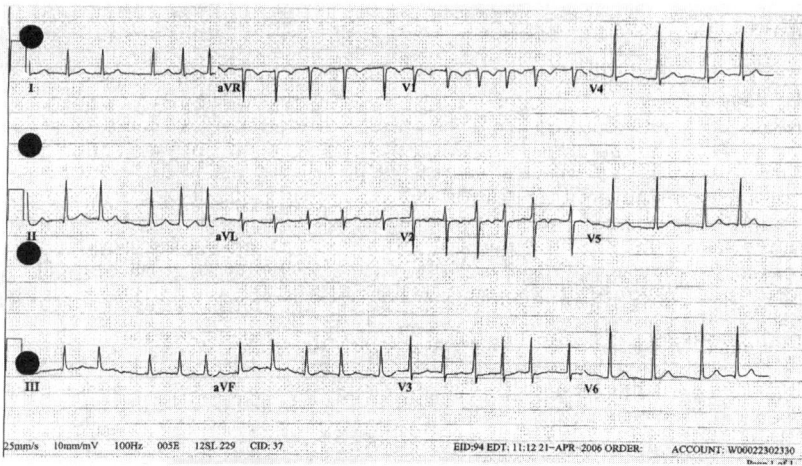

Figure 9.5-1. Atrial fibrillation: note the characteristic irregularity in the R-R intervals and the absence of well-defined P waves preceding the QRS complexes.

Treatment

Immediate management of AF depends on the hemodynamic status of the patient. If unstable, immediate synchronized cardioversion is indicated. If stable, management decisions that need to be made when managing AF include:

- Whether to attempt to restore and then **maintain sinus rhythm,** that is, **adopt a rhythm control strategy,** or
- How to optimally **control ventricular rate** both acutely and long-term, that is, **adopt a rate-control strategy,** and
- How to **minimize the risk of thromboembolism** both in the pericardioversion and long-term settings

Depending on a patient's age, presenting symptoms, medical history, comorbidities, and previous response to AF therapy, the following questions can help guide individual treatment decisions:

- Does the patient have symptoms that would benefit from maintenance of sinus rhythm?
- Is he or she a candidate for anticoagulation therapy?
- What are the potential long-term risks of antiarrhythmic drug therapy versus the risks of focusing on rate control and allowing the arrhythmia to persist?

For many years, the accepted strategy to manage AF was to routinely restore sinus rhythm with cardioversion and then maintain it with antiarrhythmic drugs. Recent studies (AFFIRM, RACE, PIAF, STAF, CAFE) have, however, shown that rhythm- and rate-control strategies were equivalent with respect to mortality and stroke rates. There were fewer hospitalizations, fewer adverse drug effects, and lower costs with rate-control strategy. The patients included in these studies were primarily elderly patients with recurrent or persistent AF or at high risk for recurrent AF who were minimally symptomatic and without significant heart failure. These trials also demonstrated that rhythm control does not prevent AF-related stroke. Based on these studies, the following extrapolations as to the **goals of treatment** can be made:

- Rate control is to be considered the first-line strategy in elderly patients with persistent or recurrent AF who are at high risk for thromboembolic events.
- Rhythm-control strategy may be appropriate in younger patients with a first episode of AF or paroxysmal AF, in patients at low risk of thromboembolism, patients with persistent AF that remain symptomatic despite rate control, and in patients with heart failure.
- Patients at **high risk for thromboembolism need to be anticoagulated with warfarin,** unless contraindicated, regardless of whether a rhythm- or rate-control strategy is pursued.

Rate Control

Rate control may be achieved by either pharmacologic or nonpharmacologic means. The recommended ventricular rate in patients with AF is 60 to 80 bpm at rest and less than 110 bpm with daily activities. Despite optimal control of the resting ventricular rate, some patients with AF will have excessive tachycardia and symptoms of palpitations and dyspnea with their usual daytime activities.

- **Pharmacologic rate control.** For patients with AF in acute settings who do not have decompensated heart failure or the Wolff–Parkinson–White (WPW) syndrome, arteriovenous (AV) nodal blocking agents such as beta-blockers, diltiazem, and verapamil are the most effective drugs.
  - **Beta-blockers** are preferred in patients with ischemic heart disease and those with high sympathetic tone such as in the postoperative period, hyperthyroidism, alcohol withdrawal, pulmonary embolism, pericarditis, or systemic infection.
  - **Diltiazem or verapramil** may be particularly useful in patients with contraindication to beta-blocker use such as reactive airways disease.
  - **Digoxin** is less useful in acute settings because of its slow onset of action. However, in patients with decompensated heart failure, it is the initial drug of choice due to the negative inotropic effect of beta-blockers and calcium-channel blockers.

Patients with minimal symptoms may initially be treated with **oral short-acting preparations** with dose titration and then converted to the appropriate dose of an extended-release preparation once their ventricular rate is controlled. Acutely symptomatic patients may require **intravenous administration** of one of these medications that can later be converted to an extended-release preparation. Intravenous dosages for beta-blockers and calcium-channel blockers are described in the latter section on supraventricular tachycardias. Loading regimens for digoxin vary between 0.25 and 0.50 mg intravenously in repeated doses up to 1.0 to 1.5 mg over 8 to 24 hours. Usual maintenance doses range between 0.125 and 0.5 mg PO daily. Caution needs to be exercised in patients with renal dysfunction to avoid digitalis toxicity.

- **Nonpharmacologic rate control.** Surgical measures are indicated in patients with permanent AF who do not respond or continue to be symptomatic with pharmacologic rate/rhythm control. These include AV node ablation with placement of a pacemaker, burst or dual-site atrial pacing and implantable atrial defibrillator, maze procedure to interrupt re-entrant circuits in the left atrium and percutaneous radio-frequency ablation of arrhythmogenic foci around the junction of the pulmonary veins and left atrium.

Rhythm Control

The main advantages to restoring sinus rhythm are that it returns the heart to normal functioning and prevents the progressive atrial remodeling associated with persistent AF, in addition to alleviating symptoms of AF.

- **Restoration of sinus rhythm.** About 50% to 60% of patients whose duration of AF is less than 48 hours will cardiovert spontaneously. An attempt to restore sinus rhythm in patients who do not do so may be made either by electrical cardioversion or the use of antiarrhythmic drugs. Cardioversion is to be preceded and followed by adequate anticoagulation as discussed in the following section.
  - **Electrical cardioversion.** This is performed using synchronized direct current (DC) cardioversion starting with low energy levels. Before cardioversion, all antiarrhythmic drug levels should be titrated to their therapeutic ranges, digoxin levels should be checked to exclude digoxin toxicity, and patients with hyperthyroidism should be functionally euthyroid to limit the likelihood of recurrence. This is usually the treatment of choice in patients with AF who are hemodynamically unstable.
  - **Pharmacologic cardioversion.** This can be achieved using class IA (procainamide, quinidine), IC (flecainide, propafenone), and III (amiodarone, sotalol) drugs. This is usually reserved for patients with highly symptomatic, persistent AF. Due to the propensity for proarrythmic effects, initiation of antiarrhythmic agents is preferably done in the inpatient setting with continuous ECG monitoring, especially in the presence of structural heart disease of left ventricular (LV) dysfunction. Some of the commonly used antiarrhythmic drugs are as follows:

- Quinidine usage has markedly decreased due to the associated risk of torsades de pointes. When used, the dose is 300 to 600 mg SR every 8 to 12 hours.
- Propafenone is usually started at a dose of 150 mg every 8 hours and may be gradually increased to a maximum daily dose of 900 mg. It is contraindicated in patients with LV dysfunction and conduction defects.
- Flecainide has a 1-year efficacy rate of about 50% in preventing AF. The initial dose is 50 mg twice daily to a maximal daily dose of 400 mg. It is also contraindicated in the presence of LV dysfunction and heart failure.
- Amiodarone is relatively slow acting and is useful in the setting of acute ischemia, acute MI or LV dysfunction. It has a 1-year efficacy rate of about 70% in preventing AF. It has a long half-life of 2 months that makes it hard to reverse its toxicity. Long-term use may be associated with bradycardia, pulmonary, liver, optic nerve and thyroid toxicity. Lower maintenance doses of 200 to 400 mg per day are preferred.
- Dofetilide is a new antiarrhythmic drug and is complicated to administer but offers an alternative if amiodarone is contraindicated.
- Sotalol is commonly used for AF prophylaxis rather than cardioversion. Efficacy varies widely depending on the severity of heart disease. It is started at a dose of 80 mg twice daily to a maximal daily dose of 500 to 600 mg.

■ **Maintenance of sinus rhythm.** This may be achieved by continuing antiarrhythmics as noted above or by surgical means. The main risks linked to pharmacologic rhythm-control strategies are a lack of efficacy with ongoing AF that goes undetected and potentially lethal proarrythmic effects, including torsades de pointes. The former is linked to the increase in stroke risk associated with the discontinuation of anticoagulation when sinus rhythm was believed to have been restored.
  ■ **Nonpharmacologic** measures to rhythm control that are being currently used include:
    - Burst or dual-site **atrial pacing and implantable atrial defibrillation**
    - **Maze procedure** to surgically interrupt re-entrant circuits in the left atrium that requires open heart surgery
    - **Percutaneous radiofrequency ablation** is a catheter-based procedure that uses radiofrequency energy for **pulmonary vein isolation (PVI)** from the left atrium and ablation of arrhythmogenic foci in and around the junction of the pulmonary veins and left atrium. Despite its high efficacy rate and low recurrence of AF, its use is still limited by the associated complications.

Minimizing Thromboembolic Risk

Prevention of of Thromboembolism in patients with atrial fibrillation undergoing cardioversion:

  ▥ Step 1. For patients with AF of ≥48 hours or of unknown duration and are hemodynamically stable, anticoagulation (INR 2.0 to 3.0) is recommended for at least 3 week prior to and 4 week after cardioversion, regardless of the method (electrical or pharmologic) used to restore sinus rhythm.
  ▥ Step 2. As an alternative to Step 1 above, it is reasonable to perform transesophageal echocardiography (TEE) to rule out left atrial thrombus. For patients with no identifiable thrombus, cardioversion is reasonable immediately after anticoagulation with unfractionated heparin administered by an initial intravenous bolus injection followed by a continuous infusion in a dose adjusted to prolong the activated partial thromboplastin time to 1.5 to 2 times the reference control value. This is continued until successful transition to oral anticoagulation with Warfarin to a target INR of 2.0 to 3.0 oral anticoagulation is then continued for at least 4 weeks post cardioversion. For patients in whom thrombus is identified by TEE, oral anticoagulation (INR 2.0 to 3.0) is recommended for at least 3 weeks after restoration of sinus rhythm, and a longer period of anticoagulation may be appropriate even after apparently successful cardioversion, because the risk of thromboembolism often remains elevated in such cases.
  ▥ Step 3. For patients with AF of more than 44-hour duration requiring immediate cardioversion because of hemodynamic instability, heparin should be administered concurrently (unless contraindicated) as mentioned in step 2. Thereafter, oral anticoagulation (INR 2.0 to 3.0) should be provided for at least 4 weeks, as for patients undergoing elective cardioversion.

- Step 4. For patients with AF of less than 48-hours duration associated with hemodynamic instability (angina pectoris, myocardial infarction [MI], shock, or pulmonary edema), cardioversion should be performed immediately without delay for prior initiation of anticoagulation.

Chronic Anticoagulation Therapy:

- Step 1. Anticoagulation recommendations for atrial flutter are the same as those for atrial fibrillation.
- Step 2. Antithrombotic therapy, using antiplatelet agents or Vitamin K antagonists, to prevent thromboembolism is recommended for all patients with AF, except those with lone AF or contraindications.
- Step 3. The selection of the antithrombotic agent should be based upon the absolute risks of stroke and bleeding and the relative risk and benefit for a given patient. The 2006 guideline recommendations for risk stratification and antithrombotic drug prescription are as follows:

Low Risk	No risk factors
Asprin, 81 to 325 mg daily	
Intermediate Risk	One moderate-risk factor
Asprin, 81 to 325 mg daily	
or, Warfarin (INR 2.0–3.0)	
High Risk	Any high-risk
factor, or	
Warfarin (INR 2.0–3.0)	>1 moderate risk factor

*High-risk factors-Prior stroke, TIA or systemic embolism
*Moderate-risk factors-Age >75 years, Hypertension, Diabetes mellitus, Heart failure or impaired left ventricular systolic function.
*Excluded populations include patients with reversible causes of AF, pregnant patients, patients with prosthetic valves or mitral stenosis and contraindications to antithrombotic therapy.

SUPRAVENTRICULAR TACHYCARDIAS

General Principles

Supraventricular tachycardia (SVT) refers to arrhythmias with three or more complexes at a rate exceeding 100 bpm where the focus originates in the AV junctional area above the bundle of His. Re-entry phenomena account for the majority of these dysrrhythmias.

Diagnosis

Clinical Presentation

Patients often describe sensations such as heart pounding or racing. They have regular or skipping beats and may become anxious. There is generally no association with activity. Episodes are usually well tolerated in young people in the absence of any coexistent heart disease. In elderly individuals and in those with pre-existing cardiac disease, the clinical presentation can be acute with hypotension, angina, and pulmonary edema.

Physical Examination

A complete physical examination should be undertaken with emphasis on the cardiovascular system. Evaluation is identical to that described for AF.

Laboratory Studies

- **Electrocardiographic findings.** Patients in whom SVT is suspected should have a 12-lead ECG with a rhythm strip lasting at least 2 to 3 minutes. If P waves are difficult to distinguish due to the rate of the tachycardia, leads aVF and V_1 may be helpful.
- **Ambulatory 24-hour electrocardiographic monitoring (Holter monitoring).** A Holter monitor or event monitor may be considered if the resting ECG is normal and the history is suggestive of a dysrrhythmia.
- **Additional studies.** Laboratory studies may also include the following depending on the clinical situation—electrolytes, calcium, magnesium, hemoglobin, arterial blood gases, thyroid function, toxic screen, and drug level.
- **A TTE** to determine structural heart disease as discussed before.

Classification of SVT

SVT may be classified according to the regularity of the rhythm, the width of the QRS complex, and the relationship of the P waves to the QRS complex. SVT can be narrow (QRS complexes less than 120 ms) or wide (QRS complexes greater than 120 ms). Wide-complex SVT arises when ventricular activation occurs with bundle branch block aberrancy or in the presence of pre-excitation. SVT can further be classified into regular or irregular SVT based on the R-R interval.

- **Regular rhythm SVT.** The R-R interval is consistent and equal. A differential diagnosis of tachycardia mechanisms can further be generated on the basis of the **R-P interval,** the time interval between the peak of an R wave and the subsequent P wave, during the tachycardia. Identification of the specific type of SVT assists in therapy.
- **Short RP tachycardias** have an R-P interval that is less than 50% of the R-R interval. These include:
  - **"Typical" AV nodal re-entrant tachycardia (AVNRT).** This occurs in patients who have functional dissociation of their AV node into "slow" and "fast" pathways. Conduction proceeds antegrade down the slow pathway, with retrograde conduction up the fast pathway. Atrial and ventricular excitation occur concurrently with every tachycardia circuit. On a 12-lead ECG, P waves are often hidden within the QRS complexes and are not visible, or they are buried at the end of the QRS complexes. This is usually an abrupt-onset tachycardia lasting seconds to hours; it accounts for 50% to 60% of all regular narrow QRS tachycardia.
  - **Orthodromic AV re-entrant tachycardia (O-AVRT)** is an accessory pathway– mediated re-entrant rhythm that occurs when anterograde conduction to the ventricle takes place through the AV node and retrograde conduction to the atrium occurs through an accessory pathway. P waves are seen shortly after the QRS complexes.
  - **Sinus tachycardia or ectopic atrial tachycardia** associated with first-degree AV block. The two rhythms differ with respect to the P wave axis and morphology. Here, the P wave after each QRS complex is actually conducting to the subsequent QRS complex with a prolonged PR interval.
  - **Junctional tachycardia** arises from the AV junction. The electrical impulses conduct to the atrium and ventricle simultaneously and therefore, as in typical AVNRT, P waves may not be easily discernible. This is commonly seen in children after surgical correction of congenital heart defects. In adults, it is commonly seen after mitral or aortic valve surgery, with acute MIs or in digitalis toxicity.
- **Long R-P tachycardias** have an R-P interval that is greater than 50% of the R-R interval. These include:
  - **Sinus tachycardia.** The P waves conduct to the subsequent QRS complexes with normal PR intervals. Typically it does not exceed 170 bpm. Onset and termination are gradual. It is often a reflection of extracardiac abnormalities, such as infection, hypovolemia, anxiety, pain, hyperthyroidism, acute severe anemia, and fecal impaction.
  - **"Atypical" AVNRT occurs** when anterograde conduction proceeds over the fast AV nodal pathway with retrograde conduction over the slow AV nodal pathway in patients with dual AV nodal physiology. As the retrograde conduction to the atrium is slow, the P wave is inscribed well after the QRS complex.
- **WPW syndrome** includes the presence of pre-excitation on a 12-lead ECG with symptoms or documentation of SVT. This results from anterograde activation of the ventricle via an accessory pathway as well as the AV node, resulting in a short PR interval together with a delta wave slurring the upstroke of the QRS complex. The most common form seen is an **orthodromic AVRT.** This can at times degenerate into AF.
- **Atrial flutter.** Atrial flutter is often a regular, narrow QRS tachycardia. It is a rhythm characterized by an atrial rate of 240 to 350 bpm, commonly with variable AV block (2:1, 3:1, or 4:1) causing a ventricular response of 70 to 150 bpm. The characteristic flutter waves (sawtooth) are best seen in leads II, II I, aVF, and V_1.

Irregular Rhythm SVT

- AF (refer to previous section)
- Multifocal atrial tachycardia is an irregular SVT characterized by three or more different P-wave morphologies on a 12-lead ECG. Frequently, PR intervals are variable. It is

often associated with chronic obstructive pulmonary disease, heart failure and may be potentiated by concomitant therapy with theophylline. Therapy is targeted at the underlying pathology.

Treatment

- Regular, narrow-complex SVT
  - **Vagal maneuvers.** Carotid sinus massage, Valsalva maneuver, gagging, and a baroreceptor reflex may be tried. If carotid sinus massage is used, auscultation should be performed first to rule out the presence of a carotid bruit. Massage should not exceed 10 seconds and should be done unilaterally.
  - **Pharmacotherapy** with drugs that slow or block the AV node can be used to acutely terminate SVTs that require the AV node as an integral part of the re-entrant tachycardia and to slow the ventricular rate in AF, atrial flutter, and atrial tachycardias.
    - Adenosine is very effective in the treatment of SVTs (excluding AF and atrial flutter). It is given by rapid (1 to 3 seconds) IV push (6 mg) via an antecubital vein followed by a 10 to 30 mL saline flush. A lower initial dose (3 mg) should be used if a central vein is used. If this is not successful, a 12-mg dose followed by 18 mg may be given in 1 to 2 minutes. Toxicities include prolonged asystole in patients with sick sinus syndrome and second or third degree AV block. Side effects such as facial flushing, dyspnea, and chest pressure are usually of brief duration.
    - Verapamil is dosed at IV boluses of 5 to 10 mg over 2 to 3 minutes and can be repeated in 15 to 30 minutes if necessary.
    - Diltiazem can be given as an IV bolus of 0.25 mg per kg over 2 minutes, with a repeat bolus of 0.35 mg per kg if needed. This can be followed with a continuous infusion initiated at 10 mg per hour that can then be titrated to the desired effect.
    - Metoprolol is dosed at 5 mg intravenously and may be repeated in 5 minutes.
  - **Electroconversion.** For patients who do not respond to pharmacotherapy or vagal maneuvers and who are unstable (i.e., hypotensive), synchronized cardioversion is recommended. Electrical conversion recommendations are identical to AF.
  - **Radiofrequency ablation** offers definitive cure for many SVTs and, given their high success rate and low complication rates, antiarrhythmic drugs are now rarely indicated for the treatment of SVTs.
- **WPW.** AV nodal blocking agents must be avoided, as they may facilitate conduction over the accessory pathway and increase the ventricular rate paradoxically, initiating VF. Hemodynamic compromise should be treated with prompt DC cardioversion. The therapy of choice is ablation of the accessory pathway. Pharmacologic therapy is reserved for patients who are unable to undergo an ablation procedure and is targeted at slowing conduction and prolonging refractoriness of the accessory bypass tract with class Ia, Ic, and III antiarrhythmic agents.

References

1. Levine HJ, et al. Antithrombotic therapy in valvular heart disease. *Chest* 1992; 102[Suppl]:426S.
2. European Atrial Fibrillation Trial Study Group. Optimal oral anticoagulant therapy in patients with nonrheumatic atrial fibrillation and recurrent cerebral ischemia. *N Engl J Med* 1995;333:5.
3. Fihn FD, et al. A multicenter randomized trial in patients treated with warfarin. *J Gen Intern Med* 1994;9:131.
4. Go AS, et al. Warfarin use among ambulatory patients with nonvalvular atrial fibrillation: the anticoagulation and risk factors in atrial fibrillation (ATRIA) study. *Ann Intern Med* 1999;131:927–934.
5. Che J. Cardiac arrhythmias. *Washington manual of medical therapeutics.* 2004:158–169.
6. Glatter, Herweg, Jaffe. Atrial fibrillation. *Patient Care* 2006;Jan:58–66.
7. Stulz B. Atial fibrillation: A Therapeutic update. *Emerg Med* 2006;Apr:35–43.
8. Zipes DP, Camm AJ, Broggrefe M, et al. Atrial fibrillation. *J Am Coll Cardiol.* 2006 Sep 5;48(5):e247–346.

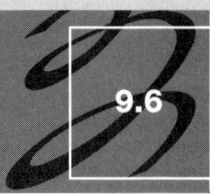

9.6 VENTRICULAR DYSRHYTHMIAS
Dan Brewer

GENERAL PRINCIPLES

Patients with frequent premature ventricular contractions (PVCs) or nonsustained ventricular tachycardias (VTs) but no other evidence of heart disease should be reassured that they have an excellent prognosis. If treatment is needed for symptomatic palpitations, β-blockers should be used.

Patients with complex ventricular dysrhytmias after myocardial infarction and those with diminished ventricular systolic function and either sustained VT or inducible VT (on electrophysiologic study, or EPS) are at high risk for cardiac death. They should be investigated for reversible ischemia and other factors that may exacerbate their rhythm disturbances. These patients should all receive β-blockade if tolerated. Those at highest risk should receive EPS and consideration of an ICD. Empirical therapy with antiarrhythmic medications is almost never appropriate because of the increased mortality associated with these agents.

Definition
Ventricular dysrhythmias are abnormal electrical conductions that arise in the ventricle. They range from simple premature ventricular beats to VT to ventricular fibrillation (VF).

Epidemiology
Almost all people have some premature ventricular beats. Complex dysrhythmias are most common in patients with cardiomyopathies, with those having the lowest ejection fractions at greatest risk.

Classification
VTs are characterized by their morphology and duration.

- Morphology
  - Monomorphic VT: Each ventricular beat is identical.
  - Pleomorphic VT: More than one pattern of monomorphic VT is present.
  - Polymorphic VT: The shape of the ventricular beat changes from beat to beat.

- Duration
  - Salvos: 3 to 5 beats.
  - Nonsustained VT: More than 6 consecutive beats, less than 30 seconds.
  - Sustained VT: More than 30 seconds or any time period with hemodynamic compromise.

Pathophysiology
VTs may be the result of a re-entrant conduction mechanism or due to abnormal automaticity of ventricular myocytes. This may occur due to hypoxia, electrolyte abnormality, or scarring from myocardial infarction.

Etiology
The most common etiology of VT/VF in developed nations is ischemic cardiomyopathy. Other cardiomyopathies, as well as congenital diseases such as Brugada syndrome or the long QT syndrome can also cause VT/VF.

DIAGNOSIS

Clinical Presentation
Patients with VT/VF may be resuscitated survivors of a sudden death episode. Many asymptomatic or minimally symptomatic patients are identified while being monitored in

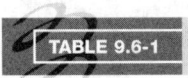

TABLE 9.6-1	Some Common Drugs That Lengthen the QT Interval

Phenothiazines, especially chlorpromazine
Tricyclic antidepressants
Class IA cardiac drugs
 Quinidine, procainamide, disopyramide
Class IC cardiac drugs
 Flecainide, encainide, sotalol

the hospital postmyocardial infarction or for congestive heart failure. Palpitations and syncope/presyncope are the most common symptoms.

History
Palpitations
Patients frequently present to family physicians complaining of palpitations. A very small minority of these will have a serious ventricular dysrhythmia as the underlying cause. Historical features that make an underlying cardiovascular cause more likely include corresponding chest pain or dyspnea, a known history of coronary disease, or multiple risk factors for atherosclerosis.

In a patient with palpitations, a careful history of the character, timing, and associated symptoms should be taken. A history of prescription (Table 9.6-1) and over-the-counter drugs, caffeine intake, alcohol and tobacco use, and anxiety is often very helpful. Illicit drugs such as amphetamines and cocaine may cause palpitations.

Syncope
A careful history of any syncopal episode may give a clue to the underlying cause. In general, syncope of cardiac origin is more likely to be sudden and associated with an injury at the time of the fall, whereas vasovagal syncope is usually preceded by warning symptoms of nausea, warmth, or lightheadedness. In vasovagal syncope, protective reflexes usually remain intact during the fall. Vasovagal syncope is much more common than syncope on the basis of VT/VF.

Exercise-induced syncope in a young person should prompt an investigation for hypertrophic cardiomyopathy. This is the most common cause of sudden death in young athletes.

Physical Examination
Physical examination in the patient who is suspected of having VT/VF should focus on **evidence of heart failure, ventricular outflow obstruction, and atherosclerotic vascular disease.** This examination should include careful palpation and auscultation of the heart searching for an **S₃ gallop.** The regularity of the cardiac rhythm should be assessed. The pulmonary examination may show evidence of pulmonary edema (rales in the dependent fields). The general examination should include evaluation for jugular venous distention and dependent peripheral edema. The character of peripheral arterial pulses should be assessed.

Laboratory Studies
- **Electrolytes.** Electrolyte disturbances can cause VT/VF. Hypokalemia is the most common abnormality, but hypocalcemia and hypomagnesemia have also been implicated in causing this problem.
- **Drug levels.** Any patient who takes digoxin should have the drug level and electrolytes checked. Digoxin toxicity most commonly causes pleomorphic VT, and this is much more common in the presence of hypokalemia. Theophylline toxicity can also cause VT.
- **Metabolic parameters.** Hypoxemia and metabolic acidosis can cause or aggravate ventricular dysrhythmias, particularly in acutely ill patients.

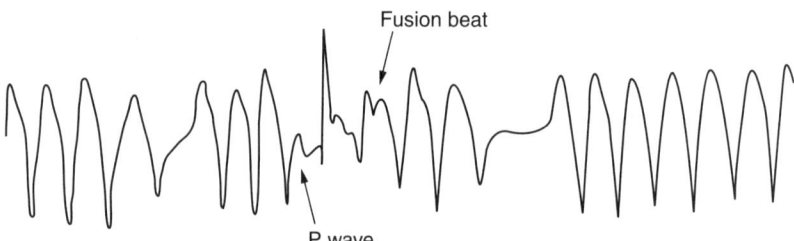

Figure 9.6-1. Ventricular tachycardia. (Courtesy of Freeman Rawson, MD, University of Tennessee, Knoxville.)

Imaging

- **Electrocardiography.** It is unusual to capture VT on a 12-lead electrocardiograph (ECG), but an office ECG during an asymptomatic period may give important clues to the underlying diagnosis of palpitations and syncope. A resting ECG cannot rule out serious disease. The tracing should be examined for signs of ventricular irritability (PVCs), pre-excitation (a delta wave of early ventricular depolarization), ventricular hypertrophy, and ischemic disease. PVCs are characterized by premature wide complexes (more than 120 ms) followed by a compensatory pause before the next ventricular beat. Patients with a pre-existing bundle branch block pattern or Wolf–Parkinson–White syndrome may have a wide complex SVT, so prior tracings should be examined if they are available. The QT interval should be carefully measured as well.
- **Distinguishing ventricular tachycardia from supraventricular tachycardia (SVT).** If the ECG shows a wide complex (>QRS 120 ms) tachycardia, a systematic approach may be taken to determine if the tachycardia is of supraventricular or ventricular origin (an example of VT is shown in Figure 9.6-1):
- Is there an absence of RS complex in all precordial leads?
- If there is an RS complex, is the RS interval greater than 100 ms in any precordial lead?
  - This is measured from the start of the R wave to the nadir of the S wave.

- Is there AV dissociation?
  - Evidenced by independent P waves or fusion beats.
  - Does morphology of lead V_6 favor VT?
  - qR or QS pattern.

- Are any of the three morphologic criteria for VT present in leads V_1, V_2?
  - R wave longer than 30 ms in V_1 or V_2. Notched S wave.
  - More than 60 ms to nadir of S wave.

- An affirmative answer to any of the five questions suggests VT rather than SVT with aberration.
- **Evaluation for ischemia.** A majority of patients with VT/VF have ischemic cardiac disease as the underlying etiologic factor (see Chapter 9.2). For this reason, most patients should undergo an evaluation for reversible ischemic disease. The specific test (exercise stress test, exercise or pharmacologic stress with nuclear imaging or echocardiography, cardiac catheterization, or positron emission tomography) should be chosen on the basis of the patient's level of risk, ability to exercise, and baseline ECG as well as the expertise and preference of the performing physician.
- **Echocardiography.** Some measure of left ventricular function is required in assessing the patient with VT/VF who is potentially at high risk for complications. The most commonly used and readily accessible test in most settings is the calculated ejection fraction obtained from an echocardiogram. The echocardiogram can also evaluate possible valvular heart disease and show focal wall motion abnormalities suggestive of ischemic cardiac disease.

Monitoring

Holter Monitor/Event Monitor

Holter monitoring is often the first step in evaluation of palpitations. This test creates a continuous ECG recording for 24 hours and allows the physician to see the cardiac rhythm that is present at the time of the patient's symptoms. It is important that the patient fill out the diary of symptoms that occur during wearing of the monitor. A normal Holter tracing at the time of symptomatic palpitations has an excellent negative predictive value (it nearly rules out serious VT/VF as the cause). On the other hand, PVCs are a very common finding on a Holter monitor, and minor abnormalities, especially if the patient is asymptomatic, should not be overinterpreted.

If the patient's symptoms are infrequent and there is concern that they will not occur during the time a Holter monitor is worn, an event monitor can be used. This device is triggered at the time the patient's symptoms occur and provides a continuous ECG. This increases the likelihood of capturing a symptomatic episode, but event monitoring is significantly more expensive than Holter monitor testing.

Critical Care Telemetry Monitoring

Many serious ventricular dysrhythmias are diagnosed in the hospital while monitoring a patient in the first few days after a myocardial infarction. Routine monitoring of continuous ECGs for such patients is now standard and the immediate treatment of VT/VF in the postinfarct period has been a major part of the reduced mortality of myocardial infarction since the introduction of coronary care units. Patients with acute myocardial infarction should have routine continuous electrocardiographic monitoring in the initial stage of their hospital care.

Patients in the hospital for exacerbation of congestive heart failure should also receive continuous monitoring. They are at increased risk of VT/VF and they often have asymptomatic dysrhythmias.

Surgical Diagnostic Procedures

- **Cardiac catheterization.** Cardiac catheterization is often required to delineate the extent of coronary disease. The cardiac output and pressure measurements obtained at the time of catheterization are generally considered to be the most accurate measurements of left ventricular function available. Cardiac catheterization and EPS can be performed at the same time.
- **EPS.** The gold standard for evaluating a patient with known or suspected VT/VF is an EPS. This is an invasive test similar to a cardiac catheterization in which multiple electrical leads are threaded to the endocardium to map electrical impulses and to induce dysrhythmias with applied electrical impulses. VTs are characterized as inducible or noninducible and suppressible or nonsuppressible (with medication) at the time of EPS. Inducible sustained VT is an indication of increased risk for sudden death in patients with reduced ejection fraction. Some VTs can be cured by ablation at the time of EPS.

Staging

- **Risk stratification.** Strategies to define which patients are at highest risk for death from VT/VF are still being refined. The most effective treatment is prevention by placement of an implantable cardiac defibrillator (ICD), but this is expensive and has significant morbidity associated with it. Reduced ejection fraction and known prior episodes of symptomatic VT/VF are clearly high-risk factors. For other patients, it is still unclear if inducibility at EPS, abnormal signal averaged ECG (SAECG) or other factors will be best at identifying those at highest risk (Figure 9.6-2).

TREATMENT

- **Emergency treatment.** Patients who present with VT/VF in an emergency setting (cardiac arrest, sustained VT with hemodynamic compromise) should be treated according to current Advanced Cardiac Life Support (ACLS) protocols. The 2005 revisions of the ACLS protocol emphasize effective ventilation and chest compressions. The protocol no longer recommends "stacked shocks" as the initial treatment of hemodynamically unstable patients.

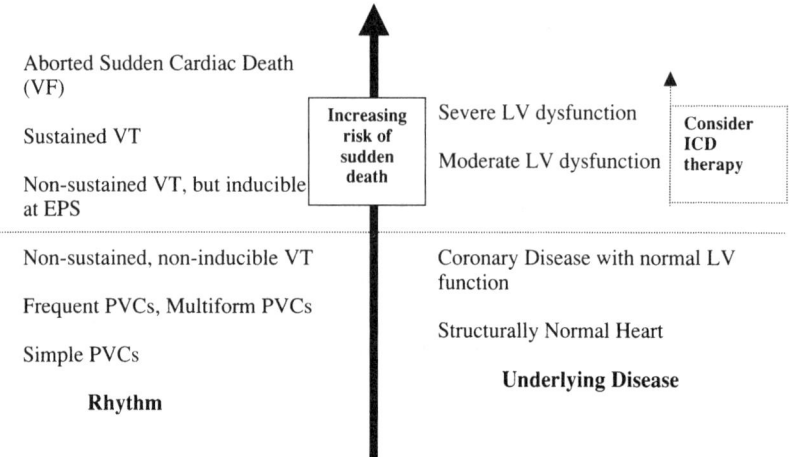

Figure 9.6-2. Risk stratification of patients with ventricular dysrhythmias.

■ **Hemodynamically unstable patients.** Patients with witnessed cardiac arrest or VT/VF and hemodynamic instability should be electrically defibrillated without delay with power according to the manufacturer's recommended settings. After the first attempt at cardioversion/defibrillation, effective cardiopulmonary resuscitation (CPR) should be instituted. Those who have been unconscious for an unidentified period of time may receive five cycles of CPR (about 2 minutes) prior to attempted defibrillation.

■ **Patients with polymorphic ventricular tachycardia (torsades de pointes)** should be given an intravenous infusion of 1 to 2 g of magnesium.

■ **Patients with wide-complex tachycardia but adequate blood pressure.** Patients with a wide-complex tachycardia who maintain an adequate blood pressure should be treated as though they have VT unless it is known with certainty that the rhythm is supraventricular. There are many guidelines that attempt to distinguish between VT and supraventricular tachycardia (SVT) with aberrant conduction on the basis of ECG criteria, but physicians caring for patients in emergency situations should ignore this distinction and manage all wide-complex tachycardias as if they are VT.

• The 2005 guideline recommends **amiodarone 150 mg** as the first agent for a stable patient with a wide-complex tachycardia that is believed to be VT. This is given as an IV infusion over 10 minutes. Alternative agents include procainamide and sotalol. Lidocaine is no longer considered to be a first-line agent in VT/VF. It is particularly important to remember to **go immediately to electrical cardioversion if the patient's hemodynamic status begins to deteriorate or** if the rhythm deteriorates to ventricular fibrillation.

Behavioral

Patients with palpitations should be instructed to reduce caffeine and eliminate smoking. They should discontinue any medications that may be contributing to the symptoms if possible. Such medications include theophylline and sympathomimetic agents such as pseudoephedrine.

Medications

β-Blockers

β-blockers have significant antiarrhythmic properties and have been shown to reduce mortality for patients with ischemic heart disease and congestive heart failure. The benefit

TABLE 9.6-2	Classification of Antiarrhythmic Drugs
Type 1A	Quinidine, disopyramide, procainamide
Type 1B	Lidocaine, tocainide, mexiletine, phenytoin
Type 1C	Flecainide, encainide
Type II	β-Blockers
Type III	Amiodarone
Type IV	Calcium-channel antagonists

of β-blockade increases with the patient's risk for adverse events. β-blockers also may have the effect of decreasing symptomatic palpitations in low-risk patients. They should be the first pharmacologic treatment considered for both symptomatic palpitations in patients with structurally normal hearts and for patients with life-threatening ventricular dysrhythmias. All patients with known coronary disease and/or congestive heart failure should receive β-blockers unless there is intolerance or a specific contraindication.

Antiarrhythmics

Patients whose dysrhythmias are not controlled with β-blockers may be candidates for amiodarone. **Amiodarone** is a type III antiarrhythmic and is the only antiarrhythmic other than β-blockers that has been shown to be no worse than placebo in causing excess mortality in clinical trials. Its effects on overall survival in high-risk patients are uncertain, however. Amiodarone and/or β-blockers are sometimes used to help reduce the number of inappropriate activations of ICDs.

There are many other antiarrhythmic medications that are available, but they all have potential for proarrhythmic effect and may cause increased mortality in treated patients. For this reason, their use has fallen out of favor. These should be used only with caution in carefully selected patients. The classification of antiarrhythmics is shown in Table 9.6-2.

Surgery

Patients with ischemic heart disease and VT/VF may benefit from revascularization (either angioplasty or bypass surgery) to correct the ischemia.

Special Therapy

Implanted Cardiac Defibrillators

ICDs are used in the treatment of patients with life-threatening ventricular dysrhythmias who are at high risk for sudden death. These devices are physically similar to pacemakers. They have an implanted power source beneath the skin of the chest and electrical leads connected to the heart, which can sense VT/VF and deliver either overdrive pacing or electrical defibrillator shocks in response to sustained dysrhythmias. **In clinical trials that have randomized patients to ICDs or antiarrhythmic drugs, the ICDs have consistently been better at improving survival in high-risk patients.** ICDs have been shown to be better even in patients who appear to have adequate suppression of their dysrhythmias with medication.

The disadvantages of ICDs are that they are invasive, expensive, and occasionally may give shocks to patients who are still conscious. They may also increase the incidence of severe heart failure.

Referrals Patients who are potential candidates for ICD therapy should be referred to an electrophysiologist for further evaluation.

The American College of Cardiology and the American Heart Association list the following as **Class 1 recommendations for ICD therapy:**

- Secondary prevention in patients with heart failure and reduced left ventricular ejection fraction (LVEF) who have a history of cardiac arrest, ventricular fibrillation, or hemodynamically destabilizing ventricular tachycardia.
- Primary prevention in patients with an LVEF of less than or equal to 30% and New York Heart Association (NYHA) functional class 2 or 3 symptoms while undergoing

optimal medical therapy, and a reasonable expectation of survival with good functional status for at least 1 year. Those patients with ischemic etiology should be at least 40 days post-MI.

Counseling Patients with risk for VT/VF should receive aggressive cardiac risk factor management according to their underlying disease(s) and risk profile. This may include counseling about exercise, smoking cessation, and low-fat diet. Aggressive management of lipids, blood pressure, congestive heart failure, and diabetes are also warranted.

Patient Education Patients with a device should be educated about topics such as air travel, use of various types of power equipment, and keeping emergency information on their person at all times. Extensive educational material is typically available from the manufacturer.

Follow-Up Patients who have had an ICD placed need a routine schedule of follow-up to investigate the correct functioning of the device. Some of this follow-up can typically be accomplished by telephonic monitoring. Patients who do not receive a device need close monitoring of their underlying illness(es). Those who take amiodarone need specific monitoring for adverse drug effects.

Results Patients at high risk for VT/VF who are treated with an ICD have a relative risk reduction for death of about 30% compared to placebo or antiarrythmic medications alone.

Complications Potential complications of amiodarone include bradycardias, pulmonary fibrosis, and thyroid dysfunction. Complications of ICDs include inappropriate shocks, operative morbidity, and a possible increase in severity of heart failure.

References

1. Hunt SA, Abraham WT, Chin MH, et al. ACC/AHA 2005 guideline update for the diagnosis and management of chronic heart failure in the adult: a report of the American College of Cardiology/American Heart Association Task Force on Practice Guidelines (Writing Committee to Update the 2001 Guidelines for the Evaluation and Management of Heart Failure). *Circulation* 2005;112:e154–e235.
2. Gregoratos G, Abrams J, Epstein AE, et al. ACC/AHA/NASPE 2002 guideline update for implantation of cardiac pacemakers and antiarrhythmia devices: summary article: a report of the American College of Cardiology/American Heart Association Task Force on Practice Guidelines (ACC/AHA/NASPE Committee to Update the 1998 Pacemaker Guidelines). *Circulation* 2002;106:2145–2161.
3. Echt DS, Liebson PR, Mitchell LB, et al. Mortality and morbidity in patients receiving encainide, flecainide or placebo. The Cardiac Arrhythmia Suppression Trial. *N Engl J Med* 1991;324:781–788.
4. 2005 American Heart Association guidelines for cardiopulmonary resuscitation and emergency cardiovascular care. *Circulation* 2005;112(24 Suppl):IV1–203.
5. Bardy GH, Lee KL, Mark DB, et al. for the Sudden Cardiac Death in Heart Failure Trial (SCD-HeFT) Investigators. Amiodarone or an implantable cardioverter-defibrillator for congestive heart failure. *N Engl J Med* 2005;352:225–237.
6. Smith SC, Allen J, Blair SN, et al. AHA/ACC guidelines for secondary prevention for patients with coronary and other atherosclerotic vascular disease: 2006 update. *Circulation* 2006;113:2363–2372.
7. Bardy GH, Lee KL, Mark DB, et al. Amiodarone or an implantable cardioverter-defibrillator for congestive heart failure. *N Engl J Med* 2005;352:225–237.
8. Moss AJ, Zareba W, Hall WJ, et al. Multicenter Automatic Defibrillator Implantation Trial II Investigators. Prophylactic implantation of a defibrillator in patients with myocardial infarction and reduced ejection fraction. *N Engl J Med* 2002;346:877–883.

VENOUS THROMBOSIS AND THROMBOPHLEBITIS

9.7

Mitchell S. King, Linda F. Chang

GENERAL PRINCIPLES

Deep venous thrombosis (DVT) and subsequent embolism of clot to the pulmonary circulation, termed pulmonary embolism (PE), are potentially life-threatening conditions that require prompt diagnosis and treatment to limit the associated morbidity and mortality. This condition accounts for up to 200,000 deaths per year and is the third leading cause for cardiovascular death.[1,2]

Venous thrombosis most commonly affects the veins of the lower extremities under conditions associated with Virchow triad—namely, venous stasis, endothelial injury, or a hypercoaguable state. Locally, the acute formation of clot can be associated with pain and edema and long term with chronic venous stasis, edema, and leg ulcerations. Embolism of the clot can lead to obstruction of the pulmonary arteries, acute right heart failure, cardiovascular collapse, and death. Superficial thrombophlebitis, although generally not life-threatening, can arise under similar conditions and pose a risk for development of DVT as well as cause considerable patient discomfort.

DEEP VENOUS THROMBOSIS

Clinical Presentation

A high index of clinical suspicion is necessary for the diagnosis of DVT.

- **The history** may include lower extremity aching, swelling, or feeling of warmth. A search for risk factors, such as obesity, trauma, surgery, recent hospitalizations or travel, family history or personal history of DVT, congestive heart failure, pregnancy, and oral contraceptive pill (OCP) use, should be included.
- **The physical examination** may be normal or may include findings of lower extremity swelling, tenderness, warmth, or palpable venous "cords."

Diagnostic Testing

Laboratory Findings

- d-Dimer laboratory testing may be used to exclude DVT in patients without risk factors or in higher-risk patients along with a negative venous duplex scan (99% sensitive, specificity 50%).[1,2]
- A complete blood count (CBC), prothrombin time (PT), and partial thromboplastin time (PTT) should be obtained in anticipation of starting anticoagulant therapy.
- In patients younger than 40 years, without apparent risk factors, or with recurrent or family history of DVT, consider assessment for protein C deficiency, protein S deficiency, antithrombin III deficiency, lupus anticoagulant, hyperhomocysteinemia, and the genetic mutations for factor V Leiden and prothrombin 20210. Interpretation of these laboratory results must take into account current usage of heparin, warfarin (Coumadin), or OCPs as well as the presence of renal or liver disease, disseminated intravascular coagulation, pregnancy, and acute arterial or venous thrombosis.

Venous Imaging

- Duplex venous scanning has become the test of choice to assess the patient for DVT. This test is noninvasive and less sensitive for calf vein thrombi, which are not thought to be clinically significant unless they propagate proximally, which occurs approximately 20% of the time. Serial testing over several days can be done to evaluate the patient for the possibility of proximal propagation of calf vein thrombosis.[2]

- Venography is the standard by which the other tests are measured, but it is invasive and carries with it a risk of contrast sensitivity and of developing DVT as a result of the procedure. Consider using venography in the setting of a high clinical suspicion when the noninvasive test results are negative or when the clinical suspicion is very low and the noninvasive test results are positive.

PULMONARY EMBOLISM
Clinical Presentation
- **History.** A patient with PE may present with nonspecific symptoms, such as dyspnea, palpitations, and a sense of impending doom, or with more classic symptoms of chest pain, cough, hemoptysis, symptoms consistent with DVT, or cardiovascular collapse.
- **Physical findings** are also nonspecific. The most common physical findings are tachypnea, tachycardia, and signs consistent with DVT.

Diagnostic Testing
Laboratory Findings
- Arterial blood gases should be obtained and may reveal a low or normal pO_2 and pCO_2.
- A CBC, PT, and PTT should be ordered in anticipation of use of anticoagulants.
- d-Dimer laboratory testing may be used to exclude PE in patients without risk factors or in higher-risk patients along with a negative chest computed tomography (CT) scan or ventilation–perfusion (V/Q) scan.
- See below for workup of the hypercoagulable state.

Imaging
- **Chest radiography** findings with PE are nonspecific and may show effusions, atelectasis, localized infiltrates, or decreased vascular markings, or they may be normal.
- **Spiral CT scan** of the chest (sensitivity 87%, specificity 91%) has become the preferred test in many centers because of its availability and ability to examine other structures within the chest. It is the test of choice in patients with abnormal chest x-rays who would be expected to have abnormal V/Q scans. With high-risk patients and normal CT scans, additional testing should be considered to exclude DVT/PE.[3,4]
- **Ventilation–perfusion scanning** is the test of choice in diagnosing PE in patients with normal chest x-rays and absence of underlying pulmonary disease. Findings are reported as normal, low, intermediate, or high probability of PE based on the presence or absence of mismatched wedge-shaped perfusion defects. If the findings are nonconfirmatory or discordant with the level of clinical suspicion, d-dimer testing and duplex scanning may be helpful, or invasive testing with pulmonary arteriography may be indicated.
- **Pulmonary arteriography** is the gold standard test for diagnosing PE, and, if positive, shows clot obstruction of one or more pulmonary arteries. This invasive test exposes the patient to contrast material and may be less readily available, depending on the availability of personnel.
- **Magnetic resonance imaging (MRI)** is being studied for its role in diagnosing PE. Currently availability and technical limitations preclude its use for diagnosing PE.[5]

TREATMENT OF DVT AND PE
Oxygen, intravenous fluids, ventilator support, and other supportive measures should be provided as indicated by the clinical status of the patient.

Anticoagulants
Initial Treatment
- **Unfractionated heparin** (UFH) or low-molecular-weight heparin (LMWH) is the immediate drug of choice for treating DVT and PE and should be initiated when the diagnosis is suspected, unless there are contraindications to its use, such as increased risk of bleeding or heparin sensitivity.[6,7]
  - It is critical to achieve a therapeutic aPTT within 24 hours of diagnosis to minimize the chances of thrombus extension or recurrent DVT or PE.

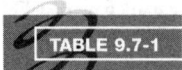

TABLE 9.7-1	Heparin Dosing,[1] Nomogram for Adjustment of IV Heparin[a]	
PTT	**Drip rate**	**Bolus**
<35 s	Increase 4 U/kg/h	Rebolus 80 U/kg
35–45 s	Increase 2 U/kg/h	Bolus 40 U/kg
46–70 s	Maintain current	
71–90 s	Decrease 2 U/kg/h	
>90 s	Decrease 4 U/kg/h	Hold infusion for 1 h
UFH subcutaneous administration		
17,500 units bid with aPTT value 6 hours after morning dose; adjust additional doses for aPTT 1.5–2.5 times control		
LMWHs		
Enoxaparin (Lovenox)	1 mg/kg twice daily or 1.5 mg/kg once daily	
Dalteparin (Fragmin)	200 IU/kg as single daily dose or divided into bid dosing	
Tinzaparin (Innohep)	175 IU/kg daily	

[a]Initial bolus 80 U/kg. Initial drip at 18 U/kg.
Source: Modified from Ref 15.

- Therapeutic range for: UFH-aPTT range of 46 to 70 seconds, which is equivalent to antifactor Xa activity of 0.3 to 0.7 IU per mL, LMWH-antifactor Xa activity of 0.6 to 1.0 IU per mL in twice a day dosing or 1.0 to 2.0 IU per mL for once a day dosing regimen.
- Dosing UFH. Can be given IV or SC administration, a weight-based nomogram has been developed to assist with attaining this goal (Table 9.7-1).
  - LMWH. Can be dosed once or twice a day without laboratory monitoring for most patients. For obese, pregnant, renal compromised individuals, dose adjustment based on the antifactor Xa level.
- Laboratory monitoring UFH. aPTT monitoring every 6 hours until therapeutic and a stable PTT has been attained for continuous administration. For SC administration, aPTT should be drawn at 6 hours after the morning administration and adjust the dose to achieve a 1.5 to 2.5 times prolongation. LMWH-anti-Xa activity peaks at 4 hours after the SC administration of a weight-adjusted dose regimen; therefore, the assay should be performed at this time. While the patient is on heparin, a CBC should be obtained every 2 to 3 days to monitor for thrombocytopenia. Mild degrees of thrombocytopenia (more than 100,000 platelets per high-power field) occur commonly with heparin therapy. More severe degrees of thrombocytopenia may be associated with arterial thrombosis and may require cessation of heparin therapy.
- Duration of therapy with UFH or LMWH should be at least 5 days and can be discontinued after the international normalized ratio (INR) is in the therapeutic range for 2 days.
- Adverse reactions and management:
  - Bleeding. Major bleeding at 0.8% per day and minor bleeding at 2% per day. Intravenous protamine sulfate at 1 mg per 100 units of UFH up to a maximum of 50 mg or 1 mg per 100 antifactor Xa units of LMWH should be given for major bleeds.
  - Thrombocytopenia. Platelet counts drop to less than 150,000 in up to 30% of patients on UFH therapy and it usually occurs within the first 5 days of therapy. This will level back to normal with continued therapy. However, heparin-induced thrombocytopenia (HIT) is a serious adverse drug reaction and requires immediate intervention. It is mediated by immunoglobulin antibodies directed against the heparin–platelet factor 4 complex. Patients should be evaluated for HIT when platelet counts drop by more than 50% or below 100,000. HIT occurs in 3% of patients receiving UFH and less than 1% of patients on LMWH.[8] Platelet counts should be monitored every 2 to 3 days.

- Pregnancy. Drug of choice is adjusted-dose LMWH throughout pregnancy or IV UFH (usual bolus and maintenance protocol) for at least 5 days, followed by adjusted-dose UFH or LMWH for the remainder of the pregnancy.[9] Neither UFH nor LMWH is secreted into breast milk and can be safely administered to nursing mothers if prolonged anticoagulation is needed.

Outpatient DVT Management

With the availability of LMWH, outpatient DVT management has been found to be safe and cost-effective.[10,11] The protocol is similar to inpatient therapy, using LMWH for short-term anticoagulation until warfarin is within the therapeutic range. Candidates must be hemodynamically stable, without renal failure, not at high risk for bleeding, have a supportive home environment, and access to daily clinical laboratory monitoring until the INR is therapeutic.

Other Treatments

- New anticoagulants. Direct thrombin inhibitors such as lepirudin, argatroban, and bivalirubin are approved as an alternative for patients with or at high risk for HIT. Fondaparinex and danaparoid sodium are approved for thromboprophylaxis with major orthopaedic surgeries such as hip replacement.
- Thrombolytic therapy is not recommended for the treatment of DVT or PE in most patients. The exception is for patients with massive ileofemoral DVT at risk of limb gangrene secondary to venous occlusion or hemodynamically unstable PE patients. The recommended means to administer the thrombolytic is intravenously.
- Inferior vena caval filter is recommended in patients with a contraindication to anticoagulant therapy.
- Pulmonary embolectomy should be considered in unstable patients with massive PE who may not be candidates for thrombolytics.

Long-Term Treatment

Warfarin is the drug of choice for long-term treatment in most patients with DVT or PE and it can be initiated concurrently with the first day of heparin therapy. Initial dose is 5 mg daily and a lower dose is recommended for elderly patients because of their increased pharmacodynamic response.[12] A loading dose is not necessary due to the long half-lives of the clotting factors.

- Laboratory monitoring. PT should be obtained daily initially. After a therapeutic value has been achieved, PT INR may be obtained twice weekly until stabilized and thereafter weekly to monthly.
- Duration of therapy. The range can be from 3 to 12 months with a target INR of 2.5 (INR range 2.0 to 3.0) for the majority of patients. If the INR is outside of the desired therapeutic range, the recommendation is to adjust the dose up or down in increments of 5% to 20% of the total weekly dose of warfarin. Tables 9.7-2 and 9.7-3 present specific duration of therapy and management of suboptimal therapeutic values.

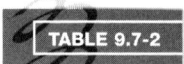 **TABLE 9.7-2**   **Recommended Duration of Anticoagulation for DVT/PE[13]**

Patient conditions	Duration
First episode due to reversible risk factor	3 months
First episode of idiopathic DVT/PE or associated with thrombophilic condition	6–12 months
Episode of PE with antiphospholipid antibodies or two or more thrombophilic conditions	12 months to indefinite
Concurrent cancer or 2 or more	Indefinite
UFH subcutaneous administration	
Episodes of DVT/PE	

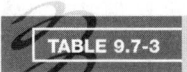

TABLE 9.7-3	**Management of Elevated INR Values[13]**
Elevated INR but <5.0; no significant bleeding	Lower or omit dose; if only minimally elevated, no dose reduction may be needed
INR ≥5.0 and <9.0; no significant bleeding	Omit 1–2 doses; monitor frequently; when therapeutic, resume at lowered dose; if urgent surgery planned, vitamin K$_1$ may be given (2–4 mg orally) with expected reduction in INR in 24 hours
INR ≥9.0; no significant bleeding	Hold warfarin; administer vitamin K$_1$ (5–10 mg orally) with expected drop in INR in 24–48 hours; monitor INR frequently; when INR therapeutic, resume warfarin at lowered dose
Serious or life-threatening bleeding with any INR value	Hold warfarin; administer fresh frozen plasma (FFP) or prothrombin complex concentrate (PCC) along with vitamin K$_1$ (10 mg by slow IV infusion); repeat FFP or PCC as needed based on INR; may repeat vitamin K$_1$ every 12 hours

- **Complications.** Bleeding and warfarin-induced skin necrosis are the two major complications. Warfarin has many clinically significant drug–drug or drug–food interactions and these can affect PT values.
- **Pregnancy.** Warfarin is absolutely contraindicated in pregnancy.

DVT Prophylaxis

- **Risk factors** for development of DVT include obesity, trauma, surgery (particularly lower extremity orthopedic surgery), prior history of or family history of DVT, OCP use, congestive heart failure, malignancy, and pregnancy. Identifying risk factors and assessing the degree of risk for the patient are the first steps in providing appropriate prophylaxis (Tables 9.7-4 and 9.7-5).

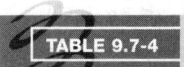

TABLE 9.7-4	**Risk Factors for Deep Venous Thrombosis[14]**

Surgery (esp. lower-extremity orthopedic surgery)
Personal or family history of deep venous thrombosis
Trauma
Obesity
Congestive heart failure
Malignancy
Pregnancy
Medications (e.g., oral contraceptives, tamoxifen, and related medications)
Immobility
Advanced age
Inflammatory bowel disease
Nephrotic syndrome
Myeloproliferative disorders
Smoking
Varicose veins

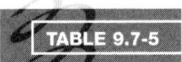

TABLE 9.7-5 Risk for DVT Without Prophylaxis[14]

Patient group	DVT prevalence, %
Medical patients	10–20
General surgery	15–40
Major gynecologic surgery	15–40
Major urologic surgery	15–40
Neurosurgery	15–40
Stroke	20–50
Hip/knee arthroplasty, hip fracture surgery	40–60
Major trauma	40–80
Spinal cord injury	60–80
Critical care patients	10–80

■ **Recommendations** are shown in Table 9.7-6. For high-risk patients, consideration should be given to evaluating for DVT prior to hospital discharge or, for orthopaedic surgical patients, empirically continuing anticoagulant therapy for 6 weeks.[8]

Superficial Thrombophlebitis

Generally occurs in the lower extremity in association with trauma, infection, or varicose veins. It manifests as a tender cord or knot with some surrounding erythema. In the upper extremity, it is most commonly seen with intravenous cannulation. In the absence of inciting causes, consideration should be given to evaluation for malignancy or an underlying hypercoagulable state. Treatment involves use of heat, elevation, and nonsteroidal antiinflammatory medications. If the process appears to be extending to the thigh and the saphenofemoral junction, anticoagulation and ligation or excision of the vein may be necessary. If extension into the deep system is a concern, duplex scanning should be performed to assess the need for additional anticoagulant therapy.

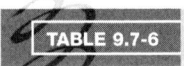

TABLE 9.7-6 Recommendations for Deep Venous Thrombosis Prophylaxis[14]

Age <40 years with no risk factors	No need to use any specific prophylaxis other than early and persistent ambulation
Low-risk medical and surgical patients	Gradient stockings alone or with SC heparin 5000 U q8–12h, starting 2 h preoperatively or on hospital admission. Therapy may continue until patient is ambulatory or discharged
Moderate-risk medical and surgical patients	Pneumatic compression stockings placed in the operating room and continued until patient is ambulatory, with SC heparin (as above) or LMWH
High-risk patients (includes knee and hip surgery)	LMWH (fonadaparinux or warfarin) along with gradient or pneumatic compression stockings

SC, subcutaneous.

References

1. Blann AD, Lip GYH. Venous thromboembolism. *BMJ* 2006;332:215.
2. Andrews EJ, Fleischer AC. Sonography for deep venous thrombosis: current and future applications. *Ultrasound Quart* 2005;21:213.
3. Quiroz R, et al. Clinical validity of a negative computed tomography scan in patients with suspected pulmonary embolism. *JAMA* 2005;293:2012.
4. van Strijen MJL, et al. Diagnosis of pulmonary embolism with spiral CT as a second procedure following scintigraphy. *Chest* 2003;13:1501.
5. Kanne JP, Lalani TA. Role of computed tomography and magnetic resonance imaging for deep venous thrombosis and pulmonary embolism. *Circulation* 2004;109S:I15.
6. Buller HR, et al. Antithrombotic therapy for venous thromboembolic disease: the seventh ACCP Conference on Antithrombotic and Thrombotic Therapy. *Chest* 2004; 126:401.
7. Hirsch J, Raschke R. Heparin and low-molecular-weight heparin: the seventh ACCP Conference on Antithrombotic and Thrombolytic Therapy. *Chest* 2004;126:188.
8. Spinler SA. New concepts in heparin-induced thrombocytopenia: diagnosis and management. *J Thromb Thrombolysis* 2006;21(1):17.
9. Bates SM, et al. Use of antithrombotic agents during pregnancy: the seventh ACCP Conference on Antithrombotic and Thrombolytic Therapy. *Chest* 2004;126:627.
10. Segal JB, et al. Outpatient therapy with low molecular weight heparin for the treatment of venous thromboembolism: a review of efficacy, safety, and costs. *Am J Med* 2003;115:298.
11. Merli G. Anticoagulants in the treatment of deep vein thrombosis. *Am J Med* 2005; 118(8A):13S.
12. American Geriatrics Society Guideline. The use of oral anticoagulants (warfarin) in older people. *JAGS* 2002;50:1439.
13. Ansell J, et al. The pharmacology and management of the vitamin K antagonists: the seventh ACCP Conference on Antithrombotic and Thrombolytic Therapy. *Chest* 2004;126:204.
14. Greets WH, et al. Prevention of venous thromboembolism: the seventh ACCP Conference on Antithrombotic and Thrombolytic Therapy. *Chest* 2004;126:338.
15. Raschke RA, Reilly BM, Guidry JR, et al. The weight-based heparin dosing nomogram compared with a "Standard care" nomogram: a randomized control trial. *Ann Intern Med* 1993;119:874–881.

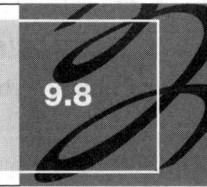

PERIPHERAL ARTERIAL DISEASE
Cecilia A. Gutierrez

9.8

GENERAL PRINCIPLES

Definition

The American Heart Association defines peripheral arterial disease (PAD) as atherosclerosis affecting the lower extremities. PAD is a manifestation of systemic atherosclerosis and carries significant morbidity and mortality. Patients with PAD have the same relative risk of death as patients with known coronary artery disease (CAD) or cerebrovascular disease. Thus, they need to be treated aggressively to reduce risk of cardiovascular events.

Anatomy

Disease that affects lower extremities involves the following arteries: aortoilliac, aortic bifurcation, common iliac, external iliac, femoral, popliteal, tibial, and dorsalis pedis.

- Following the anatomical distribution of blood flow, PAD affecting the aortoilliac arteries causes pain in buttocks and hips; disease of the common femoral or aortoilliac causes pain in the thighs; disease of the superficial femoral causes pain in the upper two thirds of the calves; disease of the popliteal vessels affect the lower third of the calves. PAD in the tibial and peroneal arteries cause foot pain.

■ Vessel location, anatomy, as well as severity of disease affect the options for revascularization.

Epidemiology

It is estimated that PAD affects 8 to 12 million people in the United States. PAD is underdiagnosed and undertreated due to disease unawareness and because symptoms may mimic other common conditions.

Classification

Arterial vascular disease (AVD) refers to noncoronary atherosclerosis, which includes: cerebrovascular disease, aortic disease, renal disease, and peripheral arterial disease.

Etiology

The risk factors for PAD are the same as for atherosclerosis.

■ Traditional risk factors: The presence of CAD or cerebrovascular disease makes patients more prone to PAD. Cigarette smoking and diabetes carry the highest risk for PAD. Hypertension, dyslipidemia, particularly low high-density lipoprotein (HDL) and high triglycerides, and hypercoagulability are important risk factors.

■ Novel risk factors for atherosclerosis. Lipoprotein (a), apolipoprotein (apo) A-1, apo B-100, high-sensitivity C-reactive protein (CRP), fibrinogen, and homocystine are new identifiable risks for atherosclerosis. Their roles in PAD are being investigated.

■ Genetic predisposition for collagen synthesis (Marfan syndrome, Ehler–Danlos IV syndrome) and inflammatory diseases (Takayasu artertitis) are rare, but carry significant risks for PAD.

Mechanism of Injury

The development of atherosclerosis is a complex process. Many factors are at play and interact in the process of plaque formation. Lipid abnormality leads to fatty deposition in the vessel's intima. Local vessel conditions such as oxidative stress, vascular smooth muscle activation, activation of the inflammation cascade, release of mediators of inflammation, endothelial dysfunction, vessel damage by shearing forces, all contribute to plaque rupture, platelet activation, and thrombosis. Eventually, blood vessel injury ensues, leading to vessel remodeling, thrombosis, compromised blood flow, and ischemia to tissues.

DIAGNOSIS

Clinical Presentation

About 30% of patients present with classic symptoms of claudication, which is the development of pain triggered by exercise and resolved by rest. Some patients have no symptoms while the majority present with vague and nonspecific symptoms: leg heaviness, achiness, fatigue when walking, numbness, etc. Occasionally, patients present with acute occlusion (a cold, cyanotic, and pulseless extremity); when they do, it is a medical emergency.

History

Medical history is focused on assessing symptoms, functional capacity and determining the existence of PAD risk factors: presence of cardiovascular disease (myocardial infarction, stroke, transient ischemic attack), cigarette smoking, hypertension, DM, dyslipidemia, and family history of arterial disease.

Physical Examination

A complete physical exam is warranted, with special attention to cardiovascular system: blood pressure in both arms. Cardiac exam: heart rate, rhythm, presence of murmurs, jugular venous distention (JVD), and carotid bruits. Lungs: auscultation. Abdomen: palpation and auscultation for bruits. Evaluation of peripheral circulation: palpation of all peripheral pulses, assessment of capillary refill and presence of signs of circulatory compromise (skin atrophy, loss of hair, nail changes), presence of skin ulceration or coolness.

Diagnostic Studies

■ Routine studies: Complete blood count (CBC), comprehensive metabolic panel, fasting blood sugar, and lipid profile. If the suspicion of PAD exists, an ankle brachial index (ABI) is the first and most useful test to order.
■ The ABI is the ratio of the systolic ankle blood pressure to the systolic brachial artery pressure, both measured in the supine position using Doppler.
  ■ A normal ABI is 0.9 to 1.3. ABI correlates well with disease severity and patient functional state. An ABI <0.9 has a 90% sensitive and 95% specificity for PAD. An ABI <0.4 correlates with pain at rest and ulceration and an ABI <0.2 is associated with ischemic gangrenous extremities.
  ■ ABI can also be measured during a treadmill test (5 minute at 2 mph and 12 degree incline). Ankle pressure <50 mmHg indicates PAD.
  ■ A normal ABI does not completely rule out PAD (patients may have an abdominal aneurysm or may have toe disease).
  ■ The presence of significant media arterial calcinosis makes ABI not reliable due to decreased compressibility of the vessel. Medial calcinosis is common in patients with diabetes. ABI >1.3 is suspicious for medial calcinosis. In these patients, toe pressures and Doppler waveforms are more useful.
■ Toe systolic pressure index (TSPI). Measured by strain-gauge or plethysmographic technique. Normally, TSPI should be >0.60 ± 0.17. Absolute values <30mmHg in patients with ulcers predict poor healing prognosis.
■ Segmental pressures. It is the serial measurement of pressures along the leg. A drop of 20 mmHg compared to opposite leg is significant.

Imaging Studies

■ Duplex Ultrasound and Doppler
  ■ It measures the velocity of flowing blood in arteries and veins and provides quantification of the degree of stenosis. As a vessel narrows, the velocity increases. It identifies stenosis and occlusion with 92% to 95% sensitivity and 97% to 99% specificity. Vessels are classified as normal; 1% to 19% stenosis, 20% to 49% stenosis, 50% to 99% stenosis, and occluded.
  ■ It allows measurement of intima-media wall thickness, which correlates with atherosclerosis.
  ■ Doppler waveform. Blood flow in normal vessels has a triphasic waveform: Forward systolic peak, reverse flow (early diastole), and forward flow (late diastole). As vessels narrow, the reverse flow is lost.
  ■ It is also useful in monitoring aneurysm progression as well as surveillance of graft patency.
■ Angiography and magnetic resonance angiography (MRA) are considered the gold standard as diagnostic tools and in the planning for revascularization.
  ■ Angiography. It is invasive, uses contrast material, carries higher morbidity, and is more expensive than MRA. However, it allows immediate angioplasty if indicated.
  ■ MRA. It is noninvasive, uses contrast agents that are not nephrotoxic, it does not use ionizing radiation, and it provides detailed anatomy of disease. It is superior to computed tomography (CT) angiography but cannot be used in patients with pacemaker or other metallic objects.
  ■ Recent advances in MRA, such as "time of flight" techniques, which allows removal of background tissue signals, and new three-dimensional (3D) MRA provide images close to the angiograms.
  ■ 3D MRA is currently used only in patients with collagen vascular disease and vascular inflammatory conditions.
■ CT angiography. Provides good images and is used to diagnose aortic dissecting aneurysm as well as postoperative surveillance for leaks. It uses ionizing radiation and nephrotoxic contrast agents.

TREATMENT

The goals of treatment are: (1) to decrease risks factors for PAD, and (2) to improve functional status by decreasing claudication, improving exercise tolerance, decreasing limb pain, preventing skin ulceration and amputation.

Behavioral Therapy

- Smoking cessation. All efforts must be made to help patients stop smoking. Smoking cessation decreases pain and slows disease progression. Patients must be counseled at each visit about cessation and be offered nicotine replacement therapies, alone or in combination with Wellbutrin (bupropion).
- Exercise. Prescribed walking regimen of 30 minutes three times a week significantly improves symptoms of claudication and improves functional status. The benefit of exercise is not fully understood; it is not just due to development of collateral circulation, but due to improved muscle biochemistry (energy utilization, endothelial function) and gait.

Medications

- Antiplatelets drugs. Aspirin 81 to 325 mg daily or Clopidogrel 75 mg per day reduces the risk of fatal and nonfatal cardiovascular events in patients with PAD.
- Cilostazol. A phosphodiesterase III inhibitor that inhibits platelet aggregation and improves quality of life of patients with PAD. Usual dose is 100 mg bid, and 50 mg bid if patient takes calcium-channel blockers. It cannot be used in patients with heart failure.
- Pentoxifylline, 1.2 g per day has been used in patients with PAD. It is thought to improve rheology of red blood cells (RBC), but its benefits are questionable.

Treatment of Risk Factors

- Hyperlipidemia. Lipid reduction using statins decrease disease progression. The benefit is likely due to plaque stabilization and improvement of endothelial function. The National Cholesterol Education Program Adult Treatment Panel III (NCEP/ATPIII) recommends treatment with target goal of low-density lipoprotein (LDL) < 100 mg per dL and triglycerides < 150 mg per dL.
- Blood pressure reduction
  - Angiotensin-converting enzyme inhibitors (ACEI) have positive effect on PAD beyond blood pressure lowering effect and are recommended in patients with PAD.
  - β-Blockers reduce cardiovascular events, so their use is encouraged in patients with PAD, except in patients with severe disease.

Endovascular Intervention

- Percutaneous transluminal angioplasty (PTA). It is the reopening of blood vessel via balloon angioplasty that causes "a controlled" medial artery dissection. Advances in techniques, wires, and stents have expanded the role of PTA in treating PAD.
  - Indication: Loss of tissue, rest pain, persistent symptoms in spite of conservative therapy, or progressive disease.
  - Generally done in patients who have localized disease, short segment, noncalcified lesions in large vessels. Most commonly used in vessels above the inguinal canal such as aortoilliac vessels. It can be done with or without stent placement.
  - Indicated in patients not able to tolerate surgery and for those who need saphaneous vein for cardiac revascularization.
  - Not recommended for popliteal or femoral disease due to risk for dissection and restenosis.
  - Risks: Dissection, restenosis, groin hematoma, and pseudoaneurysm.
- PTA can be repeated, and it does not preclude subsequent surgical revascularization if needed.

Surgery

- Arterial bypass surgery is considered the gold standard in revascularization due to long-term patency.
  - It carries significant morbidity and mortality due to its invasiveness and need for general anesthesia.

- Outcomes are affected by patient's age, gender, smoking, and comorbid conditions, particularly diabetes and hypertension.
- Indicated in patients with disabling claudication and to prevent limb loss due to ischemia.
- Indicated for patients with diffuse disease, long lesions, and those who have severe and progressive disease.
- It is the best choice for infrainguinal vessel disease.

Patient Education and Counseling

Patients need to be educated on the deleterious effects of smoking and sedentary lifestyle. All efforts must be made to improve patient's compliance with treatment of blood pressure, lipids, and diabetes.

Monitoring

The progression of PAD is variable and unpredictable. However, the higher the risk factors, the higher the likelihood of progression. Patients with disease need to be monitored for disease progression in order to identify and treat complications promptly.

Referral

Patients with severe and progressive disease should be referred to a vascular surgeon.

SPECIAL CONSIDERATIONS

- Patients with known history of Marfans syndrome, Ehler–Danlos syndrome, and those affected by Takayasu arteritis need to be screened regularly for the development of aneurysms and other symptoms of PAD. Patients with these conditions need to be under the care of a cardiologist and followed closely.

References

1. ACC/AHA Guidelines for the management of patients with peripheral arterial disease (lower extremity, renal, mesenteric, and abdominal aortic). *JACC* 2004;109:2595. Available online at http://www.acc.org/clinical/guidelines/pad/summary.pdf.
2. Graeme J, et al. Medical treatment of peripheral arterial disease. *JAMA* 2006;295:547–553.
3. Belch J, et al. Critical issues in peripheral arterial disease detection and management: a call to action. *Arch Intern Med* 2003;163:884.
4. Hiatt W. Medical treatment of peripheral arterial disease and claudication. *N Engl J Med* 2001;344:1608.
5. van den Bosch M, et al. Peripheral arterial disease. *Lancet* 2002;23;359(9311):1070.
6. Lesho E. Management of peripheral arterial disease. *Am Fam Physician* 2004;69: 525–533.
7. Lawson G. The importance of obtaining ankle-brachial indexes in older adults: the other vital sign. *J Vasc Nurs* 2005;23(2):46–51.
8. Third report of the National Cholesterol Education Program (NCEP) Expert Panel on detection, evaluation, and treatment of high blood cholesterol in adults (Adult Treatment Panel III). *Circulation* 2002;106:3143.
9. Schillinger M, Exner M, Mlekusch W, et al. Statin therapy improves cardiovascular outcome of patients with peripheral artery disease. *Eur Heart J* 2004;25(9):742–748.
10. Yusuf S, Sleight P, Pogue J, et al. Effects of an angiotensin-converting-enzyme inhibitor, ramipril, on cardiovascular events in high-risk patients. The Heart Outcomes Prevention Evaluation Study Investigators. *N Engl J Med* 2000;342:145.
11. Stewart K, Hiatt W, Regensteiner J, et al. Exercise training for claudication. *N Engl J Med* 2002;347:1941.
12. Tucker De Sanctis J. Percutaneous interventions for lower extremity peripheral vascular disease. *Am Fam Physician* 2001;64:1965.

Respiratory Problems

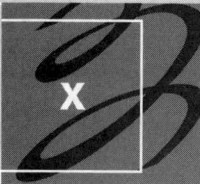

X

ASTHMA
Elisabeth L. Backer

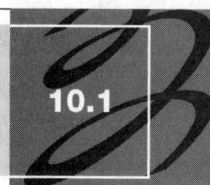

10.1

GENERAL PRINCIPLES

Definition
Asthma is a chronic inflammatory disorder of the airways involving various cells (especially mast cells, eosinophils, and T lymphocytes), which is marked by recurrent episodes of wheezing, chest tightness, breathlessness, and cough, occurring particularly at night or in the early morning. Asthma is associated with an increase in airway responsiveness to a variety of stimuli, leading to widespread, but variable airflow limitation, which may revert spontaneously or with treatment.[1-3]

Pathophysiology
- A genetic predisposition has been recognized, while atopy is the strongest identifiable predisposing factor. Episode triggers include airway inflammation and hyperresponsiveness of sensitive patients to inhaled allergens (house dust mites, cockroaches, cats, seasonal pollens).
- Nonspecific precipitators include exercise, upper respiratory tract infections, rhinitis/sinusitis, postnasal drainage, aspirations, gastroesophageal reflux disease (GERD), weather changes, and stress, while selected individuals react to aspirin and nonsteroidal anti-inflammatory drugs (NSAIDs).[3]
- Exposure to environmental tobacco smoke (or to various agents in the workplace) is a common trigger.

DIAGNOSIS

Clinical Presentation
Patients may present with intermittent or chronic symptoms of airway obstruction (breathlessness, cough, wheezing, chest tightness). Symptoms and signs may vary widely in terms of intensity and frequency. The classic triad consists of cough, shortness of breath, and wheezing.[2] Symptoms may occur infrequently or continuously, spontaneously, or secondary to triggers. There may be a circadian rhythm with symptoms worse at night; nadir between 3 and 4 A.M.

Physical Findings

Patients may present with diffuse wheezing (varying pitches, tones, and timing) heard bilaterally; prolonged expiration. There may be contributing findings, which would include allergic rhinitis, nasal polyps, hives, eczema, atopic dermatitis. Patients may use accessory muscles, be found to have pulsus paradoxus, and present with globally reduced breath sounds in severe airway obstruction.[2,3]

Classification of Severity

- Mild intermittent asthma: Symptoms equal or less than twice a week; otherwise asymptomatic and normal peak expiratory flow (PEF) between exacerbations; nocturnal symptoms equal or less than twice a month; forced expiratory volume in 1 second (FEV_1) or PEF equal or greater than 80% of predicted.
- Mild persistent asthma: Symptoms more than twice a week, but less than once a day; nocturnal symptoms more than twice a month; FEV_1 or PEF greater than 80% of predicted.
- Moderate persistent asthma: Daily symptoms; daily use of inhaled short-acting beta-2-agonist; nocturnal symptoms more than once a week; FEV_1 or PEF greater than 60% but less than 80% of predicted.
- Severe persistent asthma: Continual symptoms; limited physical activity; frequent exacerbations; frequent nocturnal symptoms; FEV_1 or PEF equal or less than 60% of predicted.

Laboratory Tests and Imaging

Peak Flow

Peak flow is a simple test measuring airflow during maximal exhalation. It is important to have establishment of baseline and zone scheme (red <50%, yellow 50% to 80%, green >80% of predicted/personal value). PEF is usually lowest upon awakening, highest before midpoint of waking day (diurnal variation). PEF <200 mL per minute indicates severe airflow obstruction.[3] PEF is used to monitor trends in lung function.[2]

Spirometry Measures FEV₁ and Forced Vital Capacity (FVC)

The degree of airway obstruction defined by percent of predicted FEV_1 achieved:

- >80%: Borderline obstruction
- 60% to 80%: Mild obstruction
- 40% to 60%: Moderate obstruction
- <40%: Severe obstruction

An increase in FEV_1 ≥12% (or increase in FVC ≥15%) postbronchodilator therapy suggests reversible airway obstruction/asthma.[2]

Bronchoprovocative Testing

Useful if asthma is suspected and spirometry is nondiagnostic, or if patient presents with atypical asthma symptoms. It is done in pulmonary function test (PFT) labs, using metacholine or histamine. A negative metacholine challenge argues against asthma diagnosis.

Other Tests

- Chest x-ray (CXR) is almost always normal, but may show hyperinflation/bronchial wall thickening. It is indicated in patients with atypical symptoms, or to exclude complications.[3]
- Blood tests are used to investigate allergic basis of disease (elevated eosinophil count/immunoglobulin E, IgE).
- Allergy testing consists of skin testing (most accurate for aeroallergens, not for foods) or radioallergosorbent test (RAST; more expensive, lesser sensitivity).[2]
- Other: Further evaluations for GERD or sinusitis may be helpful.

Differential Diagnosis

In children, consideration should be given to foreign body aspiration, cystic fibrosis, viral bronchiolitis, tracheomalacia. In young adults, the differential includes bronchiectasis, pulmonary embolism, GERD, sarcoidosis, vasculitides. In older adults the common diagnoses of chronic obstructive pulmonary disease (COPD), congestive heart failure (CHF) should be considered. Psychiatric causes that mimic asthma include conversion disorder and vocal cord dysfunction.

The differential diagnosis of persistent cough in cases of normal CXR and lung functions: postnasal drip, GERD, postviral tussive syndrome, medication-induced cough (angiotensin-converting enzyme inhibitors, ACE-I). These conditions are normally not associated with diffuse wheezing.

Comorbid conditions commonly include seasonal allergic rhinitis/conjunctivitis, perennial rhinitis, recurrent/chronic sinusitis, postnasal drip, and nasal polyps.

TREATMENT

Treatment includes initial spirometry and follow-up testing every 6 to 12 months; routine monitoring of symptoms and lung functions (PEF) at home. It is important to control trigger factors (allergens, respiratory infections, irritants, chemicals, physical activity, emotional stress). Consideration should be given to pneumococcal vaccination and annual influenza vaccinations.

Pharmacologic Treatment[2]

A stepwise approach to therapy is recommended by the 2002 update of the National Asthma Education and Prevention Program Expert Panel Report.[4] The aim of treatment is to maintain control of asthma with minimum amount of medication, thereby decreasing the risk of adverse effects.

Mild Intermittent Asthma

- Short-acting bronchodilator (inhaled beta-2-agonist) as needed for symptom relief[5]
- Mast cell-stabilizing agents (cromolyn/nedocromil) can be used prior to exercise to prevent bronchoconstriction.[6,7]

Mild Persistent Asthma

- Low-dose inhaled steroids, metered-dose inhalers (MDIs) versus multidose dry powder inhalers[8]
- Use of spacer device to optimize delivery and minimize oropharyngeal deposition
- Reduction of dose by 25% to 50% over several months if patient remains asymptomatic
- Short-acting inhaled bronchodilator as needed for symptom relief.[9]
- Trial of leukotriene-modifying agents (montelukast)—response may vary
- Long-acting inhaled beta-2-agonists (salmeterol)—less efficacious than inhaled steroids[10]; use if incomplete response to low-dose inhaled steroids
- Alternative choice to inhaled steroids: mast cell-stabilizing agents (less effective)

Moderate Persistent Asthma

- Medium- to high-dose inhaled steroids (fluticasone, budesonide)
  - Side effects possible; limit oropharyngeal/gastrointestinal absorption via mouth rinses
  - Use lowest dose needed to maintain asthma control[2]
- Combination with long-acting inhaled bronchodilator (salmeterol) if needed[2]
- Trial of leukotriene modifying agents as additional "controller" agent—patients may be able to reduce inhaled steroid dose
- Long-acting oral bronchodilators (theophylline, albuterol tablets)—effective with regular anti-inflammatory therapy, but frequent side effects and narrow therapeutic window limit usefulness

Severe Asthma

- High-dose inhaled steroids and long-acting inhaled bronchodilator
- Possible addition of theophylline and leukotriene modifiers—dosage limitations due to toxicity risk
- Oral corticosteroids if needed, at minimum dosage
- Optimal use of multiple concomitant "controllers"—no data available[2]

Management of Acute Asthma Exacerbation[11]

- Inhaled beta-2-agonist (and inhaled anticholinergic)
- Systemic corticosteroid (oral or intravenous)
- Oxygen
- Monitor FEV_1 or PEF, O_2 saturation, pulse
- Hospitalization if severe exacerbation, high-risk patient, or incomplete/poor response to initial treatment

SPECIAL CONSIDERATIONS

■ Complications include exhaustion, dehydration, airway infection, cor pulmonale, tussive syncope, pneumothorax, and acute respiratory failure (hypercapnea/hypoxia). The death rate is increasing worldwide (especially in urban minorities).

■ Patient education leads to decreased hospitalizations, improved daily functioning, and increased patient satisfaction linked to:
  ■ Active comanagement and use of written action plan (monitoring of symptoms and lung functions)
  ■ Understanding of and adherence to medication
  ■ Knowledge of treatment plan for deteriorating condition or emergency situation[2,12]

References
1. Global Initiative for Asthma Management and Prevention. NHLBI/WHO workshop report, U.S. Department of Health and Human Services. Bethesda, MD: NIH; 1995; Pub 95-3659.
2. www.uptodate.com.
3. Tierney LM, et al. *Current medical diagnosis and treatment.* Lange Medical Books, McGraw-Hill, NY; 2002:278–290.
4. National Asthma Education and Prevention Program Expert Panel Executive Summary report: guidelines for the diagnosis and management of asthma—update on selected topics 2002. NIH, NHLBI, Publication 02-5075, 2002 (full text: www.nhlbi.nih.gov/guidelines/asthma/asthgdln.pdf).
5. Nelson HS. Adrenergic bronchodilators. *N Engl J Med* 1995;333:499.
6. Woolley M, et al. Duration of protective effect of terbutaline sulfate and cromolym sodium. *Chest* 1990;97:39.
7. Bundgaard A, et al. A comparative study of the effects of two different doses of nedocromil and placebo. *Allergy* 1988;43:493.
8. Barnes PJ. Inhaled glucocorticoids for asthma. *N Engl J Med* 1995;332:868.
9. Drazen JM, et al. Comparison of regularly scheduled with as-needed use of albuterol in mild asthma. Asthma Clinical Research Network. *N Engl J Med* 1996; 335:841.
10. Verberne AA, et al. One year treatment with salmeterol compared with beclomethasone in children with asthma. *Am J Respir Crit Care Med* 1997;156:688.
11. Cline DC. Practical approaches to treating acute bronchospasm. Postgraduate Medicine Special Report; Dec 2005;9–17.
12. Gibson PG, et al. Self-management education and regular practitioner review for adults with asthma. *Cochrane Database Syst Rev* 2000;CD001117.

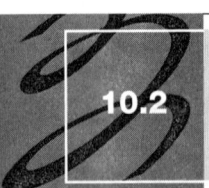

10.2 ACUTE BRONCHITIS AND PNEUMONIA
William J. Hueston

ACUTE BRONCHITIS

General Principles
Acute bronchitis is one of the most common diagnoses made in primary care practices. Symptoms of acute bronchitis can mimic asthma in acute stages. For patients in the early stages of acute bronchitis, pulmonary function tests may be indistinguishable from those of patients with asthma. As the bronchitis improves, patients are sometimes left with a lingering postbronchitic syndrome that may resemble asthma or, more specifically, cough-variant asthma (see Chapter 10.1).

Diagnosis
Clinical Presentation
Patients with either acute bronchitis or pneumonia usually present with a productive cough but may also complain of pleuritic chest pain, shortness of breath, occasional hemoptysis, and fever (usually less than 101°F). In most cases, acute bronchitis symptoms are preceded or accompanied by symptoms of an upper respiratory tract infection. On physical examination, wheezes or diffuse rhonchi may be present. The presence of localized rales should raise the possibility of pneumonia.

Laboratory or Radiologic Evaluation
Unless the patient has an underlying chronic pulmonary disease or appears seriously ill, there is little benefit from evaluating arterial blood gases, white blood cell counts, sputum Gram stains or culture, or routine chest radiograph.

Differential Diagnosis
In addition to suspecting pneumonia in patients with a cough, one should consider sinusitis and asthma in patients presenting with a productive cough and wheezing. Particularly in younger patients, symptoms of recurrent or chronic bronchitis may be indicators of underlying asthma and warrant further evaluation.

Treatment of Acute Bronchitis
Antibiotic Use
There is little evidence to support the use of routine antibiotics in previously healthy patients with acute bronchitis. Patients with underlying asthma, cystic fibrosis, chronic obstructive pulmonary disease (COPD), or another illness that would predispose to immunoincompetence may benefit from antibiotic administration using such medications as erythromycin (e.g., erythromycin ethylsuccinate, or EES, 400 mg qid or 800 mg bid), trimethoprim–sulfamethoxazole (Bactrim, Septra) 1 double-strength tablet bid, or cephalexin (Keflex), 250 mg qid.

Bronchodilators
Because patients with acute bronchitis often present with wheezing and have reversible changes on pulmonary function tests, the use of aerosolized bronchodilating agents, such as albuterol (Proventil), one to two puffs qid for 7 to 10 days, may be useful for reducing the duration of symptoms and returning patients to their usual activity earlier.

Postbronchitic Syndrome
Patients who have experienced acute bronchitis may continue to cough for several months following their acute illness. This cough is usually unproductive and may be exacerbated by exercise, changes in temperature or humidity, or other factors that instigate airway reactivity. In these patients, continued treatment with albuterol or a similar β^2-agonist agent may help the airway reactivity and reduce the cough. Eventually, these symptoms subside totally and the bronchodilator can be discontinued.

PNEUMONIA
General Principles
Many bacterial organisms are responsible for pneumonia in ambulatory patients, although in most cases a specific bacterium is not found. The morbidity of pneumonia in patients with bacterial etiologies and the increased mortality among older patients and those with underlying pulmonary diseases make the timely diagnosis and proper management of pneumonia in ambulatory patients important.

Diagnosis
Clinical Presentation
Patients with pneumonia present with a productive cough, sometimes with hemoptysis. Pleuritic chest pain, shortness of breath, tachypnea, and fever may also accompany the cough. Some patients, especially children and elderly patients, may present without a cough and with vague, poorly defined symptoms, such as fever, nausea, or abdominal pain. Patients often have rales in the affected area, although with consolidation rales may not be present. With consolidation, the only physical findings may be decreased breath sounds

and egophony. Decreased breath sounds may also be noted in patients with associated pneumonic pleural effusions.

Laboratory and Radiologic Evaluation

The diagnosis of pneumonia is confirmed by chest radiography. Both posteroanterior and lateral views should be taken when possible to help localize the area of infiltrate. A sputum specimen for Gram stain and culture can often be helpful in directing the selection of antibiotic. In patients with underlying pulmonary diseases, arterial blood oxygen concentration should be evaluated by blood gas analysis or pulse oximetry. For patients who appear ill, a white blood cell count and differential may be useful for following the progress of recovery, and a blood culture should be strongly considered.

Presentation in Elderly Patients

Older patients may not exhibit any of the usual signs and symptoms of pneumonia. Many older individuals have nonspecific symptoms, such as anorexia, confusion, or falls, as early signs of pneumonia. Because of the high mortality in the geriatric population, pneumonia should be considered in all older patients who are exhibiting acute changes in their mental status or general health.

Treatment

Individualizing Management

Many previously healthy individuals with acute pneumonia can be managed on an outpatient basis. However, based on the increased mortality from pneumonia among patients with certain risk factors, hospital admission should be strongly considered for patients with chronic pulmonary diseases, patients with cirrhosis, those showing significant hypoxia or hypotension, elderly patients, and those with impaired immunocompetence. In addition, patients with signs of compromise, such as tachypnea (respiratory rate over 30) or hypotension, should be hospitalized.

Antibiotic Selection

The difficulty in obtaining sputum specimens from some patients makes empirical treatment with antibiotics the recommended management of all pneumonias encountered in the primary care setting. In addition, recent growth in the number of *Streptococcus pneumoniae* strains that are resistant to penicillin and other commonly used antibiotics makes antibiotic selection very important. The American Thoracic Society and the Infectious Disease Society have issued recent guidelines to assist with antibiotic selection for low- and high-risk patients.[1]

■ **Treatment with low risk for drug-resistant *Streptococcus pneumoniae* (DRSP).** Initial antibiotic selection should be based on Gram stain results. In the absence of an adequate specimen, for previously healthy patients, antibiotics should be chosen to cover the most common community-acquired agents. For ambulatory patients, empirical therapy with an extended spectrum macrolide such as azithromycin (Zithromax), 500-mg single dose followed by 250 mg daily, or a fluoroquinolone with enhanced pneumococcal activity (such as gatifloxicin, levofloxacin, or moxifloxacin) will be effective against the most common bacterial organisms as well as atypical agents. In heavy smokers and patients with underlying COPD, consideration should be given to using a drug that is also effective against *Haemophilus influenzae*, such as second-generation cephalosporins or clarithromycin (Biaxin, 500 mg bid), or a fluoroquinolone with enhanced pneumococcal activity all of which are effective against *Mycoplasma, S. pneumoniae*, and *Legionella*. Patients with underlying chronic pulmonary disease or with other risk factors, such as institutional residence, alcoholism, or other debilitating illness, may require broader Gram-negative coverage with a second- or third-generation cephalosporin, such as cefuroxime (Zinacef) 750 mg IV or IM q8h. In these patients, the addition of a macrolide to cover *Legionella* and other atypical organisms should be considered. In cases where fever and symptoms persist, a follow-up chest film may be useful to evaluate for a potential empyema. In addition, patients who are not improving with empirical therapy should be suspected of having DRSP and should be treated accordingly (see below).

- **Inpatient treatment with high risk for DRSP.** Risk factors for infection with DRSP include recent hospitalization; use of β^2-lactam antibiotics in the previous 3 months; severe underlying illness such as malignancy, chronic renal failure, or advanced liver disease. In patients with higher risk for DRSP, initial therapy should be started with either a fluoroquinolone with enhanced pneumococcal activity (such as levofloxacin or ofloxacin) or, in critically ill patients, with vancomycin. Fluoroquinolones with enhanced *S. pneumococcus* activity demonstrate good activity against intermediate-resistance *Streptococcus* but not against highly resistant statins. Vancomycin should be used for highly resistant strains or in critically ill patients where resistance status is unknown.

Follow-Up

In patients with lobar or segmental pneumonias that do not clear with antibiotic therapy, further evaluation with computed tomography may be advisable to evaluate for an obstructing tumor. In addition, because of the increased possibility of an underlying tumor associated with pneumonia in patients older than 40 years, a follow-up chest film is indicated in 4 to 6 weeks in such individuals.

Special Consideration

Because of the increased morbidity associated with pneumonia in certain risk classes, patients with underlying asthma, COPD, and threatened immunocompetence (including prior splenectomy, cardiac or renal disease, or age greater than 65) should receive a pneumococcal vaccine and yearly influenza vaccinations (See Chapter 1.4). *Smoking cessation should be discussed with patients with asthma, COPD, or other conditions placing them at risk for bronchitis and pneumonia.*

Reference

1. Bartlett JG, Dowell SF, Mandell LA, et al. Practice guidelines for the management of community-acquired pneumonia in adults. *Clin Infect Dis* 2000;31:347–382.

CHRONIC OBSTRUCTIVE PULMONARY DISEASE 10.3

Joshua J. Raymond, John M. Heath

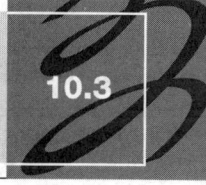

GENERAL PRINCIPLES

Chronic bronchitis and emphysema are the two clinical manifestations of chronic obstructive pulmonary disease (COPD). Airway dilatation, reduction of bronchial inflammation, and relief of hypoxia are key aspects of management. Cigarette smoking cessation is the key to avoid disease progression. Cigarette smoking causes 99% of COPD, though only 20% of smokers will develop COPD. The differing susceptibility of smokers to COPD is thought to relate in part to variability in their adaptive response to cumulative oxidative stress.[1,2] COPD is currently the 4th leading cause of U.S. mortality and the 12th leading cause of chronic disability. By 2020, COPD is estimated to be the 3rd leading cause of disability worldwide.[3]

COPD is the clinical syndrome resulting from airflow obstruction due to long-term lung tissue damage. COPD classically is grouped into two clinical manifestations:

- Chronic bronchitis. Characterized pathologically by an increase in submucosal secretory glands along bronchial walls that demonstrate inflammatory changes. The chief clinical feature is coughing episodes with sputum production lasting at least 3 months in duration and occurring over 2 consecutive years.
- Emphysema. Characterized pathologically by the loss of lung elasticity and destruction of alveolar walls. The chief clinical feature is progressive shortness of breath.

The clinical features of COPD are cough, sputum production (especially with chronic bronchitis) and progressive dyspena (especially with emphysema). Unlike the dyspena caused by the short-term airway obstruction occurring in asthma, COPD obstructive changes are less reversible. Important psychologic symptoms and functional limitations include withdrawal, isolation, and depression.

DIAGNOSIS

Clinical Findings

Airflow obstruction results in progressive hyperresonance on lung field percussion. Prominent accessory muscle use is accompanied by diminished breath sounds on auscultation. Classically described appearances of "blue bloater" and "pink puffer" are end-stage presentations of COPD.

Right-sided heart failure caused by hypoxemia and pulmonary hypertension leads to peripheral edema and dyspnea in chronic bronchitis. Failing respiratory muscles and decreasing lung supportive structures cause patients with emphysema to make prolonged puffing efforts to attempt to maintain lung expansion. Both appearances share prolonged expiration and decreased airflow.

Laboratory Tests

Pulmonary function testing demonstrates a characteristic pattern of reduced airflow, with forced expiratory volume at 1 second (FEV_1) less than 70% of the predicted value. Radiographic findings on chest x-ray can include hyperinflation of lung fields with resulting flattening of the diaphragms, an increase in the anteroposterior (AP) diameter of the chest cavity, and hyperlucency of peripheral lung fields. Patients with chronic bronchitis may also have infiltrates during periods of active infection, atelectasis-related to mucus trapping; pneumothorax, or pneumomediastinum can also be seen in critical hypoxic presentations. Arterial blood gas analysis can show hypoxia and hypercapnia. Testing for alpha-1-antitrypsin deficiency should be considered in younger patients with COPD without a smoking history.

Differential Diagnosis Considerations

During acute exacerbations, consider decompensated congestive heart failure, pneumonia, pulmonary embolism. During insidious presentations factors may include alpha-1-antitrypsin deficiency and cystic fibrosis.

TREATMENT

Smoking cessation is the only intervention proven to slow the accelerated decline in lung function causing COPD. Overall treatment goals relieve symptoms, decrease pulmonary inflammation, and improve oxygenation.[4]

Medication, Oxygen, and Surgery

- Bronchodilator therapy with sympathomimetic agents such as beta-2 receptor agonists relax airway smooth muscle and relieve air hunger.[4]
- Long-acting preparations such as salmeterol (Serevent) are given twice daily and decrease the frequency of acute exacerbations.
- Short-acting beta-2 agonists such as albuterol (Proventil, others) provide immediate relief from acute bronchospasm and are recommended for use as rescue agents delivered by either metered-dose inhalers or nebulizers.
- Anticholinergic bronchodilators inhibit the parasympathetic drive to the bronchial smooth muscle, resulting in bronchodilation. Examples include:
  - Tiotropium bromide (Spiriva) is a once daily inhaled agent that achieved 24-hour muscarinic blocker blockade for prolonged improvement in lung volume preservation.
  - Ipratropium (Atrovent) is a short-acting anticholinergic agent available in both inhaler or nebulizer form that can be combined with beta agonists for enhanced bronchodilation.
- Corticosteroid administration, by inhalation (Pulmicort, others), oral (Predinsone, others), or parental routes (Decadron, others) of administration are controversial in COPD treatment; guidelines recommend inhaled corticosteroid be considered for patients with moderate to severe airflow limitation whose symptoms persist despite optimal bronchodilatory therapy.[5]

- Theophylline may be added if symptoms continue despite combined inhaler therapies. Frequent monitoring of drug levels and concerns for adverse reactions and drug–drug interactions often limit theophylline use.
- Vaccination against pneumococcal and influenza should be offered to all patients.
- Correction of hypoxia is critical for morbidity reduction in COPD management.[4] Current Medicare continuous oxygen supplementation reimbursement guidelines require an arterial pO_2 of 55 mmHg or less on room air, clinically diagnosed cor pulmonale plus a room air pO_2 of 55 to 59 mmHg, or a hematocrit of 55% or greater. Nighttime use is critical to prevent cardiac arrhythmias and pulmonary hypertension. Oxygen can be supplied through compressed gas, liquid reservoirs, or room air concentration devices and delivered via mask or nasal cannuli that incorporate demand-flow devices.
- Surgical interventions, such as lung volume reduction surgery (surgical removal of hyperinflated but poorly perfused areas of lung) or single lung transplantation, have resulted in improved measures of quality of life and function in highly selected patients.

Supplemental Therapies

- Pulmonary rehabilitation can improve exercise capacity, reduce dyspnea, and decrease the number and length of hospitalizations for acute exacerbations and is most appropriate for patients with COPD with preserved functional capacity for some exertion and otherwise cardiac status.[6]
- Nutritional support for the increased respiratory effort for labored breathing.[7]
- Complications include respiratory failure leading to progressive hypercapnea and decreased mental alertness. Hypoxemia leads to increasing pulmonary vascular pressures, secondary polycythemia, and ischemia complications of extremities and internal organs.
- Patient education including smoking cessation is by far the single most important educational element in COPD management. It is important that the patient know the proper inhaler technique for each of the differing medication devices. Facilitating expectoration to reduce fatigue and breathing exercises can improve airflow between exacerbations.[8]

SPECIAL CONSIDERATIONS

Close communication between patient, family, and health care provider reduce unnecessary hospitalizations.[9] Facilitating the frank discussions among the patient and the family about the use of mechanical ventilation, cardiopulmonary resuscitation, and other advance treatment wishes by the health care provider team during periods of relative disease stability can help guide the treatment intensity decisions during periods of clinical decompensations when communication with the patient directly may be compromised.

References

1. Fabbri LM, Hurd SS. Global strategy of the diagnosis, management and prevention of COPD. *Eur Respir J* 2003;22:1–12.
2. Wright JL, Levy RD, Churg A. Pulmonary hypertension in COPD: current theories of pathogenesis and their implications for treatment. *Thorax* 2005;60:605–609.
3. Global Initiative for Chronic Obstructive Lung Disease, http://www.goldcopd.com/Guidelineitem.asp. Accessed on February 10, 2006.
4. National Collaborating Centre for Chronic Conditions. Chronic obstructive pulmonary disease. National clinical guideline on management of chronic obstructive pulmonary disease in adults in primary and secondary care. *Thorax* 2004;59(Suppl 1):1–232.
5. Bonay M, Bancal C, Crestani B. The risk/benefit of inhaled corticosteroids in chronic obstructive pulmonary disease. *Expert Opin Drug Saf* 2005;4:251–271.
6. Griffiths TL, Burr ML, Campbell IA, et al. Results at 1 year of outpatient multidisciplinary pulmonary rehabilitation: a randomized controlled trial. *Lancet* 2000;355:362–368.
7. Nutritional guidelines for people with COPD: Cleveland Clinic Foundation Health Information Center, http://www.clevelandclinic.org/health/healthinfo/docs/2400/2411.asp. Accessed on February 10, 2006.
8. Pulmonary health/exercise and care: National Emphysema Foundation, http://www.nef-usa.org/pulhthex.jsp.
9. Pulmonary rehabilitation: a team approach to improving the quality of life: American College of Chest Physicians, http://www.chestnet.org/patients/guides/pulmonary/.

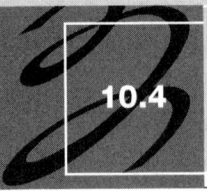

10.4 TUBERCULOSIS

Michelle Anne Bholat, Patrick T. Dowling

GENERAL PRINCIPLES

Tuberculosis (TB), a chronic, necrotizing infection, is caused by the **Mycobacterium tuberculosis** bacillus. It is spread primarily through an airborne route when an individual with pulmonary **disease** coughs, talks, or sneezes. The hallmark of this most successful pathogen, which infects one third of the world's population, is the ability to persist in the form of a long-term asymptomatic infection. This is referred to as **latent TB infection (LTBI).** In the competent host, cellular immunity maintains the latent status in most; however, 10% of those with infection go on to develop active **disease**. Each year approximately 9 million people develop active **disease** worldwide claiming almost 2 million lives. As such, TB remains a leading infectious cause of death and the greatest killer of women in child-bearing years.

The archetypal disease of poverty, over 90% of cases occur in the developing world. After many years in decline in the United States, the incidence rates began climbing in 1985 but have decreased yearly since 1992. The highest rates are found among elderly people as well as ethnic and racial minorities in many U.S. urban areas with recent immigrants. Although **foreign born (FB)** persons account for only 12% of the U.S. population they represent almost 55% of all with active disease. **Among Asian Americans with TB, 94% are FB; among Hispanics, 74% are FB. The converse is true among blacks as 74% are U.S. born.** Five countries of origin account for the greatest number of cases among FB: **Mexico (26%), Philippines (12%), Vietnam (8%), India (8%), and China (5%).** These epidemiologic data are important for screening purposes. Although pulmonary disease is the most common clinical presentation, approximately 15% of patients have an extrapulmonary form of disease. Hematogenous spread may result in miliary TB, so named because of its characteristic millet-seed appearance on chest radiographs (CXRs). Patients with HIV infection have an extremely high rate of both pulmonary and extrapulmonary disease. Furthermore, extrapulmonary involvement tends to increase in frequency **in the setting of a compromised immune system.**

Endogenous reactivation of **LTBI** as opposed to new primary infection **(exogenous reinfection)** accounts for the majority of cases of active disease in the United States. Individuals with advanced HIV infection are the exception to this because they have unusually high rates of primary infection. Chronic medical conditions, outlined in Table 10.4-1, as well as corticosteroid use and immunocompromised states (HIV) are important predisposing factors for reactivation.

An 80-year-old live attenuated vaccine, the bacillus Calmette-Guerin **(BCG),** derived from *Mycobacterium* bovine, is still administered to over half the infants in the world. Although it does not prevent TB disease, it can reduce **TB meningitis** and **miliary TB** in young children.

DIAGNOSIS OF DISEASE

History and Physical Examination

- Although some patients may be asymptomatic, most present with chronic nonspecific symptoms, such as cough, fever, night sweats, weight loss, lassitude, and hemoptysis. Extrapulmonary disease may present as a fever of unknown origin. On examination, patients often appear chronically ill with weight loss. Apical rales may be present.

Laboratory Studies

- Diagnosis depends on CXR findings and identification of the acid-fast bacillus **(AFB)** from the sputum.

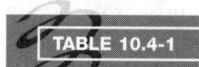

TABLE 10.4-1 Relative Risk for Developing Active Tuberculosis by Selected Clinical Conditions

Clinical condition	Relative risk (%)
Silicosis	30
Diabetes mellitus	2.0–4.1
Chronic renal failure/hemodialysis	10.0–25.3
Gastrectomy	2–5
Jejunoileal bypass	27–63
Solid-organ transplantation	20–74
Carcinoma of head or neck	16

- **Radiographic findings.** Classically, the CXR reveals fibrocavitary lesions of the upper lobes (apical and posterior segments); however, a varied picture may be present, with infiltration, miliary nodules, or an effusion; or it may be normal, especially with disseminated disease. HIV-infected patients tend to have atypical CXRs or normal CXRs **as immunosuppressed individuals may lack the cellular immune response that causes cavitation.**
- **Bacteriologic evaluation.** Sputum smears for **AFB** are available immediately but are limited by a sensitivity of 55% and a specificity of 99%; a nucleic acid amplification system test **(NAAT)** provides rapid confirmation that the infecting mycobacteria are *M. tuberculosis*. Cultures, which typically take 6 to 8 weeks, have a sensitivity of 81% and a specificity of 98%; **these percentages are lower** with noncavitary disease. The use of a liquid medium system can provide information in 7 to 14 days. *M. tuberculosis* can also be cultured from the blood; bacteremia has been reported in 14% of patients with TB.
- **Surgical and invasive diagnostic tools.** Bronchoscopy with transbronchial biopsy can provide immediate diagnosis in smear-negative cases, but because of its risks and expense it should be reserved for selected cases (e.g., HIV-infected patients), primarily to exclude other diagnoses.
- **Tuberculin skin testing (TST).** For more than a century the Mantoux test, which involves the injection of 0.1 mL of intermediate-strength purified protein derivative (PPD) intradermally, has been used in the diagnosis of TB. It cannot distinguish between past infections and current disease, or reactions due to previous BCG vaccination. The test is interpreted at 48 to 72 hours by measuring the degree of maximum **induration,** not **erythema; it is acceptable to read the skin test up to 96 hours.** A negative test result does not exclude the disease **and active disease must be ruled out before treating for LTBI.** Although anergy testing may provide prognostic information for immunocompromised individuals, it is no longer recommended. Unless additional diagnostic testing is employed, a positive reaction in those who previously received **BCG** should be assumed to be secondary to exposure as opposed to the BCG as reactivity to that vaccine wanes with time **(see 1B5 QuantiFERON-TB Gold, below).** Three cutoff levels for determining a positive **TST** reaction are based on sensitivity, specificity, and prevalence of tuberculosis in different groups:
  - A ≥5-*mm* induration for HIV-positive individuals, recent contacts with persons with active TB, individuals whose CXR findings are consistent with old healed TB (fibrotic change), and patients with organ transplants and other immunosuppressed patients receiving more than 15 mg per day of prednisone for more than 1 month.
  - A ≥10-*mm* induration for recent immigrants (within the last 5 years) from high-prevalence countries; low-income minority populations; residents and employees of correctional facilities, nursing homes, and shelters; health care workers; injection drug users, individuals with chronic medical conditions (see Table 10.4-1); and children younger than 4 years or infants, children, and adolescents exposed to adults in high-risk categories.
  - A ≥15-*mm* induration for persons with no risk factors for TB.

The **QuantiFERON-TB Gold Test (QTF-G)** is a whole blood assay approved by the FDA in 2005 as a new diagnostic test for TB. It is not subject to reader bias as the case may be with the **TST** and is not affected by prior **BCG** vaccination.

TREATMENT OF ACTIVE TUBERCULOSIS

Outpatient management of individuals suspected of **active** TB should be considered. Hospitalization is recommended if the patient is incapable of self-care or poses an infectious risk to others. Hospitalized patients suspected of having TB should be placed in respiratory isolation until **sputum** results become available or they have completed 2 weeks of treatment with clinical response. Public health officials must be notified **to locate any contacts and to ensure compliance and follow-up of these exposed individuals.**

Chemotherapy

Successful treatment requires multidrug therapy aimed at the *Mycobacterium* species susceptible to the chosen drugs; they must be taken on a regular basis with an adequate number of doses for a sufficient period of time. It is now recommended that all patients be treated with four drugs for 2 months daily. The drugs include isoniazid (INH), rifampin (RIF), pyrazinamide (PZA), and ethambutol (ETH) or streptomycin. **Children, pregnant women, and adults at risk for INH-induced neuritis should receive pyridoxine (vitamin B$_6$) daily as follows: (a) adult prophylaxis at 25 to 100 mg per day and (b) pediatric prophylaxis at 1 to 2 mg/kg/day.** Because compliance over long periods of time with several drugs is difficult, directly observed therapy **(DOT)** should be considered. Consultation with public health is strongly recommended; reporting of active disease cases is mandatory. The following are current national recommendations:

- **Confirmed or suspected active tuberculosis cases.** These should be treated with a four-drug regimen until the results of mycobacterial cultures and sensitivities have been obtained. Administer daily INH: children, 10 mg per kg; adults, 300 mg; RIF: children, 10 to 20 mg/kg/day; adults, 10 mg/kg/day to a maximum dose of 600 mg per day; PZA: children 20 to 30 mg/kg/day; adults, 25 mg/kg/day to a maximum of 2 g per day; ETH: children and adults, 15 to 25 mg/kg/day. Streptomycin should be substituted for ETH in very young children. If there is no resistance to INH and RIF, both PZA and ETH are discontinued after 2 months if repeat sputum cultures are negative and there is improvement in the patient's clinical condition. INH and RIF are continued for an additional 4 months for a total treatment course of 6 months. If the patient remains symptomatic, or if a follow-up smear or culture result remains positive after 2 months of therapy, therapy with INH/RIF should be continued for total of 9 months and consultation is recommended. (See joint document ATS/CDC in references for detailed discussion of options.)
- **HIV-infected patients.** Three possible regimens that include RIF-based treatments have been recommended by the U.S. Centers for Disease Control and Prevention. However, RIF is contraindicated when the patient is receiving protease inhibitors (PIs) or nonnucleoside reverse transcriptase inhibitors (NNRTIs). In its place are 6-month rifabutin-based treatments and 9-month streptomycin-based regimens, which may be used on such patients. The use of streptomycin is contraindicated in pregnant women. **(Consult the public health department for recommendations.)**
- **Multidrug-resistant tuberculosis (MDR),** defined as disease that is resistant to both INH and RIF. Patients should be treated with a regimen that includes three or four drugs to which the tuberculosis isolate is susceptible. Combinations with levofloxacin and moxifloxacin appear promising. Consultation with public health department and CDC is recommended.
- **Extrapulmonary disease.** Treatment is the same as above for active tuberculosis but is continued for 9 months. Due to a paucity of data, the recommendation is that miliary TB, bone or joint TB, and TB meningitis in children and infants require 12 months of therapy with public health consultation (Chapter 6.3).
- **Pregnancy and lactation.** Use INH, RIF, and ETH for 9 months with pyridoxine, 25 mg per day. Streptomycin should be avoided because of ototoxicity to the fetus; PZA is not recommended because its teratogenicity is unknown. Lactating women who are taking antituberculous medication should breastfeed before ingesting their medication. Bottle supplementation should be used for the first feeding after dosing. (For infants

whose mothers were treated for active TB during pregnancy and who are themselves on INH for treatment of LTBI, bottle-feeding is recommended.)

Monitoring for Adverse Reactions

Liver enzymes, bilirubin, creatinine, and a complete blood count/platelet count should be obtained as baseline information before implementing the standard regimens. If PZA is to be used, uric acid should be obtained. If ETH is included in the regimen, obtain baseline and monthly visual acuity as well as red–green perception testing to detect drug-induced optic neuritis. Patients should be seen monthly and monitored clinically for adverse effects. For individuals with abnormal baseline studies, follow-up studies are indicated. In those with normal baseline studies, follow-up laboratory testing should be done only if drug toxicity is suspected.

Evaluation of Response to Treatment

Repeated sputum examinations, beginning with weekly smear quantitation, are desirable until sputum conversion is documented. More than 85% of patients on INH and RIF with positive cultures convert to negative after 2 months. If sputum remains positive after 2 months, drug susceptibility studies should be repeated, and DOT should be implemented. CXRs are less valuable than sputum examinations for evaluation and should not be routinely performed.

TARGETED TUBERCULIN TESTING AND TREATMENT OF LATENT TB INFECTION

- Change in nomenclature. The term **treatment of LTBI** replaces what was once referred to as **preventive therapy** and **chemoprophylaxis.**
- Recommendations for targeted tuberculin testing. Targeted tuberculin testing is indicated to identify individuals at high risk for TB who would benefit by treatment of LTBI. These groups include individuals at risk for recent infection (lower socioeconomic status or recent immigrant from high-incidence country) with *M. tuberculosis* and those who are at risk for progression to active TB (based on presence of medical condition). Interpretation of the three cutoff points for determining a positive tuberculin skin test reaction as noted above. **According to recent CDC recommendations, TST should only be performed in persons who belong to at least one of the high-risk groups noted below, as "a decision to test is a decision to treat."** Routine screening of other persons, including children not belonging to high-risk groups, is discouraged. A notable exception are individuals receiving antitumor necrosis factor alpha products **(anti-TNFs) such as infliximab (Remicade) for rheumatoid arthritis or Crohn disease.** They should be screened for LTBI before anti-TNFs initiated. Anergic patients with HIV infection should be treated if they are close contacts, previously had a positive skin test, or are members of a group in which the prevalence of TB is at least 10% (Table 10.4-2).

| TABLE 10.4-2 | Treatment Regimens for Latent Tuberculosis Infection |

Drug	Duration (mo)	Interval	Rating[a] HIV−	Rating[a] HIV+
INH	9	Daily	A	A
		Twice weekly	B	B
INH	6	Daily	B	C
		Twice weekly	B	C
RIF	4	Daily	B	B

INH, isoniazid; RIF, rifampin.
[a]A, preferred; B, acceptable alternative; C, offer when A and B cannot be given. In situations in which rifampin cannot be used (e.g., HIV-infected persons receiving protease inhibitors), rifabutin may be substituted.

■ Reducing progression from LTBI to active disease. Whereas 90% of active cases of TB in non-HIV-infected individuals are secondary to endogenous reactivation, treatment that diminishes or eradicates the bacterial population in "healed" or radiographically invisible lesions is an important means of reducing this progression. Since 1965, INH for 6 to 12 months has been the mainstay of therapy of individuals with LTBI infection, reducing the rate of reactivation by at least 70%. However, adherence to therapy has been problematic because of the long duration of therapy and concerns about toxicity. Latest recommended therapy is 9 months of INH for all given either daily or **twice a week** by **DOT**. RIF, up to 600 mg per day, for 4 months is recommended as an alternative in contacts of patients with INH-resistant TB. **RIF-PZA is no longer a recommendation because of fatal hepatoxicity.** Anergic patients or those with a previous history of a positive PPD and HIV infection should be treated if they are close contacts. Before initiating treatment, physicians must ensure that active disease is ruled out. After that the decision to treat hinges on an analysis of risks and benefits.

■ For pregnant, HIV-negative women, INH given daily or twice weekly for 9 months is recommended. For women at risk for progression of LTBI to disease, especially those who are infected with HIV or who have likely been infected recently, initiation of therapy should not be delayed on the basis of pregnancy alone, even during the first trimester. For women whose risk for active TB is lower, some experts recommend waiting 3 months postpartum because of the risk of INH hepatotoxcity.

■ **Risk of therapy.** Treatment of LTBI is usually indicated, regardless of age, in patients who belong to high-risk groups. INH is associated with hepatitis, the incidence of which is age related beginning after age 19 and increasing significantly after age 35. Extensive use of alcohol may enhance this association. Fatal INH-associated hepatitis has been reported. The risk is highest among women, particularly black and Hispanic women; it may also be increased during the postpartum period. Baseline studies are indicated in individuals at high risk for hepatotoxicity, such as those with HIV infection, alcoholism, chronic liver disease, pregnancy, or postpartum status. Patients should be monitored monthly and liver function tests obtained if clinically indicated. INH should be discontinued if liver enzymes reach three times the upper limit of normal levels in symptomatic patients or five times the upper limit of normal levels in asymptomatic patients. Because INH may increase the serum level of phenytoin (Dilantin), a decreased dosage of the latter may be necessary. Women receiving RIF and oral contraceptives should be advised to use a backup method of contraception to avoid pregnancy. Pyridoxine, **25 to 100 mg per day,** is recommended in high-risk **adults to reduce the risk of INH-induced peripheral neuropathy.**

NONTUBERCULOUS

Nontuberculous mycobacteria **(NTM)** are ubiquitous and are responsible for producing cutaneous, pulmonary, lymphatic, and disseminated disease.

■ **Disseminated *Mycobacterium avium* complex (MAC) disease** is the most common bacterial infection in patients with AIDS, occurring in 20% to 40% and is the most common cause of NTM pulmonary disease worldwide. In those with HIV, it is rare with CD4 counts greater than 100; it should be suspected in HIV-infected persons with CD4 counts below 50. The prognosis of patients with MAC, like other opportunistic infections, has improved significantly due to several factors, including the use of highly active antiretroviral therapy (HAART) regimens. Prophylaxis with a macrolide agent such as clarithromycin or azithromycin is indicated in patients with CD4 counts below 50.

■ ***Mycobacterium kansasii,*** the second most common nontuberculous mycobacteria pulmonary disease, presents with variable and nonspecific signs and symptoms. Diagnosis is based on clinical, radiographic, and bacteriologic criteria as well as measures to exclude other pulmonary disease, including TB. Pulmonary disease caused by *M. kansasii* responds to most TB regimens. Consultation with local health department experts is recommended (see Chapter 19.4).

References
1. American Thoracic Society/Centers for Disease Control. Treatment of tuberculosis. *MMWR* 2003;1–77, www.cdc.gov/mmwr/preview/mmwrhtlm/rr5211a1.html.

2. ATS/CDC/Infectious Disease Society of America. Treatment of tuberculosis. *Am J Respir Crit Care Med* 2003;167:603–622, www.atsjournals.org.
3. Centers for Disease Control. TB associated with blocking agents against tumor necrosis factor—California 2002–03. *MMWR* 2004;53:683–686, www.cdc.gov/mmwr.htlm/mm5330a4.htm.
4. Francis J. Curry National TB Center, www.nationaltbcenter.edu/. Excellent comprehensive site with teaching modules.
5. ATS/CDC. Targeted tuberculin testing and treatment of latent tuberculosis infection. *MMWR* 2000;49(RR06):1–54, www.cdc.giv/epo/mmwr.
6. ATS/CDC Controlling TB in the US. *MMWR* 2005;54(RR12);1–81, www.cdc.gov/mmwr/preview.mmwrhtlm/rr5412al.htm.
7. CDC. Fatal liver injuries associated with Rifampin and PZA for LTBI and revisions in ATS/CDC recommendations—U.S., 2001 *MMWR* 2001;50:733–736. www.cdc.gov/mmwr.
8. Blumberg HM, Leonard MK, Jasmer RM. Update on the Treatment of TB and LTBI. *JAMA* 2005;293:2776–2784, www.jama.com.
9. Potter B, Rindfleisch K, Kraus CK. Management of active TB. *Am Fam Physician* 2005;72:2225–2235, www.aafp/org/afp.xml.
10. UpToDate. General Principles of the treatment of TB, www.Uptodate.com.

LUNG CANCER

Kenneth F. Kessel, William T. Leslie,
Daniel G. Hunter-Smith

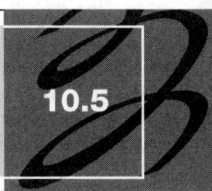

GENERAL PRINCIPLES

Epidemiology and Pathology

Primary cancer of the lung is the leading cause of cancer mortality in the United States in both men and women, with estimated cancer deaths in 2006 of 90,330 for men and 72,130 for women. Histologically, primary lung cancer is divided into two categories, small cell lung cancer (SCLC) and non-small cell lung cancer (NSCLC).

Adenocarcinoma and squamous cell carcinoma are the two major types of NSCLC. This categorization is useful for clinical staging, treatment, and prognosis. Histological types vary between men and women as follows: SCLC: 18.4% versus 22.6%; NSCLC: adenocarcinoma 33.2% versus 44.7%, squamous cell 36.3% versus 21.4%. The median age for lung cancer diagnosis is 66 for both sexes. Lung cancer has been declining in men since 1975, when the male/female incidence ratio was 3.56. This ratio changed to 1.56 in 1999.

- **Screening.** At present, there are no accepted screening methods for lung cancer. The National Cancer Institute and a European group have opened randomized studies of computed tomography (CT) scan screening for lung cancer. Mortality data should be available by 2010. Studies of CT scan screening seem to demonstrate a higher detection rate of early-stage cancers. It is not known if iatrogenic complications will offset mortality gains and whether CT scan screening is economically feasible for the general population or should be restricted to high-risk patients only.
- **History and clinical presentation.** Risk factors, especially active or passive smoking exposure, must be obtained. Industrial or home exposure to radon, asbestos, and other airborne particulate matter may also be relevant. Family members who are first-degree relatives of a patient with lung cancer have been shown to have a 2.4-fold increase in risk for developing lung cancer. The most common presenting signs and symptoms of lung cancer are cough (50%), hemoptysis (20%), dyspnea (30%), chest pain (25%), bone pain (20%), and weight loss (30%).

DIAGNOSIS

Physical Examination

Frequently, the examination is unremarkable. However, patients may present with bronchial obstruction causing fever, coarse rales, egophony, decreased breath sounds, and dullness to percussion over the obstructed area. Patients presenting with an unexplained pleural effusion have a 45% chance of malignancy.

Special Studies and Staging

Metastatic spread to regional or distant sites is present in three quarters of patients at the time of diagnosis. The histology is obtained by fine needle or bronchoscopic biopsy. Abdominal CT and bone scans are performed to identify or rule out distant metastases. One of six stages for NSCLC is determined (0, I, II, IIIA, IIIB, and IV) based on the tumor, node, metastasis (TNM) system. SCLC is rarely surgically resectable. Because of its propensity for brain metastasis, a brain magnetic resonance imaging (MRI) is obtained as part of the staging work up of SCLC.

COMPLICATIONS OF LUNG CANCER

- **Complications due to tumor extension or metastasis.** Paralysis of the cervical sympathetic nerve due to tumor invasion resulting in upper eyelid ptosis, pupillary constriction, anhydrosis, and flushing of the affected side of the face is known as **Horner syndrome.** A tumor near the apex of the lung can involve the brachial plexus resulting in Horner syndrome plus muscle atrophy and neurtic arm pain on the affected side. This is known as **Pancoast syndrome.** Compression of bronchial tubes by tumor extension commonly causes obstructive pneumonia. Compression of the superior vena cava causes facial swelling, rubor, and neck vein distention, and is called superior vena cava syndrome.
- **Paraneoplastic syndromes associated with NSCLC**
    - **Hypercalcemia.** This is most commonly seen with squamous cell carcinoma. It can be caused by ectopic secretion of parathormone as well as bone metastases and results in polyuria, dehydration, constipation, and mental confusion. Treatment consists of vigorous saline hydration and furosemide to restore a urinary output of 2 L per day. Thiazide diuretics must be avoided. Pamidronate (Ardia) may be given to rapidly lower serum calcium.
    - **Hypertrophic pulmonary osteoarthropathy.** This is associated with adenocarcinomas. Manifestations include clubbing of the fingers, joint and bone pain, and elevated alkaline phosphatase. The condition improves with nonsteroidal anti-inflammatory drugs (NSAIDs) and treatment of the tumor.
    - **Spinal cord compression. Severe back pain associated with motor and sensory loss related to the spinal cord level of compression. Treatment with IV dexamethasone (4 to 6 mg q 6 hours) should be given urgently, followed by radiation therapy or surgical decompression.**
- **Paraneoplastic syndromes associated with SCLC**
    - Syndrome of inappropriate excretion of antidiuretic hormone (SIADH). The initial therapy includes fluid restriction with the possible addition of demeclocycline (Declomycin) 150 to 300 mg qid. SAIDH improves with treatment of the tumor.
    - **Eaton Lambert syndrome.** This presents with myasthenia-like neurologic changes. Sensory neuropathies or limbic encephalothies may also occur.

TREATMENT

Surgical

Curative surgery is only possible for early stages of NSCLC (stages 0, I, II, and possibly IIIA). Patients with the following complications are not surgical candidates: superior vena cava syndrome, tumors closer than 2 cm to the carina, low pulmonary reserve, comorbid disease with unacceptable surgical risk, involvement of the pericardium, heart, esophagus, or great vessels and SCLC unless discovered as an isolated pulmonary nodule. Patients who are candidates for surgery should be evaluated with preoperative pulmonary function tests.

Radiation

This therapy is reserved for patients with localized NSCLC and for palliation of bone or spinal metastases. Radiation is also part of the definitive treatment of SCLC.

Chemotherapy

A combination of two chemotherapy drugs is more active than a single agent, but no additional benefit is seen when a third agent is added. Several doublets of chemotherapy appear to be equally active. A new class of drugs, the epidermal growth factor receptor (EGFR) inhibitors, can cause a dramatic regression of NSCLC in 10% to 20% of patients. Patients who are most likely to respond to EGFR inhibitors such as erlotinib (Tarceva) are women, nonsmokers, patients of Asian ethnicity, and those with bronchoalveolar cancer. Response rates have been correlated with specific mutations in the EGFR gene. The most common side effect is an acneiform rash, and patients who develop a severe rash are more likely to respond to the treatment. A monoclonal antibody to the vascular endothelial growth factor (VEGF), called bevacizumab (Avastin), is commercially available. In patients with advanced SCLC, the addition of bevacizumab to chemotherapy results in a significant improvement in survival. Patients with squamous cell histology were excluded because of an increased incidence of fatal hemoptysis.

Follow-Up

The estimated overall 5-year survival rates for patients with NSCLC by stage are IA, 66%; IB, 53%; IIA, 42%; IIB, 36%; IIIA, 10%; IIIB, 12%; IV, 4%. The 5-year survival rate of SCLC is 22% for limited disease and 1% for extensive disease.

References

1. Jemal A, et al. Cancer statistics, 2006. *CA* 2006;56(2):106–130.
2. Mulshine JL, et al. Lung cancer screening. *N Engl J Med* 2005;352:2714–2720.
3. Pisters KMW. Adjuvant chemotherapy for non-small-cell lung cancer. *N Engl J Med* 2005;352:2640–2642.
4. Leslie WT, Bonomi PD. Novel treatments in non-small cell lung cancer. *Hematol Oncol Clin North Am* 2004;18:245–267.
5. Dowell JE, et al. Epidermal growth factor receptor mutations in non-small cell lung cancer: a basic science discovery with immediate clinical impact. *Am J Med Sci* 2006;331(3):139–149.
6. Fu JB, et al. Lung cancer in women. *Chest* 2005;127:768–777.
7. Spiro SG, Silvestri GA. One hundred years of lung cancer. *Am J Respir Crit Care Med* 2005;172(5):523–529.
8. Schiller JH, et al. Comparison of four chemotherapy regimens for advanced non-smallcell lung cancer. *N Engl J Med* 2002;346:92–98.
9. Yang P, et al. Clinical features of 5,628 primary lung cancer patients: experience at Mayo Clinic from 1997 to 2003. *Chest.* 2005:128(1):452–462.

Gastrointestinal Problems 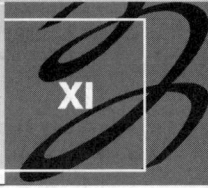 XI

PEPTIC ULCER DISEASE AND GASTRITIS
Alan M. Adelman
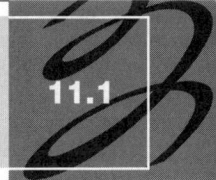 11.1

PEPTIC ULCER DISEASE

General Principles

Peptic ulcers may involve any portion of the upper gastrointestinal (GI) tract, but most ulcers are found in the stomach and duodenum. Duodenal ulcers are approximately three times as common as gastric ulcers. *Helicobacter pylori* (HP) is the major cause of peptic ulcer disease (PUD). A rare cause of PUD is Zollinger–Ellison syndrome.

Diagnosis
Clinical Presentation

Although PUD may occur or recur in the absence of pain, epigastric discomfort is the most common presenting symptom. Associated symptoms may include fullness, belching, bloating, heartburn, food intolerance, nausea, or vomiting. Severity and description of the pain is variable and correlates poorly with size or number of ulcers. The clinical presentation of PUD overlaps with that of other causes of epigastric discomfort (gastroesophageal reflux disease, nonulcer or functional dyspepsia, gastric cancer, cholelithiasis, and coronary artery disease).

Physical examination usually reveals only epigastric tenderness. Findings such as a succussion splash (gastric outlet obstruction), abdominal rigidity (perforation), or hemepositive stools (bleeding) are suggestive of complications of PUD.

Laboratory Studies[1]

■ Testing for *H. pylori*. There are several ways to test for HP. Serologic testing offers the easiest way of testing for HP and avoids the need for an endoscopy. Finger-stick testing, quantitative serologic testing, and enzyme-linked immunosorbent assay (ELISA) testing are available. A urea breath test can also be used to determine the presence of HP. If an ulcer is diagnosed endoscopically, a rapid urease test (*Campylobacter*-like Organism, or CLO; Delta West, Bentley, West Australia) is the quickest means to determine HP. To test for cure, a urea breath test (4 weeks after therapy), a falling ELISA titer (1, 3, and 6 months after therapy), or CLO at repeat endoscopy can be used.

- Quick serologic or finger-stick testing is a qualitative procedure for office use. Average sensitivity is 67% to 88% and specificity is 75% to 91%.
- Qualitative serologic testing cannot document eradication of HP.
- ELISA is a quantitative assay. Average sensitivity is 86% to 94% and specificity is 78% to 95%. Although a rapid decrease in the titer indicates cure, the titer may fall slowly over 12 to 18 months even in successfully treated patients.
- Urea breath testing requires a breath sample. Average sensitivity is 90% to 96% and specificity is 88% to 98%. This test will probably become the test of cure when it is widely available.
- Rapid urease testing requires a mucosal biopsy. Average sensitivity is 88% to 95% and specificity is 95% to 100%.
- Histologic testing requires a biopsy specimen and special stains. Average sensitivity is 93% to 96% and specificity is 98% to 99%.
- Culture requires a mucosal biopsy. Average sensitivity is 80% to 98% and specificity is 100%. Culture and drug sensitivities are important when drug resistance is suspected.

- Upper endoscopy should be performed as the initial study in patients with complications of PUD, patients with signs of systemic disease, patients 45 years of age or older, and patients who have failed empirical therapy. The main advantage of endoscopy is its capacity to obtain biopsy specimens for pathology and testing for HP.
- Double-contrast upper GI studies can reliably diagnose both duodenal and gastric ulcers, but the false-negative rate can exceed 18%, whereas the false-positive rate is 13% to 35%.

Therapy

General approach to the assessment of PUD.[2,3] First, patients with complications of PUD (bleeding, gastric outlet obstruction, perforation), patients with signs of systemic disease (anemia, significant weight loss), or patients with persistent or recurrent pain should be evaluated by upper endoscopy and managed immediately (see Chapter 11.3). Patients ≥45 years of age should also be considered for prompt endoscopy and management. Second, medications that can cause epigastric discomfort should be discontinued. In particular, patients should be questioned about the use of nonsteroidal anti-inflammatory drugs (NSAIDs), both prescription and over the counter. All other patients should be tested for HP and, if positive, should be treated with HP-eradicating agents.

The therapy is determined by the presence or absence of HP. Antibiotic treatment is given to patients who are positive for HP. The addition of a histamine receptor antagonist (HRA) or proton pump inhibitor (PPI) hastens relief of pain. PPIs such as omeprazole (Prilosec) also have anti-HP action and are included in some anti-HP regimens. Patients with HP-negative ulcers are treated with traditional antacid agents alone. The value of treating nonulcer dyspepsia patients with HP infection remains to be determined.

- **Regimens for H. pylori.**[1] Several regimens have been shown to be equally effective. The following regimens are given for 7 days. The PPI is to be given for an additional 3 weeks following the antibiotics.
  - PPI (standard dose), amoxicillin 1000 mg bid, and clarithromycin (Biaxin) 500 mg bid (the combination of lansoprazole, clarithromycin, and amoxicillin is available as Prevpac)
  - Bismuth 2 tabs qid, metronidazole 500 mg tid, tetracycline 500 mg qid, PPI (standard dose)

- **Traditional agents**
  - H_2RA. Cimetidine (Tagamet) 400 mg bid, famotidine (Pepcid) 20 mg bid, nizatidine (Axid) 150 mg bid, and ranitidine (Zantac) 150 mg bid are equally effective. Cimetidine appears to be associated with the highest incidence of side effects and drug interactions.
  - PPIs. Omeprazole (Prilosec) 20 mg daily, lansoprazole (Prevacid) 15 mg daily, rabeprazole (Aciphex) 20 mg qd, and pantoprazole (Protonix) 40 mg qd are more potent acid inhibitors than HRA.

■ Sucralfate (Carafate), 1 g qid, is effective in healing peptic ulcers. There are no significant side effects, but the size of the tablet and frequency of administration are potential drawbacks.

■ Antacids. Antacids are effective in healing ulcers, but their use is limited by the number of doses required. Aluminum hydroxide/magnesium hydroxide/simethicone antacids (Maalox extra strength, Mylanta double strength), 2 tablets qid, are unlikely to produce constipation or diarrhea. Phosphate depletion can occur with antacid use in malnourished patients, and hypermagnesemia can result in patients with chronic renal failure.

■ Dietary therapy is limited to the elimination of foods that exacerbate symptoms, and the avoidance of alcohol and coffee (with or without caffeine). Both alcohol and coffee increase gastric acid secretion.

■ Cessation of cigarette smoking speeds ulcer healing. In HP-negative ulcers, smoking cessation decreases the risk of recurrence.

■ Combination therapy. There is no evidence that combination therapy of traditional agents (e.g., sucralfate and an HRA) hastens healing.

Special Consideration
Refractory or Recurrent Ulcers
Eradication of HP reduces the rate of recurrence of peptic ulcers in individuals with HP-positive ulcers. In patients with a refractory or recurrent ulcer and documented HP, several issues should be considered. The use of NSAIDs should be discontinued. Compliance with medication should be reviewed. Resistant HP has been reported, necessitating retreatment with a different antibiotic regimen. In patients with a gastric ulcer, cancer should be considered. Zollinger–Ellison syndrome should be considered in patients with severe or multiple ulcers, large gastric mucosal folds, or unexplained diarrhea and steatorrhea.

Maintenance Therapy
Smokers, patients with recurrent non-HP ulcers, elderly patients, and patients with a history of a bleeding ulcer should receive maintenance therapy with an HRA at half the usual dose at bedtime (e.g., ranitidine 150 mg hs).

GASTRITIS/GASTROPATHY
General Principles
Gastritis/gastropathy is a collection of disorders characterized by damage to the gastric mucosa. Gastritis represents the presence of inflammation, whereas in gastropathy inflammation is absent. These disorders can be either acute (associated with acute injury secondary to NSAID use, stress, alcohol, bile acids) or chronic (autoimmune, HP). Since gastropathy associated with NSAID use is the most common form encountered by physicians, this section deals specifically with NSAID-related gastropathy.

Diagnosis
Presentation
Pain is much less common than in PUD. Usually patients are asymptomatic unless blood loss is appreciable. Life-threatening GI bleeding may be the initial presentation. Anorexia, nausea, or vomiting may be present, although dyspeptic symptoms do not correlate well with endoscopic findings.

Risk factors for development of NSAID gastropathy include age older than 60 years, previous history of ulcers with or without complications, concomitant use of corticosteroids, high doses of NSAIDs, and extended use of NSAIDs. Other potential factors may include alcohol consumption and smoking. Concurrent use of anticoagulants increases the risk of GI complications.

Physical examination. Physical findings are usually absent unless the patient presents with bleeding.

Laboratory studies. Anemia is usually the initial finding, prompting further radiologic or endoscopic evaluation.

Treatment[4]

- Discontinue use of NSAID. Reduce or discontinue other risk factors.
- Medication. HRA and PPI have been shown to be effective in healing gastric ulcers secondary to NSAID use. PPI is the drug of choice as cotherapy if the NSAID cannot be discontinued.
- If the patient has PUD and found to be positive for HP, then treatment for HP is recommended.

Special Consideration

Prevention

Use other analgesics such as acetaminophen. If switch cannot be made, reduce the dose of NSAID. Misoprostol is used in patients who have a history of ulcers, especially with bleeding as a complication. A PPI may be used as an alternative for individuals who cannot tolerate misoprostol.

References

1. Institute for Clinical Systems Improvement. Dyspepsia and GERD. Bloomington, MN: Institute for Clinical Systems Improvement (ICSI); 2004 Jul. Accessed 6/28/2006 at http://www.icsi.org/knowledge/detail.asp?catID=29 & itemID=171.
2. American Gastroenterological Association. Medical position statement: evaluation of dyspepsia. *Gastroenterology* 2005;129:1753.
3. Delany B, Ford AC, Forman D, et al. Initial management strategies for dyspepsia. [Systematic Review] Cochrane Upper Gastrointestinal and Pancreatic Diseases Group. *Cochrane Database Syst Rev* 2, 2006.
4. Lanza FL and the members of the Ad Hoc Committee on Practice Parameters of the American College of Gastroenterology. A guideline for the treatment and prevention of NSAID-induced ulcers. *Am J Gastroenterol* 1998;93:2037.

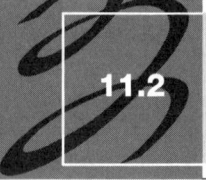

11.2 GASTROESOPHAGEAL REFLUX DISEASE
James W. Simmons

GENERAL PRINCIPLES

Epidemiology

- **Gastroesophageal reflux disease (GERD)** incorporates either characteristic symptoms or histopathologic alteration resulting from the refluxation of gastric contents into the esophagus.[1] The prevalence is difficult to predict. One has to assume that heartburn is an indicator of GERD. Many patients self-manage symptoms. An estimated 7% of adults experience symptoms of heartburn daily and 36% or more experience symptoms monthly.[1]
- The prevalence of the complications of GERD is even more difficult to predict. Symptoms do not always predict pathology, and pathology may be present in the absence of typical symptoms.[1]

Complications

- **Esophagitis** refers to tissue damage to the mucosa. Estimated to be absent in 55% to 81% of patients with typical GERD, but esophagitis is present in 48% to 81% with pathologic acid exposure by pH monitoring.[1] **Peptic stricture** occurs in 8% to 20% of patients with esophagitis.[1] **Barrett esophagus** is a **condition** in which the stratified squamous epithelium of the esophagus is replaced by metaplastic columnar epithelium (intestinal metaplasia) with the presence of goblet cells. This condition carries a **risk for progression to esophageal adenocarcinoma.** Although risk of developing cancer is 30 to 125 times higher than the general population, absolute risk of progression to cancer is low at 0.5% to 1.4% per year depending on the extent and location.[1,2] Severity of **symptoms** does not necessarily correlate with the presence or severity of any of these complications.

- **Atypical complications of GERD** commonly include laryngitis, hoarseness, noncardiac chest pain, chronic cough, and exacerbation of asthma. Many will respond to acid suppressive therapy, but it may take higher doses for a longer duration to notice an improvement.[1]

- **The cause of GERD is the breakdown of the barriers to reflux of gastric contents** including the physical barriers of the lower esophageal spincter (LES) and the crural diaphragm, esophageal peristalsis to clear the refluxate, and swallowed saliva to dilute the acid.

- **Factors that may increase the likelihood of reflux** include hiatal hernia, esophageal peristaltic dysfunction, hyposalivation, delayed gastric emptying, impaired tissue resistance, and **transient LES relaxations** not associated with a swallow. The last is felt to be the most significant factor.[1,3]

- **Specific foods, drugs, or habits** may also contribute to GERD either by decreasing the LES pressure or acting as a direct irritant. These include tobacco, alcohol, caffeine, chocolate, citrus fruits, tomato-based foods, fatty foods, onions (especially if uncooked), and peppermint. Common medications that can decrease LES pressure are nitrates, calcium-channel blockers, theophylline, morphine, Demerol (meperidine), Valium (diazepam), and barbiturates.[1]

Clinical Presentation

The most common **symptoms of GERD** are **heartburn, regurgitation,** and **dysphagia. Heartburn** is characterized as a burning sensation behind the sternum that may radiate upward toward the neck. **Regurgitation** is effortless and associated with the presence of a sour or burning fluid in the pharynx or mouth that may contain undigested food particles. **Dysphagia** can be caused by a stricture, peristaltic dysfunction, or mucosal inflammation but may not be associated with any identifiable abnormality.[1]

Less common symptoms include water brash, globus sensation, and odynophagia. Odynophagia may be more commonly associated with pill or infectious esophagitis.[1]

Symptoms are more commonly induced after eating, when in the recumbent position, during exercise or any other activity that increases intra-abdominal pressure. Quality of life has been shown to decrease as symptoms increase in severity and frequency.[1]

DIAGNOSIS[1,4]

There is no gold standard and, oftentimes, history may be sufficient. Further evaluation is warranted if symptoms are unresponsive to treatment, are chronic, atypical, or accompanied by **alarm symptoms** such as **dysphagia, odynophagia, gastrointestinal bleeding, anemia,** or **weight loss.**

- **Endoscopy** is often used as the initial study to evaluate for the presence of complications of GERD as well as exclude other diseases. Even if symptoms are well controlled, endoscopy may be indicated if patients have had chronic, untreated symptoms as their risk for Barrett esophagus is higher.

- A **double-contrast barium swallow** can **help** to identify strictures or esophageal ulcers but may miss other complications.

- **Ambulatory pH monitoring** is the best method to study the actual amount of reflux occurring in a patient. It is helpful in correlating symptoms with esophageal acid exposure especially if symptoms are atypical or if typical symptoms are refractory to treatment.

- **Esophageal manometry** can help to document effective peristalsis, especially in patients in whom antireflux surgery is being considered. It is also used to help accurately place pH probes.

TREATMENT OPTIONS[1,4]

- **Lifestyle modifications** should be discussed although their implementation has no proven efficacy at this point. Modifications typically include elevation of the head of the bed, weight loss, decreasing meal size and fat intake, avoiding recumbancy for 3 hours after a meal, and avoiding the aforementioned foods, habits, and medications that may contribute to GERD.

- **Antacids.** Many are available over the counter, are useful for milder cases of GERD, and provide a relatively immediate onset of action.
- **Antisecretory therapy.** Although hypersecretion of acid is not the underlying problem of GERD, acid suppression has been shown to be the mainstay of therapy for GERD.
- **Histamine type-2 receptor antagonists (H₂RAs)** are **now** available over the counter and have been shown to decrease acid secretion, particularly fasting and during sleep. Onset of action is more rapid than proton pump inhibitors (PPIs), so they are useful when taken before activities that are known to produce reflux. Use is limited by rapid development of tachyphylaxis and inability to suppress meal-related acid effectively.
- **PPIs suppress** acid secretion more effectively than H₂RAs. They are more effective if taken 30 minutes prior to a meal. Rebound hypersecretion of acid can occur with discontinuation of use. Some PPIs suppress acid production to a greater degree than others. Higher doses are more likely to be effective. Long-term data show PPIs are safe for chronic use.
- **Prokinetic therapy** can **control** symptoms and promote healing similar to H₂RAs; however, PPIs are more effective and safer than the current prokinetic agents. Metoclopramide is currently the only agent approved for use, but frequent central nervous system side effects limit its regular use.
- **Antireflux surgery** helps to re-establish the antireflux barrier. This is done by a partial or total fundoplication in which the gastric fundus is wrapped around the lower esophagus. Fundoplication can be as effective or superior to medical therapy. Indications to consider surgery include (a) failed medical therapy; (b) patient unwilling to take or intolerant of PPI therapy; (c) persistent symptoms secondary to regurgitation.

Special Consideration of Treatment Strategies[1,4]

- **Nonerosive GERD** management focuses on symptom relief. Initial management is directed by the severity, type, and duration of symptoms. Mild, short-term disease may respond to a conservative step-up strategy starting with lifestyle changes, antacids, or H₂RAs, whereas more severe disease will likely require PPIs. Some may be able to treat symptoms on an intermittent basis, but many will require long-term therapy that has been shown to be appropriate and effective. If symptoms are not controlled by high-dose PPIs, then an alternative diagnosis should be considered.
- **Erosive GERD** usually requires PPI therapy for healing. Continuation of acid suppression is usually necessary to prevent relapse. Maintenance doses required to maintain remission are usually similar to doses required to heal esophagitis, so a step-down strategy is often not recommended. Chronic acid suppression has been shown to decrease the recurrence of peptic esophageal strictures, but no therapy has at this point been shown to prevent the incidence or prevent the progression of Barrett esophagus.

References

1. Kahrilas PJ, Pandolfino JE. Gastroesophageal reflux disease and its complications, including Barrett's metaplasia. In Feldman M, Friedman LS, Sleisenger MH, eds. *Sleisenger and Fordtran's gastrointestinal and liver disease.* Philadelphia: Saunders; 2002:599–622.
2. Eisen GM, et al. The relationship between gastrointestinal reflux disease and its complications with Barrett's esophagus. *Am J Gastroenterol* 1997;92:27–31.
3. Mittal RK, Balaban DH. The esophagogastric junction. *N Engl J Med* 1997;336: 924–932.
4. DeVault KR, Castell DO, and the Practice Parameters Committee of the American College of Gastroenterology. Updated guidelines for the diagnosis and treatment of gastroesophageal reflux disease. *Am J Gastroenterol* 1999;94:1434–1442.

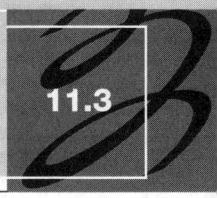
GENERAL PRINCIPLES

Definition
Upper gastrointestinal (UGI) bleeding occurs from the UGI tract.

Epidemiology
UGI bleeding is a common clinical problem, with an annual incidence of 50 to 150 per 100,000 of the population. Mortality from UGI bleeding is about 10% and may reach 35% in patients hospitalized for another medical condition. Patients over age 80 account for 25% of all UGI bleeds and 33% of UGI bleeds occurring in hospitalized patients. Most episodes of nonvariceal bleeding (80%) are self-limited and require only supportive therapy, but if bleeding is continuous or recurrent, the mortality is 30% to 40%. Surgery may be required in 15% to 30% of patients.

Etiology of UGI Bleeding (Table 11.3-1)
Peptic ulcers (50% of cases), gastritis/duodenitis, esophageal varices, gastroesophageal mucosal tears, and esophagitis account for 90% of cases. Other causes include gastric tumors, hematobilia, hiatal hernia, aortointestinal fistula, vascular malformations, vasculitis, and Dieulafoy lesion (submucosal arterial malformation).

- **Peptic ulcer disease (PUD)** is the most common cause of UGI bleeding. Duodenal or gastric ulcers caused by *Helicobacter pylori* are common causes of UGI bleeding. There is a synergistic risk of ulcer bleeding in patients using nonsteroidal anti-inflammatory drugs (NSAIDs). Although pain is the usual presenting symptom, 10% of patients present with UGI bleeding.
- **Gastritis** is associated with using NSAIDs (and selective cyclo-oxygenase inhibitors) and alcohol, severe systemic disease, major trauma, burns, and ventilator use. These conditions also increase the risk of bleeding from underlying PUD.
- **Esophageal varices** occur in patients with cirrhosis who have portal hypertension. Bleeding is more likely in patients with advanced cirrhosis and large varices. Concomitant PUD, gastritis, or Mallory–Weiss tears in alcoholic patients may also cause hemorrhage.
- **Gastroesophageal (GE) mucosal tears (Mallory–Weiss).** Hemorrhage results from mucosal laceration of the GE junction induced by retching or vomiting. Patients are often heavy alcohol users, and 30% use aspirin or NSAIDs. Tears may also occur from coughing, severe asthma attacks, seizures, cardiopulmonary resuscitation, and straining at stool.
- **Other causes.** Blood dyscrasias, vasculitis, connective tissue diseases (CTDs), and hereditary hemorrhagic telangiectasia (Osler–Rendu–Weber disease) may rarely be the cause of UGI bleeding. Hematobilia occurs secondary to trauma, injury, or vascular malformations of the liver or biliary tree. Aortoduodenal fistulas and large ectatic submucosal arteries (Dieulafoy lesion) or arteriovenous malformation (AVMs) may cause massive hemorrhage. Gastroesophageal reflux disease (GERD), cancer, and infections such as cytomegalovirus (CMV), herpes, or *Candida* may cause UGI bleeding but more usually cause chronic blood loss. Rarely, large hiatal hernias may cause blood loss as a result of linear mucosal tears. Even more rarely, gastric cancer, lymphoma, polyps, and other tumors of the stomach or small intestine may cause UGI bleeding.

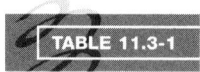

TABLE 11.3-1   Causes of Upper Gastrointestinal Bleeding

Common
Gastritis (erosive due to NSAIDs)
Peptic ulcer disease
Gastroesophageal mucosal tears
Cancer (carcinoma, lymphoma, polyps)

Rare
Infections (CMV, herpes, *Candida*)
GERD
Aortoenteric fistula
Blood dyscrasia
Vasculitis
Hemorrhagic telangiectasia
Pancreatic cancer
Uremia

CMV, cytomegalovirus; GERD, gastroesophageal reflux disease; NSAID, nonsteroidal anti-inflammatory drug.

DIAGNOSIS

Clinical Presentation

Clinical presentation depends on the location, source, and acuity of the bleed.

- Acute UGI bleeding often presents with bloody vomiting. Blood from a recent bleed is usually bright red. Bleeding from varices is usually abrupt and massive. Melena (black, tarry, malodorous stools) usually is the result of UGI bleeding or lesions of the small intestine if GI transit time is prolonged. Hematochezia (maroon or bright red blood per rectum can be the presenting symptom in up to 15% of cases of UGI bleeding. A history of alcohol abuse, cigarette smoking, or NSAID use may often exist.
- Chronic or unrecognized UGI bleeding may present with pallor, dizziness, dyspnea, iron deficiency anemia, or occult blood in stool.
- Physiologic responses to UGI bleeding
  - In acute UGI bleeding, the physiologic response depends on the rate and extent of hemorrhage.
    - Blood loss less than 500 mL is usually asymptomatic, except in elderly patients with coronary artery or chronic lung disease.
  - Rapid blood loss results in decreased cardiac output reflex, vasoconstriction, and increased peripheral resistance. Orthostatic hypotension indicates a reduction in blood volume of more than 20%. Lightheadedness, confusion, nausea, sweating, fainting, and thirst are commonly associated with blood loss.
  - When blood loss approaches 40% of blood volume, shock occurs, with tachycardia, hypotension, pallor, and cold clammy extremities.
  - Hemoglobin levels do not give a useful estimate of the volume of hemorrhage in the acute setting, and levels may be normal despite significant blood loss.
  - Chronic blood loss may be asymptomatic or present with signs and symptoms of anemia, hyponatremia, and hypoalbuminemia as a result of retention of hypotonic fluid to replenish intravascular volume.

History and Physical Examination

These identify the cause in only 50% of cases.

- **Prior history** of PUD or dyspepsia may suggest ulcer bleeding. A history of medication and alcohol use should be elicited. Symptoms of cirrhosis may suggest variceal bleeding. Bleeding from other sources (e.g., frequent nosebleeds, bruising) may suggest a coagulopathy.

- **Examination.** Epigastric tenderness is suggestive of PUD. Hepatosplenomegaly may occur in liver disease or malignancy. A rectal examination may reveal melena, but stool may be normal in patients with minimal or recent bleeding.
- **Laboratory studies.** If blood loss is rapid, the hematocrit may not reflect the magnitude of loss because equilibration with hemodilution requires 8 hours. The blood urea nitrogen may be elevated due to blood protein breakdown to urea by intestinal bacteria and reduced glomerular filtration rate. Histologic examination or culture of endoscopic specimens can be diagnostic for *H. pylori* infection. Serologic assays of *H. pylori*—specific IgG levels parallel the diagnostic accuracy of invasive tests. Urealabeled breath tests may be equally accurate.

TREATMENT

Always begins with resuscitation, restoration of intravascular volume, correction of hemoglobin loss, and treatment of pathophysiologic changes.

- **Resuscitation.** Vital signs should be monitored frequently and fluid replaced rapidly. Intravenous access using two wide-bore cannulae should be gained. Crystalloids (normal saline or Ringer solution) or fresh frozen plasma should be used until blood is available. Military antishock trousers may be required to correct shock. For unstable cardiac patients, central venous or pulmonary wedge pressures should be measured, with a goal of keeping blood pressure and pulse stable and maintaining urinary output at more than 40 mL per hour. Blood replacement is especially important in elderly patients and those intolerant of hypoxia. Intravenous proton pump inhibitor therapy (bolus followed by constant infusion of 8 mg/hour) may reduce the risk for rebleeding when endoscopy is also performed.
- **Gastric lavage through a nasogastric (NG) tube** can localize bleeding proximal to the ligament of Treitz. NG suction removes gastric fluid, blood, and swallowed air and can control nausea and vomiting. It has, however, been shown to be ineffective in achieving hemostasis and is **no longer** recommended as a first-line intervention. The presence of blood or "coffee-grounds" on NG aspiration confirms an UGI source whereas a clear aspirate reduces the likelihood of an UGI source. If endoscopy is to be scheduled in the next several hours, then NG placement is not necessary.

Specific Therapeutic Interventions
Peptic Ulcer Bleeding
- Medications: Antacids should be initiated empirically. Intravenous H_2 blocker therapy with 20 mg of famotidine IV q12h, or 40 mg of pantoprazole is the regimen of choice. Famotidine (20 mg PO q12h) and nizatidine (150 mg PO q12h) are alternatives for stable patients. Gastric acid pump inhibitors, such as omeprazole (20 mg/day PO), lansoprazole (30 mg PO q12h), and pantoprazole (40 mg/d PO) are widely used. Cytoprotective agents, such as sucralfate (1 g PO before meals and bedtime) and prostaglandins (misoprostol 200 μg PO q6h), are helpful in treating PUD. Their use in acute bleeding has not been studied. If *H. pylori* infection is diagnosed, treatment with regimens that include bismuth, subsalicylate/omeprazole, clarithromycin/tetracycline, and metronidazole are usually effective (see Chapter 11.1).
- Laser photocoagulation and electrocautery under direct endoscopic visualization may rapidly control active ulcer bleeding.
- Infusion of epinepherine in quadrants around the bleeding point and then into the bleeding vessel achieves hemostasis in 95% of cases (if endoscopic hemostasis fails). Fibrin glue and human thrombin may be the most effective injection materials.
- Mechanical devices "endoclips" may be an option for major bleeding ulcers, especially for arterial tears.
- Surgery is indicated if hemorrhage is brisk or sustained for longer than 6 to 12 hours, or if shock is not controlled by resuscitation. Patients with rapidly bleeding or recurring gastric ulcers may be surgical candidates. Surgery usually involves under-running the ulcer and pyloroplasty.

Gastritis and Gastric Erosions
Antacids and H_2 receptor blockers reduce the incidence of hemorrhage from stress ulcers. Misoprostol is effective in preventing gastritis due to NSAIDs. Sucralfate and omeprazole

are also effective for patients with prior UGI bleeding who require continued NSAIDs. Laser and electrocautery under direct visualization may control persistent bleeding.

Variceal Bleeding

May be completely controlled by endoscopic injection of a sclerosing agent, thrombin, epinepherine, or other agents. Noninvasive pharmacologic treatment aimed at causing splanchnic vasoconstriction and thus reducing portal pressure (vasopressin, somatostatin, propranolol). Thermal modalities or mechanical (banding, sewing, hemoclips, and endoloop) techniques often effectively control bleeding. Acute bleeding may be abated by balloon occlusion with a Sengstaken–Blakemore tube followed by definitive therapy within 48 hours. Recurrent bleeding may be prevented by periodic endoscopic sclerotherapy. Propranolol given twice daily (at a dose that reduces the heart rate by 25%) decreases portal pressure, although the response is nonuniform.

Arteriovenous Malformations

When actively bleeding, AVMs are best treated with electrocautery. Mallory–Weiss tears usually stop bleeding spontaneously but may require cautery or injection therapy.

Stress Gastritis

Prophylaxis using antacids, H_2 receptor blockers, omeprazole (or other proton pump inhibitors), or sucralfate decreases the incidence of bleeding. Acid reduction therapy may allow for bacterial colonization of the respiratory tract and possible pneumonia. Sucralfate does not alter gastric pH and is associated with a lower rate of nosocomial pneumonia.

Surgery

Esophagogastroduodenoscopy (EGD) has replaced barium studies for diagnosing UGI bleeding because of its greater accuracy and the potential for therapeutic interventions.

- In stable patients, EGD is usually indicated to locate the bleeding source, arrest hemorrhage, and make a definitive diagnosis.
- Persistent UGI hemorrhage is an indication for immediate EGD. If bleeding is heavy, the source may not be identified. Patients with cirrhosis should have EGD because there may be more than one source of hemorrhage. Patients with visible bleeding vessels or varices are candidates for endoscopic treatment.
- Angiography. If bleeding continues and EGD fails to reveal the source, angiography may be useful in diagnosing bleeding from varices, vascular ectasias, and aneurysms. Angiography also may be useful in the management of esophageal varices and Mallory–Weiss tears and in the embolization of bleeding ulcers or tumors in patients who are not surgical candidates.

SPECIAL CONSIDERATIONS

Bleeding from varices has a high recurrence rate and mortality (50% to 70%). Peptic ulcers with visible vessels have a rate of rebleeding of up to 50%. Other prognostic indicators include severity of the initial bleed, age (older patients have a higher mortality), concomitant disease, ulcer diameter greater than 2 cm, and the requirement for emergency surgery. The risk of rebleeding is reduced by treating *H. pylori,* prescribing proton pump inhibitors, cotreating patients who are prescribed NSAIDs with a proton pump inhibitor, and consideration of using somatostatin or octreotide.

References

1. Huang CS, Lichenstein DR. Nonvariceal upper gastrointestinal bleeding. *Gastroenterol Clin North Am* 2003;32:1053.
2. Esrailain E, Gralnek IM. Nonvariceal gastrointestinal bleeding: epidemiology and diagnosis. *Gastrorenterol Clin North Am* 2005;34:589.
3. Ferguson CB, Mitchell RM. Non-variceal upper gastrointestinal bleeding. *Ulster Med J* 2006;75(i):32.
4. Dallal HJ, Palmer KR. Upper gastrointestinal haemorrhage. *BMJ* 2001;323:1115.
5. Ferguson CB, Mitchell RM. Nonvariceal upper gastrointestinal bleeding: standard and new treatment. *Gastroenterol Clin North Am* 2005;34:607.

6. Manning-Dimmitt LL, Dimmitt SG, Wilson GR. Diagnosis of gastrointestinal bleeding in adults. *Am Fam Physician* 2005;71(7);1339.
7. Palmer K. Management of haemetemesis and melaena. *Postgrad Med J* 2004;80:399.
8. Gisbert JP, Khorrami S, Carbello F. *H. pylori* eradication therapy vs antisecretory non-eradication therapy for the prevention of recurrent bleeding from peptic ulcer. *Cochrane Collaboration* 2006;2.

CHOLELITHIASIS AND CHOLECYSTITIS
Edward C. Vincent

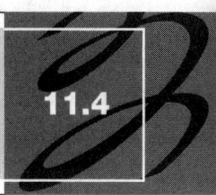

11.4

ASYMPTOMATIC CHOLELITHIASIS

General Principles
Definition
Incidental asymptomatic gallstones are usually discovered by abdominal ultrasonography (US) for unrelated symptoms or disease.

Anatomy
- The gallbladder is a pear-shaped sac 7 to 10 cm long, 30 to 50 cc capacity.
- A distended gallbladder can contain up to 300 cc bile.
- The gallbladder is lined by columnar epithelium that contains cholesterol and fat globules.

Epidemiology
- Gallstone disease affects 10% to 15% of the U.S. population.
- The incidence is lower (5%) in Asians and Africans and higher (up to 70%) in Native Americans.
- Incidence increases with age: 25% of persons over age 65 affected.
- Cholelithiasis is twice as common in women than in men.
- Other risk factors include:
  - Pregnancy or multiparity
  - Rapid weight loss, bariatric surgery, prolonged fasting, or weight "cycling"
  - Positive family history (2.2 times increase)
  - Body mass index (BMI) >30 (3.7 times increase)
  - Drugs: For example, estrogen, oral contraceptives, octreotide, clofibrate, ceftriaxone
  - Comorbid diseases: For example, diabetes mellitus, cirrhosis, biliary stasis

Pathophysiology
- Conjugated bile salts, lecithin, and cholesterol comprise 80% to 95% of solids dissolved in bile.
- Cholesterol microcrystal precipitation results in gallstone formation.

Etiology
Gallstones may occur due to high biliary cholesterol secretion, defective formation of vesicles, cholesterol crystal nucleation factor excess, deficiency of antinucleating factors, or delayed gallbladder emptying.

Diagnosis
Clinical Presentation
Asymptomatic gallstones usually discovered incidentally by abdominal US or laparotomy for nonbiliary tract disease.

History
Unremarkable except for risk factors noted above

Physical Examination
Unremarkable

Laboratory Studies
Unremarkable

Imaging
Abdominal US demonstrates gallstones

Monitoring
- Most persons with "silent" stones can be managed expectantly, as only 1% to 2% become symptomatic each year.
- 60% to 70% of patients with "silent stones" never develop symptoms.

Treatment
Protocol
- Recommendations for the treatment of gallstones have been developed by the Society for Surgery of the Alimentary Tract and are available from the National Guideline Clearinghouse web site (http://www.guideline.gov/summary/summary.aspx?ss=15& doc_id=5513&nbr=&string=).

Surgery
- Consider cholecystectomy once symptoms begin as recurrent pain or complications develop in 70% to 80%.
- Complications (cholecystitis and pancreatitis) are more likely after symptom onset.
- Also consider cholecystectomy for patients with a calcified ("porcelain") gallbladder or who undergo laparotomy for unrelated conditions.

Counseling
- Patients should be advised to seek medical care if they develop symptoms of acute or chronic cholecystitis or cholangitis (see below).
- Patients should see a surgeon within a few weeks if symptoms are mild or acute pain has resolved.
- Patients with significant right upper quadrant (RUQ) tenderness, fever, leukocytosis, and/or jaundice should be evaluated the same day.

Patient Education
- For a simple patient education handout from the American Academy of Family Physicians, Familydoctor.org, see "Gallstones: What Are They and How Are They Treated?" available on the Internet at http://familydoctor.org/555.xml.
- More detailed patient education handouts on gallstones are available from the American Gastroenterological Association, Patient Center web site (http://www.gastro.org/wmspage.cfm?parm1=688) and the National Institutes of Health, National Digestive Diseases Information Clearinghouse (http://digestive.niddk.nih.gov/ddiseases/pubs/gallstones/index.htm).

ACUTE CHOLECYSTITIS
General Principles
Definition
The patient presents with RUQ or epigastric pain, fever, leukocytosis, due to gallbladder inflammation, usually associated with gallstone disease.

Epidemiology
10% of persons with gallstones develop acute cholecystitis.

Pathophysiology
- Initial obstruction of cystic duct by gallstone causes increased gallbladder intraluminal pressure, distention, and wall edema that leads to ischemia and inflammation.
- Inflammatory response is mediated by protaglandins.
- Gallbladder distention and inflammation results in visceral and peritoneal pain.
- Biliary infection may be a factor in some patients with acute cholecystitis; however, not all patients with acute cholecystitis have infected bile.

Etiology

- Acute cholecystitis is thought to be caused by obstruction of cystic duct in combination with production of inflammatory mediators such as lysolecithin, phospholipase A, and prostaglandins.
- Gallstones present in 90% to 95% of patients with cholecystitis.
- 5% to 10% have no gallstones (acalculous cholecystitis)—these patients are more likely to be critically ill from trauma or sepsis.

Diagnosis

Clinical Presentation

Patients with acute cholecystitis usually appear moderately ill, are febrile, and complain of nausea and upper abdominal pain.

History

- Patients relate a history of rapid onset of severe, cramping, unrelenting RUQ, or epigastric abdominal pain.
- Longer pain duration (more than 4 to 6 hours) helps distinguish acute from chronic cholecystitis.
- Pain may radiate to back or right scapula.
- Low-grade fever, nausea, vomiting often present.
- 75% have experienced previous episode of similar pain.
- Patients may note onset of pain after a meal, but postprandial pain, dyspepsia, bloating, flatulence, and fatty food intolerance not specific for gallstone-related pain.

Physical Examination

- Vital signs show fever and tachycardia.
- RUQ or epigastric tenderness and guarding is usually present.
- Murphy sign (inspiratory arrest while palpating RUQ) is 90% predictive of acute cholecystitis.
- Gallbladder palpable in 20% of patients.

Laboratory Studies

- Leukocytosis of 12,000 to 15,000 cells per mm^3 often noted but white blood count (WBC) can be normal.
- WBC > 20,000 cells per mm^3 suggests complication such as perforation, gangrene, or cholangitis.
- Mild increases in the serum transaminase, amylase, and alkaline phosphatase.
- Unless common bile duct stones present, total serum bilirubin usually less than 4 mg per dL.

Imaging

Imaging usually necessary as no single symptom, physical finding, or laboratory test can establish or exclude diagnosis of acute cholecystitis. Abdominal radiographs ("plain films") seldom help diagnose cholecystitis but may exclude other conditions. Radionucleotide cholescintigraphy with hepato-iminodiacetic acid (HIDA scan) is 90% to 95% sensitive and specific for acute cholecystitis when abnormal (nonvisualization of gallbladder in spite of normal visualization of liver and bile ducts).

US usually performed before HIDA scan as it is more readily available and is 95% sensitive and specific for diagnosing gallstones, but only about 85% sensitive and specific for diagnosing acute cholecystitis. HIDA scan is test of choice in patients who have gallstones seen on US but atypical presentation, or in patients with typical presentation but nondiagnostic US. A major disadvantage of HIDA scan is high false-positive rate in a patient who is fasting or receiving parenteral alimentation, or who has severe liver disease. Computed tomography (CT) or magnetic resonance imaging (MRI) may identify gallstones when US cannot because of overlying fat or bowel gas, but are rarely used due to added time and expense.

Pathologic Findings

Thick, red, gallbladder wall with subserosal hemorrhages, with mucosal hyperemia with patchy necrosis at pathologic examination. Pericholecystic fluid may be present. Ischemia and necrosis of the gallbladder is present in 5% to 10%.

Differential Diagnosis

Biliary colic, peptic ulcer, pancreatitis, acute hepatitis, appendicitis, right kidney disease, right-sided pneumonia, or pleurisy, Fitz–Hugh–Curtis syndrome, subhepatic or intra-abdominal abscess, perforated viscus, myocardial ischemia may be confused with cholecystitis.

TREATMENT

Medications

- IV opioid or IM nonsteroidal anti-inflammatory drug (NSAID) analgesic is given once diagnosis established.
- IM NSAIDs (e.g., ketorolac 30 to 60 mg) may favorably alter disease progression by interfering with inflammatory response.
- Intravenous antibiotics, although controversial, are usually given (e.g., ampicillin/sulbactam or ampicillin plus gentamicin or third/fourth-generation cephalosporin plus metronidazole or fluoroquinolone plus metronidazole).
- Patient should fast, and nasogastic tube placed if significant vomiting or gastric distention.

Surgery

Cholecystectomy should be performed within 24 to 72 hours in most patients with acute cholecystitis, as further delay increases hospital length of stay and risk of emergency operations without improving mortality or complication rate. Patients with peritonitis or whose condition deteriorates should be evaluated for immediate surgery. Laparoscopic cholecystectomy is procedure of choice for uncomplicated acute cholecystitis. Patients with pancreatitis, peritonitis, sepsis, coagulopathy, gallbladder cancer, or cholecystoenteric fistula may need open cholecystectomy. Intraoperative cholangiography often performed as risk of choledocholithiasis at least 15%, and should be done in all patients with elevated serum bilirubin or signs/symptoms suggesting biliary obstruction. Cholecystostomy (percutaneous gallbladder drainage and stone removal) is an option for patients who are poor surgical candidates.

Special Considerations

- Common complications of acute cholecystitis include gallbladder perforation (3% to 10%) and gangrene (2% to 30%).
- Common bile duct stones (choledocholithiasis) may cause cholangitis (see below).
- Male gender, advanced age, and comorbid diseases such as diabetes are risk factors for complications.
- Emphysematous cholecystitis is a rare but serious condition with a 15% mortality; elderly patients or patients with diabetes are at highest risk for emphysematous cholecystitis.
- Mortality from acute cholecystitis treated with laparoscopic cholecystectomy is about 0.1%.

CHRONIC CHOLECYSTITIS

General Principles

Definition

Right upper quadrant or epigastric pain ("biliary colic"), without fever or leukocytosis, due to obstruction of the cystic duct by gallstones.

Epidemiology

Approximately 25% of persons with gallstones eventually develop chronic cholecystitis.

Pathophysiology

Obstruction of cystic duct by gallstone causes increased gallbladder intraluminal pressure, which results in visceral pain.

Etiology

Chronic cholecystitis thought to be caused by obstruction of cystic duct by gallstones.

Diagnosis

Clinical Presentation

Patients with chronic cholecystitis are usually mildly ill appearing, afebrile, and complain of nausea and upper abdominal pain.

History
■ Patients have a rapid onset of mild to moderate, dull, cramping RUQ or epigastric abdominal pain.
■ A shorter pain duration (1 to 5 hours) helps distinguish chronic from acute cholecystitis.
■ The pain may radiate to back or right scapula.
■ Nausea, diaphoresis is often present; fever is usually absent.
■ The onset of pain is often late at night or early morning.
■ Patients may note onset of pain after a meal, but postprandial pain, dyspepsia, bloating, flatulence, and fatty food intolerance are not specific for gallstone-related pain.
■ Patient is usually well between attacks.

Physical Examination
■ Examination usually normal between attacks. Vital signs may show tachycardia during attack.
■ Mild RUQ or epigastric tenderness during attack. Murphy's sign not present.

Laboratory Studies
Lab studies are usually normal.

Imaging
■ US is test of choice as it is 95% sensitive and specific for diagnosing gallstones.
■ Abdominal radiographs ("plain films") seldom help diagnose chronic cholecystitis as only 10% of gallstones have enough calcium to be radio-opaque, but may be useful to exclude other conditions.
■ CT or MRI may identify gallstones when the US cannot because of overlying fat or bowel gas, but are rarely used due to added time and expense.
■ CT and oral cholecystography (OCG) are occasionally used to evaluate patients who are candidates for medical dissolution therapy with oral bile acids.

Monitoring
Patients with chronic cholecystitis should see a surgeon within a few weeks to be evaluated for cholecystectomy.

Pathologic Findings
Pathologic changes vary from normal gallbladder with minor chronic inflammation to shrunken nonfunctioning gallbladder with transmural fibrosis and adhesions to adjacent organs. Pathology may not correlate with symptom severity.

Differential Diagnosis
Acute cholecystitis, peptic ulcer, pancreatitis, acute hepatitis, appendicitis, right kidney disease, right-sided pneumonia or pleurisy, Fitz–Hugh–Curtis syndrome, subhepatic or intra-abdominal abscess, myocardial ischemia all should be considered.

Treatment
Medications
■ Medical management may be considered for patients with chronic cholecystitis who are poor operative candidates or who decline surgery.
■ Dissolution therapy may be attempted with oral bile acids such as ursodiol (Actigall) or chenodiol (Chenix).
■ Contact dissolution with methyl-*tert*-butyl ether (MTBE) and stone fragmentation with extracorporeal shock wave lithotripsy (ESWL) are not Food and Drug Administration (FDA)-approved and generally not available in United States.
■ Oral bile acids must be taken daily over several months.
■ Optimal stones for dissolution by oral bile acids are radiolucent, less than 10 mm in diameter, "float" when viewed by US or OCG, and have low density and minimal calcifications on CT.
■ Gallbladder must be functioning, as noted by OCG or HIDA scan.
■ Because of these restrictions, only about 15% of patients with chronic cholecystitis are candidates for dissolution treatment.
■ Complete dissolution rates average 40% to 60% after 12 to 24 months in carefully selected patients.

■ After stopping oral therapy gallstones recur within 5 years in 25% to 50% of successfully treated patients; therefore, most are advised to continue maintenance therapy to reduce gallstone recurrence.

Surgery

■ Most patients with chronic cholecystitis should be considered for elective cholecystectomy, as risk of recurrent symptoms and complications within 2 years is 70%.
■ Laparoscopic cholecystectomy is the procedure of choice in most instances.
■ Patients who decline surgery or for whom surgery poses unacceptable risks should be referred to a gastroenterologist.

Results

Preoperative pain relieved in 90%, but 15% will develop new pain symptoms after surgery so only 75% have long-term pain relief. Only 50% of patients with preoperative nonpain symptoms (e.g., indigestion, fatty food intolerance, diarrhea) have symptom relief after surgery. Persistent nonpain symptoms more likely if diarrhea, fatty food intolerance, age <40, or both pain and nonpain symptoms present preoperatively.

Counseling

While waiting for surgery, patients with chronic cholecystitis should avoid large or fatty meals.

Special Considerations

■ Persistent RUQ pain, chills, fever, or jaundice suggests choledocholithiasis, cholangitis, or other biliary tract disease.
■ Pain with elevated serum liver enzymes or bilirubin with dilated bile duct suggests choledocholithiasis, sphincter of Oddi dysfunction, or stenosis.
■ Pregnant patients with chronic cholecystitis usually wait until after delivery to have surgery unless they develop jaundice, pancreatitis, acute cholecystitis, or severe or unrelenting pain.
■ Patients who are treated for obesity with bariatric surgery may benefit from prophylactic cholecystectomy or oral bile acid therapy (e.g., ursodiol) to prevent gallstone formation.
■ Complications if cholecystitis is left untreated: Cholangitis, pancreatitis, acute cholecystitis, gallstone ileus, and Mirizzi syndrome (common hepatic duct obstruction due to extrinsic compression from stone impacted in cystic duct or Hartmann pouch).

CHOLEDOCHOLITHIASIS AND ACUTE CHOLANGITIS

General Principles

Definition

Patients with choledocholithiasis—common bile duct (CBD) stones—may be asymptomatic but usually present with some variation of Charcot triad. Charcot triad (acute cholangitis) consists of RUQ pain, fever/chills, and jaundice. Charcot triad with altered mental status and hypotension (Reynold pentad) defines acute suppurative cholangitis and mandates emergency fluid resuscitation, antibiotics, and biliary drainage via endoscopic sphincterotomy (ES), percutaneous transhepatic catheterization, or surgery.

Anatomy

There are five extrahepatic bile ducts: (a) left hepatic, (b) right hepatic, (c) common hepatic, (d) cystic, and (e) common (CBD). CBD enters duodenum through sphincter of Oddi. CBD 7 to 11 cm long with a 5 to 10 mm diameter.

Epidemiology

In patients with cholelithiasis, 10% to 15% of those younger than age 60 and 20% to 25% older than age 60 have CBD stones.

Pathophysiology

Bile ducts normally kept sterile by continuous bile flow and by antibacterial substances in bile (e.g., immunoglobulins). Biliary tree obstruction from CBD stone reduces antibacterial defenses, increases small bowel bacterial colonization, and facilitates bacterial contamination. Exact route and cause of infection are unknown. Organisms commonly cultured (from bile) in patients with cholangitis are *Escherichia coli*, *Enterococcus*, *Klebsiella*, *Enterobacter*, and *Bacteroides fragilis*.

Etiology

Stones from gallbladder pass through cystic duct into CBD and become trapped at some point in the CBD duct causing biliary tree obstruction. Biliary obstruction is necessary but not sufficient to cause cholangitis. Partial obstruction is more likely to cause cholangitis than complete obstruction. Obstruction from CBD stone is more likely to cause cholangitis than obstruction from neoplasm.

Diagnosis

Clinical Presentation

CBD stones may be silent (discovered incidentally on US imaging) or symptomatic (obstructive jaundice, cholangitis, or gallstone pancreatitis).

History

CBD stone pain is similar to biliary colic with nausea/vomiting, and jaundice. The symptoms may be intermittent.

Physical Examination

- The physical examination may be normal. Epigastric or RUQ tenderness and mild icterus are common.
- Fever, altered mental status, and hypotension are ominous findings.

Laboratory Studies

Elevated serum bilirubin, alkaline phosphatase, and transaminases in most, but about one third of patients with CBD stones have normal liver chemistries. Leukocytosis usually occurs if cholangitis is present, with blood cultures recommended if suspected cholangitis.

Imaging

- Dilated CBD (>8 mm in diameter) on US or CT in patient with gallstones, jaundice, and biliary pain suggests CBD stones.
- MRI cholangiopancreatography (MRCP) is 95% sensitive and 89% specific for choledocholithiasis.
- Endoscopic ultrasound (EUS) may provide additional imaging information.

Surgical Diagnostic Procedures

Endoscopic retrograde cholangiopancreatography (ERCP) or intraoperative cholangiography is gold standard for diagnosing CBD stones. ERCP usually reserved for patients with clinically suspected cholangitis or symptomatic CBD stones who are likely to require therapeutic intervention.

TREATMENT

Medications

- For pain, give IV opioid analgesic once diagnosis established.
- In patients with cholangitis correct fluids, electrolytes, and coagulopathy (vitamin K deficiency from prolonged jaundice or low platelets from sepsis).
- Broad-spectrum IV antibiotics if suspected cholangitis, for example, ampicillin (500 mg q6h IV) with gentamicin (1.5 mg/kg q8h) ± metronidazole (500 mg q6h) or ciprofloxacin (250 mg IV q12h) or third/fourth-generation cephalosporin (e.g., cefoperazone, 1 to 2 g IV q12h).
- Alternative antibiotic regimen for severely ill patients is mezlocillin, 3 g IV q4h plus either metronidazole or gentamicin or both.
- Patient should fast, and nasogastric tube placed if significant vomiting or gastric distention.

Surgery

- Patients with symptoms who are suspected to have CBD stones should have either preoperative ERCP with sphincterotomy followed by cholecystectomy or an intraoperative cholangiogram with common bile duct exploration (choledochotomy).
- If choledochotomy is performed, a T tube is left in place. Patients with acute cholangitis should undergo biliary drainage via endoscopic sphincterotomy (treatment of choice for most), percutaneous transhepatic catheterization, or surgery.

- Most patients who have intact gallbladders and successfully treated CBD stones or acute cholangits should be referred for cholecystectomy as the risk of recurrent problems is high (~50%).

Special Considerations

- Prognosis for mild to moderate cholangitis treated with antibiotics and biliary drainage is fair.
- Mortality rate for severe cholangitis/Reynold pentad remains high (~50%).
- Complications of ERCP with endoscopic sphincterotomy (ERCP/ES) include pancreatitis, bleeding, stone impaction, and perforation.
- Percutaneous transhepatic catheterization and surgery have higher morbidity and mortality rates than ERCP/ES and should only be considered in patients in whom ERCP/ES fails or is not possible.

References

1. Afdhal NH. Acute cholangitis. In: Rose BD, ed., UpToDate Online Version 14.1. Waltham, MA, 2006. Available at www.uptodate.com. Accessed June 14, 2006.
2. Afdhal NH. Epidemiology of and risk factors for gallstones. In: Rose BD, ed., UpToDate Online Version 14.1. Waltham, MA, 2006. Available at www.uptodate.com. Accessed March 1, 2006.
3. Bellows CF, Berger DH, Crass RA. Management of gallstones. *Am Fam Physician* 2005;72:637–642.
4. Friedman LS. Liver, biliary tract, & pancreas—diseases of the biliary tract. In: Tierney LM, McPhee SJ, Papadakis MA, eds. *Current medical diagnosis & treatment*. 45th ed. New York: Lange Medical Books/McGraw-Hill; 2006. Available at www.statref.com. Accessed March 1, 2006.
5. Margenthaler J, Schuerer D, Whinney R. Acute cholecystitis. *Clin Evid* 2004;12: 571–580.
6. Lublin M, Crawford DL, Hiatt JR, et al. Symptoms before and after laparoscopic cholecystectomy for gallstones. *Am Surg* 2004;70:863–866.
7. Nunes D. Nonsurgical treatment of gallstone disease. In: Rose BD, ed. UpToDate Online Version 14.1. Waltham, MA, 2006. Available at www.uptodate.com. Accessed June 14, 2006.
8. Oddsdottir M, Hunter JG. Gallbladder and the extrahepatic biliary system. In: Brunicardi FC, ed. *Schwartz's principles of surgery*. 8th ed. New York: McGraw-Hill; 2005. Available at www.statref.com. Accessed March 1, 2006.
9. Trowbridge RL, Rutkowski NK, Shojania KG. Does this patient have acute cholecystitis? *JAMA* 2003;289:80–86.
10. Yusoff IF, Barkun JS, Barkun AN. Diagnosis and management of cholecystitis and cholangitis. *Gastroenterol Clin North Am* 2003;32:1145–1168.
11. Zakko SF, Afdhal NH. Clinical features and diagnosis of acute cholecystitis. In: Rose BD, ed. UpToDate Online Version 14.1. Waltham, MA, 2006. Available at www.uptodate.com. Accessed March 1, 2006.
12. Zakko SF, Afdhal NH. Treatment of acute cholecystitis. In: Rose BD, ed. UpToDate Online Version 14.1. Waltham, MA, 2006. Available at www.uptodate.com. Accessed March 1, 2006.
13. Zakko SF. Uncomplicated gallstone disease. In: Rose BD, ed. UpToDate Online Version 14.1. Waltham, MA , 2006. Available at www.uptodate.com. Accessed March 1, 2006.

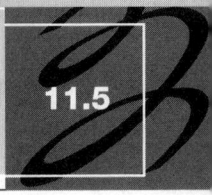

GENERAL PRINCIPLES

Definition

Hepatitis is defined as inflammation of the liver. It can be caused by drugs, toxins, metabolic and autoimmune diseases, pregnancy, and many other conditions. The disease can range from mild and subclinical to severe and rapidly progressive. Viral hepatitis accounts for the majority of cases of acute hepatitis in the United States. This condition is caused by both nonhepatotropic and hepatotropic viruses. The nonhepatotropic viruses cause clinical manifestations by infecting many organs and are usually self-limited, except in immunocompromised hosts. There are five nonhepatotropic viruses and all are members of the herpes family of viruses: Epstein–Barr virus (EBV), varicella-zoster virus (VZV), herpes simplex virus (HSV) type 1 and type 2, and cytomegalovirus (CMV). The hepatotropic viruses produce varying degrees of clinical manifestations (which may be hepatic and extrahepatic), complications, and progression to chronicity. The hepatotropic viruses include A, B, C, D, and E and are taxonomically diverse, belonging to five different viral families. New hepatitis viruses have been identified and may explain what previously had been characterized as non–A–E viral hepatitis. Approximately 5% to 20% of cases of acute and chronic hepatitis are not explained by A–E agents.[1] In the clinical diagnosis of viral hepatitis it is essential to specify the etiologic agent due to important implications in prognosis, management, epidemiology, patient education, and prevention.

Classification and Epidemiology

Nonhepatotropic Viruses

- **Epstein–Barr virus.** EBV is the etiologic agent associated with infectious mononucleosis, a viral syndrome occurring mostly in adolescents or young adults. EBV may also cause hepatitis. Clinical signs include exudative pharyngitis, periorbital edema, hepatosplenomegaly, and rash. Most cases are associated with mild transaminase elevation and less than 10% of cases present with jaundice. The diagnosis can be made in the office with a complete blood count showing a predominance of atypical lymphocytes and a positive heterophile antibody (Monospot) test. However, the Monospot test can be negative in the first 7 to 10 days of the acute illness. EBV is not thought to cause chronic hepatitis in the immunocompetent host. Treatment of persons with infectious mononucleosis is supportive. Upper airway compromise can be a concern in the acute phase of the illness.
- **Varicella-Zoster virus.** VZV causes the clinical conditions of chickenpox (primarily a disease of children) and herpes zoster (a reactivation of the latent varicella infection). Subclinical hepatitis may be common in childhood chickenpox but overt hepatitis does not usually occur, except as part of a widely disseminated viremia usually in the setting of immune compromise. Acyclovir should be administered to patients with disseminated varicella and associated hepatitis.
- **Herpes simplex virus.** HSV-1 and HSV-2 rarely cause hepatitis but can affect immunosuppressed patients undergoing a liver transplant. Fulminant hepatic failure associated with disseminated intravascular coagulation can occur in this setting. Prophylactic use of acyclovir can prevent this type of infection in liver transplant patients.
- **Cytomegalovirus.** CMV causes few symptoms in the average patient but is the most common opportunistic viral infection of the liver graft. Ganciclovir has reduced the severity of CMV infection in patients who have had recent liver transplantation.

Hepatotropic Viruses

The hepatotropic viruses infect both immunocompromised and immunocompetent hosts. Five agents have been studied most completely: the hepatitis A, B, C, D, and E viruses. These viruses have been classified according to modes of transmission and chronicity of infection. The hepatitis A and E viruses comprise the enterically transmitted group that cause only acute hepatitis, whereas viruses B, C, and D are the parenterally transmitted viruses that cause both acute and chronic infections. The chronic syndromes, thought to be associated primarily with hepatitis B, C, and possibly D, can lead to chronic hepatitis, cirrhosis of the liver, and hepatocellular carcinoma. These five agents are genetically unrelated and each can produce an acute illness of variable severity. Infections resulting from these different viruses share a number of common clinical features but can be distinguished by serologic markers. Two newer agents, hepatitis F and G viruses, are currently being reviewed.

- **Enterically transmitted hepatotropic viruses**
  - **Hepatitis A virus (HAV).** HAV is a small, 27-nm, RNA virus that belongs to the enterovirus family. Inactivation of the virus from contaminated items can be achieved by immersion in boiling water for 1 minute, contact with formaldehyde and chlorine, or ultraviolet radiation. HAV is the most common cause of acute hepatitis in the United States. However, incidence has declined substantially since licensure of vaccination in 1995. Globally, areas with high prevalence include North Africa and the Middle East. Moderate prevalence is found in Central and South America, southern Africa, and India. In the United States the highest prevalence is in the western region with Missouri, Texas, Colorado, Arkansas, and Montana having the highest rates between 1987 and 1997.[2] HAV infection can occur sporadically or in an epidemic form. HAV is transmitted primarily by fecal contamination and oral transmission through person-to-person contact or ingestion of contaminated water. Parenteral transmission is also possible, especially in intravenous drug users, but is much less common. In the United States, communities with high rates of HAV infection are often relatively well defined either geographically or culturally and include American Indian, Alaskan native, and selected Hispanic or migrant communities. However, due to the improvement of living conditions in underdeveloped countries, fewer children are infected, leading to a larger population of adults who lack protective antibodies against HAV. The incubation period is 15 to 45 days (average 4 weeks). The virus is excreted in the stool during the first few weeks of the illness prior to onset of symptoms. The mortality rate, usually from fulminant hepatitis, is very low (0.1%).
  - **Hepatitis E (HEV).** HEV virus is a single-stranded RNA virus and resembles HAV in transmission and cause. It is the major etiologic agent of enterically transmitted non-A, non-B hepatitis worldwide. The source of infection is usually contaminated water, and epidemics are frequently observed after a rainy season. The highest rates of disease are in young to middle-age adults. In the United States, all reported cases have occurred in travelers returning from endemic regions, and there has been no secondary transmission.

- **Nonenteric hepatotropic viruses**
  - **Hepatitis B virus (HBV).** HBV is a 42-nm, double-stranded DNA virus that replicates by reverse transcription. HBV is the most important cause of acute and chronic liver disease worldwide. Approximately 45% of the world population lives in areas of high prevalence of chronic HBV infection (and 7% to 8% of the population in these areas is hepatitis B surface antigen, HBsAg, positive); 43% of the world's population lives in areas with moderate prevalence (2% to 7% HBsAg-positive), and 12% in low-prevalence areas (less than 2% HBsAg positive). Lifetime risk of acquiring infection can be as high as 60% in high-prevalence areas. HBsAg is the primary component of hepatitis B vaccine. Administration of the vaccine induces a protective antibody that provides long-term immunity. The core of the hepatitis B virus contains hepatitis B core antigen (HBcAg), hepatitis Be antigen (HBeAg), DNA-dependent DNA polymerase, and a single molecule of partially double-stranded DNA. HBeAg is thought to be a degradation product of the HBV core. In the United States the most important route of HBV transmission is by sexual contact with an infected person. Injection of illegal drugs is also an important route. Other percutaneous exposures include tattooing, body part piercing, and acupuncture. Medical

personnel injured by sharp objects on the job are also at high risk. Chronically infected mothers can transmit HBV to their infants, but this route of infection has fallen since we have been screening all pregnant women prenatally for HBV infection, giving hepatitis B immune globulin (HBIG) to infected newborns, and recommending that HBV vaccine be given universally to all infants born in America.

■ **Hepatitis D (delta) virus.** HDV is a defective single-stranded RNA virus that requires the helper function of the HBV envelope protein or HBsAg to replicate. HDV cannot exist and replicate without a pre-existing chronic or acute HBV infection. Patients with acute HBV infection and concomitant HDV infection have a more severe acute illness with the risk of fulminant hepatitis ranging from 2% to 20%. Chronic HBV carriers who acquire HDV infection have a much higher incidence of cirrhosis (approaching 70% to 80%, compared to 15% to 30% chance of cirrhosis with chronic HBV infection alone). Modes of transmission for HDV are similar to those of HBV although sexual transmission is less efficient for HDV. Perinatal HDV transmission is rare. Immunoglobulin M (IgM) and IgG antibody to HDV is detectable in most patients with HDV infection but generally declines to undetectable levels after infection resolves. HDAg is detectable in about 25% of patients with HDV infection and it disappears following infection resolution (as does the HBsAg in HBV infections). As no therapy exists to prevent HDV superinfection, prevention depends primarily on risk factor reduction through education concerning contaminated needles. The geographic distribution of HDV is different from that of HBV, with South America having the highest HDV endemicity. Currently, the HDV epidemic that began in the 1970s seems to be coming to an end.[3]

■ **Hepatitis C virus (HCV).** HCV is an enveloped single-stranded RNA virus. HCV has the ability to mutate within an infected host such that heterogeneous variants, called quasi-species, can exist simultaneously in one infected person. At least six groups of genetically distinct HCVs have been isolated, each with a number of closely related subtypes. Patients infected with HCV mount an immune response to specific sites on the virus, but pre-existing antibodies do not recognize mutations in the viral genome. The mutant genome subsequently escapes detection and this appears to be the mechanism by which HCV maintains chronic infection.[4] Percutaneous exposures from an infected blood or organ donor and injection drug use are the most efficient modes of transmission, with an overall prevalence of 60% following these exposures. Hemodialysis and needle stick exposures and receiving untested blood products prior to 1990 are other significant risks. Sexual or household exposure to an HCV-positive contact, having multiple sex partners, and vertical transmission to an infant from an HCV-infected mother are other risk factors, but the magnitude of these risks has not been established.

Pathophysiology and Mechanism of Injury

Infection with the hepatitis viruses is associated with inflammation and necrosis of the liver cells resulting in hepatocellular degeneration and regeneration. However, none of the hepatitis viruses is directly cytopathic to the hepatocytes. Host immunologic reactions against the hepatitis viruses replicating in the liver cells are thought to play a role in all forms of the disease. A strong immune response related to viral factors and particularly to host genetic factors may result in rapid clearance of the virus but also in massive hepatic necrosis causing fulminant hepatic failure. Liver biopsy is used to assess the degree of liver damage but is generally not helpful in distinguishing the different types of acute hepatitis, as the histology is quite similar.

DIAGNOSIS

Clinical Presentation and Laboratory Studies

Most viral infections are asymptomatic, especially in younger individuals, and are marked only by increased aminotransferases. When symptomatic, initial features are nonspecific and include malaise, fatigue, anorexia, nausea, vomiting, abdominal discomfort, and occasionally right upper quadrant pain or arthralgias. The prodromal symptoms last for 3 to 4 days or even up to 2 to 3 weeks and may be followed by an icteric (jaundiced) phase of varying severity.

■ **HAV infection.** The illness caused by HAV infection usually has an abrupt onset of symptoms that include fever, malaise, anorexia, nausea, abdominal discomfort, dark urine, and jaundice. Diarrhea is more common in HAV infection than in other forms of viral hepatitis. The likelihood of symptoms from HAV infection correlates with age with 70% of HAV-infected children younger than 6 years being asymptomatic. Signs and symptoms usually resolve within 2 months, but 10% to 15% of symptomatic patients have prolonged or relapsing symptoms lasting up to 2 months. In infected persons, HAV replicates in the liver causing the hepatitis as manifested by serum aminotransferases (aspartate aminotransferase and alanine aminotransferase) increasing variably between 10 and 100 times normal. This rise precedes the rise in bilirubin but does not correlate with the extent of hepatocyte damage. Peak infectivity occurs in the 2-week period during the elevation of liver enzymes before the rise in bilirubin. During this time, concentration of virus in the stool is the highest and declines after jaundice appears (bilirubin higher than 2.5 mg/dL). Serum bilirubin may rise to levels of 2.0 to 20.0 mg per dL. Children can shed HAV virus in their stool for several months after the onset of clinical disease. Chronic shedding of HAV in the stool does not occur, but adults with relapsing infection can shed for up to 6 months. Hypoglycemia, elevated prothrombin times, and persistent jaundice correlate with severe disease. The overall mortality rate of HAV infection is less than 1% and is associated with fulminant hepatitis. Consumption of hepatotoxic chemicals, such as alcohol and acetaminophen, early in the illness and certain underlying conditions, such as glucose-6-phosphate dehydrogenase deficiency and sickle cell disease, are associated with the highest bilirubin levels. The diagnosis of HAV infection is made by finding IgM antibody to HAV (IgM anti-HAV) in the acute-phase or early-convalescence-phase serum. IgG antibody to HAV (IgG anti-HAV) can be detected in the convalescent phase of the disease and persists for life, conferring lifelong immunity.

■ **HEV infection.** There are no distinctive clinical features for infection with HEV. The disease is usually mild and self-limiting. No evidence of chronic infection has been detected with hepatitis E. HEV mortality is low except in pregnant women in which the mortality rate may be as high as 10% to 30%. Both IgM and IgG antibody to HEV are elicited following HEV infection. No serologic tests for diagnosis of HEV infection are available in the United States, except in research laboratories.

■ **HBV infection.** HBV develops insidiously with an incubation period averaging 120 days. Constitutional symptoms are more severe than with HAV infection. These include anorexia, malaise, nausea, vomiting, abdominal pain, and jaundice. About 10% to 20% of HBV-infected patients develop a serum sickness reaction with high fever, rash, arthralgias, and arthritis during the incubation period. Most acute HBV infections resolve, but some patients develop a fulminant hepatitis, which may be fatal. This may cause hepatic failure with confusion in association with ascites as well as elevation of the bilirubin and prothrombin time. With early and aggressive support, patients often survive without sequelae. HBsAg is found in serum 30 to 60 days after HBV infection. The corresponding antibody (anti-HBs) is responsible for long-term immunity and develops after infection resolves or with immunization. HBeAg, detectable in the serum of HBV-infected patients, correlates with viral replication and high infectivity. Antibody to HBeAg correlates with loss of viral replication and lower infectivity. An understanding of these markers for HBV infection is essential for proper diagnosis and management of HBV disease. This is summarized in Table 11.5-1. Persistent HBsAg positivity correlates with chronic HBV infection. It is therefore important to document the disappearance of this antigen from the serum after an acute HBV infection. About 10% of HBV-infected patients are HBsAg-positive after 6 months, but a full 50% of these become HBsAg-negative by 12 months. The younger a person is at the time of acute HBV infection, the more likely that person is to be HBsAg positive. A neonate has a 90% chance of being HBsAg-positive for life unless the neonate receives HBIG. A child who contracts HBV at age 5 has a 25% to 50% chance of developing chronic infection whereas in an adult the risk is less than 10%.

■ **HCV infection.** The acute phase of HCV infection is often mild and the patient usually remains anicteric or even asymptomatic. The most important feature of HCV infection is its chronicity. Between 70% and 80% of infected individuals develop chronic active

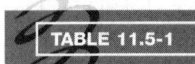

TABLE 11.5-1	Test for Markers for Hepatitis B Virus Infection
Test	**Comment**
HBcAg	No commercial test
HBsAg	Surface antigen of HBV, first serologic marker to appear
HBeAg	HBV replication and infectivity
IgM anti-HBcAg	Marker of recent acute infection
Anti-HBs	Vaccine immunity or resolved infection
Anti-HBe	Antibody indicates low infectivity better outcome
HBV, hepatitis B virus.	

hepatitis or cirrhosis. Some go on to develop hepatocellular carcinoma. The diagnosis of HCV infection is made by the detection of HCV antibody in the serum of infected persons. This antibody is detectable by 5 to 6 weeks postexposure in 80% of infected patients and by 12 weeks in 90%. Because this enzyme immunoassay (EIA) can be positive in other inflammatory conditions of the liver, false positives can be decreased through the use of a more specific, supplemental recombinant immunoblot assay (RIBA) antibody test for HCV. Alternatively, the diagnosis of acute HCV disease can be made 1 to 2 weeks after infection through detection of HCV RNA using reverse transcriptase polymerase chain reaction (RT-PCR) techniques (though this test is not widely available).

TREATMENT AND PREVENTION

- **Hepatitis A.** No specific treatment for HAV infection exists, but supportive care with attention to fluid and electrolyte balance is indicated in severe cases. HAV infection is the most common vaccine-preventable illness reported in the United States. The hepatitis A childhood immunization strategy has been implemented incrementally and the current recommendation is vaccination of all children nationwide.[5] All children should receive hepatitis A vaccine between 12 to 23 months of age with initial shot followed by a booster in 6 months. Immune globulin (IG) provides protection against HAV infection through possible transfer of antibody. Persons who have been recently exposed to HAV and were not previously vaccinated should be administered a single intramuscular (IM) dose of IG (0.02 mg/kg) as soon as possible, but not more than 2 weeks after the last exposure. People vaccinated with at least one dose of hepatitis A vaccine more than a month prior to exposure do not need IG. However, IG is indicated in the following situations for postexposure prophylaxis after exposure to a known infected person: (a) unvaccinated household and sexual contacts and anyone else with close personal contact such as babysitters; (b) unvaccinated staff and attendees of daycare centers; (c) household contacts of daycare attendees in diapers; (d) common-source food handlers if a food handler in a restaurant has been diagnosed with HAV. If hepatitis A vaccine is recommended for a person getting the IG, it can be given simultaneously at a separate site.
- **Hepatitis E.** The treatment of HEV is supportive in nature. Prevention relies primarily on the provision of clean water supplies and prudent hygienic practices while traveling. Prototype vaccines in animals have not been successful in preventing virus excretion in the stool.
- **Hepatitis B.** The treatment of HBV infection is not curative because in chronic infections treatment rarely produces permanent remission. The goals of therapy are long-term suppression of viral replication and prevention of end stage liver disease. Markers of successful therapy include HBeAg negativity, decreased or undetectable levels of HBV DNA, and lack of disease progression. The immune modulator interferon-α was approved for treatment of HBV infection in 1992 and works by affecting viral replication and upregulating cytokines involved in the response to infection. It is poorly tolerated by many patients and contraindicated in patients with decompensated cirrhosis, neutropenia, thrombocytopenia, severe uncontrolled depression, and current alcohol or

drug abuse.[6] Treatment has been improved by the introduction into clinical use of the nucleoside analogues lamivudine and adefovir dipivoxil. They are better tolerated and can be administered orally. Lamivudine has been intensively studied and is highly potent against HBV. This agent increases the loss of HBeAg and has brought about marked improvement in liver chemistries and liver histology. The major limitation has been the emergence of lamivudine-resistant strains. Adefovir dipivoxil, which was approved for the treatment of HBV infection in 2002, is effective in suppressing HBV strains that have developed resistance to lamivudine.[6] Twice yearly transaminase testing allows assessment for hepatitis activity. Patients with chronic HBV infection also benefit from measurements of serum α-fetoprotein and liver sonography at 6- to 12-month intervals, screening for the development of cirrhosis and hepatocellular carcinoma. If an adult patient with chronic HBV infection feels good and eats well, deterioration is unlikely; however, if signs of deterioration develop, liver biopsy is indicated to assess disease activity. For prevention, a comprehensive hepatitis B elimination strategy has been updated by the Advisory Committee on Immunization Practice and includes the following:

- Screen all pregnant women for HBsAg and provide HBIG and HBV vaccine to all children born to these mothers.
- Provide HBV vaccine to all infants as part of their routine childhood vaccination schedule.
- Provide catch-up vaccination for children in high-risk groups including Alaskan natives, Pacific islanders, and infants from countries with high prevalence of HBV.
- Provide hepatitis B vaccine to adolescents, including previously unvaccinated children and adolescents in high-risk groups.
- Vaccinate adults in high-risk groups including:
  - Adults with a sexually transmitted disease (STD) history who have had more than one sexual partner in the previous 6 months
  - Household contacts of a person with chronic HBV infection
  - Health care and public safety workers who have exposure to blood in the workplace
  - Clients and staff of institutions for the developmentally disabled
  - International travelers spending more than 6 months in countries with high rates of HBV
  - Injection drug users
  - Sexually active homosexual and bisexual men
  - Recipients of clotting factor concentrates

- **Hepatitis C.** Children and HCV patients treated early in the disease with interferon alone or in combination with ribavirin appear to do better than those treated later in the disease. However, all HCV-positive patients with liver enzyme elevation should undergo liver biopsy. Treatment with interferon has resulted in normalization of serum transaminases in about 50% of HCV-positive patients. This normalization appears to be higher in patients with liver inflammation who have not yet developed significant cirrhosis. Genotype testing may also be important in the treatment of HCV infection since those patients with HCV genotype non-1b have higher response rates. Despite initial enthusiasm for interferon, permanent remissions do not occur in more than 75% of treated patients and the side effect profile with interferon is quite high.[7] Combination of interferon and ribavirin is approved for patients who have relapsed following interferon treatment alone. Chronic HCV infection is the most common indication for liver transplantation in the United States. Recurrence of HCV is almost universal, however, because most patients are viremic at the time of transplantation. Research is ongoing into how to prevent infection and subsequent destruction of the transplanted organ. Most studies of chronic HCV infection have excluded patients with HCV–HIV coinfection, but small research trials indicate that the effectiveness of treatment of HCV in such patients correlates directly with the activity of the HIV infection. Better response to interferon correlates with higher CD4 counts and a healthier immune system. Prevention through risk factor reduction is clearly the most effective treatment. No vaccine is currently available and IG is not effective in the treatment of HCV infection. Fortunately, the incidence of HCV disease has declined 75% between 1989 and 1993. This decline actually started in the mid-1980s when the AIDS epidemic forced changes in blood donor selection practices. It has continued since the early 1990s when HCV antibody testing became widely available. A continuing drop today is thought to be due to safer needle-use practices among injection drug users. Patient education (particularly in patients who inject drugs), frequent testing in high-risk populations, ongoing surveillance of donated blood products, and rapid treatment when HCV infection with liver inflammation is diagnosed remain the cornerstones of therapy.[8]

References
1. Deka N, Sharma MD, Mukerjee R. Isolation of the novel agent from human stool samples that is associated with sporadic non-A non-B hepatitis. *J Virol* 1994;68:7810.
2. U.S. Centers for Disease Control and Prevention. Hepatitis surveillance report no. 60. Atlanta, GA: U.S. Department of Health and Human Services, Public Health Services; 2005.
3. Hadzyannis SJ. Decreasing prevalence of hepatitis D virus infection. *J Gastroenterol Hepatol* 1997;12:745.
4. Moyer LA, Mast EE, Alter MJ. Hepatitis C: routine serologic testing and diagnosis. Part 1. *Am Fam Physician* 1999;59:79–88.
5. U.S. Centers for Disease Control and Prevention. Prevention of hepatitis A through active or passive immunization: recommendations of the Advisory Committee on Immunization Practices (ACIP). *MMWR* 2006;55:1–23.
6. Lin KW, Kirchner JT. Hepatitis B. *Am Fam Physician* 2004;69:75–82.
7. Moyer LA, Mast EE, Alter MJ. Hepatitis C: preventive counseling and medical evaluation. Part 2. *Am Fam Physician* 1999;59:349–354.
8. Alter MJ, Mast EE, Moyer LA, et al. Emerging infectious diseases, hepatitis C. *Infect Dis Clin North Am* 1998;12:13–22.
9. U.S. Centers for Disease Control and Prevention. Prevention of hepatitis A through active or passive immunization. Recommendations of the Advisory Committee on Immunization Practices (ACIP). *MMWR* 1999;48:1–37.
10. Recommendations for prevention and control of hepatitis C virus (HCV). Infection and HCV related chronic disease. *MMWR* 1998;47(RR-19).
11. Bacon B, Di Bisceglie A. *Liver disease, diagnosis and management* Chrchill Livingstone, Philadelphia. 2000.

PANCREATITIS AND PANCREATIC CANCER
Scott W. Hughes

11.6

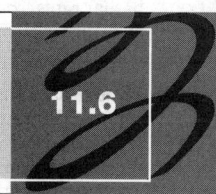

PANCREATITIS

General Principles

Definition
Pancreatitis is a common clinical disorder encountered in primary care. Yearly, there are more than 220,000 hospitalizations for this disease in the United States, with mortality as high as 10% to 30% in severe cases.[1]

Acute and chronic pancreatitis are distinguished from each other in that chronic pancreatitis results in permanent structural changes in the pancreas that lead to exocrine and endocrine dysfunction.[2]

Classification
Acute pancreatitis is classified as either mild with minimal organ dysfunction/uneventful recovery or as severe, which is associated with organ failure and/or local complications such as necrosis, ulcers, or pseudocyst.[3]

Pathophysiology

The hallmark of pancreatitis is a severe inflammatory reaction that can extend beyond the pancreas and lead to systemic inflammatory response syndrome, organ failure, and death. Several pathways to tissue damage in acute pancreatitis are theorized:

- Intracellular activation of trypsin and other digestive enzymes
- Increased intracellular calcium levels, causing increased cellular damage and death
- Vasospasm and subsequent tissue ischemia
- Neurogenic mechanisms causing vasoconstriction and edema
- Possible Coxsackie virus infection, especially in alcoholic pancreatitis[4]

Etiology

Biliary causes remain the most common in acute pancreatitis accounting for about 40% of cases. Excessive alcohol accounts for approximately 20% of cases, with the remainder of acute cases associated with a variety of causes, including post–endoscopic retrograde cholangiopancreatography (ERCP), drug induced, hypertriglyceridemia, trauma, and post-surgical.[3] In chronic pancreatitis, alcohol accounts for nearly 70% of cases. A further 20% are considered idiopathic, with the remainder associated with diseases like cystic fibrosis, pancreatic tumors, autoimmune diseases, genetic defects, and congenital anomalies.[2]

Diagnosis

Clinical Presentation

Pancreatitis usually presents with severe epigastric abdominal pain, nausea, vomiting, and fever. The pain can also radiate to the back. Pain onset is typically sudden with gallstone pancreatitis and may be less abrupt and more poorly localized with other causes.[1]

History

A history of cholelithiasis, alcoholism, or lipid disorders, particularly familial hypertriglyceridemias, is important. For any patient with prior pancreatitis with appropriate symptoms, chronic pancreatitis should be high on the differential diagnosis. Certain drugs, such as azathioprine, sulfonates, estrogens, tetracyclines, valproic acid, and thiazide and furosemide diuretics, can cause pancreatitis, as can blunt abdominal trauma.

Physical Examination

On physical examination, patients with pancreatitis can have tender left upper quadrant, basilar rates from pleural effusion, erythematous skin nodules from fat necrosis, and Cullen and Turner signs. Abdominal rigidity, diminished bowel tones, and hypotension may also be present.

Laboratory Studies

Initial Diagnosis. Serum amylase and lipase remain the initial laboratory evaluations of choice in the initial evaluation of suspected pancreatitis. Amylase greater than three times the upper normal limit is considered highly specific for the diagnosis of acute pancreatitis. Trypsinogen-2 plasma levels are also highly specific for the diagnosis of acute pancreatitis; however, the test is not widely available.[1,5] Lipase-to-amylase ratio and alanine aminotransferase (ALT) and/or aspartate aminotransferase (AST) can help distinguish between alcohol-induced pancreatitis and gallstone pancreatitis, but overall sensitivity is low for both evaluations. Carbohydrate-deficient transferrin (CDT) is an emerging test to evaluate for both chronic alcoholism and alcohol-induced pancreatitis but it is not widely available at this time.

Prognosis. Numerous systems have been developed to help determine the severity of pancreatitis. Ranson criteria have been widely used; however, their utility is limited in that the score cannot be used until the 48-hour point where multiorgan failure may have already developed. C-reactive protein levels, while very sensitive and specific for prediction of severe pancreatitis, also are not valid until the 48-hour point. The APACHE II scoring system has come into more widespread use recently as it provides an immediate prognostic score on admission and can be followed serially to follow improvement or deterioration. The APACHE II system can be modified by adding one point for a body mass index (BMI) between 25 and 30 and two points for a BMI more than 30. The combination is commonly referred to as the APACHE-O system and has a significantly higher positive predictive value (PPV) than the APACHE II system alone. Computed tomography (CT) scan can also be used to compute the CT severity index (CTSI), which is useful in predicting complications or death, especially when the CTSI is greater than or equal to 7.[6]

Imaging

CT, magnetic resonance imaging (MRI), ultrasonography, and ERCP all offer specific advantages in the diagnosis and management of pancreatitis. CT can offer a specific CT grade for pancreatitis that can provide prognostic information. MRI can offer early evidence of duct disruption. Ultrasonography is best at identifying gallstones and bile-duct dilatation. ERCP remains the most accurate test for diagnosing or ruling out biliary causes of acute pancreatitis.[1]

Treatment

Treatment goals are mainly supportive because no specific medical or surgical therapy can directly limit the pancreatic autodigestion or inflammatory processes. Goals of therapy are aimed at relief of symptoms, prevention or correction of complications, and correction of underlying cause if possible. The mainstay of treatment is pain management, aggressive intravenous hydration; correction of electrolyte imbalances, particularly low serum calcium; and putting the pancreas at rest by decreasing gastric secretions. Nasogastric suction and routine use of H_2 blockers are no longer recommended as multiple studies have not demonstrated benefit for either therapy.[7] With mild acute pancreatitis, prognosis is excellent and most patients can be discharged in 3 to 5 days. Treatment for severe acute pancreatitis is focused around two primary objectives: providing supportive therapy and limiting the severity of pancreatic inflammation and necrosis.[8] Admission to the intensive care unit (ICU) or a step-down unit may be warranted especially if patients are elderly, obese, require ongoing volume resuscitation, or have substantial pancreatic necrosis.[9] Emergent surgery to ERCP to invasive central monitoring may be required in these patients. Currently, antibiotic therapy is not recommended for mild or severe cases of pancreatitis; however, studies are ongoing.[1] The final aspect of therapy is nutritional support, using either enteral or parenteral nutrition.[1]

PANCREATIC CARCINOMA

Pancreatic carcinoma is the fourth leading cause of cancer death in the United States, and it was estimated that 31,860 Americans would be diagnosed in 2004 and that 31,270 would die from the disease.[10] It has a very poor prognosis, with a 2-year survival rate of 10%.[11]

General Principles

Definition

The vast majority of pancreatic malignancies arise from the exocrine pancreas and are histologically adenocarcinomas. Most of these arise from the pancreatic ductal system.[12]

Pathophysiology

The specific pathways and alterations in tumor suppressor genes and oncogenes remain a mystery in pancreatic cancer as much as with most cancers. Current research is focusing on the Notch and Hedgehog pathways for both understanding of the disease and for potential future treatment.[13]

Etiology

There are few well-established risks associated with pancreatic cancer. Those with the strongest association include cigarette smoking, familial history, chronic pancreatitis, and type II diabetes. Risks not firmly established due to inadequate data include obesity, gallbladder disease, dietary factors, physical inactivity, and occupational exposures.[12]

Diagnosis

Clinical Presentation/History

Weight loss, jaundice, pain, anorexia, nausea, vomiting, and weakness are common symptoms. Dark-colored urine and clay-colored stools are also common symptoms.[10]

Physical Examination

Physical examination findings may be normal with exception of jaundice, bruising, and weight loss. A nontender, distended, palpable gallbladder may also be present as well as nonspecific signs of liver obstruction, left supraclavicular lymphadenopathy, and recurrent superficial thrombophlebitis.

Laboratory Evaluation

Serum bilirubin and alkaline phosphatase levels may be elevated, but are not diagnostic. CA 19-9 levels may help confirm the diagnosis in symptomatic patients but lack the sensitivity and specificity to screen asymptomatic patients.[10]

Imaging

Dual-phase helical CT is becoming the imaging methodology of choice in diagnosis of pancreatic cancer with a sensitivity at 98% in detecting both pancreatic cancers and distant metastases—allowing for diagnosis and staging information simultaneously. If clinical suspicion is high and CT is negative, endoscopic ultrasonography should be performed next, with a sensitivity of 92% and a specificity of 100%.[10]

Treatment

Palliative

Treatment of nonresectable pancreatic cancer is focused around palliative care. Pain, weight loss, obstructive jaundice, pancreatic insufficiency, gastric outlet obstruction, depression, and fatigue are many of the symptoms the patient may have during the course of the disease.

- **Pain.** Pain management can present severe challenges as the tumor commonly invades the celiac and mesenteric plexi. Early care is focused around nonsteroidal anti-inflammatory agents and then to oral or transdermal narcotic agents. These may be insufficient as the disease progresses requiring advanced techniques such as a celiac block. Radiation therapy and chemotherapy may also assist in pain control.
- **Obstructive jaundice.** Biliary decompression can be accomplished by surgical bypass or endobiliary stenting.
- **Weight loss.** Cachexia and weight loss can be associated with fatigue, weakness, and poor quality of life. Initial management is generally with supportive nutrition. Anorexia can be effectively treated with agents such as megesterol acetate, medroxyprogesterone acetate, and dexamethasone. Metoclopramide and dronabinol are also potent appetite stimulants.
- **Pancreatic insufficiency.** About 65% of patients with pancreatic cancer will have some degree of fat malabsorption and 50% will have some degree of protein malabsorption. Enzyme therapy has been shown to ameliorate many of the symptoms associated with these problems and has been shown to result in weight gain in these patients.
- **Gastric outlet obstruction.** Affects approximately 10% to 20% of patients who survive more than 15 months. Most of these do not require surgical bypass and can be treated with prokinetic drugs such as metoclopramide once physical obstructions have been ruled out.
- **Depression and fatigue.** Occurs in 47% to 71% of patients, especially as disease advances. Typical treatment includes selective serotonin-reuptake inhibitors (SSRIs) and tricyclic antidepressants (TCAs), with SSRIs offering fewer side effects while TCAs offer additional analgesia benefit. Fatigue can be treated in many ways, including erythropoietin (EPO) for anemia and with psychostimulants such as methylphenidate.[14]

Chemotherapy

Chemotherapy is aimed at inhibition of tumor growth and spread, but it has not proved curative. There are multiple different agents available currently with gemcitabine still the chief chemotherapy agent. There are also several protocols that combine gemcitabine with other agents, generally with only minimal improvement in survival. Many newer agents with specific pathway targets are being tested and include gene therapy agents, immunotherapy agents, and signal transduction inhibitors. However, effective treatment remains an elusive goal.[15]

Surgery

Surgical resection provides the only opportunity for cure. About 15% to 20% of patients have surgically resectable disease at the time of diagnosis. The most common surgical treatment for carcinoma is Whipple resection, which involves the gastric antrum, the entire duodenum and proximal 15 cm of jejunum, the head of the pancreas, the gallbladder, and the distal bile duct. Pylorus-preserving pancreatoduodenectomy has similar long-term survival benefits and offers shorter operative times and decreased blood loss. Distal pancreatectomy is performed in patients with resectable cancer in the body or tail of the pancreas.[10]

References
1. Whitcomb DC. Acute pancreatitis. *N Engl J Med* 2006;354:2142.
2. Gupta V, Toskes PP. Diagnosis and management of chronic pancreatitis. *Postgrad Med J* 2005;81:491.
3. Pitchumoni CS, Patel NM, Shah P. Factors influencing mortality in acute pancreatitis. *J Clin Gastroenterol* 2005;39:799.
4. Pandol SJ. Acute pancreatitis. *Curr Opin Gastroenterol* 2005;21:538–543.
5. Smotkin J, Tenner S. Laboratory diagnostic tests in acute pancreatitis. *J Clin Gastroenterol* 2002;34(4):459–462.
6. Triester SL, Kowdley KV. Prognostic factors in acute pancreatitis. *J Clin Gastroenterol* 2002;34(2):167–176.
7. Munoz A, Katerndahl DA. Diagnosis and management of acute pancreatitis. *Am Fam Physician* 2000;62(1):164–174.
8. Werner J, Feuerbach S, Uhl W, et al. Management of acute pancreatitis: from surgery to interventional intensive care. *Gut* 2005;54:427.
9. Nathens AB, et al. Management of the critically ill patient with severe acute pancreatitis. *Crit Care Med* 2004;32(12):2524.
10. Freelove R, Walling AD. Pancreatic cancer: diagnosis and management. *Am Fam Physician* 2006;73(3):485–492.
11. McKenna S, Eatcock M. The medical management of pancreatic cancer: a review. *The Oncologist* 2003;8:149–160.
12. Michaud DS. The epidemiology of pancreatic, gallbladder, and other biliary tract cancers. *Gastrointestinal Endosc* 2002;56(6 Suppl):S195–200.
13. Lomberk F, Fernandez-Zapico ME, Urrutia R. When developmental signaling pathways go wrong and their impact on pancreatic cancer development. *Curr Opin Gastroenterol* 2005;21:555–560.
14. El Kamar FG, Grossbard ML, Kozuch PS. Metastatic pancreatic cancer: emerging strategies in chemotherapy and palliative care. *Oncologist* 2003;8:18–34.
15. MacKenzie MJ. Molecular therapy in pancreatic adenocarcinoma. *Lancet Oncol* 2004;5:541–549.

DIVERTICULAR DISEASE

Anne Walsh

11.7

GENERAL PRINCIPLES

Diverticulosis is an acquired anatomic condition in which gastrointestinal mucosa protrudes through weak areas of muscularis where feeding arteries penetrate. These outpouchings occur predominantly in the sigmoid colon but can be found in any portion of the gastrointestinal (GI) tract. Colonic diverticulosis is prevalent in westernized countries and incidence increases with age, affecting about one third of people by age 60 and nearly two thirds by age 80. In rural Africa, the condition is nearly absent, and in Asia, although seen in only 20% of the population, diverticulosis predominantly affects the right colon. Risk factors include low dietary fiber intake, decreased tensile strength of the colon wall, abnormal colonic motility, visceral hypersensitivity, and genetics. The condition is found incidentally in 80% of patients, who remain asymptomatic. The 20% of patients with diverticulosis who present with symptoms such as abdominal pain or hematochezia and are considered to have *diverticular disease*.[1]

SYMPTOMATIC DIVERTICULOSIS

Diagnosis

Clinical Presentation

Patients with painful diverticulosis tend to be younger than those without symptoms and typically present with colicky or aching left lower quadrant pain of short duration, which is typically worse after meals and better after bowel movements.

Examination

The examination may be completely normal or reveal some degree of left lower quadrant tenderness but no evidence of peritoneal irritation, inflammation, or mass.

Laboratory and Imaging

All laboratory studies, including complete blood count (CBC), complete metabolic panel (CMP), erythrocyte sedimentation rate (ESR), and urinalysis (UA) are normal. Diverticula are often found incidentally on barium enema or computerized tomography (CT); colonoscopy is the "gold standard" diagnostic test to confirm the presence and location of diverticula, but a definitive diagnosis of painful diverticulosis is a diagnosis of exclusion.

Differential Diagnosis

Irritable bowel syndrome (IBS) may present similarly and often occurs concomitantly. IBS is diagnosed by specific Rome III criteria (>3 months, with onset at least 6 months previously of recurrent abdominal pain or discomfort associated with two or more of the following: improvement with defecation, and/or onset associated with a change in frequency of stool, and/or onset associated with a change in stool form).[2] Diverticulitis, inflammatory bowel disease (IBD), gynecologic pathology, and other serious causes of acute abdominal pain should be ruled out.

Treatment

Treatment includes increasing dietary fiber to the recommended 25 to 35 g per day; add a fiber supplement such as psyllium hydrophilic mucoid (Metamucil, Konsyl, Hydrocil; 1 tbsp. one to two times daily), which decreases intraluminal pressure and improves stool caliber and consistency. For patients who dislike standard fiber mixes or complain of gas with psyllium, there are a variety of products available containing methylcellulose, calcium polycarbophil, and other vegetable fibers; also available are "clear" mixes (Metamucil, Citrucel, Benefiber, Fiber-Sure, Unifiber), chewable tablets (Equalactin, Benefiber, FiberChoice), caplets/capsules (Metamucil, Citrucel, Fibercon), and wafers (Metamucil). Advise patients to add fiber gradually to minimize bloating; recommend that patients take fiber supplements with an 8-oz glass of water and increase their overall water consumption. Fiber improves symptoms and reduces the risk of diverticulitis.[1] If needed, an antispasmodic such as hyoscyamine (Levsin SL) 0.125 mg can be used for relief of abdominal pain. Educate patients to avoid stimulant laxatives such as senna, cascara, aloe, and bisacodyl due to the risk of dependence, and give patients accurate educational materials about how to manage their condition.

DIVERTICULAR BLEEDING

Diagnosis

Clinical Presentation

Bleeding from diverticula is usually painless, may be occult or massive, and occurs as a result of rupture of the vasa recta on the dome of the diverticulum, most commonly in the right colon. Most patients are over age 60 and have concomitant medical conditions.

Examination

The examination may be normal or show evidence of hypovolemia, depending on the extent of bleeding. There is usually little or no abdominal tenderness. Rectal examination demonstrates hematochezia or stool that is positive for occult blood.

Laboratory and Imaging

CBC may reveal anemia, and iron studies may be low, although in acute bleeding, the results may be normal. In patients with brisk bleeding and those who cannot tolerate colonoscopy, the site of bleeding may be identified with a radionuclide scan, dynamic enhanced helical CT, or by arteriography (best with a bleeding rate of >0.5 to 1 mL/min) first, but colonoscopy is the preferred method of evaluation due to a higher diagnostic yield and fewer complications.[3]

Differential Diagnosis

Bleeding is not typically associated with diverticulitis; angiodysplasia (of small bowel or colon, especially in patients over age 65), ischemic colitis, neoplasm, and inflammatory conditions must be considered.[4] Hemorrhoidal bleeding is rarely massive; rectal varices should be considered in patients with end-stage liver disease.

Treatment

In up to 80% of patients, bleeding stops spontaneously with only supportive treatment, although the risk of rebleeding is as high as 38%.[3] Endoscopic interventions include submucosal epinephrine injection, tamponade, and bipolar coagulation. Endoclips, banding, and laser photocoagulation may also be tried. Patients with severe bleeding may be treated with transcatheter embolization or intra-arterial vasopressin for up to 24 hours if the site of bleeding is known. Patients who are unable to tolerate continued bleeding, who fail medical management, or who suffer from repeated episodes should be considered for surgery because up to 50% of patients with two episodes of bleeding will have additional rebleeding.[3]

DIVERTICULITIS

Diagnosis

Clinical Presentation

This localized infection is a result of micro/macroscopic perforation of a diverticulum due to erosion of its wall from increased intraluminal pressure and/or inspissated food particles. Patients present with abdominal pain (most often left-sided) and may have fever, chills, abdominal distention, nausea, anorexia, dysuria, and occasionally vomiting.

Examination

There may be relatively few findings if the inflammation is isolated to the pericolic fat, or findings of acute peritonitis may be evident. In early diverticulitis, temperature may be normal, or a low-grade fever may be present. On abdominal examination, there are varying degrees of tenderness with or without rebound. In the presence of abscess or fistula, a mass may be palpable. Immunosuppressed patients may show few findings on initial physical examination, even in the presence of overt perforation.

Laboratory and Imaging

CBC in mild or early disease is normal or may reveal leukocytosis. ESR may be elevated. UA can show microscopic hematuria and pyuria from irritation of the ureter or from vesicocolic fistula formation. Stool is positive for occult blood in up to 25% of patients. Plain film radiographs of the abdomen may reveal free intraperitoneal air if perforation occurs, and abdominal ultrasonography can show thickened bowel, but abdominal CT is the imaging test of choice. In addition to confirming the presence and location of bowel wall thickening and inflammation within the pericolic fat, CT can reveal any abscess, fistula, peritonitis, or obstruction. Water-soluble contrast enema is sensitive and specific for diverticulitis but less well tolerated. Colonoscopy should be performed to confirm disease presence and extent, as well as to rule out colon polyps or cancer, but only after the patient's symptoms are completely resolved, typically several weeks after the acute episode.[5]

Differential Diagnosis

Ischemic colitis, colon cancer, obstruction, volvulus, inflammatory bowel disease, nephrolithiasis, penetrating ulcer, and appendicitis, especially in patients with right-sided pain, must all be considered. In patients at risk, pelvic inflammatory disease, ectopic pregnancy, and ovarian cancer should also be ruled out.

Treatment

A reliable patient with mild symptoms can be managed on an outpatient basis. The patient should be started on a clear liquid diet. Antispasmodic medications and analgesics may be used judiciously for symptom relief. Oral antibiotics should target both aerobic Gram-negative organisms and anaerobes and are given for 7 to 10 days based on severity of symptoms, previous history, and comorbidities. First-line therapy is ciprofloxacin (Cipro) 500 mg PO BID (may substitute amoxicillin-clavulanate or trimethoprim-sulfamethoxazole) plus metronidazole (Flagyl) 500 mg PO TID (may substitute clindamycin).[5] As symptoms improve, diet may be advanced to low residue until the patient has recovered. When well, recommend increased dietary fiber intake (and/or supplements) to reduce the chance of recurrence.[1] The recommendation to avoid nuts, seeds, and popcorn is controversial; no clinical trial has been done to prove any relation to the pathogenesis of diverticulitis. However, some patients with diverticulitis have clearly linked the ingestion of these foods with acute attacks; therefore, this recommendation may be made on a patient-specific basis.[6]

Patients with more severe signs and symptoms, the immunocompromised, and frail elderly patients may require inpatient management with bowel rest and intravenous hydration plus antibiotics. Coverage for Gram-negative aerobes and anaerobes may be achieved with clindamycin or metronidazole plus a quinolone or third-generation cephalosporin. An aminoglycoside can be added if there is a concern about antibiotic resistance or if *Pseudomonas* infection is suspected. Effective single-agent treatment options include piperacillin/tazobactam (Zosyn) or ticarcillin/clavulanate (Timentin). The combination of an aminoglycoside and metronidazole is also effective.[5] Analgesics can be given as needed, but nonsteroidal anti-inflammatory drugs have been associated with a higher incidence of perforation and should be avoided.

Special Considerations

Patients with *complicated diverticulitis*, that is, those who develop perforation, abscess, fistula, or obstruction, and those who are septic, immuocompromised, or fail medical management, are candidates for surgery. In patients with abscesses, CT-guided needle drainage may delay the need for emergent surgery and allow the performance of an elective single-stage bowel resection. Previous guidelines recommend elective resection after two episodes of acute diverticulitis due to the high risk of recurrence and complications, but a recent study shows that this recommendation is not be based on current evidence and may be unnecessary.[7] In the past, surgical treatment of complicated diverticular disease comprised a two- or three-stage procedure that included colostomy. Presently, resection is often accomplished in a single, laparoscopic procedure without colostomy; a laparoscopic approach is best suited for patients whose acute episode has resolved or in those without peritonitis.[5,8]

References

1. Petruzziello L, Iacopini F, Bulajic M, et al. Uncomplicated diverticular disease of the colon. *Aliment Pharmacol Ther* 2006;23:1379–1391.
2. Drossman D. The functional gastrointestinal disorders and the Rome III process. *Gastroenterology* 2006;130:1377–1390.
3. Young-Fadok T, Pemberton J. Colonic diverticular bleeding. UpToDate, accessed July 4, 2006.
4. Saab S, Jutabha R. Approach to the adult patient with lower gastrointestinal bleeding. UpToDate, accessed July 4, 2006.
5. Young-Fadok T, Pemberton J. Treatment of acute diverticulitis. UpToDate, accessed July 4, 2006.
6. Thompson G. Nuts, seeds, and diverticula. In Diverticulosis, Publication 176, International Foundation for Functional Gastrointestinal Disorders, Milwaukee, 2003–04.
7. Chapman JR, Dozois EJ, Wolff BG, et al. Diverticulitis: a progressive disease? Do multiple recurrences predict less favorable outcomes? *Ann Surg* 2006;243:876–883.
8. Kaufman H. (Chief, Division of Colorectal/Pelvic Floor Surgery and General Surgery, USC University Hospital, Keck School of Medicine-University of Southern CA). Update in medicine: current issues in gastroenterology, presentation and personal communication, Los Angeles, CA, July 8, 2006.

IRRITABLE BOWEL SYNDROME
L. Peter Schwiebert

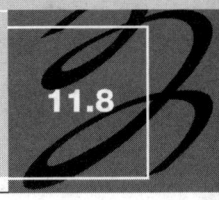
11.8

GENERAL PRINCIPLES

Definition

Irritable bowel syndrome (IBS) is chronic abdominal discomfort and abnormal bowel habits not otherwise explained. Three sets of diagnostic criteria have defined IBS (Table 11.8-1). In pediatric patients with recurrent abdominal pain severe enough to interfere with normal activity, 44.9% meet Rome II criteria.

Epidemiology

While up to 70% of patients with IBS do not consult a health care provider, **prevalence estimates** range from 3% to 25%; most studies suggest a 10% prevalence in the general population and a female-to-male ratio of approximately 3:1. Symptoms of IBS are among the top ten reasons patients consult primary care physicians. IBS has **significant comorbidities** — gastrointestinal (up to 87% of those with IBS meet criteria for functional dyspepsia, and 46% have gastroesophageal reflux disease, GERD), nongastrointestinal (48% of patients with fibromyalgia, 50% with chronic pelvic pain, 51% with chronic fatigue syndrome, and 64% with temporomandibular joint dysfunction have IBS). Compared to controls, patients with IBS have a significant increase in abdominal surgery (appendectomy, hysterectomy, cholecystectomy) and psychiatric disorders (54% to 94% incidence of anxiety, depression, somatization). Various estimates place the annual cost of IBS to sufferers in the United States at up to $20 billion (physician visits, medications, lost productivity), which is comparable to or exceeds the cost of other common chronic conditions (e.g., asthma, hypertension, and heart failure).

DIAGNOSIS

History

Historical features diagnose IBS (Table 11.8-1), coupled with absence of findings suggesting organic/structural disease (i.e., onset of symptoms after age 50, severe diarrhea, nocturnal symptoms, unintended weight loss, hematochezia, or family history of inflammatory bowel disease/celiac sprue/malignancy). **Sensitivity, specificity, and predictive value positive values** for the three sets of criteria are, respectively, 42% to 90%, 70% to 100%, and 74% for Manning; 65% to 84%, 100%, and 69% to 100% for Rome I; and 49% to 65%, 100%, and 69% to 100% for Rome II. Rome II criteria are easier to recall than Manning or Rome I, but are less sensitive and may underestimate IBS prevalence. Rome and Manning criteria were developed and tested at referral centers; many primary care physicians are unfamiliar with these criteria and therefore less confident diagnosing IBS than their specialist colleagues. **Symptoms** (diarrhea, constipation, dyspepsia, remission) in patients with IBS **characteristically fluctuate,** with up to a third changing subtype (diarrhea vs. constipation predominant) over a 12-week period.

Laboratory Studies

In patients meeting IBS criteria, the American College of Gastroenterology Functional GI Disorders Task Force concluded that **routine diagnostic testing is not supported by the literature,** as the likelihood of an abnormal result is no different comparing those with IBS and controls. The only possible exception is to test for celiac sprue (serum transglutaminase) or lactase deficiency in patients with IBS whose diarrhea improves with dietary modification.

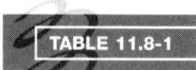 TABLE 11.8-1	Criteria for Irritable Bowel Syndrome

Manning criteria
At least two of the following symptoms:
Abdominal pain eased after bowel movement
Looser stools at onset of pain
More frequent bowel movements at onset of pain
Abdominal distention
Mucus per rectum
Feeling of incomplete evacuation

Rome I symptom criteria for IBS
At least 3 months of continuous or recurrent symptoms of the following:
Abdominal pain or discomfort:
  Relieved with defecation, or
  Associated with a change in frequency of stool, or
  Associated with a change in consistency of stool
Plus
Two or more of the following, at least on one fourth of occasions or days:
  Altered stool frequency (>3 bowel movements per day or <3 bowel movements
    per day), or
  Altered stool form (lumpy/hard or loose/watery stool), or
  Altered stool passage (straining, urgency, or feeling of incomplete evacuation), or
  Passage of mucus, or
  Bloating or feeling of abdominal distention

Rome II symptom criteria for IBS
At least 12 weeks or more, which need not be consecutive, in the preceding 12 months of
  abdominal discomfort or pain that has two of three features:
  Relieved with defecation; and/or
  Onset associated with a change in frequency of stool; and/or
  Onset associated with a change in form (appearance) of stool

TREATMENT

Treatment for IBS is symptomatic and individualized, depending on the impact of symptoms on quality of life. Evaluating the efficacy of interventions is challenging, given a placebo response as high as 70%, especially in those whose symptoms wax and wane.

Behavioral/Counseling

In a review of 10 controlled studies, 3 found cognitive–behavioral therapy (CBT) results in improvements similar to or greater than medication therapy; those most likely to benefit from CBT include individuals significantly distressed with symptoms, open to a psychologic explanation, willing to be actively involved in management, and who have already undergone appropriate interventions. Those less likely to benefit from CBT include individuals with a diagnosable psychiatric disorder, high trait anxiety, female gender, or absence of symptom-free days.

Medication

Medications for IBS include traditional, symptom-directed treatments, medications targeting global symptoms, and complementary alternative medications (CAM) (Table 11.8-2).

- **Traditional medications** have been unsatisfactory to many patients with IBS, leading to doctor-shopping and experimentation with multiple therapies.
- **Medications targeting global symptoms.** Currently these medications are typically reserved for women failing traditional therapy, because of the cost and potential side effects of global therapy. However, in terms of global symptom relief as well as

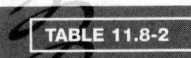 **TABLE 11.8-2**   **Medications for IBS**

Class	Examples	Dosing	Indications	SOR (no. of studies)	Comments
Traditional (symptom-focused)					
Tricyclics	Amitriptyline Imipramine Nortriptyline	10–75 mg HS 10–75 mg HS 10–75 mg HS	Abdominal pain; no more effective than placebo for global symptoms	B(6)	Anticholinergic side effects (sedation, blurred vision, constipation, dry mouth, urinary retention)
Antispasmodics	Dicyclomine Hyoscyamine		May improve abdominal pain; no benefit for global systems	B(16)	Risk of constipation
SSRIs	Paroxetine	5–20 mg day	Treat comorbid anxiety/ depression; decrease abdominal pain and improve quality of life	B(16)	
Antidiarrheal	Loperamide	2–4 mg up to qid	May decrease diarrhea/fecal urgency; similar to placebo for global symptoms	B(3)	Caution with alternating diarrhea and constipation; constipation and paralytic ileus may occur
Laxatives: osmotic	Polyethylene glycol Lactulose	17 g bid	Chronic constipation; no published controlled trials with IBS	—	Abdominal cramping; osmotics better tolerated than stimulant laxatives
Laxatives: stimulant	Senna, Bisacodyl	187 mg daily 5–10 mg daily	Chronic constipation; no published controlled trials with IBS		
Stool softeners	Docusate sodium	100 g bid	Chronic constipation; no published controlled trials with IBS		

(continued)

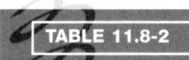

| TABLE 11.8-2 | Medications for IBS *(Continued)* | | | | |

Class	Examples	Dosing	Indications	SOR (no. of studies)	Comments
Bulking agents	Methylcellulose, Psyllium, Calcium polycarbophil		Improved nonspecific outcomes (constipation); ease of stool passage; satisfaction with bowel movements	B(13)	Calcium poly carbophil and methylcellulose cause less gas/bloating than others
Medications targeting global symptoms					
5-HT₃ receptor antagonist	Alosetron	1 mg bid	Diarrhea-predominant IBS in women	A(4)	
Complementary alternative medicines					
Neomzzycin			Treatment for 1 week improved abdominal pain, diarrhea, constipation	A	No documented improvement in global symptoms
Peppermint oil			Some improvement in abdominal pain	B	No documented improvement in global symptoms
Guar gum			Abdominal pain/bowel alternatives	B	Better tolerated than fiber
Probiotics (lactobacillus)			Abdominal pain, flatulence	C	Two studies with small numbers

Key: bid, twice daily; HS, bedtime; qid, four times daily; SOR, strength of recommendation.

potential decreased frequency of office visits and trials of other medication, the cost–benefit equation may reflect more favorably on global medications than may initially appear.

Referral

Referral of individuals with IBS to a gastroenterologist is appropriate only if the diagnosis is in question or if the patient presents with features of organic/structural disease.

Patient Education

Patient education in individuals with IBS is foundational to effective management. This includes **reassurance and a comprehensible explanation** of the underlying physiology (pathophysiology of IBS, including discussion of the role of stressors and psychiatric influences). Scant evidence supports **dietary manipulation** in IBS; however, patients may benefit from limiting intake of ethanol, caffeine, sorbitol, and fats. As increased dietary fiber is an initial intervention in most patients with IBS, it is helpful to gradually titrate upward the amount of fiber and consider using soluble fiber (oat bran, methylcellulose) to minimize abdominal pain and bloating.

References

1. Holten KB, Wetherington A, Bankston L. Diagnosing the patient with abdominal pain and altered bowel habits: is it irritable bowel syndrome? *Am Fam Physician* 2003;67(10): 2157–2162.
2. Lembo AJ. A 54-year-old woman with constipation-predominant irritable bowel syndrome. *JAMA* 2006;295(8):925–933.
3. Holten K. Irritable bowel syndrome: minimize testing, let symptoms guide treatment. *J Fam Prac* 2003;52(12):942–950.
4. Hulisz D. The burden of illness of irritable bowel syndrome: current challenges and hope for the future. *JMCP* 2004;10(4):299–309.
5. Cash BD, Chey WD. Review article: irritable bowel syndrome—an evidence-based approach to diagnosis. *Aliment Pharmacol Ther* 2004;19:1235–1245.
6. Walker LS, et al. Recurrent abdominal pain: symptom subtypes based on the Rome II criteria for pediatric functional gastrointestinal disorders. *J Pediatr Gastroenterol Nutr* 2004;38:187–191.
7. Cremonini F, Talley NJ. Irritable bowel syndrome: epidemiology, natural history, health care seeking and emerging risk factors. *Gastroenterol Clin North Am* 2005;34:189–204.
8. Viera AJ, et al. Management of irritable bowel syndrome. *Am Fam Physician* 2002; 66(10).
9. Longstreth GF. Definition and classification of irritable bowel syndrome: current consensus and controversies. *Gastroenterol Clin North Am* 2005;34:173–187.
10. Schooff M, Stelter C. Tegaserod in patients with irritable bowel syndrome. *Am Fam Physician* 2004;70(11).
11. Hutton J. Cognitive behaviour therapy for irritable bowel syndrome. *Gastroenterol Hepatol* 2005;17:11–14.

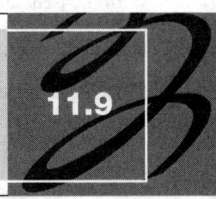

INFLAMMATORY BOWEL DISEASE
Robert Ross

11.9

GENERAL PRINCIPLES

The term inflammatory bowel disease (IBD) collectively includes the processes of Crohn disease (CD) and ulcerative colitis (UC), which are chronic, relapsing, and remitting inflammatory conditions of the gastrointestinal (GI) tract. The incidence of IBD in developed countries is approximately 3 per 100,000 to 16 per 100,000 population, the prevalence 0.1% to 0.2%. The most common age of presentation is from adolescence to 30 years with a smaller increase in incidence in the 50 to 80 year age group.

Pathology

CD is characterized by a granulomatous, transmural inflammatory infiltrate located at any level of the GI tract from mouth to anus, most commonly found in the ileocecal area. CD is a patchy, noncontinuous process. UC is limited to the colon, usually involves only the superficial layers of the bowel, and is continuous in nature. UC virtually always involves the rectal mucosa.

Etiology

The pathogenesis of IBD remains obscure. The prevailing belief is that IBD is heterogeneous with several genetic and environmental factors playing a role. The final manifestation of the process is mucosal inflammation presenting with a wide variety of symptoms.[1]

DIAGNOSIS

Clinical Presentation

Crohn Disease

The most common presentation is ileitis, which may manifest only as diarrhea and abdominal pain, or may include systemic features such as anorexia, fevers, weight loss, anemia, increased white blood cell count, erythrocyte sedimentation rate, or C-reactive protein levels. Bloody diarrhea usually indicates colonic involvement. The disease may also present as small bowel obstruction or localized peritonitis accompanied by fever, abdominal pain, and leukocytosis. This presentation is often mistakenly diagnosed as an acute appendicitis or diverticulitis. Less common presentations include refractory oral ulceration, perianal fistula or abscess, gastroduodenal disease (dyspepsia, anorexia, nausea and vomiting, epigastric pain), intra-abdominal abscess, or symptoms of enterovesical fistula (urinary tract infection, fecaluria).

Alternative diagnostic considerations in CD include appendicitis, cecal diverticulitis, *Yersinia enterocolitica* infection, ileocecal tuberculosis, giardiasis, small bowel lymphoma, the vasculitis associated with Behçet syndrome, and cecal carcinoma. CD confined to the colon may be confused with UC. In patients experiencing mainly weight loss and diarrhea, diseases associated with malabsorption (celiac sprue) are possibilities. In women, gynecologic disease should be considered.

Ulcerative Colitis

Patients experience symptoms of proctitis, including rectal bleeding, urgency, and tenesmus. Occasional incontinence of stool is seen in >50%. Rectal disease may cause constipation and hard stools streaked with blood. Patients with severe colitis develop bloody diarrhea (>6 to 10 bowel movements/day), fever, weight loss, volume depletion, and anemia. At presentation in an adult, 55% will have proctitis alone, 30% left sided colitis, and 15% will have more extensive disease. In children, disease involvement is usually more extensive.[2] The differential diagnosis of UC includes infectious colitis (discussed in the next section), ischemic or radiation colitis, and CD limited to the colon. Irritable bowel syndrome (IBS) often mimics the presenting symptoms of UC and CD, but never causes rectal bleeding or a positive fecal occult blood test.

Physical Examination

May reveal right lower quadrant tenderness or the sensation of a mass in patients with active CD. The presence of left lower quadrant tenderness in a patient with rectal bleeding should always raise the possibility of active UC. Patients with severe UC or toxic megacolon will appear acutely ill with abdominal tenderness, dehydration, tachycardia, hypotension, and often fever. In the rare case of perforation, peritoneal signs and/or abdominal rigidity will be present. Rectal examination should be performed, to check for rectal tenderness and the presence of blood. The perianal region and oral mucosa should be examined, as up to one third of patients with CD will develop perianal disease, and many will have oral ulcers.

Diagnostic Tests

Laboratory Testing and Cultures

Autoantibodies—anti-OmpC; anti-*Sacharomyces* (ASCA); antineutrophil cytoplasmic antibodies (pANCA)—have become commercially available for the diagnosis of IBD. In children and young adults, the overall sensitivity of the antibody panel was 65% for CD and 76% for UC, with a specificity of 94%. Currently, these tests should probably only be used as an adjunct to conventional testing.[3] Accurate diagnosis rests with the analysis of the clinical presentation, the omission of infectious causes that may mimic IBD, and choosing the most appropriate study. The physician must obtain a complete history, including foreign travel, exposure to food-borne illness, and antibiotic agents. Stool samples should be obtained for culture of *Salmonella, Shigella, Campylobacter, Yersinia, Escherichia coli* O157:H7, and enteroinvasive *E. coli*; examination for ova, cysts, and parasites; and testing for *Clostridium difficile* toxin. In a patient who has rectal intercourse, rectal cultures for gonorrhea and chlamydia should be obtained. HIV testing should be considered, as opportunistic GI tract infections can present with diarrhea, weight loss, and abdominal pain. Stool testing for *Giardia lamblia* antigen may help determine the cause of chronic diarrhea and abdominal pain. In the acutely ill and toxic patient who is having moderate or severe rectal bleeding, diarrhea, and/or abdominal pain, complete blood count, electrolytes, albumin, amylase, and type and screening or cross-matching of blood products is mandatory.

Endoscopy

Sigmoidoscopy is the first diagnostic test to perform in the patient with bloody diarrhea. Direct examination of the rectal and sigmoid mucosa with biopsy is possible. It is often difficult to determine the etiology of colonic inflammation based on appearance, and the physician usually must wait until cultures and pathology are available before diagnosing IBD. Caution is advised in performing sigmoidoscopy during severe colitis, because of complications. Biopsy in this situation is safe, however.

CD can be diagnosed by colonoscopy, especially if the ileocecal valve can be traversed (ileoscopy) and the terminal ileum examined. This is often the only method of diagnosing early ileal or colonic CD. Colonoscopy is also an effective method of assessing the extent of UC, which can be useful in determining if systemic or local therapy is appropriate. Colonoscopy is almost never warranted during bouts of severe colitis or in the patient with toxic megacolon, although there is debate about the safety of the exam in this situation. Typically, there is a cobblestone appearance of the colon in CD, with areas of normal mucosa between involved areas. In UC, inflammation is continuous with erosions and friability apparent. However, in about 10% of sufferers, the differentiation between CD and UC is impossible based on clinical presentation and extensive testing. In the future, wireless capsule endoscopy may become the preferred method of visualizing and diagnosing CD.

Radiography

If severe colitis or obstruction is suspected, a three-position abdominal series should be obtained (upright chest film, abdominal decubitus, and flat plate or kidney, ureters, bladder, KUB, views) to rule out perforation, obstruction, or toxic megacolon. Toxic megacolon is diagnosed when the diameter of the colon on the flat plate exceeds 5.5 cm. In CD, the terminal ileum is best viewed via a peroral pneumocolon exam. This gives a double-contrast view of the ileum. Other studies include a single-contrast small bowel follow-through examination, and enteroclysis (small bowel enema) in which a catheter is introduced into the proximal jejunum, followed by either air or methylcellulose. This is the procedure of choice if more proximal disease is suspected. In UC, the best test is the air-contrast barium enema (not during severe disease or toxic megacolon). If complications such as intra-abdominal abscess are suspected, then an abdominal CT scan should be ordered. The role of MRI and labeled white cell scans is not well defined.

TREATMENT (TABLE 11.9-1)

Hospitalization

With severe symptoms, abnormal vital signs, severe colitis, intra-abdominal abscess, or other complications, management should occur in the hospital setting. The patient should be given intravenous (IV) rehydration, left nil per oral (NPO), and receive IV therapy (usually with high dose steroids) as soon as the diagnosis is made. In these cases it is prudent to seek consultation from a gastroenterologist or surgeon.

Consultation is also advised for patients who do not respond to initial outpatient management, or develop complications such as fistula, obstruction, or abscess.

Outpatient

Local therapy of proctitis and sigmoid disease (mild to moderate) should be attempted before using systemic treatment. Patients with CD should discontinue the use of oral contraceptives and smoking. Patients with UC conversely may benefit from the use of transdermal nicotine

TABLE 11.9-1 Inflammatory Bowel Disease: Management Options

Local agent	UC indications dose	CD indications dose	Contraindication	Side effects
Hydrocortisone (HCT) Enema (Cortenema) 100 mg	Enema (100 mg) Proctitis, sigmoid disease single agent in mild disease, supplement to systemic treatment 1 appl qhs × 21 days	For CD of lower colon/rectum, same doses as with UC	Obstruction, local abscess, perforation, peritonitis, recent anastamosis, fistulas Sensitivity to drug/class, infections	Local irritation, rectal bleeding, systemic absorption Serious side effects not reported
HCT Foam (Cortifoam) 90 mg	As with HCT enema 1 appl pr qd–bid × 2–3 weeks, then qod	For CD of lower colon/rectum, same doses as with UC	See HCT enema	See HCT enema
HCT Suppositories 100 mg	As with HCT enema	For CD of lower colon/rectum, same doses as with UC	See HCT enema	See HCT enema
Mesalamine suppositories (Rowasa) 500 mg	As with HCT but more effective 500 mg PR bid	As with HCT but more effective 500 mg PR bid	Sensitivity to drug/class, obstruction, local abscess, perforation, peritonitis, fistulas	Local irritation, rectal bleeding
Mesalamine enemas (4 g/60 mL)	As with HCT but more effective 1–4 g/day PR maintenance 1–4 g qod	As with HCT but more effective 1–4 g/day PR maintenance 1–4 g qod	See mesalamine suppositories	See mesalamine suppositories
Systemic agent				
IV steroids HCT (Solu-Cortef) Methylprednisolone (Solu-Medrol)	Effective for remission induction only HCT 300 mg/day Methylprednisolone 40–60 mg/day	Effective for remission induction only HCT 300 mg/day Methylprednisolone 40–60 mg/day	Drug sensitivity Relative with infections, caution if congestive heart failure, diabetes, tuberculosis, hypertension	Adrenal insufficiency, psychosis, immunosuppression, peptic ulcer, osteoporosis, others
PO steroids Prednisone (Deltasone) CIR budesonide for CD of ileum	As with IV steroids Prednisone 40–60 mg/day	As with IV steroids Prednisone 0.25–0.75 mg/kg/day CIR budesonide 9 mg PO qam	See IV steroids	See IV steroids

Drug	Dosing	Indication/comments	Contraindications/cautions	Side effects
PO sulfasalazine (Azulfidine 500 mg tabs)	Remission induction 2–6 g/day (1 g qid), maintenance 2–4 g/day; administer with folate. 4–1 mg/day	Effective in ileocolonic disease only—induction 3–5 g/day (1 g qid) maintenance 3 g/day; administer with folate 0.4–1 mg/day	Hypersensitivity to drug/class/sulfa/salicylates, renal/hepatic dysfunction, porphyria, obstruction, caution G6PD deficiency	Poorly tolerated esp. at high doses (GI) rashes, Stevens-Johnson syndrome, hemolytic anemia, GI, headache, pancreatitis, hepatitis, sperm ab.
PO mesalamine 5-ASA (Asacol-ileo-colonic release 400 mg. Pentasa 250 mg-jejunum to colon)	Remission induction 4–4.8 g/day (Asacol 1200 mg qid) Maintenance 400–800 mg qid, prob. ineffective	Remission induction Asacol 1–1.2 g qid, Pentasa 1 g qid, better for proximal disease? maintenance same as remission effectiveness?	Hypersensitivity to drug/class, caution in impaired renal function	Anaphylaxis, confusion, headache, GI, pharyngitis, dizziness, asthenia, others
PO antibiotics Metronidazole (Flagyl) ± Ciprofloxacin (Cipro)	N/A	Effective in remission alone or in combination—first choice for perianal disease. Flagyl 250 mg qid ± Cipro 500 mg bid	Hypersensitivity to drug/class, pregnancy, caution with central nervous system disorder	GI, seizures, rash, photosensitivity, liver function test elevation, neuropathy and antabuse reaction with flagyl, tendonitis with Cipro
Methotrexate (intractable Crohn remission induction)	Role is unclear	25 mg IM weekly; effective in remission induction in refractory disease and reduction of steroid doses by 50%	Hypersensitivity to drug/class, pregnancy, breastfeeding, immunodeficiency alcohol abuse, caution with renal/hepatic dysfunction	Ulcerative stomatitis, anemia, leucopenia, thrombocytopenia Immune suppression
Infliximab	Varying doses and regimens Most often 5 mg/kg IV infusion	Varying doses and regimens; most often 5 mg/kg IV infusion; most effective Rx for fistulizing CD	Hypersensitivity to drug/class or murine proteins Active infection Congestive heart failure NYHA III, IV Caution with seizure, hematologic disorder, latent tuberculosis, multiple sclerosis, elderly	Fever, chills, myalgias, H/A, fatigue Sepsis, pneumonia, opportunistic infections, hepatotoxicity, serum sickness-like reaction, bone marrow suppression

(Nicoderm, Habitrol). IBD sufferers should avoid the use of nonsteroidal anti-inflammatory drugs (NSAIDs). Systemic agents effective in IBD include 6-mercaptopurine (6-MP, Purinethol), azathioprine (AZA, Imuran), methotrexate, cyclosporin (in UC only), and antitumor necrosis factor antibody (infliximab). Infliximab is especially effective in patients with complications of CD. A variety of experimental treatment approaches (CDP571, IL10, omega-3 diets, probiotics) are being tested. If the use of newer systemic agents is considered or complex therapy is necessary, this is best undertaken after consultation. Once remission occurs, maintenance therapy should be considered. However, recent meta-analysis has shown that oral 5-ASA agents and steroids are ineffective in maintaining remission, particularly in CD.[4] Better-tolerated agents, such as mesalamine (Asacol, Rowasa, Pentasa) and olsalazine (Dipentum), are at least as effective as sulfasalazine in UC. Symptomatic therapy for diarrhea (codeine, loperamide, imodium) is contraindicated in severe disease and megacolon.

Special Considerations
Local (GI)
UC can lead to toxic megacolon resulting in perforation and intra-abdominal sepsis. CD may cause fibrosis, stricture, intestinal obstruction, fistulas, and intra-abdominal abscesses, as well as perianal disease. Colonic mucosa that is involved with IBD is more likely to develop dysplasia and carcinoma. With extensive colonic involvement by CD, the rate of malignant transformation is probably similar to that seen with UC.[5] The frequency of screening for carcinoma in IBD is controversial, but after 8 years of disease it is prudent to perform colonoscopy and biopsy regularly. This recommendation is based on indirect evidence only.[6]

Systemic
Extraintestinal manifestations of IBD include ocular changes of episcleritis and uveitis, reactive arthropathy with ankylosing spondylitis seen in 5% of patients, and the dermatologic manifestations of erythema nodusum and pyoderma gangrenosum. There is an increased incidence of nephrolithiasis, especially in CD. A serious complication, seen most often in UC, is sclerosing cholangitis.

Patient Information
An excellent source for patient information is Crohn's & Colitis Foundation of America, 386 Park Avenue South, 17th Floor, New York, NY 10016, 800-932-2423. Internet address: www.ccfa.org.

References
1. Yamada T, ed. *Textbook of gastroenterology*. 4th ed. Philadelphia: Lippincott Williams & Wilkins; 2003.
2. Ghosh S, Shand A, Ferguson A. Ulcerative colitis. *BMJ* 2000;320:1119–1123.
3. Zholudev A, Zurakowski D, Young W, et al. Serologic testing with ANCA, ASCA, and anti-OmpC in children and young adults with Crohn's disease and ulcerative colitis: diagnostic value and correlation with disease phenotype. *Am J Gastroenterology* 2004;99:2235–2241.
4. Akobeng AK, Gardener E. Oral 5-ASA for maintenance of medically-induced remission in Crohn's disease. *Cochrane Database Syst Rev* 2006:2.
5. Sharon R, Schoen RE. Cancer in inflammatory bowel disease. An evidence-based analysis and guide for physicians and patients. *Gastroenterol Clin North Am* 2002;31:237–254, 2002.
6. Collins PD, Mpofu C, Watson AJ, et al. Strategies for detecting colon cancer and/or dysplasia in patients with inflammatory bowel disease. *Cochrane Database Syst Rev* 2006:2.

11.10

GENERAL PRINCIPLES

Anorectal disease and hemorrhoids are commonly seen within primary care practice. A disciplined approach with completion of an abdominal examination, rectal palpation, and anoscopy, when tolerated, will help avoid the grave error of delaying or missing a diagnosis of colon cancer, a cause of more than 50% of all litigation against primary care for GI disease.[1] Once cancer, which can coexist with benign conditions, has been excluded, more than 90% of anorectal complaints can be managed in the primary care office.[2]

ANAL FISSURES

General Principles

Definition

A fissure is a crack or linear tear in the anal mucosa in the distal anal canal usually found in the posterior midline of the skin. The posterior anal commissure is the most poorly perfused part of the anal canal. In patients with hypertrophied internal anal sphincters, this blood supply is lessened further, thus rendering the posterior midline of the anal canal relatively ischemic.

Anatomy

They are frequently located anterior or posterior to the anus.

Pathophysiology

Fissure persistence is due to the repeated cycle of pain and reinjury of the tear from the passage of stools as well as subsequent spasm of the internal sphincter muscle.

Etiology

Unknown. Fissures are commonly attributed to the passage of a hard stool or explosive diarrhea.

Diagnosis

Clinical Presentation

Fissures generally produce pain and bleeding associated with defecation.

History

The patient will often report a recent passage of a **hard stool or explosive diarrhea** with acute onset of severe **pain on defecation** as well as red blood on the toilet paper.

Physical Examination

Lateral retraction to spread the buttocks apart allows visualization of the fissure.[3] Patients are often too uncomfortable to tolerate a digital rectal examination or anoscopy. These evaluations may be delayed until the fissure is healed or the pain has lessened; however, an examination under anesthesia should be considered if the diagnosis is in doubt or the patient does not respond to treatment.

Differential Diagnosis

Fissures **off the midline** should prompt consideration of other medical disorders such as inflammatory bowel disease, anal carcinoma, acquired immune deficiency syndrome (AIDS), tuberculosis, occult abscesses, leukemic infiltrates, herpes, or syphilis.[4] Screening laboratories may be helpful in these instances.

Treatment

The mainstay of anal fissure treatment (like that of hemorrhoids) begins with increased **fluid** and **fiber** ingestion, the use of warm **sitz baths,** and if necessary, the use of **stool softeners** such as docusate sodium. These measures result in healing of up to 50% of symptomatic fissures, more than in untreated patients and have no side effects.[5]

Medications
Acute fissure **pain** can be managed with local anesthetics (lidocaine hydrochloride 2% jelly) as well as topical nitrates; however, according to a Cochrane review, nitrates are only marginally associated with a healing rate superior to placebo.[6]

Surgery
Lateral internal sphincterotomy is the procedure of choice. A small percutaneous incision is made into the internal sphincter, cutting muscle fibers without entering the anal canal. This technique is simple and effective, but the potential for permanent incontinence exists.

Referrals
Cancer can coexist with benign conditions such as hemorrhoids and so a complete assessment is needed for patients whose bleeding source is in doubt.

Follow-Up
Anal fissure pain may prevent a thorough exam on initial diagnosis; a complete examination to exclude cancer and assess source of bleeding is required in follow-up.

ANORECTAL ABSCESSES AND FISTULAS

General Principles
Definition
Abscesses and fistulas both begin as an **infection in the anal gland** crypts and progress to a localized collection of pus. An anal fistula is an abnormal connection from an abscess to the anal canal or external skin.

Clinical Course
As an abscess enlarges, its anatomic location determines its classification and eventual treatment need (Table 11.10-1). Fistulas form in up to 50% of all untreated perianal abscesses.[7]

Anatomy
Most abscesses extend down toward the skin to become a **perianal abscess.** The lesser encountered abscesses are **ischiorectal, submucosal,** and **supralevator** (Table 11.10-1).

Pathophysiology
Usually 8 to 10 anal glands are located circumferentially within the anal canal at the level of the dentate line; blockage of anal glands permits the growth of bacteria, which may ultimately lead to the formation of an abscess.

Etiology
An acute **infection in the anal glands,** which progresses to a localized collection of pus, an abscess, and can lead to a chronic fistula-in-ano. Other causes include Crohn disease, trauma, tuberculosis, foreign bodies and fissures that bore into the anal muscle, hematologic malignancy, actinomycosis, anal surgery.

Clinical Presentation
Dependent on the size and location of the abscess (Table 11.10-1).

Diagnosis
History
Swelling, throbbing, and continuous pain are the most common symptoms.

Physical Examination
Abscesses may cause pain, erythema, and swelling or no abnormal findings, if the abscess is in the intersphincteric or ischiorectal space.[8]

Imaging
In elusive cases, intra-anal ultrasound examination under anesthesia may be needed.

Surgical Diagnostic Procedures
An examination under anesthesia may be required.

TABLE 11.10-1	**Management Recommendations for Patients with Anorectal Abscesses**	

Type/classification	Presentation/physical exam/tests	Treatment goals
Perianal abscess—most abscesses track down toward the skin	Pain and swelling at the anal verge external to the dentate line	Incision and drainage with the aide of a drainage catheter, gauze, or seton in the office under local anesthesia
Ischiorectal abscess— grows through the external sphincter and into the fat of the ischiorectal fossa	1. May also be seen or produce pain overlying the buttocks away from the anal verge 2. **No abnormality may be appreciated on examination.** Intrarectal ultrasound should be considered	**Nontoxic appearing patient:** Incision and drainage as an outpatient if the **abscess** points to the perirectal skin area **Toxic appearing patient:** Incision and drainage should be performed in **the operating theater**
Submucosal abscess— tracks cephalad between the inner circular and outer longitudinal muscle layers of the anorectal wall	The patient complains of anal pain, and **a highly painful bulge can be palpated within the rectum**	Treatment options include surgical drainage into the rectum under general or spinal anesthesia
Supralevator abscess— abscess can arise from cryptoglandular anal disease or from an abdominal suppurative condition	Can arise from: 1. **Anal disease** or 2. An **abdominal suppurative condition** (pelvic inflammatory disease, diverticulitis, ruptured appendicitis) Consider imaging and **endoscopy or barium enema,** which may reveal a bulge in the rectal mucosa	Important to identify and treat the process leading to abscess formation as well as to relieve the abscess itself by surgical drainage Pelvirectal **abscesses** are **drained in the operating room** through an intra-anal incision rather than through the ischiorectal space

Pathologic Findings
An abscess may originate in the intersphincteric space because the anal glands terminate there. The abscess then can travel up, down, or circumferentially around the anus.

Classification
Abscesses are classified according to their location (Table 11.10-1).

Differential Diagnosis
The differential diagnosis also includes a pilonidal sinus, hidradenitis suppurativa, carcinoma, Bartholin gland abscess, and lymphoma.

Treatment
Anal abscesses should be drained in a timely manner. Lack of fluctuation should not be a reason to delay treatment. Antibiotics may have a role in special circumstances including valvular heart disease, immunosuppression, extensive cellulitis, or diabetes.

Medications
Antibiotics are an unnecessary addition to routine incision and drainage of uncomplicated perianal abscesses.[7] Antibiotics are reserved for patients who are immunocompromised or who have diabetes, or who have signs of systemic infection, such as high fever.

The American Heart Association advises preoperative antibiotics before incision and drainage of infected tissue in patients with prosthetic cardiac valves, previous bacterial endocarditis, complex congenital heart disease, surgically constructed systemic pulmonary shunts or conduits, congenital cardiac malformations, acquired valvular dysfunction (e.g., rheumatic heart disease), hypertrophic cardiomyopathy, and mitral valve prolapse with valvular regurgitation and/or thickened leaflets.[9]

Surgical Management

Incision and drainage on discovery using a cruciate incision (in the shape of a plus sign) should be made as close to the anal orifice as possible. Direct compression of the tissues expresses the pus, and a gauze, seton, or mushroom catheter can be placed to drain the abscess cavity.

Referrals

Large or high abscesses require drainage in the operating room.

Complications

- **Fistula.** About 50% of abscesses that drain spontaneously or following surgery develop into a fistula.[7] Fistulas often require complicated and extensive surgical procedures and are best referred to a specialist for treatment. Physicians should not probe fistulas in the office setting. Hospitalization and intravenous antibiotics are reserved for patients who are immunocompromised or diabetic or who have signs of systemic infection, such as high fever.

- **Protocol.** Flexible sigmoidoscopic examination is indicated to evaluate the mucosa of the distal colon for signs of inflammatory bowel disease. The index of suspicion for Crohn disease is increased by a history of episodes of diarrhea, abdominal cramping, and weight loss, and the appearance, location, and multiplicity of the fistulas.

ANAL WARTS, POLYPS, AND NEOPLASMS

Anal Condylomas

General Principles

- **Definition.** Warts are caused by the human papillomavirus (HPV), the most common sexually transmitted viral infection in the United States.[10]
- **Epidemiology.** About 1% of sexually active people have anal warts.
- **Etiology.** About 30 HPV types primarily infect the squamous epithelium of the lower anogenital tracts.
- **Pathophysiology.** It is speculated that most squamous cell cancers of the anal area are caused by HPV.[11]
- **History.** Anal intercourse is a causative factor in many (up to 80%) but not all patients. Symptoms of anal warts include pruritus, bleeding, anal wetness, and pain. Frequently, the warts are asymptomatic.

Diagnosis

- **Physical examination.** They are characterized by many small raised points, in contrast to the flat *condylomata lata* of secondary syphilis.
- **Monitoring.** Infection with HPV has been associated with an increased risk of cervical and anal cancers.[12]
- **Differential diagnosis.** Secondary syphilis.

Treatment

- **Medications.** Treatments include topical podofilox, topical 5% 5-fluorouracil (5-FU), interferon injections, cryosurgical destruction, electrosurgical ablation, surgical excision, or laser ablation. Multiple treatment modalities exist, but even when bulky lesions have resolved, the virus remains.
- **Surgery.** Surgical excision and cautery yield the highest success rate. Laser seems to offer no advantage over cautery. Cure rates of 63% to 91% are reported. Disadvantages include the need for anesthesia and the presence of bioactive HPV in cautery-induced fumes.
- **Protocol.** Topical 5-FU cream and serial examinations, rather than extensive excision, have been advocated in HIV-positive patients with dysplasia.[13] Excision is reserved for patients with obvious lesions of the skin.

- **Risk management.** Clinical or latent infection with HPV may lead to the development of anal cancer.
- **Patient education.** Condoms are very (but not completely) effective in preventing transmission of HPV. Patients should be advised to use condoms with new partners.
- **Follow-up.** Anal Pap smears can be performed to examine for anal dysplasia associated with HPV. Anogenital warts infections in immunocompromised patients are more aggressive and more often dysplastic.
- **Special considerations.** In HIV-positive patients, dysplasia and histologic evidence of HPV can occur in the absence of gross warts.[13]

Management of Polyps and Neoplasms

Anal polyps are common benign growths that may represent residual from prior hemorrhoids or fistulas. Condylomas or tumors also can appear as a polyp, and so **uncertain lesions** in the anal canal **should be biopsied. Anal malignancies** are less common, but basal cell carcinoma, squamous cell carcinoma, melanoma, or prolapsed rectal carcinoma all can occur.

PRURITUS ANI

General Principles

- **Definition.** Pruritus ani is excessive and often intractable anal itching from multiple causes.
- **Pathophysiology.** Pruritus ani may be idiopathic or secondary to an underlying disorder (infection, allergies, stool leakage), and specific treatment leads to resolution of symptoms.
- **Etiology.** Although poor hygiene may lead to pruritus ani, overzealous cleansing and application of medications also can produce itching. Other causes include contact dermatitis, such infections as pinworms (*Enterobius vermicularis*) and chronic *Candida* infection; parasites, systemic diseases (diabetes mellitus), diet (coffee, cola, chocolate, milk, beer, and others), and some medications.

Diagnosis

History

Thorough history and physical examination are required. It has been said that dietary factors, especially coffee, may be the most common culprit. Men are more commonly affected in a ratio of 4:1.

Physical Examination

A rectum and sigmoid colon examination should be performed noting the pattern of irritation (symmetrical vs. asymmetrical). Any abnormal skin should be biopsied.

Surgical Diagnostic Procedures

Anoscopy and endoscopy.

Pathologic Findings

On anoscopy, a symmetrical pattern of anal irritation is usually a diet-induced pruritis, whereas asymmetrical patterns of anal irritation are caused by infectious sources. Leakage of stool or mucus due to fecal incontinence, prolapse of the rectum, or hemorrhoids can cause irritation and itching.

Differential Diagnosis

Pruritus ani is poorly understood. Underlying premalignant lesion such as Bowen disease or Paget disease may cause similar symptoms and should be excluded.

Treatment

Behavioral

A program of gentle, but effective hygiene should be promoted. Drying the anal skin can help prevent skin maceration and further itching. Wiping gently with wet facial tissue or baby wipes is recommended. Avoiding soap and a washcloth in the shower may help. The patient should be instructed to use plain water and his or her hand to wash the perineum in the tub or shower. Creams or emulsifying ointments may be used instead of soap.[14] Perfumed soaps and astringents should be avoided. A cotton ball placed by the anus and changed several times a day will absorb moisture and create a drier environment. A diet high in fiber with plenty of fluids (similar to the diet for hemorrhoids) is recommended. Potential dietary culprits such as coffee, tea, and chocolate should be eliminated during this trial period.

Medications

Some patients have been effectively treated with topical antifungals and low-potency steroids. A limited amount of 1% hydrocortisone cream can be used. Patients should be warned that chronic use of hydrocortisone will thin the anal skin and may lead to more problems. Intradermal injection of methylene blue has been used successfully for the treatment of intractable idiopathic pruritus ani that has not responded to any other measures.

Referrals

The physician should be aware that a previously overlooked underlying problem may be the cause of the pruritis. Assistance from a dermatologist also may be helpful and should be considered.

ANORECTAL INFECTIONS

General Principles

Definition

Infections causing the rectal and anal tissues to become inflamed.

Etiology

It is usually sexually transmitted with the highest risk from anal intercourse.

Diagnosis

Clinical Presentation

Infectious proctitis can produce rectal discomfort, pruritis, rectal discharge, tenesmus, and bleeding, genital or anorectal ulcers, other mucocutaneous lesions, lymphadenopathy, and skin rash.

History

Patient may report anorectal pain, severe rectal pain after a bowel movement, rectal discharge, constipation, and/or anorectal itching/burning. Proctitis occurs predominantly among persons who participate in receptive anal intercourse.

Physical Examination

Rectal: mucopurulent discharge, ulcerations, warts or vesicular lesions, inguinal lymphadenopathy, and red skin rash may be noted on exam.

Laboratory Studies

Swab and culture of anal canal, dark-field microscopy (test for syphilis), VDRL or RPR blood test for syphilis, rectal biopsy, urethral or cervical cultures can also be helpful. Viral culture or antigen detection of herpes lesions *Neisseria gonorrhoeae, Chlamydia,* and syphilis testing DNA-based assays for detecting gonococci have been studied extensively in urogenital specimens, but their role in gonococcal proctitis is less clear. Positive tests should be confirmed with a fluorescent treponemal antibody-absorbed (FTA-Abs) test.

Surgical Diagnostic Procedures

Anoscopy and endoscopy.

Treatment

If an anorectal exudate is found on examination, or if polymorphonuclear leukocytes are found on a Gram-stained smear of anorectal secretions, the following therapy may be prescribed pending results of additional laboratory tests. Ceftriaxone 125 mg IM in a single dose, or ciprofloxacin (Cipro) 500 mg single dose orally. If a **Chlamydia infection is not ruled** out, azithromycin 1 g orally in a single dose or doxycycline 100 mg orally twice a day for 7 days. If syphilis is suspected, penicillin G (injection), tetracycline, or azithromycin should be considered. Patients with suspected or documented herpes proctitis should be managed in the same manner as those with genital herpes, for example, acyclovir, valacyclovir (Valtrex), famciclovir (Famvir). If painful perianal ulcers are present or mucosal ulcers are seen on anoscopy, presumptive therapy should include a regimen for treating genital herpes.

Risk Management
Partners of patients with sexually transmitted enteric infections should be tested for the index diseases.

Follow-Up
Follow-up should be based on specific etiology and severity of clinical symptoms. Reinfection may be difficult to distinguish from treatment failure.

HEMORRHOIDS

General Principles

Definition
Hemorrhoids can be divided into those below the dentate line in the greatly enervated anoderm, the external hemorrhoids, and those above the dentate line, the internal hemorrhoids.

History
A targeted history on the nature, duration, and severity of symptoms, dietary fiber intake, and bowel habits should be gathered. A history of rectal bleeding should prompt a family medical history to evaluate the possibility of familial colorectal neoplastic syndromes and the need for a more extensive colon evaluation.[15] Complete colon evaluation with colonoscopy or barium enema with flexible sigmoidoscopy is typically indicated for patients with rectal bleeding who meet the indications for colonic evaluation (Table 11.10-2).

Thrombosed External Hemorrhoids

- **Definition.** When external hemorrhoids become thrombosed, patients may experience extreme pain and bleeding with defecation.
- **Pathophysiology.** External hemorrhoids may thrombose spontaneously, possibly secondary to straining at stool or heavy lifting. The exact etiology remains unknown.

Diagnosis
- **History.** The patient often complains of a rapid onset of a palpable and painful perianal lump.
- **Physical examination.** On visual inspection, a tender mass at the external anal opening is appreciated.

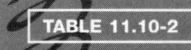

TABLE 11.10-2	Indications for Complete Colonic Evaluation

Age	Last normal endoscopy	Family history
50 years old	No complete colonic exam **within 10 years**	N/A
40 years old or older	No complete colonic exam **within 10 years**	**Single first-degree relatives** with colorectal cancer or adenoma diagnosed at age >60
40 years old or older	No complete exam within **3 to 5 years**	**Two or more first-degree relatives** with colorectal cancer or adenomas
Positive fecal occult blood Iron deficient anemia for screening people with possible genetic mutations	Use colonoscopy, instead of barium enema, for diagnostic evaluation of patients with positive findings on other screening tests	N/A

Adapted from the Multi-Society Task Force on Colorectal Cancers.[20]

Treatment

- **Surgery**
    - **Surgical management of thrombosis.** Acutely swollen and tender thrombosed external hemorrhoids may be surgically removed if the physician encounters the lesions in the first 72 hours after onset. An elliptic excision may be performed to unroof the hemorrhoid. Once the entire clot is excised, the physician can leave the wound open with gauze placed over the area to collect drainage or alternatively, the wound is closed with a buried subcuticular absorbable suture.

- **Nonoperative.** After 72 hours, the discomfort of the procedure probably outweighs the relief provided from the surgery. In this circumstance, avoidance of constipation, patient analgesia, and ice or sitz baths to the perineum may result in more rapid symptom relief than will surgical excision.[16]
- **Patient education.** Instructions on high-fiber diet, stool softeners, warm sitz baths, and anal hygiene.

Internal Hemorrhoids

General Principles

- **Definition.** The anal cushions are blood-filled sacs that reduce the effects of stool passing through the anal canal. With the chronic passage of hard stool or straining, the anal cushions can lose their fibrocollagenous support. The cushions then dilate and prolapse into the anal canal, thus becoming hemorrhoids.
- **Classification.** Table 11.10-3.

Diagnosis

- **Clinical presentation.** Internal hemorrhoids are painless and occur above the dentate line.
- **History.** The major symptoms of internal hemorrhoids are painless bleeding and protrusion. Patients may report the sensation of a lump or complain of bright red blood coloring the tissue or commode water. Hemorrhoids can prolapse and stain a patient's underwear, and increased anal moisture leading to itching.
- **Physical examination.** The diagnosis of internal hemorrhoids is made with the beveled anoscope. Internal hemorrhoids occur in three consistent positions in the anal canal. With the patient in the left lateral position, the physician usually examines the patient from the right side of the table with the patient's head to the left. The three locations for internal hemorrhoids are the right posterior position (10 o'clock position in the canal), right anterior position (2 o'clock position in the canal), and left lateral position (6 o'clock position in the canal).

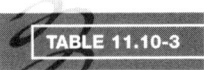 **TABLE 11.10-3** | **Classification, Presentation, and Treatment of Internal Hemorrhoids**

Grade	Presentation	Treatment
First degree	Internal hemorrhoids **do not** protrude through the anal orifice	Dietary management Fluid and fiber intake Avoid straining
Second degree	Internal hemorrhoids protrude through the anus but **spontaneously reduce**	Anal hygiene/sitz baths/moistened toilettes
Third degree	Internal hemorrhoids protrude and must be **manually replaced** into the rectum	Rubber band ligation Infrared coagulation Bipolar diathermy (electrosurgery) Hemorrhoidectomy
Fourth degree	Hemorrhoids **protrude permanently and cannot be replaced**	Hemorrhoidectomy is the surgical procedure of choice

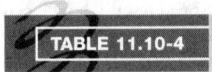

TABLE 11.10-4	Management Recommendations for Patients with Fissures or Hemorrhoids

1. Take nonprescription ibuprofen (three 200-mg tablets three times a day with food) and acetaminophen (two tablets every 6 h) if needed for discomfort. Avoid taking narcotics (such as codeine), which can produce further constipation.

2. A sitz bath (soaking in a tub of warm water) for 20 min several times a day can reduce discomfort and promote healing of the tissues.

3. Use stool softeners for at least 2 weeks to promote softer stools and to allow the tissues to heal. Start with nonprescription docusate sodium (two 100-mg capsules two times a day) and increase the dosage if you remain constipated.

4. Drink at least five to six full glasses of water or fluid daily.

5. A daily stool bulking agent will promote softer stools and improved colon health. Psyllium or methylcellulose powder (1 tablespoon) can be taken in a glass of orange juice daily to make these substances more palatable. Most patients experience bloating, gas, or cramping with the bulking agents initially, but generally this resolves after 2 weeks. You can use simultaneous stool softeners when starting the bulking agents.

6. Do not use enemas or place anything in the rectum for the next 2 weeks. Local application of ointments, creams, or pads to the anal tissues is permitted.

7. The National Institutes of Health recommends at least five servings of fresh fruits and fresh vegetables daily. A proper diet can promote soft stools and reduce the chances of recurrent anal disease.

8. Because stool in the rectum rapidly becomes dried out, do not delay going to the bathroom when you feel the rectum fill. Do not sit for long periods on the toilet or strain on the toilet. Please remove all reading materials from the bathroom.

Treatment

- **Medications.** When dietary manipulation does not work, more aggressive treatment is needed. These measures can apply to **grades 1, 2, and 3 internal hemorrhoids** (Table 11.10-4). Unless the patient has **fourth-degree internal hemorrhoids,** aggressive nonsurgical treatment is usually tried. (Most patients with **fourth-degree hemorrhoids** require surgical intervention.)

- **Surgery.** Internal hemorrhoids are most often managed medically (Table 11.10-3). Patients who fail conservative treatment can be considered for surgical intervention. Surgical excision of internal hemorrhoids often is painful and expensive. Surgical or laser excision of internal hemorrhoids has been largely replaced by other outpatient treatment modalities.

- **Nonoperative. Rubber band ligation** of internal hemorrhoids has been performed for many years. One or two small latex rings are placed at the base of the hemorrhoid, resulting in necrosis and sloughing of the hemorrhoid in the following week. The equipment for banding is inexpensive, but the procedure can produce moderate discomfort. Banding also rarely can produce pelvic sepsis, a life-threatening condition. In a meta-analysis of 18 prospective, randomized trials, rubber band ligation was found to be the most effective of the office procedures. It is associated with a lower recurrence rate, but more overall pain than sclerotherapy or infrared coagulation.[17,20]

- **Special therapy.** Infrared coagulation is an office technique for first-, second-, and third-degree internal hemorrhoids. A 0.7-cm light tip applies the infrared energy to the superior aspect of the internal hemorrhoid. A 1.25- to 1.5-second pulse of energy produces an eschar that tethers the hemorrhoid to the underlying tissues. Three to five exposures to each hemorrhoid generally reduce blood flow and shrink the lesion.

- **Other treatment modalities.** Bipolar diathermy (electrosurgery) produces a similar effect on the hemorrhoid as the infrared treatment. A low-voltage galvanic probe also is used for office treatment of hemorrhoids. These office treatments produce similar healing rates and are well tolerated. Cryotherapy and sclerotherapy generally have been abandoned for these newer, and safer, modalities.

■ **Referrals.** Surgical evaluation is recommended for recalcitrant hemorrhoids or fourth-degree hemorrhoids.

■ **Counseling.** A high-fiber diet with 25 to 30 g of daily fiber should be introduced gradually into the diet and accompanied by six to eight glasses of fluid daily. Patients are encouraged to read the package regarding the amount of fiber per serving; for instance, a bowl of bran cereal can have 5 to 7 g of dietary fiber per serving.[19] Fiber supplementation with psyllium or hydrophilic colloid may be added to achieve the optimal amount of daily fiber.

References

1. Gerstenberg and Plummer. *Gastrointestinal Endosc* 1993(39):132.
2. Pfenninger JL. Common anorectal conditions: Part II. Lesions. *Am Fam Physician* 2001;64(1). Available online at www.aafp.org/afp.
3. Lund JN, Scholefield JH. Aetiology and treatment of anal fissure. *Br J Surg* 1996; 83(10):1335–1344.
4. Koutsky LA, Galloway DA, Holmes KK. Epidemiology of genital human papillomavirus infections. *Epidemiol Rev* 1998;10:122–163.
5. Gough MJ, Lewis A. The conservative treatment of fissure-in-ano. *Br J Surg* 1983; 70:175–176.
6. Orsay C, Rakinic D, Perry B. Practical parameters for the management of anal fissures (revised). *Dis Colon Rectum* 2004;47:2003–2007.
7. Standards Practice Task Force, The American Society of Colon and Rectal Surgeons, Whiteford MH, et al. Practice parameters for the treatment of perianal abscess and fistula-in-ano (revised) Disease of the Colon Rectum 1996 Dec; 39(12):1361–1372.
8. Janicke DM, Pundt MR. Anorectal disorders. *Emerg Med Clin North Am* 1996; 14:757.
9. Dajani AS, Taubert KA, Wilson W, et al. Prevention of bacterial endocarditis. Recommendations by the American Heart Association. *Circulation* 1997;96:358–366.
10. Broker TR. Structure and genetic expression of papillomaviruses. *Obstet Gynecol Clin North Am* 1987;14:329–348.
11. Franco EL. Epidemiology of anogenital warts and cancer. *Obstet Gynecol Clin North Am* 1996;23:597.
12. Franco EL, Rohan TE, Villa LL. Epidemiologic evidence and human papillomavirus infection as a necessary cause of cervical cancer. *J Natl Cancer Inst* 1999;91:506–511.
13. Karamanoukian R, DeLaRosa J, Cosman B, et al. Conservative management of anal squamous dysplasia in patients with human immunodeficiency virus. *Dis Colon Rectum* 2000;43:A5.
14. Dasan S, Neill SM, Donaldson DR, et al. Treatment of persistent pruritus ani in a combined colorectal and dermatological clinic. *Br J Surg* 1999;86:1337.
15. Church J, Simmang C. Practice parameters for the treatment of patients with dominantly inherited colorectal cancer (familial adenomatous polyposis and hereditary nonpolyposis colorectal cancer). *Dis Colon Rectum* 2003;46:1001–1012.
16. Cataldo P. Practice parameters for the management of hemorrhoids (revised). *Dis Colon Rectum* 2005;48:189–194.
17. MacRae HM, McLeod RS. Comparison of hemorrhoidal treatment modalities: a meta-analysis. *Dis Colon Rectum* 1995;38:687–694.
18. Orkin BA, Schwartz AM, Orkin M. Hemorrhoids: what the dermatologist should know. *J Am Acad Dermatol* 1999;41:449.
19. Winawer S, et al. Colorectal cancer screening and surveillance: clinical guidelines and rationale—update based on new evidence. *Gastroenterology* 2003 Feb;124:544–560.

COLORECTAL CANCER
Eugene Orientale, Jr., Michael J. Cascio

11.11

GENERAL PRINCIPLES

Colorectal cancer (CRC), one of the most prevalent cancers in the Western world, is the second most common cause of cancer-related death in the United States. For men, CRC is the third most common cancer after prostate and lung cancer. For women, CRC is the third most common cancer after breast and lung cancer.[1]

Epidemiology

The disease has a high prevalence (4% to 5% lifetime incidence), passes through a long asymptomatic yet detectable phase, and has a high cure rate when detected at an early stage (90% survival at 5 years). In addition, CRC has a high mortality rate when advanced disease occurs (less than 10% at 5 years with metastatic disease). Thus, CRC is ideally suited to prevention and early detection programs, which are discussed at the end of this chapter.

Pathophysiology

Colonic polyps are of two general types.

- Hyperplastic polyps sometimes cannot be distinguished from other polyps solely on the basis of endoscopic appearance. They are sessile, 10 mm or less, and tend to occur in the distal colon. A smooth and uniform appearance may uniquely distinguish these lesions. On gross inspection small (less than 5 mm) hyperplastic polyps are often referred to as "diminutive" and need not be biopsied or ablated.
- Neoplastic polyps are mucosal outgrowths that may be broadly based or pedunculated. Although most polyps do not undergo neoplastic transformation, most CRCs originate from polyps through a 10- to 15-year process. Polyps undergo metaplastic transformation approximately 40% to 60% of the time. Three cell patterns are recognized.
  - Adenomatous polyps (tubular or glandular cell pattern) are histologically arranged in densely packed tubular glands and are the least malignant adenoma.
  - Villous (papillary cell pattern) polyps are arranged in fingerlike projections and are less common than tubular adenomas. A villous polyp has a higher malignant potential; if larger than 2 cm, it has a 50% chance of containing invasive cancer.
  - Mixed adenomatous–villous polyps have mixed-cell patterns and are common in large tumors. The risk for malignancy depends on the size and percentage of the villous cell pattern.

- **Colorectal cancer**
  - Histologic classification is of value for prognosis and treatment selection.
    - Adenomatous CRC is the most common neoplasm and is further differentiated by grade (poorly, moderately, and well differentiated). As with other neoplasms, poor differentiation in histologic specimens is associated with worse prognosis.
    - Mucinous CRC is an uncommon form that secretes abundant extracellular mucin and has a poor prognosis.
    - Signet ring CRC (linitis plastica) is composed of cells distorted by intracellular mucin into a signet ring shape. It is typically associated with metastasis at the time of diagnosis.
  - The Dukes classification, though somewhat less precise than the tumor–necrosis–metastasis (TNM) scheme, is commonly used because of its simplicity (Table 11.11-1). Prognosis is directly related to depth of invasion.[2]

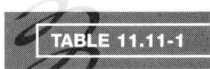

TABLE 11.11-1	Dukes Classification Scheme for Colon Cancer	
Stage	Description	5-yr survival (%)
A	Confined to the bowel wall	90
B	Through the wall and locally invasive (no lymph node involvement)	60–80
C	Metastasis to regional lymph nodes	20–50
D	Distant metastasis (peritoneum, liver)	5

From Fry R, Fleshman J, Kodner I. Cancer of the colon and rectum. *Clin Symp* 1989;41:2, with permission.

DIAGNOSIS

- **Risk factors.** These include advancing age, male sex, personal history of CRC or polyps, family history, cigarette smoking, inflammatory bowel disease, and familial genetic syndromes (familial polyposis and hereditary nonpolyposis colorectal cancer).[3] Diets that are low in fiber or high in fat or alcohol also correlate with increased risk for CRC.
- **Presentation.** There is a lack of correlation between duration of symptoms at diagnosis and survival. Early detection can be both elusive and challenging, with more than 65% of patients presenting with advanced disease.
  - Bleeding is most commonly occult, but patients also can present with melena or hematochezia.
  - Pain may be secondary to intestinal obstruction or metastasis.
  - Altered bowel movements range from diarrhea to obstipation. In elderly individuals, any change in bowel habits should prompt diagnostic consideration.
  - Constitutional complaints include fatigue, malaise, fever, and weight loss.
  - Metastatic disease may present with jaundice, pruritus, and ascites (liver); respiratory complaints (lung); or pathologic fracture (bone).
  - Weight loss, anemia, and a palpable mass comprise the triad often associated with a proximal lesion.
  - Asymptomatic presentation is not uncommon.

TREATMENT

- **Polyps.** Because polyps have malignant potential, they should be biopsied or removed at the time of colonoscopy. Larger sessile polyps sometimes require either surgical or piecemeal colonoscopic resection. Polypectomy is performed with the use of wire snare or biopsy forceps technique, both of which may be accomplished with concomitant electrocautery.
- **Cancer.** Management varies according to histology, location, and stage.
  - Colonoscopy with polypectomy may obviate the need for surgery. In some cases, even large biopsy-proven cancerous lesions can be removed in piecemeal fashion.
  - Surgery is the general treatment for cancers beyond Dukes stage A. The goal is complete removal or destruction of neoplastic tissue with maximal preservation of surrounding tissues.
  - Adjuvant chemotherapy with 5-fluorouracil plus leucovorin for stage II CRC is used but its benefit is controversial. Evidence reported by the American Society of Clinical Oncology (ASCO) shows that there is no convincing evidence that therapy with adjuvant cytotoxic chemotherapy benefits patients with stage II disease.[4]
  - Radiation can be of benefit in the management of rectal cancer and advanced CRC and in palliation for patients with unresectable disease.

■ Surveillance with cancer markers or colonoscopy has not demonstrated any improvement in survival rate. Carcinoembryonic antigen (CEA) is nonspecific and thus not useful for screening. For existing CRC, CEA may be used as a marker for disease recurrence every 3 months for the first year after resection, and then every 6 months for 2 more years. Colonoscopy is generally performed at 6- to 12-month intervals and 2 years postresection.

SPECIAL CONSIDERATIONS AND PREVENTION

■ **Diet.** A low-fat, high-fiber diet reduces the risk of CRC. Additional supplementation with folate may further reduce risk.

■ **Aspirin.** The daily use of aspirin has been shown to both decrease the incidence of CRC and the occurrence of metastasis.[5]

■ **Screening.** Screening for adenomatous polyps in an aggressive and systematic manner has proved effective in the prevention of CRC. Family physicians with full colonoscopic skills may play an integral role in the containment of this common cancer.

■ **Screening modalities:** 0

   ▪ **Digital rectal examination (DRE).** DRE is not considered a cost-effective means of detecting CRC. Less than 10% of CRCs arise within the reach of the examining finger. At age 40 years, DRE should be commenced as screening for prostate disease, not CRC. DRE should precede a flexible sigmoidoscopy or colonoscopy. Stool guaiac testing has a high false-positive rate if performed with DRE and should be withheld.

   ▪ **Fecal occult blood testing (FOBT).** Annual screening of asymptomatic individuals after age 50 is effective (sensitivity 72% to 88%, specificity 98%, and positive predictive value 10% to 17%) and decreases CRC mortality by up to 33%.[6] FOBT is usually performed on stool specimens acquired on each of three consecutive bowel movements. Any positive test should prompt a diagnostic workup. False positives can be caused by consumption of red meat, turnips, horseradish, vitamin C, and certain medications (aspirin, nonsteroidal anti-inflammatory drugs), as well as benign conditions, such as diverticulosis or hemorrhoids.

   ▪ **Flexible sigmoidoscopy.** This office procedure, performed with a 60-cm scope, is capable of screening from the rectum to the splenic flexure. It can diagnose up to two thirds of colonic lesions and has been shown to reduce CRC mortality by 60% to 80% at a fraction of the cost of colonoscopy.[6] Patient acceptability and compliance are significant issues. The procedure is embarrassing for some patients and requires an uncomfortable bowel preparation that might involve a liquid diet, laxative, electrolyte purge solution, or enema prior to the procedure. Conscious sedation is not required and complications are uncommon, with intestinal perforation occurring about once in 5000 to 10,000 examinations. The U.S. Preventive Services Task Force (USPSTF) currently recommends routine screening every 5 years beginning at age 50. The combination of annual FOBT and periodic flexible sigmoidoscopy is a cost-effective means of CRC detection in the general population.[7]

   ▪ **Air contrast barium enema (ACBE).** This radiologic procedure allows visualization of the entire colon. Patient compliance and acceptability are comparable to that of flexible sigmoidoscopy. It has limitations in evaluation of the rectum and sigmoid colon but can be useful for proximal lesions. ACBE has a sensitivity of only 48% for large, 1-cm polyps and 41% for >6-mm polyps. Specificity ranges from 99% for large cancers to 90% for large polyps.[8] There are no current recommendations to use ACBE as a routine screen for CRC. ACBE is over twice the cost of flexible sigmoidoscopy and has a similar complication profile, but can be useful in patients who refuse endoscopy.

   ▪ **Colonoscopy.** This method remains the final common pathway of all other positive screening tests. With adequate bowel preparation, it is almost 100% specific and 95% sensitive for detection of neoplasm. Biopsy or polypectomy can be performed. A bowel preparation is always necessary, and conscious sedation improves patient acceptability. Use as a primary screening tool remains controversial, and high cost has precluded widespread implementation. Many family physicians are now acquiring skills in full colonoscopy, which ultimately may be a significant factor in the early detection of CRC.

- ■ **Virtual colonoscopy.** Also called computed tomographic colonography. This method uses x-rays and computers to produce two- and three-dimensional images from the rectum to the lower end of the small intestine and then displays them on a screen. However, if a polyp or growth is found using this method, a colonoscopy would need to be done for removal or biopsy of the lesion.[9] It is not yet considered a cost-effective means of screening for CRC.
- ■ **Genetic testing of stool.** Studies are being done to find new ways to recognize DNA mutations in cells found in stool samples. New cells replace cells from the lining layer of the colon and rectum, which are constantly shed into the stool. Finding intact-appearing DNA that lacks the changes of apoptosis in stool samples may be useful in finding colorectal cancers.[10] Recommendations for screening may be brought forward after more research is done to confirm accuracy.

References

1. U.S. Department of Health and Human Services, Centers for Disease Control and Prevention. Colorectal cancer, fast facts. Available online at www.cdc.gov/colorectalcancer/basic_info/fast_facts.htm. Accessed May 18, 2006.
2. Fry R, Fleshman J, Kodner I. Cancer of the colon and rectum. *Clin Symp* 1989;41:2.
3. American Cancer Society. Detailed guide, colon and rectum cancer. What are the risk factors for colorectal cancer? Available online at www.cancer.org. Accessed May 18, 2006.
4. Benson AB III, Schrag D, Somerfeld MR, et al. American Society of Clinical Oncology recommendations on adjuvant chemotherapy for stage II colon cancer. *J Clin Oncol* 2004;22(16)3408–3419.
5. Kahn MJ, et al. Chemoprevention for colorectal carcinoma. *Hematol Oncol Clin North Am* 1997;11:4.
6. Mandel JS, Bond JH, Church TR, et al. Reducing mortality from colorectal cancer by screening for fecal occult blood. *N Engl J Med* 1993;328:1365–1371.
7. Centers for Disease Control And Prevention. Colorectal cancer screening fact sheet. Available online at www.cdc.gov/colorectalcancer/for_healthcare/screening_fact_sheet.htm. Accessed May 18, 2006.
8. Rockey D, Paulson E, et al. Analysis of air contrast barium enema, computed tomographic colonography, and colonoscopy: prospective comparison. *Lancet* 2005;365(iss 9456, 22):305–311.
9. Fenlon HM, Nunes DP, Schroy III PC, et al. A comparison of virtual and conventional colonoscopy for the detection of colorectal polyps. *N Engl J Med* 1999;341(20): 1496–1503.
10. Dong SM, Traverso G, Johnson C, et al. Detecting colorectal cancer in stool with the use of multiple genetic targets. *J Natl Cancer Inst* 2001;93(11):858–865.

Renal and Urologic Problems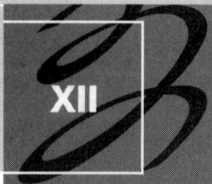

CYSTITIS AND BACTERIURIA
John E. Delzell, Jr.
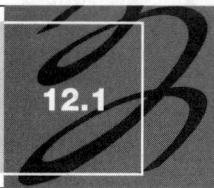

GENERAL PRINCIPLES

Definition

Lower urinary tract infections (UTIs) are common complaints in the family physician's office. Cystitis and UTIs account for 5% of all visits by women to family physicians, and at least 10% to 20% of all women will experience a UTI in their lifetimes.[1]

Significant bacteriuria is defined as the growth of greater than 10^5 colony-forming units (CFU) per milliliter obtained on routine urine culture. Cystitis is defined as urine infection without evidence of upper tract involvement.[2]

Anatomy

Cystitis is an infection of the bladder and may include infection of the distal ureters and urethra. Because of its close proximity to the vagina, cystitis will present with symptoms that are similar to vulvovaginitis.

Epidemiology

Most episodes of cystitis occur in young, sexually active women. Fortunately, people in this category are also the least likely to experience serious consequences as a result of a UTI. Pregnant women are the one exception to this as they may be at risk for sequelae such as preterm labor, pyelonephritis, or preterm delivery. Cystitis is less common in men, infants, and children and in these patients may be related to a structural abnormality.

Classification

- Asymptomatic bacteriuria
- Uncomplicated cystitis
- Pyelonephritis
- Complicated urinary tract infection (see special considerations)

Etiology

Approximately 80% of individuals with lower UTI and cystitis will have an infection from *Escherichia coli*. Other causative agents include *Proteus mirabilis, Klebsiella pneumoniae, Staphylococcus saprophyticus, Pseudomonas aeruginosa, Enterobacter aerogens,* enterococci, and Group B streptococci.[2,3]

DIAGNOSIS

Clinical Presentation

Although a definitive diagnosis of UTI requires a urine specimen with a culture, a good history can often identify patients with a likely diagnosis of cystitis. The history is also useful in distinguishing from other causes of dysuria, such as sexually transmitted disease (STD), gynecologic disorders, and mechanical or chemical irritation. History is helpful when trying to distinguish cystitis and lower UTIs from pyelonephritis and upper UTIs. Empiric antibiotics after the history can be a cost-effective method of treating cystitis.[4]

History

The history should include a complete description of the symptoms, including the onset and duration of dysuria; urinary urgency, hesitancy, and frequency; urinary incontinence; hematuria; and suprapubic pain. Systemic symptoms or their lack should be included such as fever, chills, nausea and vomiting, costoverbral angle discomfort. There should be a complete review of systems, with particular focus on gynecologic symptoms such as vaginal discharge, vaginal pain, or irregular menstrual bleeding.

The record should also include a medical history that encompasses a sexual history; a gynecologic and obstetrical history; a medication history; past infections and other relevant medical history; and a family history.

Patients should be asked to describe any personal history that includes activities that might cause mechanical or chemical irritations such as bubble baths, vaginal douching, or scented tampons or pads.

Physical Examination

Patients with cystitis often have a normal physical examination. The exam should be used to help distinguish between upper and lower UTIs. Examination should include temperature, blood pressure, and pulse. A pelvic examination should be performed if indicated by the history.

Laboratory Studies

The gold standard test is the urine culture and sensitivity. Significant bacteriuria has been defined as 10^5 CFU per mL. Lower colony counts may be used for patients with symptomatic infections.[5]

Urine dipstick for leukocyte esterase, nitrites, protein, or occult blood may be used to aid in the diagnosis of UTI. Taken together, the urine dipstick has 98% sensitivity and 19% specificity but has a 98% negative predictive value.[6] The lower sensitivity of individual portions of the dipstick makes them less useful separately.

Differential Diagnosis

- Pyleonephritis
- Chlamydia urethritis
- Gonococcal urethritis
- Candidal vulvovaginitis
- Trichomonal vaginitis
- Chemical urethritis from soaps, tampons, douches, or spermicidal
- Atrophic vaginitis

TREATMENT

Behavioral

Patients should be instructed in proper amounts of fluid intake as well as frequency of urination. Urination after sexual intercourse should also be discussed.

Medications

Many patients will respond to symptomatic treatment with phenazopyridine (100 to 200 mg PO TID). Antibiotic therapy can be divided into single-dose, short-term, long-term, and suppressive/prophylactic treatment. For most patients with uncomplicated cystitis, single-dose or short-term therapy is appropriate.

Single-Dose

- Fosfomycin, 3 g mixed in 4 oz of water
- Trimethoprim/sulfamethoxazole (160 mg/800 mg), 2 tabs PO

Short-Term (3-day)

- Cephalexin (500 mg), 1 tab PO bid
- Ciprofloxacin (100 to 250 mg), 1 tab PO bid
- Lomefloxacin (400 mg), 1 tab PO QD
- Nitrofurantoin (50 mg), 1 tab PO every 6 hours
- Nitrofurantoin SR (100 mg), 1 tab PO bid
- Norfloxacin (400 mg), 1 tab PO bid
- Ofloxacin (200 mg), 1 tab PO bid
- Trimethoprim (100 mg), 1 tab PO bid
- Trimethoprim/sulfamethoxazole (160 mg/800 mg), 1 tabs PO bid

A 3-day course of antibiotics is as effective as longer courses in patients with acute, uncomplicated cystitis.[7] Longer-term treatment (7-day) is appropriate for patients who do not respond to a 3-day regimen. Treatment length of 7, 10, or even 21 days may be appropriate for patients with complicated infection, recurrent infection, or pyelonephritis. Prophylaxis or suppression should be considered in women with three or more infections in a year. Options include: patient-initiated therapy, postcoital prophylaxis, or daily prophylactic therapy.

Special Therapy

The use of *Lactobacillus* as a vaginal suppository may decrease the risk of recurrent urinary tract infection.[8] Use of *Vaccinium macrocarpon* (cranberry juice) may help to prevent and decrease the risk of UTIs by inhibiting bacterial adherence to the bladder wall.[9] Postmenopausal women may benefit from the use of vaginal estrogen therapy.

Referrals

Patients with recurrent infections or those who do not respond to therapy should have further evaluation of their urinary tract. This may include cystoscopy, ultrasonography, intravenous pyelography, or retrograde ureterography. Referral to a urologist or urogynecologist is appropriate for these patients.

Patient Education

Medication Instructions

All patients receiving drug treatment should receive instruction in proper use of antibiotics and potential adverse effects from the medication. These effects could include drug reactions or allergies, decreased effectiveness of birth control pills while taking antibiotics, and the risk of development of yeast vaginitis while on antibiotics.

Follow-Up

Patients should return to the doctor if symptoms have not resolved or markedly improved within 48 hours of starting antibiotic treatment. Warning signs would include fever, chills, vomiting, or flank pain.

Complications

The most common complication of untreated cystitis is the development of upper urinary tract infection such as pyelonephritis. Symptoms of pyelonephritis include fever, chills, nausea or vomiting, flank pain, and elevated white blood count. Other potential complications include renal abscess, peritonitis.

SPECIAL CONSIDERATIONS

These recommendations are intended for uncomplicated cystitis and bacteriuria. Complicated urinary tract infections require a different approach.

■ Immunocompromise (e.g., HIV, chemotherapy)
■ Urinary tract obstruction, acute or chronic (e.g., nephrolithiasis)
■ Neurogenic bladder
■ Congenital anomalies
■ Chronic catheterization
■ Recent instrumentation of the urinary tract
■ Age (<10 years or >65 years)
■ Pregnancy

References

1. Berg AO, Soman MP. Lower genitourinary infections in women. *J Fam Pract* 1986; 23(1):61–67.
2. Stamm WE, Hooton TM. Management of urinary tract infections in adults [review] [60 refs]. *N Engl J Med* 1993;329(18):1328–1334.
3. Johnson JR, Stamm WE. Urinary tract infections in women: diagnosis and treatment. *Ann Intern Med* 1989;111(11):906–917.
4. Fenwick EA, Briggs AH, Hawke CI. Management of urinary tract infection in general practice: a cost-effectiveness analysis. *Br J Gen Pract* 2000;50(457):635–639.
5. Stamm WE, Counts GW, Running KR, et al. Diagnosis of coliform infection in acutely dysuric women. *N Engl J Med* 1982;307(8):463–468.
6. Wild SH, Sadler M. Negative predictive value of urine dipstick testing. *Br J Gen Pract* 2000;50(456):579.
7. Norrby SR. Short-term treatment of uncomplicated lower urinary tract infections in women. *Rev Infect Dis* 1990;12(3):458–467.
8. Reid G, Bruce AW, Taylor M. Influence of three-day antimicrobial therapy and lactobacillus vaginal suppositories on recurrence of urinary tract infections. *Clin Ther* 1992; 14(1):11–16.
9. Avorn J, Monane M, Gurwitz JH, et al. Reduction of bacteriuria and pyuria after ingestion of cranberry juice. *JAMA* 1994;271(10):751–754.

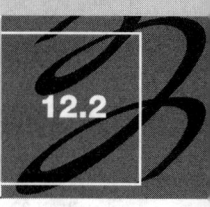
GENERAL PRINCIPLES

Definition

Hematuria means "blood in the urine." There are two types: **gross** (i.e., a visible change in urine color caused by blood) and **microscopic.** Any gross hematuria is abnormal. Microscopic hematuria is defined differently in each laboratory, but in general is accepted to be more than 3 red blood cells (RBCs) per high-powered field under the microscope.

Anatomy

Bleeding can originate at any point in the urinary tract, from the kidney, renal vasculature, ureter, bladder, prostate, or urethra.

Epidemiology

Adults

The prevalence of gross hematuria: No prevalence studies have been done. Microscopic hematuria is found in 0.19% to 21% depending on the population.

Children

Gross hematuria is found in 1.3 cases per 1,000 urgent care visits. Microscopic hematuria is present in 4% of children aged 8 to 15 in one study.

Pregnant Women

Microscopic hematuria: Up to 20% were dipstick positive once during their pregnancy in one study.

Pathophysiology

The cause of hematuria depends on the location of the bleeding. This is generally broken down into glomerular and nonglomerular bleeding. Damage to the glomerulus through inherited or acquired disease causes leaking of blood through the basement membrane. In this situation the RBCs often become dysmorphic, or mix with mucoproteins in the glomerulus to form red cell casts. In contrast, urinary RBCs from nonglomerular bleeding have a normal appearance. Lack of RBC casts or dysmorphic RBCs does not rule out a glomerular source of bleeding. Significant proteinuria (>300 mg/24 hours) may help support a glomerular source of blood loss. The causes of hematuria are listed in Table 12.2-1.

DIAGNOSIS

Clinical Presentation

Gross Hematuria

Both adults and children will likely present for evaluation soon after their first episode of gross hematuria, because it is usually perceived as frankly abnormal. Patients may note bright red blood in their urine, or on the toilet paper. Or they may note a darkening of the color of their urine to a mahogany or "cola" or "tea" colored. It is important to find out if the patient experienced pain with the hematuria. Abdominal or flank pain, dysuria, urinary frequency and urgency may be seen with urolithiasis, a common cause of gross hematuria. Lower UTIs (i.e., cystitis, urethritis) may present with gross hematuria, especially in adults. Painless gross hematuria in children is more likely to be glomerulonephritis, hypercalciuria, or IgA nephropathy. In adults, neoplasm and benign prostatic hypertrophy are the leading causes of gross hematuria (21% to 41% and 12.5%, respectively).

423

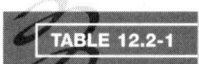

TABLE 12.2-1	Causes of Hematuria in Adults and Children

Glomerular

IgA nephropathy	Goodpasture syndrome
Idiopathic hypercalciuria (in children)	Wegener granulomatosis
Hemolytic uremic syndrome (HUS)	Alport syndrome
Henoch-Schonlein purpura (HSP)	Thin basement membrane nephropathy
Glomerulonephritis	
Lupus nephritis	
Membrano proliferative	
Mesangial proliferative	
Postinfectious (strep, viral)	

Interstitial

Polycystic kidney disease	Acute tubular necrosis
Infection: pyelonephritis, tuberculosis, schistosomiasis	Acute interstitial nephritis
	Hyperuricosuria
Hypercalciuria	
Nephrolithiasis	

Neoplastic

Renal cell carcinoma	Wilms tumor
Transitional cell carcinoma	Rhabdoid tumor
Prostate cancer	Congenital mesoblastic tumor
Angiomyolipoma	

Vascular

Renal artery/vein thrombosis	Arteriovenous malformation
Sickle cell disease/trait	Coagulopathy, congenital or acquired
Platelet disorder	Hemophilia A or B
Malignant hypertension	

Lower urinary tract

Calculi (ureteral, bladder)	Trauma
Benign prostatic hypertrophy	Prostatitis
Cystitis (bacterial, viral, drug)	Endometriosis
Urethritis	Epididymitis
Foreign body	Urethral stricture
Posterior urethral valves	

Other causes

Exercise-induced	Sexual intercourse
Menstrual contamination	

Microscopic Hematuria

Microscopic hematuria is generally discovered in one of two ways. Some patients may present with flank pain or irritative voiding symptoms, which prompt a urine dip to be performed in the office. Others may be asymptomatic and have a urine dip performed for screening reasons, such as preoperative, or at a well-child exam. Microscopic hematuria is considered abnormal when it is present in two out of three properly collected urine samples (i.e., midstream, clean catch). Causes of false positives include menstruation, recent sexual activity, and vigorous exercise, and these activities should be avoided at the time of repeated urinalysis. It should be noted that a single positive urine microscopy with casts, significant proteinuria, or in a patient with high-risk factors for transitional cell carcinoma (Table 12.2-2) should begin the evaluation for the source of hematuria without waiting for confirmatory urinalysis.

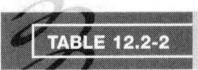

TABLE 12.2-2	Risk Factors for Transitional Cell Carcinoma of the Urinary Tract

Age >40 years

Smoking history

Occupational exposure to dyes or chemical (aromatic amines, benzenes)

Prior/current treatment with cyclophosphamide

Phenacetin abuse

History of pelvic irradiation

History

The following key points should be obtained in the history:

- **Urine color.** Yellow urine with red clots (lower tract disease) versus dark, "cola" or "tea" colored and uniform in nature (glomerular bleeding).
- **Timing.** When did the blood appear during urination? Early in void suggests urethritis, end of void suggests trigonitis.
- **Other symptoms**
  - Fever (infection, systemic disease, tumor)
  - Gastrointestinal symptoms (HUS, HSP)
  - Recent upper respiratory illness (IgA nephropathy, postinfectious nephritis)
  - Skin infection (poststreptococcal nephritis)
  - Cough (Goodpasture, Wegener)
  - Rash (vasculitis)
  - Edema or sudden weight gain (nephropathy)
  - Irritative voiding symptoms (calculi, cystitis, urethritis, bladder tumor)
  - Unexplained weight loss or night sweats (cancer, tuberculosis)

- **Medical history**
  - Prior instrumentation of the urinary tract history of umbilical cord instrumentation in infants
  - Sickle cell disease or trait
  - Prior genitourinary cancer
  - Prior history of gross hematuria
  - Nephrolithiasis
  - Sexual history
  - Menstrual history
  - Recent trauma

- **Medication history.** Medications that cause acute interstitial nephritis, such as:
  - Cyclophosphamide
  - Nonsteroidal anti-inflammatory drugs (NSAIDs)
  - Penicillins, cephalosporins
  - Anticonvulsants
  - Diuretics
  - Oral contraceptive pills

- **Social history**
  - Tobacco use
  - Occupational exposure to aromatic amines and benzenes
  - Travel to areas endemic for tuberculosis or schistosomiasis

- **Family history**
  - Hearing loss (Alports syndrome)
  - Renal failure (Alport, IgA nephropathy)
  - Kidney stones
  - Blood disorders (sickle cell disease, hemophilia, platelet disorders)
  - Cerebral aneurysms

Physical Examination

Important physical exam findings may include fever, hypertension, rash, joint tenderness or swelling, abdominal or flank tenderness or mass. In men, a genitourinary exam, including examining the urethra for lesions, and a prostate exam for nodules or signs of prostatitis is essential. For women, a pelvic exam should be performed to look at the periurethral area for lesions and to rule out a vaginal source of bleeding. In children, growth should be assessed, as failure to thrive may be a symptom of chronic renal disease.

Laboratory Studies

Urinalysis

■ Dipstick. The initial laboratory study for suspected hematuria is a urinalysis, usually done by dipstick. This test is highly sensitive, detecting as few as 1 to 2 RBCs per high-powered field. However, the specificity is low due to many false positives. The dipstick test records the reaction of hemoglobin with hydrogen peroxide and a chromagen. Therefore, hemoglobinuria, myoglobinuria, and very dilute urine that causes lysis of RBC can cause false positives. False negatives are caused by vitamin C ingestion, urinary pH < 5.1, or a urinary dipstick that has had prolonged exposure to air before using.

■ Microscopy. Unless the patient clearly has symptoms of cystitis, and the urinalysis suggests this by revealing pyuria, a positive urine dipstick test should always be confirmed by microscopy. This will confirm the actual number of RBCs, as well as evaluate the sample for evidence of dysmorphic RBC and RBC casts.

■ Proteinuria. Another important finding on urine dipstick is the presence of proteinuria. Protein at greater than 300 mg per 24 hours (roughly correlating to 3+ on dipstick) is suggestive of a renal source of the hematuria. Any proteinuria noted on dipstick should be further evaluated with a spot urine protein to creatinine ratio or a 24-hour urine collection for protein.

Urine Cytology

Urine cytology is helpful in adults to assess for transitional cell carcinoma (TCC). The sensitivity is 66% to 79%, and the specificity is 95% to 100%. The sensitivity is increased for high-grade tumors, and is limited in its ability to detect low-grade tumors or renal cell carcinoma. Table 12.2-2 outlines risk factor for TCC, and cytology should be obtained in these patients, or as part of the workup in adults with microscopic hematuria who will not undergo cystoscopy.

Other Urine Tests

Urine eosinophils can help evaluate for acute interstitial nephritis. Children with painless gross hematuria should have a 24-hour urine for calcium ordered, since hypercalciuria is found in 22% of children with this presentation. Urine culture should be sent to confirm infection if fever, irritative voiding symptoms, or suprapubic tenderness are present. If the patient has a travel history to areas that are endemic for tuberculosis or shistosomiasis, consideration of special cultures to screen for these organisms should be made.

Blood Tests

These are influenced by the patient's age, symptoms, and history. All patients with possible glomerulonephritis should have a serum creatinine and CBC drawn. Other tests for glomerulonephritis include antinuclear antibody, antistreptolysin antibody, complement levels, antiglomerular basement membrane antibody titers, and antineutrophilic cytoplasmic antibody titers. Serum IgA can be ordered if IgA nephropathy is suspected.

Imaging

The most controversial issue in evaluating hematuria is the type of imaging study to use initially. The imaging workup varies somewhat based on the patient's age, presenting symptoms, cost, and availability.

Children (Figure 12.2-1 and Figure 12.2-2)

■ Renal and bladder ultrasound is the recommended first imaging study in children. It can detect many urinary tract abnormalities, such as hydronephrosis, nephrocalcinosis, renal masses > 3 cm, and evaluate the renal parenchyma.

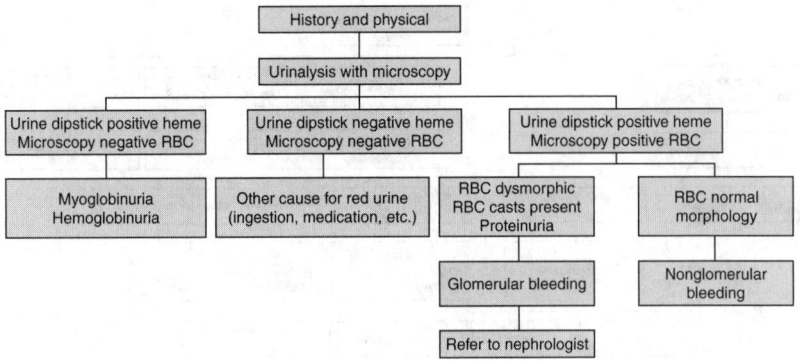

Figure 12.2-1. Hematuria in children.

- Computed tomography (CT) is useful in detecting urolithiasis, especially in the ureters, and is more sensitive for masses than ultrasound.
- Intravenous urography (IVU) used to be the initial imaging study for evaluating the urinary tract. This is now generally used more in conjunction with renal ultrasound if CT scanning is not available.

Adults (Figure 12.2-3)
- Noncontrast CT has the highest sensitivity for detecting nephrolithiasis.
- Contrast CT has better sensitivity than renal ultrasound or intravenous urography for detecting small renal masses. It also will detect vascular malformations, abscesses, and characterize a larger renal mass (i.e., simple vs. complex cyst). The drawbacks to CT scanning include high cost, limited availability, and exposure of patient to radiation.

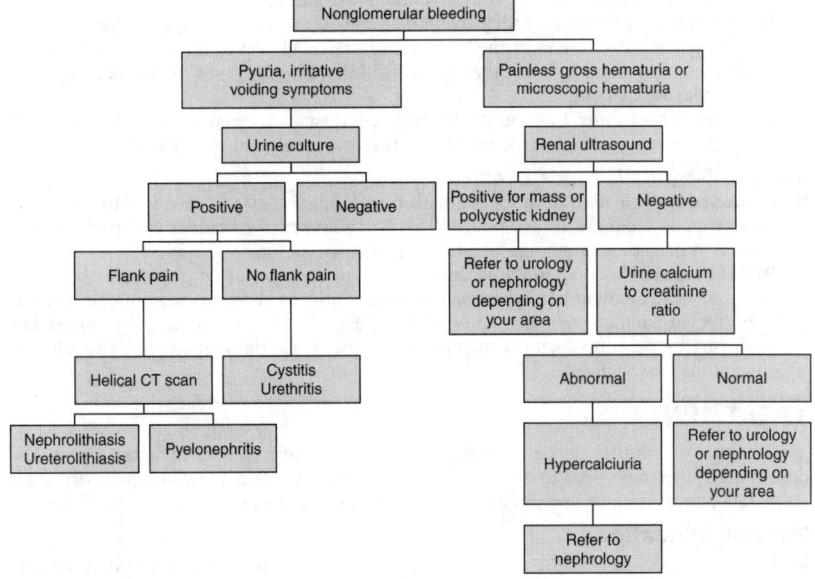

Figure 12.2-2. Nonglomerular bleeding in children.

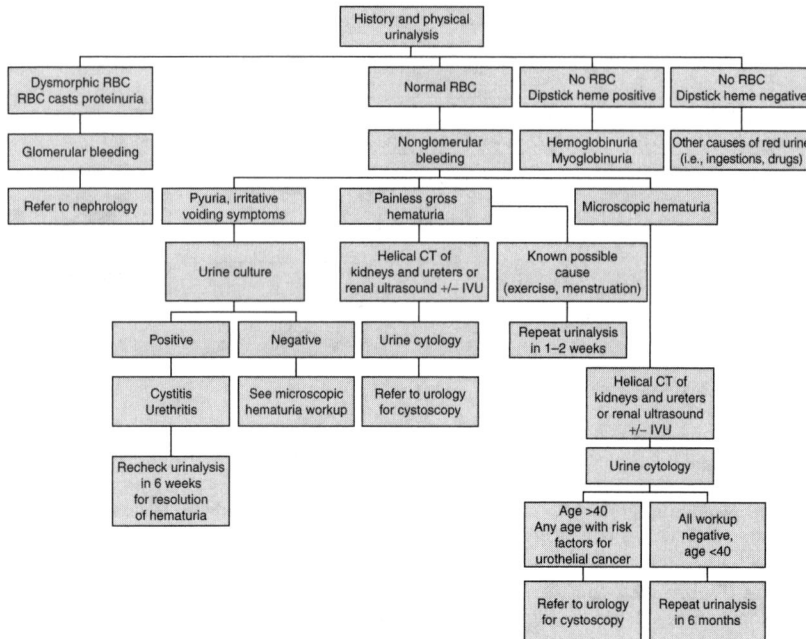

Figure 12.2-3. Hematuria in adults.

- Renal ultrasound will detect renal masses >3 cm, hydronephrosis, and nephrolithiasis/nephrocalcinosis, although the sensitivity is somewhat less than CT scan. The advantages include lower cost, and it is noninvasive in nature.
- Intravenous urography is readily available, and is superior to CT scan for detecting transitional cell carcinoma of the kidney and ureter. However, its sensitivity for renal masses less than 3 cm is lower than CT scan. Like CT, it exposes the patient to potentially nephrotoxic contrast.
- For those who cannot tolerate intravenous contrast (i.e., renal insufficiency, contrast allergy), the best evaluation for hematuria is renal ultrasound coupled with cystoscopy.

Surgical Diagnostic Procedures
- **Cystoscopy.** This used both for evaluation and diagnosis via biopsy. It is the best way to accurately diagnose transitional cell is carcinoma of the bladder and urethra. It is limited in detecting carcinoma *in situ* by its invasive nature.
- **Renal biopsy.** This may often be done as part of the workup of glomerular bleeding, especially if the patient has hypertension, proteinuria, or elevated creatinine. It is rarely indicated in isolated microscopic hematuria, even if the differential diagnosis is IgA nephropathy or thin basement membrane disease, since the biopsy results would not change the management.

TREATMENT
Treatment of hematuria depends on the cause. Isolated microscopic hematuria generally does not require treatment. In evaluations that uncover abnormalities in laboratory studies or imaging studies, or in a patient with symptoms, treatment is based on the diagnosis.

Patient Education
- Patients with gross hematuria should be reassured that it is uncommon to become anemic from urinary tract bleeding. Very little blood will make urine red, about one fifth of a teaspoon in 2 pints of urine.

■ Patients with isolated microscopic hematuria should be educated to include this as part of their medical history, as some people may have undiagnosed disease such as early transitional cell carcinoma, IgA nephropathy, or thin basement membrane disease, which could progress to renal dysfunction.

Follow-Up

Follow-up should be specific to the diagnosis. The follow-up for patients with isolated microscopic hematuria is somewhat controversial. One accepted approach would be to re-evaluate the patient every 6 to 12 months, looking for the development of hypertension, proteinuria, and a decline in renal function. In addition, adults with risk factors for urothelial cancer should also consider having urine cytology performed every 6 months, with a cystoscopy every year.

References

1. Pan CG. Evaluation of gross hematuria. *Pediatr Clin North Am* 2006;53(3).
2. Grossfeld GD, et al. Evaluation of symptomatic microscopic hematuria in adults: the American Urological Association best practice policy. Part I. *Urology* 2001;57(4):599–603.
3. Grossfeld GD, et al. Evaluation of symptomatic microscopic hematuria in adults: the American Urological Association best practice policy. Part II. *Urology* 2001;57(4):604–10.
4. Yadin O. Hematuria in children. *Pediatr Ann* 2004;23(9):474–478.
5. Mcdonald MM, et al. Assessment of microscopic hematuria in adults. *Am Fam Physician* 2006;73(10):1748–1754.
6. Sugimura K, et al. Microscopic hematuria as a screening marker for urinary tract malignancies. *Int J Urol* 2001;8(1):1–5.
7. Thompson IM. The evaluation of microscopic hematuria: a population-based study. *J Urol* 1987;138(5):1189–1190.
8. Vehaskari VM, et al. Microscopic hematuria in school children: epidemiology and clinicopathologic evaluation. *J Pediatr* 1979;95(5):676–684.
9. Brown MA, et al. Microscopic hematuria in pregnancy: relevance to pregnancy outcome. *Am J Kidney Dis* 2005;45(4):667–673.
10. Carter WC III, Rous SN. Gross hematuria in 110 adult urologic hospital patients. *Urology* 1981;18(4):342–344.
11. Cohen RA, Brown RS. Microscopic hematuria. *N Engl J Med* 2003;348(23):2330–2338.
12. Lee LW, Davis E Jr. Gross urinary hemorrhage: a symptom not a disease. *JAMA* 1953;153(9):782–784.
13. Greene LF, et al. Study of five hundred patients with asymptomatic microhematuria. *JAMA* 1956;161(7):610–613.
14. Fatica R, Fowler A. Office evaluation of hematuria. Cleveland Clinic Disease Management Project; 2003. Available online at www.clevelanclinicmeded.com/diseasemanagement/nephrology/hematuria/hematuria1.htm.
15. Pena D. Hematuria. eMedicine. Available online at .www.emedicine.com/ped/topic951.htm.

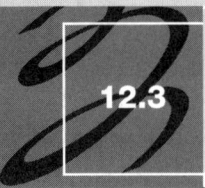

12.3 PYELONEPHRITIS
Kathryn W. Hare

$\mathcal{P}$yelonephritis is characterized by bacterial invasion of the renal parenchyma. Presenting signs and symptoms may include the classic signs of cystitis, as well as flank pain, costovertebral angle tenderness, fever, general malaise, nausea, vomiting or prostration. Pyelonephritis can have many complications if untreated, including bacteremia and sepsis (more often when there is underlying pathology or debilitation), which necessitates early diagnosis and presumptive therapy.

GENERAL PRINCIPLES

Definition

Pyelonephritis is defined as a **bacterial infection of the upper urinary tract** and, more specifically, the renal parenchyma and renal pelvis. This topic is often discussed in conjunction with other urinary tract infections (UTIs, i.e., cystitis, urethritis, and prostatitis) because they share similar pathophysiology and bacterial etiologies.

Epidemiology

Although pyelonephritis is less common than other UTIs such as cystitis, **acute cases occur roughly 250,000 times a year** and are estimated to be responsible for roughly 100,000 hospitalizations each year. The incidence of pyelonephritis increases during pregnancy and is 1% to 2% of all pregnancies.

Classification

Pyelonephritis can be differentiated into two categories: **uncomplicated and complicated.** An **uncomplicated** case of pyelonephritis would be where the infection is caused by **a known pathogen in an immunocompetent adult with a normal urinary tract and renal function.** A **complicated** case of pyelonephritis would include one of the following: **an unusual pathogen, an immunocompromised host, an elderly or very young patient, an abnormality in the urinary tract or in renal function.**

Pathophysiology

Pyelonephritis is thought to be caused by the **ascension of bacteria up through the urethra and bladder, finally reaching the kidney.** Infection may reach the kidneys hematogenously, but this usually occurs in debilitated, chronically ill, and immunocompromised patients. In men, hypertrophy or infection of the prostate can predispose to UTIs. Metastatic staphylococcal or fungal infection may spread from distant foci in the bone or skin.

Etiology

There are many different pathogens that can cause pyelonephritis. *Escherichia coli* is the most common pathogen, causing more than 80% of infections. Because older patients are more likely to have catheter use or instrumentation, *E. coli* causes less than 60% of acute pyelonephritis cases in this population. These patients are more likely to end up with Gram-negative infections with bacteria such as *Klebsiella, Serratia, Pseudomonas,* and *Proteus.* Other common bacterial agents include *Enterobacter, Staphylococcus saphrocyticus,* and *Enterococcus.*

DIAGNOSIS

Clinical Presentation

Some combination of the following signs and symptoms is usually present, but in elderly or compromised patients, any or all may be absent: **fever, flank pain, costovertebral angle tenderness, general malaise, nausea, vomiting, prostration, urinary frequency and/or urgency, dysuria, suprapubic pain, bacteriuria, pyuria, and hematuria.**

History

Adults typically present with **fever, low back pain, costovertebral angle pain, and general malaise.** They may also often present with **nausea, vomiting, or diarrhea.** A significant proportion of adults present only with lower tract symptoms: **frequency, dysuria, urgency, and suprapubic discomfort.** In infants, small children, and elderly people, the presentation may be vague, with irritability, lethargy, altered mentation, anorexia, and, eventually, dehydration. **Onset may be insidious, or acute**—as, for example, following traumatic removal of an indwelling catheter over a chronically infected prostate—and may be associated with sepsis. Again, keep in mind that in elderly or immunocompromised patients, fever may be the only presenting symptom and there may be no localizing symptoms at all.

Physical Examination

There are several key things to look for on physical exam. During the checking of vitals, look for **fever and tachycardia.** During the abdominal exam, palpate the mid and lower abdomen, and percuss the flank of the patient to assess tenderness. Look for **tenderness on deep pressure in one or both costovertebral angles, which is suggestive of upper tract disease.** Suprapubic tenderness on exam tenders to suggest lower tract infection. With male patients you want to differentiate an upper tract infection from urethritis or prostatitis. The penis should be gently milked to look for urethral discharge, and a rectal exam should be performed to look for a boggy prostate. If a woman is also complaining of vaginal discharge, a vaginal exam would be appropriate.

Laboratory Studies

- **Urinalysis.** You should **perform a dipstick urine on every patient in whom you suspect pyelonephritis.** Unless there is obstruction, urinalysis should show **pyuria** (positive leukocyte esterase and/or nitrites), usually **bacteriuria**—opinions vary on how many colony-forming units (CFU) per mL constitute a positive test—and often **hematuria, white cell casts, and proteinuria.** If a patient has lower counts of bacteria on microscopy, they may still have pyelonephritis, especially if they are pregnant or if they are male.
- **Urine cultures** are **positive in 90% of patients with acute pyelonephritis** and culture specimens should be obtained before initiating treatment so that the culture can be used to guide or evaluate treatment. Cultures typically grow more than 10^{-5} organisms per milliliter, but, particularly with fastidious or nosocomial organisms, 10^{-3} organisms per milliliter may be consistent with renal infection. *E. coli*, other Enterobacteriaceae, *Staphylococcus saprophyticus*, and *Enterococcus* still account for more than 90% of cases. *Klebsiella, Enterobacter,* and *Proteus* are becoming more common. Sexually transmitted disease (STD) pathogens are common in at-risk populations. *Serratia, Pseudomonas,* and *Staphylococcus epidermidis*, as well as other unusual organisms, are primarily nosocomial.
- **Blood cultures** are not necessary unless you are uncertain of the diagnosis, the patient is immunosuppressed, or a hematogenous source is suspected.
- **Complete blood count** (CBC) usually shows leukocytosis with left shift but is not necessarily required in the initial workup.
- **Other laboratory findings.** Elevated blood urea nitrogen (BUN), creatinine, erythrocyte sedimentation rate (ESR), C-reactive protein (CRP), and electrolyte disturbances may be found in more severe disease.

Imaging

Ultrasonography (US) is indicated if **obstruction, stones, or hydronephrosis is suspected.** If US is nonspecific, consider computed tomography (CT). Intravenous pyelogram (IVP) is relatively contraindicated.

Monitoring

With outpatient treatment, you should monitor patients within 72 hours after beginning therapy to see if they have defervesced or experienced an improvement in their symptoms. If there has been no improvement in symptoms, you should reassess the patient and consider admitting him or her the hospital. If the fever is still present after 96 hours, another urinalysis and urine culture would be appropriate to assess bacterial sensitivity and to guide a change in therapy.

Classification

When working up a patient with pyelonephritis, it is important to assess the severity of the infection, as this will determine whether the patient needs inpatient or outpatient management. An uncomplicated case would be where the patient is stable in the sense of being only moderately ill and still able to take fluids and medication by mouth. In this case, the patient may be treated with oral antibiotics on an outpatient basis, or given a loading dose of parenteral antibiotics initially, and sent home to finish the course with oral treatment.

When deciding whether to admit a patient or not, there are several indications for inpatient treatment. Absolute indications include persistent vomiting, progression of uncomplicated UTI, suspected sepsis, uncertain diagnosis, and urinary tract obstruction. Relative contraindications include a patient over age 60, poor social support, anatomic urinary tract abnormality, immunocompromised (diabetes, sickle cell disease, malignancy, transplant patient).

Differential Diagnosis

Some of the conditions that may have a similar clinical picture include **kidney stones, urinary tract obstruction, renal infarction, renal vein thrombosis, hemorrhage into a renal tumor or cyst, abdominal pathology (cholecystitis, empyema, peptic ulcer, pancreatitis, appendicitis), pelvic inflammatory disease, basal pneumonia, herpes zoster, and referred pain from a lesion of the vertebrae.**

TREATMENT

Behavioral

Patients should be advised to increase their fluid intake to at least 1500 mL per day.

Medications

- **Outpatient treatment. 7 to 14 days of an oral fluoroquinolone** is the recommended treatment for outpatient therapy given that these drugs have **good absorption in the gastrointestinal (GI) tract and good kidney penetration.** Studies have shown that oral fluoroquinolone use is nearly as effective as the intravenous (IV) preparation of fluoroquinolones. Other drugs that may be used as alternatives for susceptible bacteria are **oral amoxicillin-clavulanate potassium (Augmentin), a cephalosporin, or trimethoprim-sulfamethoxazole (TMP-SMX).** It should be noted that TMP-SMX is a fraction of the cost of the newer drugs.
- **Inpatient treatment.** Three recommended treatments for initial inpatient treatment are (all parenteral): **(a) a fluoroquinolone, (b) an aminoglycoside with or without ampicillin, or (c) an extended-spectrum cephalosporin with or without an aminoglycoside.** If a urine culture shows Gram-positive cocci, ampicillin-sulbactam, with or without an aminoglycoside, is recommended. Once the patient is afebrile, clinically stable, and is tolerating medications and fluids by mouth, you may discharge the patient to home and finish with oral antibiotics. Patients who are immunosuppressed may require 21 days of antibiotic therapy.
- **Adjunctive therapy. Hydration and pain relief are also key components of therapy for pyelonephritis.** For pain relief, use oral or parenteral narcotics for the first 48 hours. For severe dysuria, give phenazophyridine (Pyridium), 200 mg tid PO. If severe pain

persists after 48 hours, or fever after 96 hours, consider imaging. If nausea and vomiting are present, give PO or per rectum (PR) antiemetics. If fever is present, give acetaminophen PO or PR. Nonsteroidal anti-inflammatory drugs are best avoided as these drugs may impair renal function.

■ If someone is advanced to the stage of **sepsis,** you want to **aggressively rehydrate, administer parenteral antibiotics, and initiate anticipatory management of potential cardiorespiratory collapse** (shock).
■ **Cost considerations.** It should be noted that TMP-SMX is a fraction of the cost of the newer drugs. Oral therapy with any drug is invariably cheaper than parenteral therapy.

Surgery
Obstructed pyelonephritis is a closed space infection (abscess) and requires **immediate urologic drainage.**

Patient Education
Instruct patients in appropriate prophylactic measures. **Fluid intake should be at least 1,500 mL per day** to enhance recovery, avoid obstruction from urinary sediment, and reduce reinfection in patients with urinary tract abnormalities or catheters. Anticipate a preventive or suppressive program in the case of recurrence. For women, anticipate symptoms of candidal infections.

Follow-Up
All patients should receive another urine culture following treatment with antibiotics to assess the success of treatment. Generally this is done 1 to 2 weeks after finishing antibiotic therapy. If symptoms never abate, or if they return during treatment, another urine culture should be repeated promptly.

Complications
■ **Treatment failure.** Initial failure of a patient to defervesce in 96 hours should be evaluated for complicating factors.
  ■ Diagnosis can usually be established by **renal US and CT scan.**
  ■ If obstruction or perinephric abscess is present, **surgical drainage and combination parenteral therapy** with β-lactam antibiotic and aminoglycoside are indicated.
■ **Failure of bacteriologic cure.** In the case of failure of bacteriologic cure or early relapse within 1 month, take the following actions:
  ■ Diagnosis can be made via urinalysis, culture and sensitivity testing, and renal panel.
  ■ Treat with a **14- to 30-day treatment course with a culture-determined antibiotic.**
■ **Multiple recurring infections:**
  ■ Diagnosis can be made via **US for anatomical abnormalities, by renal scan for differential function, or by IVP.**
  ■ Treat with 3- to 6-month suppression therapy with nitrofurantoin, 50 mg per day (more than 50 years of use has resulted in minimal resistance), or TMP-SMX, half a tablet per day, or norfloxacin (Noroxin), 400 mg per day. Suppression therapy often allows for restoration of normal defense mechanisms.

SPECIAL CONSIDERATIONS
■ **Children with recurring infections**
  ■ Evaluate for reflux or structural abnormalities with **US and renal scanning or voiding cystourethrography.**
  ■ Suppression therapy is appropriate if a minor degree of reflux or anatomical anomaly is present. Surgery may be indicated but is usually unnecessary. The goal of treatment is prevention of symptoms, scarring, and stone formation.
■ **Pregnancy**
  ■ Pyelonephritis in pregnancy can cause many severe complications, including **transient renal insufficiency (occurs in more than 25% of women), preeclampsia, gestational hypertension, preterm labor and delivery, respiratory insufficiency, septic shock, disseminated intravascular coagulation.**

- Pregnant women should be screened for **asymptomatic bacteriuria** during weeks 12 to 16 and, if positive, **treated with 3 to 5 days with an oral cephalosporin, nitrofurantoin, or TMP-SMX** to avoid pyelonephritis later in pregnancy. TMP-SMX should be avoided at term because of the possibility that sulfonamides increase risk of neonatal kernicterus.
- Hospitalize if the patient is not clearly stable. **Quinolones are not approved.** If infection is recurrent, suppress with nitrofurantoin 100 mg per day.

- **Geriatric patients**
  - Evaluate for **stones, prostatic obstruction, or incomplete bladder emptying with urinalysis, catheterization for residual, and imaging as indicated.**
  - Review hygiene.
  - Consider estrogen deficiency if the patient is postmenopausal.
  - Consider chronic bacteriuria.
  - **Expect multiple and resistant organisms.**
  - Consider *Candida* infection in debilitated patients.
  - Consider other predisposing factors, such as malnutrition, incontinence, immobility, and drugs.
  - **The treatment should be specific to the problem.** Address underlying factors, and consider suppression for chronic bacteriuria if the patient has had an episode of pyelonephritis with uremia or sepsis.

- **Nosocomial infections.** Therapy should cover *Pseudomonas aeruginosa, S. epidermidis, S. aureus,* and *Serratia marcescens.*
- **Sexually active patients.** For treatment, consider *Trichomonas vaginalis, Neisseria gonorrhoeae, Chlamydia trachomatis,* and *Ureaplasma.*
- **In-dwelling catheters.** Treatment consists of removal of the catheter or suppression. Rotate suppression antibiotics every 6 months and expect resistant organisms. **Sterile insertion of catheters is key,** as are **avoiding long-term catheterization if possible,** using intermittent catheterization, closed drainage systems, and silver-alloy-coated catheters. Suppression prevents sepsis but not bacteriuria.
- **Urosepsis**
  - **Consider predisposing factors.**
  - Consider suppression if predisposing factors are not resolvable.
- **Prostatitis** (see Chapter 12.4)
  - Diagnosis is based on **physical examination findings or demonstration of high concentration of bacteria in prostatic secretions or post-massage urine sample.**
  - Treatment. Administer TMP-SMX or a quinolone for 1 to 3 months. If bacteria are not identified, treat with doxycycline, 100 mg bid, for 14 to 30 days.
- **Epididymitis. Evaluate for STD.** Treatment requires a 30-day course of medication.
- **Stones.** To diagnose, follow closely for persistence of urea-splitting organisms, such as *Proteus mirabilis.*
- **Women with frequent recurrences.** Treat with a single dose of nitrofurantoin, 50 mg, or a half-tablet of TMP-SMX, or 100 mg of TMP on mornings after sexual intercourse.
- **Renal failure.** Use ceftriaxone, a quinolone, or aztreonam.

References
1. McCarthy E. Inpatient utilization of short-stay hospitals, by diagnosis: United States— 1980. Hyattsville, MD: National Center for Health Statistics; 1989.
2. Pinson AG, Philbrick JT, Lindbeck GH, et al. ED management of acute pyelonephritis in women: a cohort study. *Am J Emerg Med* 1994;12:271–278.
3. Zhanel GG, Harding GKM, Guay DRP. Asymptomatic bacteriuria: which patients should be treated? *Arch Intern Med* 1990;150:1389–1396.
4. Ramakrishnan K, Scheid DC. Diagnosis and management of acute pyelonephritis in adults. *Am Fam Physician* 2005;71(5):933–942.
5. Nickel JC. The management of acute pyelonephritis in adults. *Can J Urol* 2001;8 (Suppl 1):29–38.

6. Mombelli G, et al. Oral vs intravenous ciprofloxacin in the initial empirical management of severe pyelonephritis. *Arch Intern Med* 1999;11:159:53–58.
7. Wing DA. Pyelonephritis. *Clin Obstet Gynecol* 1998;41(3):515–526.
8. Sloane P, et al. *Essentials of family medicine.* Philadelphia: Lippincott Williams & Wilkins; 1998.

EPIDIDYMITIS AND PROSTATITIS
Douglas S. Parks

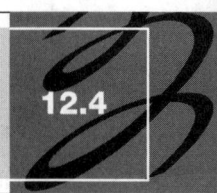

12.4

*E*pididymitis and prostatitis are infections of the male urinary tract usually caused by extension of infection from the urethra or the bladder. Infections are typically caused by usual urinary tract and sexually transmitted disease (STD) pathogens. The most likely pathogen and empiric therapy are predicted based on the patient's age.

EPIDIDYMITIS

Bacterial infection of the epididymis usually caused by an ascending urethritis.

General Principles
Epidemiology
In men >35 years old, most commonly urinary tract pathogens such as enteric organisms like *Escherichia coli* cause epididyitis. In men <35 years old, sexually transmitted pathogens, such as *Neisseria gonorrhoeae* and *Chlamydia trachomatis* are more common. History of urethral instrumentation or unprotected insertive anal intercourse makes enteric bacteria more likely. History of STD in a sex partner makes STD pathogens more likely.

Diagnosis
Clinical Presentation
The patient usually complains of rapid onset of unilateral scrotal pain, often radiating up the spermatic cord to the groin and possibly the flank. Pain is followed within 3 to 4 hours by unilateral swelling, redness, and induration of the scrotum. Testis then swells to twice normal size. Patient often has fever up to 40°C (104°F).

History
Frequently, patients have a history of recent urethritis.

- **Physical examination** reveals an exquisitely tender, swollen epididymis, which early on is adjacent to a normal testis. Within a few hours, the testis also swells, until it is not possible to differentiate between epididymis and testis by palpation. Reactive hydrocele may develop. Elevating the scrotum above the symphysis (Prehn sign) may reduce pain.
- **Laboratory studies** should include clean-catch urine for culture if enteric organisms suspected or urethral swab for Gram stain and testing for GC and *Chlamydia* if STD suspected.
- **Differential diagnosis.** Testicular torsion. If testicular torsion is missed, testis may be lost within 6 hours. Torsion is uncommon in men >25 years old. It has an abrupt onset and is frequently accompanied by nausea and vomiting. There may be a history of similar episodes with spontaneous resolution. On examination early, only testis is tender. Swelling and edema develop quickly, making it impossible to differentiate testis from epididymis. Prehn sign reveals increased pain in torsion. If any question of torsion,

prompt surgical consultation is indicated to prevent loss of testis. Ultrasonography may be useful to determine whether swelling is in testis or epididymis. Technetium scans show increased uptake in epididymitis and decreased in torsion.

Treatment

- **Medications.** Empiric antibiotics should be started promptly after obtaining appropriate lab studies. In patients at risk for enteric bacteria, antibiotics appropriate for cystitis (such as trimethoprim–sulfamethoxazole, a cephalosporin, or a quinolone) should be administered until culture results are available. In those at risk for STDs, an appropriate antibiotic (such as ceftriaxone, 250 mg IM, followed by doxycycline, 100 mg bid for 10 days, or ofloxacin, 300 mg bid for 10 days) should be started.
- **Supportive care.** Includes bed rest, scrotal elevation, and pain control. Ice may help within first 48 hours. For severe pain, consider infiltration of spermatic cord with local anesthetic, such as 1% bupivacaine or 1% lidocaine.
- **Follow-up.** Improvement should be noted in 3 days. Lack of improvement should be cause for re-evaluation of therapy. Any recent sexual partners (contact within 30 days) of men with STD epididymitis should be evaluated and treated.
- **Patient education.** Avoid STDs, urethral instrumentation, and unprotected insertive anal intercourse.

PROSTATITIS

An inflammation of the prostate gland.

General Principles
Definitions

- **Acute bacterial prostatitis** is an acute, usually Gram-negative, bacterial infection of the prostate, often accompanying an acute bacterial cystitis.
- **Chronic bacterial prostatitis** is an indolent infection of the gland, which may be a cause of recurrent cystitis.
- **Nonbacterial prostatitis** is chronic inflammation of the gland, with no identifiable cause.
- **Prostatodynia** is a clinical diagnosis with irritative voiding symptoms and pelvic pain, no evidence of inflammation in prostatic secretions.

Classification

- NIH classification system:
  - **Category I:** Acute bacterial prostatitis
  - **Category II:** Chronic bacterial prostatitis
  - **Category III:** Chronic pelvic pain syndrome that includes **IIIA:** Inflammatory (same as nonbacterial prostatitis in traditional scheme) and **IIIB:** Noninflammatory (same as prostatodynia)
  - **Category IV:** Asymptomatic inflammatory prostatitis, which refers to asymptomatic prostatitis found incidentally on biopsy

Diagnosis

- **Clinical presentation.** Patients with **Category I** present with short history of perineal pain, dysuria, urinary frequency, hesitancy, urgency, and nocturia. Pain frequently radiates to sacrum and down penis and sometimes to rectum. Urinary retention may occur. Hematuria or a purulent urethral discharge may be present. Fever is usually present, sometimes with chills and muscle aches. In severe cases, patient may be septic. In **Category II,** symptoms are minor and except for intermittent exacerbations, may be absent. Is difficult to diagnose on clinical grounds alone; high index of suspicion should be maintained. The only symptom of **Category II** may be recurring cystitis. **Category IIIA** presents in the same way as Category II, and **Category IIIB** presents mostly with pain and irritative symptoms, such as weak stream and frequent voiding.
- **Physical examination. Category I** reveals a tender boggy prostate. Should not massage prostate because of risk of bacteremia and sepsis. In **Category II** prostate is usually soft and boggy. In **Category III** prostate may be tender.

■ **Laboratory studies** include clean-catch urine for culture. May need urethral cultures if evidence of urethritis. Blood cultures if high fever or evidence of sepsis. In **Category II,** urinalysis may be negative. Urine culture may be negative, but expressed prostatic secretions or ejaculate may show >15 leukocytes per high-power field, and cultures usually positive. **Differential cultures:** first, 10 mL of urine in a void (VB_1), 10 mL from midstream (VB_2), expressed prostatic secretions (EPS) obtained by prostate massage, and 10 mL of urine following massage (VB_3) are obtained and examined microscopically and cultured. If VB_1 shows highest numbers of white blood cells (WBCs) and colonies on culture, urethritis is diagnosed. If VB_2 is highest, cystitis is more likely. If EPS or VB_3 (or both) is highest, Category II is confirmed. Category IIB shows WBCs, but culture results are negative. Category IIIB shows neither WBCs nor positive culture results.

■ **Differential diagnosis** includes cystitis and urethritis as well as differentiating the categories of prostatitis. Differential cultures may be necessary. An alternate screen in patients with no evidence of urethritis is pre- and postmassage test. Urine specimens obtained before and after prostatic massage and then compared for presence and amount of bacteria and leukocytes. This is the same as comparing VB_2 and VB_3 and is nearly as accurate.

Treatment

Treatment is guided by the results of cultures.

■ **Medications.** Most infections are due to common urinary pathogens, and treatment is selected on that basis. Severe **Category I** is treated with parenteral antibiotics followed by 3 to 4 weeks of oral antibiotics. Less severe infections are treated with oral antibiotics only. In acute phase, nearly all antibiotics penetrate inflamed prostate. Penetration of the gland is a problem in **Category II.** Treatment should continue for a minimum of 4 weeks, and often 6 weeks. Antibiotic choices include trimethoprim–sulfamethoxazole (double-strength bid), norfloxacin (400 mg bid), ciprofloxacin (500 mg bid), or ofloxacin (200–400 mg bid). Following treatment, cultures should be repeated. **Category III** (most common form of prostatitis) is hard to treat. A few patients respond to an empiric trial of an antibiotic for atypical bacteria (e.g., *Ureaplasma* and *Chlamydia*), such as doxycycline, erythromycin, or a quinolone. **Category III** with irritative symptoms may respond to an α-adrenergic blocking agent, such as prazosin (1 to 2 mg/day or bid), terazosin (5 to 10 mg/day), or finasteride (5 mg/day).

■ **Nonoperative.** Supportive treatment includes rest, analgesics (nonsteroidal anti-inflammatory drugs often helpful), hydration, and stool softeners. Warm sitz baths may provide relief. For urinary retention, consider suprapubic bladder drainage. Foley catheter causes increased risk of sepsis. **Category III** may improve with avoidance of caffeine, alcohol, and spices.

Reference

1. Hua VN, Schaeffer AJ. Acute and chronic prostatitis. *Med Clin North Am* 2004; 88(2):483–494.

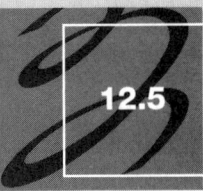

BENIGN PROSTATIC HYPERPLASIA
Kalyanakrishnan Ramakrishnan

GENERAL PRINCIPLES
General Knowledge
Benign prostatic hyperplasia (BPH) is a nonmalignant enlargement of the prostate gland associated with aging and clinically distinguished by progressive development of lower urinary tract symptoms (LUTS).[1] Hyperplasia begins in the median lobe of the prostate, and extends to involve the lateral lobes. The prevalence of *histologically diagnosed* BPH increases from 8% in men aged 31 to 40, to more than 80% in men older than age 80.[2] Its prevalence, *based on clinical criteria,* varies from 4.3% to 19% in the community.

Pathogenesis and Pathophysiology
- Age-related increased estrogen/androgen ratio in the serum and prostatic tissue. Prostatic tissue may revert to an embryonic state that survives longer, and is unusually sensitive to various growth factors.
- Hereditary and genetic susceptibility is contributory.
- BPH increases bladder outflow resistance, compresses the prostatic urethra, thins the urinary stream, and increases residual urine. Chronically increased intravesical pressure causes bladder wall hypertrophy, trabeculation, sacculation, formation of diverticula, stone formation, and infection (cystitis, pyelonephritis). Secondary hydroureter, hydronephrosis, renal calculi, and chronic renal insufficiency develop in untreated BPH. Risk of BPH is increased by saturated fat intake, heart disease, and the use of beta blockers. Severe BPH needing surgery is more common in African-Americans.[2,3]

DIAGNOSIS (EVALUATION)
History
The patient may have symptoms including urinary frequency, nocturia, hesitancy, urgency, and weak urinary stream that appear slowly and progress gradually over a period of years. Hematuria may occur from "vesical piles." There is poor correlation between symptom severity and size of prostate.[4] The American Urological Association (AUA)/International prostate symptom score (IPSS) is useful in measuring treatment outcomes (Figure 12.5-1).[5]

Physical Examination
Examination should include an abdominal, genital, and digital rectal examination (DRE), and a focused neurologic examination (to exclude neurogenic bladder). Check for renal angle tenderness, hypogastric tenderness or a mass (distended bladder), hernia, epididymo-orchitis, urethritis, prostate size, tenderness and consistency and presence of nodules, induration, and asymmetry.[5] The DRE has a low positive predictive value (17.8%; range 5.0% to 33.1%), average sensitivity (53.2%; range 49.0% to 69.2%), but higher overall specificity (83.6%; range 18% to 99.5%) for detecting prostate cancer.[6]

Laboratory and Imaging
- **Urinalysis.** Useful in detecting proteinuria (renal disease), hematuria, infection (bacteriuria, nitrite, and esterase positive), casts (renal disease), and crystals (calculus). Hematuria may also indicate calculus, chronic renal disease, or malignancy in elderly patients.
- **Serum chemistry.** Blood urea nitrogen, serum creatinine, and prostate-specific antigen (PSA). PSA is elevated in BPH, prostatitis, and prostate cancer. PSA has a low positive predictive value (25.1%; range 17.0% to 57.0%), moderate sensitivity (72.1%; range 66.7% to 100.0%), and high specificity (93.2%; range 63.1% to 100.0%) for prostate cancer.[6]

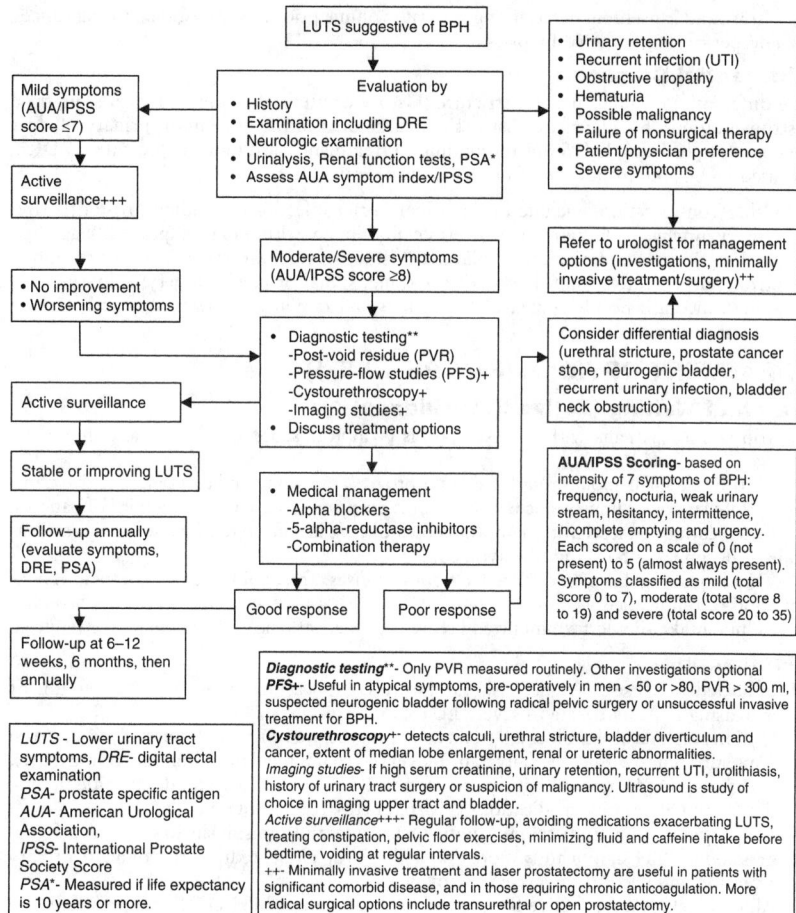

Figure 12.5-1. Diagnosis and management of benign prostatic hyperplasia.

- **Maximal urinary flow rate.** If greater than 15 mL per second excludes clinically important bladder outlet obstruction due to BPH.
- **Measurement of postvoid residual urine (PVR)** by in-and-out catheterization, ultrasound, or cystography. Large PVR correlates with severe BPH and chronic renal insufficiency, but does not predict need for surgery.[7,8]
- **Pressure-flow studies** during voiding measured through transvesical or transurethral insertion of a catheter. Useful in patients with atypical symptoms, preoperatively in men below 50 years or over 80 years, high PVR (over 300 mL), suspected neurogenic bladder, following radical pelvic surgery or unsuccessful invasive treatment for BPH.[4,9]
- **Cystourethroscopy.** Detects calculi, urethral stricture, bladder diverticulum and cancer, extent of median lobe enlargement, and through retrograde pyelography, assesses renal or ureteric abnormalities.
- **Imaging studies.** Useful in men with high serum creatinine, urinary retention, recurrent urinary tract infection, urolithiasis, history of urinary tract surgery, or suspicion of urothelial malignancy.[9] Ultrasound is the modality of choice in imaging the upper urinary tract and urinary bladder. Plain radiographs identify urolithiasis. Transrectal prostate

ultrasound is useful in determining prostate volume prior to surgery, diagnosing cancer, and performing targeted biopsies.

Differential Diagnosis

The differential includes urethral stricture (history of urethral trauma, urethritis, urethral instrumentation), bladder neck obstruction, carcinoma of the prostate or urinary bladder (hematuria, persisting LUTS not responding to treatment, hard nodular prostate on DRE, elevated PSA), and urolithiasis (pain, hematuria, graveluria).

■ Other considerations include lower urinary tract infections including prostatitis (frequency, urgency, abdominal pain, perirectal pain, constitutional symptoms, boggy and tender prostate) and neurogenic bladder (history of cerebral or spinal injury or tumor, stroke, degenerative joint disease of the spine, spinal or pelvic surgery; urinary retention or incontinence; focal neurologic deficits on examination; cystoscopy and pressure flow studies useful).

TREATMENT OPTIONS (FIGURE 12.5-1)

Watchful Waiting (Active Surveillance)

Appropriate for patients with mild symptoms (symptom score less than 7) and minimally enlarged prostate.[9–11]

Involves regular monitoring for disease progression, which indicates more active treatment. Stabilization or improvement in symptoms over time is seen in nearly a third of patients.

Medications exacerbating symptoms or inducing urinary retention (sedating antihistamines, decongestants) should be avoided.

Voiding at regular intervals, pelvic floor exercises, and avoidance or treatment of constipation recommended.

Fluid intake should be minimized before bedtime, caffeine and alcohol intake reduced.

Medication

■ Indicated in those at higher risk for future complications: PSA $\geq$1.5 ng per mL or increasing PSA, moderate to severe LUTS, and prostate size $\geq$30 cc.[11]

■ Options include alpha-blockers (terazosin 1 mg titrated to 5 to 10 mg daily, doxazosin 1 mg, titrated to 4 to 8 mg daily, tamsulosin 0.4 to 0.8 mg daily, alfuzosin 10 mg daily), and 5-alpha reductase inhibitors (finasteride 2.5 to 5 mg daily and dutasteride 0.5 mg daily), and alternative medications (saw palmetto 160 mg twice daily).

■ Long-term combination therapy with finasteride and tamsulosin lowers risk of progression of BPH significantly more than either drug alone, reduces risk of acute urinary retention and need for invasive therapy.

■ Alpha-blockers are effective for short-term treatment of BPH/LUTS and provide rapid relief of symptoms (within 48 hours). They relax the prostate and bladder neck smooth muscle, reduce bladder neck obstruction, and improve urine flow by 20% to 30%. Side effects include fatigue, orthostatic hypotension, edema, rhinitis, dyspnea, headache, angina, arrhythmia, and sexual/ejaculatory dysfunction. They are contraindicated in urinary retention, prostatic bleeding, chronic renal insufficiency, and recurrent urinary tract infections.[9]

■ 5-alpha-reductase inhibitors shrink the prostate, do not require dosage titration, and need to be administered over 6 to 12 months to improve symptoms. They reduce obstructive and nonobstructive symptom scores, increase urinary flow rates, suppress BPH-related hematuria, and reduce the need for surgery (improvement maintained over 4 to 6 years). Major side effects include decreased libido and ejaculatory or erectile dysfunction.[9,11]

■ Saw palmetto is as effective as finasteride and is better tolerated, and less expensive. Adverse effects are infrequent and include mild gastrointestinal distress.

Nonsurgical Treatment (Minimally Invasive Treatment)

Useful in those with significant comorbid disease, and in patients requiring chronic anticoagulation.[9,12]

■ Transurethral needle ablation of the prostate (TUNA). Low-energy radiofrequency ablation performed under local anesthesia, which improves symptom scores and urinary flow rates in 50% to 60% of patients, with minimal complications.[9,12]

- Transurethral microwave thermotherapy (TUMT). Involves heating prostatic tissue using computer-regulated microwaves under local anesthesia. Higher-energy TUMT is useful in patients with larger glands. It improves symptom scores and urinary flow. Serious thermal injuries may result.
- Intraurethral catheters. Self-retaining devices totally contained within the urethra, introduced with a cystoscope, offering continued relief of urinary retention. Temporary biodegradable and permanent intraurethral stents may also be used.

Surgical Treatment

Absolute indications include urinary retention, recurrent infection, obstructive uropathy, hematuria, possible malignancy. Relative indications include failure of nonsurgical therapy, patient or physician preference, severe symptoms.

- Transurethral prostatectomy (TURP). Resecting the prostate under direct vision with a resectoscope loaded with a diathermy loop exposing the capsule of the prostate, and performed under general anesthesia or regional block. It results in marked improvement in symptoms and urinary flow. Complications include hemorrhage, perforation of the prostatic capsule, urinary tract infection, bladder neck obstruction, urethral stricture, and recurrent BPH.[12]
- Transurethral incision of the prostate (TUIP). Making two deep incisions distal to each ureteral orifice through the bladder neck and the prostatic adenoma toward the verumontanum, down to the capsule of the prostate. Recommended for men with bladder outlet obstruction and minimal prostate enlargement, especially those with comorbid illnesses.[12]
- Open prostatectomy. This procedure is performed infrequently (in under 5%) on patients with large prostates, who are good surgical candidates. Retropubic, transvesical, and perineal approaches exist.
- Laser prostatectomy. Ideal for patients on anticoagulants, unfit for TURP, who desire to maintain ejaculation.[9]

Follow-Up (Figure 12.5-1)

- Annual follow-up required in patients on active surveillance, and should include evaluation of symptoms, DRE, and a PSA if initially measured, and life expectancy is 10 years or more. PVR assessments are also useful.[11]
- Patients on alpha-blockers should be seen at 6 weeks to assess symptom response and side effects. If symptoms improve, patients are seen at 6 and at 12 months.
- Patients on 5-alpha-reductase inhibitors should be monitored at 12 weeks, 6 months, and then annually.
- Patients receiving minimally invasive therapies should be seen at 6 weeks, at 3 to 6 months, then annually. After more radical surgery (TURP), they should be seen at 6 weeks to discuss histology and identify early morbidity, and then at 3 months to discuss final outcome.[12]

SPECIAL CONSIDERATIONS: INDICATIONS FOR REFERRAL TO A UROLOGIST

- History of worsening LUTS, acute urinary retention, hematuria, urinary incontinence
- Palpable urinary bladder or high PVR
- Urolithiasis, recurrent urinary tract infections
- Hard and irregular prostate, elevated PSA

References

1. Wei JT, Calhoun EA, Jacobsen SJ. Benign prostatic hyperplasia. In: Litwin MS, Saigal CS, eds. *Urologic diseases in America*. U.S. Department of Health and Human Services, Public Health Service, National Institutes of Health, National Institute of Diabetes and Digestive and Kidney Diseases. Washington, DC: U.S. Government Publishing Office; 2004:NIH Pub 04–5512, PP43–70.
2. Cunningam GR, Cadmon D. Epidemiology and pathogenesis of benign prostatic hyperplasia. UptoDate 2006. www.uptodate.com. Accessed November 7, 2006.
3. Meigs JB, Mohr B, Barry MJ, et al. Risk factors for clinical benign prostatic hyperplasia in a community-based population of healthy aging men. *J Clin Epidemiol* 2001;54(9): 935–944.

4. Cunningam GR, Cadmon D. Diagnosis of benign prostatic hyperplasia. UptoDate 2006. www.uptodate.com. Accessed November 7, 2006.
5. Barry MJ, Fowler FJ Jr, O'Leary MP, et al. The American Urological Association symptom index for benign prostatic hyperplasia. The Measurement Committee of the American Urological Association. *J Urol* 1992;148(5):1549–1557; discussion 1564.
6. Mistry K, Cable G. Meta-analysis of prostate-specific antigen and digital rectal examination as screening tests for prostate carcinoma. *J Am Board Fam Pract* 2003;16(2): 95–101.
7. Rule AD, Jacobson DJ, Roberts RO, et al. The association between benign prostatic hyperplasia and chronic kidney disease in community-dwelling men. *Kidney Int* 2005;67:2376–2382.
8. Wasson JH, Reda DJ, Bruskewitz RC, et al. A comparison of transurethral surgery with watchful waiting for moderate symptoms of benign prostatic hyperplasia. The Veterans Affairs Cooperative Study Group on Transurethral Resection of the Prostate. *N Engl J Med* 1995;332(2):75–79.
9. de la Rosette JJ, Alivizatos G, Madersbacher S, et al. European Association of Urology. EAU Guidelines on benign prostatic hyperplasia (BPH). *Eur Urol* 2001;40(3):256–263; discussion 264.
10. Burnett AL, Wein AJ. Benign prostatic hyperplasia in primary care: what you need to know. *J Urol* 2006;195(3):s19–s24.
11. Cunningam GR, Cadmon D. Medical treatment of benign prostatic hyperplasia. UptoDate 2006. www.uptodate.com. Accessed November 8, 2006.
12. Cunningam GR, Cadmon D. Surgical and other invasive therapy of benign prostatic hyperplasia. UptoDate 2006. www.uptodate.com. Accessed November 8, 2006.

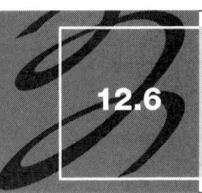

12.6

PROSTATE CANCER
Michael B. Potter

GENERAL PRINCIPLES

In the United States, prostate cancer is the most commonly diagnosed malignancy in men after nonmelanoma skin cancer. Prostate cancer is often microscopic and usually clinically silent for the life of the patient if it remains undiagnosed. However, there are enough aggressive cases to make it the third-leading cause of cancer death in American men, after lung and colorectal cancer. *Screening and treatment strategies are rapidly evolving, but remain controversial.*

Anatomy

Prostate cancer usually arises in the peripheral zone of the gland, but may also occur laterally or centrally, and is often multifocal. If it grows, it may become locally invasive, penetrating the prostate capsule, invading the seminal vesicles, spreading to pelvic lymph nodes, eventually reaching distant lymph nodes in the abdomen and beyond. Bone is usually the first site of metastasis beyond the lymph nodes, with liver and lung metastases occurring later.

Epidemiology

In 2006, there were about 234,460 new cases and 27,350 deaths from prostate cancer in the United States. This translates to one third of nonskin cancers diagnosed and 9% of cancer deaths among U.S. men. Incidence increases after age 50, with more than two thirds of prostate cancers diagnosed after the age of 65. History of prostate cancer in a brother or father doubles the risk of prostate cancer. African American men have a 60% higher incidence of prostate cancer compared to whites, whereas Asian and Hispanic Americans have lower rates than whites. African American men are also more often diagnosed with advanced disease and twice as likely as other American men to die from prostate cancer. Since the early 1990s prostate cancer screening has dramatically increased the number of prostate cancers diagnosed in the United States, with a simultaneous shift toward earlier stage at diagnosis. Meanwhile, prostate cancer deaths declined. It will not be until 2009 that the results of large ongoing randomized trials will tell us whether mortality is reduced by early detection and treatment.

Pathophysiology

Prostate cancer is thought to develop through a process in which intracellular mutations lead to transformation of normal prostate tissue into prostate intraepithelial neoplasia (PIN), which may resolve, persist, or progress to malignancy. It is not yet clear what factors cause a subset of malignancies to become aggressive and metastasize.

Etiology

Genetic markers for prostate cancer risk are not well defined, but this is an area of active research. Higher serum levels of testosterone and lower levels of vitamin D are associated with increased risk of prostate cancer. Dietary associations are being explored as well, but remain controversial. Some studies have suggested an association between prostate cancer incidence and diets that are high in fat, low in vegetables, and/or low in selenium. Recent research has focused on the possibility that chronic inflammation or viral infections of the prostate could have an important role in the etiology of prostate cancer.

DIAGNOSIS

Asymptomatic Men

Most cancers are diagnosed through screening. Screening is done with prostate-specific antigen blood testing (PSA) and digital rectal examination (DRE). The U.S. Preventive Services Task Force, American Cancer Society, and American Urological Association all advocate a discussion between doctor and patient of the potential risks and benefits of screening. Such discussions should begin at age 50 for average risk men, and during the 40s in African Americans. The importance of informed decision making is underlined by studies suggest that a substantial minority of fully informed men will decline screening.

Risks of screening include diagnosis of a clinically insignificant cancer and treatment complications such as impotence or incontinence. The benefits of screening will remain uncertain until the completion of randomized trials, but screening is unlikely to have mortality benefits for men who have a life expectancy that is shorter than 10 years. Therefore, asymptomatic screening should typically not be performed in men older than 70.

Symptomatic Men

Prostate cancer usually causes no symptoms in its early stages. When they occur, symptoms may include urinary frequency, urgency, hesitancy, or nocturia. If the cancer invades the neurovascular bundle, erectile dysfunction may result. Hematuria and hemospermia are relatively uncommon presenting symptoms. When metastatic, prostate cancer may cause bone pain or other symptoms due to distant lesions. When older men present with new symptoms of urinary obstruction or with symptoms that could be caused by bony metastases, the diagnosis of prostate cancer should be considered.

Physical Examination

DRE is part of the diagnostic evaluation for prostate cancer for symptomatic men. It is also part of the routine prostate cancer screening, although it has low sensitivity and specificity, especially when PSA levels are low. When DRE reveals an asymmetric or nodular prostate, the patient should be referred for further evaluation, regardless of PSA levels.

Laboratory Studies

PSA is a protease secreted by the prostate and helps liquefy the seminal coagulum. Serum PSA levels increase as the prostate cancer grows, disrupts the prostate-blood barrier, and metastasizes. The positive predictive value of a PSA between 4 and 10 ng per mL is in the 20% range, and is further increased at higher PSA levels. Traditionally, PSA levels below 4 ng per mL have been considered normal, but recent studies show that many men with PSA values of 2.5 to 4 ng per mL also harbor prostate cancers, some of which may turn out to be aggressive when biopsied. PSA levels should also be interpreted in the context of age.

For example, a value of 4 ng per mL may be more worrisome in a 50-year-old than a value of 5 ng per mL in a 70-year-old.

Monitoring

When PSA values are slightly elevated and DRE is normal, biopsy is sometimes deferred in favor of close monitoring of PSA values over time. In these cases, PSA may be initially repeated in a month or two and then again every 6 to 12 months. A PSA increase 1.0 ng per mL or more in 1 year is considered sufficient evidence to warrant prostate biopsy. The change in PSA levels over time is referred to as PSA velocity. PSA exists in free and bound forms in the serum, with more bound PSA secreted by glands that have disrupted cellular architecture. As the proportion of free-to-total PSA drops below 20%, the likelihood of prostate cancer increases. Therefore, free PSA is often ordered to help decide whether or not to obtain a biopsy in borderline cases. However, these strategies to improve the specificity of PSA testing prior to biopsy remain controversial. MRI is being studied as pre operative staging.

Imaging

Transrectal ultrasound (TRUS) is not an accurate screening tool, but is used to guide needle biopsies that are done for diagnostic purposes. Pelvic and abdominal computed tomography (CT) and radionuclide bone scans are ordered when there is clinical suspicion of regional or distant metastases MRI is being studied as pre operative staging.

Surgical Diagnostic Procedures

Diagnosis of prostate cancer is typically made with the aid of a transrectal core needle biopsy. Biopsies focus on abnormal areas found on DRE and TRUS and also include multiple specimens covering all areas of the gland. Benign findings are often followed by repeat biopsy when the clinical diagnosis remains in doubt. The most common side effects of prostate biopsy are transient hemospermia and hematuria.

Tumor Stage

The American Joint Committee on Cancer (AJCC) has developed a prostate cancer staging system based on the TNM (tumor, nodes, metastases) system. Stages 1 and 2 are defined, respectively, as nonpalpable and palpable tumors confined to the prostate. Stage 3 tumors extend through the prostate capsule and may involve the seminal vesicles but not the lymph nodes or other adjacent structures. Stage 4 tumors invade adjacent structures or have spread to regional lymph nodes or more distant sites.

Gleason Score

Tumors may be well differentiated or poorly differentiated at any stage, and the level of tumor differentiation, which can be graded with a score of 1 to 5, with 5 the most poorly differentiated. The Gleason score is a sum of grades for the two most prevalent patterns of differentiation seen on biopsy. A Gleason score of 4 or less is classified as a low-grade tumor. Scores of 5 to 7 are intermediate, and scores of 8 or above are high grade. Thus, a score of "2 + 1 = 3" would be low grade, and a score of "3 + 3 = 6" would be considered intermediate grade, and a score of "5 + 3 = 8" would be considered high grade. The Gleason score adds prognostic information that can be used to guide treatment decisions, especially for Stage 1 and Stage 2 tumors.

Clinical Staging

At present, approximately 90% of prostate cancers are localized at the time of diagnosis. Therefore, complete staging with bone scans, CT scans, and other imaging tests are usually reserved for patients who are clinically suspected to have a cancer that has spread beyond the prostate gland, such as in the case of a PSA > 10 ng per mL or a high Gleason score. Seminal vesicle biopsy and pelvic lymph node dissection (which can now be done laparascopically) are also sometimes used for more definitive clinical staging when needed to guide treatment.

Differential Diagnosis

In asymptomatic men with a normal DRE, a mildly elevated PSA has a relatively low specificity and may be due to benign prostatic hyperplasia (BPH), chronic prostatitis, or increased age. Local symptoms from prostate cancer can sometimes mimic BPH, and include urinary frequency, hesitancy, nocturia, and weak stream. When these symptoms develop rapidly, they may be more indicative of cancer. When infection is suspected, an empiric trial of antibiotics with repeat PSA testing after treatment is sometimes tried before referring a patient for biopsy. Clinicians should consider the possibility of metastatic prostate cancer in older men presenting with new atypical back pain or other bone pain syndromes.

TREATMENT

Watchful Waiting

Men with Stage 1 or 2 prostate cancer and a low Gleason score have a life expectancy that is unlikely to be extended by immediate treatment. These men may reasonably choose close monitoring in place of immediate treatment.

Surgery

The evidence of benefit for surgical treatment remains uncertain but seems to be accumulating for men with Stage 1 or 2 localized cancers with intermediate to high Gleason scores and who otherwise would have a life expectancy of at least 10 years. Surgery is also sometimes performed on locally invasive Stage 3 cancers though it is not considered curative in these cases. Prostatectomy is not indicated for Stage 4 cancers. To avoid surgery on Stage 4 cancers, formal staging is usually done prior to consideration of prostatectomy when the PSA or Gleason scores are high enough to be predictive of metastases. Surgery also often begins with a pelvic lymph node dissection to rule out nodal metastases on frozen section prior to prostatectomy. Even with newer "nerve-sparing" surgical techniques, postoperative impotence occurs in most men, and problems with urinary continence remain common. In cases where local invasion through the prostate capsule is found at the time of prostatectomy, additional radiation and hormonal therapy are usually offered.

Radiation

Patients with Stage 1 or 2 prostate cancer are often offered radiation therapy as an alternative to prostatectomy, especially for older patients with higher Gleason scores who desire treatment. Compared to prostatectomy, radiation has fewer complications and side effects, but randomized studies have not established its comparative efficacy to watchful waiting or prostatectomy in these patients. Prior to radiation treatment, CT and bone scans are often performed to rule out Stage 3 or 4 disease. If Stage 3 disease is suspected, hormonal therapy will often be offered in addition to radiation. Prostate irradiation is not indicated in Stage 4 disease. Short-term complications of external beam radiation include proctitis and cystitis. About one third of men experience impotence as a long-term complication. To reduce the risk of this side effect, interstitial brachytherapy, with "radioactive seeds" implanted into the prostate tissue, is sometimes used as an alternative to traditional external beam radiation, usually in Stage 1 and Stage 2 cancers.

Hormonal and Other Therapies

Prostate cancer growth is stimulated by physiologic androgens. In metastatic disease, androgen ablation can modestly improve survival and can dramatically improve symptoms of urinary obstruction and pain from bony metastases. Androgen ablation is usually achieved with orchiectomy or a gonadotropin-releasing hormone (GRH) analogue such as leuprolide. Additional androgen blockade can be provided with flutamide or bicalutamide. A variety of second-line hormonal therapies can be tried when initial antiandrogen therapy fails. Side effects of hormonal therapy include impotence, vasomotor symptoms, gynecomastia, and osteoporosis. When hormonal therapies fail, chemotherapy with docetaxel and prednisone may offer additional modest survival benefits. Symptomatic treatment for bony metastases includes bisphosphonates and targeted radiation therapy.

Referrals

Patients with persistently elevated or rising PSA and/or an abnormal DRE should be referred to a urologist for further evaluation. Treatment of prostate cancer often involves a variety of specialists, including a urologic oncologist and a radiation oncologist. Clear communication with the patient and treating physicians has the potential to help patients navigate complex diagnostic and treatment decisions.

Follow-Up

Evidence-based guidelines for follow-up of men with prostate cancer do not yet exist. Men diagnosed with localized disease who elect a watchful waiting strategy usually deserve careful monitoring, for example, PSA and DRE every 6 months and repeat biopsy at 1 year if there is evidence of disease progression. Men who have undergone prostatectomy or radiation for localized prostate cancer have a low rate of recurrence and may return to annual PSA testing after a 1 to 2 year period of more frequent testing following initial treatment. Follow-up of men who have been treated for locally invasive or metastatic disease is usually guided by specialists, but evaluation for rising PSA and symptom progression every few months is typical when monitoring for the possibility of biochemical treatment failure in these patients.

References

1. Jamal A, Siegel R, Ward E, et al. Cancer statistics, 2006. *CA Cancer J Clin* 2006;56: 106–130.
2. Harris R, Lohr KN. Screening for prostate cancer: an update of the evidence for the U.S. Preventive Services Task Force. *Ann Intern Med* 2002;137:917–929.
3. Andriole GL, Levin DL, Crawford ED, et al. Prostate cancer screening in the Prostate Lung, Colorectal and Ovarian (PLCO) Cancer Screening Trial. *J Natl Cancer Inst* 2005; 97:433–438.
4. Gann PH, Hennekens CH, Stampfer MJ. A prospective evaluation of plasma prostate-specific antigen for detection of prostate cancer. *JAMA* 1995;273:289–294.
5. Thompson IM, Pauler DK, Goodman PJ, et al. Prevalence of prostate cancer among men with a prostate-specific antigen < or = 4.0 ng/ml. *N Engl J Med* 2004;350: 2239–2246.
6. Hoffman RM, Clanon DL, Littenberg B, et al. Using the free-to-total prostate specific ratio to detect prostate cancer in men with nonspecific elevations of prostate-specific antigen levels. *J Gen Intern Med* 2000;15:739–748.
7. Smith DA, Catalona WJ. Rate of change in serum prostate specific antigen levels as a method for prostate cancer detection. *J Urol* 1994;152:1163–1167.
8. *AJCC cancer staging handbook.* 6th ed. New York: Springer; 2002:309–316.
9. Bostwick DG. Grading prostate cancer. *Am J Clin Pathol* 1994;102:S38–56.
10. Klotz L. Active surveillance for prostate cancer: for whom? *J Clin Oncol* 2005;23: 8165–8169.
11. Bill-Axelson A, Holmberg L, Ruutu M, et al. Scandanavian Prostate Cancer Group Study No. 4. Radical prostatectomy versus watchful waiting in early prostate cancer. *N Engl J Med* 2005;352:1977–1984.
12. Speight JL, Roach M. Radiotherapy in the management of clinically localized prostate cancer: evolving standards, consensus, controversies, and new directions. *J Clin Oncol* 2005;23:8176–8185.
13. Sharifi N, Gulley JL, Dahut WL. Androgen deprivation therapy for prostate cancer. *JAMA* 2005;294:238–244.

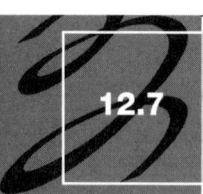

12.7 CHRONIC KIDNEY DISEASE
Joseph Hobbs

General Principles

Evidence of chronic kidney disease (CKD) is seen initially as early markers of kidney damage without changes in glomerular filtration rate (GFR) causing to damage of enough significance to cause a progressive decline in GFR. CKD is a progressive decline in kidney function over months to years caused by loss of functional units of the kidney evoked by multiple disease processes. The National Kidney Foundation Kidney Disease Outcome Quality Initiative (NKF K/DOQI) defines CKD as "kidney damage for 3 or more months as evidenced by structural and functional abnormalities of the kidney with or without decreased GFR, manifested by markers of kidney damage including abnormalities of the composition of blood (e.g., elevated serum creatinine) or urine (e.g., proteinuria) or abnormalities in imaging studies (e.g., polycystic kidneys)." CKD is a major public health problem, the prevalence of which is increasing as the population ages.

Epidemiology

The number of individuals with CKD in its earliest form is unknown but those with kidney damage substantial enough to warrant kidney replacement therapy has increased over the last two decades. African Americans, older individuals, and Native Americans have the highest rates of functional decline to levels requiring kidney replacement therapy.[1-6]

Pathophysiology

CKD is caused by primary glomerulopathies (i.e., membranoproliferative glomerulonephritis and focal and segmental glomerulosclerosis), secondary glomerulopathies caused by diabetes mellitus and systemic lupus erythematosus, tubular interstitial diseases (i.e., pyelonephritis and granulomatous interstitial nephritis), obstructive uropathy (e.g., benign prostatic hyperplasia and kidney stones), and renal vascular disease (e.g., renal artery stenosis and uncontrolled hypertension). In these settings, kidney injury and permanent functional loss are caused by an inflammatory response to both immunologic and nonimmunologic factors that cause sclerosis, which damages and destroys nephrons and ultimately leads to progressive decline in renal function. The kidneys' functional loss may initially result in adaptive responses of the remaining nephrons (i.e., hypertrophy), which depending on the amount of kidney damage may maintain and even increase GFR (i.e., hyperfiltration). This adaptive process, however, is associated with functional obstruction of postglomerular capillaries, glomerular hypertension, glomerular hypertrophy, and epithelial foot process fusion, mesangial expansion, and glomerular sclerosis of remaining nephrons, the consequences of which are progressive decline of kidney function.

Classification of CKD

The NKF K/DOQI CKD classification is stratified into five stages of sequential decrements in GFR. These advancing stages of declining GFR are associated with a greater number and severities of complications.[1,3] These stages of CKD are preceded by a category where there is no evidence of damage but there is increase risk for the development of CKD (e.g., patients with diabetes and hypertension).

- Stage 1 is "kidney damage with normal or elevated GFR" (i.e., >90 mL/min/1.73 m^2) where other early markers of kidney damage (e.g., persistent microalbuminuria or albuminuria, cystic disease of the kidney) may be present but nephron loss is not of a magnitude to decrease GFR or GFR is maintained or increased by kidney adaptive processes (i.e., hyperfiltration).
- Stage 2 is "kidney damage substantial enough to cause mild decreases in GFR" (i.e., 60 to 89 mL/min/1.73 m^2).
- Stage 3 is "kidney damage with moderately decreased GFR" (i.e., 30 to 59 mL/min/1.73 m^2).
- Stage 4 is "severely decreased GFR" (i.e., 15 to 29 mL/min/m^2).
- Finally, Stage 5 is "kidney failure" (GFR less than 15 mL/min/1.73 m^2), which is a point where renal replacement therapy is required.

DIAGNOSIS

History of Chronic Kidney Disease

Symptoms associated with CKD do not occur until the final stages (i.e., Stages 3, 4, and 5) in the disease progression and more profoundly when kidney function deterioration is substantial enough to produce uremia (i.e., GFR less than 15 mL/min/1.73 m^2). These symptoms could include generalized fatigue, findings associated with anemia, volume depletion or volume excess, and findings consistent with uremia, including encephalopathy. Many of the earlier historical findings are related to the initiating events (e.g., frequent urinary tract infections) or the underlying disease (e.g., diabetes mellitus). Early identification of CKD in asymptomatic patients or those at increased risk for CKD permits interventions aimed at enhancing the preservation of kidney function. Patients at risk for the development of CKD include those with diabetes mellitus, hypertension, vascular disease, dysproteinemia, vasculitis, chronic urinary tract infection, and immune complex–mediated glomerulonephritis (e.g., poststreptococcal infection and systemic lupus erythematosus).

History of Acute Renal Failure in Paients with CKD

Historical evidence of acute renal failure in the setting of CKD like the isolated problem frequently includes the symptoms associated with the causes of hypovolemia, which increase the risk for decreased renal perfusion and ischemic injury to the kidney. The use of nonsteroidal anti-inflammatory drugs, angiotensin-converting enzyme (ACE) inhibitors and angiotensin receptor blockers (HP_1B_S also predisposes to intrarenal hypoperfusion especially in settings where effective circulating volume is already compromised (e.g., congestive heart failure). Fever may suggest septicemia causing loss of vascular integrity and kidney hypoperfusion.[10] Patients with underlying CKD receiving diagnostic studies using contrast dyes with or without volume depletion are at risk for additional intrinsic acute renal damage, respectively. Acute skeletal muscle injury caused by prolonged hypoxemia to an extremity, severe exercise, or trauma can lead to myoglobulinemia and myoglobinuria and intrinsic acute renal failure. Renal stones, neurogenic bladder, bladder neck obstruction, or other causes of lower urinary tract obstruction can cause acute postrenal failure.[11] These acute events superimposed on the CKD accelerate kidney dysfunction.

Physical

Abnormal physical findings associated with CKD also occur late in the process (i.e., Stage 5), except those related to underlying disease processes. Late findings include edema, hypertension, pallor, easy bruising, bone pain, cardiac dysrhythmias induced by hyperkalemia, asterixis, and other neurologic manifestations of uremia. Physical evidence of hypovolemia or other causes of kidney hypoperfusion would suggest the potential of acute renal failure in the setting of CKD. Hypertension could suggest renal vascular disease and acute muscle tenderness and swelling may indicate muscle injury. Abdominal, pelvic, and prostate evaluation may reveal the source of postrenal obstruction.

Laboratory Assessment of Kidney Function

The indirect measurement of kidney filtering capacity or GFR has long been used to assess kidney function. The relationship between a declining GFR and diminishing kidney function is used to determine the severity and predict the rate of functional decline and the onset of kidney failure. Determining the serum level and the clearance of endogenously produced stable substances excreted mostly by the kidney and that are easily measured in blood and urine have been used to estimate creatinine clearance (CCr).[1,3]

Creatinine serum levels and CCr have long been surrogates for GFR estimation in clinical settings. Creatinine secretion increases with advancing CKD. However, measurement of serum creatinine levels alone to assess renal function does not account for differences caused by age, ethnicity, gender, weight, muscle mass, protein intake, or protein loss. These and other measurement variables increase the potential that serum creatinine levels and resulting GFR estimates could be inaccurate estimates of kidney function.[1,3] In spite of these limitations, serum creatinine levels and clearance performed serially over time do approximate the rate of kidney function decline in later stages of CKD. However, the time urine collections required for the measurement of CCr and the variables of patient performance over a 24-hour period make errors likely.

Studies now show that more accurate estimates of GFR, when compared to serum creatinine levels alone, can be obtained using prediction equations that not only use serum creatinine levels but age, gender, ethnicity, and weight as variable factors. The NKF K/DOQI suggests that the abbreviated modification of diet in renal disease (MDRD) study and Cockcroft-Gault equations be used in adults to estimate GFR and CCr, respectively, and the Schwartz and Counahan-Barratt equation be used in children.[1–3] The abbreviated MDRD study equation appears to provide better estimates of GFR when compared to the Cockcroft-Gault equation possibly because of the presence of the additional variables of body surface area and ethnicity. Both the Schwartz and Counahan-Barratt prediction formulas overestimate GFR in children with renal failure but provide reasonable estimates that are accurate enough for clinical purposes.[1–3]

The precision of GFR estimates using prediction formulas require a steady state of creatinine production. GFR estimates in patients with malnutrition, intake of dietary creatin, and the unsteady state of acute renal disease when using prediction equations are likely to produce unreliable GFR estimates. Prediction equations may not appropriately estimate GFR at levels approaching or exceeding normal values, in CKD Stages 1 and 2, because of the compensatory hyperfiltration in the remaining normal or less injured nephrons, which may maintain or increase GFR. A fairly significant decrease in GFR must occur for serum creatinine levels to increase beyond normal limits (e.g., 50% loss in kidney function increases baseline serum creatinine only twofold).

Because the earliest stages of CKD may not be associated with detectable changes in serum creatinine, estimates of GFR and CCr using equations may not detect the earliest phases of chronic kidney dysfunction. Therefore, there is a need to identify other markers of beginning stages of CKD to provide the earliest possible opportunity for intervention.[1,3] When the discovery of kidney dysfunction occurs as a result of routine laboratory assessments, it is necessary to determine whether the kidney disease failure is an acute process, caused by prekidney, kidney, or postkidney factors, or a chronic process.

Factors such as systemic hypertension, increased renal prostaglandins, dietary proteins, uncontrolled glycemia, phosphate retention, and hyperlipidemia contribute to the ongoing predictable decline in kidney function in this setting.[1,3,6,7]

Differential Diagnosis: Other Causes of Decreased Kidney Function

Age-Related Decline in Kidney Function

Declining kidney function with age affects the management of fluid and electrolyte disturbances and the use of potentially nephrotoxic drugs. This age-related decline in kidney function is caused by a slow, progressive sclerosis and fibrosis of functional excretory units of the kidney without evidence of primary kidney disease, resulting in a decline in CCr but with a normal serum creatinine. The normal serum creatinine occurs in part because of the decreased muscle mass of older patients, resulting in decreased creatinine production and subsequent decreased urinary creatinine excretion.

This age decline in kidney function could be as much as 1 mL/min/1.73 m² below normal baseline GFRs per year above age 20 to 30 (baseline GFR of women 8% less than men). This physiologic decline, although not called CKD, places older patients at increased risk that any kidney damage added to the age-related decrement of kidney function may have more substantial consequences, because of decreased kidney functional reserve. Age-related declines in kidney function with GFR of less than 60 mL/min/1.73 m² (no obvious precipitating events) is considered CKD.[1,3,8] Decreased kidney sodium conservation and excretion capacities in elderly individuals decreases the compensatory response to deficits or excess in the effective circulating volume. Decreased kidney water conservation in elderly individuals is caused in part by decreased pituitary responsiveness to rising osmolality and a decreased kidney responsiveness to antidiuretic hormone, thus increasing susceptibility to hypernatremia when hypotonic volume losses occur.

Acute Renal Failure

Often the causes of renal dysfunction occur acutely as isolated events or in combination with underlying CKD. The resulting acute renal failure is usually manifested as a rise in specific and nonspecific markers of kidney function based on GFR (i.e., serum creatinine and blood urea nitrogen levels, respectively). Often prolonged or severe hypovolemia, causing kidney hypoperfusion and decreased GFR, can lead to an acute decrement in renal function. This hypovolemic induced kidney dysfunction occurs without intrinsic kidney damage (i.e., prerenal acute renal failure) and with a specific type of intrinsic kidney damage, acute tubular necrosis (ATN; i.e., intrinsic acute renal failure). Prerenal acute renal failure and the hypovolemic-induced components of intrinsic acute renal failure, ATN, represent the most frequent causes of acute renal failure. Prerenal acute renal failure is usually reversible if hemodynamic support and effective circulating volume can be rapidly restored. The ischemic tubular injury of ATN causes death and shedding of renal tubular epithelial cells. These shed cells and resulting cellular casts and other debris cause decreased GFR and renal arterial vasoconstriction. Intrinsic acute renal failure can be caused by exposure to exogenous and endogenous nephrotoxins (e.g., radio contrast dyes, myoglobin, free hemoglobin, nonsteroidal anti-inflammatory drugs, aminoglyco sides, and amphotericin B), acute glomerulonephritis, acute interstitial nephritis, and acute renal vascular occlusion and postrenal obstruction (i.e., acute postrenal failure).[9]

Complications. Acute renal failure is a common occurrence, therefore, its presence must be considered in the initial evaluation of CKD when dysfunction is significant enough to produce changes in serum markers (e.g., serum creatinine) of kidney function.

Assessment of Acute Renal Failure. In CKD, when functional decline progresses more rapidly than anticipated by the reciprocal of creatinine over time, a superimposed acute process could be present. The causes of acute renal failure often result in a reversible decline in kidney function, which can result in permanent functional decline if the causes are not rapidly corrected. Acute renal failure is defined as at least a 0.5 mg per dL increase in serum creatinine and progressive decline of this magnitude per 24 hours.

Prerenal acute renal failure is usually characterized by a blood urea nitrogen (BUN) and creatinine elevation at ratios greater than 20:1, urinary sodium concentration (U_{Na}) less than 10 to 20 mEq per L, and urinary osmolalities (Uosm) greater than 450 mOsm per kg, acellular urinary sediments, and a fractional excretion of sodium (FeNa) of less than 1%. The kidney etiologic factors involved in acute renal failure cause BUN and creatinine elevation at ratios of 10:1, U_{Na} exceeding 20 to 30 mEq per L, Uosm less than 350 mOsm per kg, urinary sediment with kidney tubular cells and casts, and FeNa greater than 1%. In postkidney causes of acute renal failure, assuming bilateral obstruction, the initial findings may be similar to those of prekidney disease, but in time U_{Na} will exceed 20 to 30 mEq per L, FeNa will be greater than 2%, and urine dilution will ensue. These distinctions of acute renal failure are not present in the latter stages of CKD where salt and water handling by the kidney is severely impaired.

Assessment of Chronic Kidney Disease

Persistent detectable proteinuria suggests kidney damage which usually precedes biochemical changes. Large amounts of urinary albumin as detected by standard or albumin-specific dipsticks occurs in CKD caused by diabetes, glomerulopathies, and some tubulointerstitial processes. Standard urine dipstick to test of early morning or random urine usually detects total protein levels of 10 to 20 mg per dL and albumin-specific dipsticks detect albumin levels of 3 to 4 mg per dL. Screening for proteinuria in patients not at risk for kidney disease can be performed using standard urine dipsticks to detect total urinary protein. If the study is positive for proteinuria, then a determination of total urinary protein to urinary creatinine ratio (UP/UC) is made, which provides urinary protein levels based on corrections for differing urinary volumes assuming relative consistency of creatinine excretion. These studies can be performed on random, nontimed urine samples. These are useful tools to follow the progression of proteinuria, detect levels of proteinuria indicative of glomerular disease, and determine nephrotic-range proteinuria (e.g., U_{prot}/U_{Cr} ratio greater than 1.0 reflects urinary protein excretion greater than 3.5 g/dL). Glomerular causes of CKD results in urinary protein to urinary creatinine ratios greater than 1,000 mg per g with other causes of CKD producing proteinuria less than 1,000 mg per g.[12]

A ratio of urinary protein to urinary creatinine greater than or equal to 200 mg per g requires retesting in 3 months. If still above this level, the patient has persistent proteinuria and requires additional evaluation for CKD. For patients at risk for kidney disease, screening should be performed with an albumin-specific dipstick and, if positive, a ratio of urinary albumin to urine creatinine is performed. Repeated values greater than 30 mg per g require evaluation and treatment for CKD. In adults with CKD, albumin-to-creatinine ratio should be used to detect and quantify the degree of proteinuria. Children without diabetes should be screened for kidney disease using a standard dipstick and positive values should be quantified using ratios of total urinary protein to total creatinine.[4]

Serum creatinine elevated above the patient's normal baseline occurs when declines in GFR begin (Stage 2 and beyond). An initial doubling of baseline serum creatinine levels may represent as much as a 50% loss of kidney function even when the doubling of the serum creatinine results in levels still within normal ranges. BUN increase is at 10:1 relationship with creatinine for that portion of BUN related to declining GFR (not nonrenal cause of BUN elevation such as gastrointestinal bleeding, high protein diets, enhanced tissue destruction).

Diminished kidney capacity to concentrate urine and maximally acidify urine, as well as conserve sodium in response to decreased effective circulating volume, is an indicator of advanced CKD. Urine sediment exam may reveal red blood cells and casts in certain glomerulopathies and white blood cells and casts in kidney infections. Albumin-specific dipstick will be positive at early stages of CKD with elevated ratios of urinary albumin to urinary creatinine. If proteinuria is substantial, nephrotic range kidney albumin loss will exceed production with resulting hypoalbuminemia.

Studies to evaluate the causes of CKD can include serum protein electrophoresis for plasma cell dyscrasias, antinuclear antibody (ANA), and dsDNA antibody for systemic lupus erythematosis and consumption of serum complement for certain autoimmune glomerulopathies and antiglomerular basement membrane for Goodpasture's syndrome. Evidence of disease associated with CKD can be evaluated with studies for diabetes mellitus, HIV, thrombotic thrombocytopenic purpura (TTP), hepatitis B and C, and syphilis.[8,13]

Plain imaging may reveal evidence of nephrocalcinosis, and large kidneys caused by hyperfiltration in early disease. Renal ultrasound will also reveal presence of small echogenic kidneys in late CKD stages with normal or large kidneys in earlier stages. Ultrasound can also reveal the presence of urinary tract obstruction and abnormalities of kidney parenchyma (e.g., cysts). Computed tomography (CT) scan of the abdomen can provide better resolution of kidney structural changes. Contrasted imaging studies should be avoided. Captopril renal scans may be used in detecting the presence of renal artery stenosis at early stages of CKD.

Clinical Course of Chronic Kidney Disease

When the GFR falls below one third of normal (i.e., Stage 4), electrolyte disturbances can appear that may include hyperkalemia and metabolic acidosis. Hyperkalemia occurs because of diminished kidney potassium excretory capacity especially with acute potassium loads, even though the remaining kidney tissue and gastrointestinal tract have enhanced potassium excretion, as well as in patients with pharmacologic inhibition of distal renal tubular sites (e.g., ACE inhibitors, angiotensin II blocking agents, triamterene, amelioride) or intrinsic hypofunctioning at these distal sites (e.g., hypoaldosterone states). Volume depletion can also contribute to hyperkalemia in CKD.[8]

Metabolic acidosis usually presents as a hyperchloremic metabolic acidosis (i.e., nonanion gap) caused by declining urinary acidification capacity (i.e., type 4 renal tubular acidosis) in Stage 4 CKD but can progress to a normochloremic metabolic acidosis caused by the retention of endogenous metabolic acids (e.g., phosphates, sulfates, ammonia, urates, and hippurates) and the emergence of a large anion gap metabolic acidosis in late Stage 4 and Stage 5. Metabolic acidosis may also be absent until challenged with large fixed acid loads. Hypervolemia becomes a problem in Stage 4 but mostly prior to the institution of renal replacement therapy in Stage 5. Patients are usually not able to excrete excess loads of water or sodium, which increases the risk for hyponatremia and hypertension. Large loads of sodium and water provided acutely can cause similar problems at earlier stages of CKD.[8,13]

Through other adaptive mechanisms, the kidney is capable of maintaining sodium homeostasis in CKD but has diminished capacity to excrete sodium loads, which can lead to edema and hypertension and conserve sodium when there is a loss of effective circulating volume. Chronic and uncontrolled hypertension can accelerate the loss of functional kidney units.[8] Phosphate retention occurs early in CKD as GFR decreases. Renal phosphate retention causes a fall in serum calcium levels as does decrease intestinal calcium absorption because of decrease synthesis of 1,25,(OH)D. Hypocalcemia and hyperphosphatemia indirectly stimulates parathyroid hormone (PTH) release. PTH when chronically elevated in Stage 4 CKD can lead to renal osteodystrophy. As the functional mass of the kidney declines erythropoetin production declines. The erythropoetin decline results in decreased red blood cell (RBC) production and anemia that appears as hypoproliferative normocytic and normochromic. As uremia ensues in Stage 5 of CKD, dysfunction of platelets can result in bleeding abnormalities.[6,8,13,14]

TREATMENT OF CHRONIC KIDNEY DISEASE

Early consultation with nephrologists and kidney teams should occur to maximize the treatment of advancing CKD. In patients with established renal failure, GFR estimates should be obtained at least annually but should occur more frequently in patients with GFR less than 60 mL/min/1.73 m² (i.e., Stage 3 or greater) to determine the rate and progression of CKD. This GFR monitoring should be more frequent in patients whose rate of functional decline has been greater than predicted. More frequent measurements should also be provided for patients at risk for exposure to causes of acute GFR declines.[1-3] Diminishing the impact of factors known to cause and independently increase the rate of kidney functional decline has been shown to decrease the progression of CKD. These factors include systemic hypertension, glomerular hypertension, dietary protein intake, hyperglycemia, and possibly hyperlipidemia.[3]

Management of chronic renal disease begins with the recognition of individuals who are at risk for this problem before the presence of markers that indicate early renal dysfunction. Interventions to control hypertension and diabetes should be perceived as kidney-protective strategies. Interventions aimed at slowing the progression of CKD included control of hypertension, glycemia, and proteinuria, reducing protein intake, as well as implementing strategies for cardiovascular risk reduction to include appropriate exercise, weight loss, reduce sodium intake, control of dyslipidemias, and smoking cessation in both diabetic and nondiabetic nephropathy. Although the cardiovascular risk reduction activities have not been shown to be associated with slowing the progression of CKD, their impact on cardiovascular health is essential since patients with CKD have accelerated risk for cardiovascular disease events.[5,7,12]

Hypertension

Aggressive measures must be employed to normalize blood pressure in CKD. The ameliorating impact of blood pressure normalization on the progression of CKD occurs independently of agents used to treat hypertension. Agents used in the treatment of hypertension and early kidney disease include ACE inhibitors, angiotensin II receptor blockers, calcium-channel blockers, and diuretics, and their use must be individualized to each clinical setting. However, evidence suggests that greater renoprotective benefits are derived from the use of ACE inhibitors and angiotensin II blockers independent of their blood pressure–lowering effect in diabetic and nondiabetic nephropathies.[1] Because of the tendency for sodium retention in CKD, diuretics are frequently used to control hypertension. Thiazide diuretics (e.g., metolazone) can be effective at GFRs greater than 30 to 40 mL per minute. When GFR falls below these levels, more potent medullary loop diuretics (e.g., furosemide) should be used as resistance to thiazides ensues. To avoid the resistance to loop diuretics caused by persistent sodium reabsorption at tubular sites other than that of the loop diuretic, the addition of a thiazide is advised to enhance diuresis. The combination of loop and thiazide diuretics also delays the need for larger quantities of loop diuretics, thus decreasing the risk of ototoxicity.[15]

Strict blood pressure control is recommended for both diabetic and nondiabetic nephropathy since evidence shows that these interventions slow progression of CKD. Blood pressure targets for nondiabetic nephropathy is less than 130/85 mmHg with lower targets suggested (i.e., under 125/75 mmHg). Usually all agents can be employed to treat hypertension in patients with CKD (the exception may be dihydropyridine calcium-channel blockers that in some studies have shown high risk in kidney disease progression in diabetic and nondiabetic disease). ACE inhibitors and angiotensin II blocking agents are the choice of antihypertensive agents. Thiazide diuretics and, in advancing disease, loop diuretics may be required to lower blood pressure, reduce sodium retention of CKD, and provide additional kaluresis in response to the associated hyperkalemia.[16]

Microalbuminuria and Macroalbuminuria

Microalbuminuria in diabetes mellitus provides a window for detecting diabetic nephropathy at an earlier stage before a decline in GFR or an elevation in BUN and creatinine occurs. The use of ACE inhibitors and angiotensin II receptor blockers when microalbuminuria or macroalbuminuria is detected has been shown to slow the progression of diabetic and nondiabetic kidney disease independent of the presence of systemic hypertension.[1-3] Prospective treatment with ACE inhibitors or angiotensin receptor blockers of patients with chronic kidney disease prior to the presence of microalbuminuria or proteinuria should be considered, especially if the patient has hypertension. One must carefully monitor these agents to avoid hyperkalemia especially in advancing stages of CKD.[17-20]

Glycemic Control

Maintaining glycemic control near normal levels has been demonstrated to reduce the incidence of diabetic retinopathy and diabetic nephropathy in patients with Type I diabetes mellitus, with similar evidence mounting for Type II diabetes mellitus. Early detection and aggressive treatment of hyperglycemia together with hypertension control delays the onset of nephropathy. In diabetic nephropathy, tight glycemic control to hemoglobin A1C HbA_1c to less than 7.0% has been shown to slow the progression of CKD.[1,21]

Dietary Restriction

Patients with GFRs less than 60 mL/min/1.73 m^2 should have a formal dietary assessment with a nutritionist associated with a kidney team and several assessments when GFR is less than 20 mL per minute in nondialyzed patients. Reasonable protein restriction that avoids protein malnutrition individualized to each patient should be employed although there is no evidence to suggest any impact on the progression of chronic CKD.[22] The restriction of dietary protein to 0.80 g/kg/day and caloric intake of 30 to 35 kcal/kg/day in patients with CKD (GFR < 20 mL/min and not on dialysis) should be employed to prevent malnutrition.[7]

Renal Osteodystrophy

Patients with GFR less than 60 mL/min/1.73 m^2 should be formally evaluated for bone disease and disorders of calcium and phosphorus metabolism. Monitoring phosphate levels, restricting phosphate intake, and using non–aluminum-containing phosphate binders (e.g., calcium carbonate) to maintain near-normal (2.5 to 5.0 mg/dL) phosphorus levels (a calcium phosphorus product of less than 55 mg/dL) will ameliorate some of the negative impact of PTH elevation and calcium lowering and decrease the development of kidney osteodystrophy. Calciferol can be used to suppress PTH secretion, decrease phosphate retention, as well as increase intestinal calcium absorption. Avoid aluminum-containing binders because aluminum accumulation in CKD can contribute to the development of kidney osteodystrophy and altered mental status.[1,23]

Hyperlipidemia

Although the effect of the control of hypercholesterolemia on the progression of CKD is not known, aggressive management of hypercholesterolemia is warranted because dyslipidemias cause glomerular and interstitial injury of the kidney parenchyma in addition to their general adverse impact on the vasculature. The increase association of coronary artery disease (CAD) with patients who have CKD is a compelling reason to lower low-density lipoprotein (LDL) levels to decrease artherogenesis. The goal of therapy is LDL levels less than 100 mg per dL.[24]

Hyperkalemia

When GFR falls below 20 mL per minute (i.e., Stages 4 and 5), potassium intake should be restricted to less than 40 mEq per day. If hyperkalemia occurs, the source of excess potassium intake, decreased potassium excretion, or cellular extrusion of potassium should be eliminated. Further treatment of persistent and severe hyperkalemia is directed at antagonizing myocardial effects by using calcium gluconate, shifting potassium intracellularly with glucose and insulin or with sodium bicarbonate if metabolic acidosis is severe, removal of potassium-sparing diuretics, use of ion-exchange resins—for example, sodium polystyrene sulfate (Kayexalate)—and, in emergency settings, dialysis.

Metabolic Acidosis and Sodium and Water Hemostasis

The acidosis of kidney disease which starts in stage 4 requires the use of sodium bicarbonate when pH is less than 7.3 and serum bicarbonate concentrate (HCO_3-) is less than 22 mEq per L. Sodium restriction should be implemented based on the clinical setting, but 6 to 8 g of sodium per day creates a palatable diet. Water restriction may be required in patients who develop hyponatremia when they consume free water at rates greater than the kidney water clearance rate.

Anemia

Anemia of CKD usually starts at Stage 3. Partial correction of the anemia of CKD, which is caused by insufficient intrinsic erythropoietin production, can be achieved using recombinant human erythropoietin. Partial correction of the anemia of kidney disease improves the quality of life in predialysis and dialysis patients although there is no evidence it changes the progression of CKD. Target for treatment is a hemoglobin 11–12 mg/dL. However, other causes of anemia must also be considered. Concomitant iron deficiency anemia will impair the treatment of the anemia of CKD and will require iron replacement therapy and a search for etiology of iron loss. Monitoring markers, such as ferritin, transferrin percent, and total iron binding capacity, are useful in determining the adequacy of iron stores.[1]

Uremia

Manifestation of uremia could include anorexia, malaise, nausea, vomiting, encephalopathy, severe metabolic hyperkalemia, pericarditis, hypervolemia, and malnutrition, which would require chronic kidney replacement therapy.

Other Measures

All patients with CKD should receive pneumococcal, hepatitis B, and influenza vaccines.

Kidney Replacement Therapy

Consultation with a kidney team should occur early in the predialysis period to promote transition of patients to kidney replacement therapy in a nonurgent setting. This early contact with the kidney team ensures that patients have an appropriate understanding of the types of kidney replacement therapies available to them. The kidney team can also affect the quality of life of the predialysis kidney patient by providing specific patient education and assessments concerning medical treatment of CKD as well as treatment of associated problems (e.g., anemia). Current kidney replacement therapies include hemodialysis, intermittent peritoneal dialysis, continuous ambulatory peritoneal dialysis, and kidney transplantation. The choice of kidney replacement therapy should be individualized based on the availability of a donor kidney, the patient's desire for independence, previous abdominal surgeries, underlying medical conditions, and patient's age.

References

1. Snively CS, Gutierrez C. Chronic kidney disease: prevention and treatment of common complications. *Am Fam Physician* 2004;70(10):1921–1928.
2. Johnson CA, Levey AS, Coresh J, et al. Clinical practice guidelines for chronic kidney disease in adults: Part I. Definition, disease stages, evaluation, treatment and risk factors. *Am Fam Physician* 2004;70(5):869–876.
3. National Kidney Foundation. K/DOQI clinical practice guidelines for chronic kidney disease: evaluation, classification, and stratification. *Am J Kidney Dis* 2002;39(2 Suppl 1):S1–266.
4. Johnson CA, Levey AS, Coresh J, et al. Clinical practice guidelines for chronic kidney disease in adults: Part II. Glomerular filtration rate, proteinuria, and other markers. *Am Fam Physician* 2004;70(6):1091–1100.
5. Prevention of end-stage renal disease due to type 2 diabetes. *N Engl J Med* 2001; 345(12):910–912.
6. Hunsicker LG, Aalder S, Caggula A, et al: Predictors of the progression of renal disease in modification of diet in renal disease study. *Kidney Int* 1997;51(6):1908–1919.
7. Remuzzi G, Schieppati A, Ruggenenti P. Nephropathy in patients with type 2 diabetes. *N Engl J Med* 2002;346(15):1145–1151.
8. Verrellia M. Chronic renal failure. Accessed online November 5, 2004 at www.emedicine.com/med/topic374.htm.
9. Bellomo R, Ronco C, Kellum J, et al. Acute renal failure—definition, outcome measures, animal models, fluid therapy and information technology needs: the second international consensus conference of the acute dialysis quality initiative (ADQI) group. *Crit Care* 2004;8:R204–R212.
10. Schrier RW, Wang W. Acute renal failure and sepsis. *N Engl J Med* 2004;351(2): 159–169.
11. Agrawal M, Swartz R. Acute renal failure. *Am Fam Physician* 2000;61(7):2077–2092.
12. Levey AS. Nondiabetic kidney disease. *N Engl J Med* 2002:347(19):1505–1511.
13. Taylor RB. Chronic renal failure. In: *Manual of family practice*. Boston: Little, Brown; 1997:416–420.
14. Delmez JA, Slatopoisky E. Hyperphosphatemia: its consequences and treatment in patients with chronic renal disease. *Am J Kidney Dis* 1992;19(4):303–317.
15. Russo D, et al. The place of loop diuretics in the treatment of acute and chronic renal failure. *Clin Nephrol* 1992;38(Suppl 1):S69.
16. Brater DC. Diuretic therapy. *N Engl J Med* 1998;339(6):387–395.
17. Issue 9069 the GISEN Group (Gruppo Italiano di Studi Epidemiologici in Nefrologia) Randomized placebo-controlled trial of effect of ramipril on decline in glomerular filtration rate and risk of terminal renal failure in proteinuric, non-diabetic nephropathy. *Lancet* 1997;349:1857–1863.

18. Ruggenenti P, Perna A, Gherardi G, et al. Renoprotective properties of ACE-inhibition in non-diabetic nephropathies with non-nephrotic proteinuria. *Lancet* 1999;354: 359–364.
19. Russo D, Minutolo R, Pisani A, et al. Coadministration of losartan and enalapril exerts additive antiproteinuric effect in IgA nephropathy. *Am J Kidney Dis* 2001;38: 18–25.
20. Parving H, Lehnert H, Brochner-Mortensen J, et al. The effect of irbesartan on the development of diabetic nephropathy in patients with type 2 diabetes. *N Engl J Med* 2001;345(12):870–878.
21. Writing Team for the Diabetes Control and Complications Trial/Epidemiology of Diabetes Interventions and Complications Research Group. Effect of intensive therapy on the microvascular complications of type 1 diabetes mellitus. *JAMA* 2002;287: 2563–2569.
22. Waugh NR, Robertson AM. Protein restriction for diabetic renal disease. *Cochrane Database Syst Rev* 2000:CD002181.
23. Block GA, Port FK. Re-evaluation of risks associated with hyperphosphatemia and hyperparathyroidism in dialysis patients: recommendations for a change in management. *Am J Kidney Dis* 2000;35:1226.
24. Keane WF. The role of lipids in renal disease: future challenges. *Kidney Int* 2000; 75(Suppl 57):S27.

UROLITHIASIS
Michael A. Greene

12.8

GENERAL PRINCIPLES

- **Definition.** Urolithiasis refers to calculi (stones) in any part of the urinary tract.
- **Anatomy.** At the time of diagnosis, stones may be found in any part of the urinary tract, from papillary calcifications to the renal pelvis to the ureters to the bladder.
- **Epidemiology.** The most common stones are the calcium stones, roughly 80% of all stones.[1,2] Calcium stones are more common in men than in women and generally first occur in the third decade.[2] Uric acid stones represent 5% to 8% of all urinary calculi and are more common in men as well; this may be because gout is more common in men and half of all patients with uric acid stones have gout.[2,3] Struvite stones, which represent 10% to 15% of all urinary calculi, are more common in women, as they are often the result of urease-producing bacteria, and urinary tract infections are more common in women than in men.[2] Cystine stones are rare, only 1% of all urinary calculi, and occur in men and women with equal prevalence.
- **Classification.** Stones may be of any composition from calcium (both calcium oxalate and calcium phosphate), uric acid, struvite (magnesium ammonium phosphate), or cystine.
- **Pathophysiology.** Calcium stones are most often calcium oxalate and are thought to form secondary to any process that alters the kidney's delicate balance of prolithogenic factors and factors inhibiting the formation of stones, thus allowing a stone to precipitate out of solution in the urine. Stone-forming factors include the following: increased dietary calcium, increased dietary oxalate, decreased fluid intake, increased dietary protein (specifically from animals), increased dietary sodium, and high-dose vitamin C.[4] In addition to these easily modifiable risk factors, there are other difficult-to-modify risk factors such as hypercalciuria, hyperoxaluria, primary hyperparathyroidism, hypocitraturia, and hyperuricosuria.[1,2] Major risk factors to developing a calcium oxalate stone in addition to the preceding include prior history of a stone (likelihood of forming a second stone 50% by 50 years) and family history of stones due to both the presence of

genetic factors such as idiopathic hypercalciuria and other unknown factors.[1,2] Uric acid stones are thought to arise from saturation of urate crystals in the urine in conditions such as gout as well as simply high serum uric acid levels. Unlike calcium phosphate, calcium oxalate, and struvite stones the kidney does not have inhibitory mechanisms such as citrate in place to stop nucleation and formation of uric acid stones.[2] Struvite stones are thought to form as the result of protease-inhibiting bacteria, especially of the *Proteus* species. These stones can become quite large and have the potential to become staghorn calculi, that is, calculi that fill and obstruct the entire renal pelvis.

- **Mechanism of injury.** Stones in the renal pelvis can be an incidental finding in asymptomatic patients. Stones become painful when they become lodged in the urinary tract and the body attempts to move them along. Contraction of the ureter against the stone produces an extremely painful, colicky pain. Often, there is some bleeding associated with this, found as gross or microscopic hematuria.

DIAGNOSIS

- **Clinical presentation.** Stones present as an acute onset of colicky pain, quite severe. The pain is often unilateral and its location depends on the location of the stone in the urinary tract. The pain is often referred to the cutaneous areas T11–L2 that supply the ureter and is variably described as flank pain down to testicular or labial pain.[5] The pain moves as the stone moves and a person with previous stones may be able to tell if the stone is about to pass. Hematuria is present in up to 90% of stones, but its absence does not rule out a stone.[1] Nausea and vomiting also often accompany the pain.
- **History.** Pain is usually abrupt and severe in onset and often prompts patient to seek care in an emergency room or urgent care center within hours of onset. Patients with previous stones may simply present to their urologist or primary care physician if the symptoms are similar to stones in the past. Pain may be dulled by medications. Pain is colicky in nature, and patients will often find it difficult to find a comfortable position on the exam table and the pain is not made worse by movement.
- **Physical examination.** Patients have a lack of physical exam findings other than the pain. Tachycardia and hypertension as a result of the pain may be present. Fever is absent unless a concurrent urinary tract infection is also present. Flank pain is present, but not made worse by costovertebral angle percussion.
- **Laboratory studies.** Urinalysis looking for blood is the most helpful lab. No other abnormalities should be expected in a case of simple nephrolithiasis.
- **Imaging.** The current gold standard for diagnosis of a kidney stone is helical computed tomography (CT) scan without contrast. The specificity of a helical CT with 3 to 5 mm cuts is 98% and sensitivity 95% in one study, and specificity is consistently close to 100% in various studies.[1] CT imaging will also allow the physician to see any obstruction caused by the stone and will aid in the differential diagnosis of the pain if a stone is not present. Kidney–ureter–bladder (KUB) radiography will not demonstrate the radiolucent stones such as uric acid stones.[2] Intravenous pyelogram (IVP) is the next best choice; however, it is neither as sensitive nor as specific, and it is often a slower test. In a patient with classic symptoms, hematuria, and a lack of stone or other apparent etiology of pain, nephrolithiasis may still be suggested as the stone may simply have passed prior to the study. Such a patient should have relief of pain, however, and continued pain should prompt further investigation.
- **Monitoring.** After a stone has been diagnosed, patients may be asked to strain their urine to watch for passage of the stone.
- **Pathologic findings.** A first-time stone should be collected and sent to the pathology lab for a determination of the type of stone. The type of stone will guide treatment and strategies for prevention of reoccurrence.
- **Differential diagnosis.** An acute onset of flank or abdominal pain has a broad differential diagnosis. Renal cell carcinoma may bleed and clot off a ureter, thus producing renal colic.[1] Other illnesses that may present with vague abdominal pain but are not classically colicky in nature, such as acute appendicitis, diverticulitis, or constipation. Other colicky types of pain include biliary colic or an ectopic pregnancy. Last, renal colic may be faked by patients for secondary gain in those seeking narcotics.[1]

TREATMENT

- **Medications.** Narcotics are often required to control the pain in the acute setting. Nonsteroidal anti-inflammatory drugs (NSAIDs) are also at least as effective as opiates and both indomethacin and keterolac have been used in the acute setting. If a stone is expected to pass, the patient may be sent home with either opiate or NSAIDs for pain control. To aid in the passage of the stone, both calcium-channel blockers and alpha blockers are thought to help decrease ureteral tone and allow a stone to pass more easily.[1]
- **Surgery.** Referral to a urologist is usually reserved for those stones that are thought to have a lower likelihood of passing spontaneously. Size is the single best predictor if a stone will pass, and a stone of 4 mm or less will most likely pass on its own.[1] In one study, stones 5 to 7 mm have a passage rate of 60%.[1] Stones in the distal ureter are also more likely to pass than those proximally. A referral is also warranted if the stone is larger than 5 mm, or if a patient fails a course of 2-week outpatient therapy, or if the pain is unable to be controlled.[1]
- **Nonoperative.** Nonoperative treatments includes shock wave lithotripsy.
- **Operative.** Surgical treatment modalities include laparoscopic or percutaneous removal of the stone done by the urologist.
- **Referrals.** Urology should be involved with failed outpatient therapy, size greater than 5 mm, if acute renal failure is present, or if the pain is unable to be controlled. It should be noted that the time for passage of each stone is variable and there is no set time limit. Stones may pass in a little as a few hours, or it may take weeks. In a patient with a distal stone less than 5 mm with pain well controlled, the physician may well continue to observe for a month or more.
- **Counseling.** Patients should be instructed to strain their urine in order to determine the composition of the stone. Prevention of reoccurrence is based largely on the type of stone. For nearly all stone types, increased fluid intake is the single best suggestion to prevent recurrence. Free water, 2 L or more, taken throughout the day, will help to prevent the conditions in which supersaturation and stone formation will occur. Patients may also be counseled to modify their diet based on the type of stone found. Medications may be suggested to patients based on their metabolic profile and the type of stone, as discussed below.[4]
- **Follow-up.** For patients with recurrent calcium stones, a 24-hour urine should be collected to discover any metabolic conditions that exist that may predispose the patient to kidney stones.[4] Serum calcium and parathyroid hormone (PTH) are also helpful. These will provide the physician with information such as urine volume, urine pH, hypercalciuria, hyperuricosuria, hypocitraturia, or hyperoxaluria as well as primary hyperparathyroidism and distal renal tubular acidosis.[2,4] Thiazide diuretic may reduce the amount of calcium present in the urine. Hypocitraturia may be treated with potassium citrate.[4] Hyperuricosuria may benefit from a low purine diet and prevent the occurrence of calcium oxalate stones.[2] For patients with uric acid stones, allopurinol may be of benefit, as well as alkalinization of the urine with potassium citrate.[1,4] For patients with struvite stones, antimicrobial therapy and surveillance may be beneficial.

SPECIAL CONSIDERATIONS

- **Pregnancy.** Kidney stones can occur during pregnancy. If the pregnancy is early on, an ectopic pregnancy must be ruled out. During pregnancy, there is an increase in calcium excretion in the urine relative to urine volume, so a simple increase in glomerular filtration rate (GFR) cannot account for the increase.[7] Despite this, nephrolithiasis is a rare event. When reviewing imaging studies, it must be kept in mind that the normal pregnant patient will have a dilation of the ureters secondary to progesterone-mediated smooth muscle relaxation. Stones will often pass secondary to this relative dilation.[7] Although opiates can be used during pregnancy, NSAIDs are not routinely used in pregnancy.
- **Children.** There has been some evidence of kidney stones in children treated long term with ceftriaxone.[1] Other drugs noted to cause stones in children are allopurinol, ethylene glycol, methosyflurane, and vitamin D.[8] Metabolic disorders of children that can cause stones are primary hyperoxaluria types I and II.[9]

References
1. Curhan G, Aronson M, Preminger G. Diagnosis and acute management of suspected nephrolithiasis. www.uptodate.com. Accessed February 1, 2007.
2. Nephrolithiasis. In: Braunwald E, et al., eds. *Harrison's principles of internal medicine.* 15th ed. New York: McGraw-Hill, 2001:chap 279.
3. Gout and other crystal arthropathies. In: Braunwald E, et al., eds. *Harrison's principles of internal medicine.* 15th ed. New York: McGraw-Hill, 2001:chap 322.
4. Curhan G. Prevention of recurrent calcium stones. www.uptodate.com. Accessed February 1, 2007.
5. Moore K, Agur A. *Essential clinical anatomy.* 2nd ed. Philadelphia: Lippincott Williams & Wilkins; 2002:185.
6. Preminger G. Management of ureteral calculi. www.uptodate.com. Accessed February 1, 2007.
7. Rose B. Nephrolithiasis during pregnancy. www.uptodate.com. Accessed February 1, 2007.
8. Toxic nephropathy. In: Behrman R, et al., eds. *Nelson textbook of pediatrics.* 15th ed. Philadelphia: W. B. Saunders; 1996:chap 487.
9. In: Behrman R, et al., eds. *Nelson textbook of pediatrics.* 15th ed. Philadelphia: W.B. Saunders; 1996:chap 71.7.

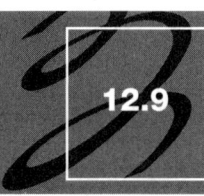

12.9 URINARY INCONTINENCE
Mary McDonald, Sarah Parrott

BACKGROUND

Urinary incontinence (UI), an involuntary, unintended leakage of urine, is a common condition affecting 13 million adults in the United States, with prevalence increasing with age. Although not a lethal condition, it is associated with great medical costs, increased risk of skin breakdown, falls, low self-esteem, social isolation, and depression. The average cost per incontinent individual in the United States is $1848 per year, primarily for incontinence supplies.

GENERAL PRINCIPLES

The cause of UI can typically be determined by the primary care provider through a thorough history and targeted physical exam. Diagnostic studies may be indicated for more complicated cases of UI, but imaging is not routinely recommended in the initial therapy. The detailed history, alone, is often telling enough to formulate a plan of care. However, the physician must remember to ask about this common condition as embarrassment associated with UI may interfere with patients volunteering this information.

Classification

The classification of UI is based on the associated pathophysiologic abnormality and patients may have features of any mixture of these types.

- **Transient UI** has abrupt onset and resolves when the underlying condition is treated. The causes of transient UI can be remembered by the mnemonic DIAPERS (delirium, infection, atrophic urethritis, pharmaceutical, excessive urinary output, restricted mobility, and stool impaction).
- **Chronic UI** can be divided into four types: Stress UI, urge UI, overflow UI, and functional UI.
  - **Stress UI** occurs when pressure within the bladder exceeds bladder sphincter pressures. These commonly occur during times of increased intra-abdominal pressure such

as with **sneezing, coughing, or changing sitting/standing positions.** Patients will describe loss of small volumes of urine and **postvoid residual volumes are usually normal (<50 mL).** Stress UI is the **most common** type and affects approximately 35% of those with UI. This common urinary complaint is essentially a sphincter disorder caused by **pelvic floor muscular relaxation** or sphincter/bladder outlet incompetence from prior instrumentation (i.e., obstetrical repair) or prostate surgery.

- A **simple bedside test** to demonstrate stress UI involves asking the patient to cough or "bear down" in supine and standing positions with the bladder filled to capacity. **Leakage of urine** indicates some degree of stress UI. The initial treatment strategy for men and women with stress UI is the **pelvic floor strengthening, or "Kegel" exercises.**
- **Pharmacologic therapy** for stress UI is currently limited. Although topical estrogen is widely used to increase urethral thickness and sensitive alpha-adrenergic receptors in the urethral sphincter, a meta-analysis of studies of estrogen effect on stress UI found no improvement in urine loss. This lack of evidence on efficacy and concerns about estrogen supplementation posed by the Women's Health Initiative make **estrogen a poor choice for the treatment of stress UI.**
- Treatments reserved for those who do not respond to pelvic floor training include placement of a **pessary** to support the bladder neck or **referral to a urogynecologic surgeon** for surgical bladder neck suspension or artificial sphincter implantation.

■ **Urge incontinence** is the leakage of often large amounts of urine and the **inability to delay voiding after the sensation of bladder fullness** is detected. Like stress UI, urge UI typically involves **normal postvoid residual volumes.** This type of UI is often associated with **neurologic disorders,** such as dementia or cerebrovascular disease. Most patients with UI, however, do not have a neurologic disease and this type is the most common form of UI experienced by older adults. This disorder is due to **detrusor hyperactivity.**
- **Pharmacologic therapy** for urge UI focuses on **anticholinergic medications,** which decrease the strength of detrusor contractions. Available anticholinergic medications include oxybutynin (Ditropan, Oxytrol) and tolderodine (Detrol). Pharmacologic therapy is limited by anticholinergic side effects, such as **dry mouth, delirium, and constipation.**
- **Nonpharmacologic therapies** for urge UI have yielded some success.
- **Scheduled toileting** at increasing intervals can aid in increasing compliance in the bladder over time. Patients can be instructed to control detrusor urge by learning to sit still and allow the bladder contraction to pass, typically less than 60 seconds, and only then move to the restroom to void. **Electrical therapy** with a sacral nerve stimulator inserted into the tissue of the lower back or buttocks may improve UI by stimulating the S3 sacral nerve and decrease detrusor muscle contractility.

■ **Overflow UI** is the frequent or continuous leakage from mechanical forces over a distended/full bladder or from other effects of urinary retention on bladder or sphincter function. **Postvoid residuals are usually high (>100 mL).** This type of UI is often a consequence of **bladder outlet obstruction** from prostatic enlargement.
- Another cause of overflow UI is **bladder hypoactivity,** referred to as **"neurogenic bladder."** This is most commonly encountered in patients with spinal cord injury, long-standing **diabetes mellitus, or vitamin B_{12} deficiency.**
- The target of medicinal therapy is relaxation of the internal urethral sphincter with **alpha-adrenergic-blocking agents.** Available alpha-blockers include terazosin (Hytrin), doxazosin (Cardura), tamsulosin (Flomax). **Orthostatic hypotension** is the typical limiting side effect of the alpha-blockers and may be less problematic with the more selective tamsulosin than the other agents.
- **Transurethral resection of the prostate** may be warranted for patients who do not respond well to pharmacologic treatment or who are limited by orthostasis.
- **Anticholinergic medications** may induce a hypoactive bladder and **medication review is crucial.** The large, hypotonic bladder continuously leaks urine. **Decompression with an indwelling Foley catheter** for 7 to 14 days may allow the

bladder to resume some contractile activity. This type of overflow UI **responds poorly to pharmacologic therapies.** Patients may successfully manage their voids by being taught to do **intermittent straight catheterization** several times a day. A less desirable course of therapy is the **insertion of a chronic indwelling catheter.**

■ **Functional UI** occurs in patients with **normal bladder function from some extrinsic cause.** Detrusor and sphincter function are intact, but the patient is either **unable to recognize the urge to void or is physically unable to get to the toilet on time.**

• **Debility, dementia, delirium, and cerebrovascular disease** are common causes of functional UI. There is **no available pharmacotherapy** for functional UI. Treatment focuses on **scheduled toileting and the use of incontinence supplies.** Chronic indwelling catheterization is not suggested but may be warranted when **perineal or sacral wounds** are present.

References

1. Weiss BD. Diagnostic evaluation of urinary incontinence in geriatric patients. *Am Fam Physician* June, 1998.
2. Moore KN, Gray M. Urinary incontinence in men: current status and future directions. 2004;53(6).
3. Rohner TJ Jr, Rohner JF. Urinary incontinence in America: the social significance. In: O'Donnell, PD, ed. *Urinary incontinence.* St. Louis: Mosby; 1997:4–6.
4. Artibani W, Cerruto M. The role of imaging in urinary incontinence. *BJU Int* 2005;95:699–703.
5. Thomal TM, Plymat KR, Blannin J, et al. Prevalence of urinary incontinence. *BMJ* 1980;281:1243–1245.
6. Kuh D, Cardozo L, Hardy R. Urinary incontinence in middle aged women: childhood enuresis and other lifetime risk factors in a British prospective cohort. *J Epidemiol Commun Health* 1999;53:453–458.
7. Moreleand RB, Brioni JD, Sullivan JP. Emerging pharmacologic approaches for the treatment of lower urinary tract disorders. *J Pharmacol Exp Ther* 2004;308(3).
8. Fantl JA, Cardozo L, McClish DK. Estrogen therapy in the management of urinary incontinence in postmenopausal urinary incontinence. The Continence Program for Women Research Group. *Obstet Gynecol* 1996;88:745–749.
9. Rossouw JE, Anderson GL, Prentice RL, et al. Risks and benefits of estrogen plus progestin in healthy postmenopausal women: principal results from the Women's Health Initiative Randomized Controlled Trial. *JAMA* 2002;288:321–333.

Problems Related to the Female Reproductive System

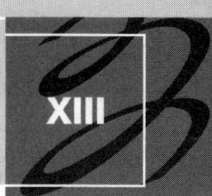

XIII

VAGINITIS AND CERVICITIS
Heather L. Paladine

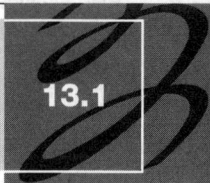

13.1

VAGINITIS

General Principles

Definition

Vaginitis represents the most common gynecologic diagnosis seen in primary care. Symptoms commonly include vaginal discharge, odor, pruritus, or irritation. The majority of cases of vaginitis are caused by bacterial vaginosis, *Candida* infections, and trichomonas. However, family physicians must consider a broad differential diagnosis for vaginitis symptoms, especially when these symptoms are recurrent or resistant to treatment. A common antecedent of these symptoms is disruption of the normal vaginal flora, which can be caused by douching, antibiotics, irritation (including vaginal intercourse), or sexually transmitted infections (STIs).

Bacterial Vaginosis

Bacterial vaginosis (BV), the most common cause of vaginitis symptoms, leads to 10% to 30% of cases of vaginitis in women of childbearing age. BV represents a change in vaginal flora from the usual *Lactobacillus* predominance to an increased growth of *Gardnerella vaginalis* and anaerobes. Although BV occurs almost exclusively in women who have been sexually active, patients can be reassured that these bacteria are not sexually transmitted, except possibly between female partners.

Diagnosis

Clinical Presentation. The classic presentation of BV is a thin, gray, homogeneous vaginal discharge. An unpleasant, fishy odor may be present. Symptoms often recur or are worse following menses or intercourse. In some women, BV may cause endometritis or pelvic inflammatory disease (PID).

Physical Examination and Laboratory Studies. Amsel criteria are used to confirm the diagnosis of BV. Three of four positive criteria are consistent with a 90% chance of BV. The four criteria are as follows:

■ Homogeneous, thin vaginal discharge
■ pH >4.5

■ Positive whiff test (fishy odor with 10% potassium hydroxide, KOH, is added to a sample of the vaginal discharge on a slide)
■ Clue cells on wet mount microscopic examination; because these bacteria are part of the normal flora, culture is not useful for diagnosis

Treatment

Many women with *Gardnerella* overgrowth (often reported on Pap tests) are asymptomatic. These women do not need treatment unless they are at risk for HIV infection (because BV can increase susceptibility to HIV) or undergoing a procedure such as hysterectomy or therapeutic abortion).

Medications. First-line treatments include:
■ Metronidazole gel 0.75% (nightly to the vagina for 5 days)
■ Clindamycin cream 2% (daily to the vagina for 7 days)
■ Oral metronidazole (500 mg twice a day for 7 days)*

Special Considerations
Recurrent Bacterial Vaginosis

■ **Definition.** Three or more episodes within 1 year, is common. Consider a longer course of oral metronidazole or a course of oral clindamycin (300 mg twice a day for 14 days).
■ **Risk management.** Prevention of BV consists of avoidance of triggers that may alter the vaginal flora, particularly douching.

Candida

Candida albicans may also be an asymptomatic part of the normal vaginal flora.

Diagnosis

Clinical Presentation. *Candida vaginitis* presents as a thick, white, "cottage cheese" vaginal discharge. Pruritus of the vagina or vulva is common; women may also experience vulvar swelling or dysuria.

Laboratory Studies

■ Microscopic examination with KOH (reveals hyphae or budding yeast forms)
■ Gram stain (more complicated to perform, will yield the same information as KOH)
■ Fungal culture (should only be considered for resistant symptoms or recurrent episodes defined as more than four episodes per year)*

Treatment

Medications. Over-the-counter (OTC) treatments, such as miconazole or clotrimazole, are available as creams or vaginal suppositories. Terconazole, tioconazole, and butoconazole are additional intravaginal therapies that are available by prescription only. Oral treatment with one 150-mg tablet of fluconazole is also a prescription first-line treatment. Although women may self-treat with OTC medications, the CDC recommends evaluation by a medical provider for symptoms that do not resolve or are recurrent within 2 months.

Recurrent or resistant infections (especially non-*albicans Candida* species) may respond better to prescription rather than OTC treatments. In these situations, treatment with oral ketoconazole (200 mg twice a day for 5 days, or daily for up to 6 months) or vaginal boric acid suppositories (600 mg daily for 14 days) can be used. Women with recurrent candidal infections should be considered for HIV and diabetes testing.

Risk Management

In studies, the percentage of women who develop symptomatic *Candida* vaginitis following antibiotic treatment is variable. Prevention includes avoidance of unnecessary antibiotics, and consideration of prophylactic treatment with antifungal medications in women with a history of frequent candidal infections who require antibiotic treatment. Probiotics

---

*Oral metronidazole may have a lower recurrence rate than vaginal treatment. Women who are treated with oral metronidazole should be cautioned to avoid alcohol intake during treatment because of the risk of a disulfiram-like reaction.
*Cultures may identify women who do not actually have *Candida* infections or who have infections with non-*albicans Candida* species. Vaginal pH is normal (acidic) in women with candidal infections.

(such as active yogurt cultures or *Lactobacillus* capsules) have not been shown to be effective for prevention or treatment of *Candida* infections, although more studies are needed. Use of combination estrogen/progesterone oral contraceptives and diaphragms have been identified as risk factors for candidal infection.

Trichomoniasis

Trichomoniasis is a protozoal infection caused by the organism *Trichomonas vaginalis*. In contrast to BV and *Candida*, *Trichomonas* is an STI.

Diagnosis

Clinical Presentation. Women with *Trichomonas vaginalis* infections typically have a profuse, yellow/green, frothy vaginal discharge with an unpleasant odor. Vulvovaginal irritation can also be present. Many of these infections are asymptomatic.

Laboratory Studies. The diagnosis is usually made by the presence of mobile, flagellated trichomonads on wet mount microscopic examination. The vaginal pH is elevated (>4.5). The classic small punctate hemorrhages on the cervix ("strawberry cervix") are present in less than 25% of infected women.

Pap tests are specific but not sensitive for infections with *Trichomonas*. Therefore, infections that are suspected based on Pap test results should be treated, but a normal Pap test does not rule out infection.

Cultures can be useful when *Trichomonas* infection is suspected despite a normal wet mount result, or to perform sensitivity analysis in recurrent infections.

Treatment

Medications. The standard treatment for *Trichomonas vaginitis* is an oral 2-g dose of metronidazole. Sexual partners should be treated as well. Resistant or recurrent infections may require a higher dose or longer duration of treatment with metronidazole; no other medication is currently available in the United States to treat trichomoniasis. Patients with an allergy to metronidazole should undergo desensitization treatment.

Risk Management. As with other STIs, *Trichomonas* infection can be prevented by abstention from sexual intercourse or a long-term monogamous relationship with an uninfected partner. Male and female condoms reduce the risk of *Trichomonas* transmission.

Atrophic Vaginitis

Atrophic vaginitis is caused by estrogen deficiency and usually occurs in postmenopausal women.

Diagnosis

Clinical Presentation. Like other forms of vaginitis, atrophic vaginitis is often asymptomatic. Symptoms include vaginal soreness or burning, dyspareunia, and occasionally bleeding or spotting.

Physical Examination. The vaginal mucosa is thin, friable, and erythematous. It can appear dry, or patients may have a thin, watery discharge.

Laboratory Studies. Vaginal pH is increased (5 to 7), and parabasal cells (small, round epithelial cells with large nuclei) can be seen on wet mount. Diagnosis is primarily based on clinical suspicion and the absence of causative organisms.

Treatment

Patients can be reassured that mild symptoms are normal and do not require treatment. Dryness can be treated with vaginal lubricants. Topical or oral estrogen replacement is used to treat more bothersome symptoms of atrophic vaginitis. Patients should improve after 1 to 2 weeks of treatment, but symptoms usually recur.

Risk Management. To prevent endometrial carcinoma, in women with uteri, oral progesterone should be used along with systemic estrogen for long-term treatment. The total estrogen dose is higher with vaginal creams than with a vaginal ring or tablet, and may result in systemic absorption. The manufacturers of topical estrogens do not recommend treatment for longer than 6 months.

Irritant/Allergic Reaction
Diagnosis
Diagnosis is based on clinical suspicion and the absence of other infections.

Clinical Presentation. Patients present with vulvar pruritus, erythema, or edema with or without vaginal discharge.

History. Common causes are soaps, detergents, perfumes, spermicides, latex condoms, hot tub or swimming pool chemicals, or synthetic fabrics.

Treatment
Behavioral. Avoidance of the irritant or allergen is the primary therapy.

Medications. Topical steroids may be used to alleviate symptoms while the trigger is being identified.

Risk Management. Patients with atopy or sensitive skin should avoid exposures, such as perfumed soaps or cleansers, to the vulva or vagina. Women with latex allergy can use polyurethane male or female condoms for contraception and STI prevention.

CERVICITIS
General Principles
Definition
Mucopurulent cervicitis is characterized by a purulent cervical discharge. A friable cervix and white blood cells on wet mount or Gram stain are also common, although there is no standard number of white blood cells that confirms the diagnosis. Postcoital bleeding, dyspareunia, and irregular vaginal bleeding are also symptoms of cervicitis. *Chlamydia trachomatis* and *Neisseria gonorrhea* are the most common causes of cervicitis; however, in some cases a specific infection is not identified.

Chlamydia
Chlamydia trachomatis is the most common bacterial STI in the United States. Infections with *C. trachomatis* are common in younger women and adolescents, and the U.S. Preventative Services Task Force recommends routine screening for *Chlamydia* in sexually active women less than 25 years old.

Diagnosis
Clinical Presentation
- As many as 80% of chlamydial infections in women are asymptomatic.
- Chlamydia cervicitis can lead to PID (in about 40% of infected women), ectopic pregnancy, and infertility.

Laboratory Studies. Diagnosis is usually made by a nucleic acid amplification test, although antigen-detection tests and culture are also appropriate. These tests can be done on samples from urine, endocervical swabs, or liquid-based Pap tests. Retesting after treatment is not necessary in nonpregnant women. Retesting within 3 weeks with a nucleic acid amplification test may yield false-positive results due to killed bacteria. However, consider rescreening high-risk patients (such as young women and teens who have previously been infected with *Chlamydia*) because of the high rates of reinfection.

Treatment
Recommended treatments for *Chlamydia cervicitis* include doxycycline (100 mg orally twice a day for 7 days) or azithromycin (1 g orally as a single dose). Alternative regimens with erythromycin, levofloxacin, or ofloxacin are also effective; please see Chapter 19.7 on *Chlamydia* infections for details.

Sexual partners should be treated as well, and women are advised to abstain from intercourse for 7 days after they and their partner have started treatment.

Risk Management. Abstention from sexual intercourse or a long-term monogamous relationship with an uninfected partner will prevent *Chlamydia* infection. Male and female condoms reduce the risk of *Chlamydia* transmission.

Gonorrhea
Diagnosis
Clinical Presentation. Many women who are infected with *Neisseria gonorrhea* are asymptomatic. In addition to mucopurulent cervicitis, gonorrhea can also cause PID, ectopic pregnancy, and infertility.

Laboratory Studies. As with *Chlamydia*, diagnosis of gonorrhea infection is usually made with a nucleic acid amplification test. Retesting after treatment is also not recommended.

Treatment
Medications. Treatment for gonorrhea infection includes any of the following: cefixime (400 mg orally), ceftriaxone (250 mg intramuscularly), ciprofloxacin (500 mg orally), ofloxacin (400 mg orally), or levofloxacin. Because many women with gonorrhea infections are also coinfected with *Chlamydia,* presumptive treatment of both organisms in women found to have gonorrhea infection is appropriate.

Risk Management. As with *Trichomonas* and *Chlamydia,* gonorrhea infection is spread by intercourse with an infected partner. Male and female condoms reduce the risk of transmission.

References
1. ACOG technical bulletin number 226—vaginitis. *Int J Gynecol Obstet* 1996;54:293–302.
2. Owen MK, Clenny TL. Management of vaginitis. *Am Fam Physician* 2004;70(11): 2125–2132.
3. Centers for Disease Control and Prevention. Sexually transmitted diseases treatment guidelines 2002. *MMWR* 2002;51(RR-6).
4. Screening for chlamydial infection: recommendations and rationale. Article originally in *Am J Prev Med* 2001;20(3S):90–94. Agency for Health care Research and Quality, Rockville, MD. Available online at http://www.ahrq.gov/clinic/ajpmsuppl/chlarr.htm.

DYSMENORRHEA AND PREMENSTRUAL SYNDROME
Pamela D. Parker

13.2

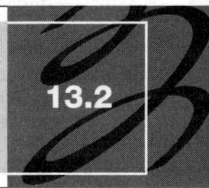

DYSMENORRHEA
General Principles
Definition/Pathophysiology
Dysmenorrhea is cramping pain associated with menstruation. Primary (functional) dysmenorrhea is a painful paroxysmal syndrome that precedes or may accompany menses. It is not associated with pelvic pathology. The pain is thought to be due to elevated levels of prostaglandins. Prior to the onset of menses, cyclic progesterone withdrawal leads to degradation of endometrial cell membranes. The cellular debris is converted to arachadonic acid, which is further metabolized by cyclo-oxygenase (COX) enzymes to form prostaglandins.[1] The prostaglandins stimulate endometrial and uterine smooth muscle contractility and promote myometrial vasoconstriction, resulting in pain.

Epidemiology/Etiology
Primary dysmenorrhea is one of the most common gynecologic complaints, thought to affect from 50% to 90% of women of reproductive age. It is a leading cause of absenteeism for women under 30 years of age and the leading cause of school absences for adolescent women.[2] Secondary (acquired) dysmenorrhea is pain that results from a pelvic abnormality. Possible etiologies include reproductive tract structural anomalies, endometriosis,

adenomyosis, uterine tumors and leiomyomata, polyps, chronic salpingitis, pelvic inflammatory disease, cervical stenosis, irritable and inflammatory bowel syndromes, and urologic disorders. Several authors have correlated dysmenorrhea with smoking cigarettes, high intake of omega-6 fatty acids, nulliparity, depression, and stress. Causation has yet to be proved in rigorous controlled studies.

Diagnosis
Clinical Presentation
Primary dysmenorrhea is characterized by symptom onset around the time of menses. Pain can be colicky or spasmodic and is usually felt in the lower abdomen, back, and thighs. Patients may also experience nausea, vomiting, diarrhea, headache, and dizziness—prostaglandin-mediated symptoms. Menstrual flow may be heavier than normal. Physical examination will be unrevealing. A pelvic examination is not initially required to make the diagnosis, especially in nonsexually active and virginal women. The diagnosis can generally be made based on history alone. If the history and physical examination are inconsistent, or initial therapies are unsuccessful, further evaluation for secondary causes of dysmenorrhea should be pursued.

Treatment
First-line therapy is either a nonsteroidal anti-inflammatory drug (e.g., naproxen, ibuprofen, mefenamic acid-nonspecific COX inhibitors) or a specific COX-2 inhibitor (e.g., celecoxib). These medications act to decrease prostaglandin production, thereby decreasing both menstrual flow and prostaglandin-mediated pain. Other pharmacologic therapies for dysmenorrhea have included oral contraceptives (either traditional or extended cycle dosing), leuprolide, danazol, depot medroxyprogesterone, levonorgestrel-containing intrauterine device, nifedipine, terbutaline, oral guaifenesin,[3] magnesium, thiamine, aspirin, B_{12}, fish oil supplements, and the Japanese herb Toki-shakayaku-san.[4] Topical heat has been shown to be more effective than placebo.[4]

Nontraditional modalities include acupuncture and acupressure, transcutaneous electrical nerve stimulation (TENS) unit therapy, and local application of unidirectional static magnets.[5] Surgery is considered the intervention of last resort. Surgical interventions include laparoscopic uterosacral nerve ablation (LUNA), presacral neurectomy, and hysterectomy. The long-term efficacy of nerve pathway interruption has yet to be proved. Despite the great prevalence of dysmenorrhea, many patients will not report symptomatology unless the provider specifically inquires. Inquiry and intervention can result in significant improvement of quality of life for these women.

PREMENSTRUAL SYNDROME
General Principles
Definition
Premenstrual syndrome (PMS) is a poorly understood psychoendocrine condition characterized by an array of somatic, cognitive, affective, and behavioral disturbances that recur in cyclic fashion during the luteal phase of the menstrual cycle and resolve with the onset of menstruation. More than 150 symptoms have been documented, varying from mild to severe enough to disrupt normal activities and interpersonal relationships. Not all cycles are associated with PMS symptoms and not all premenstrual changes should be labeled PMS.

Pathophysiology/Etiology
PMS represents a biophysiologic, endocrine phenomenon. Altered levels of various hormones have been offered as the cause for premenstrual symptomatology, including estrogen, progesterone, prolactin, growth hormone, thyroid hormone, follicle-stimulating hormone, lutenizing hormone, antidiuretic hormone, insulin, prostaglandin, and cortisol. Studies have failed to confirm any of these as absolutely causative. However, women with PMS are thought to have an altered response to normal gonadal steroids.[6] Endorphins, monoamines, and serotonin have been implicated in altered physiologic and behavioral states in humans.[7] Premenstrual symptomatology and behavior may also stem from social, psychologic, or cognitive dysfunction.

Diagnosis

Clinical Presentation

There is no typical presentation of PMS. Some of the more common physical symptoms include abdominal bloating and cramping, breast tenderness, fluid retention and weight gain, acne, cold sores, fatigue, head and muscle aches. Emotional changes include anxiety, panic, depression, heightened aggressiveness, hostility, food craving, forgetfulness, insomnia, irritability, mood lability, poor concentration, tearfulness, and reduced coping skills. In 2000, the American College of Obstetrics and Gynecology (ACOG) published a practice bulletin of 10 PMS diagnostic criteria. According to ACOG, the diagnosis of PMS requires that a woman have one or more of the affective or somatic symptoms listed. Symptoms must occur during the 5 days before menses (late luteal phase) in each of the three prior menstrual cycles; be relieved within 4 days of the onset of menses; and not recur until at least cycle day 13. The symptoms must be bothersome to the patient. They must exist in the absence of any pharmacologic therapy, hormones, alcohol, or recreational drugs. Finally, all other psychiatric or medical disroders must be excluded.[8] The American Psychological Association (APA) has included severe PMS in the *Diagnostic and Statistical Manual of Mental Disorders* 4th edition text revision (DSM-IV-TR) as an axis I diagnosis called Premenstrual Dysphoric Disorder (PMDD). For the APA diagnosis, a woman must experience 5 or more from a list a of 11 symptoms. As with the diagnosis of PMS, the symptoms must be experienced only in the luteal phase; all other diagnoses must be excluded; and the patient must have experienced them for the majority of cycles within the past year.[8]

History/Physical/Laboratory

A detailed history must be obtained, including inquiries about alcohol, tobacco, and recreational drugs. A complete physical examination must be performed. The need for in-depth neurologic or psychologic evaluation may become apparent. No specific diagnostic test is available for detecting PMS/PMDD. Laboratory investigation should be tailored to the individual patient. For example, complete blood count and thyroid studies should be considered in patients with menorrhagia or chronic fatigue. Charting the menstrual cycle and documenting symptomatology must be done for two to three cycles. Patients write down the symptoms that trouble them most and rate the severity throughout the entire menstrual cycle. Presence of luteal phase symptoms in at least two cycles, lack of follicular phase symptoms, and absence of other specific disease entities strongly suggest the diagnosis of PMS or PMDD.

Treatment

Nonpharmagologic

The clinician must individualize the treatment plan to maximize therapeutic response. Treatment should begin with a 2 to 3 month trial of lifestyle changes while the patient records symptoms. Patients and significant others must be educated about PMS. Stress management strategies should be taught. Sufficient rest should be advocated. Regular aerobic exercise has been demonstrated to alleviate some PMS symptomatology, probably due to endogenous endorphin release. A well-balanced diet with adequate protein, fiber, and complex carbohydrates is essential for everyone's good health. However, these recommendations have not been investigated in rigorous controlled studies. Caffeine, salt, excess sugar, alcohol, and recreational drugs may worsen physical symptoms and emotional lability. Multivitamins, calcium, and magnesium supplements may be helpful. Pyridoxine (vitamin B_6) may reduce fatigue, depression, and irritability in selected women. Doses higher than 50 mg per day have been associated with irreversible neurotoxicity.

Pharmacologic

If premenstrual complaints do not respond to the above, medical therapy can be initiated. Symptom logs assist the clinician in tailoring treatment to individual needs. Prostaglandin inhibitors can relieve headaches, body aches, and dysmenorrhea. Spironolactone 25 to 50 mg bid during cycle days 14 to 28 may reduce fluid retention. Danazol and bromocriptine have been utilized in the past to reduce mastalgia. However, adverse side effects limit their usefulness.

Without menstrual cyclicity, PMS cannot occur.[9] Oral contraceptives, depo-medroxyprogesterone, levonorgestrel-containing intrauterine devices (IUDs), and gonadotropin-releasing hormone agonists have been tried with variable success. Oral contraceptive pills that contain the newer progestin drospirenone (an antimineralocorticoid and antiandrogen) are effective in reducing bloating and mood changes that accompany the placebo pill week. A newer combination contraceptive pill that contains only four (rather than seven) placebo pills is expected to be even more efficacious in this regard.[10] Multiple herbs have been utilized with variable success and safety in treating premenstrual molimina. These include evening primrose oil, black current oil, chaste tree extract, black cohosh, wild yam root, dong quai, kava kava, and St. John's wort. Interactions with other medications the patient might be taking must always be considered.[11]

Selective serotonin-reuptake inhibitors (SSRIs) are the first-line drugs for treating PMDD. Treatment only during the luteal phase has been proved to be as effective as full monthly dosing, with fewer adverse side effects.[12] Alprazolam is an anxiolytic with proven effectiveness for symptoms of premenstrual tension, anxiety, irritability, and hostility. However, its addictive potential makes it a second-line treatment.

Buspirone is an effective anxiolytic that is not addictive.

PMS is a complex disorder of reproductive-aged women. Successful management requires continued communication and collaboration between patient and clinician.

References

1. Harel Z. Cyclooxygenase-2 specific inhibitors in the treatment of dysmenorrhea. *J Pediatr Adolesc Gynecol* 2004;17:75–79.
2. Sultan C, et al. Adolescent dysmenorrhea. Pediatric and adolescent gynecology evidence-based clinical practice. *Endocrinol Dev* (Basel) 2004;7:140–147.
3. Marsden JS, et al. Guaifenesin as a treatment for primary dysmenorrhea. *JABFP* 2004; 17(4):240–246.
4. Proctor ML, Farquar CM. Dysmenorrhoea. *Clin Evidence* 2005;13:2303–2325.
5. Eccles NK. A randomized double-blinded, placebo-controlled pilot study to investigate the effectiveness of a static magnet to relieve dysmenorrhea. *J Altern Complementary Med* 2005;11(4):681–687.
6. Winer SA, Rapkin AJ. Premenstrual disorders. Prevalence, etiology and impact. *J Reprod Med Obstetr Gynecol* 2006;51(4):349–357.
7. Clayton AH, et al. Exploratory study of premenstrual symptoms and serotonin variability. *Arch Women's Ment Health* 2006;9:51–57.
8. Futterman LA, Rapkin AJ. Diagnosis of premenstrual disorders. *J Reprod Med Obstetr Gynecol* 2006;51(4):349–357.
9. Sulak PJ. Ovulation suppression of premenstrual symptoms using oral contraceptives. *Am J Managed Care* 2005;11(16 Suppl):S492–S497.
10. Yonkers KA, et al. The efficacy of a new low-dose oral contraceptive with drospirenone in premenstrual dysphoric disorder. *Obstet Gynecol* 2005;106(3):492–500.
11. Kaur G, et al. Premenstrual dysphoric disorder: a review for the treating practitioner. *Cleveland Clin J Med* 2004;71(4):303–321.
12. Kroll R, Rapkin AJ. Treatment of premenstrual disorders. *J Reprod Med Obstetr Gynecol* 2006;51(4):359–370.

ABNORMAL GENITAL BLEEDING IN WOMEN AND GIRLS

Pepi Granat

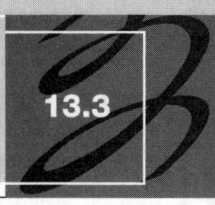

GENERAL PRINCIPLES

Definition
Abnormal genital bleeding is any blood loss from the vaginal or perineal area other than the individual menstrual pattern of flow of a premenopausal girl or woman, or the expected cyclic hormonal bleeding in a postmenopausal woman taking hormones.

Anatomy
Bleeding coming from structures surrounding the vagina, rectum, and perineum must be differentiated from uterine bleeding originating from the cervical os. Pregnancy, structural pelvic pathology such as fibroids or polyps, benign and malignant tumors, anovulation, and coagulopathies are leading causes.

Epidemiology
The incidence of genital bleeding from all causes is unclear, but abnormal uterine bleeding (AUB) accounts for nearly one third of all gynecologic visits, mostly at menarche or perimenopause. In postmenopausal women an estimate of uterine bleeding in the first 12 months is 409 per 1,000 person-years, but only 42 per 1,000 person-years 3 years postmenopause.

Classification
Urgent or Emergent
- **Nonuterine.** See below for nonurgent
- **Uterine.** See below for nonurgent

Nonurgent
- **Nonuterine.** The actual source of the bleeding may not be obvious. A laceration of the cervix, or of the vagina, especially if high in a fornix, may appear to be uterine bleeding. Urinary, rectal, or vulvar bleeding may be mistaken for vaginal bleeding.
    - Vulvar or vaginal: Infection, laceration, tumor, foreign body
    - Extravaginal: Perineal, urinary, rectal
    - Systemic/medical: Bleeding diathesis, thrombocytopenia; von Willebrand disease; liver, renal, endocrine disease

- **Uterine.** Age-grouping is important
    - Age: Premenarche—any bleeding is abnormal
    - Age: 13 to 40
        - The clinician should consider pregnancy-related causes, especially ectopic pregnancy, even when bleeding is light or moderate, and even in young and perimenopausal women. A common response of patients is, "I couldn't be pregnant; I just had my period." Once pregnancy is ruled out, the diagnosis of dysfunctional uterine bleeding (DUB), although one of exclusion, does not require total certainty before reasonable treatment for anovulation is implemented.
        - Anovulatory bleeding (DUB) is common and may be treated as such without an exhaustive search for all other causes initially, as long as there is a normal medical history, pregnancy test, complete blood count (CBC), Pap smear, and a normal bimanual pelvic examination. Although not all uterine bleeding in this group will prove to be DUB, serious pathology in the face of normal findings is unlikely. If hormonal manipulation fails, a more complete workup can follow. Over age 35, an endometrial biopsy should be done.

469

- Age: 40 and older—higher index of suspicion of neoplasm. A very different scenario pertains to the peri- and postmenopausal woman, in whom bleeding must be investigated before anovulation can be assumed.
- Age: Postmenopausal—neoplasm until proven otherwise, unless known hormonal cause.

Pathophysiology/Etiology

- Pregnancy should be considered.
- Anovulation is a common cause (DUB, defined as uterine bleeding associated with anovulation, in the absence of other pathology):
  - Physiologic: Adolescence (although 4% to 20% of adolescents have a coagulopathy underlying their abnormal bleeding), perimenopause (although abnormal bleeding must be considered neoplastic or hyperplastic until proven otherwise), lactation, pregnancy.
  - Pathologic: Hyperandrogenic anovulation (e.g., polycystic ovary syndrome, congenital adrenal hyperplasia, androgen-producing tumors), hypothalamic dysfunction (e.g., secondary to anorexia nervosa), hyperprolactinemia, hypothyroidism, primary pituitary disease, premature ovarian failure, and iatrogenic factors (e.g., secondary to radiation therapy or chemotherapy).
  - Iatrogenic or treatment-induced:
    - Estrogen withdrawal: Occurs after removal or irradiation of ovaries, or after giving and then withdrawing estrogen to a person without ovaries (midcycle bleeding can be due to preovulation drop in estrogen).
    - Estrogen breakthrough: Due to stimulation of endometrium from unopposed low- or high-level estrogen. (Low-dose estrogen produces intermittent light spotting; high-dose estrogen yields amenorrhea followed by profuse bleeding. Cyclic progesterone corrects this.)
    - Progestin withdrawal: Occurs only if there has been prior estrogen priming.
    - Progestin breakthrough: Can occur when endometrium becomes so atrophic that lack of estrogen effect yields too little and too ragged a lining for synchronous cellular events. (Estrogen replacement therapy can restore responsiveness. This occurs after months on oral contraceptives (OCs) or depoprogesterone. Adding estrogen for a week usually corrects the problem.)
- Noncyclic uterine bleeding (non-DUB)
  - Uterine leiomyoma, leiomyosarcoma, endometrial polyp(s)
  - Endometrial hyperplasia or carcinoma
  - Cervical or vaginal neoplasia
  - Endometritis, adenomyosis
  - Bleeding associated with pregnancy (threatened or incomplete abortion, trophoblastic disease, ectopic pregnancy)
  - Bleeding associated with the puerperium (retained products of conception, placental polyps, subinvolution of the uterus)
  - Coagulopathies (von Willebrand disease, platelet abnormalities, thrombocytopenic purpura)
  - Iatrogenic causes, medications, and devices—intrauterine devices (IUDs), diaphragms, pessaries
  - Systemic diseases (liver, renal, thyroid, other endocrine)
- Infection, laceration or contusion, tumor, foreign body
- Perineal, rectal, urinary disease
- Systemic medical causes: Bleeding diatheses, especially thrombocytopenia; von Willebrand disease; liver, renal, endocrine disease
- Ovulatory excessive bleeding

DIAGNOSIS/TREATMENT

Clinical Presentation

Urgent or emergent bleeding: Most common cause is pregnancy or its complications.

Assessment

When taking a history, consider ectopic pregnancy, uncontrolled hemorrhage, trauma, large degenerating fibroids, and train staff to be sufficiently alert to query and triage a patient who calls or arrives with bleeding.

Severity

■ **Rate of flow.** How heavy is the bleeding? Pad counts are unreliable because of differences of absorbency but may give a rough estimate. The patient's own opinion is probably more valid. When did it start? Is the blood bright red or dark, with or without clots? If it is heavier than she has ever seen it, if it is flowing, if brighter red than menstrual blood, and if there are clots or pieces of tissue, there might be significant hemorrhage and the patient should not wait even a short time. If she cannot get to the office immediately she should go to the nearest emergency room, by ambulance or 911. She should be instructed to retrieve any tissue passed for the purpose of analysis.

■ **Amount of flow.** A rough estimate of blood loss can be made by asking how much more bleeding than a usual period she has had since onset. (Normal menstrual blood loss is 20 to 80 cc.)

Associated Symptoms

Has there been fever, dizziness, abdominal pain, diarrhea? Any of these could signal associated pelvic infection or abscess, shock, severe loss of blood volume, dehydration, other intra-abdominal pathologic process, or bleeding tendency.

Likely Causes

Has this ever happened before? What have previous pelvic exams revealed, such as known fibroids? Does she have an IUD? Ask about abuse and trauma. What was the date of last period, or of any bleeding? Is pregnancy a possibility? Has she performed a proprietary pregnancy test? Such tests are quite reliable and results, with dates, should be noted. Any history of sexual activity presupposes pregnancy; even when the possibility is denied, a pregnancy test should be done. Postmenopausal women must be asked date of last bleeding. Find out present and recent past medication and hormone regimens (including adherence), with names and dosages. Any use of a medication, including drops, creams, and/or "natural" remedies, should be noted. Hormonally active nostrums, such as ginseng, found in drug stores, health food stores, and mail-order or Internet pharmacies, can cause bleeding.

Physical Examination

Check vital signs; do abdominal, perineal, vaginal, pelvic, and rectal exam. The exam must meticulously pinpoint the exact source, which may not be obvious.

Management

Acute, heavy bleeding requires close observation, accurate determination of the source and likely cause, and immediate therapy. Hospitalization, hydration, and transfusion may be required.

Medical

If the bleeding is uterine, intravenous conjugated estrogen (Premarin) 25 mg can be given acutely every 4 hours for 24 hours, or until bleeding stops. Also, one can give Premarin orally, 10 to 20 mg per day in divided doses. Antiemetics should be given for nausea.

Surgical

After one or two doses, if bleeding has not slowed or if patient is unstable, intrauterine balloon placement for tamponade, or dilatation and curettage (D&C) should follow.

Follow-Up

After bleeding stops, combination OC pills without placebo break, or a progestin alone, should be given for 3 to 4 months. Then cyclic OCs can be given. Anemic patients should receive iron.

Clinical Presentation–Nonurgent:

Assessment

Initial evaluation as with urgent bleeding.

History and Physical Examination

A detailed, sensitive history and physical exam with good exposure for the speculum exam, and optimal palpation of pelvic organs using bimanual and rectovaginal techniques, is crucial to finding serious and treatable pathology. A Pap smear and breast exam should be done. Obesity and hirsutism should be noted. An estimate of prior hormonal influences should be made in an attempt to classify the type of anovulation.

Basic Laboratory Tests

Should include pregnancy test (β-human chorionic gonadotropin), complete blood count (CBC) with platelets and differential, sedimentation rate or C-reactive protein, prothrombin time, partial thromboplastin generation time, thyroid-stimulating hormone, and, if indicated, ristocetin cofactor for von Willebrand disease. These will suffice to make the presumptive diagnosis and initiate treatment.

Examination Findings

Examination Findings may suggest other studies, such as endometrial biopsy or colposcopy (easily performed by many family physicians), hysteroscopy, pelvic and/or endovaginal sonography (TVS), hysterosalpingography, and saline infusion hysterosonography (SIS), usually performed by radiologists or gynecologists. Most procedures carry known risks, benefits, and advantages, and are chosen based on individual needs of the specific patient and circumstance.

Ultrasonography

If is performed in a postmenopausal woman, an endometrial biopsy is mandatory when the endometrial stripe is greater than 8 mm. An endometrial height of less than 4 mm nearly rules out hyperplasia. Between 4 and 8 mm, other features of the clinical presentation (such as persistent bleeding) and the patient's (and physician's) tolerance for uncertainty must guide the decision regarding biopsy. Usually, 5 mm is the cutoff point at which biopsy is considered essential. The situation is different in premenopausal women, in whom endometrial findings on ultrasound depend on the cycle.

Management

Treatment for specific pathology depends on the underlying cause and may be managed by the family doctor or require referral to a gynecologist, endocrinologist, or gynecologic oncologist.

Medical Management

Ovulatory, heavy periods (menorrhagia) may be managed with antiprostaglandins, or even with antifibrinolytic agents such as tranexamic acid or aminocaproic acid (Amicar). If, by exclusion or judgment, DUB is the working diagnosis, either an OC or cyclic progesterone can be used. Monophasic OCs can be used continuously, with 1-week breaks every 3 months. Natural micronized progesterone, 200 mg, can be given for 12 to 14 days, monthly. Medroxyprogesterone or norethindrone in doses of 5 or 10 mg per day (or even higher initially to stop the bleeding) for 12 to 14 days can also be used. Duration of treatment depends on circumstances of bleeding, fertility or contraceptive needs, and the age of the patient.

Surgical Management

Between medical control and the definitive cure of hysterectomy there is a wide range of options, including myomectomy, endometrial ablation via a variety of techniques, progesterone IUDs (LNG-IUS), and uterine artery embolization.

Special Considerations

■ **Structural or anatomical causes concurrent with DUB.** Fibroids, especially when large, can degenerate and be the primary source of bleeding. But fibroids are common and their presence, especially if small, does not mean that they caused the bleeding. DUB may still be the primary diagnosis, as may cancer. DUB or infection can occur with an IUD in place, which may be retained if treatment of the underlying cause is successful.

■ **Postmenopausal bleeding**
  ■ For the woman not on hormones the decision is clear. She needs a thorough investigation of the cause of the bleeding, including endometrial sampling to rule out endometrial cancer. Hysteroscopy, TVS, or SIS may be needed.
  ■ For the woman on hormones an individual decision must be made based on her prior problems and her hormone regimen.

- Patients taking unopposed estrogen should be told that they must have endometrial biopsies yearly.
- Although continuous or monthly progesterone is protective, endometrial cancer is not entirely ablated by its addition to the estrogen regime; it must be ruled out by endometrial biopsy in the face of persistent bleeding.
- Patients taking progesterone less than monthly should have endometrial sampling if bleeding is off schedule. It is reasonable to obtain an endometrial sample without prior ultrasonographic examination; the procedure is simple and yields definitive tissue, although it can also miss areas.
- Patients taking tamoxifen are at higher risk for endometrial cancer; those taking raloxifene are at lower risk.

- **Perimenopause.** Although hormonal therapy remains controversial, it is now common in perimenopause. Decision-making must take into account the special circumstances of the bleeding. In some cases, one can treat the hormonal transition as DUB or hormonal bleeding, before doing more testing. In others, endometrial sampling and/or imaging is advised. It is better to err on the side of sampling/imaging.
- **Cervical stenosis.** If endometrial biopsy is impossible, an ultrasound scan with acceptable endometrial height (less than 4 to 5 mm) may suggest therapy for DUB. If the endometrial height is greater than 8 mm, referral to a gynecologist (with probability of D&C) is indicated.

References

1. Albers JR, Hull SK, Wesley RM. Abnormal uterine bleeding. *Am Fam Physician* 2004;69:1915–1926.
2. Nicholson WK, Ellison SA, Grason H, et al. Patterns of ambulatory care use for gynecologic conditions: a national study. *Am J Obstet Gynecol* 2001;184:523–530.
3. Munro MG. Dysfunctional uterine bleeding: advances in diagnosis and treatment. *Curr Opin Obstet Gynecol* 2001;13:475–489.
4. Astrup K, Olivarius Nde F. Frequency of spontaneously occurring postmenopausal bleeding in the general population. *Acta Obstet Gynecol Scand* 2004;83:203.
5. American College of Obstetricians and Gynecologists (ACOG). Management of anovulatory bleeding. Washington, DC: American College of Obstetricians and Gynecologists (ACOG); 2000 Mar:9 pp (ACOG practice bulletin; no. 14). Current as of December 2005, based on a review of literature published that is performed every 18 to 24 months. Available online at www.guideline.gov.
6. Banu NS, Manyonda IT. Alternative medical and surgical options to hysterectomy. *Best Pract Res Clin Obstet Gynaecol* 2005;19(3):431–449.
7. Speroff L, Glass RH, Kase NG. Clinical gynecologic endocrinology and infertility. 6th ed. Philadelphia: Lippincott Williams & Wilkins; 1999:575–593.
8. Clark TJ, Barton PM, Coomarasamy A, et al. Investigating postmenopausal bleeding for endometrial cancer: cost-effectiveness of initial diagnostic strategies. *BJOG Int J O&G* 2006;113(5):502–510.

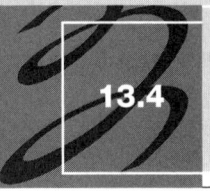

13.4 PAP SMEAR EVALUATION FOR CERVICAL CANCER
Ed Evans

GENERAL PRINCIPLES

Definition
The Pap smear is the primary detection tool for cervical cancer. Since its widespread acceptance following publication of Papanicolaou and Traut's paper in 1943,[1] developed countries using the Pap smear as screening have had dramatic drops in rates of cervical cancer.

Pathophysiology
The cervix is the inferior extension of the uterus. The vaginal (lower) portion is covered by squamous epithelium peripherally and centrally to a point referred to as the squamo-columnar junction (SCJ), where columnar (glandular) epithelium progresses from that point inward through the cervical os and into the body of the uterus. At birth, the SCJ is effaced more laterally on the vaginal portion of the cervix compared to the finding in a nonpregnant adult. A process known as squamous metaplasia results in the change from columnar to squamous epithelium between the original SCJ and the "new" SCJ. This area is referred to as the transformation zone (TZ). Virtually all cervical dysplasia and cancer occurs within the limits of the TZ, as it is the most "mitotically active" region of the cervix.

Risk factors for development of cervical cancer include human papillomavirus (HPV) exposure, early age of initiation of sexual activity, multiple sexual partners, cigarette smoking, and *in utero* diethylstilbestrol (DES) exposure. Cervical cancer results in approximately 200,000 deaths annually worldwide, about 4500 of whom are in the United States.[2] There is a dramatic difference (approximately threefold) between more and less developed countries in the incidence of cancer, primarily due to the availability of screening via the Pap smear.

It is now well established that HPV is the causative agent of cervical cancer. This sexually transmitted virus exists in over 100 "strains," most of which are not felt to be oncogenic. The known "high-risk" HPV subtypes are strains 16, 18, and about 10 others. Types 6, 11, and others are implicated as causes of condyloma. The other known risk factors for cervical cancer are known to accelerate the oncogenicity of the high-risk subtypes; in addition, acquiring a new partner who exposes the patient to new low-risk strains is known to accelerate the risk of cancer in a patient who already has high-risk strains of HPV.

HPV is transmitted when infected genital epithelial cells desquamate during intercourse and bind to basal keratinocytes in areas of microtrauma on the sexual partner. The immune response of the host is usually inadequate to kill the virus, because the virus does not kill the infected cells. It is believed that 20% of infections are handled through humoral immunity, and approximately 20% of infected patients have persistent infection despite therapy. The majority of patients, therefore, respond to therapy for warts or dysplasia with a lasting clinical remission. Patients with persistent infection may progress to low-grade disease, high-grade (cervical intraepithelial neoplasia, or CIN) disease, or invasive cancer.

DIAGNOSIS

Clinical Presentation
The great majority of patients who present with cervical cancer have had no screening for several years. The precursor conditions are imminently treatable when caught in any stage prior to invasive disease. Other than presenting for routine annual screening, patients may present with intermenstrual or postcoital bleeding, or have been referred for colposcopy because another provider has visualized a gross lesion.

History

Important aspects of the history, in addition to elucidation of risk factors mentioned above, include documentation of last menstrual period (LMP), any history of prior abnormal Pap or HPV testing, and history of prior treatment(s) for cervical disease. In older patients who may be menopausal, current or former hormone replacement therapy should be documented.

Physical Examination

Screening should begin at age 18 or at the time of first sexual intercourse, then every 1 to 3 years, depending on risk factors, up to age 65. Direct visualization of the cervix with a speculum exam is necessary for collection of a sample for Pap smear. Patients should avoid douching or intercourse for 24 hours prior to the procedure. The speculum should be warmed with water; the new thin-layer preps do not require avoidance of lubrication for insertion of the speculum, but most pathologists still feel it should be avoided when possible. Note should be taken of any bleeding that is spontaneous or induced by contact with the instruments used to collect the sample. Any lesions, such as leukoplakia and Nabothian cysts, should be documented. A through bimanual exam is a standard part of an annual evaluation, with attention to size and position of the uterus and any nodularity or masses noted in the parauterine and adnexal regions.

Laboratory Studies

Thin-layer ("thin-prep") cytology is now the standard collection technique for Pap smear. This specimen has the same sensitivity as older, conventional smears and also allows for detection of HPV in the same sample. The "broom" is centered over the cervical os and twirled with pressure against the cervix two full rotations, and then deposited into the collection medium. In patients who have had hysterectomy, the vaginal cuff is sampled. It is standard care now to request testing for high-risk HPV subtypes if "ASCUS" is found in the sample (discussed further under Pathologic Findings).

Pathologic Findings

Adequacy of the collection is noted on the pathologist's report; if endocervical cells are not detected in a patient who has a cervix, the collection should be repeated. The Bethesda system adopted in 2001[4] includes the following:

■ **Statement of adequacy of the sample**
■ **A general categorization** of the findings, benign or malignant
■ **Descriptive diagnoses** that may include benign changes (reactive, or secondary to infection). Epithelial changes may be squamous or glandular. The squamous components include atypical squamous cells of undetermined significance (ASCUS); HPV changes including "koilocytotic atypia"; low-grade squamous intraepithelial lesion (LSIL); high-grade squamous intraepithelial lesion (HSIL); and squamous cell cancer (SCC). The glandular components include atypical glandular cells of undetermined significance (AGUS), adenocarcinoma *in situ* (AIS), and adenocarcinoma.

TREATMENT

Nonoperative

Patients with Pap smears showing ASCUS with high-risk HPV subtypes present, and with LSIL, HSIL, or SCC need colposcopic evaluation. ASCUS without high-risk HPV present may continue annual cytology surveillance.[5] It is anticipated in the near future that primary screening will be accomplished with high-risk HPV testing, with simultaneous Pap and colposcopy as the first diagnostic tool in patients who are positive. Patients with glandular cell abnormalities (AGUS, AIS, and adenocarcinoma) usually benefit from referral to a gynecological oncologist, as the source of the abnormal cells could be endometrial, tubal, ovarian, or even from nongynecological abdominal metastasis.

Operative

After colposcopy with appropriate biopsies, patients with cervical intraepithelial neoplasia (CIN) 1, 2, or 3 may be appropriately managed with cervical cryotherapy or loop electrosurgical excision procedure (LEEP). If endocervical curettage (ECC) was done and was abnormal, the patient should be referred for consideration of cold knife cone (CKC) biopsy.

Counseling

With the ease and efficacy of modern techniques for the management of Pap smear abnormalities, virtually all patients can be assured that they will never develop cervical cancer if they maintain appropriate follow-up visits for any abnormalities. Counseling about the risk factors for accelerating their risk of cancer (new contacts, smoking) is appropriate.

Follow-Up

Telephone follow-up with Pap smear results is usually appropriate. Patients should be specifically told when their next screening is due. Guidelines for follow-up Pap, HPV testing, and/or colposcopy are well established by the American Society for Colposcopy and Cervical Pathology (ASCCP).[6]

Complications

Other than transient discomfort and occasional mild spotting, collection of Pap smears is not associated with any complications.

References

1. Papanicolaou GN, Traut HF. *Diagnosis of uterine cancer by the vaginal smear.* New York: Commonwealth Fund; 1943.
2. Ferris DG, Cox JT, et al. Cervical cancer: epidemiology and etiology. *Modern colposcopy textbook and atlas.* 2nd ed. Dubuque, IO: Kendal/Hunt; 2004.
3. Solomon D, Davey D, Kurman R, et al. The Bethesda System 2001: terminology for reporting the results of cervical cytology. *JAMA* 2002;287:2114–2119.
4. Wright TC Jr, Cox JT, et al. 2001 Consensus guidelines for the management of women with cervical cytological abnormalities. *J Low Gen Tract Dis* 2002;6:127–143.
5. Ferris DG, et al. Cervical screening and management of the abnormal pap. *Modern colposcopy textbook and atlas.* 2nd ed. Dubuque, IO: Kendal/Hunt; 2004:chap 18.

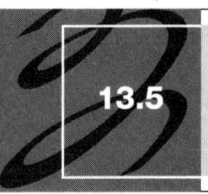

13.5 PELVIC INFLAMMATORY DISEASE
Martin A. Quan

GENERAL PRINCIPLES

Definition

Acute pelvic inflammatory disease (PID) is an ascending infection of the female genital tract involving the uterus, fallopian tubes, ovaries, and adjacent pelvic structures.

Epidemiology

- Up to 1.5 million American women are diagnosed and treated for acute PID each year.[1]
- Direct and indirect medical costs of PID and its sequelae in the United States are estimated at $10 billion per year.[2]

Pathophysiology

- PID arises from the ascent of microorganisms from the vagina and cervix into the upper female genital tract.
- Although PID commonly stems from a cervicitis caused by **Neisseria gonorrhoeae** or **Chlamydia trachomatis,** there is evidence that an imbalance in the vaginal ecosystem, such as that seen in **bacterial vaginosis,** may also play a role in initiating the ascending infection.[3,4]

Etiology

- Microorganisms recovered from the upper genital tract of women with PID include **C. trachomatis, N.** **gonorrhoeae,** and anaerobic and aerobic bacteria of the endogenous vaginal flora, including **Prevotella** species, **Bacteroides** species, **Peptostreptococcus,** aerobic **Streptococcus, Gardnerella vaginalis, Haemophilus influenzae,** and enteric Gram-negative rods.
- Epidemiologic risk factors that identify a patient at increased risk for acute PID include age less than 25 years, sexarche prior to age 16 years, multiple sexual partners, history of a sexually transmitted disease (including PID), the postinsertion period in intrauterine device (IUD) users, vaginal douching more than three or four times per month, and the presence of bacterial vaginosis.[2,5,6]

DIAGNOSIS

- As a result of the difficulty of diagnosis and its serious consequences if left untreated, guidelines for its diagnosis developed by the U.S. Centers for Disease Control and Prevention (CDC) reflect a lowering of the diagnostic threshold.[7]
- Once competing diagnoses are adequately excluded in a woman at risk for sexually transmitted diseases (STDs), the CDC recommends that a provisional diagnosis of PID be made and a therapeutic trial of antibiotics be initiated in patients who meet one or more of the following criteria on pelvic examination:
  - Cervical motion tenderness
  - Uterine tenderness
  - Adnexal tenderness
- Although not required, corroborating diagnostic laboratory, imaging, and surgical procedures should be sought in patients with an unclear diagnosis, severe symptoms, or who fail to respond to therapy.

Clinical Presentation

PID can present with a wide spectrum of nonspecific clinical symptoms and signs, ranging in degree from mild to severe.

History

- Lower abdominal pain usually described as constant and dull and of less than 14-day duration is the most common complaint reported by patients with acute PID.
- Other manifestations include abnormal vaginal discharge, abnormal vaginal bleeding, gastrointestinal upset, and dysuria.
- Right upper quadrant pain secondary to **perihepatitis (Fitz-Hugh-Curtis syndrome)** is seen in up to 10% to 15% of patients.[3]

Physical Examination

- Cervical motion tenderness and adnexal tenderness (unilateral in up to 20% of cases) are the physical findings most frequently elicited in patients with PID.
- Rebound tenderness is present in two thirds of patients, and an adnexal mass or fullness in 16% to 49% of patients.
- Although a temperature of 38.3°C or higher supports the diagnosis, it is important to be aware that fever is a variable finding present in 24% to 60% of patients.[5]

Laboratory Studies

- White blood count. A leukocytosis is present only 50% of the time.
- Erythrocyte sedimentation rate (ESR). Although classically elevated in PID, the ESR is normal (less than 15 mm/hour) in 25% of patients.[8]
- An elevated C-reactive protein (CRP) is found in 70% of patients with PID.[9]
- Examination of the male partner for the presence of urethritis can be a source of confirmatory evidence for the diagnosis of PID in 50% of cases.
- A sensitive pregnancy test should be routinely obtained in all patients with suspected PID because of the great difficulty encountered in clinically differentiating patients with PID from those with ectopic pregnancy.

■ Urine monoclonal antibody pregnancy tests and qualitative serum pregnancy tests become positive at human chorionic gonadotropin (hCG) levels as low as 25 mIU per mL and detect up to 96% of ectopic pregnancies.

■ Quantitative serum pregnancy tests detect hCG levels as low as 5 mIU per mL, and a negative test result virtually excludes the diagnosis of an ectopic gestation.[5,10]

■ The finding of **mucopurulent cervicitis** or evidence of white cells on microscopic examination of a saline preparation of vaginal fluid is seen in the great majority of patients with PID.[7,9]

■ Laboratory documentation of a cervical infection with **N. gonorrhoeae** or **C. trachomatis** corroborates the diagnosis of PID.[7]

■ Cultures have traditionally been regarded as the gold standard.

■ Nonculture tests, which offer a more rapid turnaround time than do cultures, include nuclear amplification tests and enzyme immunoassays for the detection of **Chlamydia** and **gonorrhea,** as well as immunofluorescent antibody tests for **Chlamydia.**

Imaging

■ **Transvaginal pelvic ultrasonography.** Sonographic findings supportive of the diagnosis include:

■ Thickened, fluid-filled fallopian tubes

■ Fluid in the cul-de-sac

■ A complex, multiloculated adnexal mass

■ Hyperemia on power Doppler transvaginal sonography[11,12]

■ **Magnetic resonance imaging (MRI).** MRI findings that support the diagnosis of PID include:

■ Fluid-filled tubes

■ Thickened tube walls with a dilated lumen

■ An ill-defined adnexal mass with thickened walls containing fluid[13]

Surgical Diagnostic Procedures

■ **Endometrial biopsy.** The histopathologic finding of plasma cell infiltration in the endometrial stroma obtained on biopsy confirms the diagnosis of PID[11]

■ **Diagnostic laparoscopy**

■ Diagnostic laparoscopy is regarded by many authorities as the standard for the diagnosis of acute PID.

■ Criteria required for the diagnosis include abnormal erythema and edema of the fallopian tubes and sticky exudate on tubal surfaces and from fimbriated ends.[11]

TREATMENT

■ Once the diagnosis of PID is made, 2006 CDC guidelines favor hospitalization under the following circumstances:

■ A surgical emergency, such as ectopic pregnancy or acute appendicitis, cannot be adequately excluded

■ A tubo-ovarian abscess is present

■ Pregnancy

■ Failure to respond clinically to oral antimicrobial therapy

■ Severe illness, nausea and vomiting, or high fever

■ Inability to follow or tolerate an outpatient oral regimen

Medications

Antibiotic therapy is the cornerstone of treatment for acute PID. Empirical, broad-spectrum antimicrobial therapy targeting **N. gonorrhoeae, C. trachomatis,** enteric Gram-negative facultative bacteria (including **Escherichia coli**), and certain anaerobic bacteria is recommended.

■ **Inpatient regimens.** Parenteral therapy can be discontinued as soon as 24 hours after the patient has improved clinically. Regimens suggested by the 2006 CDC guidelines are as follows:

- **Doxycycline,** 100 mg IV (or PO) q12h, plus **cefoxitin,** 2 g IV q6h (or **cefotetan,** 2 g IV q12h), followed by **doxycycline,** 100 mg PO bid for a total of 14 days.
- **Clindamycin,** 900 mg IV q8h, plus **gentamicin,** 2.0 mg per kg IV followed by 1.5 mg per kg IV q8h, followed by either **doxycycline,** 100 mg PO bid, or **clindamycin,** 450 mg PO qid, to complete 14 days of total therapy.
- **Outpatient regimens.** Suggested regimens are as follows:
  - **Cefoxitin,** 2 g IM plus **probenecid,** 1 g PO concurrently, or **ceftriaxone,** 250 mg IM, or other third-generation **cephalosporin,** IM once, plus **doxycycline,** 100 mg PO bid for 14 days **with or without metronidazole,** 500 mg PO bid for 14 days.
  - **Ofloxacin,** 400 mg PO bid or **levofloxacin** 500 mg PO qd for 14 days, **with or without metronidazole,** 500 mg PO bid for 14 days.

Surgery

- Surgical treatment has a limited role in the management of pid.
- Possible indications include the confirmation of the diagnosis in a patient failing to respond to therapy, excision of chronically infected pelvic organs, and draining of pelvic abscesses.

Nonoperative

- General supportive measures, such as bed rest, sexual abstinence until cure is achieved, hydration, and provision of antipyretics and appropriate analgesia, are recommended in the management of pid.
- Although there is no evidence that IUDs have to be removed in women diagnosed with acute pid, if the IUD is not removed CDC guidelines mandate that close clinical follow-up be provided.

Follow-Up

- Patients should be seen within 3 days after initiation of therapy.
- Patients who fail to respond require careful reevaluation of both the diagnosis and therapy.
- Male sex partners who have had contact with the patient during the preceding 60 days should be evaluated and provided empiric treatment for **Chlamydia** and **gonorrhea.**
- Patients should be provided counseling regarding safe sexual behavior, the use of condoms as a means for preventing the transmission of sexually transmitted diseases, and the advisability of HIV testing.
- Periodic screening for **Chlamydia** is recommended in sexually active women at risk for this infection, such as unmarried women 25 years of age or younger.[14,15]

Complications

- Tubal factor infertility is seen in 8% to 12% of patients after one episode of pid, 20% to 25% after two episodes, and 40% to 50% after three episodes or more.
- Chronic pelvic pain has been reported in 15% to 20% of patients after pid.
- The risk of ectopic pregnancy is increased 3- to 10-fold in a patient with a history of pid.[3,6]

References

1. Rein DB, Kassler WJ, Irwin KL, et al. Direct medical cost of pelvic inflammatory disease and sequelae: decreasing but still substantial. *Obstet Gynecol* 2000;95:397–402.
2. Crossman SH. The challenge of pelvic inflammatory disease. *Am Fam Physician* 2006; 73:859–864.
3. Banikarim C, Chacko MR. Pelvic inflammatory disease in adolescents. *Semin Pediatr Infect Dis* 2005;16:175–180.
4. Sweet RL. Role of bacterial vaginosis in pelvic inflammatory disease. *Clin Infect Dis* 1995;20(Suppl 2):S271.
5. Quan M. Pelvic inflammatory disease: diagnosis and management. *J Am Board Fam Pract* 1994;7:110.
6. Simms I, Stephenson JM. Pelvic inflammatory disease epidemiology: what do we know and what do we need to know. *STI* 2000;76:80–87.
7. U.S. Centers for Disease Control and Prevention. 2006 sexually transmitted diseases treatment guidelines. *MMWR* 2006;55(RR-11):56–61.

8. Jacobson L, Westrom L. Objectivized diagnosis of acute pelvic inflammatory disease. *Am J Obstet Gynecol* 1969;105:1088–1098.

9. Peipert JF, et al. Laboratory evaluation of acute genital tract infection. *Obstet Gynecol* 1996;87:730–736.

10. Cartwright PS, et al. Diagnosis of ectopic pregnancy. *Obstet Gynecol Clin North Am* 1991;18:19.

11. Munday PE. Pelvic inflammatory disease—an evidence-based approach to diagnosis. *J Infect Dis* 2000;40:31–41.

12. Molander P, Sjoberg J, Paavonen J, et al. Transvaginal power Doppler findings in laparoscopically proven acute pelvic inflammatory disease. *Ultrasound Obstet Gynecol* 2001;17:233–238.

13. Tukeva TA, Aronen HJ, Karjalainen PT, et al. MR imaging in pelvic inflammatory disease: comparison with laparsocopy and us. *Radiology* 1999;210:209–216.

14. Washington E, Berg AO. Preventing and managing pelvic inflammatory disease: key questions, practices, and evidence. *J Fam Pract* 1996;43:283.

15. Scholes D, et al. Prevention of pelvic inflammatory disease by screening for cervical chlamydial infection. *N Engl J Med* 1996;334:1362.

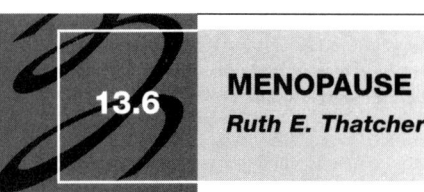

13.6 MENOPAUSE
Ruth E. Thatcher

GENERAL PRINCIPLES

Definition
Failure of ovarian follicular development in the presence of adequate gonadotropin stimulation, resulting in the cessation of spontaneous menstrual periods. A woman is considered to be postmenopausal after 1 year of amenorrhea.

Epidemiology
The average age for menopause is 51 years. Genetics, smoking, altitude, nutritional status, and percentage of body fat influence age at menopause. Hot flashes, the most common menopausal symptom, affect 75% to 85% of perimenopausal women, often beginning several years prior to menopause and persisting for up to 8 years.

Classification
Menopause may be secondary to surgical intervention or drug effect, particularly chemotherapeutic agents. Evidence of menopause before age 35 to 40 is considered premature menopause and usually necessitates a workup.

Pathophysiology
Vasomotor symptoms are believed to be triggered by estrogen withdrawal resulting in dysfunction of thermoregulatory centers of the hypothalamus. Obese women may have fewer symptoms secondary to increased estrogen production via aromatization of adipose tissue. The vaginal epithelium is estrogen dependent. As estrogen levels fall, Bartholin glands and the vaginal mucosa become atrophic. This may lead to dyspareunia and increased susceptibility to traumatic injury. Decreased libido sometimes experienced at menopause may be secondary to dyspareunia, stress, depression, concurrent medical illness, or the hormonal milieu. Estrogen deficiency may lead to decreased osteoblastic activity with increased osteoclastic activity resulting in osteoporosis and risk for fractures. Bone loss is estimated to be 1% to 5% per year for the first 5 years after menopause and about 0.5% per year thereafter.

DIAGNOSIS

Clinical Presentation

During the perimenopausal years women may experience signs or symptoms of estrogen excess or estrogen deprivation. Symptoms may include dysfunctional uterine bleeding, vasomotor flushes (hot flashes), sleep disturbance, vaginal dryness, dyspareunia, decreased libido, anxiety, dysphoria, or fatigue.

History

The history should focus on menstrual and cardiovascular history, family history of breast or uterine cancer, and risk factors for osteoporosis or coronary artery disease, as well as frequency and severity of menopausal symptoms including hot flashes and their affect on the patient's sleep pattern, work, and general well-being. Hot flashes are described as intense warmth and profuse sweating, which may be accompanied by palpitations and red blotchy skin. They last from seconds to minutes, rarely up to 1 hour, and may occur as often as 20 times per day.

Physical Examination

The physical examination should be complete, including vital signs, thyroid, cardiovascular, breast, lymphatic, and pelvic examination with Pap smear.

Laboratory Studies

Persistently elevated follicle-stimulating hormone (FSH) and leutinizing hormone (LH) levels can confirm the diagnosis of menopause. Eventually FSH will increase 10- to 20-fold, while LH will increase to three times that of premenopausal levels. The potential for ovulation exists until both FSH and LH are elevated. Laboratory testing should include evaluation of thyroid function and other tests based on findings from the history and physical examination.

Imaging

Pelvic ultrasound to assess for endometrial hyperplasia is recommended for frequent non-cyclic uterine bleeding during the perimenopause and for all uterine bleeding in post-menopausal women. **Yearly mammograms** are recommended for all women after age 50 and are especially important in women who are using hormone replacement therapy (HRT).

Surgical Diagnostic Procedures

Endometrial biopsy to rule out endometrial cancer should be performed on women with dysfunctional uterine bleeding and an endometrial stripe measuring more than 4 mm by ultrasound.

Differential Diagnosis

The diagnosis of menopause can often be made based on clinical symptoms alone. Social or personal circumstances may contribute to perimenopausal symptoms. Stressors such as onset of major illness or disability in the spouse, retirement from employment, financial insecurity, the need to care for aging parents, and separation from children may have a role in a woman's ability to cope with the physical symptoms of menopause. The differential diagnosis of vasomotor instability includes alcohol withdrawal, anxiety disorders, carcinoid tumor, epilepsy, insulin reaction, pheochromocytoma, thyrotoxicosis, and drug effects.

TREATMENT

Treatment of menopausal symptoms should be tailored to the severity of symptoms. Mild symptoms may be treated with behavioral modification, while more severe symptoms may require pharmacologic therapy. There is a significant placebo effect in the treatment of hot flashes. Controlled trials have shown a 25% reduction in the number of hot flashes with placebo treatment alone.

Behavioral

Nonpharmacologic treatments that may reduce the frequency or severity of hot flashes include good air circulation, sipping cool drinks, maintaining lower room temperatures, loose fitting or layered clothing, and avoidance of alcohol, caffeine, and spicy foods. Risk of osteoporosis may be reduced by weight-bearing and muscle-strengthening exercise, risk factor reduction (including smoking cessation and moderation of alcohol intake), and adequate nutrition including calcium 1200 to 1500 mg with vitamin D daily.

Medications

Estrogen has been used in the treatment of perimenopausal symptoms for more than 50 years. Antidepressants, anticonvulsants, and antiadrenergic agents may be utilized in patients who have a contraindication or intolerance to hormonal therapy. Estrogens, selective estrogen receptor modulators, and bisphosphonates are approved for the prevention and treatment of osteoporosis.

- **Estrogens** have a dose–response effect on hot flashes and will relieve symptoms in 75% to 90% of cases. Lower estrogen doses are usually sufficient to improve symptoms of vaginal dryness. Symptoms of urge, stress, or mixed urinary incontinence may improve with estrogen therapy. The Women's Health Initiative found that long-term estrogen therapy has beneficial effects on bone density. This benefit is offset by an increased risk of blood clots, breast cancer, stroke, and coronary artery disease. The study did not address short-term risks or benefits of HRT for treatment of menopausal symptoms. Risk of breast cancer is increased in those with a positive family history or with estrogen doses of >1.25 mg daily for more than 10 years. Yearly mammograms are necessary for all women on HRT. Contraindications to estrogen therapy include known or suspected pregnancy, undiagnosed abnormal genital bleeding, known or suspected breast cancer, liver disease, history of venous thromboembolic disease, cardiovascular disease, or stroke.
  - **Estrogen/progestin combination therapy** is necessary in patients with an intact uterus or with endometriosis remaining after hysterectomy to avoid endometrial hyperplasia and development of endometrial cancer. There is no increased benefit in hot flash reduction with combination therapy over estrogen alone. The progestin in combination therapy may be dosed in either a continuous or cyclic manner.
  - **Continuous progestin dosing** leads to breakthrough bleeding in 40% to 60% of women during the first 6 months of therapy. Endometrial biopsy is indicated for breakthrough bleeding beyond this time frame. The progestin dose may be doubled if no pathology is found on biopsy.
  - **Cyclic progestin dosing** causes less breakthrough bleeding but may worsen migraine headaches. Estrogen is given at the lowest effective dose along with a progestin for 10 days at the end of each month, for 25 days each month, or for 3 out of every 6 days of the month. Nonsmoking women still in the perimenopausal period may use low-dose oral contraceptive pills for both cycle control and treatment of vasomotor symptoms, as well as prevention of unintended pregnancy.
  - **Intravaginal estrogen** in the form of cream or tablets used daily for 2 to 12 weeks will reverse vaginal atrophy. This benefit is maintained with two or three treatments per week. Estrogens are well absorbed through the vaginal mucosa, so long-term intravaginal estrogen therapy in women who have an intact uterus or endometriosis remaining after hysterectomy must include a progestin.
  - **Plant-derived phytoestrogens** found in soy, wheat, cereals, nuts, and apples are converted to estrogens in the gut. These estrogens may have agonist and/or antagonist activity when bound to estrogen receptors. Controlled trials have shown conflicting results in the reduction of hot flashes with soy protein therapy. No difference in endometrial thickness has been observed with soy protein use.
- **Progestins without estrogen** have been shown to reduce the frequency and severity of hot flashes but may contribute to symptoms of dysphoria, anxiety, and fatigue.
  - **Megestrol acetate,** indicated for palliative treatment of advanced carcinoma of the breast and endometrium, reduces hot flashes by 75% to 80%.
  - A pilot study using **depomedroxyprogesterone** injections at 2-week intervals showed a 90% reduction in hot flashes; a Phase 3 trial is currently under way.
  - **Transdermal progesterone** cream (pro-gest), available without a prescription, has been shown to reduce hot flashes in 83% of patients.
- **Androgens. Low-dose testosterone/estrogen** combination therapy appears to control hot flash symptoms better than low-dose estrogen alone, but combination therapy

with high-dose estrogen has shown no benefit over high-dose estrogen alone. Androgen therapy improves libido, but potential side effects include virilization, worsening lipid profile, and liver toxicity.

- **Synthetic steroids. Tibolone** is a synthetic steroid whose metabolites have estrogenic, progestogenic, and androgenic activity. It has been used in Europe for prevention of osteoporosis and menopausal symptoms for the past 20 years. European studies have shown improvement in hot flash symptoms with tibolone that is comparable to estrogen therapy. Tibolone metabolites appear to have estrogenic effects on bone and the vaginal mucosa, progestogenic effects on the endometrium, and androgenic effects on the liver, while blocking formation of active estrogens in breast tissue.
- **Antidepressants. Venlafaxine, fluoxetine, citalopram,** and **paroxetine** reduce hot flashes by 50% to 67%.
- **Anticonvulsants. Gabapentin** dosed at 900 mg per day reduces hot flashes in 46% to 54% of cases. **Bellergal,** a combination of belladonna and phenobarbitol reduces hot flashes by about 50% but is not generally recommended because of the potential for addiction.
- **Antiadrenergic agents. Clonidine** therapy reduces hot flashes in 37% to 80% of cases. **Methyldopa** may reduce hot flashes, but controlled trials have shown conflicting results.
- **Vitamins and minerals. Vitamin E** (tocopherol) therapy has had anecdotal reports of improvement in hot flashes. However, no significant benefit was noted over placebo during controlled trials with 800IU/day dosing. **Calcium** supplementation of 1200–1600 mg/day with vitamin D is recommended to reduce age associated bone loss.
- **Herbal remedies. Black Cohosh,** approved for treatment of hot flashes in Germany, showed no significant benefit over placebo during controlled trials in the United States. Limiting use to less than 6 months is recommended since long-term effects are unknown. **Dong Quai** and **evening primrose** were found to have no benefit over placebo in controlled trials. **Red clover extract** controlled trials have shown conflicting results with a tendency toward mild improvement in the number of hot flashes compared to placebo.
- **Water-based lubricants** are recommended to help symptoms of vaginal dryness.

Risk Management

Risk of venous thromboembolism, breast cancer, abnormal mammograms, coronary artery disease, and stroke should be discussed with all patients prior to initiating hormonal therapy. Yearly breast exams and mammograms are recommended for all women receiving HRT.

Patient Education

Hot flash symptoms are self-limited. Mild symptoms can often be treated nonpharmacologically. Moderate to severe symptoms may require treatment with hormonal therapy, antidepressants, anticonvulsants, or antiadrenergics. Controlled trials of most herbal remedies have shown no significant benefit over placebo in the treatment of hot flashes.

Follow-Up

Follow-up in 3 to 6 months after initiation of therapy for menopausal symptoms is recommended to determine the adequacy of the regimen and review side effects. Once an appropriate regimen has been established, the patient should be evaluated yearly.

References

1. Leonetti H, Longo S, Anasti J. Transdermal progesterone cream for vasomotor symptoms and postmenopausal bone loss. *Obstet Gynecol* 1999;Aug:225–228.
2. Modelska K, Cummings S. Tiblone for postmenopausal women: systematic review of randomized trials. *J Clin Endocrinol Metab* 2002;87(1):16–23.
3. Shanafelt T, Barton D, Adjei A, et al. Pathophysiology and treatment of hot flashes. *Mayo Clin Proc* 2002;Nov:1207–1218.
4. Writing Group for the Women's Health Initiative Investigators. Risks and benefits of estrogen plus progestin in healthy postmenopausal women. *JAMA* 2002;Jul 17:321–333.
5. Nelson H, Vesco K, Haney E, et al. Nonhormonal therapies for menopausal hot flashes. *JAMA* 2006;May 3:2057–2071.
6. Pandya K, Morrow G, Roscoe J, et al. Gabapentin for hot flashes in 420 women with breast cancer: a randomized double blind placebo-controlled trial. *Lancet* 2005;Sep 3–9:818–824.

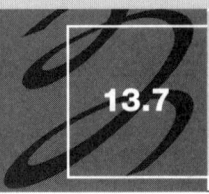

BENIGN BREAST CONDITIONS AND DISEASE

13.7

Edward J. Lewis, Steven Crossman

GENERAL PRINCIPLES

Definition

Benign breast conditions encompass a multitude of conditions united only in that cancer and precancerous lesions are excluded. Many women present to their physician for benign conditions of the breast that they perceive to be abnormal. Common complaints include pain, hypertrophy, breast lumps, breast infections, and nipple discharge. The health care provider must differentiate benign from malignant disease, reassure patients with benign conditions, manage common symptoms and conditions, and seek consultation when necessary. The provider must recognize the emotional distress common during this process and provide timely and effective communication.

Anatomy and Breast Development

The adult breast is a tear-shaped milk-producing gland supported and attached to the chest wall by the Cooper suspensory ligaments. Each breast is composed of 15 to 20 lobes, each composed of multiple lobules. Glandular milk-producing lobules drain through a series of branching ducts to the nipple, and are supported by fibrous tissue, or stroma. Typically, 6 to 10 pinhole openings on the areola each drain a duct that leads to a single lobe. Because more lobes are present in the outer quadrants, especially the upper outer quadrants, many breast conditions (including breast cancer) occur more frequently in these regions.

Breast development and change may be seen as a process of dynamic change beginning with embryonic development and continuing through the postmenopausal years. Newborns commonly have hypertrophied breast tissue caused by stimulation from maternal estrogen and progesterone. In most cases spontaneous regression occurs. Prepubertal children may develop unilateral or bilateral soft mobile subareolar nodules of uniform consistency that usually resolve spontaneously within a few months. Biopsy should be avoided as it may impair pubertal breast development. In girls puberty marks the normal onset of glandular proliferation within the breast. For most girls, breast bud development (thelarche) is the first sign of puberty (average age 11 years; range 9 to 13.4 years), while full breast development is usually the last sign. Thelarche is considered "premature" if it occurs earlier than age 8. Premature thelarche without other signs of pubertal development or accelerated growth is usually benign. No treatment is needed if medical evaluation excludes true precocious puberty, estrogen-producing tumors, ovarian cysts, or exogenous estrogen exposure. Other signs of puberty generally begin within 6 months of breast development and are completed within 4 years. Breast development may begin on one side and be asymmetrical. If there is a discrepancy in size, the left breast is usually larger. Breast development is considered "delayed" if stage 1 persists beyond 13.5 years; stage 2 persists more than 1 year; stage 3 greater than 2.2 years; or stage 4 more than 6 to 8 years.[1]

The normal breast changes in size and texture throughout the menstrual cycle as well. During the premenstrual phase, acinar cells, or the cells of the terminal duct-lobule unit, increase in number and size, the ductal lumens widen, and breast size and turgor increase. These changes reverse in the postmenstrual phase.

Gynecomastia, or the proliferation of glandular breast tissue in a male, is common in the middle phases of pubertal development and in adulthood. In puberty, this may be attributed to serum estradiol levels rising to adult levels before serum testosterone levels. Although it can be psychologically disturbing, workup is indicated only if there is rapid progression, onset before puberty, or association with true precocious puberty. More than 90% of affected boys experience regression within 3 years.

Classification of Conditions

Nipple Anomalies

The most common anomaly is polythelia, or, accessory nipple. Ectopic nipple tissue may occur at any point in the embryonic breast line, from the groin to the axilla. In many instances, an accessory nipple may be misdiagnosed as a nevus or dermatofibroma. Other nipple findings include discharge, Paget disease, and painful nipples.

Breast Infections

Infectious disease of the breast may include mastitis, abscess, or cellulitis. In evaluating and treating infections of the breast, it is important to determine if the woman is lactating.

Structural/Functional Anomalies

These changes encompass many common complaints including palpable masses as well as cyclical and noncyclical breast pain.

ASSESSMENT OF AN INDIVIDUAL WITH BREAST COMPLAINTS

History

In taking the history of the breast complaint, it is important to describe when and in what setting symptoms first occurred, any change over time, and past history of similar symptoms. Women should be asked about the relation of symptoms to the menstrual cycle. History should also include the menstrual and reproductive history (age of menarche and menopause); parity (age of the first-term pregnancy); whether currently pregnant; use of hormonal therapy or contraceptives; rapidity and amount of weight gain after menopause; whether breast self-examination is performed and any past breast surgery (with any biopsies and their results). The patient should also be queried for any family history of breast and ovarian cancers.

Examination of the Breast

- Inspection is first followed by palpation. The exam should be performed in a well-lit room and privacy is facilitated by draping parts of the body not being examined. Inspection occurs with the patient seated, arms at side; seated with hands on hips; and seated with arms above the head. Changes in size, shape, symmetry, or texture are noted. Palpation is performed with the patient supine, arms flexed at a 90-degree angle at the sides. Palpation includes supraclavicular, infraclavicular, and axillary nodes. Compression may identify a mass and/or elicit a discharge. Nipples should be examined for deviation, retraction, skin changes, or discharge.

Laboratory Evaluation

Currently, genetic screening is not part of the routine evaluation of individuals with breast-related complaints.

Diagnostic Tests[1]

- **Imaging.** Mammography is discussed elsewhere in this manual. When mammography is indicated, a "diagnostic" rather than a "screening" mammogram is obtained to evaluate women with breast complaints. Important diagnostic information may be obtained regarding a known or undetected mass. **However, a negative mammogram should never preclude biopsy of an appropriate palpable lesion.** Since mammography is unable to visualize lesions well in younger women, ultrasonography may be preferable in women under 30 years of age to differentiate whether a mass is solid or cystic and as an adjunct to aspiration or biopsy. Magnetic resonance imaging is utilized in some settings.
- **Aspiration.** A cystic lesion or lesion of uncertain nature may be aspirated both diagnostically and therapeutically.
- **Fine-needle aspiration (FNA).** FNA involves cytologic aspirate of a mass usually with ultrasound guidance. Specimen must have adequate number of epithelial cells for interpretation (sensitivity 87%).
- **Fine-needle aspiration and biopsy (FNAB).** Indications for biopsy include any suspicious lesion; bloody nipple discharge or bloody fluid following cyst aspiration;

persistent mass; suspicious skin changes; inflammatory changes unresponsive to antibiotic; suspicious axillary nodes; or suspicious microcalcifications on mammography. The sensitivity of FNAB is 60% to 98% and specificity 90% to 100%.

■ **Triple test.** The "triple test" combines physical examination, mammography, and FNAB. If all three are congruent, results are highly predictive (sensitivity 97% to 100%; specificity 98% to 100%).

■ **Open biopsy.** An open biopsy may be "excisional" (removal of the entire mass) at the same time as it establishes a definitive diagnosis. Frequently the diagnosis can be obtained without this degree of surgical intervention.

Pathologic Findings

Benign breast lesions diagnosed by the above methods may be subdivided based on the degree of risk they confer for the future development of malignancy. Such categorization is usually determined by proliferation and atypia. Lesions associated with an increased risk of developing breast cancer include any proliferative lesion, common benign lesions in patients older than 50 (such as cyst, adenosis, mammary duct ectasia fibrosis, metaplasia, fibroadenoma), mild/moderate or florid hyperplasia without atypia and simple papilloma. This risk is likely increased in patients with a strong family history of breast cancer. Findings with a small increase in relative risk include ductal hyperplasia without atypia, sclerosing adenosis, diffuse papillomas, complex fibroadenomas, and radial scars. Lesions conferring moderately increased risk include atypical ductal hyperplasia (relative risk 4.0 to 6.0) and atypical lobular hyperplasia (relative risk >10.0). Both of the aforementioned lesions also confer an increased risk for development of breast cancer in the contralateral breast.

    Emotional well-being of the patient. The evaluation of a breast complaint is extremely stressful for many women. Most patients assume that their sign or symptom indicates cancer. The provider should anticipate the emotional responses typical in patients and family members. Timely assessment, diagnostic evaluation, and consultation when necessary should be provided. It may be useful to inquire how best to assist with the period of uncertainty and how the patient would like results conveyed to her. Realistic estimates of the likely time involved in diagnosis are beneficial. Adequate time should be made available to address questions and additional methods of contact (office visits, telephone calls, or e-mail) should be offered.

BREAST PAIN

Mastalgia is an extremely common complaint among women, which may interfere significantly with quality of life. Pain without an associated mass is unlikely to be the presenting symptom of breast cancer, although evaluation may lead to the coincidental diagnosis of cancer. Mastalgia may be classed as cyclical or noncyclical, and may be acute or chronic.

■ **Epidemiology.** Mastalgia is a more common complaint in premenopausal women than in postmenopausal women. The incidence of breast pain varies based on the study group and inclusion criteria, but may range from 30% to 50% of working-aged women.

■ **Classification/etiology.** Breast pain may be classified as cyclical (2/3) or noncyclical (1/3). Cyclical breast pain commonly occurs as a result of estrogen stimulation of ductal elements, and progesterone stimulation of the stromal elements. Noncyclical causes of pain may include extramammary or chest wall pain, neuropathic pain, trauma, fat necrosis, infection, painful breast mass or cyst, and a multitude of other causes.

■ **History.** Pertinent historical details include palliative or provocative factors, quality, radiation, severity, location, and laterality. It is important to illicit timing with regard to menstrual cycle, association with oral contraceptive pills or hormone replacement use, recent birth, pregnancy, loss of pregnancy or termination. History of trauma, heavy muscular exertion, and constitutional symptoms should be sought.

■ **Physical examination.** Physical exam should be used to evaluate for mass or nipple discharge, to localize areas of tenderness, and to assess for lymphadenopathy and changes in symmetry, contour, and overlying skin.

■ **Laboratory studies and imaging.** Standard lab testing may be sought to assess for infection. Mammography or ultrasound may be useful in assessing for masses.

Noncyclical Breast Pain

- **Trauma.** Trauma may produce a hematoma or rupture of a cyst and may also lead to fat necrosis. The patient will typically complain of pain and tenderness following an injury. Mild swelling and discoloration may be present. Unless a coagulopathy is suspected, no diagnostic tests are indicated. Fat necrosis is usually caused by preceding trauma and may be more likely if there is a history of fibrocystic breast disease. Physical examination reveals localized pain, swelling, and erythema. Evaluation should be performed to exclude malignancy if symptoms persist for more than a week, although fat necrosis commonly results in a residual calcified mass.

- **Lactation-related pain.** Breast engorgement is a common cause of breast pain in new mothers. Breast engorgement usually occurs on the second or third postpartum day. Lactating women may also develop pain secondary to a galactocele or milk-filled cyst. These often resolve spontaneously.

- **Mastitis.** Both mastitis and breast abscesses almost always occur in lactating women or in women with a history of a bite or penetrating trauma. Mastitis commonly presents 1 week or more after delivery. Moderate to severe pain, tenderness, erythema, swelling, and warmth are usually localized to one breast, often to one quadrant or lobule. Axillary adenopathy may be present and there may be purulent drainage. The patient may be febrile and appear toxic. History and physical examination are diagnostic. Leukocytosis is common. Breast milk cultures are not useful and *Staphylococcus aureus* is typically causative in breastfeeding women. Treatment for mild infection includes warm compresses and 7 to 10 days on oral antibiotics deemed safe for a nursing infant (dicloxacillin 500 mg PO every 6 hours; amoxicillin clavulanate 500/125 mg tid; cephalexin 500 mg qid; or clindamycin 300 mg qid for penicillin-allergic patients). Patients should be reassessed in 48 to 72 hours. Breastfeeding should be continued on the affected breast to encourage drainage (the infant is not at risk for developing infection). Breast pumping is also appropriate.

- **Abscess.** Pitting edema over an area of inflammation and fluctuation is suggestive of abscess development. For patients with infections unresponsive to conservative management, severe infection, abscess, or deep infection, the wound should be drained and cultured. Breastfeeding should be discontinued and parenteral antibiotics (nafcillin or cefazolin) given for 2 to 3 days, followed by oral antibiotics. Nonpuerperal abscesses are usually caused by anaerobic bacteria if subareolar and by staphylococci in other locations. Nonpuerperal abscesses are treated with clindamycin or metronidazole plus nafcillin or cefazolin. If the clinical setting is atypical, the woman is not breastfeeding, or she does not improve with antibiotics, a biopsy of indurated areas to exclude an underlying cancer should be considered. Presence of a periareolar inflammatory mass, breast abscess in a nonlactating woman, or a mammary duct fistula should raise suspicion of periductal mastitis. Tobacco use is associated with an increased prevalence of this condition. Further evaluation is warrant.

Cyclical Breast Pain

- **Etiology.** Most cyclical breast pain is associated with the menstrual cycle. Pain is usually worse in the luteal phase and abates following menstruation. Most women report some degree of cyclical breast pain at some point in their lives; 11% to 30% experience severe pain that interferes with function. Cyclical breast pain is not always associated with premenstrual syndrome, but 60% of women with premenstrual syndrome (PMS) report breast pain as the predominant symptom. There is a high likelihood of spontaneous resolution of cyclical breast pain.

- **Treatment.** Watchful waiting and reassurance may be acceptable in up to 85% of patients. Breast support and analgesia with acetaminophen and ibuprofen may be beneficial. There is no evidence of benefit from dietary change. Progesterone and diuretics have also not been proved to be effective. Danazol has significant adverse effects (voice change, hirsutism, weight gain, acne), but 200 mg daily in the luteal phase (day 14 to 28) may be effective and minimize the total dose.[2] Tamoxifen 10 mg daily is efficacious as a continuous dose only during the luteal phase, but side effects limit its long-term use. Bromocriptine and gonadotropin-releasing hormone agonists have also been successfully used for severe pain but are associated with a number of side effects. However, additional therapies may include:

- Evening primrose oil 500 mg, two tablets tid, has been demonstrated efficacious in a randomized controlled clinical trial with no apparent adverse effects.
- Lowering the dose of estrogens in the treatment of postmenopausal women may be helpful, and the addition of an androgen to hormone replacement therapy (HRT) may alleviate symptoms as well.
- The use of oral contraceptives has not been well studied, but low-dose estrogen and 19-nor progestins may be effective in relieving symptoms.

Breast Mass

Benign breast masses are most commonly fibroadenomas or cysts, but must be differentiated from malignant disease. Benign breast masses will often change with the menstrual cycle, while worrisome masses are persistent throughout. Greater than 90% of palpable breast masses in women between 20 and 55 are benign. Masses may be discrete or poorly defined, but differ from the surrounding breast tissue and the corresponding area in the contralateral breast. Cancer should be excluded in a woman who presents with a solid mass. A woman with a clinically suspicious lesion should undergo mammography and/or ultrasound, and biopsy. Between 9% and 22% of palpable breast cancers will not be detected with imaging studies, with lobular carcinoma particularly difficult to detect on mammography. Characteristics of a mass that are concerning for malignancy include single lesion, hard, fixed/immobile, irregular border, and size greater than 2 cm. Any asymmetry, skin dimpling, nipple discharge, and lymphadenopathy must also be assessed. Sensitivity and specificity of physical exam for detecting cancer are reported to be 54% and 94%, respectively. The sensitivity of FNA alone has been reported to be 87%, and when combined with physical exam and imaging, the sensitivity is above 95%.

- **Breast cysts.** Cysts may be solitary or multiple, and may be difficult to differentiate from solid masses on physical exam. Cystic disease is most common in premenopausal women older than 40 years. Ultrasound may be used to differentiate solid versus cystic masses and aspiration may be both diagnostic and therapeutic. Cysts should be surgically biopsied if they contain bloody fluid, fail to resolve completely after drainage, or recur after 4 to 6 weeks. It is not necessary to send aspirated fluid for cytologic examination, however. Nonpalpable cysts identified during routine mammography do not require further evaluation or treatment.
- **Fibrocystic breast changes (FBD).** Fibrocystic changes are the most common benign condition of the breast, occurring to some extent in most, if not all, women. Most experts consider such changes to be part of the natural history of the breast as histologic changes consistent with this diagnosis may be found in 50% to 60% of asymptomatic women. Changes are most common in women 35 to 45 years old and are rare in postmenopausal women. No treatment is necessary unless the woman is symptomatic (for example, from an enlarging cyst) or if physical findings are worrisome for possible cancer.
  - **Anatomy.** Fibrocystic changes consist of an increased number of cysts or fibrous tissue in an otherwise normal breast.
  - **Epidemiology.** Fibrocystic change may be divided into three subgroups with predominant histologic characteristics and age distributions. Hyperplasia commonly occurs in women in their 20s and presents as stromal proliferation and pain in the upper and outer quadrants. Adenosis is caused by proliferation of glandular cells and presents commonly as multiple 2 to 10 mm breast nodules in women in their 30s. Cystic disease occurs more commonly in women older than 40 with the painful enlargement of multiple or solitary cysts.
  - **History.** When symptoms are present, the most common symptom is cyclical pain (mastalgia). The pain is generally bilateral, located in the upper outer quadrants, begins a few days prior to menstruation, diminishes with the onset of menses, and may be associated with an increase in breast size. Family history is common.
  - **Physical examination.** Cysts are smooth, regular, rubbery, and easily movable lumps or areas of local tenderness without a discrete mass. Cysts can range in size from 1 mm to many centimeters. Compression causes tenderness. Larger cysts are more common as women age. To assess for possible menstrual changes, it may be helpful to repeat the examination with the patient at another point in her cycle. It may be difficult to discern a cyst from a solid mass on physical exam. Pale green to brown nipple discharge may be noted in cystic disease.

- **Diagnostic evaluation.** Although fibrocystic symptoms typically differ from those associated with malignancy, if there is any doubt regarding the diagnosis or if a single mass is present, further evaluation for breast mass is needed. There is no increased risk of cancer in women with fibrocystic changes in a woman younger than 50 years unless proliferative or hyperplastic lesions with atypical epithelial cells are present on biopsy.

- **Management.** Most women do not require treatment. Treatment if necessary is focused on the predominant symptom or sign, be it a mass or pain. A well-padded support bra and loose light clothing may relieve discomfort and weight reduction is recommended in women with a body mass index greater than 30 mm per kg. Calcium may be beneficial, but many other previously recommended therapies (dietary restriction of caffeine and methylxanthines in chocolate, tea, coffee, soda, and theophylline; use of vitamins including A, E, and thiamine; and use of diuretics) have not proven efficacious in randomized controlled clinical trials. Additional management may include the following:

  - Low estrogen/high progesterone oral contraceptives may be used but the patient may not notice significant change until 1 to 2 years of use.
  - Progesterone, such as medroxyprogesterone 5 to 10 mg daily for 10 days before menses, may be given for a trial of 4 to 6 months. Side effects may include weight gain, depression, breakthrough bleeding, and lipid alterations.
  - If thyroid-stimulating hormone (TSH) is elevated even when other thyroid hormones are normal, a trial of thyroid replacement may be helpful.
  - *cis*-Linoleic acid (evening primrose oil) at a dose of 1 g every 8 hours may be beneficial. However, the benefit may not be seen for 3 to 4 months.
  - Danazol is the only pharmacologic agent approved by the U.S. Food and Drug Administration for treatment of FBD. 60% to 90% of women benefit, but significant side effects (hirsutism, amenorrhea, weight gain of 4 to 6 pounds, hot flashes, and acne) are common. Danazol is generally reserved for women with severe symptoms. Dose at 200 to 600 mg per day PO initially and then may decrease to 50 to 100 mg per day as maintenance once response is achieved. Some women benefit from 200 mg daily, given on days 14 to 28 of the menstrual cycle. Duration of treatment is usually limited to 4 to 6 months. Once danazol is discontinued the treatment response may persist for months to years.[2]
  - Tamoxifen, an antiestrogen, reduced breast pain in approximately 70% of patients within 3 to 6 months in several studies. In premenopausal women younger than 49 years, 20 mg per day was found to cause no increase in the incidence of deep venous thrombus, pulmonary embolism, stroke, transient ischemic attack (TIA), or endometrial cancer. Tamoxifen may be effective when used only during the luteal phase (days 15 to 25), but its use should be restricted to fewer than 6 months. Side effects may include hot flashes, gastrointestinal (GI) symptoms, and vaginal discharge.
  - Surgery (subcutaneous mastectomy; oophorectomy) should only be considered after medical management has failed for women with recalcitrant symptoms. Surgery may be useful for patients with one large dominant cyst.
  - Bromocriptine and luteinizing hormone-releasing agents have also been used but have significant side effects.

- **Fibroadenoma.** Fibroadenoma, the most common solid tumor, contains both fibrous and epithelial elements. These tumors occur in young women, usually within 20 years of puberty. They are more common and occur at earlier ages in black women than in white women. Multiple lesions may develop. Growth may be rapid especially at the end of a menstrual cycle and in pregnancy. Older women characteristically have a single, solitary, more slowly growing lesion. Fibroadenomas frequently calcify and may involute after menopause. Occasionally they may develop in a postmenopausal woman after administration of estrogen.

  - **History.** A painless mass is generally discovered by the patient and reported to the physician.
  - **Physical examination.** A well-defined, rubbery, mobile, nontender, 1 to 5 cm mass can generally be palpated. The usual location is in an upper quadrant.

- ■ **Diagnostic procedures.** Aspiration of the mass should be attempted. A fine-needle biopsy may be diagnostic. Mammography is not usually helpful, especially in young patients.
- ■ **Breast cancer risk.** Fibroadenomas are neither cancerous or premalignant but may require excisional biopsy to confirm the diagnosis.
- ■ **Management.** Excisional biopsy is both diagnostic and curative.

- **Cystosarcoma phyllodes** is a rapidly growing fibroadenoma that recurs if not completely excised. This tumor is rarely malignant but, because of its extreme size, simple mastectomy may be necessary to achieve complete removal.

NIPPLE ANOMALIES

Nipple Discharge

Nipple discharge is an extremely common concern in young women and most isolated complaints of discharge are of a benign origin. It is practical to divide nipple discharge into two categories based on the presence or absence of galactorrhea. Normal, healthy women commonly have some degree of clear or milky nipple discharge following pregnancy and lactation that can either spontaneously drain from the breast or be produced by palpation. This discharge may be more frequently noted just before menses or with breast stimulation as part of sexual activity. This benign discharge has a small volume and the amount does not change over time. However, characteristics of pathologic discharge include unilaterality; presence from a single duct; association with an underlying mass; spontaneous, intermittent, and persistent occurrence in a postmenopausal woman; and bloody to serosanguinous color.

- ■ **History.** History should elicit the nature of discharge, underlying mass, laterality, single or multiple duct involvement, relation to menses, color of discharge, the menopausal status of the patient, association with hormonal therapy, and whether the discharge appears spontaneously or must be expressed. The amount and type of nipple stimulation should also be explored. **Nipple discharge in a postmenopausal woman is more ominous** and is more likely to be caused by cancer.
- ■ **Physical examination.** A complete breast exam should be performed, with attention to identifying masses, underlying induration, and lymphadenopathy as well as characterizing the discharge. Warm compresses placed on the breast may enhance the ability to detect a discharge. It is important to note whether the discharge originates from one or more ducts. A "pseudo-discharge" is a stain on clothes originating from outside the breast (such as from an abrasion, eczema, or viral condition like herpes). If nipple crusting is present, Paget disease should be excluded.
- ■ **Fluid characteristics.** The characteristics of the fluid may aid in diagnosis. Green, black, creamy, or mucoid discharge is characteristic of FBD. Straw-colored discharge is most commonly due to a papilloma (which is benign histologically and has only a slight potential for malignant degeneration). Bloody or serosanguinous discharge is associated with malignancy, but may also represent bleeding papilloma or fibrocystic change with an intraductal component. Bloody discharge, or brown-green discharge suggesting old blood, should be investigated further. Cheesy discharge often results from duct ectasia, a chronic inflammatory reaction resulting in permanent distention of the major ducts. The typical patient with duct ectasia is a multiparous woman 40 years or older who notes thick, white, or discolored cheesy material draining from the nipple and noncyclical, burning breast pain. Purulent discharge could indicate an underlying mastitis.
- ■ **Diagnostic procedures:**
  - ▩ **Mammography.** A mammogram should be performed in women with abnormal discharge and may reveal abnormalities such as the presence of an associated mass.
  - ▩ **Galactography.** The role of galactography and/or ductography in a woman with a nipple discharge is controversial. A negative galactogram does not replace the need for terminal duct excision.
  - ▩ **Fluid analysis.** The discharge can be tested for the presence of blood (with a hemoccult slide). Gram staining can be performed to identify white blood cells if there is a concern for infection. Fat stain can demonstrate fat globules indicative of milk if galactorrhea is suspected. Cytologic examination of the nipple discharge is not generally useful.

- **Management.** Management includes surgical exploration of the duct and removal of the papilloma, if present.

Galactorrhea

Galactorrhea consists of a milky discharge from the breast beyond 6 months postpartum in a nonbreastfeeding woman. Although galactorrhea can have many causes, it is usually benign. It has been described in women who jog because friction between the nipple and clothing can stimulate prolactin. Athletic activities may also trigger endorphin release from the hypothalamus, which stimulates prolactin secretion. Correlation is poor between presence of lactation and serum prolactin level. Galactorrhea is not associated with an increased risk of breast cancer.

- **History.** History should include recent childbirth, excessive breast stimulation, and medication use. Additionally, it should be determined if galactorrhea is present from both nipples and from multiple ducts. Galactorrhea from multiple ducts in a nonlactating woman may occur in certain syndromes (Chiari–Frommel, Argonz–Del Castillo). Processes that inflame or irritate the chest wall such as thoracotomy, herpes zoster infection, radiation to the chest wall, burn, may also cause galactorrhea (presumably from a stimulatory increase in prolactin secretion) and should be investigated. Any associated change in menstrual pattern, such as amenorrhea or oligomenorrhea, is suggestive of a central nervous system lesion and approximately 20% of patients with galactorrhea will have a prolactin-secreting pituitary tumor. Headache or visual change may indicate the presence of an intracranial process. Conditions that affect the pituitary and/or the hypothalamus (tuberculosis and multiple sclerosis) and other chronic medical conditions (chronic renal failure, hypothyroidism, Cushing disease) may cause galactorrhea and should be explored in the past medical history.
- **Medication history.** Medications may be the cause of galactorrhea in up to 20% of patients. Drugs associated with galactorrhea include digitalis, marijuana, heroin, dopamine receptor blockers, phenothiazine, haloperidol, metoclopramide, isoniazid, antidepressants, reserpine, methyldopa, atenolol, cimetidine, benzodiazepines, amphetamines, verapamil, cocaine, progesterones, oral contraceptives, copper-containing intrauterine devices (IUDs), and others. Herbal products that can cause galactorrhea include fenugreek seed, fennel, and red clover. Post–oral contraceptive galactorrhea may occur as well where the milk production is triggered by the withdrawal of estrogen and progesterone. This usually resolves spontaneously. Some patients eventually develop radiologically evident pituitary adenomas.
- **Diagnostic evaluation.** Serum prolactin level, TSH, and renal function tests can be useful. Further endocrine workup may be indicated. If serum prolactin is greater than 75 to 100 mg per mL, brain computed tomography (CT) or magnetic resonance imaging (MRI) is necessary to rule out pituitary adenoma. Nonpituitary prolactin-producing malignancies are less common but include bronchogenic carcinomas, renal adenocarcinomas, Hodgkin disease, and T-cell lymphoma. A CT or MRI scan is necessary if serum prolactin is elevated; if serum prolactin is normal but the patient has an aberration in her menstrual pattern; or if any central nervous system symptoms or signs are present.
- **Management.** Any medication associated with galactorrhea should be withdrawn. Any thyroid abnormalities detected on workup should be treated. If serum prolactin is elevated, a workup for pituitary adenoma is indicated. If elevated serum prolactin but no pituitary adenoma is demonstrable, treatment may still be indicated to decrease the risk of hyperprolactin-associated osteoporosis. If a microadenoma is present but fertility is not desired, and the risk of osteoporosis does not warrant treatment, patients can be followed without therapy. Microadenomas may regress spontaneously and do not typically transform into macroadenomas. Serum prolactin levels can be followed every 6 months, with repeat CT or MRI every 2 to 5 years. If a macroadenoma is present, therapy is indicated to prevent further growth. Medical management consists of bromocriptine, 2.5 mg per day for 1 week, increased to 2.5 mg bid-tid, or pergolide and cabergoline. Side effects may include nausea, nasal congestion, and postural hypotension. Tumor regrowth may occur following withdrawal of the medication. Bromocriptine can be used to lower prolactin levels to normal to allow fertility and to shrink tumor size preoperatively. Transsphenoidal surgery is an option for large tumors and in patients with macroadenomas who wish to become

pregnant. However, surgical success is limited as these tumors frequently recur. Radiation may be an option for patients who are not surgical candidates.

Painful Nipples

Breastfeeding Women

Tenderness of the nipples is a common symptom when breastfeeding is initiated. Proper positioning of the baby so that the most cracked or tender portion of the breast is at the corner of baby's mouth and not aligned with the roof of the mouth or tongue and correct techniques to "break suction" are essential. Nursing position may be changed. Any engorgement should be treated. Alternate which breast is presented first and begin with the less sore one. Warm or cold compresses and crushed ice applied to nipples before nursing may be beneficial. Milk should be expressed until "let-down" occurs. Avoid petrolatum and zinc oxide. The area can be washed with warm water and can air dry with colostrum applied.

Nipples should be examined for the presence of fissures or local infection. If candidal disease is suspected, treat with topical nystatin or antifungals. Thrush or *Candida* diaper rash in the newborn or maternal *Candida* vaginitis should be treated concurrently.

A plugged milk duct can present as a white blister on the nipple following breastfeeding and a hardened area in the breast. Soak the nipple in warm water before next nursing. Gently rub a clean washcloth across the tip of the nipple. As baby nurses, massage behind the hard area to encourage milk expression.

Nonbreastfeeding Women

Nipples can develop painful localized irritation and bleeding in joggers. Small elastic bandages can be applied to the nipple before running or other athletic activities. Emollients or low-dose hydrocortisone cream may ameliorate symptoms.

A unilateral, weeping, ulcerated, irritated nipple is suggestive of Paget disease, especially in middle-aged or older women, and may be associated with an underlying ductal carcinoma. Further evaluation is necessary.

Gynecomastia[4]

Gynecomastia has a bimodal distribution. Most boys at puberty develop bilateral gynecomastia, which resolves without treatment within 3 years. It is also common for men in their 50s and 60s to experience breast enlargement. Gynecomastia associated with pain, asymmetry, rapid onset or progression, galactorrhea, and/or erectile dysfunction requires further workup. Association with precocious puberty is also a concerning sign.

Drugs and medications that can cause gynecomastia include estrogen (whether the patient is taking it himself or absorbing it from the genital skin of a partner who uses vaginal cream), anabolic steroids, corticosteroids, clomiphene, marijuana, methadone, testosterone, amphetamines, spironolactone, digoxin, reserpine, methyldopa, hydroxyzine, ketoconazole, cimetidine, tricyclic antidepressants, and phenothiazine.

Medical conditions that cause gynecomastia include cancer (testes, liver, bronchiole, stomach, or pancreas, especially the human chorionic gonadotropin (hCG)–producing neoplasms), hyperthyroidism, hypogonadism, cirrhosis, renal failure, severe pulmonary disease, Klinefelter syndrome, testicular feminization, and refeeding after starvation.

Laboratory evaluation includes thyroid function tests, renal and liver function studies; if these are normal, luteinizing hormone, hCG, estradiol, and testosterone should be obtained. If hCG is elevated, testicular ultrasonography and search for other hCG-secreting tumors should be undertaken. If estradiol is elevated, a search for an estrogen-secreting tumor should be undertaken.

Older men develop gynecomastia at an age close to that at which male breast cancer occurs. If a breast mass is felt, a combination of physical examination and FNA can establish the correct diagnosis in the majority of patients. Mammography may add little additional information.

References

1. Morrow M. Evaluation of common breast problems. *Am Fam Physician* 2000;61: 2371–2378.
2. O'Brien PM, Abukhalil IEH. Randomized controlled trial of the management of premenstrual syndrome and premenstrual mastalgia using luteal phase only danazol. *Am J Obstet Gynecol* 1999;180:18–23.

3. Copeland JA. Nipple discharge. In: Taylor RB, ed. *The 10-minute diagnosis manual.* Philadelphia: Lippincott Williams & Wilkins; 2000:236–237.
4. Andolsek KM, Copeland J. The breast. In: Taylor RB, ed. *Family medicine: principles and practice.* 5th ed. New York: Springer-Verlag; 1998:925–933.
5. Santen RJ, Mansel R. Current concepts: benign breast disorders. *N Engl J Med* 2005; 353(3):275–285.
6. Zylstra S. Office management of benign breast disease. *Clin Obstet Gynecol* 1999; 42(2):234–248.
7. Miers M. Understanding benign breast disorders and disease. *Nurs Stand* 2001; 15(50):45–55.

BREAST CANCER

Ariel K. Smits, Elizabeth Steiner

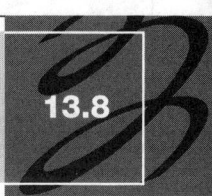

13.8

GENERAL PRINCIPLES

Definition

Breast cancer includes cancers confined to the ducts (ductal carcinoma in situ) or lobules (lobular carcinoma in situ) of the breast as well as invasive lobular and ductal tumors, inflammatory cancer, and Paget disease.

Epidemiology

Among U.S. women, breast cancer is the most commonly diagnosed cancer and the second leading cause of cancer death.[1–3] In 2005, it was projected that 211,240 U.S. women would be diagnosed with invasive breast cancer and 40,410 women would die of the disease.[1] Approximately 95% of new cases and 97% of breast cancer deaths occur in women aged 40 and older.[1] Native American and white women have the highest rates of breast cancer; African American and Asian women have lower rates.[4]

Risk factors with a relative risk of >4.0 for breast cancer include (a) female sex (>99% of breast cancer cases), (b) increasing age, (c) certain genetic mutations such as BRCA1 and/or BRCA2, (d) two or more first-degree relatives with breast cancer diagnosed premenopausally, (e) increasing breast density, and (f) personal history of breast cancer. Risk factors with a relative risk of 2.1 to 4.0 include (a) one first-degree relative with breast cancer, (b) biopsy-confirmed hyperplasia, (c) high-dose radiation to the chest, and (d) high bone density (postmenopausal). Other risk factors with lower relative risks (1.1 to 2.0) include (a) age >30 at first delivery, (b) early menarche (<12 years), (c) late menopause (>55 years), (d) nulliparity, (e) no history of breastfeeding, (f) recent oral contraceptive use or use for more than 5 years, (g) recent and long-term use of hormone replacement therapy, (h) obesity (postmenopausal), (i) personal history of endometrial, ovary, or colon cancer, (j) alcohol consumption, and (k) higher socioeconomic status.[1,5]

DIAGNOSIS

Clinical Presentation

Early-stage breast cancer is generally asymptomatic when the tumor is small and most treatable. Later-stage breast cancer most commonly presents as a painless mass.[1] Less common symptoms include breast pain, persistent changes such as skin irritation or distortion, and nipple abnormalities such as spontaneous discharge, erosion, or inversion.[1]

History

The history should include date the lump was found, prior breast problems, and possible risk factors.

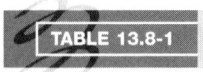

TABLE 13.8-1	Recommendations for Breast Cancer Screening from National Organizations	
Organization	**Mammography**	**Clinical breast exam**
U.S. Preventive Services Taskforce American Academy of Family Physicians	Every 1–2 years with or without CBE for women aged 40 and older [B]^a	Insufficient evidence to recommend for or against routine CBE alone [I]
American Cancer Society	Annual mammography beginning at age 40	Women in their 20s and 30s should have CBE at least every 3 years; women aged 40 and over should have a CBE annually as part of a periodic health examination
American College of Obstetrics and Gynecology	Mammograms every 1–2 years for women age 40–49 [B] Annual mammography for women aged 50 years [B]	All women should have CBE annually as part of the physical examination [C]
Susan Komen Foundation	Mammogram every 1–2 years beginning at age 40	Women in their 20s and 30s should have CBE at least every 3 years; women aged 40 and over should have a CBE annually as part of a periodic health examination
American College of Radiology/American College of Surgeons	Annual mammogram beginning at age 40	

^{a}U.S. Preventive Services Task Force grade of evidence: A: Consistent, high-quality evidence; benefits of screening substantially outweigh the harms. B: Inconsistent or fair evidence; benefits of screening are only moderately greater than the harms. C: Fair evidence; the benefits of screening are too close to the harms. I: Insufficient evidence.

Physical Examination

Clinical breast examination (CBE) is an important method for early detection of breast cancer. Expert groups differ in their recommendation for inclusion of CBE; the American Cancer Society and the American College of Radiology recommend yearly CBE with mammography (Table 13.8-1). The patient should be examined in the upright and supine positions, and the examination should be unhurried. The breast should be inspected for differences in size, retraction of the skin or nipple, and signs of inflammation. The flat surface of the fingertips should be used to palpate the breast tissue using the vertical strip, three pressure method.[6] The axillary and supraclavicular areas should be checked for adenopathy. Concerning masses are generally solitary, discrete, hard, fixed, nontender, and unilateral, but cancer cannot be excluded based solely on physical exam findings that differ from the common presentation. Other concerning findings include axillary lymphadenopathy, nipple inversion, or skin changes such as retraction.[7]

Imaging

Mammography is the major screening tool for early detection of breast cancer in women over 40. The effectiveness of screening with mammography for early detection of breast cancer has been clearly established by multiple studies.[1,3,8,9] Mammography will detect 80% to 90% of breast cancers in women without symptoms, although the sensitivity is markedly lower in women under 50. Various national organizations recommend CBE and mammography at various intervals for different age groups (Table 13.8-1).

Screening mammography of an asymptomatic woman provides two views of each breast. Diagnostic mammography is used to evaluate women with signs of symptoms of breast cancer and may include additional views or ultrasonographic imaging.

Newer imaging modalities include digital mammography, which allows computer-aided diagnosis, computer-aided interpretation of mammography, and magnetic resonance imaging (MRI) of the breasts.[7] The utility of these newer modalities has not yet been proved, however, and they are not generally recommended for routine screening.

Surgical Diagnostic Procedures

When a mass is detected by breast self-exam, CBE, or mammography, definitive diagnosis depends on tissue sampling. Breast imaging should be performed before palpable masses are biopsied because hemorrhage can distort the tissue structure. Even if the mammogram is normal, discrete, noncystic palpable masses should be biopsied. Biopsy procedures include fine needle aspiration, which generally uses a 20-guage needle to obtain samples from a solid mass for cytology. Other types of biopsies include needle localization aided by ultrasonography and stereotactic biopsy. Core biopsy uses a 14-guage or similar needle to remove cores of tissue from a mass and can be performed with ultrasound or stereotactic guidance. This procedure requires a small skin incision. Lumpectomy or open excisional biopsy may be done when needle biopsies are negative but the mass is clinically suspicious, or if there other concerning clinical features.

Pathologic Findings

Pathologic findings from breast biopsies include tumor type, *in situ* or invasive pathology, and estrogen and progesterone receptor analysis. If a tumor resection is done, surgical margins can be evaluated and, if lymph node sampling was conducted, the presence or absence of cancer cells in the lymph nodes can be determined.

Staging

Breast cancer is staged based on primary tumor size, spread to regional lymph nodes, and the presence or absence of distant metastases.[10] The staging of a tumor has a significant impact on the prognosis, treatment options, and recurrence potential of a tumor. Table 13.8-2 presents staging definitions. The most important factor in prognosis of patients with breast cancer is the axillary node status. Sentinel node biopsy is a new technique to help determine this, but without the morbidity of an axillary node dissection. Once the diagnosis has been made, a metastatic workup is done, including a complete blood count, liver enzymes, chest radiography, and, in some cases, bone scanning.

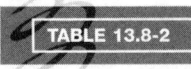

TABLE 13.8-2   Breast Cancer Staging

Stage	Tumor size	Lymph node involvement	Distant metastases
0	*In situ;* contained within the breast ductal or lobular system	No	No
I	Less than 2 cm	No	No
IIA	2–5 cm	No	
IIB	2–5 cm	Axillary nodes on same side of the body	No
IIB	More than 5 cm	No	No
IIIA	More than 5 cm	Axillary nodes on the same side of the body	No
IIIB	Any size	Tumor has spread to the chest wall	No
IV	Any size	Any lymph node involvement	Yes

TREATMENT

Surgery

Primary treatment for breast cancer is surgical resection. Types of surgery include lumpectomy, simple mastectomy, and modified radical mastectomy. Considerations for surgical therapy include not only size and histology of the tumor but also the patient's wishes. Today, modified radical mastectomy has replaced the radical mastectomy as the most common type of surgery. Breast-conserving surgery combined with radiation therapy is equivalent to a mastectomy in some cases. After surgical treatment for breast cancer, the patient may elect to undergo breast reconstruction.

Radiation

Results of randomized clinical trials indicate that radiation therapy in conjunction with surgery and chemotherapy improves long-term survival in women with lymph-node-positive breast cancer.[1]

Chemotherapy

Current adjuvant therapy for premenopausal women with positive nodes consists of various combinations of cyclophosphamide, methotrexate, 5-fluorouracil, doxorubicin, epirubicin, and paclitaxel (Taxol).[11] Multidrug therapy is more effective than single drug therapy for breast cancer treatment.[11] Tumor size, histology, and the presence of cancer in axillary nodes are considered in deciding which adjuvant therapy regimen to use.

Hormonal Therapy

Estrogen receptor–positive cancers can be treated with hormone therapy, which include tamoxifen, raloxifene, and aromatase inhibitors (letrozole, anastrozole, and exemastane). Additionally, oophorectomy or the use of gonadotropin-releasing hormone analogues can be used.[12] Hormonal therapy is commonly used but more debatable in node-negative patients. Neoadjuvant hormonal chemotherapy has been shown to reduce the annual rates of tumor recurrence and death.[12] Studies have found that using chemotherapy and hormonal therapy sequentially is more effective than using either alone for women with high-risk estrogen receptor–positive cancer.[11]

Biologic Therapy

Trastuzmab (Herceptin) is a monoclonal antibody, which directly targets the HER2/neu protein of breast tumors and offers survival benefit for some women with metastatic breast cancer.[1]

Follow-Up

Clinical follow-up should continue on a regular basis. Evaluation should include tumor marker levels, liver enzymes, chest radiography, and annual physical and pelvic examination. Although 10-year survival for early-stage lesions is 75% to 85%, women continue to die of breast cancer 15 to 20 years later.

SPECIAL CONSIDERATIONS

Pregnancy and Breast Cancer

About 2% of all breast cancers are diagnosed in pregnancy, which does not influence prognosis. If cancer is found during the first or second trimester, a mastectomy and axillary dissection should be carried out. Therapeutic abortion does not improve outcome. Third-trimester patients can be observed until delivery and then receive prompt therapy.

Carcinoma of the Male Breast

Male breast carcinoma accounts for 0.5% of all breast cancers. It too is more common in older men and can also be *BRCA1* or *BRCA2* related. Workup and treatment are similar to those for female breast cancer.

References

1. ACS. Breast cancer facts and figures 2005–2006. Available online at http://www.cancer.org/downloads/STT/CAFF2005BrF.pdf. Accessed December 22, 2005.
2. Humphrey LL, Helfand M, Chan BKS, et al. Breast cancer screening: a summary of the evidence. *Ann Intern Med* 2002;137(5):347–360.

3. CDC. Implementing recommendations for the early detection of breast and cervical cancer among low-income women. *MMWR* 2000;49(RR02):35–55.
4. Bigby JA, Holmes MD. Disparities across the breast cancer continuum. *Cancer Causes Control* 2005;16:35–44.
5. Singletary SE. Rating the risk factors for breast cancer. *Ann Surg* 2003;237(4):474–482.
6. Saslow D, Hannan J, Osuch J, et al. Clinical breast examination: practical recommendations for optimizing performance and reporting. *CA Cancer J Clin* 2004;54(6):327–344.
7. Apantaku LM. Breast cancer diagnosis and screening. *Am Fam Physician* 2000;62:596–602.
8. USPSTF. Screening for breast cancer: recommendations and rationale. *Ann Intern Med* 2002;137(5):344–346.
9. Whitman GJ. The role of mammography in breast cancer prevention. *Curr Opin Oncol* 1999;11(5):414–423.
10. Singletary SE, Connolly JL. Breast cancer staging: working the sixth edition of the AJCC cancer staging manual. *CA Cancer J Clin* 2006;56:37–47.
11. Smith IE, Chua S. Medical treatment of early breast cancer. III: chemotherapy. *BMJ* 2006;332:161–162.
12. Smith IE, Chua S. Medical treatment of early breast cancer. I: adjuvant treatment. *BMJ* 2006;332:34–37.

COLPOSCOPY
Gary R. Newkirk

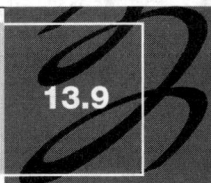

13.9

GENERAL PRINCIPLES

Diagnosis and management of genital epithelial dysplasia requires mastery of colposcopy, punch biopsy, and endocervical curettage (ECC). The colposcope is essentially a stereoscopic operating microscope combined with a bright-light source. The ultimate challenge for the colposcopist is to distinguish normal from abnormal areas and direct biopsy to allow for histologic interpretation of abnormal areas. Colposcopy with biopsy helps to identify patients who may have invasive genital malignancy requiring advanced cancer therapies and women who have premalignant changes, which frequently can be managed with outpatient procedures, such as cryotherapy or loop electrosurgical excision procedure (LEEP).

INDICATIONS FOR COLPOSCOPY

- Papanicolaou (Pap) smear indications (see Chapter 13.4)
  - Smear with dysplasia or cancer
  - Persistent unexplained atypia
  - Evidence of human papillomavirus (HPV) infection
- Suspicious visible lesion of the cervix, vagina, or vulva
- Follow-up of previously treated patients
- History of diethylstilbestrol exposure
- Colposcopy highly recommended
  - Patients with visible persistent condylomata
  - Unexplained vaginal discharge, itching, or bleeding
  - HIV-infected women
  - Intravenous drug abusers

CONTRAINDICATIONS FOR COLPOSCOPY

- Contraindications usually delay rather than prevent the examination.
- Active gonococcal, chlamydial, or trichomonal infections
- Uncooperative patient
- Heavy, active menses

BASIC CERVICAL COLPOSCOPIC FINDINGS

- Normal cervical findings
  - Squamous epithelium
  - Columnar epithelium
  - Squamous metaplasia
  - Squamocolumnar junction

- Variants of normal
  - Nabothian cysts
  - Atrophy
  - Pregnancy changes
  - Inflammatory or infectious process
  - Traumatic changes, clefts, or prior therapy

- Abnormal cervical mucosal patterns, indicating the need for biopsy
  - Leukoplakia (a white area prior to application of acetic acid, i.e., vinegar)
  - Acetowhite change (a whitening following vinegar application)
  - Punctation (a vessel pattern of small red dots usually within an acetowhite area)
  - Mosaic (a vessel pattern with the appearance of chicken-wire)
  - Atypical vessel pattern (abnormal branching, hairpins, corkscrew patterns)

BASIC PROCEDURAL STEPS FOR COLPOSCOPY OF THE CERVIX

- Perform a bimanual examination.
- Insert speculum.
- Adjust and focus colposcope initially on low power.
- Gently blot off excess mucus; apply normal saline to further clean and highlight vessel patterns.
- Apply acetic acid to allow for acetowhite changes within areas of dysplasia.
- Colposcopically examine the cervix, identifying areas of abnormality that will require biopsy.
- Lugol iodine solution may be applied to further identify abnormal areas. Lack of black staining on squamous epithelium implies dysplasia.
- Perform ECC to evaluate for occult cervical canal disease. This procedure is contraindicated in pregnancy.
- Perform punch biopsies of abnormal areas.
- Apply Monsel solution for local hemostasis.
- Carefully examine the vagina and vulva, and biopsy abnormal areas.

INTERPRETATION AND MANAGEMENT OF BIOPSY RESULTS

- Histologic diagnosis of cervical cancer requires definitive staging and advanced therapy, such as radical hysterectomy and radiation therapy.
- A positive ECC result or colposcopic evidence of significant endocervical canal involvement requires further tissue biopsy with either LEEP or cold knife conization.
- A negative ECC result (normal tissue, no dysplasia) and no colposcopic evidence of dysplasia in canal with low-grade squamous dysplasia on ectocervix biopsy can be managed with:
  - Expectant management, which requires repeat colposcopy and biopsy at 6 to 12 month intervals to rule out progression.

- Pap testing at 4 to 6 month intervals to rule out progression. Repeat colposcopy at 12 month intervals.
- Cryotherapy, LEEP, and laser ablation (for large lesions) can be considered for persistent low-grade lesions (persisting defined as dysplasia present longer than 2 years)
- Definitive treatment if dysplasia grade progresses.

- High-grade squamous dysplasia requires definitive therapy, including LEEP, laser excision, or cold cone. Cryotherapy can be performed in selected cases but never with a positive ECC. Limited ectocervical dysplasia that does not involve the canal is rarely a sole indication for hysterectomy.
- Adenomatous or glandular dysplasia on biopsy or ECC usually requires cold cone biopsy to evaluate for possible adenocarcinoma of the canal. Endometrial biopsy may also be necessary if there is suspicion of a endometrial sources of adenodysplasia.

COMPLICATIONS AND MORBIDITY OF COLPOSCOPY

- Infection or bleeding occurs in less than 1% of women.
- The most severely dysplastic tissue is not biopsied, and the degree of dysplasia is underestimated, resulting in delayed or inadequate therapy.

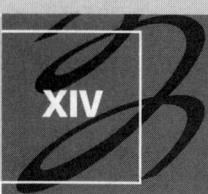

CONTRACEPTION
Carey Christiansen Ford

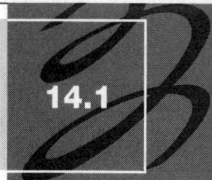

*M*any forms of contraception exist, each of which has unique benefits and disadvantages. Counseling a patient regarding birth control options should include discussion of many factors, including efficacy, convenience, duration of action, reversibility and return to fertility, effects on uterine bleeding, side effects, cost, and sexually transmitted disease (STD) protection.[1] Additionally, contraception has moral implications for some individuals that should not be overlooked. A patient's individual characteristics and medical history may also limit or influence the selection of an appropriate form of contraception and a thorough medical history and review of systems should be taken. Attention should be given to cardiovascular, gynecologic, and reproductive conditions, as well as psychologic or psychiatric conditions that might affect adherence.

NATURAL FAMILY PLANNING

This includes several methods described below of calculating the fertile time of a woman's cycle and maintaining complete abstinence during that period. Estimates of reliability vary, and for maximal effectiveness strict adherence must be followed. Advantages are lack of hormonal manipulation, cost, availability, and avoidance of artificial interventions that may contradict the beliefs of some religious and cultural groups. Disadvantages include the low rate of effectiveness compared to other methods, and the need for education to be provided in order to use it effectively.[2]

The calendar method is based on three assumptions: (a) A human ovum is capable of fertilization only for approximately 24 hours after ovulation; (b) sperm can only fertilize an ovum for about 48 hours after intercourse; and (c) ovulation usually occurs 12 to 16 days before the next menses begins. After recording six menstrual cycles the fertile period can be estimated. The earliest day of the fertile period is determined by the number of days in the shortest menstrual cycle subtracted by 18. The latest day of the fertile period is calculated by the number of days in the longest cycle subtracted by 11. Abstinence is maintained during that interval.[2]

Cervical Mucus Method

The woman attempts to predict her fertile period by examining the cervical mucus with her fingers. Under the influence of estrogen, the mucus increases in quantity and becomes progressively more elastic. After a peak day, the mucus becomes scant and dry, secondary to the influence of progesterone, and remains until the onset of the next menses. Intercourse is allowed 4 days after the cervical mucus peaks until menses begins.[2]

Symptothermal Method

This method predicts the first day of abstinence by using either the calendar method or the first day mucus is detected, whichever is noted first. The end of the fertile period is predicted by measuring basal body temperature. The basal body temperature is lowest during the follicular phase and rises in the luteal (postovulatory) phase of the menstrual cycle in response to progesterone. The rise in temperature can vary from 0.2 to 0.5°C. The elevated temperatures begin 1 to 2 days after ovulation and correspond to the rising level of progesterone. Intercourse is allowed 3 days after the temperature rise.[2]

Lactational Amenorrhea Method

While breastfeeding, a woman's fertility is typically reduced. The lactational amenorrhea method (LAM) can be relied on when three criteria are met: (a) It has been 6 months or less since delivery; (b) the woman's menstrual cycle has not returned; and (c) the infant's nutritional needs are at least 90% met at the breast. This method relies on frequent breastfeeding, both day and night, to be effective. Mechanism of action is inhibition of ovulation by elevated prolactin level. Disadvantages to this method include variability and unpredictability of the return of menses, and uncertainty of some women of the anticipated duration of breastfeeding.[3]

Abstinence

The complete avoidance of sexual intercourse. Mechanism of action is exclusion of sperm from the female reproductive tract. Advantages include STD prevention or reduction, although skin-to-skin contact without intercourse can transmit some infections. Disadvantages include lack of preparation for unanticipated intercourse, as well as difficulty maintaining the degree of willpower and self-control required.[3]

BARRIER METHODS

These methods physically prevent the union of ovum and sperm.

Male Condoms

Sheaths made of latex, polyurethane, or natural materials worn over the penis during intercourse. Effectively reduces the risk of STDs. Disadvantages include short shelf life, possibility of failure if used with oil-based lubricants, problems with correct usage, and decreased sensation.[4] Many people are allergic to latex, in which case polyurethane condoms, which are somewhat less effective, may be used.

Female Condoms

A polyurethane sheath inserted into the vagina up to 8 hours before intercourse. Provides some protection from STDs. Inner surface coated with lubricant but does not contain spermicide. May be cumbersome or uncomfortable to use, and may contribute to the development of a urinary tract infection if left in place for too long.[2]

Diaphragms and Cervical Caps

Cervical barriers inserted vaginally to prevent sperm from reaching the cervical canal. Should be used in conjunction with spermicide to increase efficacy. Advantages include absence of hormone exposure and reduced likelihood of sexually transmitted infection, but are not recommended in women at high risk of HIV exposure. Disadvantages include lower efficacy than other methods, vaginal irritation, and discomfort in some women.[1]

Intrauterine Device

T-shaped device placed in the uterus through the cervix during a simple office procedure. Two types approved for use in the United States, the copper-releasing type (ParaGard) and hormone-releasing type (Mirena). Very effective, but may be morally opposed by some patients and physicians due to potential for both pre- and postfertilization mechanisms of action. Contraindicated in those with a greater risk of developing pelvic inflammatory disease (PID) (history of PID, exposure to STDs, nonmonogamy). Nulliparous women have a higher rate of device expulsion and failure and the device may be more difficult to place.[5]

Progesterone Releasing

Levonorgestrel coating releases progesterone at 20 μg per day, causing thickening of cervical mucus, and possibly inhibiting ovulation and thinning the uterine lining. Can remain in the uterus for up to 5 years. Advantages include improvement in menorrhagia and dysmenorhea.[5,6]

Copper Releasing

Copper coating releases ions that interfere with sperm mobility and create a spermicidal environment. May be in place for up to 10 years.[5] Bleeding and dysmenorrhea may temporarily increase after insertion.[3]

COMBINED CONTRACEPTIVES

- **Oral combined contraceptive pills (OCPs).** Daily tablet containing a progestin and a synthetic estrogen. Many users rely on OCPs for their noncontraceptive benefits, including improvement in menstrual cycle regulation, acne, hyperandrogenism, dysmenorrhea, breast and ovarian cysts, premenstrual syndrome, endometriosis, and others.[7] Newer formulations exist that allow less frequent menses, with 84 active pill days and 7 placebo, rather than the standard "21 + 7" schedule. Prevent midcycle gonadotropin release and thus inhibit ovulation. Combined OCPs may be started at any time during the menstrual cycle; a barrier method is typically recommended for the first week after starting, unless started on the first day of menstrual bleeding.[8]
- **Contraindications** include uncontrolled hypertension, venous thromboembolism, coronary heart disease, cerebrovascular disease, postpartum <21 days, age >25 years, and smoke >15 to 20 cigarettes per day, headaches with focal neurologic symptoms, diabetes with vascular complications, lactation (<6 weeks), breast cancer, pregnancy, liver disease, inherited thrombophilias, anticonvulsant drug use, and undiagnosed abnormal uterine bleeding.[1,7]
- **Implanted combination contraceptives (Implanon).** A single-rod progestin implant is available in the United States. Contraception is provided for 3 years by the progestin etonogestrel. Protection from pregnancy occurs within 24 hours of insertion and fertility returns rapidly after removal. Training sponsored by the manufacturer is required before implant can be purchased or inserted.[1]
- **Ortho Evra patch.** Worn on the torso, buttocks, or upper arm, and changed weekly for 3 weeks followed by a patch-free week of bleeding similar to placebo-pill week of OCPs. Mechanism of action, benefits, risks, and contraindications to use of the patch are similar to those of combined OCPs. Conflicting data exist regarding possible increased risk of thromboembolism. May be started on first day of menses or on Sunday following first day of menses, and requires 1 week of back-up barrier method.[1]
- **NuvaRing.** Flexible plastic ring worn intravaginally for 3 weeks and removed for a 1-week interval before a new ring is inserted. Mechanism of action, benefits, risks, and contraindications to use are similar to those of combined OCPs. Should be started within the first 5 days of menses with a back-up barrier method used for the first week.[1]

PROGESTIN-ONLY CONTRACEPTIVES

Prevent ovulation by inhibiting the midcycle release of gonadotropins. Atrophic endometrium and thickened cervical mucus also protect against pregnancy by minimizing ability of a fertilized ovum to implant and decreasing sperm penetration through endocervical canal, respectively.[9]

■ Progestin-only pills. Include Micronor and Ovrette. To maintain efficacy, must be taken within 3-hour window regularly. Often prescribed to women who are breastfeeding. Unlike estrogen-containing contraceptives, no increased risk of thromboembolism.[9]
■ Depo-Provera. Medroxyprogesterone acetate given intramuscularly every 3 months. Can be started any time, as long as pregnancy is ruled out. A back-up barrier method is needed the first week. Data indicate that bone density decreases while using this medication[10]; it is unclear how much is regained. Irregular bleeding, amenorrhea, and delayed return to fertility are common side effects.[9]

STERILIZATION

Tubal Sterilization

Surgical method of preventing the ovum from being fertilized or reaching the uterine cavity by occluding or otherwise interrupting the fallopian tubes. This method is effective and permanent. There is an associated decreased risk of PID and ovarian cancer in women who have undergone sterilization procedures.[11] Drawbacks to this method include the risks inherent to any surgical procedure as well as the permanence of the procedure. Sterilization regret is highly correlated with age younger than 30 and unpredictable life events such as change in marital status or death of a child.[11] Reversal is costly and unpredictable. Also, there is an increased risk for ectopic pregnancy, should pregnancy occur.

Vasectomy

Surgical method of preventing the release of sperm in the ejaculate by disrupting the vas deferns typically with ligation and cautery. Less expensive than tubal ligation; restoring fertility after vasectomy is unreliable and expensive. Another method should be used until documentation of azoospermia, which may be about 10 weeks. Bleeding and infection are rare complications.[12]

EMERGENCY CONTRACEPTION

This typically refers to high-dose progestin in pill form used postcoitally to prevent pregnancy by preventing ovulation, altering cervical mucus, or preventing implantation of fertilized ovum. Does not interrupt an already-implanted pregnancy, and not teratogenic.[3]

■ Plan B. 75 μg levonorgestrel taken within 72 hours of intercourse, with second 75 μg tablet taken 12 hours later.[3,13] Some sources say the first tablet may actually be given within 120 hours of intercourse.[3]
■ Alternatively, combined OCPs may used. The first dose should be given within the first 72 hours after unprotected intercourse, and the second dose given 12 hours after the first dose. Many brand name OCPs can be used for emergency contraception including:
  ▪ Preven Kit. Two pills per dose (0.5 mg of levonorgestrel and 100 μg of ethinyl estradiol per dose)
  ▪ Ovral. Two pills per dose (0.5 mg of levonorgestrel and 100 μg of ethinyl estradiol per dose)
  ▪ Lo/Ovral. Four pills per dose (0.6 mg of levonorgestrel and 120 μg of ethinyl estradiol per dose)
  ▪ Nordette. Four pills per dose (0.6 mg of levonorgestrel and 120 μg of ethinyl estradiol per dose)
  ▪ Triphasil. Four pills per dose (0.5 mg of levonorgestrel and 120 μg of ethinyl estradiol per dose)
  ▪ Ovrette. 20 pills per dose (1.5 mg of levonorgestrel per dose)
  ▪ Seasonale. Four pills per dose (0.6 mg of levonorgestrel and 120 μg of ethinyl estradiol per dose)
  ▪ Alesse. Five pills per dose (0.5 mg of levonorgestrel and 100 μg of ethinyl estradiol per dose)[3,13]

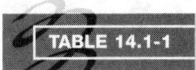

| TABLE 14.1-1 | A Comparative Summary of Available Contraceptive Methods |

| Method | Women who had an unintended pregnancy within the first year (%) | | Women who continued use at 1 yr (%) | Risks and side effects |
	Typical use	Perfect use		
No method	85	85	—	—
Spermicides	29	15	42	Allergy to spermicide
Withdrawal	27	4	43	None known
Periodic abstinence	Unknown	1–9	—	None known
Cervical cap with spermicide: parous/ nulliparous	32/16	26/9	46/57	Vaginal and bladder infections, allergy to spermicide
Diaphragm with spermicide	16	6	57	Vaginal and bladder infections, allergy to spermicide
Female condom	21	5	49	Difficult to use, vaginal and bladder infections
Male condom	15	2	53	Decrease in spontaneity, allergic reactions
Combined OC	8	0.3	68	Nausea, vomiting, headaches, dizziness, mood changes, breast tenderness, spotting, breakthrough bleeding
Patch (Ortho Evra)	0.8	0.6	68	Same as OC, application site reactions
Vaginal contraceptive ring (Nuva-ring)	0.65	0.3	68	Vaginitis, breast tenderness, spotting, bleeding
Depo-Provera injection	3	0.3	56	Menstrual changes, weight gain, headaches, mood changes
Copper IUD (Paragard)	0.8	0.6	78	Increase in menstrual flow and cramping, risk of perforation and PID after insertion
Levonorgestrel- releasing IUD (Mirena)	0.1	0.1	81	Irregular bleeding, amenorrhea, risk of perforation and PID after insertion
Female sterilization	0.5	0.5	100	—
Male sterilization	0.15	0.1	100	—

OC, oral contraceptive; IUD, intrauterine device; PID, pelvic inflammatory disease.
Adapted from Hatcher RA et al, eds. *A pocket guide to managing contraception 2004–2005.* Tiger, GA: Bridging the Gap Communications; 2005.

References
1. Zieman M. Overview of contraception (on-line). Available at: http://www.uptodate.com.
2. Samra O. Contraception (on-line). Available at: http://www.emedicine.com.
3. Hatcher R, Cwiak C, Zieman M. *A pocket guide to managing contraception.* Tiger, GA: Bridging the Gap Communications; 2005.
4. Steiner MJ, et al. Contraceptive effectiveness of a polyurethane condom and a latex condom: a randomized controlled trial. *Obstet Gynecol* 2003;101:539–547.
5. Johnson BA. Insertion and removal of intrauterine devices. *Am Fam Physician* 2005;71:95–102.
6. Herndon EJ. New contraceptive options. *Am Fam Physician* 2004;69:853–860.
7. Cerel-Suhl SL, Yeager BF. Update on oral contraceptives. *Am Fam Physician* 1999; 60(7):2073–2084.
8. Martin KA, Barbieri AR. Overview of the use of estrogen-progestin contraceptives. Available at: http://www.uptodate.com.
9. Apgar BA, Greenberg G. Using progestins in clinical practice. *Am Fam Physician* 2000;62(8)1839–1846,1849–1850.
10. Berenson AB, Breitkopf CR, Grady JJ, et al. Effects of hormonal contraception on bone mineral density after 24 months of use. *Obstet Gynecol* 2004;103:899–906.
11. Baill IC, Cullins VE, Sangeeta P. Counseling issues in tubal sterilization. *Am Fam Physician* 2003;67:1287–1294,1301–1302.
12. Dassow P, Bennett J. Vasectomy: an update. *Am Fam Physician* 2006;74:2069–2074.
13. Erdahl K, Holten K. Emergency contraception care. *J Fam Pract* 2006;55(12): 1073–1075.

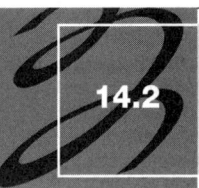

14.2 INFERTILITY
Keith A. Frey, Jennifer W. Boyden

GENERAL PRINCIPLES

The diagnosis of infertility is established after 1 year of unprotected intercourse in which a pregnancy has not been achieved. By this definition, approximately 15% to 17% of couples in the United States are affected. There are many causes of infertility, including abnormalities of any portion of the male or female reproductive system. Infertility is due to a single cause in the majority of couples, but more than one factor contributes to infertility in approximately 15% of couples. Therefore, a comprehensive diagnostic evaluation is recommended for all couples.

Common Etiology and Pathophysiology

- **Male factors.** A male cause for infertility occurs in 26% to 30% of couples. The most common male etiologic factor is a varicocele. Other causative factors include oligospermia or azoospermia, disorders of sperm function or motility (asthenospermia), and abnormalities of sperm morphology (teratospermia). Antisperm antibodies as a cause of male infertility is quite rare.
- **Ovulatory dysfunction.** Disorders of ovulation account for approximately 21% of cases of infertility. The possible causes may be grouped under four major headings:
  - **Hypothalamic anovulation** includes anatomical defects, congenital defects, psychologic trauma, anorexia nervosa, and pharmacologic agents.
  - **Ovarian anovulation** includes ovarian tumors, premature ovarian failure, ovarian dysgenesis, thyroid disease, and adrenal disease.
  - **Pituitary anovulation** includes pituitary tumors and ischemia.
  - **Integrative anovulation** includes nonpsychogenic weight disturbances and polycystic ovary syndrome.

■ **Tubal damage.** Infertility due to tubal damage or adnexal adhesions accounts for approximately 14% of cases of infertility. Tubal obstruction may result from previous episodes of salpingitis, although many cases of tubal occlusion are encountered in which no episodes of salpingitis are recalled by the patient (see Chapter 13.5). Endometriosis may result in the anatomical distortion of adnexal structures.

■ **Endometriosis.** The chronic inflammation associated with endometriosis may disrupt normal conception by interfering with ovum capture and gamete and embryo transport, or by causing tubal damage. Endometriosis is the cause of approximately 6% to 20% of infertility cases.

■ **"Unexplained" infertility.** No specific etiologic factor is identified in approximately 28% of infertile couples after an initial diagnostic survey.

DIAGNOSTIC EVALUATION

A thorough diagnostic survey of both spouses is necessary to evaluate all areas of the reproductive system. Begin the workup for women under 35 years old after 12 months of infertility and after only 6 months of infertility in women over 35 years old. A meeting with the couple early in the evaluation provides an opportunity to review reproductive biology, discuss the rationale for subsequent tests, and assess the couple's coping skills.

History

The initial assessment of the couple consists of a thorough history of each partner, taken individually, to assess current and past contributing symptoms, illness, medication, or surgery. The key elements of such a history are outlined in Table 14.2-1.

Physical Examination

As with the history, a thorough physical examination of each partner is essential. Areas of special attention for each physical are listed in Table 14.2-2.

Laboratory Studies

Each couple is evaluated with a few routine laboratory and appropriately timed studies to assess every major reproductive factor that may contribute to the infertility. This comprehensive diagnostic survey can and should be completed for the majority of couples in 3 to 6 months. The evaluation should be individualized based on the findings of the history and physical examination, but an initial survey of all major reproductive factors is necessary in all couples and can be coordinated by the family physician. The specifically timed diagnostic tests required for an infertility survey are outlined in Table 14.2-3.

■ **Male factors.** The male is evaluated with a complete blood count, urinalysis, and at least two semen analyses. Each semen analysis is performed on a fresh (within 2 hours), warm specimen obtained by masturbation after at least 2 days of abstinence. Normal results vary between laboratories but in general include a volume (2 to 5 mL), complete liquefaction within 30 minutes, sperm count (>20 million/mL), sperm motility (>50%), and morphology (>30% normal forms). Evidence of oligospermia after two or more semen analyses requires further evaluation, including blood levels for luteinizing hormone, follicle-stimulating hormone, and testosterone.

■ **Ovulatory dysfunction.** Anovulation or inconsistent ovulation may be suggested by history (irregular menses), and confirmed by an abnormally low serum progesterone levels in the luteal phase, or persistently negative home luteinizing hormone (LH) testing. If the patient is not ovulating further laboratory evaluation is needed (see Table 14.2-3). Those patients with a diminished ovarian reserve (follicle-stimulating hormone >10) should be referred to an infertility specialist.

■ **Tubal factors.** The female partner must undergo an evaluation for tubal patency. A hysterosalpingogram is obtained if the history and physical examination show no evidence of tubal damage. Otherwise, the patient is referred for laparoscopy.

TREATMENT

Treatment should not be initiated until the diagnostic survey is complete and the infertility cause or causes identified. The diagnosis should be shared with the couple together and the treatment options outlined. The workup, diagnosis, and treatment of infertility can precipitate

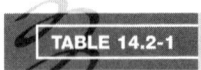

TABLE 14.2-1	Key Areas of Infertility History

Marriage
Duration of infertility
Fertility in previous relationship
Sexual techniques
Frequency of intercourse (optimal is daily around time of ovulation)
Use of coital lubricants (often spermicidal)

Adult illness
Acute viral or febrile illness in past 3 mo
Orchitis
Renal disease
Sexually transmitted diseases
Tuberculosis

Occupation and habits
Exposure to radiation, chemicals, excessive heat (e.g., hot tub)

Childhood illness
Cryptorchidism
Age at puberty

Surgery
Herniorrhaphy
Retroperitoneal surgery
Vasectomy

Review of systems
Focus on endocrine conditions
Gynecologic history
Coital frequency
Contraceptive use
Diethylstilbestrol (DES) use by mother
Douches and lubricant use
Menarche
Menses (regularity and flow)
Mittelschmerz

Drug use
Alcohol, tobacco, excessive caffeine, and other drugs
Anabolic steroids, nitrofurantoin, cimetidine

intense emotional reactions. The sensitive physician discusses such emotions as guilt, anger, self-doubt, depression, and grief. Helping the couple understand their motives for parenting can be helpful. These motives may include a desire to parent, to experience a pregnancy, to meet the expectations of others, and to promote genetic continuity. The physician should assist the couple in the development of mutual support and an adaptive "couple-coping" style. This assistance includes the discussion of sexual issues and the encouragement to nurture their intimacy. Periodic meetings with the couple to review diagnostic or treatment progress provides further opportunity to reinforce coping skills. Referral to self-help groups, such as RESOLVE, Inc. (www.resolve.org), assist the couple in broadening their support systems.

- **Male factors.** Consultation with a urologist is necessary to coordinate treatment for a varicocele or other causes of sperm dysfunction.
- **Ovulatory dysfunction.** Treatment with clomiphene should be considered for women diagnosed with anovulation. Amenorrheic and oligomenorrheic women attempting to conceive are among the most suitable patients for clomiphene. Patients with other cause

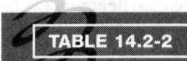

TABLE 14.2-2	Physical Examination in Infertility: Areas of Special Attention

Male	Female
Hair pattern	Breast formation and galactorrhea
Genitalia	Distribution of body fat
Meatus size and location	Hair pattern (virilization)
Prostate and seminal vesicles	**Neurologic**
Scrotum	Anosmia
Testicular size (>4 cm in long axis)	Visual fields
Varicocele (standing and with Valsalva maneuver)	**Pelvis**
Neurologic	External genitalia
Anosmia	Retrovaginal area (endometriosis)
Visual fields	Uterus and adnexa
	Vagina and cervix

for their anovulation respond best to specific therapy, such as surgery for a pituitary tumor or medical therapy for thyroid disease. The starting dose for clomiphene is 50 mg per day PO on menstrual cycle days 3 to 7. The dosage should only be increased if the patient is not ovulating. If a midluteal progesterone is greater than 10 pg per mL, continue the same clomiphene dose. If the progesterone is less than 10 pg per mL, then increase the dose of clomiphene by 50 mg per cycle until the patient is ovulating. The patient should be aware of the common side effects of clomiphene therapy: ovarian enlargement (13.9% of cases), vasomotor flushes (10.7%), abdominal or pelvic discomfort (7.4%), and multiple gestation (<5% and usually twinning). Ovulation should be expected 3 to 8 days after the treatment ends and should be confirmed by a LH home detection kit and an elevated serum progesterone on day 21. If ovulation does not occur despite clomiphene therapy, consultation with an infertility specialist is recommended.

- **Tubal damage.** Tubal deformity or blockage may require surgical correction via laparoscopy or laparotomy with tubal microsurgery, although pregnancy outcomes may be more cost effectively achieved via in vitro fertilization (IVF).

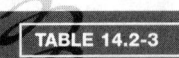

TABLE 14.2-3	Laboratory and Diagnostic Testing in Infertility

Routine laboratory tests:
Male
    CBC
    Semen analysis (at least 2)
    Urinalysis
Female
    CBC
    Pap smear
    Urinalysis

Special circumstances:
Anovulation: serum prolactin and TSH
Galactorrhea: serum prolactin and TSH
Hyperandrogenism: serum prolactin, TSH, LH, FSH, DHEA-S, 17-OH progesterone
Advanced maternal age: cycle day 3 FSH and estradiol

■ **Endometriosis.** The treatment of infertile women with endometriosis depends on the degree and location of the endometrial deposits. Conservative surgical treatment may enhance fertility by destroying endometrial implants and endometriomas. The laparoscopic cauterization of early-stage endometriosis has been shown in one study to improve pregnancy rates. Ovulation suppression by danazol, progestins, and gonadotropin-releasing hormone analogues has been shown not to be effective in the treatment of endometriosis-associated infertility. Superovulation with clomiphene or human menopausal gonadotropins has been shown to be effective in such patients.

Prognosis

The specific prognosis of infertility is difficult to determine due to the multiple etiologies. For most causes of infertility, conception will not occur without specific treatment. However, favorable pregnancy rates are reported when specific therapy is instituted. If the comprehensive diagnostic workup fails to establish a diagnosis or if appropriate treatment is unsuccessful, the physician should consider referring the couple to an infertility specialist. The options for adoption should also be discussed with the couple at this time.

References

1. Speroff L, Glass RH, Kase NG. *Clinical gynecologic endocrinology and infertility.* 5th ed. Baltimore: Williams & Wilkins; 1994.
2. Frey KA, Patel KS. Initial evaluation and management of infertility by the primary care physician. *Mayo Clin Proc* 2004;79:1439–1443.
3. Adamson GD, Baker V. Subfertility: causes, treatment and outcome. Best practice and research. *Clin Obstet Gynecol* 2003;17:169–185.
4. Jose-Miller AB, Bryden JW, Frey KA. Infertility. *Am Fam Physician* 2007;75:849–56, 857–858.

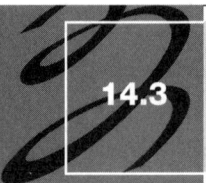

14.3 GENETIC DISORDERS AND PREGNANCY

Karen E. Muchowski, Heather L. Paladine

GENERAL PRINCIPLES

Genetic disorders in pregnancy is a complex topic for patients and providers. For most genetic conditions, the benefits of prenatal diagnosis have not been scientifically evaluated, other than the option for a patient to terminate a pregnancy affected by a genetic disorder. Patients may be concerned about possible discrimination against themselves or future offspring. Genetic counseling is recommended to clarify these issues and discuss the implications of testing for patients who are at risk. This chapter reviews the most common genetic disorders found during pregnancy, specifically the ones for which screening tests are available.

Types of Genetic Disorders

■ **Chromosome disorders** are caused by the loss, gain, or abnormal arrangement of one or more chromosomes. The incidence of these disorders in the population is about 0.2%. Down syndrome (trisomy 21) is discussed below.

■ **Mendelian disorders** are single-gene disorders caused by a mutant allele at a single genetic locus. The transmission pattern is further divided into autosomal dominant, autosomal recessive, X-linked dominant, and X-linked recessive. The incidence of these disorders is about 0.35%. Screening for cystic fibrosis, hemoglobinopathies, and Tay–Sachs disease is discussed below.

- **Multifactorial disorders** involve interactions between genes and environmental factors. The nature of these interactions is poorly understood. Screening for cardiac defects and neural tube defects (NTD) is described below.

CHROMOSOME DISORDERS: DOWN SYNDROME

Down syndrome (trisomy 21) occurs in 1 in 700 births. The risk of having a fetus with Down syndrome increases with maternal age. Affected children have variable degrees of mental retardation (mean IQ 50). About one third of the children will have congenital heart defects, and there is an increased risk of duodenal atresia and tracheoesophageal fistula. Affected children also have increased problems with hearing, vision, hypothyroidism, leukemia, cervical spine instability, and Alzheimer disease.

Noninvasive Prenatal Screening for Down Syndrome

Screening for Down syndrome includes first trimester screening (serum and ultrasound), second trimester serum screening, and second trimester ultrasound evaluation. The American College of Obstetrics and Gynecology (ACOG) recommends that all women be offered serum screening during their pregnancy. Both the first and second trimester serum screening can be accomplished relatively early in pregnancy, are simple to perform, and have high rates of sensitivity with small false-positive rates. Second trimester ultrasound is readily available but has a lower sensitivity for detection of Down syndrome.

- Early testing allows women who would choose termination of the pregnancy to do so at an earlier gestational age (when termination is safer). For women who would not choose termination, determination of the fetal abnormality allows patients to prepare for the baby and its added needs. It also allows providers to do further testing on the fetus (i.e., cardiac echo). Identification of pregnancies that have a fetus affected by Down syndrome will also assist physicians in management of the pregnancy. These pregnancies often have higher rates of pre-eclampsia, postdates pregnancy, and dysfunctional labor.
- **First trimester screening.** Serum and ultrasound markers that can be evaluated during weeks 10 to 13 of gestation. The serum markers are pregnancy-associated plasma protein A (PAPP-A) and the free unit of beta human chorionic gonadotropin (hCG). PAPP-A levels are 2.5 times lower in fetuses with Down syndrome and levels of the free unit of beta HCG are two times higher.
  - Increased nuchal translucency seen on ultrasound during weeks 11 to 13 of gestation is associated with Down syndrome, trisomy 18, and other aneuploides. The combined test (serum markers and ultrasound for nuchal translucency) is recommended and has been studied in more than 300,000 women. Published sensitivities range from 85% to 92% with false-positive rates of 5% to 6.1%. Women who have first trimester screening for Down syndrome still need to have an alpha-feto protein (AFP) level done in the second trimester for evaluation of NTDs.
  - Mathematical models of cost-effectiveness have shown that first trimester screening is more cost-effective than second trimester screening; much of the decreased cost is from fewer amniocenteses needing to be performed.

- **Second trimester screening.** The quadruple test is a serum study that evaluates AFP, HCG, inhibin A, and estriol levels. The test can be performed from 15 to 22 weeks of gestation and has a sensitivity of 85% with false-positive rates of 5% to 6%. Calculation of the serum marker levels combined with maternal age provides a personal risk score for each woman for her risk of having a fetus with Down syndrome. The screening test is considered positive if the calculated risk is greater than 1/270. This is the risk of a 35-year-old woman having a fetus with Down syndrome and is also the risk of a procedure-related loss from invasive testing for Down syndrome.
  - Incorrect gestational age is the most common reason for a false-positive result. Gestational age should always be first confirmed with an ultrasound prior to proceeding to invasive testing for an evaluation of a positive screen.
  - **Ultrasound.** Second trimester ultrasound can be used to identify major and minor structural abnormalities of the fetus that are associated with Down syndrome.

Major structural abnormalities include heart defects and duodenal atresia. However, only 20% to 30% of fetuses with Down syndrome have these defects. Minor ultrasound markers include increased nuchal fold, echogenic bowel, pyelectasis, echogenic cardiac focus, choroids plexus cysts, two-vessel cord, and absent nasal bone. Sensitivity for detection of Down syndrome is 69% with a false-positive rate of 8%.

Invasive Screening

Available both to evaluate a positive screen for Down syndrome and also as primary screening for women over the age of 35.

■ **Chorionic villus sampling (CVS)** can be performed from 10 to 13 weeks of gestation. A cannula is used to obtain a small amount of placental tissue via a transcervical (TC-CVS) or transabdominal (TA-CVS) approach. This provides a large amount of genetic material and karyotype results are often available in 48 hours.
  ▪ Risks of the procedure include spontaneous fetal loss (5.4% to 6.2%); the higher rates of loss are seen with TC-CVS. There is a 10% total fetal loss (which includes fetuses that would have been lost even without CVS procedure). The relative risk of fetal loss compared to amniocentesis is 1.3 (CI 1.2 to 1.5). However, when rates of TC-CVS are removed, the rate of loss is similar to amniocentesis. Other risks include bleeding, infection, and fetomaternal hemorrhage.

■ **Amniocentesis** can be performed as early as 13 weeks gestation, but is more commonly done after 15 weeks. A needle is introduced into the amniotic cavity and amniotic fluid is removed. Sloughed fetal cells are cultured and DNA is extracted for karyotyping. Results can take up to 2 weeks.
  ▪ Total fetal loss after amniocentesis is 6.1% with a procedure related loss of 0.6%. Membrane rupture occurs 1.7% of the time, but most of the leaks are small, resolve spontaneously, and reaccumulate within a week. Other risks include indirect fetal injury (increased rates of talipes equinovarus, 0.76% vs. 0.56% in controls), infection, and fetomaternal hemorrhage.

MENDELIAN DISORDERS

Cystic Fibrosis

Cystic fibrosis (CF) is the most common autosomal recessive disorder of Caucasians of Northern European decent. The carrier rate for a mutation is 1 in 25. Carrier rates are also high in Ashkenazi Jews (1 in 29). CF can cause abnormal pulmonary function, pancreatic insufficiency, or congenital absence of the vas deferens. The average age of survival is 40 years.

■ Serum screening can be done at any time, but ideally is best done prior to pregnancy. Because most screening tests only detect 90% of the mutations that cause CF, screening can decrease risk but not eliminate it.
■ The ACOG recommends that screening be offered to all women. Women who are not in high-risk groups (family history of CF, reproductive partner with CF, Caucasian of European descent, or Ashkenazi Jews) should be offered the test, but the decreased detectability of mutations should be discussed.
■ The fetus can be tested for CF with amniocentesis, CVS, or fetal blood sample. Issues that need to be considered include the related fetal loss associated with invasive testing. Knowledge of the diagnosis for the fetus will most likely not change the neonatal course (except for monitoring/treatment of meconium ileus). In addition, parents need to be reminded that the same genotypes often have different phenotypic presentations, which makes prediction of morbidity and mortality from CF problematic.

Hemoglobinopathies

Hemoglobinopathies have an autosomal recessive inheritance pattern. High-risk groups are people of African, Southeast Asian, and Mediterranean descent. Complete blood count (CBC) is an appropriate first-line screening test for most at-risk women. ACOG recommends that all women of African descent have hemoglobin electrophoresis.

Women with a low mean corpuscular volume (MCV) on CBC testing (less than 80 μ^3) should have hemoglobin electrophoresis to determine if they are hemoglobinopathy carriers.

Prenatal genetic testing by amniocentesis is available for sickle cell disease, and for alpha and beta thalassemia when the mutations have previously been identified in the parents. These patients can also be offered genetic counseling prior to pregnancy and preimplantation genetic diagnosis with in vitro fertilization.

Sickle Cell Disease

Sickle cell disease is the most common hemoglobinopathy; 1 out of 12 African Americans has sickle cell trait. Sickle cell trait can be detected by hemoglobin electrophoresis. If a woman who is pregnant or contemplating pregnancy tests positive, the next step is testing of the male partner. If both partners test positive, the couple should be referred for genetic counseling. Despite the relatively high prevalence of sickle cell disease, surveys have shown that most African American women of childbearing age do not understand the inheritance pattern or implications of the carrier state.

Thalassemia

Alpha thalassemia trait (alpha thalassemia minor) has two variants. In individuals of Southeast Asian descent, both α-globin genes on the same chromosome are deleted. They are at higher risk for a child with hemoglobin H disease (deletion of three of the four α-globin genes) and hemoglobin Bart (or alpha thalassemia major, deletion of all four α-globin genes). Hemoglobin H results in mild to moderate hemolytic anemia. Hemoglobin Bart can lead to hydrops fetalis, intrauterine fetal demise, and pre-eclampsia.

In individuals of African descent with alpha thalassemia trait, one α-globin gene is deleted on each copy of chromosome 16. They are not typically at risk for offspring with hemoglobin H or hemoglobin Bart. However, mild anemia is often present.

Alpha thalassemia trait will not be detected on hemoglobin electrophoresis. DNA based testing is needed for women with low MCV, no iron-deficiency anemia, and a normal hemoglogin electrophoresis.

Tay–Sachs Disease

The carrier rate for Tay–Sachs disease is 1 of 30 for people of Eastern European Jewish descent (Ashkenazi); people of French-Canadian and Cajun descent also have higher rates. Inheritance is autosomal recessive.

In this disorder, accumulation of gangliosides in the central nervous system results in progressive neurologic disease and death in early childhood.

In nonpregnant women, carrier screening can be performed by molecular or biochemical analysis. Biochemical analysis has a higher carrier detection rate, especially in low-risk populations. However, in women who are pregnant or taking oral contraceptives, serum biochemical testing may yield a false-positive result. These women should have biochemical testing on peripheral leukocytes or molecular testing. Genetic counseling is recommended for high-risk patients to determine the correct type of testing and to interpret the test results.

MULTIFACTORIAL DISORDERS

Congenital Heart Disease

Congenital heart disease (CHD) is the most common congenital anomaly, occurring in 8 of 1000 live births. Risk factors include family history of CHD, maternal diabetes, exposure to cardiac teratogens, noncardiac fetal anomalies detected on ultrasound, chromosomal abnormalities, single umbilical artery, fetal arrhythmias, nonimmune fetal hydrops, and increased nuchal translucency.

Women with risk factors should be referred for fetal echocardiography. However, the majority of CHD will occur in a low-risk population. In the United States, although routine ultrasound screening is not mandated, most women do undergo ultrasound screening during pregnancy. The detection rate of CHD on routine 18- to 22-week ultrasound is very variable, ranging from 23% to 77%.

The advantages of early detection of CHD fall into three categories: offering patients the choice of pregnancy termination, prenatal intervention, and postnatal management. Prenatal intervention is still in the experimental stages. Although postnatal management, such as delivery at a tertiary care center and preparation for early surgery, would appear to have logical benefits, the advantages of this have been difficult to demonstrate in studies.

Neural Tube Defects

NTDs are the second most prevalent congenital anomaly. In the United States, NTDs occur in 1 in 1000 pregnancies. The defects either appear in the spine (spina bifida, meningomyelocele, meningocele) or the cranium (anencephaly, which accounts for 50% of NTDs). Some NTDs are associated with genetic syndromes, but the majority are isolated defects.

NTDs most likely result from a combination of genetic and environmental influences. In a family with a child with a previous NTD, the relative risk of having another child with an NTD is 2% to 4%. Exposure to drugs that interfere with folic acid metabolism (carbamezapine, valproic acid) can cause NTDs. Maternal hyperthermia, diabetes, and obesity also increase the risk of having a fetus with an NTD. Finally, folic acid deficiency is known to increase the risk of NTDs. Preconception and early gestation (prior to 6 weeks) supplementation decreases the risk of NTDs.

Screening

Since 90% of NTDs occur in women with no prior history of having an affected fetus, it is recommended that all pregnant women be offered screening during weeks 15 to 20 of gestation.

- **Maternal serum alpha fetoprotein (MSAFP)** is elevated in 89% to 100% of pregnancies with a fetal NTD. A MSAFP greater than 2.5 multiples of the mean is 85% sensitive (5% false positive rate) for detection of all NTD and 95% sensitive (2% to 5% false positive rate) for detection of anencephaly.
- **Ultrasound** examination is 97% to 100% sensitive for the detection of NTDs and should be offered to all women with an abnormal MSAFP or women who are at high risk for a fetus with NTD.
- **Amniocentesis** allows for removal of amniotic fluid and evaluation of amniotic fluid AFP (AFAFP). Amniocentesis should be considered if the ultrasound is normal or equivocal or if the patient wishes to have karyotype determination of the fetus. If both AFAFP and amniotic acetylcholinesterase levels are abnormal, the fetus most likely has an open NTD (96% sensitivity, 0.14% false positive).

OTHER CONGENITAL ANOMALIES

The rates of ultrasound detection of anomalies vary from over 90% for major defects such as hydrocephalus and anencephaly, to just over 17% for cleft lip and palate and foot deformities. Because of this wide variability, the value of ultrasound screening for congenital anomalies is still unproven. Pregnant women should be informed about the detection rates of anomalies on ultrasound, and that many anomalies may be missed on ultrasound testing.

References

1. ACOG Committee Opinion 296, First-trimester screening for fetal aneuploidy. *Obstet Gynecol* 2004;42–44.
2. Canick, J, Messerlian GM, Farina A. First trimester screening for Down syndrome and trisomy 18. www.uptodate.com; 2006.
3. Canick, J, Messerlian GM, Farina A. General principles of second trimester maternal serum screening for Down syndrome. www.uptodate.com; 2006.
4. Wenstrom K. Cystic fibrosis: prenatal genetic screening. www.uptodate.com; 2005.
5. ACOG committee opinion 325. Update on carrier screening for cystic fibrosis. *Obstet Gynecol* 2005;106(6);1465–1468.
6. ACOG practice bulletin 64. Hemoglobinopathies in pregnancy. *Obstet Gynecol* 2005;106(1):203–211.
7. ACOG committee opinion 318. Screening for Tay–Sachs disease. *Obstet Gynecol* 2005;106(4):893–894.
8. Sharland G. Routine fetal cardiac screening; what are we doing and what should we do? *Prenat Diagn* 2004;24:1123–1129.
9. Goldberg JD. Routine screening for fetal anomalies: expectations. *Obstet Gynecol Clin North Am* 2004;31(1):35–50.
10. ACOG practice bulletin. Neural tube defects. *Obstet Gynecol* 2003;102(1);203–213.
11. Hochberg L, Stone J. Prenatal screening and diagnosis of neural tube defects. www.uptodate.com; 2006.

GENERAL PRINCIPLES

Family-centered prenatal care is the delivery of effective, efficient, accessible, safe, and economical quality care for the psychosocial, spiritual, and physical needs of the mother, child, father, and family unit. Family physicians with this philosophy view childbirth as a vital life event in the family and a foundational event in the formation of community and society. The family physician is ideally suited to provide this care, whether the family physician will deliver the baby or provide "shared prenatal care" with a delivering midwife or physician. An in-depth review of routine prenatal care is beyond the scope of this chapter; however, basic information that is frequently needed during prenatal care is provided, and Figure 14.4-1 illustrates important considerations and decision points in prenatal care.

DIAGNOSIS

History

A comprehensive history is required to provide appropriate prenatal care and distinguish between uncomplicated and higher-risk obstetrical patients. Ideally, prenatal care begins before conception and includes preventive, health-maintenance care, counseling, and screening for risks to maternal and fetal health.[1] The following components should be included:

- **Medical/surgical history.** History of diabetes, hypertension, asthma, seizure disorder, mental illness, hematologic disorders, cancer, HIV, recurrent urinary tract infections. Past surgeries. Previous history of varicella.
- Maternal care history. Past history of complicated pregnancy or delivery. History of preterm delivery; prior cervical or uterine surgery. History of fetal anatomic abnormality or intrauterine fetal demise.
- **Psychosocial history.** History of eating disorder, substance use, mood disorder, psychosis, or postpartum depression.
- Family history of medical and genetic disorders; prescription and over-the-counter medication use; substance use; history of domestic violence; history of transfusions; and immunization status. Ascertain risk for tuberculosis as well as sexually transmitted infections (STIs) or diseases (STDs) caused by HPV, HIV, hepatitis B or C, gonorrhea, *Chlamydia*, herpes, or syphilis.[2]

Physical Examination

- Initial visit. Ascertain the estimated date of delivery (EDD) based on the patient's last menstrual period (LMP). Early ultrasound is indicated to determine the EDD if there is uncertainty about the LMP.
- Examination should include height, weight, body mass index (BMI); blood pressure; screening Pap smear for women who have not been recently screened. Obtain cervical cultures for gonorrhea (GC) and *Chlamydia* (Chl) in high-risk women (age <25 years; unmarried; Black, a history of STIs or STDs, new or multiple sexual partners, cervical ectropion, and inconsistent use of barrier contraception; and living in communities with high infection rates).[3]
- Initial lab includes blood type and Rh, HIV, rubella, hepatitis B surface antigen (HBsAg), urine culture; varicella titer if unsure of history.
- All subsequent visits should include interval history and address any patient concerns or symptoms suggestive of preeclampsia or preterm labor, along with assessment of blood pressure, weight gain, fundal height, and fetal heart tones.

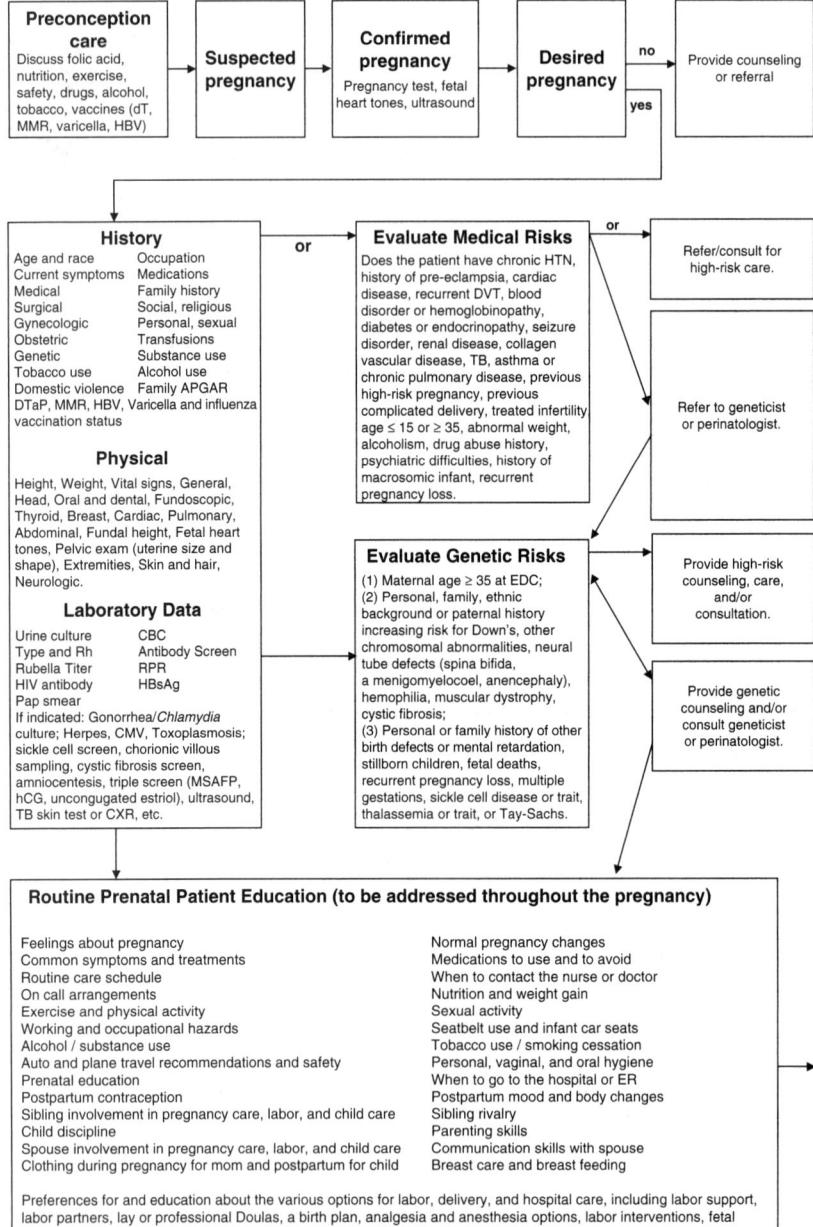

Preconception care
Discuss folic acid, nutrition, exercise, safety, drugs, alcohol, tobacco, vaccines (dT, MMR, varicella, HBV)

→ **Suspected pregnancy** → **Confirmed pregnancy**
Pregnancy test, fetal heart tones, ultrasound → **Desired pregnancy**

no → Provide counseling or referral

yes

History

Age and race	Occupation
Current symptoms	Medications
Medical	Family history
Surgical	Social, religious
Gynecologic	Personal, sexual
Obstetric	Transfusions
Genetic	Substance use
Tobacco use	Alcohol use
Domestic violence	Family APGAR
DTaP, MMR, HBV, Varicella and influenza	
vaccination status	

or

Physical

Height, Weight, Vital signs, General, Head, Oral and dental, Fundoscopic, Thyroid, Breast, Cardiac, Pulmonary, Abdominal, Fundal height, Fetal heart tones, Pelvic exam (uterine size and shape), Extremities, Skin and hair, Neurologic.

Laboratory Data

Urine culture	CBC
Type and Rh	Antibody Screen
Rubella Titer	RPR
HIV antibody	HBsAg
Pap smear	

If indicated: Gonorrhea/Chlamydia culture; Herpes, CMV, Toxoplasmosis; sickle cell screen, chorionic villous sampling, cystic fibrosis screen, amniocentesis, triple screen (MSAFP, hCG, unconjugated estriol), ultrasound, TB skin test or CXR, etc.

Evaluate Medical Risks

Does the patient have chronic HTN, history of pre-eclampsia, cardiac disease, recurrent DVT, blood disorder or hemoglobinopathy, diabetes or endocrinopathy, seizure disorder, renal disease, collagen vascular disease, TB, asthma or chronic pulmonary disease, previous high-risk pregnancy, previous complicated delivery, treated infertility, age ≤ 15 or ≥ 35, abnormal weight, alcoholism, drug abuse history, psychiatric difficulties, history of macrosomic infant, recurrent pregnancy loss.

or

Refer/consult for high-risk care.

Refer to geneticist or perinatologist.

Evaluate Genetic Risks

(1) Maternal age ≥ 35 at EDC;
(2) Personal, family, ethnic background or paternal history increasing risk for Down's, other chromosomal abnormalities, neural tube defects (spina bifida, a menigomyelocoel, anencephaly), hemophilia, muscular dystrophy, cystic fibrosis;
(3) Personal or family history of other birth defects or mental retardation, stillborn children, fetal deaths, recurrent pregnancy loss, multiple gestations, sickle cell disease or trait, thalassemia or trait, or Tay-Sachs.

Provide high-risk counseling, care, and/or consultation.

Provide genetic counseling and/or consult geneticist or perinatologist.

Routine Prenatal Patient Education (to be addressed throughout the pregnancy)

Feelings about pregnancy
Common symptoms and treatments
Routine care schedule
On call arrangements
Exercise and physical activity
Working and occupational hazards
Alcohol / substance use
Auto and plane travel recommendations and safety
Prenatal education
Postpartum contraception
Sibling involvement in pregnancy care, labor, and child care
Child discipline
Spouse involvement in pregnancy care, labor, and child care
Clothing during pregnancy for mom and postpartum for child

Normal pregnancy changes
Medications to use and to avoid
When to contact the nurse or doctor
Nutrition and weight gain
Sexual activity
Seatbelt use and infant car seats
Tobacco use / smoking cessation
Personal, vaginal, and oral hygiene
When to go to the hospital or ER
Postpartum mood and body changes
Sibling rivalry
Parenting skills
Communication skills with spouse
Breast care and breast feeding

Preferences for and education about the various options for labor, delivery, and hospital care, including labor support, labor partners, lay or professional Doulas, a birth plan, analgesia and anesthesia options, labor interventions, fetal monitoring, birth positions, episiotomy, circumcision, breastfeeding, early discharge.

Figure 14.4-1. *(continued)*

Routine care—each visit	Additional assessments
Interval History–Maternal well-being (symptoms pain); signs and symptoms of preterm labor (contractions, cramping, or bleeding); symptoms of hypertensive disorders (headache, visual c/o); or any other new problems. Exam–weight, blood pressure, fundal height, fetal heart tones.	Offer multiple marker maternal serum analyte screen at 15–18 weeks EGA. Urine C&S with urinary complaints or every trimester if history of recurrent UTI or UTI this pregnancy. Fetal anatomy ultrasound at 16–20 weeks EGA. If Rh-negative, antibody screen at 28 weeks. One hour glucose tolerance test at 24–28 weeks (earlier for prior h/o GDM). Perform rectovaginal swab for Group B streptococcus (GBS) screen at 36 weeks. Hemoglobin or hematocrit at the start of the 3rd trimester. Consider 36 week syphilis, gonorrhea, or chlamydia screen in high risk pts.

First trimester pain or bleeding. —**yes**→ Screen for ectopic or abnormal intrauterine pregnancy.

no

Other abnormal symptoms, abnormal weight gain, vaginitis, UTI, bleeding, nausea and vomiting, etc. —**yes**→ Evaluate and manage. Consultation if indicated.

no

Discrepancy between fundal height and EDC, decreased fetal motion, abnormal bleeding, abnormal fetal heart tones, etc. —**yes**→ Consider ultrasound and/or antenatal testing.

Rho(d)-negative mother. —**yes**→ Rh immune globulin at 28 weeks, if antibody screen is negative.

no

Preterm labor or rupture of membranes. —**yes**→ To L&D for evaluation and management. **labor not stopped** / **labor stopped**

no

Term labor or rupture of membranes. —**yes**→ To L&D for evaluation and management.

no

Postterm/Postdates → Antenatal testing or induction.

Preconception care ← **Postpartum care** ← **Labor and delivery**

TB = tuberculosis; UTI = urinary tract infection; C&S = culture and sensitivity; CBC = complete blood count; CMV = cytomegalovirus; c/o = complains of; CXR = chest X-ray; DTap = diphtheria, tetanus, acellular pertussis vaccine; DVT = deep venous thrombosis; EDC = estimated date of confinement (due date); EGA = estimated gestational age; ER = emergency room; GDM = gestational diabetes mellitus; HBsAG = hepatitis B surface antigen; HBV = hepatitis B Vaccine; hCG = human chorionic gonadotropin; HIV = human immunodeficiency virus; h/o = history of; HTN = hypertension; L&D = labor and delivery; MMR = measles, mumps, rubella vaccine; MSAFP = maternal serum alpha-fetoprotein; Rh = Rhesus factor; RPR = Rapid plasma regain

Figure 14.4-1

- Beginning with the start of the third trimester, visits should also include an assessment of fetal movement and abdominal palpation to assess fetal presentation at 36 weeks gestation.[2]
- It is no longer recommended to routinely perform urine tests for proteinuria and glycosuria. Evaluation of edema as assessment for pre-eclampsia.[2]

TREATMENT, INTERVENTIONS/RECOMMENDATIONS

Behavioral Counseling

- **Nutrition and weight gain.** The National Research Council recommends a 300 kcal per day increase in calories above nonpregnant levels throughout pregnancy.[4] For most patients, a well-balanced diet provides adequate nutrition during pregnancy. In general, special diets, skipping meals, and food avoidance may lead to nutritional deficiencies and inadequate weight gain during pregnancy. Recommendations for weight gain are based on a prepregnancy ideal body weight (IBW) or body mass index (BMI).[4] The average weight gain in women with a normal BMI (19 to 24.9) is 25 to 35 pounds. Women who enter pregnancy substantially below their IBW should gain a greater amount of weight during pregnancy (e.g., 28 to 40 pounds). Overweight (BMI 25 to 29.9) and obese (BMI >30) women should be advised to gain less weight during pregnancy (e.g., 15 to 25 pounds for the overweight and <15 pounds for the obese).
  - **Iron** is necessary to expand maternal red cell mass and for fetal-placental development. Iron consumption should be increased to **30 mg per day,** the amount found in most prenatal vitamins. **Dietary sources** include lean meat, whole grains, dried fruits, green leafy vegetables, and legumes, seeds, and nuts. **Vitamin C** enhances iron absorption from plant foods when taken with a meal. Women with **iron deficiency anemia** should receive an additional iron supplement of 30 to 120 mg per day until the anemia is corrected.[4] There is no evidence for routine as opposed to selective iron supplementation in populations with a low prevalence of iron deficiency.
  - **Folate** supplementation is recommended to reduce the risk of neural tube defects (NTDs). Supplemental folate is ideally recommended in the preconceptual period, as the neural tube closes between 18 and 26 days after conception. The Centers for Disease Control and Prevention (CDC) recommend all low-risk fertile women to take **400 µg of folic acid per day.** Women at increased risk for offspring with NTDs should take higher prepregnancy doses (4 mg/day): personal or family history of neural tube defect, maternal insulin-dependent diabetes, and possibly adolescents.[5] Women who are taking anticonvulsants with no personal or family history of NTDs are advised to take 1 mg of folate supplementation, but there are no large studies to confirm these dosage recommendations.[4]
  - **Calcium** is required for fetal skeletal development, particularly in the last trimester. Calcium absorption is increased during pregnancy and, if necessary, is easily mobilized from maternal stores. During pregnancy and lactation, elemental calcium intake should include at least **1000 mg per day,** divided in two doses taken with food, in women 19 to 50 years old; 1300 mg per day is recommended for girls 14 to 18 years old.[4]
  - **Proteins** are a critical part in the fetus's proper brain development. As such, pregnant women are advised to ingest an **additional 5 to 6 g of protein** daily above the nonpregnant state.[4]
  - **Vegetarian diets** may not provide adequate amounts of essential amino acids, iron, vitamin B_{12}, or complex lipids for normal embryonic development. Minor dietary alterations, such as increasing soy and dairy products, may correct these deficiencies. Consultation with a registered dietician for further recommendations is advised.
  - **Mega-vitamins and natural medications (herbs, vitamins, and supplements).** Inquire about consumption of these substances. Excessive intake of these substances may prove toxic and possibly teratogenic.
  - **Foods to limit or avoid** due to potentially adverse effects: high caffeine intake, unwashed produce, unpasteurized dairy products, undercooked meats, and fish potentially containing high levels of mercury.

- **Exercise.** At least 30 minutes of moderate exercise on most days of the week is reasonable for most pregnant women. Pregnant women should avoid activities that put them at risk for falls or abdominal injuries.
- **Immunizations.** Live-virus vaccines are generally contraindicated for pregnant women because of the theoretical risk of transmission of the vaccine virus to the fetus. If a live-virus vaccine is inadvertently given to a pregnant woman, or if a woman becomes pregnant within 4 weeks after vaccination, she should be counseled about the potential effects on the fetus; however, it is not typically an indication to terminate the pregnancy.[1]
  - Inactive influenza vaccine is **recommended** during pregnancy.
  - **Live** vaccines are contraindicated during pregnancy: **Influenza (live-attenuated), measles, mumps, rubella, varicella.**
  - The following vaccines can be safely administered if clinically indicated: **Hepatitis B, tetanus/diphtheria.**
    - Recommendations for travel and other circumstances are published at the CDC web site.[6]
- **Medications.** Few medications have been proven to be completely safe for use in pregnant women, especially in the first trimester. Benefits and risks must be carefully weighed before initiating prescription, over-the-counter, or natural medications.[1]

Patient Education

- **Breastfeeding education.** Breastfeeding education should be offered to all pregnant women at their first visit with the provider and should be encouraged throughout the pregnancy.[2]
- **Preterm labor precautions.** Pregnant women should be educated about the most common symptoms of preterm labor: low, dull backache; four or more uterine contractions per hour; increased pelvic pressure; change in vaginal discharge.[2]
- **Labor and delivery.** Pregnant women should be counseled about signs of labor, ruptured membranes, pain management, and what to expect in labor.[1]
- **Injury prevention.** Seat belts should be properly worn.

Screening

- **Substance abuse.** All pregnant women should be screened for tobacco, alcohol, and illicit substance use.[1,2]
- **Domestic violence.** Domestic violence affects a significant number of pregnant women and may put both the woman and her fetus at risk. Patients generally accept screening questions about domestic violence.[1,2]
- **Asymptomatic bacteriuria.** Perform screening urine culture and sensitivity (C&S) at the initial visit. Repeat urine C&S each trimester in patients with a history of recurrent urinary tract infections (UTIs) or UTI during their pregnancy, as well as in symptomatic patients.

Genetic Screening

- **Chorionic villi sampling** may be offered between 10 and 12 weeks EGA. It is associated with 1% to 1.5% risk of spontaneous abortion (SAB) and may be associated transverse limb defects. Amniocentesis may be offered after 15 weeks EGA and is associated with a 0.5% risk of SAB.[1]
- **Maternal serum analyte screen** should be offered at 15 to 20 weeks EGA to screen for NTDs and trisomies 21 and 18. Optimal timing is 15 to 18 weeks EGA to maximize accuracy and allow time for adequate follow-up counseling and testing.[1,2]
- **Fetal anatomy ultrasound** can be offered at 16 to 20 weeks EGA to evaluate for structural anomalies.[1,2]
- **Antibody screen** at 28 weeks EGA for Rh-negative women.
  - Administer $Rh_o(D)$ immune globulin antepartum at 28 to 32 weeks and postpartum (if the baby is Rh-positive) to prevent hemolytic disease of the newborn in subsequent pregnancies.
  - $Rh_o(D)$ immune globulin is also indicated for spontaneous or induced abortion, ectopic pregnancy, chorionic villus sampling, amniocentesis, vaginal bleeding, significant abdominal trauma, external cephalic version, and transfusion of unmatched Rh-positive blood or any platelet transfusion. For a more detailed discussion, see Chapter 14.8.

- **Gestational diabetes mellitus (GDM) screening** at 24 to 28 weeks (earlier for history of GDM). **Risk factors** include obesity, history of miscarriage or fetal death, age 40 or older, history of premature infant, family history of diabetes, polyhydramnios, history of infant with macrosomia (>4000 g) or congenital malformation, pre-eclampsia, excessive weight gain, and glycosuria.
    - **Screening** is based on risk factors. The American Diabetes Association recommends that women at risk for GDM be screened with a **50-g glucose** load given at **24 to 28 weeks** without regard to the time of day or the last meal. Women with a plasma glucose **exceeding 140 mg per dL** during a 1-hour glucose tolerance test (GTT), a fasting plasma glucose exceeding 140 mg per dL, or a random plasma glucose greater than 200 mg per dL need a 3-hour GTT.
    - **Diagnosis.** Administer a 3-hour fasting GTT with a **100-g glucose** load. **Two or more** of these plasma values (*not* fingerstick values) must be met or exceeded for diagnosis of GDM: Fasting, 105 mg per dL; 1 hour, 190 mg per dL; 2 hours, 165 mg per dL, and 3 hours, 145 mg per dL.
- **Group B streptococcus (GBS) screening.** Perform a rectovaginal swab at 35 to 37 weeks EGA. Colonized women and women with a previous child with early-onset GBS infection should be treated with intravenous antibiotics at the time of labor or ruptured membranes.
- **Screening for sexually transmitted infections.** Consider **syphilis, gonorrhea, or Chlamydia** screening at in the third trimester in high-risk patients.
- **Bacterial vaginosis.** Routine screening of all pregnant women is not recommended. In women with a history of a previous preterm birth there is some evidence that detection and treatment of bacterial vaginosis early in pregnancy may prevent some of these women from having another preterm birth.[8]

SPECIAL CONSIDERATIONS

- **Nausea and vomiting of pregnancy (NVP), also called morning sickness,** is experienced by 80% of pregnant women.
    - **Lifestyle modifications should** encourage small frequent protein meals and increased rest. Avoidance of fried and heavily seasoned food, noxious odors, and environmental stimuli should also be recommended.
    - **Nonpharmacologic treatments** include acupressure wrist bands (available over the counter), biofeedback, and self-hypnosis. Ginger suppresses gastric contractions and increases gastrointestinal motility. Ginger (250 mg oral capsules taken four times daily) significantly reduced nausea and vomiting compared with placebo in women who were <17 weeks pregnant.[4]
- **Oral pharmacologic treatments**
    - **Pyridoxine (vitamin B$_6$),** 12.5 to 25 mg tid, or pyridoxine, 25 to 50 mg PO tid-qid used in combination with doxylamine, 10 to 12.5 mg PO qd-bid. **Doxylamine** is available over the counter in 12.5-mg (Decapryn) and 25-mg tablets (Unisom Nighttime Sleep-Aid Tablets). The latter combination is contained in the prescription drug Diclectin, which is currently available in Canada.
    - **Antiemetics,** antihistamines, anticholinergics, and corticosteroids are common prescription oral medications for NVP. An algorithm for the suggested evaluation and treatment with NVP is available.[6]
    - Newer data indicate that more than 90% of women with **hyperemesis gravidarum** are infected with *Helicobacter pylori*. *H. pylori* infection may be safely and effectively treated with triple therapy (amoxicillin, metronidazole, and an H$_2$-receptor blocker) during pregnancy.
- **Vaginal bleeding** is common in early pregnancy, occurring in approximately **25%** of all pregnant patients. Any report of bleeding deserves further investigation to delineate between potentially serious and less worrisome causes.
    - Evaluation should include a physical examination, laboratory studies (quantitative b-hCG and progesterone, blood type and Rh, serology, and cultures when indicated), and ultrasound. First trimester etiologies include threatened or spontaneous abortion, ectopic pregnancy, trophoblastic disease, cervical polyps, friable cervix, trauma, or

malignancy. Bleeding that occurs in the second and third trimesters warrants immediate investigation for abnormally implanted placenta, placental abruption, or other potentially serious conditions (see Chapter 14.10).

- **Vaginal discharge** is common in pregnancy, with many women noting increased vaginal discharge during pregnancy. If this becomes symptomatic, further investigation is warranted using culture and microscopic techniques. Symptomatic monilial and chlamydial infections and bacterial vaginosis should be treated with appropriate medications.

  - Treatment of symptomatic bacterial vaginosis with oral medications reduces the risk of preterm labor more effectively than topical medications. Increased vaginal discharge or secretions may signal preterm cervical changes or labor and may warrant sterile vaginal examination.

- **Back pain** is common in pregnancy and aggravated by mechanical and hormonal factors. It occurs in up to 56% of all pregnancies, with one third of these being reported as severe. Usual recommendations include stretching and strengthening exercise, oral or topical analgesics, massage, heat therapy, or cryotherapy. Acupuncture has been demonstrated to be more effective than physiotherapy.[9]

  - Specially shaped pillows can help to reduce back pain in late pregnancy and improve sleep.[10] Up to 50% of back pain in pregnancy is caused by sacroiliac subluxation, which can be treated quickly, safely, and simply with manipulation. This results in more than 90% of treated patients reporting relief of pain and resolution of signs of sacroiliac subluxation. Readers who wish to learn the technique are referred to a review on the topic.[11]

- **Leg cramps** affect almost half of all pregnant women, particularly in the second and third trimesters of pregnancy; they mostly occur at night. Their cause is unknown, but may be associated with reduced blood levels of calcium or increased levels of phosphorus. Leg cramps may be reduced by changing position or performing **stretches** such as straightening legs, dorsiflexing ankles, massaging the calves, and walking. **Regular exercise** and supportive stockings may also help. The best evidence for pharmacologic therapy is **magnesium** lactate or citrate.[12]

- **Heartburn and gastroesophageal reflux disease (GERD):** may occur in the second to third trimesters and can be a source of significant discomfort.

  - **Nonpharmacologic interventions** include eating small, frequent meals; avoiding fried, greasy, and spicy foods; and eating slowly and chewing food well. Like nonpregnant patients with these symptoms, it is helpful to avoid lying down immediately after eating, to take walks after meals, and to drink fluids between meals.

  - **Pharmacologic agents** used to treat heartburn include:

    - **Antacids** (calcium carbonate, magnesium hydroxide and oxide, and aluminum hydroxide and carbonate). Systemic absorption of antacids is negligible; recommended doses are safe in pregnancy and lactation.

    - **Antisecretory agents** used for heartburn and GERD include the histamine H_2 antagonists and proton pump inhibitors. **The histamine antagonists**—cimetidine (Tagamet), famotidine (Pepcid), nizatidine (Axid), and ranitidine (Zantac)—are available in low strengths over the counter and, with the exception of nizatidine, are compatible with breastfeeding. Of the **proton pump inhibitors**—esomeprazole (Nexium), lansoprazole (Prevacid), omeprazole (Prilosec), pantoprazole (Protonix), and rabeprazole (Aciphex)—only omeprazole is available without a prescription.

References

1. Kirkham C, Harris S, Grzybowski S. Evidence-based prenatal care: Part I. General prenatal care and counseling issues. *Am Fam Physician* 2005;71:1307–1316. http://www.aafp.org/afp/20050401/1307.html.

2. Veterans Health Administration, Department of Defense. DoD/VA clinical practice guideline for the management of uncomplicated pregnancy. Washington, DC: Department of Veteran Affairs; 2002(Oct). Available at www.guideline.gov.(http://www.guideline.gov/summary/summary.aspx?doc_id=3847).

3. Kirkham C, Harris S, Grzybowski S. Evidence-based prenatal care: Part II. Third-trimester care and prevention of infectious diseases. *Am Fam Physician* 2005;71: 1555–1560. Available at http://www.aafp.org/afp/20050415/1555.html.
4. Nutrition in pregnancy. Up To Date Online. Updated 23 June 2005. Available only to subscribers at www.utdol.com.
5. Screening for neural tube defects—including folic acid/folate prophylaxis. In: U.S. Preventive Services Task Force. Guide to clinical preventive services. 2nd ed. Washington, DC: U.S. Department of Health and Human Services, Office of Disease Prevention and Health Promotion; 1996. Available at http://cpmcnet.columbia.edu/texts/gcps/gcps0052.html.
6. Guidelines for vaccinating pregnant women. Recommendations of the Advisory Committee on Immunization Practices (ACIP). Centers for Disease Control and Prevention, Department of Health and Human Services. October 1998 (updated July 2005). http://www.cdc.gov/nip/publications/preg_guide.htm.
7. University of Texas at Austin, School of Nursing, Family Nurse Practitioner Program. Evaluation and management of nausea and vomiting in early pregnancy (less than or equal to 20 weeks gestation). Austin, TX: University of Texas at Austin, School of Nursing; 2002 (May 19). www.guideline.gov (http://www.guideline.gov/summary/summary.aspx?ss=15&doc_id=3228&nbr=2454).
8. Sexually transmitted diseases treatment guidelines 2002. Centers for Disease Control and Prevention, Department of Health and Human Services . http://www.cdc.gov/STD/treatment/5-2002TG.htm.
9. Wedenberg K, Moen B, Norling A. A prospective randomized study comparing acupuncture with physiotherapy for low-back and pelvic pain in pregnancy. *Acta Obstet Gynecol Scand* 2000;79(5):331–335.
10. Young G, Jewell D. Interventions for preventing and treating backache in pregnancy. *Cochrane Database Syst Rev* 2000;2:CD001139.
11. Daly JM, Frame PS, Rapoza PA. Sacroiliac subluxation: a common, treatable cause of low-back pain in pregnancy. *Fam Pract Res J* 1991;11(2):149–159.
12. Young GL, Jewell D. Interventions for leg cramps in pregnancy. *Cochrane Database Syst Rev* 2000;2:CD000121.

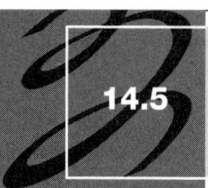

14.5 ECTOPIC PREGNANCY
Shikar Saxena

GENERAL PRINCIPLES

Ectopic pregnancy presents a major health problem to women of child-bearing age. The syndrome is considered a medical emergency and hemorrhage from ectopic pregnancy is still the leading cause of pregnancy-related maternal death in the first trimester.[1] Prompt diagnosis and treatment is a must in all patients with the diagnosed condition.

Definition

Ectopic pregnancy occurs when a fertilized ovum implants anywhere but the uterine cavity. The most common location is the fallopian tube, which accounts for 97% of all ectopic gestations. This can become a surgical emergency when there is a tubal rupture with internal bleeding.[2]

Etiology

Risk factors for ectopic pregnancy can be classified into high-, intermediate-, and low-risk factors. High degree of risk of ectopic pregnancy occurs in patients with previous ectopic pregnancy, previous tubal surgery, tubal ligation, tubal pathology, *in utero* diethylstilbestrol

(DES) exposure, and current intrauterine device (IUD) use. Intermediate risk is attributed to patients who are smokers and have a history of pelvic inflammatory disease (PID). Low risk is seen in patients who have had previous abdominal surgery or in patients who become pregnant at a young age (<18).[3,4] All the aforementioned risk factors increase the chance of tubal pathology and thus tubal pregnancy.

Epidemiology

Ectopic pregnancy occurs in nearly 2 per 100 pregnancies. The incidence has increased in the 20th century, largely due to a rise in PID. The prevalence ranges from 6% to 16% of women who go to the emergency department with first trimester bleeding.[5]

DIAGNOSIS

History

Pelvic/abdominal pain, amenorrhea, and vaginal bleeding are the classic symptoms of ectopic pregnancy. Pain is almost always present before rupture, but is highly variable in location, character, and severity.[4] The onset of pain is usually at 6 to 8 weeks gestational age. Often, there is amenorrhea followed by irregular vaginal bleeding. More than 50% may be asymptomatic before tubal rupture and have no identifiable risk factor for ectopic pregnancy, making the diagnosis difficult.[4]

Physical Examination

Signs may include localized lower quadrant tenderness with or without a palpable mass, peritoneal irritation, with guarding and rebound tenderness (suggesting tubal rupture with hemoperitoneum) or cervical motion tenderness. Signs of shock, including pallor, diaphoresis, weakness, and orthostatic pulse and blood pressure changes, may be present. Syncope occurs in up to 3% of patients.[4]

Laboratory Tests

An initial workup should include a complete blood count (CBC), quantitative β-human chorionic gonadotropin (β-HCG), and serum progestone. The β-hCG concentration in a normal intrauterine pregnancy rises until 41 days of gestation at which time it plateaus at approximately 100,000 IU per L and the mean doubling time for the hormone is from 1.4 to 2.1 days. In ectopic pregnancy, the doubling time is 3 or more days. A falling value signals nonviability. A single value is not interpretable and serial testing should only be used if the patient remains hemodynamically stable.[5]

Imaging

Transvaginal ultrasound should be the initial diagnostic test in women known to be pregnant who present with first trimester vaginal bleeding and/or pelvic pain. If the imaging study is nondiagnostic, transvaginal ultrasound findings in conjunction with serial serum β-HCG concentrations facilitate a diagnosis of ectopic pregnancy.[6]

Differential Diagnosis

This includes appendicitis, PID, ruptured corpus luteum cyst, twisted ovarian cyst, urinary tract disease, and threatened or incomplete uterine abortion. Consider concurrent problems, such as intrauterine pregnancy (IUP) and appendicitis, or IUP and ectopic pregnancy (rare, except in patients who have undergone in vitro fertilization). Also consider rare types of ectopic pregnancy, including interstitial, abdominal, cervical, ovarian, or multiple.

TREATMENT

Emergent Presentation

Emergency laparotomy is indicated if signs of intraperitoneal bleeding or shock are present. Fluids and blood transfusions are given as required. Ultrasonogrophic examination may waste critical time.

Nonemergent Presentation

- **Surgery.** Surgical management is favored if pain is prolonged for more than 24 hours, quantitative β-HCG is more than 10,000 mIU per mL, or in ectopics larger than 3.5 cm on ultrasound. Perform laparoscopy or laparotomy to remove the ectopic pregnancy and consider tubal repair.[7]

■ **Methotrexate.** Eligible patients for this treatment have a gestational sac diameter less than 3.5 cm, with no fetal cardiac activity, and no evidence of rupture on ultrasound. The current recommended regimen is a single intramuscular injection of the drug at 50 mg per m^2. Absolute contraindications include immunodeficiency, liver disease, blood dyscrasia, pulmonary disease, renal dysfunction, or peptic ulcer disease (PUD). The β-HCG level may rise for 3 to 4 days, but should then fall 15% between days 4 to 7. If this does not occur, consider a second dose of methotrexate or laparoscopy.[6,7]

Counseling

Nearly 47% of pregnancies can be managed with expectant management β-HCG should be followed weekly until undetectable, regardless of the method of treatment. Rho (D) immune globulin should be given to Rh negative women.[1]

SPECIAL CONSIDERATIONS

Maternal mortality is about 1% in the United States. Medical treatment has been shown to be as efficacious as surgical management in appropriate candidates. Complications to surgery include anesthesia risks, routine surgical risks, postoperative pain and discomfort. Methotrexate side effects are minimal and self-limiting. The most common are stomatitis and conjunctivitis.

In patients with an ectopic pregnancy, another ectopic pregnancy occurs in 6% to 12% of patients Fertility is compromised and only one third of patients will subsequently deliver a live infant. Patients should be counseled to practice "safe sex" to avoid pelvic infections. Women with a high risk of exposure to a sexually transmitted disease (STD) should avoid using an IUD. Finally, patients should be encouraged to discuss their feelings about the loss of the pregnancy and the possibility of compromised fertility in the future.

References

1. Flystra DL. Tubal pregnancy: a review of current diagnosis and treatment. *Obstet Gynecol Surv* 1998;53:320–328.
2. Kim HH, Fox JH. The fallopian tube and ectopic pregnancy. In: Ryan KJ, et al. eds. *Kistner's gynecology and women's health*. 7th ed. St. Louis: Mosby; 1999:143–165.
3. Ankum WM, et al. Risk factors for ectopic pregnancy: a meta-analysis. *Fertil Steril* 1996;65(6):1093–1099.
4. Carr RJ, Evans P. Update in maternity care. Ectopic pregnancy—primary care. *Clin Office Pract* 2000;27:169–183.
5. Murray H, et al. Diagnosis and treatment of ectopic pregnancy. *Can Med Assoc J* 2005; 173(8):905–912.
6. Yao M. Tulandi T. Current status of surgical and nonsurgical management of ectopic pregnancy. *Fertil Steril* 1997;67(3):421–433.
7. Lipsicomb GH, Bran DB. Analysis of 315 ectopic pregnancies treated with single dose methotrexate. *Am J Obstet Gynecol* 1998;178:1354–1358.

MEDICAL PROBLEMS DURING PREGNANCY
Benjamin Soloman

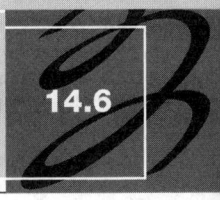

NAUSEA OF PREGNANCY

General Principles

Nausea of pregnancy is one of the most common complaints from pregnant women. It is most often managed conservatively, but may require hospitalization if vomiting is severe.

Background

Most pregnant women experience nausea and/or vomiting at some point during pregnancy. Nausea of pregnancy usually starts around 4 to 6 weeks, peaks at 8 to 12 weeks, and subsides by 20 weeks. Severe nausea and vomiting in pregnancy is called hyperemesis gravidarum. This is poorly defined, but is most often considered to be associated with clinical deterioration.

Pathophysiology

The cause of nausea of pregnancy remains unclear, but appears to be related to increased levels of female sex hormones, especially progesterone. A newer hypothesis is that it may be related to *Helicobacter pylori*.[1]

Diagnosis

The most important part of the diagnosis of nausea of pregnancy is history. Frequency and volume of vomiting as well as any weight loss is important.

Physical Examination

Physical examination to assess fluid status is also essential. Important signs are dry mucous membranes, tachycardia, orthostatic hypotension, and poor skin turgor. Weight loss greater than 5% of prepregnant weight associated with nausea and vomiting would likely fit with hyperemesis gravidarum. Vomiting of this severity increases the risk of poor fetal outcome.

Laboratory

Laboratory is done, if the history and physical exam warrant further investigation. Serum electrolytes are worth checking.

Treatment

Most nausea of pregnancy can be managed conservatively with diet modifications. A common diet recommendation is small meals up to six times daily. Also, some patients find it helpful to have a small dry snack, such as crackers, by the bedside to take before getting out of bed in the morning. Patients with hyperemesis gravidarum may require hospitalization for intravenous hydration and antiemetics. Serotonin antagonists, such as ondansetron, are currently the most commonly prescribed class of antiemetics because of their benign side-effect profile and relative effectiveness. Serotonin antagonists are, however, very expensive.[2]

Complications

Severe nausea and vomiting in pregnancy can lead to lack of maternal weight gain and subsequently low-birth-weight infants Severe electrolyte abnormalities could lead to injury or death of the fetus.

Patient Education

Patients with a significant amount of vomiting should be asked to follow their weight. They should be given tips on avoiding nausea.

APPENDICITIS IN PREGNANCY

General Principles

Pregnant women are unfortunately not immune to developing an acute abdomen. Appendicitis in pregnancy may have an alternative presentation in pregnancy with right upper quadrant pain due to displacement of abdominal contents.

Epidemiology

Appendicitis occurs in approximately 1 in 1500 pregnancies. In one series, 30% of cases occurred in the first trimester, 48% in the second trimester, and 25% in the third trimester.[3] The pathophysiology of appendicitis in pregnancy is the same as that occurring in nonpregnant patients.

Diagnosis

The key to diagnosing acute appendicitis in pregnancy is a good history and physical exam. Ultrasound may be used for imaging, but may or may not be useful. The decision to operate may need to be made on clinical judgment alone as computed tomography (CT) scans are avoided in pregnancy.

Diagnosis is based on abdominal tenderness in the right lower quadrant (85%) or right upper quadrant (20%) if after 20 weeks due to displacement of the abdominal contents. Rebound tenderness is 60% sensitive. A white blood cell count greater than 16,000 white blood cells (WBCs) per mm³ is suggestive of an infectious process as 15,000 WBCs per mm³ is the upper limit of normal in pregnancy.[4]

Treatment

Management is surgery.

Complications

Fetal loss ranges from 1% to 5% in uncomplicated appendicitis to as high as 20% in perforated appendicitis, with a maternal mortality of 4% in perforated appendicitis.

VIRAL HEPATITIS IN PREGNANCY

General Principles

Although pregnancy does not tend to change the course of chronic hepatitis, it is important to know that a pregnant patient has a chronic viral hepatitis because some measures may be taken to avoid vertical transmission.

Epidemiology

Acute hepatitis A (HAV), B (HBV), and C (HCV): each occurs in approximately 1 in 1000 pregnancies. Hepatitis D is only present if there is a chronic infection with HBV, and need not be considered in the absence of HBV. Hepatitis E (HEV) should be considered if there is a history of travel as it can be severe in pregnant women.[5]

Pathophysiology

HAV, an RNA virus, is transmitted by the fecal–oral route and selectively infects hepatocytes. This triggers a cell-mediated immune response that causes hepatocellular death. HAV has an acute course and rarely causes chronic liver disease.[6] HBV is a DNA virus that, like the other viral hepatidites, invades the hepatocytes and evokes an inflammatory response that damages the liver.[7] HCV, an RNA virus, acts by infecting the hepatocytes and causing and inflammatory response. HCV causes release of oxidants and tissue damage, leading to scaring.[8]

Diagnosis

A thorough social history is necessary to identify risk factors for hepatitis. Onset of symptoms, if any, is important as this may help to differentiate between an acute or chronic problem. Pay attention to skin and scleral color, right upper quadrant tenderness, hepatomegaly, and abdominal distention. If jaundiced with right upper quadrant tenderness, it is advisable to obtain an ultrasound to evaluate the liver and biliary tree. Hepatitis viral serologic studies should be drawn.[5]

Serum studies should include assays for immune globulin M (IgM) antibodies against HAV, hepatitis B surface antigen (HBsAg) and IgM antibody to hepatitis B core antigen (anti-HBc IgM), as well as antibodies to HCV. If negative, the above tests would rule out the most common viral hepatidites, but if clinically necessary, anti-HDV and anti-HEV assays can also be drawn.[9]

Treatment

Fortunately, 99% of patients with HAV infection recover completely without sequelae. However, the babies born to mothers infected with HAV perinatally should receive a prophylactic dose of immune globulin. Unfortunately, perinatal transmission of HBV occurs in 10% to 20% of pregnancies, but the risk can be lowered by active and passive immunization in the neonate. There is currently no commonly used therapy for HCV, HDV, and HEV in pregnant women.[10]

Complications

The most common complication is passage of the virus to the neonate. However, acute hepatitis presents a risk for fetal demise.

Patient Education

Patients should be counseled about the common sources of viral hepatitis.

HYPERTENSION

General Principles

As many women are becoming pregnant at older ages, chronic hypertension now plays a larger role in management issues in pregnant women. Patients should be screened for hypertension at every visit. They should also be screened regularly for proteinuria, a sign of pre-eclampsia.

Hypertension in pregnancy is classified into four groups: pre-eclampsia-eclampsia, chronic hypertension, pre-eclampsia-eclampsia superimposed on chronic hypertension, and gestational hypertension. Hypertension in pregnant women is defined as blood pressure greater than 140/90 measured on more than one occasion.

Pathophysiology

Most cases of chronic hypertension in pregnancy is caused by essential, or primary, hypertension. This process involves complex hemodynamics and often is associated with obesity. Pre-eclampsia is associated with abnormal immunologically mediated invasion of the trophoblast into the endometrium. This leads to altered development of placental vasculature. Because the blood flow to the placenta is altered, it releases vasoactive hormones, which cause endothelial dysfunction. In addition, the clotting cascade is triggered by the activated endothelium. These hemodynamic changes lead to hypertension and end organ damage seen in pre-eclampsia.

Diagnosis

Measurement of resting blood pressure should be a standard part of every prenatal visit. This is important because timing of onset of hypertension in pregnancy determines the category into which the disorder is classified. Other than measurement of blood pressure, the next most important screening test is a urinalysis for protein, most often by the dipstick method. If pre-eclampsia is diagnosed, other laboratory parameters that should be monitored include hemoglobin and hematocrit, liver transaminases, and platelets.

Hypertension prior to pregnancy or occurring before 20 weeks gestation is classified as chronic hypertension. Conversely, hypertension with an onset after 20 weeks is classified as either pre-eclampsia or gestational hypertension. To differentiate between pre-eclampsia and gestational hypertension, one must monitor for proteinuria, a prime feature of pre-eclampsia. As mentioned, pre-eclampsia can be superimposed on chronic hypertension and the physician must continue to monitor for pre-eclampsia regardless of the timing of onset of hypertension. Particularly severe pre-eclampsia is manifested by hemolysis, elevated liver enzymes, and low platelets, the so-called HELLP syndrome.

Treatment

Many medications have been used to control hypertension in pregnancy. Chronic hypertension in pregnancy should be treated if diastolic pressures are greater than 100 mmHg. First-line treatment is with methyldopa. Methyldopa has been used in pregnancy for many years and has been demonstrated to be safe. Although less supportive data are available for safety and efficacy in pregnancy, second-line agents include hydralazine, labetalol, and dihydropyridine calcium-channel blockers. Atenolol has also been used with some success, but it has been associated with intrauterine growth restriction, and neonatal bradycardia, respiratory depression, and hypoglycemia.

Many classes of medications have been proposed for use in pre-eclampsia, but none has led to improved maternal or fetal outcomes. In cases of severe hypertension (systolic greater than 160 mmHg or diastolic greater than 110 mm Hg), hydralazine may be used to safely decrease the blood pressure to prevent cerebrovascular accidents. Most importantly, the only definitive treatment for pre-eclampsia is delivery.[11]

Complications
When severe, pre-eclampsia can cause end organ damage to the heart, kidneys, liver, and brain. In addition, pre-eclampsia may lead to eclampsia, which is characterized as pre-eclampsia plus seizures.

Patient Education
Patients should understand the risks of hypertension in pregnancy.

THROMBOCYTOPENIA

General Principles
Although thrombocytopenia can cause bleeding, most thrombocytopenic patients are detected as such through routine laboratory screening. The workup becomes much more sensitive if combined with a thorough past medical history and family history.

The important causes of thrombocytopenia in pregnancy are idiopathic thrombocytopenic purpura (ITP) and the HELLP syndrome.

Pathophysiology
ITP is caused by an autoantibody against platelets. Coating of the platelets leads to increased splenic destruction of platelets and eventually to thrombocytopenia. HELLP is a complex inflammatory syndrome that leads to platelet aggregation and consumption.

Diagnosis
Patients with ITP may present with purpura, but most often a workup ensues only after finding thrombocytopenia on routine lab work. Alternatively, some patients may present with mild to severe bleeding. Serious bleeding does not usually occur until platelets drop below 10,000. Other blood studies that may be important if HELLP is a concern are transaminases, a peripheral smear, and a serum haptoglobin to evaluate for hemolysis. Other possible causes of thrombocytopenia are medications, transfusion-mediated, and familial thrombocytopenia.[12]

Differential Diagnosis
The diagnosis of ITP is often one of exclusion. If a brief workup for HELLP is negative, the family history is unrevealing, adverse medication reactions are unlikely, and the patient has no transfusion history, ITP is very likely.

Treatment
The first-line therapy for mild to moderate ITP is oral prednisone (1 mg/kg/day). Severe cases may require IVIG (0.4 g/kg/day for 5 days). If bleeding is severe, platelet replacement may be necessary.

Complications
The most common complications of ITP are maternal hemorrhage and fetal loss.

ASYMPTOMATIC BACTERIURIA

General Principles
Patients often can harbor bacteria in their urinary tracts without displaying any signs or symptoms. This asymptomatic bacteruria poses a risk to both the mother and the fetus.

Epidemiology

The incidence of asymptomatic bacteriuria is 4% to 8% of pregnancies. Asymptomatic bacteriuria is generally defined as 100,000 colonies per milliliter or more; however, pyelonephritis can occur even with colony counts of 20,000 to 50,000 per milliliter. The most common causative agents are *Escherichia coli*, *Klebsiella*, *Proteus*, and *Streptococcus* group B.

Pathophysiology

Many physiologic changes lead to an increased tendency for pregnant women to harbor bacteria in their urine. Progesterone can cause smooth muscle relaxation, leading to less ureteral parastalsis and urine stasis. Hormones also cause the bladder to increase its capacity. In addition, mechanical changes such as compression of the ureters by the enlarging uterus and a positional change of the bladder due to shifting of the abdominal organs can also cause urinary stasis. Any stasis of the urine provides a good culture medium for bacteria.[13]

Diagnosis

A urine dipstick is an adequate screening test for asymptomatic bacteriuria and is reasonable to do at each prenatal visit. Dipsticks positive for leukocyte esterase or nitrites should be sent for culture and sensitivity.

Asymptomatic bacteriuria is diagnosed if the colony count is 100,000 per milliliter or greater on at least two successive urine samples done early in pregnancy.

Treatment

Options include nitrofurantoin 100 mg PO at bedtime for 10 days; ampicillin or amoxicillin 500 mg PO qid for 7 to 10 days; and cotrimoxazole DS 1 tablet PO bid for 7 to 10 days. After the first trimester, cephalexin 250 to 500 mg PO qid for 7 to 10 days can be given. Repeat urine culture after treatment; if culture is still positive, treat for 2 to 3 weeks. If condition recurs, treat for 2 to 3 weeks. If the patient continues to have recurrences, give prophylactic treatment for the remainder of the pregnancy using nitrofurantoin 50 mg PO at bedtime, or amoxicillin 250 mg PO at bedtime. Regular repeat urine cultures should be done throughout the pregnancy. Screening with dipstick and culture or dipstick and subsequent culture if dipstick-positive are cost effective in preventing pyelonephritis.

Complications

About 30% of women with asymptomatic bacteriuria go on to develop pyelonephritis. Eradication of the bacteriuria reduces the risk of pyelonephritis to about 5%. In addition, treatment of asymptomatic bacteriuria has been shown to reduce the incidence of preterm labor, which is four times higher if untreated, as well as reduce the incidence of low-birth-weight infants. Cystitis is also a complication of asymptomatic bacteriuria and would be managed similarly. Often, simple cystitis requires only a 3-day course of antibiotics.

Patient Education

Patients should be educated on the importance of completing antibiotic therapy even though they may have no symptoms.

ACUTE PYELONEPHRITIS

General Principles

Acute pyelonephritis is a relatively severe infection of the urinary tract that can lead to poor outcomes of pregnancy if not properly managed.

Epidemiology

Acute pyelonephritis occurs in about 1% of pregnancies. The greatest risk factor is asymptomatic bacteriuria. The most common pathogens are *E. coli* (77%), *Klebsiella* (11%), *Proteus* and *Enterobacter* (4%), and a small number of *Streptococcus* group B–induced pyelonephritis.

Pathophysiology

If asymptomatic bacteriuria or cystitis is allowed to progress long enough, the upper urinary tract can become inflamed and infected causing acute pyelonephritis.

Diagnosis

History
Patients may present with abdominal, back, or flank pain, fever, chills, and nausea or vomiting. They may complain of dysuria or foul-smelling urine. Physical exam should include a thorough abdominal exam including test for costovertebral angle tenderness.

Laboratory Studies
Include a complete blood count (CBC) with differential, electrolytes, blood urea nitrogen, creatinine, urine analysis, and urine and blood cultures.

Differential Diagnosis
Any patient with evidence of urinary tract infection on urine dipstick with accompanying fevers, chills, and back or abdominal pain likely has acute pyelonephritis.

Treatment
Often, these patients require inpatient treatment. This is mandatory if the patient appears toxic by clinical exam. First, rehydrate the patient in order to maintain a minimum urine output of 30 mL per hour. Treat with antibiotics for 14 days, orally if not toxic. Options include cotrimoxazole DS, 1 tablet PO bid, or cephalexin, 500 mg PO q6h, or amoxicillin, 500 mg PO q6h. Intravenous options include gentamicin or tobramycin IV/IM 3 to 5 mg/kg/day divided q8h, or amikacin IV 15 mg/kg/day plus ampicillin IV 1 to 2 g q4h. If IV antibiotics are started, switch to orals if the patient remains afebrile after 3 to 4 days.[14]

Complications
If the recovery is not prompt after initiation of antibiotics, urinary obstruction, pulmonary injury, and septic shock must be considered. Obstruction could be commonly caused by renal calculi or a perinephric abcess. Obstruction can be safely evaluated by ultrasound. Respiratory insufficiency secondary to pulmonary injury occurs in 1 in 50 women with severe pyelonephritis and is treated by supportive oxygen therapy. Finally, septic shock may occur and should be suspected if patient becomes hypotensive. And, as with many other infections during pregnancy, acute pyelonephritis in pregnancy can lead to fetal demise if severe.

Patients should be educated on the importance of completing antibiotic therapy even after their symptoms subside.

DIABETES MELLITUS

General Principles
Diabetes mellitus is a serious chronic illness that can have major effects on the outcome of pregnancy. Tight glycemic control is key to avoiding complications.

Like hypertension, diabetes in pregnancy can either be pregnancy-induced or pre-existing. Gestational diabetes is defined as any type of diabetes that was first recognized during pregnancy. This means that a patient could have pre-existing type II diabetes mellitus that is first recognized during routine prenatal laboratory tests. In this case, during the pregnancy, the disorder would be called gestational diabetes and if it continued after the pregnancy it would be reclassified as diabetes mellitus type II. Gestational diabetes is common and signals patients who are at increased risk of developing type II diabetes mellitus later in life even if they were euglycemic prior to pregnancy.[15]

Pathophysiology
Gestational diabetes most often develops in the second or third trimesters, when the placenta begins to secrete hormones that cause increased insulin resistance. It is believed that patients with new-onset diabetes during pregnancy are likely predisposed to insulin resistance and that pregnancy simply pushes them over the edge into insulin resistance and hyperglycemia.

Diagnosis
Screening for gestational diabetes is important, but risk stratification is necessary. Patients who are obese, have a family history of diabetes mellitus, have a personal history of insulin

resistance or delivery of a macrosomic infant, or have glucosuria are considered at high risk for developing gestational diabetes. Patients considered low risk are younger than 25 years old, are of low-risk ethnicity, have no family history of diabetes, have a normal prepregnancy weight with normal weight gain during pregnancy, and have no personal history of insulin resistance or of macrosomic infants. Average-risk patients fall somewhere between high and low risk. Average-risk patients require screening for gestational diabetes between 24 and 28 weeks, whereas high-risk patients should be screened at the first prenatal visit.[16]

Laboratory: Screening starts with a 50-g 1-hour oral glucose challenge. A positive test is a serum glucose measurement of >140 mg per dL after 1 hour. This test does not require fasting. A positive glucose challenge followed up by a 100-g 3-hour oral glucose tolerance test. First, a fasting glucose level is measured (nml <95). Sequential serum glucose measurements are then taken 1 hour (nml <180), 2 hours (nml <155), and 3 hours (nml <140) after the 100-g dose of glucose. A positive test is determined if two or more of these measurements are above the normal range.

Treatment (Kelly)

Diet and exercise should be attempted first, but insulin is often necessary to keep blood glucose in the normal range. In addition, glyburide has been proven to be safe and effective for use in management of gestational diabetes in the second and third trimesters.

Complications: Hyperglycemia early in pregnancy has been shown to cause defects in organogenesis. During the first few weeks of gestation, when organogenesis occurs, the embryo cannot make its own insulin and maternal insulin does not cross the placenta. Thus, maternal hyperglycemia directly leads to hyperglycemia in the developing baby. For this reason, preconception glycemic control is important in diabetic women of childbearing age. Second, maternal hyperglycemia often leads to fetal macrosomia and problems with delivery as well as neonatal hypoglycemia and increased risk of neonatal death.

References

1. Quinlan JD, Hill DA. Nausea and vomiting of pregnancy. *Am Fam Physician* 2003; 68;121.
2. Flake ZE, Scalley RD, Bailey AG. Practical selection of antiemetics. *Am Fam Physician* 2004;69:1169.
3. Mahmoodian S. Appendicitis complicating pregnancy. *South Med J* 1992;85:19.
4. Richards C, Daya S. Diagnosis of acute appendicitis in pregnancy. *Can J Surg* 1989; 32:358.
5. Reyes H. The spectrum of liver and gastrointestinal disease seen in cholestasis of pregnancy. *Gastrointest Clin North Am* 1992:21:905.
6. Brundage SC, Fitzpatrick AN. Hepatitis A. *Am Fam Physician* 2006;73:2162.
7. Yim HJ, Lok AS. Natural history of chronic hepatitis B virus infection: what we knew in 1981 and what we know in 2005. *Hepatology* 2005;43:S173.
8. Choi J, Ou JH. Mechanisms of liver injury. III. Oxidative stress in the pathogenesis of hepatitis C virus. Diagnosing and treating hepatitis. Hepatitis Foundation International. Web site accessed September 13 2006. http://www.hepfi.org/living/liv_diagnosis.html#hep_A.
9. Guntupalli S, Steingrub J. Hepatic disease and pregnancy: an overview of diagnosis and management. *Crit Care Med* 2005;33:S332.
10. Frishman WH, Schlocker SJ, Awad K, et al. Pathophysiology and medical management of systemic hypertension in pregnancy. *Cardiol Rev* 2005;13:274.
11. Bussel J. Treatment of immune thrombocytopenic purpura in adults. *Semin Hematol* 2006;43:S3.
12. Connolly A, Thorp JM. Urinary tract infections in pregnancy. *Urol Clin North Am* 1999;26:779.
13. Cunningham FG, Lucas MJ. Urinary tract infections complicating pregnancy. *Bailliere's Clin Obstet Gynecol* 1994;8:353.
14. Kelly L, Evans L, Messenger D. Controversies around gestational diabetes: practical information for family doctors. *Can Fam Physician* 2005;51:688.
15. Buchanan TA, Xiang AH. Gestational diabetes mellitus. *J Clin Invest* 2005;115:485.

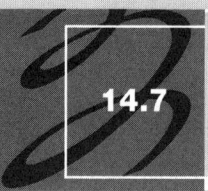

14.7 POSTDATE PREGNANCY

Brian J. Finley

GENERAL PRINCIPLES

Postdate pregnancy (PDP) is pregnancy lasting beyond 42 weeks, or 294 days from the first day of the last menstrual period. The incidence of PDP is approximately 10%.[1]

The advent of early prenatal care and accurate estimate of gestational age based on known last menstrual period, known date of conception, and early ultrasound can decrease the overestimation of postdates and therefore the need for intervention, and should be utilized more for this purpose.

DIAGNOSIS

Postdate pregnancy (PDP) is pregnancy lasting beyond 42 weeks. The most common cause of PDP is inaccurate dating of the pregnancy. Other causes include previous PDP (50% recurrence rate), history of high parity, first pregnancy, excessive maternal weight gain, and lower socioeconomic status. In rare cases, postdate pregnancy is associated with anencephaly and placental sulfatase deficiency.

Assessment of fetal well-being, necessary during the postdate period (after 42 weeks) to maintain a low risk of mortality and morbidity to the infant, includes the following:

- **Amniotic fluid volume.** Oligohydramnios is readily measured and correlates highly with perinatal morbidity and mortality in the postdate period.[2] After 41 weeks gestation, the amniotic fluid volume declines approximately 25% per week. Changes in fluid volume can occur quickly and often dramatically in the postdate period. An amniotic fluid index (AFI) less than 5.0 is an indication for delivery.[3]
- **The nonstress test (NST)** measures fetal heart rate accelerations after spontaneous movement. A reactive NST (at least two accelerations of at least 15 beats/minute above the baseline that last 15 seconds within a 10-minute window) is reassuring of fetal well-being during the postdate period, and the test should be performed biweekly after 41 weeks gestation.[4] A nonreactive NST indicates the need for further assessment of the fetus.
- **Acoustic stimulation testing,** which uses the application of low-frequency mixed vibroacoustic sound generated by an electronic larynx, can be used to test fetal well-being. A nonreactive acoustic stimulation test indicates the need for further assessment of the fetus.[5]
- **The biophysical profile** can be used to assess placental insufficiency, but data show that the biophysical profile adds little useful information to a normal AFI and a reactive NST.[6]
- There is no evidence that NST and obstetrical ultrasound to assess AFI between 40 and 42 weeks improves fetal outcomes in postdate pregnancy.[1]

TREATMENT

Treatment of postdate pregnancy remains controversial. Expectant as opposed to active management yields no difference in perinatal mortality and neonatal morbidity.

Expectant Management

- After 36 weeks, weekly office visits are done for evaluation of weight, fundal height, blood pressure, fetal movements, and cervical examination if indicated.
- Daily fetal monitoring by having mom do fetal kick counts should begin after 40 weeks. Any decrease in movement perceived by the mother should be further evaluated with an NST.

■ After 41 weeks, biweekly NSTs and weekly ultrasound for AFI assessment are indicated. A nonreactive NST indicates a need for further evaluation with a contraction stress test (CST). CST can be accomplished by using several different methods to induce contractions, that is, nipple stimulation, prostaglandins, or pitocin. The test is considered negative if there are no fetal heart rate decelerations when there are three contractions within 10 minutes. If the CST is positive, admission is indicated and delivery should be considered.

■ If clinical evaluation remains normal and the NSTs are reactive, then continued expectant management is appropriate. Once the cervix ripens (Bishop score >5 to 6), induction of labor should be considered.

■ Before 43 weeks gestation, all patients should be delivered because fetal morbidity and mortality are significantly increased.

Active Management

Active management of the PDP advocates the induction of all women who reach 41 weeks gestation without signs of ensuing labor. Women should be informed that 500 inductions are necessary to prevent one perinatal death and the induction group had lower caesarean delivery rates.[7]

■ Cervical ripening agents. Dinoprostone, a prostaglandin E2 (PGE$_2$) analogue, has been shown to improve induction outcome as well as decrease the length of induction time in patients with an unfavorable cervix. Prepidil (gel) in a standard dose of 0.5 mg administered intracervically can be used every 6 hours as needed to a maximum dose of 1.5 mg PGE$_2$ or 7.5 mL PGE$_2$ gel.[8] Cervidil (10 mg vaginal insert) is introduced into the posterior fornix of the vagina for 12 hours. Continuous fetal monitoring is recommended during use of either agent. Both agents require refrigeration and are extremely expensive. Misoprostol, a PGE$_1$ analogue, is also used for cervical ripening and labor induction (not Food and Drug Administration approved). Cytotec 25 to 50 μg inserted intravaginally into the posterior fornix used every 3 to 4 hours significantly reduces labor time. Uterine tachysystole and hyperstimulation can occur; therefore, continuous fetal monitoring is recommended. Misoprostol is temperature stable and inexpensive.[9]

■ Membrane stripping or sweeping has also been used as a method for inducing labor. Sweeping membranes somewhere between every other day and once weekly starting at 39 weeks can reduce the number of women who reach 41 weeks gestation. Risks of the procedure include membrane rupture, infection, and bleeding.[10]

■ Amniotomy, with or without oxytocin, is widely used to induce labor. Early amniotomy shortens the duration of labor and reduces the incidence of dystocia but does not reduce the need for anesthesia or caesarean section. Timing of the amniotomy is important because once it is done, the patient is committed to delivery. Amniotomy is best performed in conjunction with the administration of some agent to induce contractions, when there are regular uterine contractions and the head is well applied to the cervix.[11]

■ Oxytocin administration remains the most common form of labor induction. Various protocols exist. The use of the low-dose infusion (starting at 1.0 to 2.0 mU/minute and increasing the dose every 15 to 30 minutes with a maximum of 20 mU/min) is associated with less uterine hyperstimulation, water intoxication, and antidiuretic effect than high-dose protocols. Misoprostol is also being used for labor inductions and has been shown to shorten times to delivery and a significant decrease in caesarean when compared to pitocin but has higher rates of tachysystole and hyperstimulation.[12] Fetal monitoring should be continuous during induction to ensure fetal well-being.[13]

Complications

Complications of PDP include postmaturity of the infant, birth asphyxia, meconium aspiration, and macrosomia leading to shoulder dystocia.

■ **Complications during induction of labor** (see Chapter 14.10)
■ **Neonatal complications** include birth asphyxia, postmaturity of the infant, and meconium aspiration. Macrosomia occurs more often (3% to 7% in PDP) and is associated with an increased risk for shoulder dystocia, neurologic injuries to the shoulder girdle, and cephalohematoma. Hypoglycemia is often seen during the neonatal period in the macrosomic infant.

- **Maternal complications** include an increased incidence of postpartum hemorrhage, vaginal and rectal lacerations, endometritis, and caesarean section.

References

1. Management of postterm pregnancy. *ACOG Pract Patterns* 1997;6:1–6.
2. Marks AD, Divon MY. Longitudinal study of amniotic fluid index in post-date pregnancy. *Obstet Gynecol* 1992;79:229.
3. Jeng CJ, et al. Decreased amniotic fluid index in term pregnancy: clinical significance. *J Reprod Med* 1992;37:789.
4. Fetal heart rate patterns: monitoring, interpretation, and management. *ACOG Tech Bull* 1995;207:1–9.
5. Kuhlman KA, Depp R. Acoustic stimulation testing. *Obstet Clin North Am* 1988;15:303.
6. Vintzileos AM, Kampbell WA, Rodis JF. Fetal biophysical profile scoring: current status. *Clin Perinatal* 1989;16:661.
7. Sanchez-Ramos L, Olivier F, Delke I, et al. Labor induction versus expectant management for postterm pregnancies: a systematic review with meta-analysis. *Obstet Gynecol* 2003;101:1312–1318.
8. Sawai SK. Sequential outpatient application of intravaginal prostaglandin E gel in the management of postdate pregnancies. *Obstet Gynecol* 1991;78:1.
9. Wing D. Labor induction with misoprostol. *Am J Obstet Gynecol* 1999;181:339.
10. Cammu H, Haitsma V. Sweeping of the membranes at 39 weeks in nulliparous women: a randomised controlled trial. *Br J Obstet Gynecol* 1998;105:41.
11. Fraser WD, Turcot L, Krauss I, et al. Amniotomy for shortening spontaneous labour (Cochrane review). In: *The Cochrane Library*, Issue 2:2000. Oxford: Update Software.
12. Induction and augmentation of labor. *ACOG Tech Bull* 1991;157.
13. Sulik SM. Postdate pregnancy. In: Taylor RB, ed. *Manual of family practice*. 2nd ed. Philadelphia: Lippincott Williams & Wilkins; 2002.

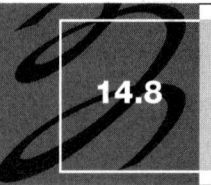

14.8 OBSTETRIC PROBLEMS DURING PREGNANCY

James W. Jarvis, Daphne J. Karel, S. Lindsey Clarke

PRE-ECLAMPSIA AND ECLAMPSIA

Pre-eclampsia is a clinical syndrome defined by the development of hypertension and proteinuria after 20 weeks of gestation. Occurring predominantly in the primipara, pre-eclampsia ranks as an important cause of maternal and fetal morbidity and mortality. Hallmark features include generalized edema, weight gain, impaired renal function, and gastrointestinal (GI) distress. In severe cases, patients may manifest central nervous system (CNS) and hepatic abnormalities with thrombocytopenia. Eclampsia refers to the new onset of grand mal seizures in the pre-eclamptic patient.

General Principles
Definitions
Pre-eclampsia is a pregnancy-specific syndrome requiring both of the following:

- Hypertension, defined as systolic blood pressure (SBP) of 140 mmHg or higher or diastolic blood pressure (DBP) of 90 mmHg or higher that occurs after 20 weeks of gestation in a previously normotensive patient. Blood pressure (BP) elevation must be documented with two measurements at least 6 hours and no more than 7 days apart.
- Proteinuria, defined as urinary excretion of 300 mg or greater of protein in a 24-hour specimen.

Eclampsia is the occurrence of one or more generalized seizures that cannot be otherwise explained in the setting of pre-eclampsia.

Epidemiology
Pre-eclampsia complicates 5% to 8% of pregnancies. Eclampsia occurs in less than 1% of pre-eclamptic patients. Risk factors for pre-eclampsia include nulliparity, prolonged interval since previous pregnancy, age greater than 35 years or less than 20 years, African American ethnicity, multiple gestation, pre-eclampsia in a previous pregnancy, chronic hypertension, pregestational diabetes, renal disease, autoimmune and connective tissue diseases, antiphospholipid antibody syndrome or other thrombophilia, obesity, and family history of pre-eclampsia in a sister or mother. Smokers have a lower risk for pre-eclampsia than nonsmokers.

Classification
Pre-eclampsia and eclampsia are classified as hypertensive disorders of pregnancy. However, hypertension is a sign rather than a cause of the underlying disease process. Pre-eclampsia may be categorized as either mild or severe (see below).

Pathophysiology
The pre-eclamptic syndrome is marked by reduced placental perfusion and abnormal function of the vascular endothelium. Vasospasm, hemoconcentration, and increased vascular permeability interfere with circulation, setting the stage for multiple-organ dysfunction.[1,2]

Etiology
The etiology of pre-eclampsia is unknown.

Diagnosis
Clinical Presentation
Pre-eclampsia may develop gradually or rapidly. Most women with pre-eclampsia have mild disease, and patients often are asymptomatic at the time of diagnosis. Others present with headaches, visual disturbances, abdominal pain, or edema. Symptoms indicate more severe disease. Pre-eclampsia or eclampsia may arise before, during, or after delivery.

- CNS disturbances include headache, visual changes, confusion, coma, hyperreflexia, stroke, and seizures (eclampsia). Visual changes consist of scotomata, diplopia, blurred vision, blind spots, and transient cortical blindness. GI disturbances include nausea, vomiting, and epigastric or right upper quadrant abdominal pain that resembles heartburn. These symptoms sometimes reflect hepatic dysfunction. Edema of the legs, hands, and face may persist after bed rest. Dyspnea due to pulmonary edema may occur.

History
At the initial prenatal visit, screen patients for risk factors for pre-eclampsia, and note complications of previous pregnancies. Beginning at 20 weeks of gestation, assess patients routinely for headache, visual disturbances, abdominal pain, and edema.

Physical Examination
Measure BP at every prenatal visit. Increases above a patient's baseline should be tracked closely. Monitor weight regularly. Patients with pre-eclampsia may gain a pound of fluid or more daily. Lower extremity edema is a common finding in normal pregnancy, but edema of the face and upper extremities is more closely associated with pre-eclampsia. Fundal height measurements that do not match dates may point to fetal growth restriction (FGR) or oligohydramnios.

Laboratory Studies
Laboratory studies are essential in assessing severity.

- Obtain baseline liver enzymes, platelet count, serum creatinine, and 12- or 24-hour urine protein measurement early in pregnancy in women at high risk for pre-eclampsia. Urine protein dipstick values of 1+ or greater at prenatal visits should prompt 24-hour urine protein collection, which remains the most accurate means of quantifying proteinuria. A random urinary protein-to-creatinine ratio of 0.2 or more is predictive of significant proteinuria.[3]

- In patients who develop hypertension after 20 weeks of gestation, measure 24-hour urine protein and creatinine clearance, as well as serum hemoglobin, hematocrit, platelets, creatinine, uric acid, hepatic aminotransferases, albumin, lactate dehydrogenase (LDH), peripheral blood smear, and coagulation studies.
- Once the diagnosis of pre-eclampsia has been established, the above tests should be repeated at least weekly to monitor for worsening of disease. More frequent testing is warranted whenever progression of disease is suspected. Severe pre-eclampsia may require testing as frequently as every 6 hours.
- Hemoconcentration with hemoglobin greater than 15 mg per dL may be present.
- The constellation of hemolysis (LDH more than 600 IU/L or total bilirubin higher than 1.2 mg/dL), elevated liver enzymes (aspartate aminotransferase greater than 70 IU/L), and low platelets (fewer than 100,000 platelets per microliter), called the HELLP syndrome, is a marker of severe disease and impending disseminated intravascular coagulation (DIC). The presence of the HELLP syndrome increases the risk of developing eclampsia.
- Prolongation of prothrombin time and activated partial thromboplastin time, elevation of fibrin degradation products and D-dimer, and consumption of fibrinogen and platelets are suggestive of DIC. However, D-dimer increases with gestational age and may be elevated in normal pregnancy.

Monitoring
Monitoring for signs of maternal and fetal compromise is critical for timing of delivery once the diagnosis of pre-eclampsia has been established.

- At each visit check maternal BP, weight, urine dipstick for protein, deep tendon reflexes, retinoscopy, and edema.
- Fetal surveillance should be performed on the following schedule:
  - Nonstress test (NST) weekly[1]
  - Biophysical profile weekly, often alternated with NST for total of two tests weekly; repeat more frequently for suspected FGR or oligohydramnios or as indicated by severity of maternal condition[1]
  - Fetal movement counts daily (more than 10 kicks daily is considered normal)
  - Ultrasound assessment of fetal growth every 3 weeks[1]
  - Doppler velocimetry for monitoring suspected FGR

Staging
Pre-eclampsia is considered severe if one or more of the following occurs:

- SBP of 160 mmHg or higher or DBP of 110 mmHg or higher on two occasions at least 6 hours apart, while the patient is on bed rest
- Urinary excretion of 5 g or greater of protein in a 24-hour specimen or 3+ or greater on two random urine samples collected at least 4 hours apart
- Oliguria of less than 500 mL in 24 hours
- Cerebral or visual disturbances
- Pulmonary edema or cyanosis
- Epigastric or right upper quadrant abdominal pain
- Impaired hepatic function
- Thrombocytopenia
- FGR

Classification
Distinguishing pre-eclampsia from chronic hypertension and gestational hypertension may prove challenging. Pre-eclampsia may be superimposed on chronic hypertension and renal disease.

Differential Diagnosis
In addition to those conditions listed above, the following conditions may be confused with pre-eclampsia and eclampsia: hepatitis, acute fatty liver of pregnancy, cholestasis, pancreatitis, migraine, cerebral hemorrhage, epilepsy, gestational and autoimmune thrombocytopenia, systemic lupus erythematosus, and thrombotic thrombocytopenic purpura-hemolytic uremic syndrome.

Treatment

Behavioral

- Ambulatory treatment is appropriate for patients with mild pre-eclampsia. Severe pre-eclampsia, disease progression, and inadequate compliance with treatment or follow-up represent indications for hospitalization.[1]
- Bed rest and dietary manipulations have shown no benefit and may exacerbate pre-eclampsia.
- If the patient is still smoking, that may prove disastrous for the pregnancy.

Medications

- **Anticonvulsants.** Magnesium sulfate is the drug of choice for the prevention and treatment of seizures in severe pre-eclampsia (BP 160/105 to 110 or higher; see above) and eclampsia. It is not indicated for mild pre-eclampsia. Start with a 4 to 6 g intravenous (IV) bolus followed by a 2 g per hour IV infusion.[1,3] Check the magnesium level 4 hours later. The desired level is 4 to 8 mg per dL. Follow reflexes, respirations, mental status, and urine output. Continue the magnesium infusion until 24 to 48 hours postpartum and until the patient is diuresing well.
- **Antihypertensives.** Initiate therapy for persistent BP of 160/105 or higher. Lower BP gradually to a goal of 140 to 155/90 to 105.[1,3]
  - Labetalol 20 to 80 mg IV every 10 minutes as needed in escalating doses up to a total of 220 mg.
  - Hydralazine 5 to 10 mg IV every 20 minutes as needed up to a total of 20 mg.
  - Methyldopa 250 mg by mouth two or three times daily (and up to 3 g daily) is standard for ambulatory treatment. Oral labetalol, hydralazine, and long-acting nifedipine also may be used.
  - Angiotensin-converting enzyme inhibitors and diuretics are contraindicated.
  - Corticosteroids, such as betamethasone 12 mg intramuscularly every 24 hours for two doses, can enhance fetal lung maturity between 24 and 34 weeks gestation.

Operative

Obstetric interventions will depend on careful perinatal management, obstetric consultation, and balancing issues such as maternal preference, gestational age, disease severity, presence of labor, cervical status, and fetal lung maturity.

- Delivery of the placenta is the ultimate treatment.
- Consider labor induction at 38 weeks gestation.[3] Deliver as soon as it is safe to do so. There is no reason to continue the pregnancy past 40 weeks, because placental blood flow may continue to fall.
- Prompt delivery always should be considered if seizures, fetal compromise, or worsening maternal disease is present.[2] Indications for delivery include severe FGR, nonreassuring fetal surveillance, oligohydramnios, thrombocytopenia, hepatic subcapsular hematoma, progressive hepatic or renal dysfunction, suspected placental abruption, persistent severe CNS or GI distress, and eclampsia.[2,3]
- Vaginal delivery is preferred. When caesarean delivery is necessary, regional anesthesia is best, except in the setting of coagulopathy.[1,3]

Referrals

Patients with severe pre-eclampsia who are remote from term are best managed in tertiary care settings or in consultation with physicians who are experienced in the management of high-risk pregnancy.[1,3]

Counseling

Pre-eclampsia recurs in approximately 20% of subsequent pregnancies. The recurrence rate may be higher in nulliparous women who develop pre-eclampsia before 30 weeks of gestation. Early-onset pre-eclampsia also is associated with thrombophilias. Consider measuring antiphospholipid antibodies, homocysteine, and proteins C and S.[2,3]

Follow-Up

Pre-eclampsia-related hypertension usually resolves spontaneously in 1 to 3.5 weeks postpartum, although some cases may take up to 12 weeks. Remember that eclampsia may occur up to 23 days postpartum. Persistent hypertension should be evaluated and treated as in nonpregnant women. Labetalol, propranolol, and long-acting nifedipine are safe pharmacologic options for breastfeeding mothers.

ALLOIMMUNIZATION OF ERYTHROCYTES IN PREGNANCY

Erythrocyte (red blood cell, RBC) alloimmunization in pregnancy has drastically diminished since 1968 but has not disappeared. The decreased incidence is due in part to smaller family sizes, but mostly due to the introduction of anti-D immune globulin, formerly referred to as $Rh_o(D)$ immune globulin. Careful attention to maternal blood typing, prior obstetric history of RBC immunization, and careful prophylaxis of the nonimmune gravida for all potential risks of feto-maternal transfusion are critical elements of managing this potentially lethal complication of pregnancy.[4]

General Principles
Definition
Alloimmunization is the development of maternal anti-D antibodies that may result in unwanted consequences for the fetus or newborn, and may occur in women who are Rh(D) negative, and rarely from an anti-ABO or other antigen.

Epidemiology
- **Major blood type antigens**
  - D or Rhesus D (formerly Rh) is the most clinically significant.
  - Other Rhesus (C, c, E, e).
  - ABO (usually not hemolytic, but 98% of all hemolytic disease is Rhesus or ABO).
  - Kell, Duffy, Kidd, Diego are other rare hemolytic antigens.
- **Population distribution.** 15% of whites are D-negative, and 8% of blacks are D-negative; 1% of Asians and Native Americans are D-negative.
- **Incidence.** 6.8 per 1000 births, with 25 per 10,000 with clinical significance.

Etiology
If an Rh negative woman is exposed to a Rhesus antigen she may develop IgG antibodies that can cross the placenta and sensitize fetal erythrocytes of an Rh-positive fetus. This may result in erythrocyte destruction, causing fetal or newborn complications.

- **Causes of alloimmunization**
  - Incompatible blood transfusion is mostly seen with non-Rh and non-ABO sensitization. Major antigens D or Rhesus D (formerly Rh) are the most clinically significant.
  - Possible clinical settings of incompatible transplacental hemorrhage are as follows:
    - Procedures: Amniocentesis, caesarean section, and, to a lesser extent, external version
    - Any antepartum bleeding
    - Abortion, spontaneous and elective
    - Molar pregnancies
    - Fetal–maternal hemorrhage. In 75% of pregnancies there is some evidence of fetal blood in the maternal circulation, most frequently less than 0.1 mL.

- **Fetal and perinatal complications** include immune hydrops fetalis (severe), anemia (mild to severe), heart failure, hyperbilirubinemia leading to kernicterus, extramedullary hematopoiesis, and fetal demise.

Diagnosis
Identify antibodies against fetal erythrocytes in the maternal circulation. Once the antibody is specifically identified, the hemolytic potential of these erythrocytes is determined.

Laboratory Studies
- Rh/ABO typing. Every pregnant patient should have Rh/ABO typing at the first prenatal visit.
- Antibody screening. Every patient must have an antibody screening; if positive, identification and titration of the antibody is essential. An indirect Coombs test is usually done to determine titers. The majority of maternal antibodies identified are nonhemolytic.

Management
- Prevention by screening and treating those at risk for alloimmunization is the key.

- D-positive (Rh-positive), O-type blood requires no therapy.
- D-negative gravidas should:
  - Receive anti-D immune globulin (Rh Ig, RhoGAM) 300 μg as a single dose at 28 to 32 weeks gestation. Consider repeat antibody screening at 28 to 32 weeks gestation to identify alloimmunization earlier in pregnancy.[4]
  - Receive anti-D immune globulin (Rh Ig, RhoGAM) 300 μg as a single dose within 72 hours of delivery when susceptible to alloimmunization (delivery of D-positive or Rh-unknown infant).[4]
  - Receive 300 μg anti-D (Rh Ig) within 72 hours of a potential transfusion (see above). Some physicians still use minidose (50 μg) anti-D.[4]
- Postpartum management should include any deliveries at risk for increased fetal–maternal transfusion (caesarean section, increased blood loss, pregnancy-induced hypertension, manual removal of the placenta). Consideration of quantification of the fetal–maternal transfusion should be done if the baby's blood type is D-positive. The Kleihauer–Betke test assesses the amount of fetal blood in the maternal circulation. If less than 15 mL of blood is transfused, give the routine 300 μg of anti-D (Rh Ig); if more than 15 mL of blood is transfused, 300 μg per 15-mL transfusion should be given.
- The patient with a positive antibody screen and an identified antigen (D, C, c, E, or e) should be treated as follows:
  - If the antibody titer is 1:16 or higher or is elevated four times baseline in monthly measurement, the following should be considered looking for evidence of fetal anemia:
    - Ultrasound, including Doppler velocimetry
    - Amniocentesis for optical density
    - Fetal blood sampling[4]
- Treatment of suspected fetal complications is usually carried out in a perinatal center.
  - Intraperitoneal fetal transfusions are effective.
  - Intravascular fetal transfusion into the umbilical vein or intrahepatic vein is also effective.
  - Plasmapheresis, corticosteroids, and promethazine have no proven benefit.
  - Delivery decisions are based on the fetal risk of immaturity versus rising hemolysis risks with continued pregnancy.
  - Fetal distress may be present, with the characteristic sinusoidal heart rate indicating repetitive decelerations. The severely distressed fetus should be delivered.

Delivery where a level II or III neonatal intensive care unit is available is essential in the sensitized mother. Fetal exchange transfusion should be readily available.[4,5]

PRETERM LABOR

Preterm labor (PTL) is a leading cause of perinatal morbidity and mortality in the United States. Of all births, 11% are complicated by PTL. Large societal costs result from neonatal intensive care and long-term treatment for complications. When developmental defects are excluded, 70% to 80% of neonatal mortality is attributable to low birth weight. Early, accurate diagnosis of PTL provides for secondary prevention of premature births. Primary prevention attempts to reduce risk factors for prematurity. Once the patient is in PTL, a comprehensive management plan is essential. Unfortunately, no current intervention has been able to significantly reduce the incidence of preterm birth and most are aimed at decreasing morbidity associated with preterm birth.[6]

General Principles
Definition
PTL is defined as contractions occurring between 20 and 37 weeks gestation and producing cervical change.

Epidemiology
As stated above, 11% of all births are complicated by PTL. PTL accounts for 70% to 80% of all neonatal mortality.

Etiology
Multifactorial. See History and Risk Management below for details.

Diagnosis of Preterm Labor
Clinical Presentation
Detecting PTL early enough for effective intervention has proven to be a challenge in practice. The patient presents between 20 and 37 weeks gestation with uterine contractions or irritability producing cervical dilatation and/or effacement.

History
Risk factors for PTL include low socioeconomic status, nonwhite race, age less than 18 or more than 40, low prepregnancy weight, prior preterm births, at least one spontaneous second-trimester abortion, absence of prenatal care, and maternal substance abuse (tobacco, cocaine), uterine overdistension, abruption, bacterial infections, and cervical incompetence.[8] Menstrual history, outpatient records, and early ultrasounds should be reviewed to confirm dates. Usually, the patient will give a history of recent or intermittent contractions with or without other signs of labor, such as pelvic pressure or bloody show.

Physical Examination
- **PTL signs.** Contractions can be palpated. A single observer should document cervical change (such as effacement or dilation) over time. Uterine measurement can provide an estimate of gestational age.
- **Routine cervical examinations.** There is no predictive advantage to routine cervical examinations in pregnant women with average risk.[6] However, these may prove useful in women with a history suggestive of incompetent cervix and should be performed in women with a complaint of preterm contractions to evaluate for cervical change.

Laboratory
Fetal fibronectin is an extracellular protein that is believed to act as an adhesive between the developing embryo and the uterine surface. It is present in vaginal secretions at implantation but disappears by 20 weeks estimated gestational age (EGA). In a patient with suspected PTL, the posterior vaginal fornix and cervix are swabbed, and the sample is sent to the lab for a fetal fibronectin monoclonal antibody assay. The negative predictive value of a negative test is greater than 90%, and a positive test is correlated with imminent delivery.[6]

Imaging
Wedging of the internal cervical os on transvaginal ultrasonography has been associated with preterm delivery, and may prove more sensitive than the digital vaginal exam.[7]

Monitoring
The U.S. Food and Drug Administration has approved home uterine monitoring in women with a history of PTL, but the cost is high and the benefit is equivocal. Hospital- or office-based monitoring can be helpful in the presence of symptoms.

Differential Diagnosis
The differential includes false labor, Braxton–Hicks contractions, incompetent cervix, and uterine irritability secondary to infection or dehydration.

Treatment
Behavioral
Bed rest and pelvic rest do not prolong pregnancy and may have adverse maternal effects.[6]

Conservative Management
- Treat underlying causes (urinary tract infection, cervicitis, dehydration, substance use).[8]
- Hydration decreases contractions, but no causal relationship has been identified. Use 500 to 1000 mL lactated Ringer solution or normal saline, followed by 125 mL per hour (if not contraindicated).

Medications
- **Tocolytic therapy**
  - **Efficacy.** Tocolytics have successfully lengthened pregnancy by an average of 48 hours, which may provide enough time to administer corticosteroids or to transfer to a tertiary care center. The decision to use tocolytics should be influenced by maternal condition, fetal size and maturity, and fetal condition.

- **Contraindications.** Contraindications include advanced labor, pre-eclampsia or eclampsia, abruptio placentae, chorioamnionitis, dead or distressed fetus, anomalies incompatible with life, fetal maturity, and maternal homodynamic instability.[7]
- **Drug dosage and comparison.** Direct comparison of tocolytics has shown them to have similar efficacy, and choice usually depends on side effects. For all tocolytics, use the minimum necessary to stop contractions, monitor for side effects, and discontinue or switch to an oral agent as soon as labor ceases. Combining tocolytics increases maternal morbidity and should be avoided.[6] Table 14.8-1 presents a list of tocolytics, dosages, and potential complications.
- **Adverse effects.** Pulmonary edema has been associated with the concomitant use of tocolytics (primarily β_2-agonists and magnesium sulfate) and corticosteroids. The

TABLE 14.8-1   Tocolytics for Management of Preterm Labor

Medication	Dosage	Precautions/ complications	Contraindications
Magnesium sulfate	4–6 g IV load, then 2–4 g/h drip, continue 12 h after contractions stop. Therapeutic level 5–8 mg/dL	Pulmonary edema toxic levels may cause profound hypotension, paralysis, tetany, cardiac arrest, respiratory depression, and renal failure Areflexia at 8–10 mg/dL, respiratory suppression at >10 mg/dL	Hypocalcemia, myasthenia gravis, renal failure
Terbutaline (β_2-agonist)	0.25–0.5 mg SC q3–4 h or 10 mg PO q2h × 24 hr, then 10–20 mg q4–6h	Hypokalemia, hyperglycemia, hypotension, pulmonary edema, tachycardia and arrhythmias, cardiac insufficiency, myocardial infarction, and maternal death	Maternal arrhythmias, uncontrolled diabetes mellitus, hypertension, or thyrotoxicosis
Ritodrine (β_2-agonist)	No longer available in the U.S.	Same as terbutaline	Same as terbutaline
Nifedipine (calcium-channel blocker)	10–20 mg PO q4–6h	Transient hypotension	Maternal liver disease
Indomethacin (NSAID)	50–100 mg PR; and/or 25 to 50 mg PO q6h	Renal failure, GI bleed, hepatitis, oligohydramnios, constriction of ductus arteriosis Possible risk of necrotizing enterocolitis and intraventricular hemorrhage in neonates	Aspirin sensitive asthma, coronary artery disease, GI bleed, renal failure, oligohydramnios, fetal cardiac, or renal anomalies
Sulindac (NSAID)	200 mg PO q12 (up to 6 doses)	Same as indomethacin	Same as indomethacin

GI, gastrointestinal; NSAID, nonsteroidal anti-inflammatory drug.

risk can be decreased by limiting fluid intake to less than 200 mL per day, restricting sodium intake to 4 to 6 g per day, monitoring serum potassium and glucose, and avoiding steroids with high mineralocorticoid potency. Do not withhold corticosteroids from PTL. For magnesium sulfate, the target serum level is 5 to 8 mg per dL. Higher levels (10 to 12 mg/dL) result in respiratory suppression. Monitor deep tendon reflexes, which disappear at levels of 8 to 10 mg per dL. The nonsteroidal anti-inflammatory drugs can cause constriction of the ductus arteriosus in the fetus and a decreased amniotic fluid index. These effects are reversible if use is restricted to a short period (24 to 48 hours). Nifedipine has few adverse effects.[6,7] Ketorolac and atosiban have been studied as tocolytics. Ritodrine is no longer being marketed.[6,8] See Table 14.8-1 for additional complications and precautions.

- **Corticosteroids**
  - **Efficacy.** Antenatal steroids given between 24 and 34 weeks EGA have been proved to reduce the incidence and severity of respiratory distress syndrome, intraventricular hemorrhage, and necrotizing enterocolitis.[7]
  - **Complications.** There have been no significant maternal or fetal complications associated with antenatal steroids. Pulmonary edema in the mother has occurred with the use of tocolytics and steroids together, but not with corticosteroid use alone, and may be due in part to increased fluid volume, multiple gestations, and/or infection. As expected, closer monitoring of gestational diabetes may be necessary after steroid administration, and steroids may mask maternal fever.[7,8]
  - **Dosage and comparison.** Corticosteroids result in significant benefits, starting within 24 hours and persisting for a week. Corticosteroids are indicated in PTL between 24 and 34 weeks EGA unless delivery is imminent. There are two accepted steroid courses, chosen for their ability to cross the placenta, their longer duration of action, and their proven efficacy in clinical trials. Higher or more frequent doses than those listed below do *not* provide any additional benefit.
    - Betamethasone: two 12-mg doses given IM 24 hours apart.
    - #160; Dexamethasone: four 6 mg doses given IM 12 hours apart.

- **Antibiotics**
  - In premature rupture of membranes, antibiotics have been shown to prolong latency and improve neonatal outcome.[7,8] Treatment of group B *Streptococcus*-positive mothers prior to delivery has been proved to decrease the incidence of neonatal sepsis.[7] Studies indicate that empiric antibiotics for prophylaxis or to cover asymptomatic colonization do not prolong the pregnancy in PTL. However, maternal infections including bacterial vaginosis, urinary tract infections, and sexually transmitted infections should be treated.[6,8]

Risk Management

Risk-scoring systems (Papiernik, Creasy) have sensitivity less than 50% and a positive predictive value of less than 20% for detecting patients who will undergo PTL, but they can be used to increase your level of suspicion and need for primary intervention.

Patient Education

All pregnant patients with signs or symptoms of labor should seek immediate medical attention. Counsel risk reduction, such as smoking cessation, proper nutrition, avoiding contact sports, and treating infections promptly.

Complications

Preterm infants have significant risk of pulmonary, neurologic, and enteral complications that require specialized medical care. Whenever possible, preterm delivery should occur in a hospital with specialized newborn care available.

References

1. ACOG Committee on Practice Bulletins—Obstetrics. *Diagnosis and management of pre-eclampsia and eclampsia.* ACOG Practice Bulletin No. 33. *Obstet Gynecol* 2002; 99:159–167.
2. Lain KY, Roberts JM. Contemporary concepts of the pathogenesis and management of pre-eclampsia. *JAMA* 2002;287:3183–3186.

3. Wagner LK. Diagnosis and management of pre-eclampsia. *Am Fam Physician* 2004; 70:2317–2324.
4. ACOG Practice Bulletin. No. 4. *Prevention of Rh D alloimmunization*, May 1999.
5. MacKenzie IZ, et al. Routine antenatal Rhesus D immunoglobulin prophylaxis: the results of a prospective 10 year study. *Br J Obstet Gynaecol* 1999;106:492–497.
6. American College of Obstetricians and Gynecologists. *Preterm labor*. Committee Opinion No. 206.Washington, DC, 1995.
7. Weismiller D. Preterm labor. *Am Fam Physician* 1999;59:593–602.
8. Egarter C, et al. Antibiotic treatment in preterm premature rupture of membranes and neonatal morbidity: a metaanalysis. *Am J Obstet Gynecol* 1996;174:589–597.

INTRAPARTUM CARE
Brian J. Finley

14.9

GENERAL PRINCIPLES

Intrapartum care of the healthy term pregnant woman is the subject of this chapter, beginning with her arrival at the labor ward in active labor.

DIAGNOSIS AND ADMISSION

History

The woman in active labor gives a history of regularly occurring contractions, of increasing frequency, length, and intensity and associated with pain in the abdomen and/or back. Establish whether she has had, and the time of, obvious or suspected rupture of the membranes. Ask whether it was clear, green (meconium), or bloody. Determine whether there has been abnormal bleeding or pain. Review her antenatal history, confirming her due date and whether there were any significant problems in this pregnancy. Review her past obstetric history, medical history, and psychosocial history, identifying problems therein that are active or relevant to her current labor (e.g., previous shoulder dystocia or caesarean section) (see Chapter 14.10).

Physical Examination

Perform a complete physical examination at the time of admission, focusing attention on the areas identified in the history as being of concern. Confirm the uterine size and the fetal lie, presentation, and position. Inspect the vulva for herpes. Confirm a history of rupture of the membranes by sterile speculum examination, pH test, and microscopic evidence of "ferning" when the fluid is air dried on a slide. Digitally examine the cervix for softness, effacement, dilatation (in centimeters), and location. Confirm a vertex presentation and ascertain its station relative to the ischial spines.

Investigations

The antenatal investigations do not need to be repeated. Draw blood for a complete blood count and draw a clot tube for cross and match if needed later. Do a urinalysis.

Problem Formulation and Plan

Assess the risk level of the pregnancy and the current labor. Make the appropriate plan for management and maternal–fetal surveillance. Assess the plan on an ongoing basis and adjust management appropriately.

LABOR MANAGEMENT

The monitoring of fetal and maternal well-being of the low-risk woman in labor does not require highly technical equipment or much intervention, but it does require close observation.

■ **Stage I,** from onset of labor to full dilatation at 10 cm, is divided into latent and active phases. The latent phase, which may be more sensitive to anesthetics and sedatives, has slow dilation until 3 to 4 cm. The active phase is characterized by more rapid dilation.

■ **Monitoring and care**

- **Maternal nutrition and position.** Allow a low-residue, low-fat diet in labor with frequent small meals (e.g., tea, fruit juice, broth, toast). Encourage upright posture, which might result in a shorter first stage and lower requirements for analgesics.

- **Fetal surveillance.** The fetus is monitored to detect and prevent problems that could lead to fetal morbidity and mortality.

   - **Amniotic fluid.** When the membranes are (naturally or artificially) ruptured, assess the fluid for the presence of meconium and blood. Meconium has been associated with increased perinatal morbidity. Blood may signify abruption. In both situations, closer surveillance may be in order.

   - **Fetal heart rate (FHR) monitoring.** The FHR should be monitored every 15 to 30 minutes, and this should be done immediately following a contraction. This can be by simple auscultation or by Doppler ultrasonography. Continuous electronic fetal monitoring (EFM) in labor results in the reduction of the rate of neonatal seizures, the long-term impact of which is unclear. EFM also leads to a significant increased rate of caesarean and operative deliveries.[1]

      - **Baseline fetal heart rate pattern.** Assess the FHR pattern for baseline rate and variability. The baseline FHR (i.e., the rate between contractions at term) is usually 120 to 160 beats per minute. FHR may be lower in the postterm infant and higher in the premature infant. Variability (the beat-to-beat variation in the FHR) may be diminished or absent in the premature or "sleeping" fetus. Otherwise, absence of variability may indicate fetal compromise. Causes include hypoxia, drug use in labor, or congenital anomalies. Tachycardia (>160 beats/min) can be caused by maternal fever, drugs, or fetal hypoxia. Other less common causes of **fetal tachycardia** include fetal hyperthyroidism, fetal anemia, fetal heart failure, and fetal tachyarrhythmias.[1] Bradycardia (<120 beats/min) can be normal in the postterm infant or indicative of severe hypoxia, maternal systemic lupus erythematosus, or fetal heart block.

      - **Periodic heart rate changes.** Document accelerations and decelerations. Accelerations of 15 to 25 beats per minute above baseline are often associated with fetal movement or contractions and are reassuring. Decelerations are of three patterns: early, late, and variable. In early decelerations, the heart rate decreases with the start of the contraction and recovers as the contraction diminishes. This type of deceleration is usually secondary to fetal head compression. Late decelerations begin as the contraction peaks. The lowest FHR is reached well after the peak of the contraction and recovery does not take place until after the end of the contraction. These may be associated with uteroplacental insufficiency and resultant hypoxia. Variable decelerations begin at no fixed time in relation to the contraction and may be the result of cord compression.

      - Management of worrisome FHR patterns is a very difficult task and causes much worry for the delivering provider. Despite a great increase in technology and knowledge, there is not one method of evaluation of the worrisome FHR that has been proved to be accurate, reliable, and readily available. Some options that may be available and may be considered for use by an experienced provider include fetal scalp acid–base sampling, fetal pulse oximetry, and fetal electrocardiogram. Appropriate management is based on the fetal scalp pH. In the case of a prolonged deceleration, change maternal position, give oxygen, and check for cord prolapse. A nonreassuring FHR pattern, poor pH, low pulse ox, change in the fetal electrocardiogram, or a prolonged deceleration may indicate the need for immediate delivery, consultation with a caesarean capable provider, or both.

■ **Progress.** Periodically assess the cervix for further dilation, effacement, and descent of the head. These examinations should not be done more often than necessary to minimize discomfort and, when the membranes have already ruptured, the risk of infection. An acceptable rate of dilatation in the active phase may be 0.5 to 1.5 cm per hour, with primiparas generally progressing more slowly than multiparas. Slow progress may be, but is not necessarily, a sign of abnormal labor. Interpret the rate of progress in the context of both fetal and maternal well-being.

■ **Pain control can be nonpharmacologic or pharmacologic.** Anything that relaxes and distracts the woman from her pain is beneficial. Maternal movement and position changes help with pain tolerance. Encourage the use of hot and cold compresses, baths, showers, or reassuring touch from her partner and labor coach.

- **Systemic drugs** include narcotics, tranquilizers, and inhalation gases. Narcotics provide reasonable analgesia but are also associated with dose-related maternal sedation, hypotension, nausea, and vomiting, and neonatal respiratory depression. If narcotics are used, always have the antagonist naloxone (Narcan) available for the infant at delivery. Dosage: Naloxone, at 0.01 mg per kg SC, IV, or endotracheally.[2]

- **Regional anesthesia** options include the epidural, spinal, and pudendal anesthetics. Epidurals generally provide more effective pain relief than narcotics or pudendal block. However, epidurals may lengthen labor and result in increased incidence of fetal malposition, increased need for oxytocics, and increased rate of operative vaginal delivery (but not of caesarean section).[3]

■ **Second stage** comprises 10 cm dilatation to delivery of the infant. Confirm full dilatation. Allow the unanesthetized woman to push in the position of her choice and according to her own urges. For women with epidural, delayed pushing up to 2 hours, unless there is an irresistible urge, visibility of head, or medical indication to shorten the second stage, may reduce the need for obstetric interventions.[4] Give her guidance and feedback on her propulsive efforts. Sustained and early bearing down may result in a slightly shorter second stage but may be associated with compromise of maternal–fetal gas exchange.[5] Auscultate every 5 to 15 minutes, following every contraction–pushing series. As long as there is progress, intervention is generally only required if there is a concern about maternal or fetal well-being.

■ **Care of the perineum.** Episiotomy should not be done unless indicated, as it does not reduce the risk of severe perineal trauma or urinary incontinence, nor does it improve perineal healing or prevent fetal trauma. Indications include relief of maternal or fetal distress or for prevention of progress by a nonyielding perineum. Time it at the last possible moment to avoid blood loss. Local anesthetic is injected into the unanesthetized perineum along the anticipated line of the incision.

■ **Spontaneous delivery of the occiput-anterior infant**

- **Delivery of the head.** Minimize perineal trauma by conducting a *controlled* delivery of the head. At crowning, guide the woman to give small, short pushes of submaximal power, and to pant between the pushes. Assist her to nudge the head out. Suctioning should be done in the presence of meconium. Allow the head to restitute.

- **Shoulders.** Check for the presence of a nuchal cord. Slip it over the head or shoulders, or double clamp and cut between the clamps. Deliver the anterior shoulder first by gentle downward traction on the head, then the posterior shoulder by upward traction. Watch and support (often by squatting yourself) the posterior perineum to control for lacerations and extensions. The rest of the infant easily follows. The cord is clamped and cut, often by the woman's partner. The vigorous infant can be placed directly on the maternal abdomen.

■ **Third stage**

■ **Delivery of the placenta.** Spontaneous delivery of the placenta almost always occurs. The signs of delivery include (a) the uterus becoming firmer, (b) a gush of blood, (c) the uterus rising in the abdomen, and (d) the umbilical cord lengthening. Maintain firm gentle traction on the cord while the abdominal hand pushes upward on the anterior wall of the uterus to prevent uterine inversion.[2] Routine administration of oxytocics may shorten the third stage and reduce the risk of postpartum hemorrhage. Dosage: Oxytocic (Oxytocin injection, USP) 10 units IM or IV should be given with delivery of the anterior shoulder or as soon as possible after that. There is a small risk of hypertension. Manual removal of the placenta is considered if the placenta is not delivered within 30 minutes.

- **Vaginal repair.** Inspect the vagina, periurethral tissues, and cervix (if anesthesia allows) for tears. Confirm the presence or absence of a third- or fourth-degree tear, and repair these first. Repair an episiotomy or tear with 2-0 absorbable suture, in the standard fashion, ensuring hemostasis and anatomical restoration, with the minimal suturing required.

- **The first hour postpartum.** Follow the woman closely for any evidence of bleeding. Check her fundus frequently, and massage if not firm. If her flow seems too fast or heavy, then manage according to postpartum hemorrhage instructions (i.e., pitocin, methergine, or hemabate). Encourage and assist with early breastfeeding.

References

1. Thacker SB, Stroup DF. Continuous electronic heart rate monitoring for fetal assessment during labor. *Cochrane Database Syst Rev* 2001;1.
2. Shankaran S, Cepeda E. Neonatal resuscitation and emergencies. In: Tintanalli JE, et al., eds. *Emergency medicine: a comprehensive study guide.* New York: McGraw-Hill; 1996:75.
3. Howell CJ. Epidural versus non-epidural analgesia for pain relief in labour (Cochrane review). In: *The Cochrane Library,* Issue 2, 2000. Oxford: Update Software.
4. Fraser WD, Marcoux S, Krauss I, et al. Multicenter, randomized controlled trial of delayed pushing for nulliparous women in the second stage of labor with continuous epidural analgesia. The PEOPLE (Pushing Early or Pushing Late with Epidural) Study Group. *Am J Obstet Gynecol* 2000;182:1165–1172.
5. Nikodem VC. Sustained (Valsalva) vs exhalatory bearing down in 2nd stage of labour. In: Enkin MW, et al., eds. Pregnancy and childbirth module. *Cochrane Database Syst Rev* 1995.
6. MacDonald SE. *Intrapartum Care.* In: Taylor RB, ed. *Manual of family practice.* 2nd ed. Philadelphia: Lippincott Williams & Wilkins; 2002.

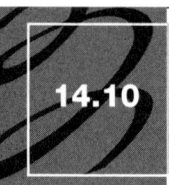

COMPLICATIONS DURING LABOR AND DELIVERY

14.10

James L. Greenwald

$\mathcal{B}$leeding occurs in the third trimester in 2% of pregnancies. Half of the significant cases of bleeding are attributable to either placental abruption or placenta previa. Premature rupture of the membranes (PROM) and dystocia are more common than the hemorrhagic complications of labor and delivery, but they rarely result in significant maternal or neonatal morbidity or mortality.

PLACENTAL ABRUPTION

General Principles

Definition

Placental abruption, or abruptio placentae, is defined as premature separation of a normally inserted placenta from the endometrium.

Anatomy

Hemorrhage occurs into the decidua basalis and usually, but not always, dissects through to the cervix. It can occur in any trimester. Early in pregnancy, abruption can manifest clinically as threatened or spontaneous abortion, and on ultrasound as a subchorionic hemorrhage. Unless the abruption occurs traumatically in an auto accident or as the consequence of uterine rupture, the bleeding source is maternal vessels.

Epidemiology
Abruption occurs in about 0.5% of all pregnancies.[1]

Classification
Abruption can be marginal, partial, or total. If the blood does not dissect through to the vagina, this is designated a concealed abruption.

Pathophysiology
Microvascular damage appears to lead abruption. This can be caused by hypertension, smoking, diabetes, infections, autoimmune, genetic metabolic anomalies such as hyperhomocyteinemia or clotting disorders. Myomas, septae, and other structural abnormalities can also increase the incidence of abruption.[1]

Etiology
Risk factors include chronic hypertension, preterm PROM, external trauma, cigarette smoking, uterine leiomyomas, and cocaine abuse. Abruption increases somewhat with increasing maternal age. Cocaine abuse is particularly important, causing at least a threefold increase in the rate of abruption. The increase in the use of this drug may in part be responsible for the increased national incidence of abruption.[2]

Mechanism of Injury
- **Maternal.** Maternal mortality is rare with modern obstetrical management, but morbidity can occur due to blood loss, disseminated intravascular coagulation and subsequent renal damage, or anemia. Most of the blood loss is maternal, but some fetal–maternal transfusions may occur leading to isoimmunization.
- **Fetal.** Abruption can lead to fetal mortality due to prematurity or stillbirth. Morbidity such as cerebral palsy may be seen infants who deliver prematurely.

Diagnosis
Clinical Presentation
Abruption may present in different ways. The classic presentation is excessive bleeding with unusually painful contractions. Concealed abruption may present with fetal distress associated with painful labor and no bleeding.

History
Abruption is often an obstetrical emergency and the clinician must be looking for symptoms that may be subtle. Most patients have abnormal bleeding, hypertonic painful contractions, or back pain. Preterm labor may be associated with abruption.

Physical Examination
Uterine tenderness, back pain, vaginal bleeding, and fetal distress may each be seen in more than half of cases. Less common but still occurring in more than 10% are hypertonic contractions, rapid progress of labor, preterm labor, and in 15% of cases, fetal demise.[2] Abruption may rarely present as shock.

Laboratory
Blood tests occasionally demonstrate renal failure and coagulation defects that are associated with increased maternal and fetal complications. Hypofibrinogenemia is found in 30% of patients with abruption and associated fetal demise (Stage III B). Coagulopathy can be rapidly detected at the bedside when a tube of whole blood takes longer than 7 to 10 minutes to form a good clot in a plain test tube. Proteinuria is also a common accompaniment of disseminated intravascular coagulation (DIC). Other maternal serum markers may be elevated such as alpha fetoprotein. Human chorionic gonadotropin has a strong negative predictive value and a normal serum hCG may help rule out concealed abruption.[1] In Rh-negative mothers, a Kleihauer Betke test may be done. This test indicates the presence of fetal cells in the maternal circulation. Although it is not helpful in diagnosing abruption, it can indicate a need to increase the dosage of RhoGam if a larger than normal fetal maternal transfusion has occurred.

Imaging
- **Ultrasound.** An ultrasound examination should be performed as soon as possible when abruption is suspected. Although a clot may not be seen in as many as 50% of cases,

the study is still useful in excluding placenta previa. A hemorrhage greater than 60 cc or 50% of the surface that attaches to the uterus is associated with a 50% mortality.[3]

- **Magnetic resonance imaging (MRI)** may detect a higher percentage of suspected cases of abruption where the diagnosis is not obvious clinically. However, lack of portability renders MRI less useful in an emergency situation.

Staging
The Sher classification[4] lists three grades that can be used to help direct management.

- Grade I mild abruption. Clot is often minimally symptomatic and discovered at the time of delivery after unexplained bleeding.
- Grade II symptomatic abruption (tender abdomen) with live fetus.
- Grade III abruption with fetal demise.
  - IIIA without coagulopathy
  - IIIB with coagulopathy

Monitoring
Continuous electronic fetal monitoring is essential if the patient is allowed to labor.

Treatment
Nonoperative
Labor may be allowed to progress if no fetal distress is noted, although rapid deterioration may be seen. Augmentation is rarely needed as blood provides a stimulant to labor.

Operative
A caesarean section is performed if there are signs of fetal distress. About half of symptomatic abruptions receive a caesarean section.[1]

Special Treatment
Coagulopathy may require replacement of blood products while waiting for the effects of the placental inflammation to reverse.

Complications
- **Maternal.** Maternal mortality is rare and may be due to shock, renal failure, or DIC. Any significant bleeding in pregnancies where the mother is at risk for anti-D isoimmunization should prompt treatment with Rh immune globulin.
- **Fetal.** Abruption is associated with a 25% to 30% perinatal mortality. Although a majority of perinatal deaths are related to extreme prematurity, intrauterine fetal demise is possible even at term related to disruption of placental function. Abruption is associated with poorer neurodevelopmental outcome in low-birth-weight infants but not in normal-weight infants.

Patient Education and Prevention
In spite of the high incidence of recurrence (12%), preventive measures are not available to lower the increased incidence of fetal demise (7%) in pregnancies with a history of abruption.

PLACENTA PREVIA
General Principles
Definition
Placenta previa occurs when the site of placental implantation impinges on the internal cervical os.

Anatomy
Bleeding from separation of the placenta in the presence of previa is a common cause of bleeding in the second and third trimesters.

Epidemiology
Placenta previa causes bleeding in about 0.5% of late pregnancies. A higher than normal rate of placenta previa is associated with previous caesarean section, previous induced or spontaneous abortion, advanced maternal age, and smoking.[3] The recurrence rate can be up to 7%.

Classification
Depending on the precise location of the placenta, the previa may be qualified as being total (completely covering the internal os), partial (partially covering), or marginal (edge of

placenta touching the os). Vasa previa, where the vessels divide before implanting on the margin and protrude through the os during labor, is a rare and often fatal variant.

Pathophysiology
Placenta previa, although it may be due to a random faulty localization of the placenta, is also associated with factors that cause damage to the vascular function or continuity of the endometrium. Up to 7% of patients with placenta previa may have an abnormal placental attachment (placenta accreta, increta, or percreta). This is especially noted in patients with repeated caesarean sections, indicating that both conditions may be related to endometrial defects. The rate of accreta may be as high as 65% after multiple caesarean sections.[1]

Etiology
Advanced maternal age, multiparity, prior caesarean section, and smoking all increase the rate of placenta previa.

Mechanisms of Injury
- **Fetal.** Perinatal fetal mortality is less than 5%, primarily due to increased premature births by caesarean section.[3] In addition to the common forms of morbidity associated with prematurity, neonatal anemia is common and related to the degree of maternal hemorrhage. Respiratory distress syndrome occurs more commonly than would be predicted by the rate of prematurity. Other effects, such as an increased incidence of congenital anomalies, may be associated with the causes of abnormal implantation. It is likely that a number of spontaneous abortions occur due to a low insertion of the placenta.
- **Maternal.** Women with placenta previa have a mortality of 0.03%, or about three times the overall U.S. rate of mortality in childbirth. Death may be due to hemorrhage from a digital exam in labor or postpartum hemorrhage from placenta accreta, increta, or percreta. These can cause exsanguination and must be anticipated especially when previa occurs with a prior caesarean section. Other complications include an increase in caesarean birth, fetal malpresentation, premature labor, and postpartum hemorrhage.

Diagnosis
Clinical Presentation
Placenta previa may present as painless bleeding in the second or third trimester or as heavy bleeding after an examiner unwittingly damages the presenting placenta or vessels.

History
The ubiquitous use of ultrasound has allowed most cases of placenta previa to be diagnosed in the antepartum period. Previa is frequently diagnosed prior to any bleeding and commonly overdiagnosed. One study of 267 patients having placenta previa diagnosed on ultrasound performed between 14 and 20 weeks gestation showed that the previa persisted to the time of delivery in only 2.5% of patients with partial or marginal previa, although it persisted in 26% of patients with total previa.[3] Placenta accreta may present as excessive bleeding in the third stage of labor due to incomplete separation. Placenta percreta and increta may also be associated with difficulty in delivering the placenta.

Physical Examination
Vaginal examination should be avoided if placenta previa is suspected before performing an ultrasound examination, due to the risk of perforating the portion of placenta that is palpable through the os. If the localization of a low-lying placenta is not clear from ultrasound a "double set up" examination may be performed in the operating room after the patient is prepared for caesarean delivery and the operative team is assembled.

Laboratory Studies
Blood tests are generally normal in the absence of anemia due to massive hemorrhage.

Imaging
- **Ultrasound.** An ultrasound should be performed with the onset of painless bleeding in pregnancy. False-positive and false-negative rates may each approach 5%. Bladder overdistention is associated with false positives, and consideration should be made to catheterizing the bladder before performing an ultrasound. Clinical judgment is important. Heavy bleeding, especially when coexisting with signs of fetal distress, should lead to an immediate delivery without taking time to perform studies.

- **MRI** can clearly outline the location of a placenta previa, but it is much more expensive and less readily available.

Monitoring
- **Antepartum.** Monthly ultrasound can be performed to document whether the placenta will move from the os, allowing normal labor.
- **Preterm.** Patients with transient minor bleeding who are not in labor may be managed in consultation with a perinatologist. Avoiding vaginal exams may increase the latent period. In preterm placenta previa prior to 36 weeks gestation without evident fetal jeopardy, authorities recommend attempting delay in delivery by avoiding vaginal examination. Reliable patients with minor degrees of bleeding who have been adequately observed for premature delivery and fetal distress may be managed at home without increased maternal or infant morbidity or mortality. In practice, few patients with symptomatic placenta previa meet these criteria.[1]
- **Term and intrapartum.** Prompt delivery should be the goal in term placenta previa. Hemorrhage and shock must be managed aggressively, and the delivering physician should be prepared to perform an emergency caesarean section or hysterectomy if bleeding from placenta accreta cannot be controlled. Continuous electronic fetal monitoring is needed when labor is allowed. Maternal hypotension should be managed with two large-bore intravenous lines, type and cross match, consideration of transfusion, and prompt delivery.

Differential Diagnosis
Physical exam and history are usually sufficient to help differentiate abruptio and previa from normal bleeding. Bleeding may also be due to trauma upon a friable cervix and the normal bloody show in early labor. DIC caused by sepsis or infection and clotting disorders are rare and may be anticipated with a prior history or signs of shock.

Treatment
Behavioral
Women who are managed expectantly are restricted from vaginal intercourse.

Medications
In preterm placenta previa prior to 36 weeks gestation without evident fetal jeopardy, authorities recommend attempting delay in delivery by tocolysis (see below). The efficacy of this reducing infant mortality or morbidity in previa or other causes of prematurity has yet to be proved by a large, prospective study.

Surgery
Caesarean section is performed if fetal distress or significant hemorrhage is evident.

Special Considerations
Regional anesthesia is less likely to exacerbate heavy bleeding than general anesthesia and is preferred for caesarean sections in patients with symptomatic previa.

PREMATURE RUPTURE OF MEMBRANES
General Principles
Definition
Premature rupture of membranes (PROM) is a loss of integrity of the fetal membranes with leakage of amniotic fluid that occurs more than 1 hour before the onset of active labor. The duration between membrane rupture and the onset of active labor contractions is defined as the latent period.

Epidemiology
PROM occurs in 5% to 10% of term and 30% of preterm deliveries.[1]

Classification
PROM may be subdivided into PROM at term or preterm (PPROM), which occurs prior to 37 weeks of gestation.

Pathophysiology
Many cases of premature rupture of membranes are thought to be due to inflammation from subclinical infections of the genital tract. The bacterial enzymes that facilitate colonization

are thought to weaken fetal membranes. Vascular damage may be a cause, as in diabetes or hypertension.

Etiology

Positive cultures of amniotic fluid are present in 30% of pregnancies with PPROM. Smoking and vaginal bleeding are associated but it is not known how. Previous PROM is a risk factor. Other risk factors include vaginal group B streptococcal colonization, cigarette smoking, hypertension, diabetes, amniocentesis, and cervical surgery during the pregnancy.

Mechanisms of Injury

- **Maternal.** Most complications are related to infection. The rate of postpartum endometritis historically approached 30%, but the widespread use of antibiotics has greatly reduced this. Abruption occurs in 5% of pregnancies with PROM.
- **Fetal.** Subclinical infection is common, but less than 10% of neonates actually develop sepsis after PROM. Most complications are related to prematurity. Although PPROM poses a significant risk of morbidity and mortality to the neonate, 75% of cases of PROM occur at term and generally run a benign course. PROM increases the frequency of neonatal sepsis from 0.1% to 1.4%. Fatalities are common in neonatal sepsis, especially in low-birth-weight infants (20% in very low-birth-weight infants vs. 12% in normal-weight infants) and those with group B streptococcal sepsis. Although an increase in the latency period in term pregnancy increases the incidence of sepsis, the neonatal mortality is unaffected. Even the presence of acute chorioamnionitis for up to 24 hours does not increase neonatal mortality in term births.[1]

Diagnosis

Clinical Presentation

Patients will notice a gush of fluid or leaking fluid prior to the onset of labor.

History

If the flow does not persist, the physician should ask the patient to examine the clothing for an odor of urine.

Physical Examination

- On examination of the vagina with a sterile speculum, a flow of fluid, sometimes containing vernix caseosa or meconium, is diagnostic, as is seeing or palpating the fetal scalp.
- Signs of acute chorioamnionitis, or acute infection complicating premature rupture, include fever and foul or cloudy amniotic fluid.
- Readiness of the cervix for labor is determined by direct observation and digital examination. Engagement of the presenting part, cervical softness, forward position of the os, dilatation, and effacement all indicate impending labor and are associated with successful oxytocin induction of labor.

Laboratory

- **Ferning.** Amniotic fluid dries with a characteristic arborization pattern, called *ferning,* seen on microscopic examination. False-positive fern test results may rarely be seen in the presence of scant fluid due to the presence of cervical mucus.
- **Nitrazine test.** This test checks for elevation of the normally acidic vaginal pH due to the presence of amniotic fluid. False-positive results are more common than with the fern test and may be caused by bacterial vaginosis or by contamination of the vaginal sample with blood, lubricant jelly, or povidone–iodine.
- **Fetal fibronectin** can be detected in a vaginal fluid sample obtained before performing a digital vaginal exam. If negative, this test is useful in ruling out a premature delivery in the next 2 weeks.
- **Chorioamnionitis** may be associated with DIC. Chorioamnionitis occurs in 3% to 25% of PROM cases. When this condition is suspected, clotting studies and measurement of renal and hepatic function should be done.
- **Amniocentesis** to evaluate pulmonary maturity may be performed in preterm PROM before 35 weeks. A decreased level of amniotic fluid glucose provides rapid confirmation of chorioamnionitis.

- **Group B streptococcal colonization** can increase morbidity and mortality. Those who have no prior testing or a negative Group B streptococcal screen should have a single swab of the vagina and rectum sent for testing.
- **Coagulation** studies and studies of renal function should be performed if signs of chorioamnionitis develop.

Monitoring
- **Fever.** In addition to frequent fetal monitoring, those with PROM need routine measures of temperature to help anticipate chorioamnionitis.
- **Hyperstimulation.** The use of prostaglandin analogues may cause hyperstimulation of the uterus. This is defined as the presence of prolonged (≥ 2 minutes) contractions, excessively frequent contractions, or tachysystole (≥ 6 in 10 minutes) and fetal distress (late decelerations or fetal bradycardia).

Treatment
Medication
- **Preterm PROM**
  - **Tocolysis.** In preterm PROM before 35 weeks tocolysis is often used but little evidence exists for its effectiveness in improving fetal outcomes. Indomethacin and parenteral terbutaline have the best evidence supporting their use in prolonging the latent period, although parenteral magnesium sulfate and ritodrine are also commonly used.[4]
  - **Corticosteroid administration** has been extensively utilized to induce the production of mature lung surfactant. There is good evidence that they are effective in reducing neonatal mortality and morbidity due to respiratory distress syndrome and intraventricular hemorrhage. A typical dose of corticosteroids is betamethasone 12 mg IM in two doses 24 hours apart.
  - **Antibiotic prophylaxis** is designed to lengthen latency through a reduction of amnionitis, but it also reduces the risk of endometritis in the event that a caesarean section is required. Antibiotic treatment in PPROM also reduces the need to treat the infant for neonatal sepsis.

- **Term PROM**
  - **Ripening the cervix.** Digital exam is performed. If the cervix is not dilated more than 2 cm, vaginal application of a prostaglandin can cut the latency period by at least half, as was shown in several studies. Cervidil, an insert impregnated with 10 mg dinoprostone (prostaglandin E), may be the preferred preparation because it can be removed in the case of hyperstimulation. Administration of misoprostol (25 to 50 μg vaginally every 3 to 6 hours to a maximum of 100 μg) is a much less expensive alternative that frequently has the advantage of resulting in regular contractions in addition to ripening the cervix. Prostaglandins are also safe and effective in the induction of labor if the cervix is ripened and not dilated beyond 5 cm.[2]
  - **Oxytocin.** Induction of labor with an intravenous infusion of oxytocin decreases latency significantly but seems not to affect the low rate of maternal or neonatal mortality in term pregnancy. Recent Cochrane Collaboration reviews indicate that induction does offer certain benefits and risks in comparison with expectant management.
  - **Antibiotic prophylaxis.** The CDC and American Academy of Pediatrics recommend treating a mother with prophylactic antibiotics if delivery is likely to occur after 18 hours of ruptured membranes, if she has delivered an infant with GBS infection previously, or if there is a fever greater than 38°C.

Counseling
The benefits—a lower risk of maternal and neonatal infection and increased maternal satisfaction—and risks—increased epidural anesthesia and internal monitoring—must be presented to the patient when oxytocin or prostaglandin is offered.[5]

Special Considerations in PPROM
- **Digital exam.** In preterm PROM, digital examination shortened the latent period from 11 to 2 days in one study. This may be avoided by assessing cervical dilatation and effacement by sterile speculum exam, vaginal or transperineal ultrasound.[1]

- **Transport.** In hospitals without neonatal intensive care units, transport of the mother if delivery is not imminent may improve neonatal mortality by 60%.[4]

DYSTOCIA

General Principles

Definition

Dystocia is defined as a delay of labor. Dystocia may occur in any of the stages of labor.

- **First stage**
  - Latent phase, where regular contractions occur prior to 4 cm dilation.
  - Active phase, with dilation from 4 to 10 cm.

- **Second stage** from full dilation until completed delivery of the infant. This includes a special case, shoulder dystocia, where delivery of the anterior shoulder is prolonged.

The Society of Obstetricians and Gynecologist of Canada[4] has a simple working diagnosis of dystocia:

- **Active phase.** When there are more than 4 hours of less than 0.5 cm per hour dilation.
- **Second stage.** When there is 1 hour with no descent during active pushing.

Anatomy

Dystocia may be due to cephalopelvic disproportion, inadequate uterine expulsive forces, or unfavorable presentation. Labor that is delayed after delivery of the head is referred to as shoulder dystocia. In shoulder dystocia, delivery is obstructed when the fetal anterior shoulder impacts the maternal pubic symphysis.

Epidemiology

- **Delayed active phase** of labor is associated with overdistention of the uterus (multiple gestation, polyhydramnios), abnormal lie, macrosomia (fetal weight more than 4500 g), hydrocephaly, obstruction of the maternal reproductive tract (pelvic contraction, tumors, developmental anomalies), and with the onset of chorioamnionitis late in labor. One retrospective study showed a higher incidence of diagnosis of cephalopelvic disproportion and subsequent caesarean section in patients receiving care from obstetrician-gynecologists than in patients of family physicians.[6] Overall, 60% of the caesarean section rate is due to dystocia.
- **Shoulder dystocia** occurs in no more than 1% of births. Shoulder dystocia is much more common in larger babies, with a rate of 5% seen in those weighing 4000 to 4500 g. More than half of cases of shoulder dystocia occur in normal weight infants and are unanticipated.

Classification

Friedman's work has been used to subdivide abnormalities in the first stage of labor:

- **Latent phase.** Prolongation of the latent phase of the first stage of labor is defined as more than 20 hours in nulliparas and more than 14 hours in multiparas.
- **Prolongation of dilatation.** In the active phase of the first stage of labor, prolonged dilatation is defined as dilatation less than 1.2 cm per hour in nulliparas and less than 1.5 cm per hour in multiparas.
- **Prolongation of descent.** This is defined as descent less than 1 cm per hour in nulliparas and less than 2 cm per hour in multiparas.
- **Arrest of dilatation** is said to occur if the patient is in the active phase of labor and no cervical change has been noted in more than 2 hours.

Mechanisms of Injury

- **Delayed first and second stage**
  - **Maternal.** The major maternal complications associated with dystocia are those related to the increased rate of operative delivery, including hemorrhage, infections, and prolongation of hospital stay. Dystocia is a contributing factor in 47% of primary cesarean sections.
  - **Neonatal.**
    - **Prolonged latent phase.** Prolonged latent phase is associated with an increased risk of depressed 5-minute APGAR scores and a need for neonatal resuscitation but without long-term sequelae.

- **Prolonged first stage.** Most of the morbidity and mortality in infants with prolonged labors is related to events occurring in the second stage. Selection of a caesarean section or use of oxytocin induction prior to the second stage does not affect the infant. Even the increase in amnionitis, which might be caused by prolonged first-stage labor in the presence of a ruptured membrane, is not likely to cause morbidity in a term infant.
- **Prolonged second stage.** Prolongation of the second stage of labor up to 6 hours did not increase morbidity in the newborn term infant. Prolonged second-stage labor is associated with an increased incidence of shoulder dystocia and should prompt alertness for the condition.
- **Assisted delivery.** Vacuum extraction is more likely to cause cephalohematoma and a potentially lethal subgaleal hematoma. Unlike cephalohematoma, the subgaleal space is not limited by suture lines and the hematoma can extend to cover the entire scalp and lead to hypotension or anemia.

■ **Shoulder dystocia**
  ▪ **Maternal.** There is an increased rate of trauma to the birth canal including lacerations and symphysis separation. Transient femoral neuropathy can be seen. These are related to the size of the fetus as well as the maneuvers performed to permit delivery.
  ▪ **Neonatal**
  - Can cause death or brain damage due to hypoxemia, as the umbilical cord is usually impacted by the fetus.
  - Clavicular and humeral fractures are more common.
  - Brachial plexus trauma occurs in 7% to 20% of infants. It occurs due to stretching of the cervical nerve roots. While some trauma may occur even prior to the delivery of the head, this damage may theoretically be increased by allowing the mother to push with shoulder dystocia or applying fundal pressure. Most cases spontaneously resolve but a few do not.
    ◦ Erb palsy affects the C5 and C6 nerve roots. The infant has impaired shoulder abduction on Moro testing but preserved hand movements.
    ◦ Klumpke palsy affects the C8 and T1 nerve roots, affects palmar strength, is often associated with upper nerve root involvement resulting in total arm paralysis, and is less common.[4]

Diagnosis
Clinical Presentation
Dystocia is seen in many common scenarios in family practice deliveries, from the primipara who dilates to 6 cm and then runs out of steam to the patient who has pushed for 2 hours and still does not have the head on the perineum to the nauseating silence that occurs when a large head retracts in spite of effective pushing.

History
It is important to document carefully that the patient is actually in active labor before making the diagnosis of prolonged active phase because the management of prolonged latent phase and that of prolonged active phase are different. It may be easy to confuse these two conditions, such as in a multipara with an elastic cervix and low pain tolerance.

Physical Examination
Serial examinations are necessary to diagnose prolongation of dilation or descent. When dystocia is suspected, creating a chart of dilation versus time ("Freidman curve") can be very helpful. Shoulder dystocia is obvious when the head delivers and then the shoulders do not promptly follow in spite of effective pushing. Often the head will be seen to retract when the mother pushes, which is called "the turtle sign."

Monitoring
Regular monitoring of the fetal heartbeat can provide reassurance when interventions are deferred.

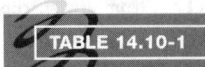 **TABLE 14.10-1**	Abnormal Labor Patterns, Diagnostic Criteria, and Treatment		
Labor pattern	**Nulligravida**	**Multipara**	**Treatment**
Prolonged latent phase	>20 h	>14 h	Rest. Consider discharging to home. If need to deliver exists, can give oxytocin if cervix dilated, if not consider prostaglandins.
Prolonged active phase	<1.2 cm/h	<1.5 cm/h	Amniotomy. Oxytocin if contractions are inadequate. If under 5 cm dilatation, consider prostaglandin.
Prolonged second stage	>1h[a]	>2 hours[a]	Oxytocin if contractions are inadequate. Consider assisted delivery.
[a]Add 1 h if epidural anesthesia.			

Treatment (Table 14.10-1)
Behavioral
The provision of trained labor support through prepared childbirth classes, the use of a doula, and one-on-one nursing have been shown to reduce the diagnosis of dystocia and the incidence of operative delivery.[4]

Medications
- **Prolonged active phase and arrest of labor.**
- **Therapeutic sleep.** Failed dilatation and descent can be managed with analgesics and hypnotics (see Section 14.9), especially in an exhausted patient who has not progressed beyond 6 cm dilatation.
- **Oxytocin** augmentation of labor can be used. Newer protocols using a higher starting dose (4 to 6 mU/min) than the usual (0.5 to 1.0 mU/min) and a shorter dosage interval (15 to 20 minutes vs. 30 to 60 minutes) have been proved safe and may shorten the duration of labor by 3 hours. Hyperstimulation is more common with these protocols and must be managed by discontinuation of oxytocin followed by reinstitution at a lower rate.
- **Analgesia** with narcotics or epidural anesthesia may help increase a mother's tolerance for prolonged labor. Epidural anesthesia is safer and more effective than narcotic analgesia, but it should be delayed until after the patient has dilated to 5 cm to reduce the associated increased risk of caesarean birth.
- **Prolonged descent in the second stage of labor.** Oxytocin augmentation is often helpful.

Surgery
- **Prolonged latent phase and failure of dilation.** Consideration for a caesarean section should be made if more serious signs of fetal distress, such as late decelerations or thick meconium, are present.
- **Arrest of descent in second stage.** Caesarean section causes less neonatal and maternal morbidity than any type of assisted delivery except outlet.

Nonoperative Management
Nonoperative management of shoulder dystocia is facilitated by use of the HELPERR[4] mnemonic. The maneuvers are performed in a rapid sequence, although not necessarily in this order.

- **H.** Call for **H**elp.
- **E. E**pisiotomy may help facilitate the maneuvers.

- **L.** The McRoberts maneuver consists of removing the mother's **L**egs from any stirrups and actively flexing them against her abdomen. This is supposed to straighten the sacrum and decrease the angle of pelvic inclination.
- **P. P**ressure. Suprapubic pressure may help disengage the shoulder. Fundal pressure increases the impaction and must be avoided. Pressure may be applied to the fetal shoulders in a side to side, rocking motion (Rubin maneuver I).
- **E. "Enter"** the pelvis for internal maneuvers. Push the fetus's anterior shoulder toward the fetal chest (Rubin maneuver II). Push the posterior shoulder from the pectoral region toward the fetus's back (Wood screw maneuver). The Wood and Rubin II maneuvers push the fetus in the same direction and can be performed simultaneously. The Wood screw can also be performed in reverse if these motions fail.
- **R.** Next try to **r**emove the posterior arm by pushing behind the humerus, sweeping the arm across the chest.
- **R. R**olling the patient onto all fours, the Gaskin maneuver, may disimpact the shoulder by increasing the pelvic width.

Other methods, which are rarely necessary, include deliberate fractures of the fetal clavicle, cephalic replacement (the Zavanelli maneuver), and symphysiotomy.

Operative Management
- **Active phase.** Routine amniotomy. According to a meta-analysis by the Cochrane Collaboration, routine amniotomy in active labor shortens the active phase by a little more than 1 to 2 hours but may result in an increased incidence of caesarean section. The reviewers recommend limiting its use to women with abnormal labor progress.[4]
- **Second stage.** Assisted delivery is required only if further progress of the second stage seems impossible and fetal distress forces rapid reaction. Assisted delivery is frequently offered for maternal exhaustion, although in the informed consent parents must be told that in instrumental delivery will occasionally harm the fetus and, strictly speaking, a caesarean section is safer.
- **Midforceps and rotation.** If the delivering physician has adequate training, midforceps delivery with rotation using a forceps may be considered when the vertex is arrested in the midpelvis in a transverse lie. If a prompt caesarean section can be performed, this is usually preferred, as vacuum or forceps deliveries with more than 45 degrees rotation or anything less than complete descent (outlet forceps) are associated with increased maternal morbidity from bleeding and damage to the pelvic sphincters.
- **Low and outlet forceps.** The following ABCDEFGHIJ[4] mnemonic is recommended to ensure proper procedure:
- **A.** Ask for help. **A**ddress the patient and her helper to provide informed consent; make sure **A**nesthesia is adequate.
- **B.** Empty the **B**ladder with a straight or Foley catheter.
- **C.** Make certain the **C**ervix is fully dilated.
- **D. D**etermine the position and anticipate the increased risk of shoulder dystocia in assisted deliveries. Rotation less than 45 degrees from occiput anterior and vertex at the pelvic floor are required for a low risk outlet vacuum extraction or forceps delivery. Special rotational forceps provide less scalp trauma and should be used only by those with special training for anything more than 45 degrees of rotation.
- **E. E**quipment should be checked and ready.
- **F.** Applying the suction cup 3 cm in front of the anterior **F**ontanelle will provide optimal flexion to allow delivery of the head. With forceps, the posterior **F**ontanelle should be 1 cm above the shanks of the forceps.
- **G. G**entle traction should be maintained throughout the duration of a push.
- **H. H**alt traction between pushes, and with vacuum if there are three pop-offs or three pulls with no progress. With forceps, elevate the handle to follow the J-shaped pelvic curve.
- **I. I**ncision. Evaluate the perineum for the need for episiotomy.
- **J.** Remove the assistive device when the **J**aw of the neonate can be reached.[4]

Counseling
- **Assisted delivery.** Complications affecting the neonate including scalp hematomas, intraocular and intracranial hemorrhage, and trauma to the maternal birth canal should limit the use of vacuum or forceps to situations where fetal distress, hemorrhage, fever,

or maternal exhaustion make a spontaneous delivery dangerous or impossible. Complications are greatly increased through improper technique or patient selection, and caesarean section should always be entertained as an alternative likely to be less harmful to the neonate.

■ **After a difficult delivery,** speak with both the patient and her family carefully explaining what has ensued and answering any questions. Studies show that the primary driver of lawsuits is not the event itself but the family's subsequent interactions with the medical staff.[5]

Protocol
Medical and nursing staff members should meet regularly to create and update protocols for prostaglandin and oxytocin induction and fetal monitoring to reduce error.

Risk Management
Comprehensive programs for training of medical professionals, such as ALSO[4,5] are available to help obstetrical units develop better interprofessional communication, practice time-sensitive emergency treatments, and promulgate evidence-based treatment.

References
1. Scott JR, et al., eds. *Danforth's obstetrics and gynecology.* 9th ed. Philadelphia: Lippincott Williams & Wilkins; 2003.
2. Cunningham FG, et al., eds. *Williams' obstetrics.* 22nd ed. Norwalk, CT: Appleton & Lange; 2005.
3. Gabbe SG, et al., eds. *Obstetrics: normal and problem pregnancies.* 3rd ed. New York: Churchill Livingstone; 1996.
4. Atwood L, Deutchman M, Bailey E, et al. *ALSO Course syllabus.* 4th ed. Leawood, KS: American Academy of Family Physicians; 2000.
5. MORE[OB] Risk management comprehensive programs such as ALSO[4] and MORE[OB] are available to professionals. Ottawa: Society of Obstetricians and Gyneacologists of Canada www.moreob.com version 2.9.3. Accessed August 1, 2006.
6. Hueston WJ, et al. Practice variations between family physicians and obstetricians in the management of low-risk pregnancies. *J Fam Pract* 1995;40:345.

POSTPARTUM CARE
Dwenda K. Gjerdingen

14.11

EARLY POSTPARTUM PROBLEMS (0 TO 2 WEEKS)

Pain

General Principles
Classification. Postpartum pain may occur in the breasts, abdomen, perineum, or at surgical sites. Perineal discomfort lasts 1 month, on average.

Diagnosis
Physical Examination. Observe for mastitis, wound dehiscence, hematoma, or infection.

Treatment
Medications
■ **Medication choices for mild to moderate pain include:**
   ■ Ibuprofen 400 to 800 mg PO q 6h
   ■ Acetaminophen 500–1000 mg PO q 6h
   ■ Acetaminophen with codeine 30 mg (Tylenol No. 3) PO q 4-6 h

■ **For severe pain, give:**
   ■ Morphine sulfate 2.5 to 10 mg SC/IM/IV q 2-6 h, or
   ■ Hydromorphone (Dilaudid) 1 to 4 mg SC/IM/IV q 4-6 h

Special Therapy

- **Perineal pain:** ice packs, tub baths, Tucks ointment
- **Breast engorgement:** apply warm packs for 20 minutes before breastfeeding, hand express or pump before nursing to soften the breast, and nurse frequently
- **Sore nipples:** ensure proper positioning and latching during breastfeeding, apply lanolin (Lansinoh) cream to nipples after breastfeeding.

Primary Postpartum Hemorrhage

General Principles

Definition. Postpartum hemorrhage is defined as a blood loss of more than 500 cc after delivery.[1]

Etiology. Causes of postpartum hemorrhage include:

- **Uterine atony (80% of cases)[1]**
- **Retained placenta**
  - Genital tract lacerations
  - Uterine rupture
  - Coagulation disorders

Diagnosis

Physical Examination. Evaluate for hypotension, examine uterus for tone, and examine cervix, vagina, and labia for lacerations.

Laboratory Studies. Obtain hemoglobin, von Willebrand factor if indicated.

Treatment

Medications. Use one or more of the following uterotonics:

- **Oxytocin 10 to 40 units in 1000 cc IV fluids, titrate rate**
- **Methylergonovine maleate (Methergine) 0.2 mg IM q2-4 h (use cautiously if hypertensive)**
- **Carboprost tromethamine (Hemabate) 250 μg IM q 90-120 minutes**
- **Misoprostol 200 μg PO plus 400 μg SL, or 800 μg per rectum**
- Also, give IV fluids or blood products (packed red blood cells) if necessary.

Surgery

- Internal iliac artery ligation or hysterectomy
- Uterine compression sutures

Nonoperative

- Treat the cause: Massage atonic uterus, remove retained placenta, replace inverted uterus, repair hemorrhaging lacerations
- Radiologic embolization of uterine arteries
- Less commonly used: Uterine tamponade with condom catheter, inflated to 250 to 500 cc normal saline[2]

Risk Management. Reduce risk of postpartum hemorrhage by actively managing the third stage of labor with a prophylactic uterotonic (oxytocin), early cord clamping and cutting, and controlled cord traction.[1]

Anemia

General Principles

Epidemiology. Anemia is seen in a majority of women in the early postpartum period, and is usually secondary to blood loss from delivery.

Diagnosis

Clinical Presentation. Although women with mild anemia are often asymptomatic, those with severe anemia may develop skin pallor, postural hypotension, tachycardia, fatigue, and weakness.

Laboratory Studies. Check hemoglobin (Hb) 24 hours after delivery, or sooner if indicated.

Treatment

Medications. For mild to moderate anemia, give ferrous sulfate 325 mg qd-bid, until Hb normalizes.

Special Therapy. For severe or symptomatic anemia, transfuse with packed red blood cells.

Endometritis
General Principles
Definition. Postpartum endometritis is defined as an infection of the endometrial lining, the myometrium, and the parametrium.[3]

Epidemiology. Endometritis develops in approximately 10% of women who have delivered by caesarean section, and 5% who have delivered vaginally.[3]

Etiology. Causal organisms include Group B *Streptococcus, Enterococcus faecalis, Staphylococcus epidermidis, Staphylococcus aureus, Prevotella bivia, Peptostreptocci* spp., *Clostridium* spp., *Gardnerella vaginalis, Escherichia coli,* and *Bacteroides* spp.

Diagnosis
Physical Examination. Physical findings include elevated temperature, tachycardia, uterine tenderness, and purulent vaginal discharge.

Laboratory Studies. Obtain white blood cells (WBC) with differential, urinalysis, electrolytes, and creatinine (also, if indicated, endometrial/vaginal cultures, blood cultures, and pelvic imaging).

Treatment
Medications. Give intravenous antibiotics until patient is afebrile for 24 to 48 hours. If symptoms have completely resolved, the patient can be discharged without oral antibiotics. Antibiotics choices include[3]:

- Piperacillin/tazobactam 3.375 g IV q 6h
- Ampicillin/sulbactam 1.5 to 3 g IV q 6h plus gentamicin 5 mg/kg IV q 24h
- Clindamycin 900 mg IV q 8h plus gentamicin 5 mg/kg IV q 24h
- Metronidazole 500 mg IV q 8h plus gentamicin 5 mg/kg IV q 24h
- If initial antibiotics fail, evaluate for resistant bacteria, pelvic abscess, or septic pelvic thrombosis.

Risk Management. Preventive strategies include limiting the number of intrapartum vaginal exams, limiting duration of labor and ruptured membranes, and using prophylactic antibiotics (e.g., first-generation cephalosporins) at the time of caesarean section.

Complications. Complications include peritonitis, pelvic abscess, dynamic ileus, bowel obstruction, and necrosis of the lower uterine segment.[3]

The "Blues"
General Principles
Definition. The postpartum "blues" is defined as a transient, self-limited mood disturbance occurring within the first 2 weeks after delivery. These episodes affect a majority of mothers, and last hours to days.

Diagnosis
Clinical Presentation. Symptoms include sadness, mood lability, crying, anxiety, insomnia, poor appetite, and irritability.

Treatment
Behavioral
- Treatment consists of support and reassurance.

DELAYED POSTPARTUM PROBLEMS (>2 WEEKS)
Fatigue
General Principles
Epidemiology. Fatigue is seen in a majority of women after childbirth, and may last for weeks to months.

Etiology. Causes include the physical sequelae of childbirth (general recovery, anemia, infections), parenting demands, postpartum hypothyroidism, or postpartum depression.

Diagnosis
Laboratory Studies
- Check Hb, thyroid-stimulating hormone (TSH), and depression screen.

Treatment
Behavioral. Treat the cause, encourage use of social supports, and curtail work and other obligations, if possible.

Postpartum Thyroiditis
General Principles
Definition. Postpartum thyroiditis is an autoimmune disorder that classically consists of a hyperthyroid phase at 2 to 6 months postpartum, followed by a hypothyroid phase at 3 to 12 months postpartum. Usually, women return to a euthyroid state by 12 months postpartum, but a minority will continue to be hypothyroid indefinitely.[4]

Epidemiology. Prevalence ranges from 1.1% to 16.7%, with a mean prevalence of 7.5%.[4]

Diagnosis
History
- Symptoms of hyperthyroidism include fatigue, palpitations, heat intolerance, and nervousness.
- Symptoms of hypothyroidism include fatigue, dry hair and skin, impaired concentration, and depression.

Laboratory Studies. TSH will be low in the hyperthyroid phase, and high in the hypothyroid phase.

Imaging. Thyroid imaging is usually unnecessary, particularly if there are no thyroid nodules and the TSH normalizes.

Treatment
Medications. If symptomatic in hyperthyroid phase, give propranolol 10 to 20 mg PO qid. If symptomatic in hypothyroid phase, give levothyroxine 25 to 50 mcg PO qd, and continue treatment either until 1 year postpartum or until mother has finished childbearing.[4]

Mastitis, Breast Abscess
General Principles
Epidemiology. Approximately 1% to 5% of nursing mothers experience mastitis and/or breast abscess.[5]

Etiology. Causal organisms include *Staphylococcus aureus* (most common), *E. coli*, *Klebsiella pneumoniae*, and *Streptococcus* species. Predisposing factors include a decrease in nursing frequency or irregular nursing, inadequate drainage, cracked nipples, and fatigue.

Diagnosis
Clinical Presentation. Clinical manifestations include fever, chills, body aches, malaise, and an inflamed breast.

Laboratory Studies. Check WBC and differential; if abscess is present, do culture and sensitivities on aspirate.

Imaging. Use ultrasound to demonstrate presence of abscess.

Treatment
Behavioral
- With mastitis, nurse frequently. If abscess is present, nurse with opposite breast.
- Alternate warm/cold compresses.
- Gently massage area affected by mastitis.
- Drink sufficient fluids.

Medications
- **Antibiotics:** Choices include cephalexin 500 mg PO qid or cefazolin 0.5 to 1.5 g IV q 6-8h; or amoxicillin-clavulanate 500/125 mg PO tid
- **Analgesics:** Acetaminophen or ibuprofen

Surgery. If abscess is present, incise and drain. Alternatively, use ultrasound guidance to aspirate small abscesses (<3 cm) or to place a drainage catheter for larger abscesses (3 cm or greater).[6]

Risk Management. To prevent mastitis, breastfeed frequently, get adequate rest, and avoid sleeping on stomach.

Marital/Partner and Sexual Changes
General Principles
Epidemiology. Most couples do not resume intercourse until about 2 months or longer after delivery. Thereafter, sexual interest and activity may be reduced for several months, and sexual problems occur fairly often. In addition, marital/partner satisfaction tends to decline after the birth of a first child, and this decline may persist until children reach school age.

Etiology. Declines in marital/partner satisfaction may be related to changing roles, increased work responsibilities, and fatigue. Factors associated with postpartum sexual dysfunction include assisted vaginal delivery, vaginal or perineal lacerations, mediolateral episiotomy, depression, and vaginal atrophy secondary to estrogen withdrawal, which may be exacerbated by breastfeeding.

Diagnosis
History. Inquire about partner relationship and sexual concerns at mother's postpartum visit.

Treatment
Behavioral. Inform parents of anticipated postpartum sexual changes, reassure them that problems often resolve, and encourage partners to continue to affirm and support one another.

Medications. For dyspareunia due to vaginal atrophy and dryness, consider vaginal lubricants or short-term use of estrogen cream.

Risk Management. To reduce the risk of perineal trauma, limit episiotomies.[7]

Postpartum Depression
General Principles
Definition. Postpartum depression is identical to major depressive disorder, except that the onset is theoretically within the first 4 weeks after delivery (practically, this could be expanded to 1 year).

Epidemiology
- Incidence over the first 3 months is 6.5% for major depression, 14.5% for major plus minor depression. Point prevalence at various intervals over the first year is 1.0% to 5.9% for major depression, and 6.5% to 12.9% for major plus minor depression.[8]

Etiology. Etiology is likely multifactorial, including genetic, hormonal, fatigue, and work/role factors.

Diagnosis
Clinical Presentation. Clinical manifestations include five or more of the following symptoms, occurring nearly every day over 2 weeks or longer: markedly depressed mood, diminished interest or pleasure, decreased or increased appetite, insomnia or hypersomnia, psychomotor agitation or retardation, fatigue, feelings of worthlessness or inappropriate guilt, decreased concentration, and recurrent thoughts of death or suicide.

History. Inquire about past history of depression, endocrine abnormalities, social situation, and suicidal/homicidal ideation.

Laboratory Studies. Check Hb and TSH.

Treatment
Behavioral. Encourage the mother to obtain social support from family and friends, and to cut back on work responsibilities, if possible.

Medications. Selective serotonin-reuptake inhibitors (SSRIs) and tricyclic antidepressants (TCAs) are both effective; however, SSRIs are first-line, due to their lower toxicity and side effects.[9] Although all SSRIs cross the placenta, SSRIs in breastfeeding women have not been associated with major congenital malformations. Of drugs currently used, sertraline, paroxetine, and nortriptyline may be the preferred choices for breastfeeding women.[10] Fluoxetine and doxepin should be avoided in breastfeeding mothers, if possible, due to potential adverse effects on newborns. Favor a previously effective drug. Antidepressants should be continued for at least 6 to 12 months (4 to 6 months beyond remission).

Counseling. Cognitive–behavioral therapy is likely as effective as antidepressant therapy.

Risk Management. Monitor for suicidal ideation. Longer maternity leaves (e.g., 3 to 6 months or more) may be helpful in preventing postpartum depression, as they have been associated with better mental health.

Follow-Up. See depressed mothers frequently (every 1 to 2 weeks) until they begin to improve. If possible, involve case manager to ensure that the patient complies with treatment and follow-up.

Complications. Complications include suicide, infanticide (rare), marital strain, and decreased work productivity.

References

1. Selo-Ojeme DO. Primary postpartum haemorrhage. *J Obstet Gynaecol* 2002;22(5): 463–469.
2. Akhter S, Begum MR, Kabir Z, et al. Use of a condom to control massive postpartum hemorrhage. *Medscape Gen Med* 2003;5(3):38. Available online at www.medscape.com/ viewarticle/459894.
3. Faro S. Postpartum endometritis. *Clin Perinatol* 2005;32:803–814.
4. Stagnaro-Green A. Postpartum thyroiditis. *Best Pract Res Clin Endocrinol Metab* 2004;18(2):303–316.
5. Leung AKC, Sauve RS. Breast is best for babies. *J Natl Med Assoc* 2005;97(7): 1010–1019.
6. Ulitzsch D, Nyman MKG, Carlson RA. Breast abscess in lactating women: US-guided treatment. *Radiology* 2004;232:904–909.
7. Flynn P, Franiek J, Janssen P, et al. How can second-stage management prevent perineal trauma? *Can Fam Physician* 1997;43:73–84.
8. Gaynes BN, Gavin N, Meltzer-Brody S, et al. Perinatal depression: prevalence, screening, accuracy and screening outcomes. Evidence Report/Technology Assessment No. 119, AHRQ Publication No. 05-E006-2. Rockville, MD: Agency for Healthcare Research and Quality; February 2005.
9. Hallberg P, Sjoblom V. The use of selective serotonin reuptake inhibitors during pregnancy and breast-feeding: a review and clinical aspects. *J Clin Psychopharmacol* 2005; 25(1):59–73.
10. Weissman AM, Levy BT, Hartz AJ, et al. Pooled analysis of antidepressant levels in lactating mothers, breast milk, and nursing infants. *Am J Psychiatry* 2004;161: 1066–1078.

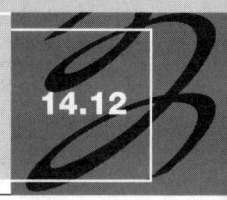

GENERAL PRINCIPLES

Advances in transvaginal sonography have markedly improved the ability to detect an early intrauterine pregnancy. The gestational sac can be found as early as 4 weeks; however, caution must be exercised as a pseudosac commonly arises during ectopic pregnancy. The presence of a yolk sac confirms the existence of an intrauterine pregnancy and can be seen as early as 5 weeks. An embryo within the gestational sac and fetal cardiac activity can generally be detected during week 6.[1]

Ultrasound imaging of the pregnant patient has become an increasingly common component of obstetrical care in the United States. The Centers for Disease Control reported in 2002 that prenatal ultrasounds were done in nearly two thirds of live births.[2] However, the use of routine prenatal ultrasound for screening purposes remains a controversial subject. Several well-designed studies, most notably the Routine Antenatal Diagnostic Imaging with Ultrasound Study (RADIUS) from 1993 found no benefits in reducing neonatal morbidly or mortality with screening exams.[1,3,4]

Currently the American College of Obstetrics & Gynecology (ACOG) supports the use of ultrasound if a specific medical question arises (i.e., Does a patient at 24 weeks who has vaginal bleeding have a placenta previa?). Casual or screening ultrasounds for fetal anomalies may be performed commonly but are not considered mandatory practice by ACOG, American Academy of Family Physicians (AAFP), or American Institute of Ultrasound in Medicine (AIUM).[1,4,5]

DIAGNOSIS

- The indications for and diagnoses derived from prenatal ultrasounds can be divided into exams done during the first or second and third trimesters of pregnancy.

Goals of First Trimester Exams

- **Confirm the presence of an intrauterine pregnancy**
    - The **gestational sac** can be found as early as **4 to 5 weeks;** however, caution must be exercised as a pseudosac may be seen that commonly arises during **ectopic pregnancy.** The echogenic (bright) borders of the true sac, also called the double decidual sac, help differentiate this.[6,7]
    - The presence of a **yolk sac** confirms the existence of an intrauterine pregnancy and can be seen as early as **5 weeks** or when the gestational sac is 10 mm or greater. If the yolk sac is greater than 6 mm or abnormally shaped, this could signal a failing pregnancy.[6-8]
    - When the maternal serum **beta-human choronic gonadatropin (hCG)** level is between 1000 and 2000 mIU per mL (by first international reference preparation) the gestational sac can be seen. This range is also referred to as the **discriminatory zone.** If the gestational sac is not seen by 2000 mIU per mL, an ectopic pregnancy must be excluded.[7,8]
    - The top priority in **vaginal bleeding** in the first trimester is to determine the location of the pregnancy. Once a viable intrauterine pregnancy is diagnosed the differential shifts from ectopic to threatened abortion, cervicitis, vaginal trauma, implantation bleed, etc. Approximately 15% to 25% of women bleed in the first trimester and half of these women go on to eventual miscarriage. However, intrauterine pregnancies identified with a heartbeat in the normal range of 110 to 160 are reassuring as most of these pregnancies (about 90%) will proceed to beyond the first trimester.[6,7]

- **Ensure fetal viability**
  - The **embryo** is the second structure to appear in the gestational sac after the yolk sac. **Fetal cardiac activity** can generally be detected by transvaginal ultrasound during **week 6** or when the **embryo is 5 mm in length**.[8] An embryonic heart rate less than 90 beats per minute in embryos less than 8 weeks is associated with an 80% rate of eventual embryonic demise.[6] A **blighted ovum (anembryonic gestation)** is diagnosed when a gestational sac of greater than 2 cm is seen without embryonic echoes. **Missed abortion** is referred to fetal death in the first trimester without expulsion from the uterus spontaneously. A combination of repeat scanning and maternal serum beta-hCG values can help determine the fetal viability.[7]
  - A sonographic assessment for fetal aneuploidy can be done in the first trimester and is often combined with maternal serum markers. **Nuchal translucency** screening, also referred to as nuchal fold scan, can detect up to 90% of fetuses with Down syndrome as well as other chromosomal and cardiac abnormalities.[9]

- **Confirm the estimated date of delivery (EDD)**
  - Evidence shows that ultrasound derived EDDs are more accurate than the last menstrual period (LMP) and physical exam, even in women with regular menstrual cycles.[10] The most accurate sonographic measurement correlating with menstrual dates is the **crown-rump-length (CRL).** This measurement is the maximum visible length of the embryo. Care must be taken not to include the umbilical cord or yolk sac in the crown rump measurement. Between 6 and 10 weeks there is little variability in embryonic size. The CRL is accurate to ±4 to 5 days of the menstrual age-derived EDD. A recent Cochrane review revealed first trimester scans are superior to last menstrual period in estimating EDD and resulted in a 70% decrease in post-term gestations with subsequent inductions.[11]
  - The **maternal hCG** value is not precise enough to use for dating purposes.[10]

- **Assess for multiple gestations**
  - Early identification of a multiple gestation is an additional benefit to first trimester scans. The Helsinki Trial from the late 1980s reported a decrease in perinatal mortality for those twins identified before 20 weeks.[3]

Goals of Second and Third Trimester Exams

- **Fetal anatomy**
  - Second trimester screening anatomy exams are typically done between 18 and 22 weeks gestation. The ability of routine ultrasound to **detect fetal anomalies** in an otherwise low-risk unselected population remains highly controversial. As mentioned above, the RADIUS study found no overall benefit in detecting the fetal anomalies in any perinatal outcome study parameter. This conflicts some with other European trials that showed a modest decrease in the neonatal morbidity and mortality. The authors concluded that this was likely due to increased number of abortions of affected fetuses.[3,12]
  - The experience of the sonographic examiner, the specific defect, the gestational age, and overall population risk are cornerstones to detection. Baseline detection rates of any type of anomaly is about 50% with central nervous system and urinary tract anomalies detection rates higher (~80%) than that of cardiac and musculoskeletal anomalies (~30% to 40%).[13,14]

- **Placental location, fetal presentation, and amniotic fluid index**
  - The placenta typically adheres to the anterior or posterior wall of the uterus. Placenta location is of concern when it approaches or covers the internal os. This is called **placenta previa** and occurs in about 5% of pregnancies. Abnormal placentation in the form of **placenta accreta, percreta,** and **increta** can be diagnosed by ultrasound as well. Sonographically, they appear as multiple placental lakes and give a "Swiss cheese" appearance.[15] These abnormal attachments of the placenta to the uterine myometrium are a significant source of maternal hemorrhage and rarely death. Even more rarely, a **vasa previa** can be detected if the ultrasound protocol includes examination of the cord insertion.[15]
  - Determining presenting fetal part is important in the management of the vaginal delivery. Leopold maneuvers and cervical exams are the standard for assessing

cephalic presentation. When there is doubt with regard to presenting part, the ultrasound is key. External cephalic version via manipulation of the maternal abdomen has decreased the number of noncephalic presentations during labor and caesarean deliveries for this reason.

- The AFI is a qualitative or quantitative analysis of the amount of amniotic fluid (fetal urine) surrounding the fetus. Various techniques including a four-quadrant approach and single deepest vertical pocket approach have been described. Normal amount is typically 8 to 18 cm. A normal AFI infers a level of reassurance of fetal well-being secondary to an adequate urine output and thus renal perfusion. The diagnosis of **oligohydramnios** (AFI <5 to 6 cm) or **polyhydrammnios** (AFI >20 to 25 cm) is diagnosed and monitored by ultrasound.[7]

- **Fetal biometry for assessment of gestational age and growth and weight**
  - During the second and third trimesters, fetal biometry is used for gestational age assessment and growth evaluation. Measurements of the fetal biparietal diameter, abdominal circumference and femoral diaphysis length are combined and compared to published nomograms to predict growth percentile. The variability of gestational age estimations, however, increases with advancing pregnancy.
  - **Intrauterine growth restriction (IUGR)** can be diagnosed if interval growth is abnormal or if the ratio of abdominal circumference to other parameters is abnormal.
  - Estimating **fetal weight** has been described using numerous measurements and formulas, attesting to the inadequacy of most of these assessments. Abdominal circumference is the most common and reliable single parameter used. However, the estimated fetal weight can differ significantly from the true birth weight.[17]

- **Assessment of fetal well-being**
  - In the latter half of pregnancy it often becomes necessary to assess fetal well-being. This can be due to acute issues like decreased fetal movement and vaginal bleeding. The most severe causes of vaginal bleeding in the third trimester include: **placental abruption, placenta previa, uterine rupture, vasa previa,** and the previously described placental attachment abnormalities (placenta accreta, increta, percreta). Ultrasound is of significant use in diagnosing these conditions **with the exception of** placental abruption where less than a quarter of cases are identified sonographically.[15]
  - Complications of pregnancy such as gestational diabetes, chronic or gestational hypertension, or pre-eclampsia may infer a greater risk to the fetus. Thus the fetus is monitored closely. The basic evaluation, a **modified biophysical profile,** includes the **AFI** (described above) and the nonstress test. The role of ultrasound is in the more in-depth **biophysical profile** that sonographically looks at four fetal parameters: fetal breathing motion, fetal activity, fetal muscular tone, and AFI. A score of either 0 or 2 points is given to each category. A score of 8 of 8 is considered reassuring.[7]

TREATMENT

- Although ultrasound has no direct therapeutic utility, it is a fundamental adjunct to the treatment of many conditions in pregnancy. For example, in the first trimester elective pregnancy termination and fetal reduction in a multiple gestation require ultrasound guidance. Amniocenteses, cordocentesis, and fetal blood transfusions all require ultrasound technology.

SPECIAL CONSIDERATIONS

- **Role of routine cervical length measurements**
  - Numerous studies have looked at the role of cervical length as a predictor for preterm delivery. Mixed results were found based on study designs and populations studied. The cervix is described as "funneled" or "funneling" when the internal os is opened and forms a funnel or beak-shaped appearance on ultrasound. Funneling is most concerning when it is persistent and occurs before 32 weeks. The appearance of funneling combined with an overall cervical length of 3 cm or less are features consistently associated with preterm delivery. Who should be scanned? High-risk women with previous preterm birth and symptomatic women with preterm contractions seemed to

benefit from cervical length monitoring. The predictive value of scanning a woman with no risk factors is very low. Studies showed that most low-risk women with a shortened cervix (less than 2.5 cm) went on to deliver after 35 weeks. ACOG recommends against routine ultrasound screening of the cervix in low-risk women but states that offering screening after 16 to 18 weeks in high-risk women is reasonable.[16,17]

- **Final thoughts from the perspective of a family medicine educator**
  - There is no doubt that obstetric ultrasound has revolutionized antenatal care. It practically seems that undiagnosed twins or unknown breech presentations at term are now exceptionally rare. Teaching the limited obstetric ultrasound to family medicine residents is considered a core skill.[18] At our residency we teach our residents limited obstetric ultrasound from both a transabdominal and transvaginal approach. We insist on an indication to be listed on the chart and documentation of up to five findings: (a) fetal lie, (b) AFI, (c) placenta location, (d) fetal number, (e) presence of fetal cardiac activity. We also insist that a statement of the limited nature of the ultrasound be documented with the patients' understanding noted.
  - In addition to the above, most of our residents reach competency in first trimester CRL measurement.
  - As our society continues to expect the latest technology the obstetric ultrasound will remain commonplace in antenatal care. Understanding its benefits and limitations is the key.

References

1. ACOG Practice Bulletin No. 58. Ultrasonography in pregnancy. *Obstet Gynecol* 2004;104:1449.
2. Martin J, et al. Births: Final data for 2002. National Vital Statistics Reports 2003.
3. Ewigman BG, et al. Effect of prenatal ultrasound screening on perinatal outcome. RADIUS Study Group. *N Engl J Med* 1993;329:821.
4. ACOG Committee Opinion No. 297, August 2004. Nonmedical use of obstetric ultrasonography. *Obstet Gynecol* 2004;104:423.
5. American Institute of Ultrasound in Medicine. AIUM standards and guidelines. Available online at www.aium.org. Accessed June 28, 2006.
6. Weiss J, et al. Threatened abortion: a risk factor for poor pregnancy outcome, a population-based screening study. *Am J Obstet Gynecol* 2004;190:3.
7. Gabbe S, Niebyl J, Senkank J et al. *Obstetrics—normal and problem pregnancies*. 4th ed. Churchill Livingstone. Elsiver Science, 2002.
8. Sohaey R. First trimester ultrasounds. Available online at http://medlib.med.utah.edu/kw/human_reprod/lectures/clin_radiology/. Accessed June 28, 2006.
9. Hulten M. Combined serum and nuchal translucency screening in the first trimester achieved 85% to 90% detection rate for Down and Edward syndromes. *Evidence-Based Healthcare* 2004;8:82–84.
10. Mongelli M, Wilcox M, Gardosi J. Estimating the date of confinement: ultraonographic biometry versus certain menstrual dates. *Am J Obstet Gynecol* 1996;174:278.
11. Neilson JP. Ultrasound for fetal assessment in early pregnancy. *Cochrane Database Syst Rev* 1998;4:CD000182.
12. Bennett KA, et al. First trimester ultrasound screening is effective in reducing post term labor induction rates: a randomized controlled trial. *Am J Obstet Gynecol* 2004;190:1077.
13. Levi S. Ultrasound in prenatal diagnosis: polemics around routine ultrasound screening for second trimester fetal malformations. *Prenat Diagn* 2002;22:285.
14. Munim S, Nadeem S, Khuwaja NA. The accuracy of ultrasound in the diagnosis of congenital abnormalities. *J Pak Med Assoc* 2006;56(1):16–18.
15. Lazebnik N, Lazebnick R. The role of ultrasound in pregnancy-related emergencies. *Radiol Clin North Am* 1004;42:315–327.
16. Ressel G. Practice guidelines: ACOG releases bulletin on managing cervical insufficiency. *AFP* 2004;69(2).
17. Taipale P, Hiilesmaa V. Sonographic measurement of uterine cervix at 18–22 weeks'(tm) gestation and the risk of preterm delivery. *Obstet Gynecol* 1998;92:902.
18. Training and credentialing of family physicians in diagnostic ultrasonography (position paper). Available online at www.aafp.org. Accessed May 3, 2006.

Musculoskeletal Problems and Arthritis

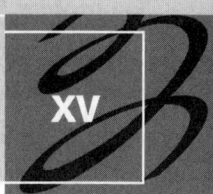

XV

OSTEOARTHRITIS
John R. Gimpel

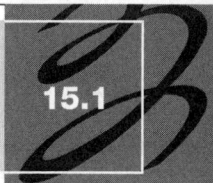

15.1

EPIDEMIOLOGY AND PATHOPHYSIOLOGY

Osteoarthritis (OA) is the most common arthritic disorder. Most healthy asymptomatic people will have developed some evidence of this degenerative process by the age of 55. Risk factors include age older than 50, injury to a joint, obesity, prolonged occupational or sports stress (especially competitive contact sports), and heredity. OA is considered to be more degenerative than inflammatory, with biomechanical and immune damage to the articular cartilage, bone, and synovium. Bone and cartilage are worn away in conjunction with synovial thickening. Bony spurs (osteophytes) form at the articular edges, with local (and generally mild) inflammation involving the joint capsule and adjacent ligaments.

DIAGNOSIS

Clinical Presentation

OA usually presents in a middle-aged or older person as mild, dull, aching pain in one or a limited number of joints. Pain typically worsens with activity, improves with rest, and can be aggravated by damp, cold weather. There are no systemic symptoms or signs. Stiffness comes from inactivity but commonly improves after about 15 minutes of exercise. Morning stiffness lasts less than 30 minutes. Patients may have joint instability or buckling. The patient complains of pain and reduced function and, in the case of knee and hip disease, difficulty walking and climbing stairs. Usually the symptoms will wax and wane over time, with increasing involvement of more joints. However, the patterns and trajectory of the disease are highly variable and often cannot be predicted.

Physical Examination

The distribution of joints affected—distal interphalangeal (DIP) and proximal interphalangeal (PIP) in the hands and feet—in OA is different from that in rheumatoid arthritis, and it is more likely than other arthritides to affect large joints such as the knee or hip, and often involves the hands and the spine as well. There will likely be boney enlargement and limitation of the range of motion of affected joints. The joint will be swollen and cool, and motion may be limited. Crepitus is a common and sensitive criterion for the disease. There

567

may be effusions in large joints. OA of the wrists, ankles, and shoulders is often the result of trauma or other secondary causes. Most commonly affected joints are the DIP and PIP joints of the hands, the thumb carpometacarpal joint, the big toe and DIP joints of the feet, the knees and hips, and the spine. Degenerative change in the spine is common, commonly with formation of osteophytes (bony spurs) at the facet joints that can produce local pain as well as compression of spinal nerve roots, causing neuropathy (weakness and sensory loss). When disc degeneration and osteophyte formation are severe, spinal canal stenosis can cause direct injury to the spinal cord in the neck or lumbar spine areas. Spinal stenosis can present with symptoms that mimic claudication.

Laboratory Findings

Synovial fluid analysis is useful in ruling out possible inflammatory arthritis, but is not often necessary in patients with OA. The erythrocyte sedimentation rate (ESR) is normal except in the rare case of erosive OA or primary generalized OA, which may have an inflammatory presentation much like rheumatoid arthritis.

Radiologic Findings

Imaging is useful primarily in monitoring disease progression rather than making a diagnosis; osteoarthritic changes are routinely found in asymptomatic patients. These findings include nonuniform loss of joint space, osteophyte formation, calcification of cartilage, cyst formation, and subchondral sclerosis. Computed tomography (CT) and magnetic resonance imaging (MRI) can be helpful to evaluate possible cervical or lumbar spinal stenosis.

TREATMENT

Obese patients should be encouraged to lose weight, especially before orthopedic surgery for joint replacement, and weight loss can improve long-term progression of OA. Twice-daily exercise programs and low-impact aerobic conditioning produce increased strength and pain reduction. Activity that causes pain lasting longer than 2 hours should be avoided. Exercise to the muscle group or groups that support particular affected joints (e.g., quadriceps for the knees) can be beneficial to reduce the wear and tear on the affected joints. The use of braces, attention to supportive shoes, and other orthotics can relieve pain from asymmetric walking patterns.

Glucosamine sulfate, which is derived from oyster and crab shells, may provide substrate for proteoglycan synthesis and have mild anti-inflammatory effects. Patients treated with glucosamine may show some improved efficacy when compared to placebo in relieving painful symptoms in some studies, though limited value after 2 to 4 months in others. However, there is limited information on the long-term efficacy and toxicity of glucosamine. The usual dosage is 1500 mg daily in three divided doses. Short-term use of glucosamine seems to be well tolerated, with the most common adverse effect of gastrointestinal discomfort occurring less than with nonsteroidal anti-inflammatories (NSAIDs).

Chondroitin sulfate, made from shark and cow cartilage, may provide some anti-inflammatory effects, and, like glucosamine, may be superior to placebo in reducing pain of OA. Likewise, chondroitin sulfate is also well tolerated by patients, and has a somewhat slower onset of action but possibly a longer duration than NSAIDs in OA. Therefore, chondroitin sulfate or glucosamine should be taken for at least 1 month before any symptom relief would be expected. The usual dose of chondroitin sulfate is 1200 mg daily in three divided doses. There is little evidence that the combination of glucosamine and chondroitin sulfate is any better than either used alone, but studies are under way.

Nonrandomized trials the following have shown some symptom relief in patients with OA: S-Adenosylmethionine (SAMe), oral avocado, and soybean unsaponifiables. There is little evidence that the use of ginger is beneficial in OA.

Medication can be given for pain relief. Acetaminophen, up to 4000 mg per day, is superior to placebo and has a similar safety profile, so it is generally considered first-line medical therapy for OA. At higher doses, acetaminophen can cause some gastrointestinal symptoms, and massive overdosages or use with excessive alcohol has been associated with hepatotoxicity. Acetaminophen may not be as effective as NSAIDs for pain reduction in people with OA of the knee and hip, but may be equal in improving function. If there is an unacceptable response to acetaminophen, NSAIDs can either be added or substituted, basing the dose on the patient response. The use of topical capsaicin (0.025% cream applied four times daily for OA affecting the knee, ankle, finger, wrist, or shoulder) may be beneficial with the minor side effects of local burning sensation. It is postulated to act as an irritant-counterirritant. Care is needed to avoid contact with the eyes. In the same fashion, topical analgesic creams (salicylate cream) may be effective for focal joint pain, and can be applied four times daily. Tramadol, a nonopioid centrally acting analgesic, can be added to NSAID therapy for short-term use to help with severe pain. Intra-articular steroid injections can be used for joints with effusion and inflammation. Another option is to use intra-articular lavage with sterile saline, which has been shown to be more effective, although more costly, than standard medical therapy.

Viscosupplementation is now being utilized widely—particularly for OA of the knees, with relatively low risks of adverse reactions. These viscous agents are injected into the joint space to replace depleted hyaluronic acid (a natural substance essential for maintaining joint fluid viscosity). Sodium hyaluronate (Hyalgan) and Hylan G-F20 (Synvisc) are given in two to five injections (2 mL) over 2 to 4 weeks. Adverse effects (e.g., pain, swelling, allergic reaction) occur in 5% of cases. Studies have confirmed short-term relief of pain and good patient-oriented evidence with viscosupplementation for OA of the knee. However, costs of the injection series are significant ($600 to $800 per course) and long-term effectiveness has not been fully established.

Patients with severe OA not responding to medication and those with intractable pain or serious functional impairment should be referred to an orthopaedic surgeon for osteotomy or arthroplasty. Fewer than one half of patients with osteoarthritis who undergo arthroscopic debridement (simple lavage or abrasion arthroplasty) will have sustained pain reduction. Long-term outcomes for joint replacement/arthroplasty are good.

Prevention

In both primary and secondary prevention of OA, the most important factor in protecting the weight-bearing joints is maintenance of an appropriate body weight. Exercise, especially for supporting joints (quadriceps for knees, abdominal muscles for lumbar spine), plays an important role, and adaptive equipment and mobility aides can reduce disability. Patients should be advised to maintain an adequate vitamin D intake.

References

1. Rice D. Musculoskeletal conditions: impact and importance. United States Bone and Joint Decade. 2000. Available online at www.usbjd.org. Accessed December 1, 2005.
2. Klippel JH, et al. *Primer on the rheumatic diseases*. 12th ed. Arthritis Foundation; Atlanta: 2001.
3. Lawrence RC, Helmick, CG, Arnett FC, et al. Estimates of the prevalence of arthritis and selected musculoskeletal disorders in the United States. *Arthritis Rheum* 1998;41: 788–799.
4. Manek NJ, Lane NE. Osteoarthritis: current concepts in diagnosis and management. *Am Fam Physician* 2000;61(6):1795–1805.
5. Morelli V, Naquin C, Weaver V. Alternative therapies for traditional disease states: osteoarthritis. *Am Fam Physician* 2003;62(2):339–344.
6. Towheed TE, Maxwell L, Anastassiades TP, et al. Glucosamine therapy for treating osteoarthritis. *Cochrane Database Syst Rev* 2005;4. Available online at www.cochrane.org. Accessed October 28, 2005.
7. Towheed TE, Hochberg MC, Judd MG, et al. Acetaminophen for osteoarthritis. *Cochrane Database Syst Rev* 2003;1:CD004257.
8. Lane NE, Thompson JM. Management of osteoarthritis in the primary care setting: an evidence based approach to treatment. *Am J Med* 1997;103:25S–32S.
9. Ike RW, Arnold WJ, Rothschild EW, et al. Tidal irrigation versus conservative medical management in patients with osteoarthritis of the knee: a prospective randomized study. *J Rheumatol* 1992;19:772–779.
10. Wen DY. Intra-articular hyaluronic acid injections for knee osteoarthritis. *Am Fam Physician* 2000;62:565–570.
11. Wen DY. Intra-articular hyaluronic acid injections for knee osteoarthritis. *Am Fam Physician* 2000;62(3):565–571.

12. Gill GS, Mills DM. Long term follow up evaluation of 1000 consecutive cemented total knee arthroplasties. *Clin Orthop Rel Res* 1999;273:276.
13. Dieppe P, Chard J, Faulkner A, et al. Total knee replacement. In: Godlee F, ed. *Clinical evidence.* 3rd ed. London: BMJ Publishing Group; 2000:536–540.
14. Hinton R, Moody R, Davis AW, et al. Osteoarthritis: diagnosis and therapeutic considerations. *Am Fam Physician* 2002;52(5):841–848.

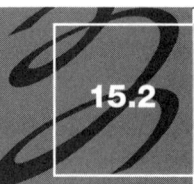

15.2 RHEUMATOID ARTHRITIS AND RELATED DISORDERS
William M. Simpson, Jr.

$\mathcal{T}$he rheumatic diseases include more than 100 diagnoses. We focus in this chapter on four commonly seen diffuse connective tissue diseases: rheumatoid arthritis (RA), juvenile idiopathic arthritis (JIA), systemic lupus erythematosus (SLE), and systemic sclerosis.

RHEUMATOID ARTHRITIS
General Principles
Definition
Rheumatoid arthritis is a chronic, systemic inflammatory synovitis affecting many joints.

Anatomy
Typically initially involves wrist, metacarpophalangeal (MCP), or proximal interphalangeal (PIP) joints.

Epidemiology
Prevalence: 5 cases per 1,000 adults, female to male ratio 3:1, prevalent age 34 to 45, after age 50, sex difference less marked.

Pathophysiology
The result of activation of proinflammatory cells that infiltrate the synovium. These cells release cytokines and tumor necrosis factor (TNF) alpha, which cause the bone and cartilage destruction.

Etiology
Unknown.

Mechanisms of Injury
As described above.

Diagnosis
Clinical Presentation
Diagnostic criteria have 90% sensitivity and specificity if more than four of the following criteria are present:

- Early **morning stiffness** for more than 6 weeks
- Arthritis involving **more than three joints** for more than 6 weeks
- Wrist, MCP, or PIP joint involvement
- **Symmetrical** arthritis
- **Rheumatoid nodule** or nodules
- Positive **rheumatoid factor** titer
- **Bony radiographic changes**

History
Usually gradual onset of joint pain with systemic symptoms (weakness, fatigue, anorexia).

Physical Examination
Symmetric joint involvement; most often hands, sometimes feet; with effusions, tenderness, restricted movement.

Laboratory Studies
Rheumatoid factor (RF) (up to 30% false negative early); anticyclic citrullinated peptide antibody (anti-CCP) in combination with RF improves both sensitivity and specificity.

Imaging
Earliest findings soft tissue swelling and periarticular osteopenia; erosions (present in up to 25% at first visit); later joint space narrowing, visible deformity.

Monitoring
At each visit, evaluate for subjective and objective evidence of active disease.

- Degree of joint pain (by visual analog scale)
- Duration of morning stiffness
- Duration of fatigue
- Presence of actively inflamed joints on exam (tender and swollen joint counts)

Differential Diagnosis
SLE, seronegative spondyloarthropathies, polymyalgia rheumatica, acute rheumatic fever, scleroderma.

Treatment
Behavioral
The patient's recognition of the chronic, progressive nature of the disease is central to healthy adjustment to the diagnosis and optimal participation by the patient in his or her therapy. The primary physician and consultants play important roles in educating the patient and family about the disease and providing longitudinal care. The Arthritis Foundation also has valuable educational materials and programs.

Medications
Joint damage begins early in the disease. Therefore, early aggressive therapy with disease modifying antirheumatic drugs (DMARDs) is advocated to prevent or delay joint destruction. Although nonsteroidal anti-inflammatory drugs (NSAIDs) may control symptoms, the opportunity to control the disease may be lost if more potent therapies are not initiated early.

NSAIDs. No NSAID is more effective than aspirin. All are associated with gastrointestinal side effects. Newer NSAIDs with selective cyclo-oxygenase-2 (COX-2) inhibition produce equivalent pain relief with somewhat reduced gastrointestinal (GI) complications compared to nonselective NSAIDs. However, placebo-controlled trials suggest increased risk of thrombotic cardiovascular events with COX-2-selective NSAIDs. The American College of Rheumatology Guidelines for the Management of Rheumatoid Arthritis recommend that physicians should weigh the potential risks and benefits of treatment with these medications (as with all drugs).

DMARDs. DMARDs should be initiated within 3 months of diagnosis. Usually used in combination with NSAIDs and often with other DMARDs if control cannot be obtained with a single DMARD.

- Methotrexate (Rheumatrex): Therapy initiated at three 2.5-mg tablets weekly. Discontinue with development of any pulmonary symptoms until they resolve. Eliminate or significantly restrict alcohol. Ensure nonpregnant state and adequate birth control. Monitor complete blood count (CBC) and liver-associated enzymes every 4 to 8 weeks. Supplement with folic acid, 1 mg per day.
- Antimalarials: Hydroxychloroquine (Plaquenil) 200 mg bid, reduced to 200 mg daily after 3 to 6 months if improved, for maintenance. Baseline retinal examination, repeated q6 months while on medication.
- Injectable gold salts: Gold sodium thiomalate (Myochrysine) and aurothioglucose (Solganol) are more effective than oral formulations. Give 10 mg IM as first dose, 25 mg for second and third doses, then subsequent doses of 50 mg per week to total of 0.8 to 1.0 g.

If improved, 50 mg q2 to 4 weeks indefinitely. CBC, platelets, and urinalysis prior to each injection.

■ Biological DMARDs. TNF-alpha inhibitors may dramatically suppress disease activity. Etanercept (Enbrel), infliximab (Remicade), and adalimumab (Humira) have been effective in reducing signs and symptoms of RA in patients whose disease is refractory to methotrexate. Other DMARDs target additional anti-inflammatory mediators (interleukin-1, T cells, and B cells). Biological DMARDs have significant safety considerations, contraindications, and costs and should be used in consultation with a rheumatologist.

Glucocorticoids. Low-dose oral glucocorticoids (<10 mg prednisone daily) and local injections of glucocorticoids are highly effective for relieving symptoms in patients with active RA. Recent evidence suggests that low-dose glucocorticoids slow the rate of joint damage, indicating disease-modifying potential. Bone protection should be undertaken with adequate calcium intake and consideration of bisphosphonates. Individual joint steroid injections should be given no more often than every 3 months.

Surgery
Patients with unacceptable levels of pain, loss of range of motion, or limitation of function because of structural joint damage should be considered for surgical treatment.

Referrals
Instruction in joint protection techniques, energy conservation, range of motion, muscle strengthening, and aerobic exercise are all important in achieving the goal of maintaining function. Physical and occupational therapists may be needed to assist with this teaching.

Protocol
Guidelines for the Management of Rheumatoid Arthritis are published by the American College of Rheumatology and are available at **http://www.rheumatology.org/publications/guidelines/raguidelines02.asp?aud=mem.**

JUVENILE IDIOPATHIC ARTHRITIS
General Principles
Definition
Persistent arthritis for more than 6 weeks with an onset at less than 16 years of age, after excluding other causes. There are seven subtypes, defined under "Classification" below.

Anatomy
Knees, ankles, wrists, and elbows are most frequently involved, but all joints can be affected.

Epidemiology
More common in girls than boys; incidence varies from 1 to 22 per 100,000, with a prevalence of 8 to 150 per 100,000.

Classification
(a) Systemic onset (previously Still's disease), (b) oligoarthritis (<4 joints involved in first 6 months), (c) polyarthritis RF (rheumatoid factor) negative, (d) polyarthritis RF positive, (e) enthesitis-related arthritis (formerly call spondyloarthropathy or inflammatory bowel syndrome related), (f) psoriatic arthritis, (g) other (fits none or >1 category).

Pathophysiology
Inflammatory mediators in joints produce joint injury and eventual destruction.

Etiology
Unknown, probably a complex of genetic traits related to immunity and inflammation.

Diagnosis
Clinical Presentation
As noted in classification.

History
Many patients complain little of joint pain, but limit or modify motion due to pain. Decreased activity, morning stiffness, and "gelling" are common.

Physical Examination

Systemic onset disease, spiking fevers, an evanescent centripetal salmon-pink rash, generalized lymphadeonopathy, and hepatosplenomegaly may occur. Oligoarticular disease lacks systemic features except iridocyclitis, which may develop in up to 60% of these patients. In polyarticular disease, multiple joint involvement without systemic symptoms occurs, but malaise, growth retardation, weight loss, mild adenopathy, and low-grade fevers are sometimes present.

Laboratory Studies

RF and antinuclear antibody (ANA) are rarely positive in systemic disease. RF-positive children with polyarticular onset have a worse prognosis and more vasculitis than those with polyarthritis who are RF negative. In oligoarticular disease of early onset (before 6 years) most are ANA positive and RF negative.

Imaging

Radiologic joint damage occurs in most patients with systemic arthritis and polyarthritis within 2 years of onset and in oligoarthritis within 5 years.

Differential Diagnosis

Trauma; malignancy; sarcoidosis; SLE; progressive systemic sclerosis; infections: viral, rickettsial, bacterial; serum sickness.

Treatment

Behavioral

Patients and families should be encouraged to seek supportive counseling to assist in dealing with a chronic illness in a child.

Medications

Systemic onset. NSAIDs (ibuprofen and naproxen are available as elixirs; tolmetin and naproxen are approved in patients as young as 2 years; ibuprofen as young as 6 months) and systemic corticosteroids.

- **Oligoarthritis.** NSAIDs, unless presenting with flexion contractures or leg length discrepancies or if unresponsive to NSAIDs in 4 to 6 weeks then intra-articular corticosteroids (triamcinolone hexacetonide). Unresponsive or with small joint involvement, treat as polyarthritis.
- **Polyarthritis, RF negative.** NSAIDs for symptom control; methotrexate started early (10 mg/m^3/week), increased to 15 mg/m^3/week, if ineffective.
- **Polyarthritis, RF positive.** Treated per protocols for rheumatoid arthritis in adults (see previous section).
- **Enthesitis-related arthritis.** Sulfasalazine may be most effective, particularly for boys over age 9, although few evidence-based data are available.
- **Psoriatic arthritis.** Can present as oligo-, poly-, or enthesitis-related arthritis and should be treated as the parallel JIA subset, since no treatment studies are available of psoriatic arthritis in children.

Special Therapy

Early consultation with physical and occupational therapy to maintain or regain muscle and joint strength, range of motion, and function.

Referrals

Early involvement of an ophthalmologist to identify and treat iridocyclitis is mandatory to prevent disability. Early involvement of rheumatologist for therapeutic decisions.

SYSTEMIC LUPUS ERYTHEMATOSUS

General Principles

Definition

The presence of four or more of the American Rheumatological Association Preliminary Criteria for SLE is a reliable indicator of the diagnosis:

- **Malar rash,** tending to spare the nasolabial folds
- **Discoid rash,** follicular plugging with alopecia and atrophic scarring in older lesions
- **Photosensitivity**
- **Oral ulcers,** classically painless

- **Nonerosive arthritis** involving two or more peripheral joints
- **Serositis**
- **Renal disorder** manifested by persistent proteinuria >0.5 g per day or cellular casts
- **Neurologic disorder** manifested by seizures or psychosis
- **Hematologic disorder,** either hemolytic anemia with reticulocytosis, leukopenia (<4000 cells/μL on two or more occasions) or lymphopenia (<1,500 cells/μL on two or more occasions) or thrombocytopenia (<100,000/μL).
- **Immunologic disorder,** antibody to double-stranded DNA or Smith antigen
- **Antinuclear antibody** (in the absence of any drugs known to be associated with "drug-induced lupus" syndrome)

Epidemiology
Female-to-male ratio is 7:1. Generally in the childbearing years. Prevalence: 20 per 100,000.

Etiology
Unknown. Autoantibodies are typically present for years before the diagnosis of SLE.

Mechanisms of Injury
Autoantibodies produce multisystem inflammatory damage.

Diagnosis
Clinical Presentation
Arthritis or arthralgia is usually the earliest symptom.

History
Almost all patients are fatigued and feel general malaise. Pleuritis, pericarditis, or a combination of both may produce chest pain. Central nervous system changes may result in subtle changes in cognitive function, depression, or seizure disorder.

Physical Examination
Approximately 85% of patients have skin, hair, and mucous membrane involvement, ranging from mild malar rash to ulcerations, patchy to diffuse alopecia and mucosal ulceration. Symmetrical arthritis, most commonly involving the PIP joint (80%), followed by wrists, knees, ankles, elbows, and shoulders. Little objective joint inflammation.

Laboratory Studies
Anemia, elevated sedimentation rate (ESR) or C-reactive protein and polyclonal gammopathy reflect systemic inflammation. ANA is positive in nearly 100% but is nonspecific. Antibodies to double-stranded DNA (anti-ds DNA) or the Smith nuclear antigen (Anti-Sm) are highly specific for SLE.

Imaging
Chest x-ray to evaluate pulmonary involvement; echocardiogram for valvular heart disease (present in 18% of patients with SLE).

Differential Diagnosis
Other connective tissue disorders (e.g., progressive systemic sclerosis, RA), neoplasm, infection.

Treatment
Behavioral
Patients with photosensitivity should avoid sunlight and use high–sun protection factor (SPF) sunscreens.

Medications
Therapy should be individualized, based on disease severity.

- Joint pain and mild serositis are generally well controlled with NSAIDs; antimalarials (hydroxychloroquine 200 to 400 mg/day) are also effective.
- Cutaneous manifestations are treated with topical corticosteroids.
- Intradermal corticosteroids are helpful for individual discoid lesions, particularly of the scalp.
- Acute illness with renal or central nervous system dysfunction, give high-dose corticosteroids, such as prednisone 1 mg/kg/day divided q12h, tapered slowly when evidence of active disease subsides. NSAIDs should be used adjunctively. Addition of antimalarials should be considered as tapering of steroids occurs. Pulsed high-dose

steroid and immunosuppressive agents are used in poorly responsive patients or those with glomerulonephritis, in consultation with a rheumatologist.

Referrals
Rheumatology for initial consultation regarding therapy and for patients poorly responsive to first-line therapy.

Patient Education
Education regarding recognition of disease flares and anticipated course of the illness.

Complications
The leading cause of death in patients with SLE is infection (one third of all deaths). Serum creatinine levels >3 mg per dL or evidence of diffuse proliferative involvement on renal biopsy are poor prognostic factors.

SYSTEMIC SCLEROSIS (SSC)

General Principles

Definition
A progressive connective tissue disorder characterized by **thickening and fibrosis of skin and variable involvement of internal organs.**

Epidemiology
4-12 cases per million; female-to-male ratio 4:1, peak onset 30 to 50.

Etiology
Unknown.

Mechanisms of Injury
Fibrotic changes in skin and visceral organs; primarily lung, kidney, and esophagus.

Diagnosis

Clinical Presentation
- **Limited SSc (lSSc) or CREST syndrome** (calcinosis, Raynaud phenomenon, esophageal motility disorders, sclerodactyly, and telangiectasia). Skin involvement limited to distal extremities or above clavicles. Lung involvement is common, sometimes leading to pulmonary hypertension.
- **Diffuse (dSSc)** has more widespread skin involvement and more common visceral involvement. Almost all have Raynaud phenomenon and esophageal disease. Monitor for pulmonary involvement and renal crisis.

History
Most present with Raynaud phenomenon and edema of fingers; arthralgias may be present. Rarely, esophageal symptoms first.

Physical Examination
- Edema of hands and feet, followed by thickening of skin of fingers (sclerodactyly).
- Digital pits secondary to Raynaud phenomenon and other findings as outlined in CREST components above.

Laboratory Studies
- Most patients positive ANA; nucleolar pattern associated with dSSc and centromere pattern with lSSc. ESR is often normal.
- Anticentromere antibody positive in 50% to 95% with limited disease (i.e., good prognosis if positive).
- Screen for visceral involvement with CBC, urinalysis, creatinine, pulmonary function tests, and diffusion capacity of carbon monoxide.

Imaging
Chest x-ray for pulmonary fibrosis, esophageal motility studies.

Surgical Diagnostic Procedures
Skin biopsy.

Differential Diagnosis
- Limited disease: Mycosis fungoides, amyloidosis, porphyria cutanea tarda, reflex sympathetic dystrophy

- Diffuse disease: Idiopathic pulmonary fibrosis, primary biliary cirrhosis, GI dysmotility problems, SLE and overlap syndromes

Treatment
Behavioral
Because of the sometimes disfiguring nature of the disease, counseling is recommended for supportive care. Protect extremities from cold.

Medications
- **Raynaud disease** should be managed with **calcium-channel blockers** (immediate or extended release) or **peripheral alpha blockers. Antiplatelet therapy** may be tried (aspirin, 81 to 325 mg/day). **Recombinant human relaxin** has been effective in small trials.
- **Penicillamine** (started at 250 mg/day and titrated up to 1 g/day) for skin changes, in addition to **moisturizing agents.**
- **Proton pump inhibitors and H2-receptor blockers** for esophageal reflux symptoms. Promotility agents may be helpful.
- **Monitor blood pressure** and make early use of angiotensin-converting enzyme inhibitors.

Surgery
Progression of disease may eventually lead to lung transplant, dialysis, or renal transplantation.

Referrals
Physical and occupational therapy to prevent and treat functional loss secondary to skin changes. Rheumatology for confirmation of initial diagnosis and continuing comanagement. Pulmonary and renal consults as needed with disease progression.

References
1. American College of Rheumatology Subcommittee on Rheumatoid Arthritis Guidelines. Guidelines for the management of rheumatoid arthritis. 2002 Update. *Arthritis Rheum* 2002;46(2):328–346.
2. Hashkes PJ, Laxer RM. Medical treatment of juvenile idiopathic arthritis. *JAMA* 2005; 294(13):1671–1684.
3. Taylor ML, Gill JM. Lupus & related connective tissue disorders. *Clin Fam Prac* 2005; 7(2):209–224.
4. Wigley FM. Scleroderma (systemic sclerosis). In: Goldman L, Ausiello D, eds. *Cecil textbook of medicine.* 22nd ed. St. Louis: Saunders; 2004;1670–1677.

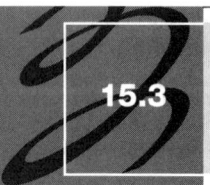

15.3 FIBROMYALGIA
Jimmy H. Hara

*F*ibromyalgia is a nonarticular rheumatologic syndrome characterized by widespread musculoskeletal pain and tenderness on palpation at characteristic sites, called tender points. Nonmusculoskeletal symptoms often accompany the nonarticular musculoskeletal pain. Fatigue, sleep disturbance, anxiety or depression, headache, irritable bowel syndrome, dysmenorrhea, and paresthesias are among the more common nonmusculoskeletal features.

DIAGNOSIS
History
Fibromyalgia occurs predominantly in women; only 5% to 20% of patients with fibromyalgia are men. The most common age of presentation is 40 to 50 years; whites predominate in most

series. The prevalence in the general population is 4% to 10%. Pain is the cardinal symptom and is widespread. According to the American College of Rheumatology, the pain must be above and below the waist, on both sides of the body, and along the axial skeleton.[1] Associated nonmusculoskeletal symptoms are commonly seen; these include fatigue, sleep disturbance (with a characteristic alpha wave intrusion on delta rhythm sleep on the polysomnogram), headache, irritable bowel syndrome, dysmenorrhea, and paresthesias. Anxiety and depression are common. There is also frequently an overlap with chronic fatigue syndrome.[2]

Physical Examination

There must be tenderness on digital palpation (using 4 kg of force, or enough to blanch the nail bed of the thumb) in at least 11 of the following 18 (nine pairs of) tender point sites:

- **Occiput:** bilaterally at the suboccipital muscle insertions a few centimeters below the nuchal ridge
- **Low cervical:** bilaterally at the anterior aspects of the intertransverse spaces at C5–C7, corresponding to the upper trapezius trigger point of Travell[3]
- **Trapezius:** bilaterally at the midpoint of the upper border of the trapezium, corresponding to the supraspinatus tendon area
- **Supraspinatus:** bilaterally above the medial border of the scapular spine, corresponding to the middle trapezius myofascial trigger point of Travell[3]
- **Second rib:** bilaterally at the second costochondral junctions, probably representing costochondritis
- **Lateral epicondyle:** bilaterally 2 cm distal to the epicondyles, probably representing lateral epicondylitis or extensor-supinator enthesitis
- **Gluteal:** bilaterally in the upper outer quadrants of the buttocks in the anterior fold of muscle and corresponding to the multifidus myofascial trigger point of Travell[3]
- **Greater trochanter:** bilaterally just posterior to the trochanteric prominence and probably representing a trochanteric bursitis
- **Knee:** bilaterally at the medial fat pad proximal to the joint line and corresponding to anserine bursitis

Laboratory Studies

There are no routine laboratory markers for fibromyalgia. Specifically, the complete blood count and erythrocyte sedimentation rate are normal. Rheumatologic serologies are not diagnostic. Although abnormalities in T-cell subsets have been described, these tests are not recommended for routine use at this time.[3]

TREATMENT

Injection

The tendonitis, bursitis, and costochondritis tender points (lateral epicondyle, trapezius, greater trochanter, knee, and second rib) may be injected with lidocaine (Xylocaine) and corticosteroid (see Chapter 15.6).

Stretch and Spray

The myofascial trigger points of Travell (occiput, low cervical, supraspinatus, and gluteal tender points) may be stretched and vapocoolant applied; alternatively, these may be injected with 0.5% procaine.[3]

Pharmacotherapy

Low-dose tricyclics, such as amitriptyline (Elavil), 10 to 50 mg per day, or cyclobenzaprine (Flexeril), 10 to 30 mg per day, are recommended (see Chapter 5.2). Likewise, selective serotonin-reuptake inhibitors, such as fluoxetine (Prozac), 10 to 20 mg per day or paroxetine (Paxil), 5 to 10 mg per day, or low-dose dual reuptake inhibitors, such as duloxetine (Cymbalta), 60 mg per day, or venlafaxine (Effexor), 75 to 150 mg per day, may be tried. Nonsteroidal drugs and tramadol (Ultram) may also prove useful for the treatment of fibromyalgia pain.[4]

Exercise

Low-impact aerobic fitness training has proved to be of benefit in fibromyalgia.[5] Gentle stretching is probably also beneficial.

Behavioral Therapy

Electromyographic biofeedback training and cognitive–behavioral therapy have proven benefit in patients with chronic fibromyalgia symptomatology.[6]

References

1. Wolfe F, Smythe HA, Yunus MB, et al. The American College of Rheumatology 1990 criteria for the classification of fibromyalgia. *Arthritis Rheum* 1990;33:160.
2. Aaron LA, Burke MM, Buchwald D. Overlapping conditions among patients with chronic fatigue syndrome, fibromyalgia, and temporomandibular disorder. *Arch Int Med* 2000;160:220.
3. Hara J. Myofascial syndromes (fibromyalgia and myofascial trigger points). In: Rakel R, ed. *Saunders manual of medical practice.* Philadelphia: WB Saunders; 2000.
4. Goldenberg DL, Burckhardt C, Crofford L. Management of fibromyalgia syndrome. *JAMA* 2004;292:2388.
5. Busch A, Schachter CL, Peloso PM, et al. Exercise for treating fibromyalgia syndrome (Cochrane Review). *Cochrane Database Syst Rev* 2002;CD003786.
6. Hadhazy VA, Ezzo J, Creamer P, et al. Mind-body therapies for the treatment of fibromyalgia. A systematic review. *J Rheum* 2000;27:2911.

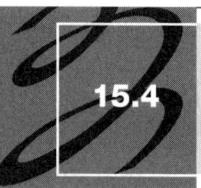

15.4

GOUT

Joseph W. Gravel, Jr., Kristen H. Goodell

GENERAL PRINCIPLES

Definition

Gout is an inflammatory disease caused by the deposition of uric acid crystals in and around joints, subcutaneous tissues (tophi), and kidneys.

Epidemiology

Gout primarily affects middle-aged men (ages 40 to 60) and postmenopausal women. The prevalence of gout has been increasing over the last two to three decades with an incidence of 1.6 per 1,000 men over 50 years of age and 0.3 per 1,000 women over 50.[1] Acute attacks of gout are less common in elderly people, in whom it may present insidiously or develop into a chronic polyarticular arthritis.

Pathophysiology

Painful gouty attacks occur when uric acid crystals, a product of purine oxidation, are deposited in joints and subcutaneous tissues. Hyperuricemia is a marker for gout, but they are not one and the same; each can exist without the other. Approximately 40% of patients have normal uric acid levels during an acute episode of gout.[2] However, the risk of gout is proportional to the degree and duration of hyperuricemia. Defined as uric acid levels greater than 8 mg per dL in men and more than 7 mg per dL in women, hyperuricemia is present in about 5% of the U.S. male population, of whom 5% will develop acute gout. Levels normally rise during puberty in men and in women after menopause. It normally takes 20 to 30 years of hyperuricemia before a patient has his first episode of gouty arthritis. Primary hyperuricemia results from inborn errors of metabolism, either reduced excretion (90% of patients) or increased production (10%) of uric acid. Secondary hyperuricemia associated with gout is the result of other diseases or drug therapies that raise uric acid levels.

Etiology

Gout is historically associated with overeating and alcoholic binges. Risk of gout increases with increasing body mass index (BMI) and with weight gain over time. Weight loss, on the other hand, is protective against gouty attacks. Presence of hypertension is strongly associated with gout independent of renal failure and diuretic use.[3] High levels of purine-rich seafood and meat consumption may precipitate gout whereas consumption of dairy products is protective. Increased consumption of purine-rich foods has no effect on clinical gout.[4] Ethanol metabolism increases serum lactate, which blocks renal uric acid excretion, leading to gouty attacks. Other factors provoking gouty attacks include rapid changes (either up or down) in serum uric acid levels, infection, surgery, renal failure, diuretic use, and emotional stress.

DIAGNOSIS

Clinical Presentation

Acute gout typically presents as an acutely painful monoarticular arthritis that may progress to chronic arthritis after years of progressively more severe and frequent episodes interspersed with variable symptom-free periods. The first metatarsophalangeal (MTP) joint is involved in 50% of initial acute gouty attacks (podagra), and 75% to 90% of patients with gout have first MTP involvement eventually. This is probably due to the propensity of the first MTP to microtrauma and its relative coolness compared with the rest of the body. Gout severity ranges from vague aches and pains of low-grade polyarticular gout to dramatic attacks of extreme monoarticular pain to chronic polyarticular arthritis. Even in untreated gout, acute attacks resolve within several days to weeks.

Timing of gouty attacks is quite variable and unpredictable. After an initial gouty arthritis attack, it may be weeks or decades before the next one. However, gout recurs within 1 year in more than half of patients. As time passes, gouty attacks tend to occur more frequently, with less time between attacks, greater severity, and polyarticular involvement; in addition, the attacks take longer to respond to therapy. For unknown reasons, gouty attacks may be slightly more common in spring.

Gout in elderly people is often polyarticular and involves upper extremity joints (especially proximal interphalangeal joints and distal interphalangeal joints) and is associated with subcutaneous tophaceous deposits on the fingers, toes, and elbows. This may be misdiagnosed as rheumatoid arthritis.[5]

Women present 70% of the time with polyarticular disease rather than the classic monoarticular arthritis seen in men.[6]

Physical Examination

During acute gouty attacks, pain, swelling, redness, and exquisite tenderness develop suddenly in the joint and often the surrounding area. The heel, ankle, knee, midtarsal joints, and olecranon bursa can all be initially involved but less frequently than the first MTP. In chronic gout, joint swelling, deformity, and disability may all be present.

Laboratory Studies

There are no laboratory studies that are pathognomonic for acute gout. However, negative joint cultures and hyperuricemia contribute to the presumptive diagnosis.

Imaging

There are no imaging studies that are diagnostic of acute gouty arthritis. The classic radiographic finding of chronic gout is sharply marginated erosions proximal to the joint space with an overlying rim of cortical bone. Uric acid calculi can be seen as filling defects on intravenous pyelograms.

Diagnostic Surgical Procedures

Definitive diagnosis of gout requires aspiration of synovial fluid or tophi with pathologic examination.

Pathologic Findings

In acute gout, needle-shaped urate crystals are found inside synovial fluid phagocytes or free within tophaceous deposits. These are strongly negatively birefringent under a polarized microscope lens. The calcium pyrophosphate crystals of pseudogout are, on the other hand, weakly positively birefringent and rhomboid.

Classification

- **Acute gout** describes acute painful attacks of arthritis induced by urate crystal deposition. During the intervals between acute gouty attacks, patients with early gout are virtually asymptomatic.
- **Intercritical gout** describes these symptom-free periods. Urate crystals can be aspirated from quiescent joints during these interval periods; therefore, the finding of urate crystals during an acute episode provides little reassurance of a nonseptic cause, and antibiotic therapy should be based on clinical presentation, Gram stain, and culture.[7] Crystals remain present in joints as long as hyperuricemia persists; when serum uric acid levels are reduced to normal, urate crystals slowly dissolve and finally disappear from the joint.
- **Chronic tophaceous gout** has become increasingly rare due to more widespread drug treatment for hyperuricemia and gout. Tophi without prior episodes of gouty arthritis are unusual because they normally occur after gout has been present for more than 10 years. Tophi can occur anywhere but tend to occur in the helix of the ear, proximal ulnar surface of the forearm, olecranon, Achilles tendon, prepatellar bursa, or near active joints. Presumptive diagnosis of acute gout can be made based on clinical signs and symptoms and a significant response to colchicine or nonsteroidal anti-inflammatory drugs (NSAIDs).
- **Secondary gout** is caused by overproduction or underexcretion of uric acid due to drugs or other disease processes. Overproduction of uric acid occurs in myeloproliferative and lymphoproliferative disorders, polycythemia, hemolytic anemia, multiple myeloma, and other malignancies. Renal disease, diuretics, low doses of salicylates, chronic lead intoxication ("saturnine gout"), nicotinic acid, alcohol, ethambutol, and pyrazinamide all cause underexcretion of uric acid. Acute uric acid nephropathy occurs primarily in patients undergoing chemotherapy for hematologic or myeloproliferative disorders and can be prevented by several days of allopurinol administration and adequate hydration before initiation of chemotherapy (see Chapter 18.4).

Differential Diagnosis

Gout can be misdiagnosed as inflammatory osteoarthritis, particularly given that erosions on radiographs are seen in both conditions (see Chapter 15.1). Gout may be mistaken for rheumatoid arthritis because tophi may resemble rheumatoid nodules and rheumatoid factors often become weakly positive as people age (see Chapter 15.2). It may be difficult to differentiate cellulitis or septic arthritis from gout, particularly when a low-grade fever, leukocytosis, redness, or desquamation is present. The term pseudogout, for calcium pyrophosphate deposition disease, belies the difficulty in clinically differentiating it from gout. For definitive diagnosis, joint fluid must be aspirated for culture and a search for urate crystals.

TREATMENT

Medications

- **NSAIDs** are considered by most to be the drugs of choice for acute gouty attacks due to their efficacy and the fact that they have relatively few side effects. They are effective, particularly if used at initial high (maximal) doses with rapid tapering over 2 to 8 days. However, 12 to 24 hours may be needed before clinical improvement is seen. How soon NSAID therapy is instituted after onset of symptoms is more important than which NSAID is chosen. NSAIDs can cause gastrointestinal (GI) toxicity (nausea, abdominal discomfort, GI bleeding, peptic ulcer disease), nephrotoxicity, and central nervous system side effects (headache, dizziness, confusion), and therefore must be used with caution, especially in elderly patients or in patients with underlying disease. Indomethacin has been used for years and is effective at a dose of 50 mg PO q8h for 2 days followed by a tapering dose during the next week. All NSAIDs are about equally effective, although long-acting NSAIDs may be less so.
- **Colchicine** terminates most acute gout attacks within 6 to 12 hours; however, it is limited by its GI side effects and is often poorly tolerated by elderly people. Colchicine is much more effective if given within the first 12 to 24 hours of an acute attack. Its mechanism of

action is not entirely known but apparently reduces the inflammatory response to urate crystals and diminishes phagocytosis. It is normally given 0.6 mg PO every 1 to 2 hours until symptoms abate, GI symptoms (cramps, diarrhea, vomiting) preclude further use, or the maximum total daily dose is reached. Possible bone marrow toxicity limits the total dose for a single day to 4.8 mg (less if the patient has hepatic or renal disease). Because of the oral colchicine GI side effects, IV colchicine is sometimes used; the clinical response is faster with fewer GI complaints, but the IV form can cause neuropathy, myopathy, bone marrow suppression, and, in rare cases, death. The dose is 2 mg diluted in 20 mL saline and injected slowly over 5 minutes into a freely flowing IV line; extravasation or infiltration can result in painful tissue necrosis. A dose of 0.5 to 1 mg IV may be repeated every 6 hours up to 4 mg total for a single attack. No additional colchicine should be given for the following week to patients given the full 4-mg IV dose. Colchicine should be used prophylactically when initiating uric acid–lowering therapy to prevent precipitating an acute gouty attack. The optimal duration of prophylaxis is unknown, but it can usually be stopped after the uric acid level is brought down to a normal range for 2 months. Colchicine, 0.6 mg bid, is usually started several days before the urate-lowering agent is started.

- **Corticosteroids** are normally used in cases when NSAIDs or colchicine cannot be tolerated or are ineffective. Prednisone, 40 to 60 mg per day PO, can be given for 3 to 5 days and then tapered over 10 days, but many patients rebound when it is discontinued. Rebound can be avoided by using colchicine prophylactically, 0.6 mg PO bid, which should then be discontinued 6 to 8 weeks later. In patients with gout involving only one or two joints or who are unable to tolerate oral therapy, intra-articular corticosteroid injections are useful. These usually result in resolution of an acute gouty episode within 12 to 24 hours.

- **Allopurinol** (Zyloprim) is a xanthine oxidase inhibitor that decreases production of uric acid. For patients with recurrent gouty attacks, renal stones, renal damage, or asymptomatic uric acid levels greater than 12 mg per dL or those who are undergoing cancer chemotherapy or taking cyclosporine after transplantation, uric acid–lowering therapy should be initiated. Allopurinol is effective in most patients regardless of the source of hyperuricemia (overproduction or underexcretion) because it produces a more soluble metabolite. A 24-hour urinary uric acid determination to differentiate urate overproduction from underexcretion is therefore unnecessary in most patients. Allopurinol is also better tolerated than uricosuric agents, has fewer drug–drug interactions, is effective in patients with renal failure or nephrolithiasis, and is used in a single daily dose. In patients receiving chemotherapy, allopurinol should be used when daily uric acid excretion exceeds 800 mg per 24 hours in male patients and 750 mg per 24 hours in female patients. Allopurinol may be started at 100 mg daily with food and increased at weekly intervals by 100 mg until a serum uric acid level of 6 mg per dL or less is attained. The average effective dose for mild gout is 200 to 300 mg per day, although some patients need 400 to 600 mg per day, particularly those with tophaceous gout or those on cancer chemotherapy. Enough fluids should be taken to keep daily urine output greater than 2 L. If an acute attack occurs while taking allopurinol, the dose should be maintained as is and the attack treated as usual (e.g., NSAIDs, colchicine). In elderly patients, a starting dose of 50 to 100 mg on alternate days, to a maximum daily dose of 100 to 300 mg based on the patient's creatinine clearance and serum urate level, decreases the risk of hypersensitivity reactions.[8] Life-threatening hypersensitivity reactions involving skin, kidney, and liver occur rarely but are being recognized with increasing frequency. The most frequent adverse reactions to allopurinol are skin rash, GI reactions (diarrhea, nausea, and alkaline phosphatase, aspartate aminotransferase, and alanine aminotransferase elevations), and acute attacks of gout, which can be minimized by proper use. Renal function must be monitored in patients taking thiazide diuretics. Allopurinol may also cause a rash in patients taking ampicillin or amoxicillin, and it may potentiate anticoagulants.

- Uricosuric drugs block renal tubular reabsorption of uric acid. As with allopurinol, they should never be started during an acute attack but should be maintained if an acute attack occurs when the patient is already on them. Before using these agents, a 24-hour urine for creatinine clearance and urine uric acid should be performed, as uricosuric drugs are ineffective for a glomerular filtration rate less than 50 mL per minute and can increase the risk of urate stones if the urinary uric acid is already elevated (800 mg/24 hours). Urate stone formation can be minimized if patients maintain a high fluid intake and alkalinize the urine. These include probenecid and sulfinpyrazone.

- **Probenecid** (Benemid) is started at 250 mg bid for 1 week and then 500 mg bid. The dose is increased by 500 mg every 1 to 2 weeks until the serum urate level is normal or the 24-hour uric acid excretion is not above 800 mg. The usual effective dose is 1.0 to 1.5 g per day. Probenecid is well tolerated. It should not be used with salicylates that antagonize its action. It can raise plasma levels of penicillin, sulfonylureas, and NSAIDs. In patients with glucose-6-phosphate dehydrogenase deficiency, it can cause hemolytic anemia.

- **Sulfinpyrazone** (Anturane) is started at 100 mg bid with meals and advanced to full maintenance dosage (200 mg bid) within 1 week. Maximum dosage is 400 mg bid. Upper GI disturbance is the most common side effect. It has similar efficacy and toxicity to probenecid.

- **Febuxostat** is a novel nonpurine selective inhibitor of xanthine oxidase, which has been proved to more effectively reduce serum uric acid levels at doses of 80 or 120 mg given PO once daily than allopurinol at its commonly used dose of 300 mg per day. However, it produced more acute gout flares when not used with colchicine. In addition, the rates of discontinuation were significantly higher in both the 80-mg febuxostat group and the 120-mg febuxostat group than in the allopurinol group.[9] Moreover, four deaths occurred in the febuxostat groups as compared with none in the allopurinol group. At the present time, this medication is not commercially available in the United States and continues to be investigational.[10,11]

- **Adrenocorticotropic hormone** has been used with success at doses of 40 to 80 units IV or IM q12h for 2 to 3 days when other measures fail, including combination therapy with NSAIDs, colchicine, and/or corticosteroids.

Special Therapy

Although not commonly used in practice, one preliminary study in 12 patients suggested that regular prophylactic phlebotomy, performed to maintain total body iron at near iron-deficiency levels is effective in markedly reducing the incidence and severity of gouty attacks.[12]

Counseling

Although no randomized controlled trials have proved the effectiveness of counseling patients on decreasing the frequency of attacks of gout, it is prudent for the physician to counsel patients with a gout history about factors known to worsen the course of the disease. Counseling should suggest dietary decrease in meat and seafood, an increase in dairy product consumption. Advice on weight loss may also be beneficial.

Risk Management

While there are multiple disease states that increase risk of gouty attacks, the presence of gout generally does not increase risks for other diseases or have multiple complications. One exception to this is in the kidney, namely, interstitial renal disease and nephrolithiasis. Men with gout have a twofold increased risk for developing kidney stones compared to men without gout. Therefore, it may be prudent to counsel men to increase fluid intake and decrease salt consumption to modify this risk factor.[13]

References

1. Uderwood M. Gout. *Clin Evidence* 2005;13:1435–1444.
2. Schlesinger N, Baker DG, Schumacher HR. Serum uric acid during bouts of acute gouty arthritis. *J Rheumatol* 1997;24:2265–2266.
3. Choi H, Atkinson K, Karlson E, et al. Obesity, weight change, hypertension, diuretic use, and risk of gout in men: the health professionals follow-up study. *Arch Intern Med* 2005;165:742–748.
4. Choi H, Atkinson K, Karlson E, et al. Purine-rich foods, dairy and protein intake, and the risk of gout in men. *N Engl J Med* 2004;350:1093–1103.
5. Sturrock RD. Gout: easy to misdiagnose. *BMJ* 2000;320:132–133.

6. Lally E, Ho G, Kaplan S. The clinical spectrum of gouty arthritis in women. *Arch Intern Med* 1986;146:2221.
7. Johnson JR. Diagnosis of intercritical gout. *Ann Intern Med* 2000;132:843.
8. Fam AG. Gout in the elderly. Clinical presentation and treatment. *Drugs Aging* 1998;13:229–2439.
9. Becker M, Palo W, Joseph-Ridge N. Febuxostat versus allopurinol for gout. *N Engl J Med* 2006;354(14):1532.
10. Becker M, Schumacher R, Wortmann R, et al. Febuxostat, a novel nonpurine selective inhibitor of xanthine oxidase: a twenty-eight day multicenter phase II randomized double-blind placebo-controlled dose-response clinical trial examining safety and efficacy in patients with gout. *Arthritis Rheum* 2005;52:916–923.
11. Becker M, Schumacher H, Wortmann R, et al. Febuxostat compared with allopurinol in patients with hyperuricemia and gout. *N Engl J Med* 2005;353(23):2450–2461.
12. Facchini F. Near-iron deficiency-induced remission of gouty arthritis. *Rheumatology* 2003;42:1550–1555.
13. Kramer H, Choi H, Atkinson K, et al. The association between gout and nephrolithiasis in men: the health professionals' follow-up study. *Kidney Int* 2003;62:1022–1026.

OVERUSE INJURIES
Ted C. Schaffer

15.5

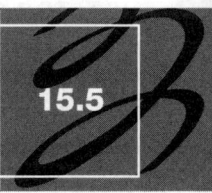

GENERAL PRINCIPLES

Definition
Overuse injuries occur when forces over time applied to a bone, muscle, tendon, or ligament exceed the ability of those tissues to adapt to the forces. Repetitive microtrauma leads to local tissue damage in the form of cellular and extracellular degeneration, and most likely occurs when there is a sudden change in mode, intensity, or duration of activity.

Anatomy
Overuse injuries generally occur on the extremities.

Epidemiology
- More than 50% of pediatric sports injuries are overuse injuries.
- More than 50% of occupational illnesses involve overuse from repetitive motion injuries.

Pathophysiology
The muscle-tendon unit is the most common site of injury, but other structures such as bone, cartilage, ligament, bursa, and fascia may be involved. In children, the growth plates are also vulnerable to the stress of repetitive injury.

Etiology
Etiology is multifactorial, leading to a pathway of repetitive microtrauma and local tissue injury.

- **Intrinsic factors** are characteristics inherent to an individual's body. These include muscle inflexibility, muscle weakness, joint laxity, previous injury, anatomic malalignment, and lower extremity asymmetry. Frequently a deficit in one body area may affect function in another region.
- **Extrinsic factors** include equipment malfunction, training errors, environmental conditions, biomechanical errors, and ergonomic problems. Modification of both intrinsic and extrinsic factors is key for injury treatment and prevention.

TREATMENT APPROACH

- The **initial treatment** aim is to reduce the inflammatory process with relative rest and ice.
  - **Ice.** Applied for 15 to 30 minutes every 2 to 6 hours as necessary.
  - **Nonsteroidal anti-inflammatory drugs (NSAIDs).** Controversial in acute injury—may reduce inflammation, but may also slow inflammatory-mediated healing.
  - **Modalities** such as iontophoresis may reduce initial inflammation.
  - **Corticosteroid** injection may reduce inflammation. Diagnostic information is obtained if injection of local anesthetic (1% lidocaine or 0.5% bupivocaine) reduces local pain. Side effects include subcutaneous fat atrophy or necrosis, depigmentation, hyperpigmentation, tendon rupture, accelerated joint destruction, or infection.

- **Definitive treatment** includes identification and modification of predisposing risk factors.
  - Exercises, especially eccentric exercises, to address deficits in strength, flexibility, and proprioception
  - Correction of biomechanical abnormalities, such as poor throwing motion
  - Addressing poor ergonomics such as chair height or computer screen adaptation
  - Orthoses useful for specific gait disorders
  - Addressing incomplete rehabilitation of any previous injury

ROTATOR CUFF TENDINOPATHY

Diagnosis

Clinical Presentation

This is the most common cause of nontraumatic shoulder pain in both children and adults. Pain is frequently insidious and there is often a nocturnal component. In adults, impingement of the supraspinatus tendon as it courses beneath the subacromial arch is the most common cause of tendinopathy.

Physical Examination

Pain with shoulder abduction is the most common finding. Provocative maneuvers with forward flexion and internal rotation (Hawkin or Neer signs), which force the humerus into the subacromial space, will often reproduce symptoms.

Imaging

Radiographs are helpful in excluding other causes of persistent shoulder pain including calcific tendonitis, glenohumeral arthrosis, and bone tumors. A supraspinatus outlet view is helpful to evaluate the bony morphology of the anterior acromion. For diagnostic uncertainty or for treatment nonresponders, magnetic resonance imaging (MRI), potentially with gadolinium contrast, is useful to help treatment.

Treatment

Nonoperative

Initial treatment includes ice, a limited course of NSAIDs, and avoiding aggravating factors. A subacromial corticosteroid injection combined with local anesthetic may confirm symptom source and reduce pain. More definitive therapy involves maximizing glenohumeral motion, stabilizing the scapulothoracic articulation, strengthening the rotator cuff, and addressing biomechanical or ergonomic errors.

Operative

For adults with persistent impingement symptoms, referral for surgery to remove boney impingement may be necessary.

EPICONDYLITIS

Diagnosis

Clinical Presentation

This is the most common overuse problem of the elbow. Pain, often insidious, is present over the affected epicondylar region. Excessive wrist extension precedes lateral epicondylitis while excessive wrist flexion precedes medial epicondylitis. Lateral epicondylitis is more common than medial epicondylitis.

Physical Examination

With lateral epicondylitis, "tennis elbow," pain radiates distally along the extensor forearm muscles. Symptoms are reproduced with wrist extension while the forearm is pronated. Resisted supination may also reproduce symptoms. With medial epicondylitis, "golfer's elbow," pain is commonly elicited with resistance to wrist flexion and forearm pronation. There may also be reduced grip strength. Imaging is rarely of help in confirming the diagnosis.

Treatment

Nonoperative

Initial treatment includes ice with friction massage, relative rest and a short course of NSAIDs. Avoiding pronation activities ("palms up") may be useful in lateral epicondylitis. A counterforce brace distal to the affected epicondyle may be useful. When pain persists, a corticosteroid injection at the site of maximal tenderness may control symptoms. Care should be exercised in a medial epicondyle injection to avoid infiltrating the ulnar nerve. Rehabilitation should include stretching and strengthening, especially eccentric strengthening of the forearm musculature, and biomechanical or ergonomic modifications.

Operative

Surgical intervention is rarely indicated for these disorders.

CARPAL TUNNEL SYNDROME

Diagnosis

Clinical Presentation

This is an entrapment neuropathy caused by compression of the median nerve between the transverse carpal ligament and the flexor tendons of the wrist. Symptoms of pain, paresthesias, or numbness occur in the sensory distribution of the median nerve, especially the index finger. It may be bilateral in up to 50% of cases. It is common in middle-aged women and in workers with repetitive manual labor. Tasks requiring a strong grip with risk flexion and extension or that have vibration exposure are at greatest risk. The majority of patients experience pain sharp enough to awaken them from sleep. The syndrome affects up to 3% of the population, and is three times as common in women as men.

Physical Examination

Pain in the distribution of the median nerve can often be elicited with percussion of the median nerve (Tinel test) or hyperflexion of the wrist (Phalen test). In severe cases there will be thenar atrophy. diagnostic confirmation can be made with electrophysiologic testing (EMGs).

Imaging

Wrist radiographs are rarely of help, although a special carpal tunnel view can rule out other anomalies such as a fracture of the hook of the hamate.

Treatment

Nonoperative

Initial identification of aggravating causes, including work modification, may be all that is needed for mild cases. Up to 50% of cases resolve spontaneously. Other early interventions may include nocturnal or job-specific splinting and a trial of NSAIDs, although there is little evidence-based support for these interventions. Direct injection of corticosteroid into the carpal tunnel often alleviates symptoms initially but long-term benefit is less certain.

Operative

For refractory cases or when there is EMG evidence of moderate to severe nerve compression, median nerve decompression by incision of the transverse carpal ligament is recommended.

DE QUERVAIN TENOSYNOVITIS

Diagnosis

Clinical Presentation

de Quervain disease is inflammation of the first dorsal compartment of the wrist (the extensor pollicis brevis and abductor pollicis longus) as it courses over the radial styloid. Excessive repetitive hand motion, especially involving radial and ulnar wrist deviation, is a frequent cause.

Physical Examination
Pain is exquisitely reproduced by sharp ulnar deviation of the hand with the thumb either extended or flexed (Finkelstein maneuver).

Imaging
Imaging is rarely of help in making the diagnosis. Degenerative arthritis of the first carpalmetacarpal joint may be seen but this problem manifests pain in a different location.

Treatment
Nonoperative
Initial treatment includes ice, relative rest, NSAIDs, and a thumb spica splint. Iontophoresis may also be useful as an early modality. If symptoms persist, local corticosteroid injection into the tendon sheath is frequently beneficial.

Operative
When nonoperative treatments fail to alleviate symptoms, surgical release of the compartment may be necessary.

TRIGGER FINGER
Diagnosis
Clinical Presentation
Trigger finger involves a stenosing tenosynovitis of the flexor tendons of the hand. Although the complaint may be of pain at the proximal interphalangeal (PIP) joint, the problem is located at the palmar surface of the metacarpophalangeal (MCP) joint.

Physical Examination
Most commonly there is inflammation at the A1 pulley, the first of five pulleys that guide the flexor tendon into the finger. A locking or triggering may occur as the stenosed tendon becomes trapped in the pulley.

Treatment
Nonoperative
Treatment is directed at tendon sheath injection with a corticosteroid. For persistent or recurrent symptoms, a second injection with application of a trigger-finger splint is helpful.

Operative
For patients who do not respond to injection, surgical release of the pulley will be necessary.

PATELLOFEMORAL PAIN SYNDROME (PFS)
Diagnosis
Clinical Presentation
PFS or patellofemoral dysfunction refers to anterior knee pain arising from the patellofemoral joint. Symptoms can range from mild activity-related knee pain to severe pain limiting ordinary daily routine. In general there is a dull aching anterior knee pain exacerbated by activities that require repetitive knee flexion or prolonged sitting.

Physical Examination
The "theater sign" is anterior knee pain produced by prolonged sitting with the knees flexed. Provocative maneuvers of the ligaments or menisci will be negative. Pain at the inferior pole of the patella is present with patellar tendonitis, or "jumper's knee." This condition occurs in athletes involved in running or jumping and is treated similarly to PFS.

Imaging
Radiographs are most helpful in excluding other diagnoses such as osteochondritis dessicans. a patellar or "sunrise" view, which shows tilting of the patella, most commonly to the lateral side, is suggestive but not diagnostic of PFS.

Treatment
Nonoperative
Treatment should be aimed at reducing pain and eliminating predisposing risk factors. Activities with significant quadriceps loading, such as stair climbing, should be minimized. After a brief period of relative rest, ice, and NSAIDs, a rehabilitation program should aim at correcting lower extremity deficits in flexibility, strength, and proprioception. Abnormal foot biomechanics, such as excessive pronation, should be addressed. Patellar taping techniques to correct malalignments may reduce symptoms.

Operative
Surgery is rarely needed for PFS treatment. In refractory conditions, release of the lateral retinaculum can be considered.

ANSERINE BURSITIS
Diagnosis
Clinical Presentation
The anserine bursa is located on the medial aspect of the proximal tibia, deep to the insertion of the semitendinosis, gracilis, and sartorius tendons. Inflammation is most common among overweight elderly women.

Physical Examination
There is tenderness at the anserine bursa, located on the proximal medial aspect of the tibia. This location helps differentiate the problem from actual joint disease.

Treatment
Nonoperative
A corticosteroid injection into the bursa usually resolves the symptoms and differentiates anserine bursitis from degenerative joint disease symptoms.

PREPATELLAR BURSITIS "HOUSEMAID'S KNEE"
Diagnosis
Clinical Presentation
Chronic inflammation of the prepatellar bursa results from recurrent trauma, such as repetitive kneeling.

Physical Examination
Acute trauma may also lead to immediate swelling of the prepatellar bursa, as can underlying infection. If infection is suspected, aspiration for Gram stain and culture should be performed.

Treatment
Nonoperative
Protective padding is an essential part of treatment in recurrent cases. When infection is suspected, antibiotics should be instituted after cultures are obtained. Chronic inflammation may respond to a corticosteroid injection, but there is some risk of infection.

Operative
For refractory cases, surgical excision of the bursa may be necessary.

SHIN SPLINTS
Diagnosis
Clinical Presentation
Both the name and exact cause of this entity, which is common among runners, dancers, and other athletes, continues to generate controversy. Pain is often worse after the activity, but worsens with increased activity levels. Contributing intrinsic factors include biomechanical abnormalities and deficits in flexibility and strength of the lower extremity. Extrinsic factors include inadequate or excessively worn footwear, insufficient warmup, uneven or hard running surfaces, and rapid advancement of a training regimen.

Physical Examination

The diagnosis is based on diffuse pain and tenderness at the posteromedial aspect of the tibia (the medial tibial stress syndrome) or, less commonly, the anterolateral aspect of the tibia (the anterior tibialis stress syndrome).

Imaging

Radiographs are useful primarily to rule out other disorders such as tibial or fibular stress fractures.

Treatment

Nonoperative

Initial treatment includes relative rest, ice massages, and NSAIDs. Occasionally symptoms can persist for weeks, especially if the athlete continues at high levels of activity. At times total rest, including cessation of all athletic activities, is necessary to resolve symptoms. Definitive treatment also includes identification of those intrinsic and extrinsic risk factors that caused symptoms, and a gradual increase to premorbid activity levels.

CHRONIC COMPARTMENT SYNDROME

Diagnosis

Clinical Presentation

The patient presents with a history of pain with activity, worsening with increased activity and relieved by rest. In contrast, the pain of shin splints is often relieved with activity and worsens after the activity. The most common locations are the anterior compartment, with pain on the anterolateral leg and dorsum of the foot, and the deep posterior compartment, with posteromedial and instep pain.

Physical Examination

Generally normal. The diagnostic test for confirmation is measurement of compartment pressures before and after exercise.

Treatment

Nonoperative

If activity with a chronic compartment syndrome is not curtailed, ("pushing through the pain"), there may be prolonged muscle weakness and persistent pain for several days. Initial treatment includes rest and analgesics. With persistent symptoms, compartment pressure testing will be necessary.

Operative

For refractory cases with elevated compartment pressure or for rare cases of acute compartment syndrome, a surgical fasciotomy is indicated.

PLANTAR FASCIITIS

Diagnosis

Clinical Presentation

Heel pain is caused by inflammation of the thick aponeurosis that arises from the os calcis and inserts distally on the proximal phalanges. The pain is typically most intense upon arising in the morning, with symptom improvement with activity. Risk factors include obesity, excessive foot pronation, poor lower extremity flexibility, planus or cavus feet, and calf weakness. Patients may be active or sedentary.

Physical Examination

There is frequently a single area of severe pain slightly anterior to the medial calcaneal tubercle. The exact origin of plantar fascial pain is controversial, but most likely the pain emanates from an enthesopathy or nerve entrapment rather than from bone pathology.

Imaging

Radiographs are of little diagnostic help. Although 50% of patients with plantar fasciitis show heel spurs on the anterior calcaneus, this finding is also present in up to 19% of asymptomatic individuals.

Treatment

Nonoperative

Initial measures should include relative rest, appropriate shoe support including shoe inserts, and calf stretching. As a second step, custom-made night splints, physical therapy, and steroid injection may be helpful. Extracorporeal shock therapy may be effective is select populations, such as runners with chronic heel pain.

Operative

In rare cases, surgical intervention is needed to relieve symptoms.

ACHILLES TENDONITIS

Diagnosis

Clinical Presentation

Patients complain of pain and swelling in the Achilles tendon, usually 4 to 7 cm proximal to the calcaneal insertion, in a watershed area of relatively poor vascular supply. Activity will exacerbate the pain.

Physical Examination

Dorsiflexion of the foot or local palpation reproduces the symptoms, and the patient may walk with a limp.

Treatment

Nonoperative

Ice, NSAIDs, relative rest, and gentle stretching of the calf should be the first treatments. Early referral for physical therapy should be added to address flexibility, resolve strength deficits, and correct biomechanical abnormalities.

STRESS FRACTURES

Diagnosis

Clinical Presentation

When repetitive weight-bearing activity causes the boney architecture to exceed a given threshold, a stress fracture will occur. Risk factors include sudden increases in training regimen or activity level, osteopenia, poor biomechanics, and hormonal factors. In general, women are more susceptible than men.

History

There is a gradual increase in pain that resolves with rest. If untreated, the pain will occur with lower levels of activity, and eventually with rest. Approximately 90% to 95% of stress fractures involve the lower extremity, although specific sports can be associated with upper injuries (rowing: rib fractures; throwing: arm/ulnar fractures).

Physical Examination

There will be point tenderness over the bone in lower leg injuries. In upper leg fractures, the pain may be more ill-defined. The most common sites for injury are the tibia, the second and third metatarsals, and the fibula.

Imaging

Radiographs are often normal until 2 to 4 weeks from symptom onset, when reactive sclerosis of the bone appears. Bone scan may provide diagnostic confirmation as early as 72 hours from symptom onset, but early findings may be inconclusive. MRI is an expensive but very accurate diagnostic tool, with detection as early as 24 to 48 hours from symptoms.

Classification

Stress fractures can be divided into high-risk and low-risk fractures based on their potential for long-term morbidity (Table 15.5-1). High-risk fractures have greater potential for complications such as delayed union, nonunion, bone displacement, or fracture completion. Orthopaedic consultation is advisable for these injuries, which require individualized and prolonged management.

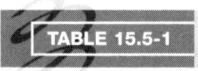

| | | **TABLE 15.5-1** | **Stress Fracture Identification** | | |

Location	Frequency	At risk for long-term morbidity	Physical finding	Immediate treatment
Second and third metatarsals	Common	No	Localized tenderness	Rest; symptomatic
Proximal fifth metatarsal	Occasional	Yes	Localized tenderness	Nonweight bearing, casting vs. surgery
Tarsal navicular	Occasional in track and field	Yes	Midfoot pain	Nonweight bearing, casting
Proximal tibia	Common	No	Localized tenderness	Rest; symptomatic
Distal tibia	Common	No	Localized tenderness	Rest; symptomatic
Midtibial anterior cortex	Rare	Yes	Anterior shin pain	Prolonged rest; occasionally surgery
Fibula	Common	No	Localized tenderness	Rest; symptomatic
Femoral shaft	Occasional	No	Thigh pain	Rest; symptomatic
Femoral neck	Rare	Yes	Groin pain	Nonweight bearing, orthopaedic referral

Treatment

Nonoperative

Immediate treatment for low-risk stress fractures includes relative rest, ice, and analgesics. Pain relief should be expected within 1 to 2 weeks. Nonweight-bearing activities, such as swimming or stationary biking, and muscle stretching should be encouraged until pain resolution indicates healing; then a gradual increase in activity level can be resumed along with appropriate counseling and review of the training regimen to prevent injury recurrence. The average return to activity with low-risk stress fractures is 8 weeks, with a range of 3 to 14 weeks.

Operative

Once a high-risk stress fracture is suspected, activity should be very limited until an accurate diagnosis is made and orthopaedic consultation is obtained. Occasionally surgery may be indicated (Table 15.5-1).

SPECIAL CONSIDERATIONS—OVERUSE SYNDROMES IN CHILDREN

Osgood–Schlatter Condition

Diagnosis

Clinical Presentation. This traction apophysitis at the patellar insertion on the tibial tuberosity is a common complaint among peripubertal adolescents. Caused in part by longitudinal forces created by rapidly growing bones, Osgood–Schlater disease is associated with increased physical activity.

Physical Examination. There is localized edema and tenderness over the tibial tuberosity.

Imaging. Imaging is needed only in refractory cases, primarily to rule out other problems such as bone tumors.

Treatment

Nonoperative. Several days or weeks of relative rest, along with analgesics, reduce symptoms to a manageable level. A boney prominence may remain due to residual fragmentation of the upper tibial epiphysis. Improvement in lower extremity flexibility and reduction of quadriceps loading, especially stair walking, will help reduce symptoms. For refractory cases several weeks of prolonged rest may be necessary.

Sever Condition
Diagnosis
Clinical Presentation. This is a calcaneal apophysitis, similar to Osgood–Schlatter disease, which occurs primarily in adolescent male soccer players.

Physical Examination. Inflammation at the insertion of the calcaneal apophysis leads to localized pain, tenderness, and swelling, which may be aggravated by activity.

Treatment
Nonoperative. Treatment includes ice, relative rest, calf stretching, and often a temporary heel lift.

Little League Elbow
Diagnosis
Clinical Presentation. This term describes a group of overuse elbow injuries that result from repetitive stresses in the skeletally immature thrower. It most commonly involves baseball pitchers. The most common problems are fragmentation/avulsion of the medial epicondyle, stress reaction to the apophysis of the medial epicondyle, osteochondrosis of the capitellum, and olecranon apophysitis. Contributing factors include improper warmup, poor throwing mechanics, and throwing of curve balls.

Physical Examination. There is pain with the throwing motion and usually localized tenderness over the medial epicondyle.

Imaging. Radiographs are important to exclude bone abnormalities associated with little league elbow.

Treatment
Nonoperative. Rest, ice, and occasionally a short course of NSAIDs are the first therapies. When symptoms subside, the patient may play a less-demanding position (e.g., first base) as long as he or she is pain free while throwing. Stretching and strengthening of the muscles of the forearm, shoulder, and scapulothoracic musculature are the mainstay of rehabilitation. Return to pitching should be framed in months, not days or weeks.

Operative. Osteochondrosis of the capitellum often requires further diagnostic workup and may necessitate surgical intervention.

Spondylolysis
Diagnosis
Clinical Presentation. Up to 50% of back pain in adolescent athletes may be caused by a vertebral defect in the pars interarticularis. The defect can be unilateral or bilateral, and is thought to be due to repetitive hyperextension of the posterior spine in such activities as gymnastics, ballet, offensive lineblocking in football, volleyball, and soccer. The problem most commonly affects the fourth and fifth lumbar vertebrae. The patient presents with activity-related back pain exacerbated by hyperextension.

Physical Examination. The best test is pain reproduced with ipsilateral single leg hyperextension (the "stork test"). Other findings may include hyperlordotic posture, decreased range of motion, and hamstring tightness.

Imaging. Initial studies should include a full lumbar series with anteroposterior (AP), lateral, and oblique films. On the oblique view, spondylolysis will manifest as a "Scotty dog collar," which is a complete fracture through the pars interarticularis. Radiographs may also demonstrate spondylolisthesis, which is the anterior displacement of a vertebral body on another. When spondylolysis is suspected but initial x-rays are negative, other more sensitive tests can be ordered including a single photon emission computed tomography (SPECT) scan, an MRI, or a CT scan.

Treatment
Nonoperative. Accepted treatment includes relative rest, analgesics, and bracing. Bracing should be continued until the patient is completely asymptomatic or there is radiographic

evidence of complete healing. In some cases this may take up to 9 to 12 months. Physical therapy should focus on flexion, hamstring stretching, and core strengthening. The goal with prolonged treatment is to prevent nonunion and subsequent spondylolisthesis.

Operative. Whereas treatment for low-grade spondylolisthesis, up to 50% slippage, is similar to spondylolysis, more severe grades will likely require surgical spine stabilization.

References

1. Akhtar S, Bradley MJ, Quinton DN, et al. Management and referral for trigger finger/thumb. *Br Med J* 2005;331:30.
2. Andrews JR. Diagnosis and treatment of chronic painful shoulder: review of nonsurgical interventions. *Arthroscopy* 2005;21:333.
3. Cassas KJ, Cassettari-Ways A. Childhood and adolescent sports-related overuse injuries. *Am Fam Physician* 2006;73:1014.
4. Cole C, Seto C, Gazewood J. Plantar fasciitis: evidence-based review of diagnosis and therapy. *Am Fam Physician* 2005;72:2237.
5. Diehl JJ, Best TM, Kaeding CC. Classification and return-to-play considerations for stress fractures. *Clin Sports Med* 2006;25:17.
6. LaBella C. Patellofemoral pain syndrome: evaluation and treatment. *Primary Care Clin Office Pract* 2004;31:977.
7. Rausch WG, Hergan DJ. Treatment of stress fractures: the fundamentals. *Clin Sports Med* 2006;25:29.
8. Wilder RP, Sethi S. Overuse injuries: teninopathies, stress fractures, compartment syndrome, and shin splints. *Clin Sports Med* 2004;23:55.
9. Wilson JJ, Best TM. Common overuse tendon problems: a review and recommendations for treatment. *Am Fam Physician* 2005;72:811.

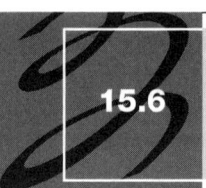

15.6   ARTHROCENTESIS AND JOINT AND SOFT-TISSUE INJECTIONS

Michael J. Henehan

$\mathcal{T}$he removal of joint fluid (arthrocentesis) and intra-articular or soft-tissue injection of medication are common primary care procedures. The indications and techniques for these procedures are outlined in this chapter.

INDICATIONS

Arthrocentesis (Figure 15.6-1)

- **Diagnostic.** Arthrocentesis can be helpful in evaluating a joint effusion of uncertain etiology. The differential diagnosis includes septic arthritis, aseptic inflammation (rheumatologic process), degenerative changes, and traumatic effusion (hemarthrosis).
- **Therapeutic.** In rare instances, repetitive joint aspiration is indicated to relieve pain and restore joint range of motion. In general, treatment of the underlying problem is preferred because the joint fluid will often reaccumulate rapidly, and repeated arthrocentesis increases the risk of a joint infection.

Intra-Articular and Soft-Tissue Injection (Figure 15.6-2)

- **Diagnostic.** Intra-articular and soft-tissue injection can be helpful in differentiating the source of pain.
- **Therapeutic**
  - Therapeutic injections relieve inflammation in tendon sheaths, bursae, muscles, and joints in inflammatory, noninfectious arthropathies.

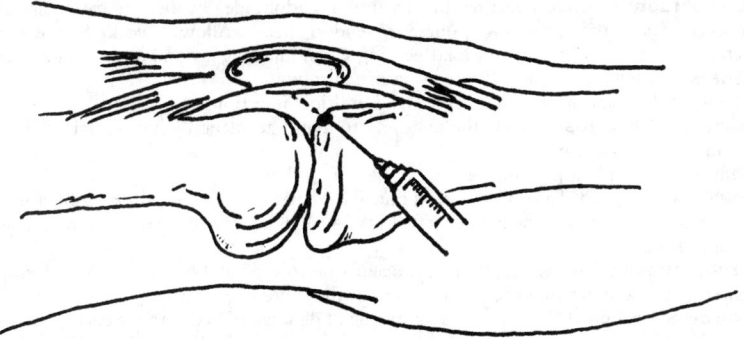

Figure 15.6-1. Arthrocentesis of the knee.

■ Therapeutic injections provide adjunctive therapy for joints and soft-tissue inflammation not responsive to systemic therapy.

RISKS AND RISK MANAGEMENT

■ **Intravascular injection.** Always aspirate back before injecting. If blood is aspirated, redirect the needle and proceed again.

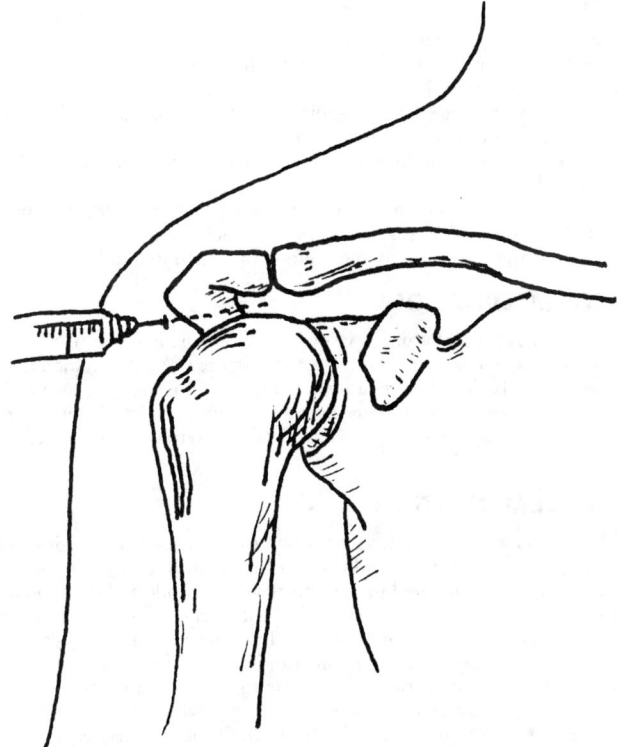

Figure 15.6-2. Injecting the subacromial space: lateral approach.

- **Tendon rupture.** Avoid injecting directly into a tendon. Ideally, the medication should be injected into the surrounding bursa or tendon sheath. Allow 2 weeks before reinjecting or permitting significant load bearing when injecting around large tendons.
- **Hypersensitivity.** Ask about allergies before injecting.
- **Infection.** Use sterile technique, and avoid multiple injections.
- **Anatomical hazards.** Review the anatomy to avoid accidentally hitting nerves, large blood vessels, or organs.
- **Hematoma.** Apply a pressure dressing.
- **Postinjection pain.** Pain occurs in about 5% of patients. It is thought to be a local inflammatory response. The pain usually lasts 24 to 36 hours and occurs within hours of the injection.
- **Tissue atrophy.** Fat degeneration can occur due to the catabolic properties of corticosteroids. The more superficial the injection, the more likely atrophy is to occur.
- **Skin discoloration.** This is usually a lightening of pigmentation due to the corticosteroid. The change is most pronounced in dark-skinned individuals. It is most likely to occur with superficial injections.

CONTRAINDICATIONS TO JOINT INJECTION

- Suspicion of septic arthritis or bacteremia
- Coagulopathy
- Cellulitis overlying the site of the injection
- More than three steroid injections in a weight-bearing joint during a 12-month period (relative contraindication)

SUPPLIES

- Antiseptic solution (e.g., povidone–iodine)
- Syringes. A 10- to 30-mL syringe is used for arthrocentesis, and a 3- to 10-mL syringe for joint or soft-tissue injection.
- Needles. A 16- to 18-gauge 1.5-in. needle is used for arthrocentesis, and a 25-gauge 1.5-in. needle for joint or soft-tissue injection.
- Medication. Local anesthetic may be used prior to arthrocentesis. Steroid and anesthetic are used for intra-articular or soft-tissue injection.
- Other supplies. Specimen containers, gauze pads, sterile gloves, sterile drapes, and plastic strip bandages are needed. A sterile hemostat is helpful to grasp the needle hub if the syringe must be removed to empty the aspirate or switch to another syringe.

SELECTING MEDICATIONS

For diagnostic trials, 1% lidocaine (Xylocaine) alone is injected; 0.5% bupivacaine (Marcaine) can be used if a longer anesthetic effect is desired. If inflammation is suspected, a steroid may be added. Typically, either a long-acting steroid is injected, such as betamethasone (Celestone Soluspan), or an intermediate-acting steroid, such as methylprednisolone acetate (Depo-Medrol). Lidocaine, bupivacaine, and the steroid can be mixed in the same syringe.

VISCOSUPPLEMENTATION

Injection of hyaluronan and hylan derivatives into the knee joint is emerging as an acceptable treatment option for patients with knee osteoarthritis. Recent studies show at least a moderate beneficial effect compared to placebo. The magnitude and duration of the effect varied with different studies, but 5 to 13 weeks postinjection is when the greatest benefit is observed. The mechanism of action is unclear. Intra-articular injection given weekly for 3 to 5 weeks is the usual protocol. The number of injections varies with the product used. Complications and complication rates are similar to other intra-articular injections with the exception of a slight increased incidence of synovitis with some products. The importance of molecular weight in terms of side effects and product effectiveness remains controversial. Preparations typically come in prefilled syringes and the injection technique is similar to that used with injection of corticosteroids as outlined below. Since the material is very viscous, a large bore needle (18 to 20 gauge) is needed for the injection. Cost of a course of treatment typically ranges from $400 to $800 for the medication.

TECHNIQUE

Arthrocentesis

- Obtain informed consent.
- Use sterile technique, including sterile skin preparation.
- Decide what equipment and medication you will need and have it available before you start the procedure.
- Synovial fluid can be very viscous, and a large-bore needle (i.e., 18-gauge) is needed to aspirate the fluid.
- When using a large-bore needle, local anesthetics are helpful; 1% lidocaine superficially injected using a 27- or 30-gauge needle (i.e., a tuberculin needle and syringe) provides adequate anesthesia. Ethyl chloride sprayed on the skin immediately before inserting the needle can also be helpful.
- During aspiration of a joint, the fluid generally flows easily. If fluid is not immediately aspirated on entering the joint, the needle can be gently repositioned while suction is maintained on the syringe.
- If the joint is to be injected after aspiration, leave the needle in place and change the syringe to inject the medication. This ensures that you are injecting into the joint. A sterile hemostat is helpful in removing the needle from the syringe while keeping the needle positioned in the joint.
- The total volume of fluid (anesthetic and steroid) as well as the steroid dose depends on the joint size. In general, smaller joints require less steroid and a smaller injection volume (Table 15.6-1).
- If there is no joint effusion to aspirate and only a steroid/lidocaine preparation is to be used, joint injection can be completed using the technique described above with the exception that a smaller bore needle (typically 25 gauge 1½ in. for larger joints or a 27 gauge ½ in. for small joints) can be used. Preinjection local anesthetic is usually not necessary when using a small-gauge needle.

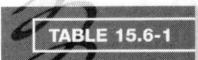 **TABLE 15.6-1** **Volume of Injections and Steroid Dosages**

Structure to be injected	Total volume of injection (lidocaine + steroid)	Dose of steroid
Small joints (e.g., digits, acromioclavicular joint)	0.5–1.0 mL	Betamethasone (or equivalent), 0.5–2 mg; methylprednisolone (or equivalent), 4–10 mg
Soft-tissue structures (e.g., tendon sheaths, carpal tunnel)		
Medium joints (e.g., ankle, elbow)	1–5 mL	Betamethasone (or equivalent), 2–4 mg; methylprednisolone (or equivalent), 20–40 mg
Soft-tissue structures (e.g., subacromial space, trigger points, bursae, epicondylitis)		
Large joints (e.g., knee)	3–10 mL	Betamethasone (or equivalent), 4–6 mg; methylprednisolone (or equivalent), 30–80 mg

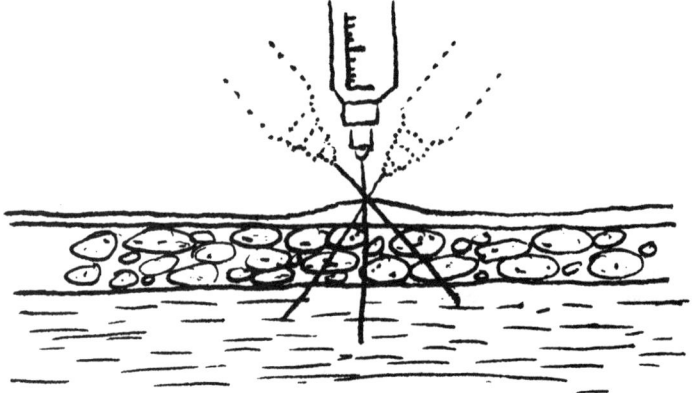

Figure 15.6-3. Repositioning the needle when injecting soft-tissue structures.

Soft-Tissue Injection

- Obtain informed consent.
- Use sterile technique, including sterile skin preparation.
- Decide what equipment and medication you will need and have it available before you start the procedure.
- Local anesthetic is generally not needed to inject a joint or soft-tissue structure.
- During injection of a soft-tissue structure or joint, the fluid should flow easily. If it does not, you may be injecting into the tendon or may not be in the joint. Gently reposition the needle and attempt to inject again. Always aspirate before injecting to avoid undesired intravascular injection of medication.
- Soft-tissue injections work best when the fluid is infiltrated into several parts of the inflamed area. This can be done by fanning out the injection (Figure 15.6-3). With this technique, the needle is repositioned by bringing the needle tip back to just below the skin surface and then passing it back into a different location within the inflamed tissue. Part of the steroid preparation is injected with each repositioning.

SYNOVIAL FLUID ANALYSIS

Typically includes appearance, characteristic of mucin clot, cell count, glucose, Gram stain, culture, and crystal studies (Table 15.6-2). Additional studies that may be helpful in some situations include fungal studies as well as measurement of lactate dehydrogenase, complement, rheumatoid factor, and antinuclear antibodies.

TABLE 15.6-2	**Synovial Fluid Analysis**		
Characteristic	**Normal**	**Inflammatory**	**Septic**
Color	Clear	Yellow	Cloudy
Viscosity	High	Low	Low
White blood cell count (mm^3)	0–200	2,000–50,000	>50,000
Neutrophils (%)	<25	Variable	>65

References

1. Pfenninger JL. Joint and soft tissue aspiration and injection. In: Pfenninger JL, ed. *Procedures for primary care physicians.* St. Louis: CV Mosby; 1994:1036–1054.
2. Steinbrocker O, Neustadt D. *Aspiration and injection therapy in arthritis and musculoskeletal disorders.* New York: Harper & Row; 1972.
3. Genovese MC. Joint and soft-tissue injection. *Postgrad Med* 1998;103:2.
4. Bellamy N, et al. Viscosupplementation for the treatment of osteoarthritis of the knee. *Cochrane Database Syst Rev* 2006;2:CD005321.

Dermatologic Problems 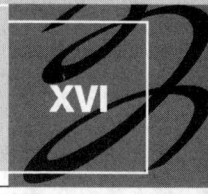 XVI

PYODERMA AND CELLULITIS
Michael L. O'Dell

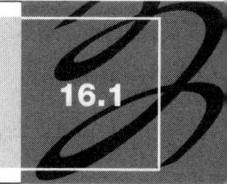 16.1

GENERAL PRINCIPLES

Definition
Pathogenic bacteria occasionally invade the skin with impetigo, ecthyma, erysipelas, cellulitis, folliculitis, furuncles, or carbuncles occurring as a result.

Anatomy
Skin comprises two layers: the epidermis, which is a superficial and avascular layer comprised of stratified squamous epithelium; the dermis, a vascular layer with such structures as nerves, hair follicles, and sebaceous glands.

Epidemiology
Skin infections are quite common and a busy family practice is likely to encounter several cases each week.

Classification
Skin infections are generally classified according to traditional names, which in turn are defined by causative bacteria, the depth of the infection, how generalized the infection is, and what skin structures are primarily infected.

Pathophysiology
Skin infections may be caused by many different bacteria, but the most common are *Staphylococcus aureus* and streptococci (predominantly Groups A and G). *Haemophillus influenza* Type B (HIB) was previously a common causative bacteria, but is in decline due to immunization. Most skin infections are confined to the epidermis and dermal layers. More serious infections involve the subcuticular space as well.

Etiology
Most skin infections are related to a break in the skin due to a puncture, abrasion, or laceration. Often this break is due to a minor trauma not even noted by the patient.

IMPETIGO

Diagnosis

Clinical Presentation

The patient generally presents with a complaint of a rash, and sometimes with complaints of itching or pain in the affected area and fever.

History

An antecedent history of a break in the skin may be present. In children, a history of exposure to another infected child is sometimes noted.

Physical Examination

Small-vesicle impetigo begins with small, reddened macules progressing to water-filled vesicles surrounded by a band of erythema. A honey-colored crust follows rupture of the vesicle. *Streptococcus* infection is often the cause of small-vesicle impetigo. Sporadically and sometimes as an epidemic, impetigo predates poststreptococcal nephritis. *Staphylococcus aureus* infection may cause small-vesicle impetigo as well. Bullous impetigo begins as a large flaccid blister or blisters. The blister quickly becomes filled with cloudy, purulent-appearing fluid. Occasionally, staphylococcal scalded skin syndrome accompanies bullous impetigo. A necrotic center is a potential sign of methicillin-resistant *S. aureus* (MRSA) infection.

Laboratory

Lab studies are generally not necessary.

Treatment

Behavioral

Good hygiene speeds healing and helps prevent spread of the illness.

Medications

In most instances, impetigo is preferentially and effectively treated topically with mupirocin (Bactroban) tid for 5 days. Systemic therapy is needed in immunosuppressed patients, those with extensive disease, patients with eczema, or those who live in communities that are experiencing an outbreak of poststreptococcal nephritis. MRSA is now the predominant isolate in many communities. MRSA that is community acquired generally remains sensitive to trimethoprim-sulfamethoxazole (note this agent is ineffective against streptococci), clindamycin, quinolones, or vancomycin.[1] Hospital associated infection is generally multidrug resistant. Due to resistance, erythromycin, b-lactams, and antistaphylococcal penicillins are of limited usefulness.

ECTHYMA

Diagnosis

Clinical Presentation

This illness is associated with debility and poor nutrition. It is most common in immunocompromised patients.

History

A small bullous lesion, generally on the lower extremities, is followed by a lesion with an adherent crust. Finally, a slowly healing ulcer appears.

Physical Examination

A deeply ulcerated lesion, with an adherent crust, is noted on a lower extremity.

Laboratory

Culture should be obtained. Ecthyma is often due to *Pseudomonas aeruginosa,* but may be associated with many other organisms, including fungi and herpes simplex virus.

Treatment

Behavioral

Nutrition needs should be addressed.

Medication

Treatment should include conservative debridement and antibiotics based on culture results.

FOLLICULITIS, FURUNCLES (BOILS), AND CARBUNCLES

Diagnosis

Clinical Presentation
These illnesses are associated with infection in a hair-bearing area. These lesions are more common in adolescents and in patients with diabetes, poor hygiene, seborrhea, or immunodeficiency.

History
Redness in an area surrounding a hair shaft progresses to a pustule or abscess. There may be associated pain, particularly with larger abscesses. Fever is only rarely present and usually heralds the onset of cellulitis. A special form of folliculitis, hot tub folliculitis, occurs with use of a poorly maintained hot tub.

Physical Examination
Folliculitis is present when there is a redness and a small perifollicular abscess associated with a single hair follicle. Multiple hairs may have a similar appearance. A furuncle is present when there is a tender, fluctuant lesion extending into the subcuticular space but still associated with a single hair follicle. A carbuncle is present when there is a collection of furuncles that intercommunicate with each other. This finding is generally on the nape of a male over the age of 40.

Laboratory
Folliculitis lesions may be cultured by removing the roof of the pustule and collecting the contents of the pustule for culture: *S. aureus* is often a cause. Culture is generally not useful for larger abscesses associated with furuncles and carbuncles: infection is generally polymicrobial.

Differential Diagnosis
Hidradenitis suppurativa is an inflammatory process involving the apocrine gland areas (axilla and groin primarily), that is chronic and progressive. This illness may have a similar appearance to furuncles initially, but the lesions are deeper, recurring, and chronic. A family history of hidradenitis suppurativa may be present.

Treatment

Behavioral
Improving hygiene often aids in prevention of recurrence, especially among athletes. Hot tub folliculitis can be prevented by learning about how to properly maintain the hot tub.

Medications
Folliculitis in a limited area responds well to topical mupirocin. *S. aureus* is a common causative agent, and systemic therapy should reflect current resistance patterns as noted for impetigo treatment above. Hot tub folliculitis, although related to *Pseudomonas aeruginosa,* is a self-limited disease: systemic treatment is reserved for patients who are immunocompromised or with systemic signs. Furuncles and carbuncles must be incised and drained. Carbuncles, due to their extensive septa and intercommunications, are generally referred to a surgeon. Although it is common to prescribe antibiotics after incision and drainage, there is little evidence that this practice improves outcomes: drainage is largely curative.

ERYSIPELAS AND CELLULITIS

Diagnosis

Clinical Presentation
Erysipelas and cellulitis are common infections in all age groups, races, and genders. A break in the skin may precede the onset of these illnesses. Injuries in brackish water may signal *Vibrio* infection. Patients with facial cellulitis and poor oral hygiene may have an odontogenic source of infection. A patient with facial cellulitis and a preceding complaint of sinusitis may have a source of infection in the sinus. Patients with underlying illnesses or who are immunocompromised may have unusual infections.

History
The patient experiences rapidly spreading redness and warmth in the affected area. Any skin surface can be involved, with extremities and the face more commonly affected. Fever often accompanies the onset, especially in cellulitis.

Physical Examination
Erythema and warmth is present in the affected area. Erysipelas tends to remain confined to the epidermis and dermis creating a very distinct, palpable border. The affected area is brightly red, almost violaceous, in color. Lymphangitic streaking is common. Cellulitis is often pinkish in color with an indistinct border due to infection of subcuticular spaces. Tenderness and swelling in draining lymph nodes is common in both illnesses. The presence of facial cellulitis should prompt a careful oral examination and search for submental or retropharyngeal swelling: either finding is ominous. In facial cellulitis, note should be made of any redness near the orbit. Proptosis, chemosis, or pain on moving the eye may indicate orbital cellulitis, a significant and life-threatening illness.

Treatment
Medication
Systemic therapy is generally required. Patients with facial infections and many patients with lower extremity infection will require admission for effective therapy. Inpatient therapy should be with vancomycin and or a quinolone. Note that most quinolones achieve adequate blood levels when taken orally and there is more cost and little advantage to intravenous administration. In outpatients, the resistance patterns in the community should be taken into account. In general, MRSA should be considered present and therapy should be initiated with a quinolone or clindamycin, although third-generation cephalosporins and penicillinase-resistant penicillins (PSRP) remain useful in some regions. Children are more likely than adults to have HIB, which responds well to second- or third-generation cephalosporins. Patients with cellulitis following injury in brackish water should receive doxycycline or a quinolone and may require an aminoglycoside if significantly ill.

Surgery
Patients with odontogenic infections may require dental surgery and those with submental or retropharygeal space infection require drainage to prevent airway compromise. Orbital cellulitis may require drainage.

Referral
Patients with dental abscess and odontogenic infection require oral surgery attention. Patients with submental or retropharygeal infection require ear, nose, and throat (ENT) referral. Patients with orbital cellulitis require ophthalmology and ENT referral.

Complications
Lower extremity erysipelas or cellulitis may damage lymphatic channels and lead to persistent edema and recurring episodes of cellulitis in the affected area. Orbital cellulitis can spread to the central nervous system or result in cavernous sinus thrombosis. Odontogenic facial infections may spread to the submental or retropharyngeal space resulting in airway collapse.

Reference
1. King MD, Humphrey BJ, Wang YF, et al. Emergence of community-acquired methicillin-resistant *Staphylococcus aureus* USA 300 clone as the predominant cause of skin and soft-tissue infections. *Ann Intern Med* 2006;144:309–317.

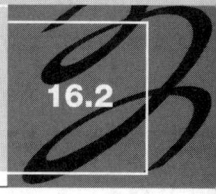

FUNGAL INFECTIONS OF THE SKIN

16.2

Lars C. Larsen, Valerie B. Laing

TINEA INFECTIONS

Tinea infections are caused by the dermatophytes: *Trichophyton, Microsporum,* and *Epidermophyton.* Infections may be subacute or chronic and are usually not invasive. These fungi selectively inhabit the keratin in the skin, hair, and nails. Tinea infections are not highly contagious.

Clinical Presentation

Infections commonly involve the scalp (*T. capitis*), body (*T. corporis*), groin (*T. cruris*), feet (*T. pedis*), hands (*T. manuum*), face (*T. faciei*), and nails (*T. unguium;* onychomycosis). Annular erythema with scaling is characteristic. Edema, plaques, pustules, and vesicles may be present in varying degrees. Onychomycosis is characterized by elevation of the distal nail, with subungual thickening and crumbling.

Diagnosis

Diagnosis is based on the clinical presentation of lesions and confirmed by examination of a potassium hydroxide preparation of skin scrapings, nail debris, or broken hair. Scrapings from a leading edge of inflammation yield the highest results. Scalp infections caused by *Microsporum* species (less than 25% of cases in the United States) may fluoresce blue-green with Wood light examination. Fungal cultures are reserved for cases in which the diagnosis is in doubt. Documentation of cure in scalp infections and justification for prolonged systemic therapy in onychomycosis are additional indications for cultures.

Management

Oral antifungal medications are necessary for the management of tinea capitis and most cases of onychomycosis. Topical agents are usually adequate for most other tinea infections, with oral medications occasionally required for extensive involvement or after failure of topical agents. Ancillary measures to avoid heat and moisture and increase exposure to air are beneficial.

- **Tinea capitis.** Oral treatment with griseofulvin for 4 to 6 weeks in adults (or until culture is negative; ultramicrosize tablets, 375 mg/d); children older than 2 years: microsize suspension for 6 to 8 weeks, 20 to 25 mg/kg/day (maximum dose 1000 mg/day). Other effective treatments include terbinafine for 2 to 4 weeks (children: 10 to 20 kg, 62.5 mg/day; 21 to 40 kg, 125 mg/day; more than 40 kg, 250 mg/day; adults: 250 mg/day); itraconazole (Sporanox) for 4 weeks (children: 5 mg/kg/day; adults: 200 mg bid); or fluconazole (Diflucan) for 3 to 4 weeks (children: 3 to 6 mg/kg/day). Concurrent twice-weekly shampooing (Head & Shoulders, Selsun Blue, or Nizoral) may reduce spore shedding.
- **Tinea corporis, tinea cruris, tinea pedis, tinea manuum, tinea faciei.** Topical medication until 2 weeks after the rash clears is curative for most infections. Tinea pedis typically requires a longer course of treatment. Oral therapy may be necessary for extensive, refractory, or recurrent disease. First-line medications effective against tinea include the following over-the-counter (OTC) medications: those containing terbinafine (e.g., Lamisil; 1% cream, spray, solution; bid) and butenafine (e.g., Lotrimin Ultra, Mentax; 1% cream daily for 14 days; bid for 7 days for tinea pedis). Naftifine (e.g., Naftin; 1% cream, gel; daily for 14 days) remains a prescription medication. Other OTC and prescription medications that are only slightly less effective include those containing clotrimazole (Lotrimin, Mycelex, clotrimazole; 1% cream, solution; bid for 2 to 4 weeks), econazole (Spectazole, econazole; 1% cream; daily for 2 to 4 weeks), miconazole (Lotrimin AF spray, Micatin, Monistat-Derm, miconazole; 2% cream, spray, powder; bid for 2 to 4 weeks), oxiconazole (Oxistat; 1% cream, lotion; bid for 2 to 4 weeks),

sulconazole (Exelderm; 1% cream, solution; bid for 3 to 4 weeks), ketoconazole (Nizoral, ketoconazole; 2% cream; bid for 2 to 6 weeks), and ciclopirox (Loprox, ciclopirox; 0.77% cream, gel, suspension; bid for 2 to 4 weeks). Sertaconazole (Ertaczo; 2% cream; bid for 4 weeks) is also used to treat tinea pedis. Medications containing undecylenic acid and tolnaftate are inexpensive, but are significantly less effective. Oral medication regimens for adults: tinea corporis/cruris—terbinafine (Lamisil)(250 mg/day × 2 weeks), itraconazole (100 mg/day × 2 weeks or 200 mg/day × 1 week), fluconazole (150 mg once weekly × 2 to 3 weeks), or ultramicrosize griseofulvin (375 mg/day × 2 to 4 weeks); tinea pedis/manuum/faciei—terbinafine (250 mg/day × 2 weeks), itraconazole (100 mg/day × 4 weeks or 400 mg/day × 1 week), fluconazole (150 mg once weekly × 4 weeks), or ultramicrosize griseofulvin (750 mg/day × 4 to 8 weeks).

■ **Onychomycosis.** Treatment regimens include oral terbinafine (adults, single daily dose, 250 mg/day for 6 weeks for fingernails, 12 weeks for toenail infections), itraconazole (Sporanox; adults, 200 mg daily for 6 weeks for fingernails, 12 weeks for toenail infections or 200 mg bid for 1 week each month for 2 months for fingernails, 3 months for toenail infections), or fluconazole (adults, 150 mg once weekly for 6 to 12 months, until the abnormal nail has grown out). Topical medications for control of infection contain ciclopirox (Penlac nail lacquer, applied daily at bedtime up to 48 weeks).

Prevention

Preventive measures include wearing of loose undergarments, wearing of cotton socks or sandals, avoidance of other occlusive clothes, and tight control of blood sugar in persons with diabetes. Sharing of contaminated combs and hairbrushes should be discouraged.

CANDIDAL INFECTIONS

Superficial candidal infections of the skin and mucous membranes may be acute or chronic and are most often caused by the fungus *Candida albicans*. Infection often indicates abnormalities of the epithelium or host immunologic system that are associated with moist, warm, and macerated skin; antibiotic therapy; or systemic conditions, such as diabetes mellitus and HIV infection. Candidiasis is not highly contagious.

Clinical Presentation

Common sites for infection include the mouth (thrush), angles of the mouth (angular cheilitis, perlèche), between moist skin folds (intertrigo), in diaper areas of infants (diaper dermatitis), on the glans and prepuce of the penis (balanitis), and in periungual skin and nails (paronychia). Skin infections typically present as erythematous plaques with "satellite" papules or pustules, or both; maceration, fissures, and exudate may be present. Lesions involving the mucous membranes include erythematous plaques and superficial erosions covered with creamy white exudate.

Diagnosis

Diagnosis is based on the typical clinical presentation of lesions and is confirmed by microscopic examination of a potassium hydroxide preparation of exudate, skin, or mucosal scrapings. Fungal pseudohyphae and spores are readily identified. Culture for the presence of candidal species is rarely needed.

Management

Topical antifungal agents are the mainstay of treatment for candidal infections of the skin and mucous membranes. It is also important to avoid heat and moisture, unnecessary antibiotic or corticosteroid therapy, and use of cornstarch. Blood sugar in persons with diabetes should be tightly controlled. Systemic antifungal therapy is generally reserved for chronic and resistant infections, systemic infections, and for prophylaxis in immunocompromised hosts.

■ **Thrush.** Most patients can be treated with nystatin oral suspension. Treat for 10 to 14 days or until 2 days after lesions clear; dosage for infants is 1 mL in each side of mouth qid; adult dosage is 4 to 6 mL in each side of mouth qid held as long as possible or clotrimazole oral troches (10 mg five times per day for 14 days). Treatment of adults with fluconazole (200 mg PO single dose or 100 mg/day × 5 days) or itraconazole (200 mg PO single dose) and children with fluconazole (3 mg/kg × 7days) are alternatives.

■ **Intertrigo, perlèche, diaper dermatitis, balanitis, paronychia.** OTC topical medications include creams, ointments, solutions, or sprays containing miconazole (Micatin, Monistat) or clotrimazole (Lotrimin AF; Mycelex OTC 1%). Prescription medications include those containing clotrimazole (Lotrimin 1% cream, lotion, solution; apply bid), ciclopirox olamine (Loprox 1% cream, lotion; apply bid), miconazole (Monistat-Derm 2% cream; apply bid), ketoconazole (Nizoral 2% cream, apply daily), and econazole (Spectazole 1% cream; apply daily). Zimycan (Vusion) is a new ointment for *Candida* diaper dermatitis that provides an effective barrier protection to the skin of zinc oxide and petrolatum while delivering an anticandidial agent of 0.25% miconazole. If maceration is present in intertrigo or diaper dermatitis, soaks with Burow solution for 15 to 20 minutes tid can be helpful. If a systemic agent is required in extensive intertrigo, fluconazole, or itraconazole (100 mg/day × 7 to 4 days) may be used.

Prevention

Preventive measures include wearing loose cotton undergarments, frequent diaper changes, conservative use of antibiotics and corticosteroids, tight control of diabetes, exposure of moist areas to air (also, blow drying with cool air after bathing), and well-fitted dentures to prevent drooling. Aggressive treatment of oral, penile, vaginal, and perirectal infections may prevent transmission to sexual partners.

TINEA VERSICOLOR (PITYRIASIS VERSICOLOR)

Tinea versicolor results from infection of sebum-producing skin follicles by yeasts in the genus *Malassezia*. Infection is common and is often chronic and recurrent. It is exacerbated by warm humid weather and use of oils on the skin. Tinea versicolor is not highly contagious.

Clinical Presentation

A fine scale covering lighter-colored skin is characteristic, with small circular lesions coalescing to involve large areas. It often becomes noticeable in the summers when the surrounding skin tans. Macules, plaques, and erythema may be present. Lesions vary in color and can be hypopigmented (white) or hyperpigmented (pink, tan, brown, or black). Although the upper chest, arms, and back are commonly affected, lesions may also be found on the face and intertriginous areas.

Diagnosis

Diagnosis is based on the clinical presentation of skin lesions and is confirmed by microscopic examination of a potassium hydroxide preparation of skin scrapings, which yields characteristic "spaghetti and meatballs" hyphae and spores. Culture for *Malassezia* is rarely needed.

Management

Selenium sulfide suspension (e.g., Selsun Blue, Exsel) may be used for acute or prophylactic therapy. Acute therapy includes application of a 2.5% suspension (prescription) for 10 to 20 minutes per day for 7 days or a single overnight application, repeated in 1 week. Prophylaxis with daily 5-minute applications of 1% (OTC) or 2.5% suspensions is useful, particularly in warm weather. Although more expensive, acute therapy for 2 to 4 weeks with other topical agents (see above) is effective. Oral ketoconazole, 400 mg taken once is an alternative for extensive or bothersome infections. Patients should work up a sweat 1 hour after the dose and not bathe immediately afterward. Itraconazole (200 mg daily × 7 days) and fluconazole (300 mg taken twice 1 week apart or 400 mg taken as a single dose) are also effective.

Prevention

Skin oils should be avoided. Prophylactic therapy with selenium sulfide suspension usually prevents clinically significant recurrences in susceptible individuals.

References

1. Chan YC, Friedlander SF. New treatments for tinea capitis. *Curr Opin Infect Dis* 2004;17;97–103.
2. Crespo-Erchigo V, Florenzio VD. Malassezia yeasts and pityriasis versicolor. *Curr Opin Infect Dis* 2006;19:139–147.

3. Gupta AK, Batra R, et al. Skin diseases associated with *Malessizia* sp. *JAAD* 2004;51 (5):785–798.
4. Gupta AK, Tul O. Dermatophytes. Diagnosis and treatment. *JAAD* 2006;54(6):1050–1055.
5. Thomas B. Clear choices in managing epidermal tinea infections. *JFP* 2003;52(11): 850–862.

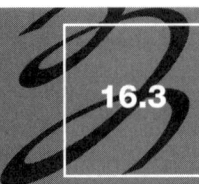

16.3 PEDICULOSIS AND MITE INFESTATIONS
Jeffrey G. Jones

ediculosis is an infestation with head lice (*Pediculus humanus* var. *capitis*), body lice (*P. humanus* var. *corporis*), or crab lice (*Phthirus pubis*). Hundreds of types of mites can cause symptoms in humans, the most common of which is scabies, an infestation with *Arcoptes scabiei* var. *hominis*. Mites or their products may be an important source of allergic reactions in people or they may cause symptoms by feeding and causing a pruritic dermatitis, as in the case of chiggers (Trombiculid mites), among many others.[1]

CLINICAL MANIFESTATIONS

- **Pediculosis**
  - **Pediculosis capitis.** Head lice infest millions of children. The infestation is transmissible by close contact or fomites, and small epidemics in schools are common. There is frequently a secondary infection with pustules, crusting, and cervical adenopathy. The infestation is found most commonly on the back of the head, the neck, and behind the ears.
  - **Pediculosis corporis.** Body lice infestation is uncommon, but when it does occur, it most often affects adults. The lice live on clothing, where they are generally found, along with eggs. Infestation is associated with poor hygiene, and is frequently seen in the homeless population. Patients complain of itching and often have red pustules, 2 to 4 mm in diameter on an erythematous base. Chronic infestation leads to skin thickening and diffuse pigmentation. They may be a vector for the diseases of epidemic typhus, relapsing, and trench fever.[2]
  - **Pediculosis pubis.** Crab lice is a sexually transmitted infestation, with at least 30% of affected persons having at least one other sexually transmitted disease.[3] The majority of patients complain of pruritus. The infestation may spread to other thick hair, including eye lashes and axillary hair.

- **Scabies and chiggers**
  - **Scabies.** Mite infestation results from direct skin contact with an infected person or fomites. Scabies is ubiquitous, and pruritis is the most common symptom. On examination, burrows in the web spaces between the fingers, wrists, hands, feet, genitals, and waistline area are seen. The mite almost never affects the head and neck region in adults. Discrete vesicles and papules are frequently seen in similar locations. Secondary infection with pustules, nodules, and regional adenopathy may develop. Norwegian, or **crusted scabies,** refers to the hyperkeratotic lesions found in immunosuppressed people, and is highly contagious.
  - **Chiggers.** The larval Trombiculid mite feeds on many hosts, including humans. The bites present as intensely pruritic, grouped erythematous papules, usually on the lower extremities, and often in areas of constricted clothing. They may mimic scabies nodules, and can spread rickettsial infections in Asia.[4]

DIAGNOSIS

Pediculosis

- Head and pubic lice can be seen on the individual hairs by careful visual examination or under the microscope. The use of a fine-toothed comb (nit comb) aids in their detection.
- Nits, the eggs attached to hairs, are indicative of infestation by head and pubic lice.
- Examination of seams of clothing may reveal body lice and their eggs.

Scabies

The diagnosis is suspected when burrows are found or when dermatologic features in the characteristic locations are present. The definitive diagnosis is made with identification of the mite, egg, egg casing, or feces. The diagnosis can be aided by the following techniques.

- With a magnifying lens, the burrows can be seen in the typical locations. The dark spot at the end of the burrow is the mite. It can be removed with a needle and examined under the microscope.
- By adding a drop of potassium hydroxide to a slide with a skin scraping, better visualization of the mite, egg, egg casing, and feces is often possible.
- Apply mineral oil to a suspicious lesion to improve the yield. After the application of the mineral oil, scrape the lesion and look for mites, eggs, egg casings, or feces with and without potassium hydroxide.
- If burrows are not obvious, apply ink to a suspicious area of rash. After washing off the ink with alcohol, any area that remains stained represents a burrow. This area can be scraped with a scalpel and the material examined.

Chiggers

This condition is diagnosed by the characteristic history of being in grassy areas and location of lesions.

TREATMENT

Drug resistance is becoming a problem for all classes of topical peduculicides. Occluding oils and plant oils may prove to be important treatment modalities as resistance increases. Ivermectin (Stromectol), 200 µg per kg, a broad-spectrum antihelmintic, is useful as an off-label treatment against lice and scabies.[5] It is not ovicidal, so a second dose must be given after 7 to 12 days.

- **Pediculosis**
  - Lindane (Kwell, Scabene) cream, lotion, and shampoo may be effective in treating head, body, and pubic lice. The shampoo should be left on the hair for 5 to 10 minutes prior to rinsing. After treatment, nits will remain and should be removed with a fine comb (nit comb). When the eyelashes are involved, careful manual removal is necessary. The lotion and cream should be applied over the entire affected area, washed off after 10 minutes, and repeated in 7 to 10 days. Lindane should be avoided in children younger than 2 and pregnant or lactating women.[6]
  - Pyrethrum (Rid, A-200) is available as shampoos, sprays, and gels and should be used as described with lindane.
  - Permethrin (Nix creme rinse, Elimite) is useful in the management of head and pubic lice. As in management with lindane, the nits must be removed with a nit comb.
  - Malathion 0.5% (Ovide) lotion is an alternative for refractory pediculosis. It has ovicidal activity, and is applied to the affected area and washed out 8 to 12 hours later.

- **Scabies.** Topical steroids and antihistamines may be used to help control itching. Retreatment of nonresponsive patients after 1 to 2 weeks with an alternative regimen is recommended.[6]
  - Lindane (Kwell, Scabene) 1% lotion or cream should be applied over the affected area and left on for 8 to 12 hours. Repeat application 7 to 10 days after the initial application is often necessary. Use of lindane should be avoided in children younger than 2 and in pregnant or lactating women.
  - Permethrin (Elimite) 5% cream is considered the drug of choice by many experts and, as with lindane, should be applied to the affected area and left on for 8 to 12 hours.

▓ Crotamiton (Eurax) 10% cream should be applied daily, left on for 8 to 14 hours, and reapplied once a day for 5 days. This may be less effective than lindane or permethrin.
▓ Sulfur 6% precipitated in ointment applied thinly to all areas nightly for 3 nights is effective. The old ointment should be washed off prior to application.

PREVENTION

■ All close contacts of individuals infected with pediculosis or scabies should be treated concomitantly.
■ All clothing, bed linens, and towels should be washed and dried in a hot cycle or dry cleaned.
■ Education regarding institution of adequate hygiene is important.

References
1. Lane RP, Crosskey RW, eds. Medical insects and arachnids. London: Chapman & Hall; 1993.
2. Goddard J. *Physician's guide to arthropods of medical importance.* 4th ed. Boca Raton, FL: CRC Press; 2002.
3. Chapel TA, Katta R, Kuszmar T. Pediculosis pubis in clinic for treatment of sexually transmitted disease. *Sex Transm Dis* 1979;6:257.
4. Jones JG. Chiggers. *Am Fam Physician* 1987;36(2):149.
5. Heukelbach J, Feldmeier H. Ectoparasites—the underestimated realm. *Lancet* 2004;363: 889.
6. Centers for Disease Control and Prevention. Sexually transmitted diseases treatment guidelines 2002. *MMWR* 2002;51(RR-6):67.

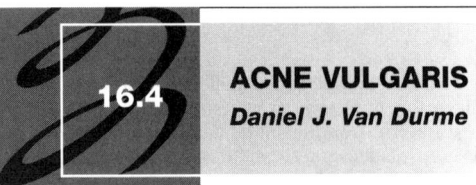

16.4 ACNE VULGARIS
Daniel J. Van Durme

GENERAL PRINCIPLES

Definition
A very common follicular disorder, particularly in adolescents.

Anatomy
Blocked pilosebaceous unit that leads to retained sebum and distention (comedones), inflammation (papules and pustules), or hypertrophy of sebum glands (nodules and cysts).

Epidemiology
Extremely common—found in about 85% of patients between 15 and 24 years old.

Classification
Mild (noninflammatory): primarily comedones; moderate (inflammatory): primarily papules and pustules; severe (nodulo-cystic): primarily nodules and cysts.

Pathophysiology and Etiology
Hypercohesive keratinocytes that block follicular opening of pilosebaceous unit. This may be idiopathic or aggravated by androgens. The organism *Propionibacterium acnes* may proliferate and lead to inflammation.

DIAGNOSIS

Clinical Presentation
Patients may present with a wide range of severity, sometimes very distressed over minimally visible lesions and at other times with minimal distress over marked physical findings.

Physical Examination

Most commonly found on the face, but may include the back, shoulders, and anterior chest wall; these areas should be examined to determine the extent of the disorder.

Differential Diagnosis

Acne vulgaris starts with microcomedones that then develop into comedones, papules, and pustules. In the absence of comedones, one should consider acne mechanica, steroid acne, or rosacea.

TREATMENT

Behavioral

Avoid excess scrubbing of the skin, this can aggravate the condition; acne is not due to poor hygiene. There is no good evidence that diet affects acne. Avoid "picking" or "popping" as these can increase the likelihood of scarring.

Medications

Choice of medication is based on several factors: (a) the predominant lesion and skin type, (b) the distribution of lesions, (c) the patient's preferences that will affect compliance, and (d) some degree of trial and error.

■ **Benzoyl peroxide** preparations (soaps, lotions, gels) used once or twice a day are an excellent starting point for all types of acne. There are many preparations available over the counter or as a prescription. The strengths range from 2.5% to 10%, with increased drying of the skin associated with higher concentrations (there is no increase in efficacy). The water-based preparations are also less drying.

■ **Mild or comedonal acne.** This is best treated with a topical retinoid, such as tretinoin, adapalene, or tazarotene applied thinly at bedtime. Always start with the lowest dose and increase strength over several weeks or months as needed and as tolerated. Erythema and irritation are common at first and can be minimized by decreasing frequency to every other day or every third day as needed. The gel and alcohol forms are more drying, and stronger. They are best used in patients with relatively oily skin or when creams fail. Azelaic acid has keratolytic, antibacterial, and anti-inflammatory properties and has shown efficacy with both mild and moderate acne. It may lead to hypopigmentation, which can be advantageous in those prone to postinflammatory hyperpigmentation, but can be a problem in ethnic groups with more skin pigment.

■ **Moderate or inflammatory (papular and pustular) acne.** This calls for the addition of antibiotics. Oral and topical agents can be used, depending on how widespread the lesions are and whether the patient prefers oral or topical therapy. Topical antibiotics are applied thinly bid after washing (with benzoyl peroxide agent) and drying the skin. Common preparations are available as solutions, gels, lotions, ointments, and creams, including erythromycin, clindamycin, and sulfacetamide. Choice of the vehicle should depend on the patient's skin type. Those with oily skin may do better with the drying effects of gels and solutions, whereas those with dry skin may do better with the moisturizing effects of lotions, creams, and ointments. Topical erythromycin and clindamycin are most effective when used with benzoyl peroxide and there are commercial preparations that combine these into one. Oral antibiotics are indicated when lesions are widespread (making topical application impractical) or severe. First-line agents include tetracycline or erythromycin at 1 g per day in divided doses. Tetracycline may cause photosensitivity, and qid dosing on an empty stomach makes compliance difficult. Gastrointestinal (GI) upset can be common with erythromycin, and increasing resistance is noted with this agent. Minocycline 50 to 100 mg qd-bid, or doxycycline 50 mg (occasionally 100 mg) qd-bid, and less commonly trimethoprim–sulfamethoxazole 160/800 mg bid can be helpful. Oral agents are generally stronger than topical agents and can be used when topicals fail.

■ **Nodulocystic acne,** the most severe form of acne vulgaris, can cause emotional and physical scarring. Treatment starts with judicious use of the agents above, but the condition can often be resistant to these therapies. When this happens, oral isotretinoin may be indicated; see special considerations below.

■ **Oral contraceptives (OCs).** Several OCs are Food and Drug Administration (FDA)-approved for use in acne. These have low doses of estrogen and nonandrogenic progestins, such as norgestimate, levonorgestrel, or desogestrel. Therapy must be used for 2 to 4 months to see effects.

Counseling

The potential physical disfigurement from acne, whether temporary from the current lesions or from scarring, can be extremely distressing for the adolescent who is developing a self-image and who may be very self-conscious. The psychologic trauma from acne for a developing adolescent should not be underestimated and general supportive counseling can be very helpful. This is also a valuable time to teach adolescents about self-care and responsibility for their own health.

Patient Education

Acne is controlled (not cured) with medications. The patient will need to continue to use treatments to prevent new lesions even after the current lesions have resolved. Treatments are designed to prevent new lesions far more than clearing existing lesions. Thus, topical treatments should be applied all over the affected area, not just on the lesions themselves. Some patients notice an initial worsening with treatment before it improves. They need to be warned of this so they do not stop medications prematurely.

Follow-Up

Expect 4 to 8 weeks to see significant improvement with most treatments. Recommend follow-up about every 6 weeks until the optimal regimen has been determined, then every 2 to 3 months for maintenance and adjustments.

Results

Most acne can be well controlled with some combination of medications as listed above. It may take time to determine the ideal regimen, but patients should be reassured that there are extremely effective treatments to control this condition. Nevertheless, optimal treatment may never make the skin look "completely normal."

Complications

Scarring from deep lesions or from self-inflicted picking at lesions.

SPECIAL CONSIDERATIONS

Isotretinoin can be *tremendously effective* in cases of severe, recalcitrant, nodulocystic acne. This agent is also *highly* teratogenic, and has numerous side effects, including myalgias, arthralgias, epistaxis, xerosis, liver function elevation, hyperlipidemia, and leukopenia. Frequent monitoring of bloodwork is advised. In order to obtain isotretinoin, the prescriber, pharmacy, and patient must receive specific information through an FDA program called iPLEDGE and become registered (www.ipledgeprogram.com). The numerous administrative burdens and potential complications with this medicine have led many family physicians to stop prescribing this medicine and refer these patients to a dermatologist.

References

1. *Management of acne.* Summary, Evidence Report/Technology Assessment: Number 17. AHRQ Publication No. 01-E018, March. Rockville, MD: Agency for Healthcare Research and Quality; 2001. Available online at http://www.ahrq.gov/clinic/epcsums/acnesum.htm.
2. Webster GF. Acne vulgaris. *BMJ* 2002;325:475.
3. Haider A, Shaw JC. Treatment of acne vulgaris. *JAMA* 2004; 292:726.
4. James WD. Acne. *N Engl J Med* 2005;352:1463.
5. Liao DC. Management of acne. *J Fam Pract* 2003;52:43.

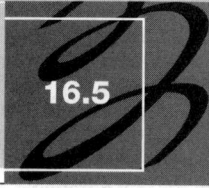

COMMON DERMATOSES

Rhonda A. Sparks, Brian Coleman,
Kalyanakrishnan Ramakrishnan

16.5

ermatologic problems are commonly encountered in the primary care setting. This chapter reviews the diagnosis and management of seven of the most common dermatoses encountered in clinical practice.

PSORIASIS

General Principles

Definition

Psoriasis is a life-long papulosquamous dermatologic disorder characterized by chronic recurrent bouts of characteristic erythematous papules and scaling plaques.

Anatomy

Psoriasis may be ubiquitous in its distribution. In children under age 2 it may present as a diaper rash.[1]

Epidemiology

Psoriasis affects between 1% and 3% of the population. It is found equally in men and women, and usually presents in the second or third decade of life, but may be seen in infants and elderly people. Psoriasis is much less common in African Americans, Native Americans, and Asians than in whites.[2]

Classification

Several forms of psoriasis, as defined by morphology and location, exist.

- **Chronic plaque psoriasis** is the most common morphologic presentation.
- **Guttate psoriasis** (multiple, small, droplike) usually develops prior to age 20, and is usually preceded by a streptococcal or viral upper respiratory tract infection.
- **Generalized pustular psoriasis** is a rare, serious, and sometimes fatal variant. Patients develop fever, malaise, diarrhea, and leukocytosis. This form of psoriasis may be precipitated by withdrawal from systemic steroids.
- **Erythrodermic psoriasis** is another rare and potentially fatal form of psoriasis, occurring in patients with previously stable, chronic psoriasis. Light-sensitive psoriasis is usually precipitated by solar exposure (in some patients hypersensitive to ultraviolet light).
- **Psoriasis of the scalp** presents with characteristic plaques that are more difficult to treat as they are anchored to the scalp by hair.
- **Psoriasis of the palms and soles** may be a distinct entity marked by exclusive involvement of the palms and soles or involvement (though uncommon) as part of a generalized eruption.
- **Pustular psoriasis** of the palms and soles cause deep pustules of the central palm and central sole of the foot.
- **Keratoderma blennorrhagicum** is a form of psoriasis that develops in patients with Reiter syndrome.
- **Psoriasis inversus** affects less common areas including the axillae, groin, submammary folds, and other intertriginous areas.
- **HIV-induced psoriasis** may have an atypical clinical presentation, and an unusually severe course.

Pathophysiology

Typical psoriatic plaques show characteristic changes including hyperproliferation of epidermal keratinocytes and hyperkeratosis, and infiltration of immunocytes along with

611

angiogenesis, with resultant thickening and scaling of the erythematous skin. Mitotic activity of keratinocytes is greatly increased.[2]

Etiology

A genetic predisposition to psoriasis is postulated, although the exact pattern of inheritance is unclear. It appears that genetic predilection in combination with environmental factors precipitates the disease. Symptoms of psoriasis usually improve during summer, which may reflect the presumed positive effect of sunlight. Of patients with childhood psoriasis, 71% have a positive family history.[2]

Mechanisms of Injury

Physical trauma may trigger the appearance of psoriatic lesions, and is referred to as Koebner phenomenon.

Diagnosis

Clinical Presentation

Characteristic dermatologic lesions of psoriasis are red, scaling papules that coalesce into larger plaques. The classic scale of psoriasis is silvery white. There may be small, pinpoint areas of bleeding known as Auspitz sign. The plaques of psoriasis may become thick, especially on the scalp. Psoriasis without scaling is most common in the intertriginous areas, where it can appear as smooth, red, or macerated plaques. Psoriasis affects the extensor surfaces more commonly than the flexures and, in its most common form, spares the palm, soles, and face. Severe psoriasis may be a presenting finding in HIV infection. Psoriatic nail changes and psoriatic arthritis are the most common extracutaneous manifestations of psoriasis, and occur in 5% to 20% of patients with psoriasis.[2] Scalp lesions are seen in approximately 50% of patients with psoriasis.

History

Approximately 30% of patients with psoriasis have their first episode before age 20.[1] In many cases, the initial presentation is that of guttate psoriasis—psoriatic rash developing after a streptococcal or viral upper respiratory infection. Guttate psoriasis may resolve spontaneously, with recurrence of chronic plaque psoriasis common. Pruritis is variable. Response to treatment is often temporary. Exacerbations and remissions are usual. Psoriatic arthritis is more common in patients with severe dermatologic disease. Medications may also precipitate or exacerbate the disease. These include lithium, quinidine, clonidine, iodine, indomethacin, some beta-blockers, terfenadine, nonsteroidal anti-inflammatory drugs (NSAIDs), angiotensin-converting enzyme (ACE) inhibitors, interferon-alpha, interleukin-2, isotretinoin, and anti-malarial agents.

Physical Examination

Psoriasis most commonly presents with noninflammatory, well-defined, localized plaques involving the extensor surfaces of the elbows, the scalp, the gluteal cleft, and the nails of both the hands and feet. If these occur in intertriginous areas, they may appear inflamed (i.e., bright red and shiny). If a plaque resolves, the skin demonstrates a temporary brown or white macule. The joints may exhibit asymmetric arthritis of one or more joints of the fingers and toes, most often the proximal interphalangeal (PIP), distal interphalangeal (DIP), metatarsophalangeal, or metacarpophalangeal joints. The joint may be red, warm, painful, and exhibit soft tissue swelling known as "sausage finger." Range of motion may be decreased. Nail changes, including pitting, yellowing, and severe nail dystrophy, are most commonly seen among patients with joint involvement. Ocular involvement occurs in some patients with psoriatic arthritis. Uveitis, which is the most common manifestation, may present with insidious visual impairment or with acute, painful red eye.

Laboratory Studies

Laboratory tests are of limited value in this disease. If guttate psoriasis is suspected, throat cultures may be obtained to rule out streptococcal infection. There is a high incidence of positive, antistreptolysin O (ASO) titers in this group.[1] If psoriatic arthritis is suspected, other rheumatologic causes of arthritis should be ruled out. Rheumatoid factor levels are usually normal, although a small percentage of patients with psoriatic arthritis will have mild elevations.[1] Erythrocyte sedimentation rate (ESR), white blood cell counts (WBC), and uric acid levels may show mild elevation but have limited predictive value in the diagnosis of psoriatic arthritis.

Imaging
The most severe form of psoriatic arthritis is arthritis mutilans, which classically presents with marked deformity and destruction of the digits on radiograph.

Monitoring
The ESR is the best laboratory test to monitor disease activity.

Surgical Diagnostic Procedures
In rare instances, when the diagnosis is not apparent on clinical presentation, punch biopsy of skin lesions may be diagnostic.

Classification
Diagnostic classification is based on morphology and location of psoriatic lesions (see above). For treatment options, patients are classified according to percentage of body surface affected by psoriasis. Patients with less than 20% of body surface involvement can be managed with topical therapy. Patients with greater cutaneous involvement require more aggressive therapy.

Differential Diagnosis
Seborrheic dermatitis is commonly confused with psoriasis. Chronic eczema with lichenification may present with thickened plaques, and should be included in the differential diagnosis. Other considerations include superficial fungal infections, lichen planus, pityriasis rosea, squamous cell carcinoma, and cutaneous T-cell lymphoma.[3]

Treatment
Behavioral
A positive correlation between the severity of psoriatic symptoms and psychologic stress has been demonstrated. Stress reduction techniques are, therefore, useful in some patients.[1]

Medications
Disease control, including decreasing frequency and exacerbations, should be the goal of therapy. The mainstay of treatment in mild psoriasis (less than 20% cutaneous involvement) is topical therapy with or without ultraviolet light exposure. Most common topical treatments include topical steroids, calcipotriene (Doponex), tazarotene (Tazorac), anthralin, and tar. Topical steroids provide rapid response and control itching and inflammation. Disadvantages include tolerance and skin atrophy. Efficacy may be increased by using occlusive dressings. Calcipotriene produces long remissions but may cause severe irritation and burning. Tazaratene (a retinoid) can also be very irritating to the skin. Efficacy of these medications may be enhanced, and irritation decreased, by concomitant topical steroid use. Anthralin can be used in short bursts, and is effective for scalp psoriasis. It is most effective on chronic, noninflamed plaques, and when used with ultraviolet light (UVB) therapy. Tar solutions are effective in only a small percentage of patients and are best combined with UVB light. There appears to be no benefit of adding ultraviolet therapy to topical steroids.[1] Regimens including ultraviolet therapy require major commitment of time and money making them less accessible.

Therapeutic options for severe psoriasis (involving greater than 20% of the cutaneous surface) include ultraviolet light (UVB) and tar solutions as well as the use of psoralens, along with exposure to long-wave ultraviolet light (PUVA). PUVA therapy is effective for symptomatic control of severe and disabling plaque psoriasis, but requires significant time commitment, and is not effective for scalp lesions. Because of concerns with long-term exposure and toxicity, PUVA is most appropriate for patients older than 50 years of age. Other treatment options for severe psoriasis include methotrexate, acitretin, and cyclosporin. Methotrexate and cyclosporin are effective in psoriatic arthritis but are of limited value secondary to hepatotoxicity and nephrotoxicity, respectively.[1] Combining PUVA with UVB, calcipotriene, tazaratene, acitretin, or methotrexate improves efficacy, and decreases cost and adverse effects of treatment.

Recent advances in psoriasis research have provided biologic agents that target key mechanisms in the pathogenesis of psoriasis. Three agents, currently approved by the Food and Drug Administration for the treatment of psoriasis, include alefacept, efalizumab, and etanercept. These agents bind to specific cells and do not have multiorgan adverse effects as seen with acitretin, cyclosporine, or methotrexate.[2] Rotation of these available therapies for severe psoriasis may minimize toxicity, and allow for effective long-term treatment.

Referrals

Treatment of severe psoriasis and frequent exacerbations and medications used in their management require frequent monitoring, best accomplished through specialized dermatologic care. If psoriatic arthritis is suspected, rheumatologic referral is recommended.

Patient Education

Patients should be informed of the chronic nature of this disease. Environmental factors, medications, and stress exacerbating psoriasis should be avoided.

Follow-Up

Frequent follow-up is important to determine effectiveness of treatment. Some systemic therapeutic agents require special testing to avoid medication side effects.

ACNE ROSACEA

General Principles

Definition

Rosacea is a chronic acneiform dermatologic disorder characterized by erthyema, edema, papules and pustules, and telangiectasia, usually affecting middle-aged individuals, with periods of remission and exacerbation.[4]

Anatomy

Rosacea common involves the central face area including the nose, forehead, cheeks, and sometimes periorbital and eyelid areas. Hyperplasia of the soft tissue of the nose (rhinophyma) may occur in long-standing rosacea.

Epidemiology

Rosacea most commonly occurs between the ages of 30 and 60 years of age, although it has rarely been reported in younger individuals. It is relatively common among individuals with light hair and eye color, fair skin, and patients who have a history of experiencing blushing or flushing.

Classification

Rosacea disorders are divided into four broad subtypes to guide diagnosis and treatment:

- Erythematotelangiectatic characterized by flushing, stinging, and burning
- Papulopustular (classic), characterized by small papules and pinpoint pustules
- Phymatous, characterized by marked skin thickening and surface nodularities
- Ocular, characterized by blepharitis and conjunctivitis[5]

A fifth type—glandular, characterized by sebaceous gland hyperplasia—has been proposed.

Pathophysiology

The cardinal features include erthyema, edema, papules and pustules, and telangiectasia.[4]

Etiology

The cause of rosacea is unknown. Infection with the hair mites *Demodex folliculorum* and *D. brevis* may be contributory. One study found an increased frequency of *Helicobacter pylori* infection,[5] but current literature does not support this to be a causative factor.

Diagnosis

Clinical Presentation

The earliest manifestations include facial erythema and fine telangiectasia typically involving the cheek. This may progress to a papular or cystic rash involving the cheeks, nose, or forehead. Patients may also present with ocular symptoms.

History

Patients with rosacea usually have a history of recurrent flushing, precipitated by hot or spicy foods, alcohol consumption, temperature changes and extremes, or emotional stimulus. Symptoms may also be brought on or aggravated by sun exposure, but solar skin damage is not a prerequisite for the development of rosacea.[4] Later in the disease process, patients may develop hyperplasia of sebaceous glands with accompanying papules, pustules, and nodules resembling acne vulgaris. Ocular symptoms may develop alone or in association with skin lesions, and may include burning, foreign body sensation, meibomian gland dysfunction, blepharitis, conjunctivitis, or episcleritis. Cystic lesions of the nose can occur late in the disease, mostly in middle-aged men.

Physical Examination

Classic skin findings include **erythema** of the forehead, cheeks, and nose. Close inspection may reveal telangiectasias. These may be accompanied by papules, pustules, nodules, and cysts. Comedones are not characteristic of rosacea. Granuloma formation, characterized by hard papules or nodules, may be severe and most apparent on the nose, representing rhinophyma. Ocular involvement may present with mild conjunctivitis, conjunctival hyperemia, telangiectasia of the lid, blepharitis, and chalazion. The National Rosacea Society Expert Committee recommends the presence of one or more of the following primary features for diagnosis:

- Flushing (transient erythema)
- Nontransient erythema
- Papules and pustules
- Telangiectasia

The following secondary features may appear with primary features:

- Burning or stinging
- Plaque
- Dry appearance
- Edema
- Ocular manifestations
- Peripheral location
- Phymatous changes[5]

Laboratory Studies

Laboratory studies are not helpful in diagnosis.

Surgical Diagnostic Procedures

Diagnosis of rosacea is clinical. Punch biopsy may be helpful if diagnostic uncertainty is present.

Differential Diagnosis

Differential diagnosis includes acne vulgaris, seborrheic dermatitis, carcinoid syndrome, systemic lupus erthymatosus (SLE), and chronic topical steroid use. Rosacea is differentiated from acne vulgaris by the absence of comedones, and from SLE by the presence of papules and pustules. Seborrheic dermatitis usually has prominent scales. Carcinoid syndrome is rare and may cause brief flushing. The cutaneous effects of chronic topical steroids can be indistinguishable from rosacea but resolves with its discontinuation.

Treatment

Behavioral

Control of symptoms is the goal of therapy.

Medications

The three topical medications approved by the Food and Drug Administration for rosacea include topical solutions of **metronidazole,** several brands of **sodium sulfacetamide with sulfur,** and **azelaic acid gel.** Metronidazole, either alone or combined with oral antibiotics, is frequently used for initial therapy to decrease inflammation and erythema. The azelaic acid gel is as effective as metronidazole, although its use is limited by skin irritation. Sodium sulfacetamide is less effective than metronidazole and azelaic acid gel. Topical agents should be used for at least 4 weeks before assessing effectiveness. If symptoms persist after initial topical therapy, tretinoin cream may be useful in papular or pustular lesions, and may be combined with topical antibiotics. Oral antibiotics may be necessary for nodular rosacea or in patients with ocular involvement. Effective oral antibiotics include **tetracycline, doxycycline, erythromycin,** and **minocycline.** Maintaining remission with **topical metronidazole** is required after initial therapy. **Oral clonidine** and **beta-blockers** have been used with some success in flushing associated with rosacea.[5]

Surgery

Vascular laser therapy and light therapy may be useful in telangiectasias.

Special Therapy

Minimizing sun exposure is important . Broad-spectrum sunscreen should be applied daily. Some sunscreens can cause irritation and trigger rosacea. Silicon-based preparations are the best. A combination sunscreen and 1% metronidazole is now marketed in Canada. Cosmetic sensitivity is a common feature of rosacea and therefore cosmetic use should be minimized. Astringents and camphor-containing products should also be avoided.[6]

Referrals

Referral to a dermatologist is indicated if response to topical and oral therapy is inadequate. Referral to an ophthalmologist is recommended if ocular rosacea is suspected.

Patient Education

See Special Therapy.

Follow-Up

After initial treatment, follow-up is required in 6 to 8 weeks to determine treatment efficacy.

Complications

Patients with rosacea can develop ocular symptoms that include subnormal tear production, corneal vascularization, and infiltration. Visual acuity may be affected.

ATOPIC DERMATITIS

General Principles

Definition

Atopic dermatitis (AD) is a chronic, inflammatory skin condition commonly seen in people with a personal or family history of allergic rhinitis or asthma. It is commonly referred to as "eczema." In modern usage, AD and atopic eczema are used interchangeably, and both are acceptable.[7]

Anatomy

AD occurring in infants usually involves the cheeks and spares the perioral and perinasal areas. In childhood (2 to 12 years), it most commonly affects the flexure surfaces including the antecubital fossae, neck, wrists, and ankles. In adults (older than 12 years) AD involves the flexures but also may involve the hands and periorbital area.[8]

Epidemiology

The prevalence of AD has steadily increased over the past 50 years, and now affects more than 10% of children.[9] More than 60% of patients present before the first year of life. It is rare in adults.[7]

Classification

Classification is based on age—infant phase (0 to 2 years), childhood phase (2 to 12 years), and adult phase (12 years and older).

Pathophysiology

The epidermis in AD shows spongiosis and a damaged stratum corneum. This breakdown of the normal barrier exposes patients to environmental irritants, antigens, and infectious agents. Atopic patients exhibit reduced cell-mediated immunity, high concentrations of serum immunoglobulin E (IgE), and a high incidence of IgE-mediated responses on skin testing. They also have a predominance of a specific T cell that causes high concentrations of serum IgE, eosinophilia, and the initial inflammatory response.[9]

Etiology

The precise immunologic mechanism involved in the development of AD is unclear. Allergic triggers such as some foods, dust mites, and animal dander have been implicated. AD-associated food allergies are more common in childhood while airborne allergens are more commonly associated with AD in adults. Other triggers may include temperature change and sweating, excessive washing, contact with irritating substances, and decreased humidity.[8]

Diagnosis

Clinical Presentation

In infants, typical skin lesions include scaling on erythematous papules involving cheeks. These lesions may also affect the extremities or trunk, sparing the diaper area. In children, intensely pruritic patches more commonly affect the flexure surfaces of the arms and legs. Adults present with a distribution of lesions similar to children but may also have lesions on the hands and eyelids.

History
Patients with AD usually have symptoms from childhood. Many patients with AD also exhibit symptoms of allergic rhinitis and/or asthma. Lesions are intensely pruritic. Patients may have history of recurrent bacterial, fungal, and viral skin infections. Food allergies in children and airborne allergens in adults may trigger AD flares.

Physical Examination
Acute lesions of AD are usually vesicles and may have exudate. More chronic lesions usually demonstrate thickened skin, increased skin markings (lichenification), and excoriated papules and plaques. The flexure areas most commonly involved include antecubital and popliteal fossae, wrists, and forearms. Severe cases may affect any skin surface, although lesions of the axillae, gluteal, or groin area are uncommon. Scratching, leading to destruction of melanocytes, results in areas of hypopigmentation. Associated clinical findings may include severe xerosis, development of ichthyosis, keratosis pilaris, hyperlinear palmar creases, and atopic pleats (appearance of an extra line on the lower eyelid, also known as Dennie–Morgan infraorbital fold).[8]

Laboratory Studies
Allergy testing may be of benefit to identify triggers causing AD flares.

Surgical Diagnostic Procedures
Punch biopsy may be indicated if clinical diagnosis is obtuse.

Differential Diagnosis
Differential diagnosis of AD includes contact dermatitis, seborrheic dermatitis, drug reactions, psoriasis, and scabies. In infants the rare disorders Wiskott–Aldrich syndrome and hyperimmunoglobulin E syndrome should be considered.

Treatment
Behavioral
Management of AD requires a comprehensive approach that addresses skin inflammation as well as elimination of exacerbating factors. Contact with wool, excessive heat, and other irritants should be minimized. Airborne allergens and allergenic foods must be identified and avoided. Skin hydration is key and skin must be moisturized by the application of non-irritating, hydrophobic lubricating agents.[11]

Medications
Acute flares of AD may require potent **topical corticosteroid** preparations for 7 to 10 days. **Tar preparations** can help control pruritus and resolve inflammation, decreasing the need for topical corticosteroids. **Antihistamines** also control pruritus. Nonsedating antihistamines may have some anti-inflammatory effects. **PUVA** or **UVB** phototherapy are options in patients resistant to conventional measures. Ongoing therapeutic trials using immunomodulators show promise.[11] **Oral immunosuppressants** such as methotrexate or azathioprine may be considered in severe AD but should be avoided in children. **Oral corticosteroids** should be reserved for severe flares not responding to topical therapy.

Referrals
Referral to a dermatologist is appropriate if the diagnosis is uncertain, in patients failing to respond to conventional therapy, or if systemic immunosuppressive agents are considered necessary.

Protocol
Disease management should be considered in three phases: (a) Induction of remission, (b) maintenance, and (c) rescue from flares. Induction of remission usually requires steroids while emollients are critical for maintenance therapy. Rescue from flares involves treatment of secondary infections with oral antibiotics and avoiding exposure to triggers.

Follow-Up
Patients should be followed regularly to assess treatment efficacy.

Complications
Complications of chronic steroid use include skin atrophy, telangiectasia, striae, steroid rosacea, acne, hypopigmentation, and delayed wound healing.[11]

Special Considerations
Dealing with this chronic disease may result in emotional sequelae, but AD is not an emotional disorder as previously thought.

ALLERGIC AND IRRITANT CONTACT DERMATITIS
General Principles
Definition
Allergic contact dermatitis (ACD) is an inflammatory skin reaction that follows absorption of some antigen applied to the skin and recruitment of previously sensitized antigen-specific T lymphocytes. Irritant contact dermatitis (ICD) is an inflammatory skin reaction that results from direct epidermal damage produced by contact with an irritant and is not immunologic. ICD can affect any person at any time if the irritant and exposure are sufficient, while ACD requires a susceptible individual with prior sensitization by the allergen. Systemic contact dermatitis (SCD) is an inflammatory skin reaction that occurs in a previously sensitized person, following exposure to the allergen by ingestion, inhalation, or injection (e.g., patients allergic to poison ivy may develop a diffuse inflammatory skin reaction following ingestion of raw cashew nuts, which are chemically related to the specific allergen of poison ivy).[12]

Anatomy
Site of exposure of the suspected allergen is usually congruent with the distribution of the rash (under a watchband, elastic waistband, or shoe). Plants usually produce linear lesions at the site of contact. Half of all ACD involves the hands.[13] ACD usually affects the dorsum of the hand, where the skin is thinner. ACD secondary to allergens applied to the head will usually involve the hairline or ears, and spares the scalp, where the skin is thick. Airborne allergens, which can be transferred from the hands to the eyes and face, and cosmetics may cause facial involvement. The torso and groin are affected in the area of application of the allergen. Involvement of the oral mucosa is rare, but may occur with dental implants. Genitalia is commonly involved secondary to transfer of the allergens from hands.

Epidemiology
CD constitutes 80% of contact dermatitis. Industrial workers are at high risk for occupational skin exposure.

Classification
Contact dermatitis is classified as ICD, ACD, or SCD (see definition).

Pathophysiology
Unlike most clinical allergic diseases, which involve an immediate hypersensitivity response, ACD is a delayed (cell-mediated) hypersensitivity reaction that depends on previous sensitization in susceptible individuals. ICD results from direct epidermal damage. SCD involves systemic re-exposure following previous sensitization to an allergen applied topically.

Etiology
ACD is caused by exposure to common contact allergens including poison ivy, poison oak, poison sumac, nickel (the most common metal allergen), topical medications (neomycin and bacitracin), latex and rubber chemicals, formaldehyde, and balsam of Peru (most common fragrance implicated in ACD).

Diagnosis
Clinical Presentation
ACD presents as an acute pruritic eruption.

History
History should be directed at uncovering contact allergens—specifically work-related exposure, plant exposure, household products, jewelry, clothing, and cosmetics. The timing of an eruption may be as brief as 8 hours (common with plant exposure) and as remote as 1 week after exposure. Pruritus is uniformly present in ACD.

Physical Examination

The acute phase of ACD involves erythema, edema, and vesicles. Vesicles may coalesce to form bullae. Vesicles contain clear fluid and rupture spontaneously during the subacute stage (most common presentation). Vesicles are then replaced by papules, which develop crusting and scaling. Secondary bacterial infection may occur. As the papulovesicular lesions resolve, the chronic stage involving lichenification and scaling occurs.[13]

Laboratory Studies

Patch testing is the gold standard for diagnosis of ACD. It involves reproducing ACD by applying the same or a cross-reacting allergen (23 allergens known to be responsible for 80% of ACD) on a small area of the patient's skin. Patch testing is indicated when inflammation persists despite avoiding the offending agent. Reaction is noted at 48 hours and 4 to 7 days. A negative test does not rule out ACD as sufficient concentration of allergen may not be provided with standard testing.[12]

Staging

Lesions may present in acute, subacute, or chronic stages (see Physical Examination).

Differential Diagnosis

The differential diagnosis includes atopic dermatitis, seborrheic dermatitis, nummular eczema, dishydrotic eczema, photocontact dermatitis, psoriasis, T-cell lymphoma, and bacterial, fungal, or viral skin infections.

Treatment

Behavioral

Central to ACD prevention and treatment is identifying specific allergens and avoiding contact with them. If the allergen cannot be avoided, wearing a protective barrier is recommended.

Medications

Initial treatment of vesicles and erythema includes cold compresses, which should be used for 15 to 30 minutes initially during the acute stage. Erythema may respond to topical corticosteroids. Hydroxyzine and diphenhydramine control itching. If dermatitis is severe or widespread, involves mucous membranes, or is unresponsive to initial therapy, **systemic corticosteroids** should be used. ACD due to plant allergens require 10 to 21 days of treatment with **topical or oral corticosteroids** to prevent rebound dermatitis.[14]

Referrals

Referral to a dermatologist if the diagnosis is unclear or if the patient is unresponsive to conventional therapy.

Patient Education

See Behavioral.

Follow-Up

Patients should be instructed to follow-up if rash does not resolve or worsens, as rebound dermatitis is possible and may be more severe than the initial eruption.

Special Considerations

The appearance of new lesions remote from the initial eruption, seen in plant contact dermatitis (Rhus dermatitis), may be confused with active spread of the disease. Contrary to popular belief, vesicle fluid does not contain allergen and cannot spread the inflammation.

SEBORRHEIC DERMATITIS

General Principles

Definition

Seborrheic dermatitis (SD) is a chronic, inflammatory papulosquamous skin disease, characterized by erythema and scaling.

Anatomy

The term "seborrhea" suggests the anatomic distribution of this disorder, which is predominantly in areas where sebaceous glands are abundant—the scalp, face, and upper trunk. Seborrhea also tends to present under mustaches and beards, eyebrows, and nasolabial folds. In infants, seborrhea commonly affects the scalp and is termed "cradle cap."[15]

Epidemiology
In infants, seborrhea usually presents in the first 3 months of life. In adults, seborrhea is most commonly seen between 30 and 60 years of age.

Classification
Seborrhea is classified by age as **adolescent and adult SD** and **infant SD**. Infant SD may have a classic scalp distribution, or may be generalized. Generalized infant SD is associated with immunodeficiency and warrants further diagnostic evaluation.

Etiology
The etiology of SD is unknown. *Malassezia furfur* (formerly *Pityrysporum ovale*) has been implicated, but both genetic and environmental factors seem to influence the onset and course of the disease.[16] Other possible causes include hormones, nutritional deficiencies, and a neurogenic cause (based on the association with parkinsonism and other neurologic syndromes).[17]

Diagnosis
Clinical Presentation
Patients with SD typically present with erythema and mild epidermal hyperproliferation leading to scaliness. The erythema of SD is usually pink-red rather that bright red as in psoriasis.[15] SD in infants is not usually pruritic, whereas adult SD has varying degrees of pruritus.

History
The onset of seborrhea in infants is usually in the first 3 months of life with scalp involvement. Adults present with an itchy red rash. Patients may have a history of "dandruff" (mild seborrhea), with progression and worsening of symptoms. Symptoms may be worse in the winter with dry indoor environments. Sunlight may cause some patients to flare while promoting improvement in others. SD is a chronic disease in adults, with periods of remission and flares.

Physical Examination
SD of the scalp presents as mildly greasy scaling and erythema. Blepharitis may also be present. On the chest, SD presents with follicular and parafollicular papules with scales. In infants, SD presents with thick scales and erythema of the vertex of the scalp.[17] If lotions or oils have been applied to the scalp, SD may appear intensely erythematous without scales.

Laboratory Studies
Fungal cultures and potassium hydroxide (KOH) preparations may be indicated in resistant cases.

Pathologic Findings
Histologically, SD reveals focal parakeratosis, with few neutrophils, moderate acanthosis, spongiosis, and nonspecific inflammation of the dermis. The most characteristic finding is neutrophils at the tips of dilated follicular openings.

Differential Diagnosis
SD of the scalp and face should be differentiated from tinea capitis, psoriasis, atopic dermatitis, impetigo, and rosacea. SD involving the trunk should be differentiated from pityriasis versicolor and pityriasis rosea. Underlying immunodeficiency should be suspected in generalized SD in infants, especially if associated with diarrhea and weight loss.[17] Immunodeficiency should be suspected in adults who present with severe, recalcitrant cases of SD.

Treatment
Behavioral
Emotional stress has been linked to SD flares.

Medications
Effective treatment options include keratolytics, antifungals, and anti-inflammatory agents. Keratolytics induce sloughing of cornified epithelium. Salicylic acid, zinc pyrithione, and tar shampoos are effective for lesions involving the scalp and face. Treatment of infantile SD requires milder formulations. Shampoos may be used two to three times per week. Anti-inflammatory topical agents and shampoos such as fluocinolone shampoo and cream are also effective. Patients may apply a topical steroid once or twice a day with a shampoo.

Topical calcineurin inhibitors have anti-inflammatory and antifungal properties. Most antifungal agents are effective against *Malassezia* species associated with SD. Ketoconazole and selenium sulfide shampoos are commonly used. Ketoconazole preparations should be avoided in infants.[17]

Special Therapy
Seborrheic blepharitis may respond to cleansing of the eyelashes with baby shampoo and cotton-tipped applicators as the use of ketoconazole in this area is controversial.

Referrals
Referral to dermatology is typically required only in recalcitrant or very severe cases.

Patient Education
Patients should be educated that this is a chronic disorder that may require continued maintenance therapy.

Special Considerations
SD is the most common cutaneous manifestation of AIDS.[16] Severe intractable or extensive seborrhea should prompt evaluation for HIV infection.

PITYRIASIS ROSEA
General Principles
Definition
Pityriasis Rosea (PR) is an acute, self-limiting papulosquamous skin eruption, preceded by a viral illness in 69% of patients.[18]

Anatomy
PR typically involves the trunk and proximal extremities, but in rare cases may involve the arms, legs, and face. An inverse presentation, involving the extremities, is rarely seen.

Epidemiology
The average age of patients affected with PR is 23, with most cases occurring between 10 and 35 years of age. PR occurs most often in the spring and fall.

Classification
The initial phase involves appearance of the "herald patch," followed 7 to 14 days later by a generalized eruption—the "eruptive phase."

Etiology
The etiology of PR is unclear, although an infectious agent is likely. This is supported by the fact that PR occurs in clusters, rarely recurs, and is preceded commonly by a prodromal illness.

Diagnosis
Clinical Presentation
Typical presentation is a prodromal viral illness (headache, malaise, pharyngitis), followed by the herald patch and subsequent smaller salmon-colored lesions of the eruptive phase.

History
Many patients will report an upper respiratory illness a few weeks prior to the rash. The herald patch is typically seen on the torso or proximal arm. Then, 7 to 14 days later, similar smaller oval lesions appear on the trunk and proximal extremities. The majority of patients (over 75%) will also report pruritus. The rash of PR resolves spontaneously in 5 to 8 weeks.[19]

Physical Examination
The herald patch is a 2- to 10-cm ovoid erythematous, raised patch with a peripheral collarette of fine scales. Subsequent eruption involves similar 5- to 10-mm salmon-colored lesions with a characteristic distribution following lines of cleavage (Christmas tree pattern). Lesions may be excoriated.

Laboratory Studies
Physicians may perform KOH testing to rule out tinea. Serologic testing for syphilis is a consideration in appropriate clinical settings.

Pathologic Findings

Histologically, PR demonstrates parakeratosis with or without acanthosis, spongiosis, a perivascular infiltrate of lymphocytes and histiocytes.

Differential Diagnosis

Psoriasis, secondary syphilis, tinea corporis, Lyme disease, HIV seroconversion illness, and drug eruptions (e.g., hepatitis B vaccine, interferon, captopril, clonidine) should all be considered.[17]

Treatment

Behavioral

Patients should be counseled that PR is a self-limited illness.

Medications

PR, as it is self-limited, requires only symptomatic treatment. Oral antihistamines, topical agents (steroids and calamine) may be used for relief of pruritus. Systemic steroids may be used in extensive lesions with severe pruritus, but may lengthen the course of the illness.

Special Therapy

PR may be alleviated by UVB phototherapy or natural sunlight exposure if started in the first week of symptoms.

Referrals

Consider referral to dermatology for variable lesion morphology, or if lesions are more extensive or last longer than expected.

Patient Education

Educate patients about etiology (unknown), infectivity (very low), relapse (uncommon), and complications (rare).

Follow-Up

Patients should be instructed to follow up if rash persists longer than 3 months.

Complications

Complications are rare, but postinflammatory hyperpigmentation or hypopigmentation may occur.[17]

SUPERFICIAL FUNGAL INFECTIONS

General Principles

Definition

Fungal dermatoses are superficial spreading infections of cutaneous surfaces caused commonly by dermatophytes.

Anatomy

Common areas affected by fungal dermatoses are scalp (hair and hair follicles), trunk, groin, feet, nails and nail beds of fingers and toes.

Epidemiology

Dermatophyte infections usually affect otherwise healthy individuals. Patients with compromised immunity are particularly susceptible to severe and persistent infections. Approximately 20% of the U.S. population has a dermatophytic infection. Tinea pedis is the most common dermatophyte infection. Tinea cruris is more common in males. Tinea capitis is most common in children 6 to 10 years of age.

Classification

Dermatophyte infections are classified according to the area affected, including the scalp (tinea capitis), hair (tinea barbae), trunk, face, and limbs (tinea corporis), inguinal area (tinea cruris), pedal interdigital area (tinea pedis), and nails of the hands and feet (tinea unguium).[20]

Pathophysiology

Dermatophytes are usually present in the dead cornified layers of the skin. Dermatophytes are able to metabolize keratin, a protein resistant to most other organisms, as a nutrient source.

Etiology
Three types of dermatophytes cause the majority of infections: epidermophyton, trichophyton, and microsporum.

Diagnosis
Clinical Presentation
Tinea capitis and tinea barbae present with an erythematous scaly, well-demarcated patch. This patch will spread over a period of weeks to months, and then remain stable and persistent. Multiple lesions may exist and lesions may coalesce and become nodular and tender on the scalp (kerion). Tinea corporis and tinea cruris present as pruritic, circular, erythematous scaling lesions that spread centrifugally. Tinea pedis (also called athlete's foot) presents as erythematous, intensely pruritic, and sometimes macerated areas on the plantar and interdigital spaces (onychomycosis and tinea unguium).

History
Patients usually report the gradual onset of a scaling, erythematous, maculopapular rash. Lesions typically spread centrifugally. Lesions may improve spontaneously then worsen, remain stable for years, or spread rapidly. Tinea cruris and tinea pedis may become macerated in intertriginous areas. Pruritus is variable; intense in tinea pedis. Tinea unguium may initially appear as yellow or dark discoloration, followed by thickening of the nails, and erythema and scaling of the surrounding skin.

Physical Examination
Tinea corporis and tinea cruris exhibit macular erythematous patches with partial central clearing and serpiginous, irregular advancing borders. Tinea pedis presents with erythematous scaling lesions in the web space of the toes and on the soles. Tinea capitis may present with papules, pustules, plaques, or nodules of the scalp. Involved regions of the scalp may show areas of alopecia.

Laboratory Studies
KOH preparation aids in the diagnosis. Scraping of the affected skin or extracted hair is placed in KOH solution and visualized under direct microscopy. Characteristic findings include the presence of fungal spores and hyphae. The nail plate of the toenails may be infected by nondermatophytes (e.g., mold species). Fungal culture may therefore be necessary before initiating treatment.

Classification
There are three main classes of fungal dermatoses: dermatophytoses of keratinized epidermis (tinea facialis, tinea corporis, tinea cruris, tinea manus, tinea pedis), dermatophytoses of nail apparatus (onychomycosis, tinea unguium), and dermatophytoses of hair and hair follicles (tinea capitis, tinea barbae).

Differential Diagnosis
PR, secondary syphilis, atopic dermatitis, palmoplantar psoriasis, and seborrheic dermatitis should be considered.

Treatment
Behavioral
Avoidance of occlusive footwear that promotes sweating and frequent use of antifungal sprays may help prevent recurrence of tinea pedis.

Medications
Tinea corporis ("ring worm") responds well to topical antifungals. Therapy should be extended for 7 to 14 days after resolution of symptoms to prevent relapse.[21] Twice daily use of topical agents such as miconazole, clotrimazole, ketoconazole, and econazole is usually effective. Oral antifungals are recommended for extensive or recalcitrant tinea corporis. Tinea cruris usually responds to topical and powdered antifungals. Therapy should be continued for 2 to 3 weeks. Less than 20% of cases of tinea unguium respond to topical therapy.[21] Available oral medications include terbinafine, itraconazole, and fluconazole. Itraconazole and fluconazole may be used in pulse doses. Some authorities recommend continuing therapy until nail changes associated with infection have resolved.[21]

Referrals
Dermatology referral is recommended for severe or persistent eruptions.

Patient Education
Use of powder containing miconazole or tolnaftate to areas prone to fungal infections after bathing.

Follow-Up
Patients should be instructed to follow up if symptoms do not resolve with appropriate treatment as recurrence is common.

Complications
Severe nail dystrophy may result from untreated tinea unguium. Macerated areas, specifically of chronic tinea pedis and onychomycosis, may lead to secondary bacterial infections, especially in patients with diabetes.

Special Considerations
Tinea incognito refers to a superficial dermatophyte infection that is inappropriately treated with topical steroids. Lesions may appear intensely red without the classic scales of a tinea infection.

References
1. Habif TH. Psoriasis and other papulosqualous diseases. In: *Clinical dermatology*. 4th ed. Philadelphia: Mosby; 2004:209–239.
2. Schon MP, Boehncke W-H. Medical progress: psoriasis. *N Engl J Med* 2005;18: 1899–1912.
3. Khachemoune A, Guillen S. Psoriasis: disease management with a brief review of new biologics. *Dermatol Nurs* 2006;18:40–43,49.
4. Habif TH. Acne rosacea. In: *Clinical dermatology*. 4th ed. Philadelphia: Mosby; 2004: 198–202.
5. Goldstein BG, Goldstein AO. Rosacea. UpToDate Online 14.2 (www.utdol.com/utd/content/topic.do?topickey=pri_derm/6783&type=A&selectedTitle=1~40). Accessed September 10, 2006.
6. Pelle MT, et al. Rosacea: II. Therapy. *J Am Acad Dermatol* 2004;51:499–512.
7. Simpson EL, Hanifin JM. Atopic dermatitis. *Med Clin North Am* 2006;90:149–167.
8. Habif TH. Atopic dermatitis. In: *Clinical dermatology*. 4th ed. Philadelphia: Mosby; 2004:105–128.
9. Shaw JC. Atopic dermatitis (eczema). UpToDate Online 14.2 (www.utdol.com/utd/content/topic.do?topickey=pri_derm/2326&type=A&selectedTitle=1~40). Accessed September 10, 2006.
10. Leung DYM, et al. Allergic and immunologic skin disorders. *J Am Med Assoc.* 1997; 278:1914–1923.
11. Hengge UR, et al. Adverse effects of topical glucocorticosteroids. *J Am Acad Dermatol* 2006; 54:1–15.
12. Habif TH: Allergic contact dermatitis. In: *Clinical dermatology*. 4th ed. Philadelphia: Mosby; 2004:84–103.
13. Mark BJ, Slavin RG. Allergic contact dermatitis. *Med Clin North Am* 2006;90:169–185.
14. Craig K, Meadows SE. What is the best duration of steroid therapy for contact dermatitis (rhus)? *J Fam Pract* 2006;55:166–167.
15. Shaw JC. Overview of dermatitis. UpToDate Online 14.2 (http://www.utdol.com/utd/content/topic.do?topicKey=pri_derm/2219&type=A&selectedTitle=1~10). Accessed September 13, 2006.
16. Habif TH. Psoriasis and other papulosqualous diseases. In: *Clinical dermatology*. 4th ed. Philadelphia: Mosby; 2004:242–245.
17. Schwartz RA, Janusz CA, Janniger CK. Seborrheic dermatitis: an overview. *Am Fam Physician* 2006;74:125–130.
18. Habif TH. Ch. 8. Psoriasis and other papulosqualous diseases. In: *Clinical dermatology*. 4th ed. Philadelphia: Mosby; 2004:246–249.
19. Stulberg, DL, Wolfrey, J. Pityriasis rosea. *Am Fam Physician* 2004;69:87–91.

20. Habif TH. Superficial fungal infections. In: *Clinical dermatology.* 4th ed. Philadelphia: Mosby; 2004:409–439.
21. Vander Straten MR, Hossain MA, Ghannoum MA. Cutaneous infections: dermatophytosis, onychomycosis, and tinea versicolor. *Infect Dis Clin North Am* 2003;17: 87–112.

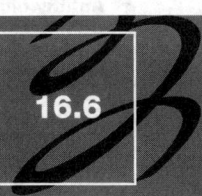

URTICARIA
William A. Alto

16.6

GENERAL PRINCIPLES

Definitions

- **Urticaria** is a common and reversible skin eruption characterized by multiple, palpable, circumscribed, erythematous, blanchable, pruritic papules (wheals) and plaques ranging in size from 2 mm to 30 cm.
- **Angioedema** occurs abruptly on the skin and mucous membranes, may or may not be erythematous, and seldom itches.
- They are classified by their time course as acute or chronic (lasting more than 6 weeks) and by the presumed inciting agent or mechanism.

Pathophysiology

- **Urticaria** involves the superficial dermis, angioedema, the deep dermis, and subcutaneous tissue.
- They result from **vasodilation and increased vascular permeability** caused by the release of mast cell mediators of inflammation, such as histamine and other vasoactive substances.
- Mechanisms are autoimmune, immune complement, and nonimmune mediated.

DIAGNOSIS

Clinical Presentation

- **Acute urticaria/urticarial** wheals develop rapidly over 15 minutes and dissipate within 90 minutes to 24 hours, rarely lasting 48 hours. As lesions resolve new crops appear, and the patient may mistakenly report that the individual "hives" have been present for days or weeks.
- **Physical urticarias** are provoked by skin stimulation, resulting in mast cell degranulation. Duration is brief, lasting only 30 to 60 minutes.
- **Angioedema** has indistinct borders, typically involves the mouth, lips, larynx, tongue, the genitalia, and mucosa of the gastrointestinal tract, and lasts 2 to 3 days.
- **Angiotensin-converting enzyme (ACE) inhibitor angioedema** does not have associated urticaria.

History

- **A careful history** often identifies the cause.
- **Gastrointestinal angioedema** causes abdominal pain.
- **Oral angioedema** may result in airway obstruction.

Physical Examination

- **Physical urticarias** can be identified by application of the offending agent or force.
- **Urticarial vasculitis** is an indicator of underlying disease and must be differentiated from the acute and chronic urticarial wheals. Urticarial vasculitis is suggested by the presence of painful wheals lasting more than 24 hours, wheals with underlying purpura, or those with residual hyperpigmentation.

- **Angioedema** frequently accompanies the urticarial wheals of chronic, cold, or solar urticaria.

Laboratory Studies

- **Radioallergosorbent testing (RAST)** is occasionally helpful.
- **Direct challenge tests** may be life threatening.
- **Elimination diets** are unwieldy.
- **Antithyroid antibodies** may be found in chronic urticaria with an associated thyroiditis.
- **Complement assays** are used to diagnose hereditary angioedema.
- **An autologous serum inoculation test** may help in the diagnosis of chronic urticaria.

Surgical Diagnostic Procedures

- **Suspected urticarial vasculitis** merits a biopsy.

Classification

- **Allergic urticaria** is immunoglobulin E (IgE) mediated (type 1 hypersensitivity).
- Direct contact, ingestion, or inhalation of an allergen causes hives.
- **Typical allergens** include grasses, pollens, insect toxins, drugs, foods, or simultaneous infections.
- **Medications** commonly associated with urticaria include penicillin, cephalosporins, sulfonamides, aspirin, nonsteroidal anti-inflammatory drugs, and vaccines.
- **Foods** frequently linked with transient urticaria are eggs, nuts, shellfish, strawberries, chocolate, and tomatoes.
- **Infectious agents** include hepatitis and Epstein–Barr virus, bacterial, and intestinal parasites.
- **Children with atopic dermatitis** are more likely to have urticaria.
- **Physical urticarias** comprise 20% to 30% of chronic urticarias.
- **Dermatographism** is the most common physical urticaria.
- **Cholinergic urticaria** is characterized by small (1- to 3-mm) pruritic papules with blanched centers. Physical exercise, hot showers, fever, and anxiety are antecedent stimuli.
- **Uncommon** (cold) and rare (solar, localized heat, delayed pressure, vibratory, and aquagenic) causes of urticaria can be identified by application of the offending agent or force.
- **Delayed-pressure urticaria** has a 4- to 6-hour lag time between the stimulus and the appearance of a wheal, which may last several hours.
- **Chemical or contact urticarias** do not involve IgE release.
- **Drugs** can cause the direct release of histamine in susceptible individuals: aspirin, amphotericin B (Fungizone), dextromethorphan, opiates, buproprion, selective serotonin-reuptake inhibitors (SSRIs), polymyxin B (Aerosporin), scopolamine (Transderm Scop), and radiographic contrast-containing iodine.
- Nonimmunologic urticaria does not require prior exposure to the offending agent. It has a gradual onset over hours and makes up 90% of drug-associated urticaria.
- Certain foods, including spoiled mackerel and tuna, may cause urticaria because of their high histamine content (scombroid poisoning).
- **Chronic urticaria** is frequently caused by an autoimmune disorder with an autoantibody to a receptor on mast cells and basophils.
- **Less common** causes of chronic urticaria include food or food additive allergies (less than 1%), psychologic stress, medications, and, rarely, parasitic infections.
- **Focal infections,** candidiasis, and undiagnosed malignancy are rarely, if ever, the cause of chronic urticaria.
- **Angioedema** is most commonly an adverse reaction to drug therapy.
- ACE inhibitors (ACE I) cause angioedema without hives (Kinin pathway). One half of patients present during the first week on the medication.
- **Hereditary autosomal dominant angioedema is rare** (less than 0.4%). Penetrance is variable and acquired cases occur so that a family history may not be helpful. If the fourth component of complement (C4) is low, then the diagnosis should be confirmed with an assay of C1 esterase inhibitor, which is also low.

Differential Diagnosis

- **Erythema multiforme (EM)** may be confused with large urticarial wheals. EM has an acute onset and typically evolving target lesions that last at least 7 days and fade by 4 weeks.

- **Insect bites** may occasionally resemble urticaria. The patient's history and location of the lesions will help clarify the etiology.
- **Mastocytosis** (urticaria pigmentosa, solitary mastocytoma, systemic disease, and mastocytosis with associated hematologic disorders) is characterized by histamine and other vasoactive substances released from overabundant mast cells. Urticaria and flushing are common symptoms.
- **Dermatitis herpetiformis and bullous pemphigoid** can occasionally resemble urticaria. They are longer lasting.
- **Pruritic urticarial papules and plaques of pregnancy (PUPPP)** is a fixed rash.
- **Angioedema** could be confused with facial cellulitis or the edema of superior vena cava syndrome.

TREATMENT

- A thorough **history** coupled with knowledge of frequently implicated triggers can help prevent further attacks.
- **Local therapies** that provide symptomatic relief include cool compresses, topical antipruritics such as doxepin cream (Zonalon), and 1% menthol in aqueous cream.
- **Antihistamine therapy** with H_1 receptor blockers is more effective for acute urticarias. Regular dosing around the clock offers better control. Older antihistamines are effective but not well tolerated at higher doses except at bedtime.
- **Nonsedating antihistamines** are frequently given, occasionally in higher than recommended doses. Drug interactions should be considered at higher dosages.
- **Histamine H_2 blockers** are sometimes helpful when treatment with H_1 blockers is inadequate, but they are seldom effective alone.
- **Corticosteroids** given as an oral taper are more rapidly effective than antihistamines.
- **Management of chronic urticaria** is less satisfactory because the autoimmune etiology may ultimately necessitate immunosuppressive therapy. Androgens, corticosteroids, cyclosporine, intravenous immunoglobulins, and plasmapheresis have been used with success.
- Evaluation and treatment is usually coordinated by dermatologists.
- Patients should be advised to avoid aspirin, and other nonsteroidal anti-inflammatory agents and opioid narcotics.
- Angioedema patients may require intubation. Epinephrine, first-generation antihistamines, and corticosteroids have been used.
- Fresh frozen plasma has been effective in ACEI-induced angioedema.
- Complement deficiency associated angioedema is treated with androgens.

References

1. Baxi S, Dinakar C. Urticaria and angioedema. *Immunol Allergy Clin North Am* 2005;25: 353–367.
2. Kaplan AP. Chronic urticaria: pathogenesis and treatment. *J Allergy Clin Immunol* 2004; 114:465–473.
3. Kaplan AP, Greaves MW. Angioedema. *J Am Acad Dermatol* 2005;53:373–387.
4. Kazel M, Sabroe R. Chronic urticaria: an etiology management, and current and future treatment options. DRUGS:2004;64:2515–2536.

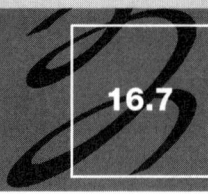

STASIS DERMATITIS, STASIS ULCERS, AND DECUBITUS ULCERS

16.7

Kristy D. Edwards

STASIS DERMATITIS

Stasis dermatitis (SD) is the chronic skin changes of eczema, hyperpigmentation, edema, and lipodermatosclerosis that arise as a complication of venous hypertension. Venous hypertension is caused by faulty venous valves in the legs.

Anatomy
Normal veins have a series of valves in them that help control the flow of blood return from the superficial to the deep veins of the lower extremity. When these valves malfunction venous hypertension occurs resulting in SD.[1]

Classification
SD is a chronic and progressive condition that is one stage of the grading system for chronic venous disease. Chronic venous insufficiency is graded by CEAP (clinical, etiologic, anatomic, pathologic) classification: Class 0: No signs or symptoms of venous disease; Class 1: Reticular veins and telangiectasias; Class 2: Varicose veins; Class 3: Edema; Class 4: SD changes; Class 5: SD with healed ulcer; Class 6: SD with active ulceration.[2]

Pathophysiology
Vein valves can be permanently damaged due to venous thrombosis, infection, trauma, surgery, or anything that increases venous pressure such as obesity or prolonged standing. Damaged veins result in dependent edema and venous incompetence.

Diagnosis
Clinical Presentation
SD is found in the lower extremities because of their dependent location. Early signs of SD are ankle edema at the end of the day, worsening varicose veins, or pruritus. Subacute and chronic eczematous (dry, flaking, or peeling erythematous skin) changes can occur followed by hemosiderin deposition resulting in reddish brown pigmentation and fibrosis of the subcutaneous tissue resulting in the leg appearing as an inverted wine bottle known as lipodermatosclerosis. Often patients present for the first time with a stasis ulcer.[3]

History
Because of the chronicity of SD you may obtain a history of progressive edema and increasing pigmentation. Past history of vein harvesting for cardiac artery bypass graft (CABG) or venous stripping may increase your suspicion of SD.

Physical Examination
Findings will often include dilated veins, edema, eczema, inflammation, and hemosiderosis. An assessment for lower extremity pulses is essential to evaluate for mixed venous and arterial disease.

Differential Diagnosis
Distinguishing SD from cellulitis, contact dermatitis, and tinea corporis can be difficult. The chronic nature of this condition will help in the diagnosis. Careful history will exclude contact irritants and a simple potassium hydroxide test will differentiate SD from tinea infection.

Treatment
Behavioral
Treatment of SD requires significant lifestyle changes. Control of the edema associated with SD is essential. Elevation of the legs whenever possible and avoidance of prolonged standing can improve dependant edema.

Medications

Antibiotics that cover skin flora should be used if concomitant cellulitis is diagnosed. Topical application of emollients or midpotency steroids can help alleviate the dryness.

Nonoperative

Compression is the mainstay of treatment for venous hypertension and SD.[3] Gradient compression stocking provide the greatest pressure (20 to 40 mmHg) around the ankle and gradually decrease proximally. If stockings are too difficult for the patient to place consider zipper or velcro aided leggings or bandage wraps. Multilayered compression bandages are more expensive than single-layer bandages but they provide faster healing. In severe cases, intermittent pneumatic compression pumps should be considered.

Prevention

Prevention of chronic edema prevents SD. The general population should exercise regularly, interrupt prolonged periods of sitting or standing with walking, and elevate the legs whenever possible.

STASIS ULCER

A stasis ulcer (SU) is a chronic ulcer commonly located on the distal medial aspect of the lower leg and is associated with SD.

Clinical Presentation

SU are often preceded by SD and relatively minor trauma. SU are typically shallow and stay the same size but they can suddenly enlarge with increased edema or infection.

Imaging

Venous duplex ultrasonography and ankle:brachial index (ABI) are useful studies performed to delineate the degree of arterial or venous disease.

Pathologic Findings

In nonhealing ulcers a tissue culture or biopsy may be necessary to determine infection or malignancy.

Differential Diagnosis

Of ulcers occurring on the lower extremity, 90% are caused by venous, arterial, or neuropathic disease.[3] Ulcers of the lower extremity are often caused by more that one etiology; therefore, the diagnosis can be complicated. Arterial ulcers are associated with pain, decreased pulses, and cool extremities. Neuropathic ulcers are often associated with diabetes and loss of sensation in the lower extremities. Neuropathic ulcers occur over pressure points and are surrounded by a thick callous. Infection, neoplasm, and vasculitis are other more rare causes of lower extremity ulcers.

Treatment

SU treatment is prolonged, taking weeks to months to heal typical SU. There is a high rate of recurrence of SU.

Medications

Directed antibiotics should be used in venous ulcers that are infected as diagnosed by a quantitative tissue biopsy culture.

Nonoperative

Compression therapy is recommended as with SD. However, before aggressive compression therapy is initiated, arterial disease should be excluded.

Operative

Artificial skin grafting and skin grafting are often considered in SU that fail to respond to compression therapy and other treatment modalities.

Prevention

Preventive is the key. Reducing edema and SD also reduces the incidence of SU.

DECUBITUS ULCER

Decubitus ulcers (DUs) are localized areas of tissue destruction caused by prolonged pressure usually over a bony prominence.

Anatomy

DUs typically occur over bony prominences such as sacrum, ischial tuberosities, trochanters, ankles, and heels.

Classification

DUs are classified using a staging system. They are staged as follows:

- **Stage 1:** Nonblanchable erythema seen over intact skin
- **Stage 2:** Ulceration of epidermis, dermis, or both
- **Stage 3:** Ulceration extending to the subcutaneous layer
- **Stage 4:** Ulceration extending to muscle, bone, and/or supporting tissues[5]

Pathophysiology

The major contributing factors resulting in DUs are pressure, shear, friction, and moisture. The effects of pressure are determined by the intensity and duration of the pressure and the tissue's tolerance to the pressure. Pressure, especially over a bony prominence, causes soft tissue compression and interferes with the tissue blood supply. Shear forces exert force parallel to the skin causing stretching or tearing of underlying blood vessels and reducing the amount of pressure necessary to cause tissue ischemia. Shear forces can occur when the head of a patient's bed is elevated causing the patient to sit on an incline for a prolonged period of time. Shear and friction are increased with mild to moderate moisture.

Clinical Presentation

DUs typically occur in elderly individuals, but can occur in patients with significant neurologic disease. Patients are at increased risk for developing DUs if the are immobile, incontinent, have poor nutrition, poor circulation, and/or profound sensory deficits.

Differential Diagnosis

Includes SU, arterial disease ulcers, neuropathic ulcers, and less commonly neoplasm, vasculitis, or infection.

Treatment

Assessing and correcting risk factors is the goal of treatment in stage 1 ulcers. Stage 2 ulcers are typically treated using an occlusive dressing and avoiding all pressure to the area. Stage 3 and 4 ulcers are treated based on the degree and severity of the ulcer. Presence of necrotic tissue, exudates, or evidence of infection usually requires debridement. This can be performed using enzymatic, mechanical, or surgical techniques. Although not all DUs require management by a wound care specialist, a wound care consult may be necessary in advanced stage 3 and stage 4 ulcers. In some patients, advanced DUs can be managed with skin grafts or flap closures.

Prevention

Prevention is the key for high-risk patients. Knowing the factors that increase DU risk and utilizing a prediction tool (i.e., Norton or Braden scales) allows early initiation of prevention measures. Minimizing pressure with pressure-relieving devices and repositioning schedules as well as maintaining good nutrition and decreasing moisture can help prevent DUs.

References

1. Simon D. Management of venous leg ulcers. *BMJ* 2004;328:1358–1362.
2. Beebe H. Classification and grading of chronic venous disease in the lower limbs. a consensus statement. *Eur J Vasc Endovasc Surg* 1996;12:487.
3. Habif T. Stasis dermatitis and venous ulcers. In: *Skin diesase diagnosis and treatment.* Mosby, Philadelphia: 2005:56–63.
4. London N. Ulcerated lower limb. *BMJ* 2000;320(7249):1589–1591.
5. Resnick NM. Geriatric medicine. In: Fauci AS, et al., eds. *Principles of internal medicine.* New York: McGraw-Hill; 1998:42–43.

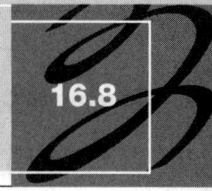

SKIN CANCERS

General Principles

Definition

Skin cancers are the most commonly diagnosed cancers in this country, accounting for one third of all cancers. The majority are preventable and curable. Basal cell carcinoma (BCC) is the most common (800,000 cases per year), followed by squamous cell carcinoma (SCC) (200,000 cases per year) and malignant melanoma (MM) (66,000 cases per year). MM accounts for the majority of skin cancer deaths (8500 deaths per year), and its incidence has doubled in the last decade.

Etiology

Predisposing factors for all types of skin cancer include fair skin (blonde hair, blue eyes), poor tanning ability, and a predilection to burn, especially severe sunburns in childhood. However, all individuals are at risk with excessive exposure to ultraviolet (UV) light from solar radiation. UV light damages epidermal DNA. About 20 to 30 years of exposure is required to induce tumor development. Tanning booths use UVA light, a longer wavelength than UVB, but there is no evidence to support the use of tanning booths to acquire a protective tan, and tanning booth exposure adds to the lifetime dose of UV radiation. Additionally certain occupational exposures (coal tars, creosote, arsenic compounds, radium) increase risk.

Special Considerations

Prevention

Skin cancers are preventable. Patients should be counseled to avoid sun exposure and use broad-spectrum sunscreens (those that screen UVB and UVA rays) with a minimal sun protection factor (SPF) of 15. Sunscreens have been shown to prevent BCC and SCC in animal models, but they appear to be ineffective in preventing MM. In addition, these cancers are curable if detected early and treated promptly. Patients' skin should be examined periodically, and high-risk individuals should be instructed in regular self-examinations.

NONPIGMENTED CANCERS

Basal Cell Carcinoma (BCC)

There are three main clinical types:

- **Nodular:** Most common, also known as ulcerative or rodent tumor. This begins as a nodule that ulcerates as the tumor progresses.
- **Superficial:** Tend to occur on the trunk and can be multiple. They are flat and reddish pink but typically have a thready border consistent with BCC.
- **Sclerosing** (morphea-like): Least common of the BCCs. These plaque-like lesions are somewhat indurated, ivory colored, and telangiectatic, but they do not always have a thready border.

Diagnosis

Clinical Presentation. BCCs are found in areas of sun exposure, with 90% occurring on the head or neck. Look for raised nodular lesions with central ulceration surrounded by a pearly or thready border with telangiectasias. The surrounding skin is often wrinkled or sagging, secondary to loss of normal thickness and elasticity from chronic sun damage.

Treatment

If BCCs are excised when smaller than 2 cm, there is a less than 5% likelihood of recurrence; if they are larger than 2 cm when excised, 20% will recur within the first year. Less than 0.1% of BCC will metastasize, but they cause local destruction.

Squamous Cell Carcinoma (SCC)

SCC is a disease of the elderly (mean age 70 years), although it can be seen in younger individuals. SCC can be thought of as a continuum of disease, including actinic keratosis (AK) and carcinoma *in situ* (Bowen disease; BD), both of which involve atypia of the epithelial keratinocytes.

- **Actinic keratosis.** Characterized by localized nests of atypia and dysplasia within the keratinocytes. AK (also known as solar keratosis) is common in elderly individuals and is seen in most areas of chronic sun exposure (face, back of hands, forearms). AKs are circumscribed, rough lesions with indistinct margins. Size ranges from pinpoint to plaque-like nodules of varying colors, and occasionally the nodules are scaly, with skin horns. Clinically, it can be difficult to tell whether a lesion is an AK or an SCC, but because SCC represents an invasion into the dermis, these lesions are firmer, indurated, and adherent to the underlying dermis. Approximately 20% of AKs slowly transform into SCC; therefore, they should be removed or, at the very least, followed closely.
- **Bowen disease.** Atypia encompasses the full thickness of the epidermis. With SCC, there is invasion into the dermis. BD is characterized by an erythematous, hyperkeratotic, scaly plaque with sharp irregular borders and erosions or ulcerations on the surface. The condition is often seen on areas of skin that are not exposed to sun. BD can be mistaken for a patch of psoriasis or eczema. Like AK, these lesions can transform into SCC, so they must be managed or followed closely.

Etiology

SCCs are associated with environmental exposures (arsenic, petroleum, and smoking) and inflammatory dermatoses (discoid lupus, chronic osteomyelitis, hidradenitis suppurativa, chronically draining pilonidal sinus, severe burns, leg ulcers, and psoriasis managed with methotrexate); in addition to the usual risk factors. Renal transplant patients who are on chronic suppression are at higher risk. The link between chronic inflammation and immune suppression is unclear. A viral etiology is postulated, possibly human papillomavirus (HPV 5).

Diagnosis

Clinical Presentation. SCCs are nodular to plaque-like with a variety of colors. Frequently, there is ulceration and scaling. Occasionally, SCC can be verruciform. About 2% to 3% of lesions metastasize to the local or regional lymph nodes. The main morbidity is from local destruction.

Treatment

There are three underlying principles for treating BCC and SCC:

- Remove the cancerous tissue
- Preserve normal tissue and function
- Achieve an optimal cosmetic result

Surgery

Management of AK and BD consists of removal. Destruction is appropriate for lesions that are smaller than 2 cm and not in areas that would present problems should there be a recurrence or growth (i.e., around eyes, nose, and mouth). Surgical excision with a 2- to 3-mm margin is an excellent way to manage BCC and SCC. Not only is the lesion removed, but the specimen can confirm the diagnosis and determine whether the skin margins are clear of tumor. Occasionally, BCC occurs in areas that are difficult to excise, in which case referral may be necessary to achieve complete excision. A shave or punch biopsy would be appropriate to confirm the diagnosis prior to referral.

Destructive means include:

- Electrodesiccation and curettage
- Cryosurgery (topical liquid nitrogen is acceptable; be aware that unlike the case of pre-cancerous lesions, liquid nitrogen treatment, alone, is not sufficient and a cryoprobe must be used to achieve sufficient depth of freeze to destroy the tumor)
- Acetic acid applications
- 5-Fluorouracil (Efudex) and dermabrasion (5-fluorouracil is not the optimal therapy and should be reserved for patients, such as nursing home residents, who would find it difficult to come to the office for a procedure)
- Tretinoin (Retin-A): Has shown promise in the management of small AKs
- Imiquimod (Aldara): Used for BD
- Photodynamic therapy (PDT) with topical 5-aminolevulinic acid can be used for multiple AK and BD, especially for those with sensitivity to 5-fluorouracil

For larger lesions, those located in high-risk areas, or recurrent lesions, it would be appropriate to refer for Mohs surgery. This is a specialized technique whereby the lesion is removed in a slowly enlarging, concentric pattern. The margins are examined under frozen section, and tissue is removed until there is microscopic confirmation that the margins are clear.

Patient Education
Patients should be counseled to avoid further sun exposure.

PIGMENTED CANCERS

Benign Lesions

Acquired Nevus

Common nevi, or moles, change predictably over time, beginning as a simple lentigo, transforming into junctional nevi, compound nevi, and, finally, intradermal nevi. Frequently, moles involute and disappear.

Simple lentigos are not related to solar exposure and can be seen anywhere on the body. They arise in early childhood and are less than 5 mm, round, macular, brown or black, with smooth or slightly jagged edges. Simple lentigo should be distinguished from ephelides (freckles). Ephelides are the result of increased production of melanin by melanocytes in response to sunlight, whereas lentigo consists of a number of melanocytes clumping together. Junctional nevi remain small and are similar in appearance to simple lentigo but may contain hair. They arise in childhood or early adolescence in sun-exposed areas of skin.

During later adolescence or early adulthood, melanocytes migrate through the epidermal–dermal junction, creating a compound nevus. As these cells cross the junction, nevi rise above the surface of the skin. These well-circumscribed papules remain smaller than 6 mm in circumference, are tan to brown, and have a smooth or rough surface. Occasionally, there is hair growth. The final stage is that of the intradermal nevi. As the melanocytes migrate to the dermis, the nevi lose pigmentation to become flesh-colored papules and may disappear. Progression other than these normal stages should be considered suspicious. Indeed, any new mole that develops after age 40 should be evaluated closely.

Congenital Nevus

This lesion is present at 1% of all births, although some authorities manage any pigmented lesion seen within the first year of life as a congenital nevus. Small congenital nevi (<3 cm) have a 1% to 2% chance of malignant transformation during the individual's lifetime, doubling the underlying risk of MM. Giant congenital nevi (>20 cm) have a 4% to 8% risk of malignant transformation. Treatment is controversial, and options include careful observation with removal for suspicious changes or removal when the child is old enough to undergo a procedure under local anesthesia.

Dysplastic Nevus

This lesion has variations of color (tan, brown, pink, red, or blue) and size; many dysplastic nevi are larger than 7 mm with irregular, distinct borders. Dysplastic nevi are markers for MM-prone individuals, who have a lifetime risk of developing melanoma of 6%. This risk increases substantially if two family members have MM (up to 100% in some studies).

Dysplastic nevus syndrome refers to the development of multiple lesions (100 or more). Normal individuals have 25 to 40 acquired nevi. Dysplastic nevus syndrome is probably an inherited familial disorder.

These patients need to be followed periodically (every 3 to 12 months), with biopsy of the worst-looking lesions. Total-body photographs or spot photographs can be used to follow particular lesions. In all, 20% of melanomas arise from dysplastic nevi. Patients must be counseled to avoid the sun and to use SPF-15 sunscreen.

A shave biopsy is not appropriate for pigmented lesions. The depth of the lesion is an important prognostic indicator and is essential to future management of the disease. A punch biopsy is fine if it can encompass the whole lesion. However, if one merely punches the worst-looking area of the pigmented lesion, it is possible to miss malignant cells elsewhere in the lesion. Therefore, these lesions should be managed with excisional biopsy techniques.

Solar Lentigo
Solar lentigo (liver or age spots) is a benign indicator of sun-related damage to skin. Classically, uniform tan or brown macules are seen on the back of the hand and forearms of older individuals. Treatment is not necessary, although patients frequently request therapy because of cosmetic concerns. Tretinoin and "bleaching" creams, such as hydroquinone (Melanex), can be used. The benefits of cryotherapy and laser treatment must be weighed against the potential for scarring.

Seborrheic Keratosis
Commonly seen in older individuals, this is a sharply demarcated, verrucal, warty, raised lesion with brown, black, and tan coloring and a waxy appearance. It appears to be stuck onto the skin and varies in size from a few millimeters to several centimeters. Lesions are typically seen on the face, neck, and trunk. Seborrheic keratosis is an autosomal dominant trait. Onset occurs in the 40s and progresses slowly. Lesions are occasionally seen as firm, dark black nodules, which should raise suspicion of nodular melanoma. Like lentigos, no treatment is necessary, unless there is a concern about cosmetics. Simple destructive methods (cryosurgery, curettage, etc.) are appropriate.

Malignant Melanoma
Etiology
Genetic predisposition, excessive UV light exposure (including severe childhood sunburns), and having multiple nevi (as few as 20 nevi increases the risk; individuals with more than 200 nevi are at highest risk). If there is a family member with MM, other members have a 2% to 8% increased risk. This is primarily a disease of whites, although people of color have a higher mortality rate as they tend to be diagnosed at a more advanced stage. The majority of MMs arise de novo. The median age of diagnosis is 53 years and there is a slight male predilection; however, it is the most common cancer in women between 25 and 29 years of age.

Diagnosis
Physical Examination.   Remember the ABCDE evaluation for MM. Lesions that possess these characteristics (listed below) should be watched closely or biopsied. A lesion need not possess all characteristics to be an MM.

> **A = Asymmetry.** A line drawn through the middle does not create matching halves.
> **B = Border.** Uneven scalloped or notched edges.
> **C = Color.** Variable shades of brown or black and hues of blue, gray, white, pink, or red.
> **D = Diameter.** Size greater than 6 mm (the diameter of a pencil).
> **E = Elevation** (or Evolving). A flat lesion that begins to rise above the skin surface, or a change over time in lesion.

Staging.   In 2002 the American Joint Committee on Cancer (AJCC) revised the staging criteria that are based on several factors, including tumor thickness (Breslow depth), anatomic level of invasion (Clark level), presence of ulceration and lymph node involvement. Stage 1 disease is localized to the skin (>90% 5-year survival); stage 2 is for deeper lesions though still localized to the skin, but without lymph node involvement (45% to 80%

5-year survival depending on the substage); stage III disease indicates that the regional lymph nodes are involved (24% to 70% 5-year survival depending on the substage); stage IV disease is for distant metastasis, often bone or central nervous system (<20% 5-year survival).

Classification. MMs are classified as four types:

- **Superficial spreading MM:** Majority (70%) of MMs.
- **Nodular MM:** 15% of MMs; does not follow the ABCD criteria, but may elevate. These present as black nodules and tend to invade early.
- **Lentigo maligna melanomas:** 5% of MMs; arise from a precursor lesion known as a lentigo maligna or Hutchinson freckle, which is a large pigmented macule seen in sun-exposed areas. These have a good prognosis because they tend to spread superficially before invading.
- **Acral–lentiginous MMs:** 5% of MMs; arise on the hands or feet and are the most common type seen in Asians and blacks. Often they are not observed until late in progress because they are hidden on the soles of the feet, between the toes, or underneath a nail.

Treatment
Surgery. For lesions that are thinner than 1 mm, a 1-cm margin is required; for thicker lesions, a 2-cm margin is sufficient. When removing a lesion that is suspicious for MM, use an elliptic incision with 1-cm margins. Should the biopsy reveal a lesion thicker than 1 mm, a wider re-excision of the area is necessary. Lesions thinner than 1 mm are associated with a >95% 10-year survival rate. Lesions thicker than 4 mm have a <45% 10-year survival rate.

Lymph node exploration is not necessary for lesions thinner than 1 mm, although any suspicious nodes should be explored. As it is not possible to know the depth of the lesion before obtaining the biopsy, a careful history and physical are crucial to search for any changes in regional lymph nodes before obtaining a biopsy as reactive changes maybe induced by the biopsy procedure. Sentinel node (SN) biopsy is helpful as a negative SN obviates the need for further lymph node exploration. The technique is to inject vital blue dye around the melanoma or biopsy scar (if planned for a wider re-excision); this is followed by lymphoscintigraphy (nuclear medicine mapping) to identify the regional draining lymph nodes, which are then excised and examined for disease. No baseline studies are required for superficial MM (<1 mm), unless there are signs of metastasis; for lesions with greater depth, a baseline chest x-ray and lactate dehydrogenase (LDH) levels are useful. These can be used for surveillance on a 3- to 12- month basis depending on the stage, and S-100 protein levels may also be used as a tumor marker for those with metastasis. Interferon (IFN) alpha-2b is the only approved adjuvant therapy, and it shows some promise in treating stages IIB, IIC, and III. Additionally, experimental adjuvant therapy is being explored with melanoma vaccines.

References
1. Cancer facts and figures. Atlanta, GA: American Cancer Society; 2006.
2. Early diagnosis of cutaneous melanoma: revisiting the ABCD criteria. *JAMA* 2004; 292:2771–2776.
3. Jeffes EW, Tang EH. Actinic keratosis: current treatment options. *Am J Clin Dermatol* 2000;1(3):167–179.
4. Rubin AI, Chen EH, Ratner D. Current concepts: basal-cell carcinoma. *N Engl J Med* 2005;353(21):2262–2269.
5. Rigel DS, Carucci JA. Malignant melanoma: prevention, early detection, and treatment in the 21st century. *CA Cancer J Clin* 2000;50:215–236.
6. Tucker MA, Halpern A, Holly EA, et al. Clinically recognized dysplastic nevi: a central risk factor for cutaneous melanoma. *JAMA* 1997;277:1439.
7. Balch CM, Soong SJ, Atkins MB, et al. An evidence-based staging system for cutaneous melanoma. *CA Cancer J Clin* 2004;54:131–149.
8. Spence AR, Franco EL, Ferenczy A. The role of human papillomaviruses in cancer: evidence to date. *Am J Cancer* 2005;4(1):49–64.
9. Cummins DL, Cummins JM, Pantle H, et al. Cutaneous malignant melanoma. *Mayo Clin Proc* 2006;81(4):500–507.
10. Piepkorn M, Weinstock MA, Barnhill RL. Theoretical and empirical arguments in relation to elective lymph node dissection for melanoma. *Arch Dermatol* 1997;133:995.

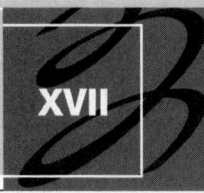

OBESITY
Meg Hayes
17.1

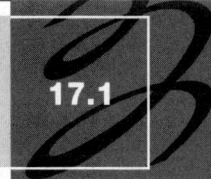

OVERVIEW

Obesity has increased in prevalence in both sexes, in all age groups and races, and at all educational levels over the past 30 years in the United States. Obesity increased from 12% of the population in 1991 to 17.9% in 1998.[1] Data collected from 1999 to 2002 estimate that nearly one third of U.S. adults are obese (27.6% of men and 33.2% of women) and one in six children and adolescents is overweight. Increased prevalence of excessive weight is noted among all age, gender, and racial/ethnic groups.[2] Obesity is associated with increased risk of death in all adult age groups for all categories of death.[3] Obesity substantially raises the risk and morbidity from the metabolic syndrome (insulin resistance syndrome) type 2 diabetes mellitus, coronary artery disease, hypertension (HTN) and stroke, dyslipidemia, osteoarthritis, obstructive sleep apnea, gallbladder disease, menstrual irregularities, hirsutism, stress incontinence, and cancers of the colon, kidney, gallbladder, prostate, breast, and endometrium.[4]

Metabolic Syndrome

Obesity is associated with insulin resistance, particularly in the case of abdominal obesity. Insulin resistance increases the risk of developing type 2 diabetes mellitus. The resulting hyperinsulinemia, hyperglycemia, and adipocyte cytokines are thought to lead to vascular endothelial dysfunction, hyperlipidemia, hypertension, and vascular inflammation promoting atherosclerotic cardiovascular disease.

The World Health Organization proposed a set of criteria for defining the metabolic syndrome in 1998:

■ A fasting plasma glucose >110 mg per dL, or a plasma glucose 2 hours after an oral glucose tolerance test >200 mg per dL, or hyperinsulinemia, defined as the upper quartile of a measure of insulin resistance in the nondiabetic population.

Plus at least two of the following:

■ Abdominal obesity, defined as a waist-to-hip ratio of >0.90, a body mass index (BMI) ≥30 kg per m^2, or a waist girth ≥94 cm (37 in.).

637

- Dyslipidemia, defined as serum triglyceride ≥150 mg per dL or high-density lipoprotein (HDL) cholesterol <35 mg per dL.
- Blood pressure ≥140/90 mmHg or the administration of antihypertensive drugs.

The metabolic syndrome has been associated with several obesity-related disorders including fatty liver disease, chronic renal disease, polycystic ovarian syndrome, obstructive sleep apnea, and increased risk of cognitive decline and dementia. Given this high burden of disease, the American Heart Association and the National Institutes of Health have supported two major therapeutic goals[5]:

- Treat underlying causes (overweight/obesity and physical inactivity) by intensifying weight management and increasing physical activity.
- Treat cardiovascular risk factors if they persist despite lifestyle modification.

The U.S. Preventive Services Task Force (USPSTF) recommends that clinicians screen all adult patients for obesity and offer intensive counseling and behavioral interventions to promote sustained weight loss for obese adults (B recommendation).[6]

CLINICAL ASSESSMENT

Assessment of body fat, risk factors, and patient motivation provides the basis for development of appropriate treatment plan.

Body Mass Index

The USPSTF found good evidence that BMI is reliable and valid for identifying adults at increased risk for mortality and morbidity due to overweight and obesity. The BMI calculation is a simple-to-use, indirect measure of body fat. It provides relative weight adjusted for height as a correlation of body fat content for adults. This measurement should not be used to evaluate growing children, frail elderly individuals, pregnant or lactating women, individuals with high muscle mass, or patients with disorders that preclude obtaining an accurate measurement of height.

$$BMI = [weight(pounds)/height\ inches)^2] \times 704.5\ or\ Weight(kilograms)/height(meters)^2$$

Underweight: BMI <18.5	Obesity Class I: BMI 30.0 to 34.9
Normal: BMI 18.5 to 24.9	Obesity Class II: BMI 35.0 to 39.9
Overweight: BMI 25.0 to 29.9	Obesity Class III: BMI ≥40

Waist Circumference (WC) and Waist-to-Hip Ratio (WHR)

Excess abdominal fat is a risk factor independent of obesity for development of health problems, including type 2 diabetes, hypertension, and cardiovascular disease.[7] For adults, a BMI of 25 to 34.9, with a WHR > 1.0 or WC > 102 cm (40 in.) in men or WHR > 0.8 or WC > 88 cm (35 in.) in women, identifies patients at **high risk** for development of obesity-associated comorbidity.

Risk Status

Comorbidities compound the health risks associated with obesity. Comorbidities are usually exacerbated by excessive weight and improved with weight reduction.

- Patients with coronary or peripheral atherosclerotic disease, type 2 diabetes mellitus, and obstructive sleep apnea are at **very high risk** for disease complications and mortality.
- Other obesity-related diseases include osteoarthritis (especially knee, hip, and back), gastroesophageal reflux disease, infertility, urinary stress incontinence, cholelithiasis, idiopathic intracranial hypertension, and lower extremity venous stasis.
- Patients with three or more of the following are classified at **high risk:** tobacco abuse, hypertension, hypercholesterolemia, impaired fasting glucose, family history of premature coronary heart disease.
- Conditions that promote weight gain include such pre-existing illnesses as Cushing disease and hypothyroidism; medications such as olanzepine, paroxetine, valproate, carbamazepine, gabapentin, steroid hormones including contraceptives and glucocorticoids, Paroxetine and tricyclic antidepressants; psychologic factors such as depression; tobacco cessation, and menopausal period associated with an average 5-lb weight gain.

Patient Motivation

Factors that allow the patient to successfully enter into a weight reduction program include motivation, previous history of weight loss, social support, capacity and willingness to engage in physical activity.

TREATMENT

Goals of a weight loss program are to prevent additional weight gain, reduce body weight, and maintain lower weight over time. Initially set a 4- to 6-month goal for weight reduction of 10% or a reduction of BMI by two units. As targets are met the patient may maintain the reduced weight or set a new goal of weight reduction. Either strategy should include permanent behavior modification including stress reduction and self-monitoring. Treatment options are employed based on the BMI and adjusted risk:

BMI 18≤25, no adjusted risk:	Healthy diet and physical exercise
BMI 25≤27, moderate risk:	As above plus low calorie diet
BMI 27≤30, high risk:	As above
BMI 30≤35, very high risk:	As above plus medication and very low calorie diet
BMI 35≥40, extremely high risk:	As above and consider surgical interventions when obesity-related comorbidities are present
BMI 40+, extremely high risk:	As above plus surgical interventions

Calorie Reduction

■ A decrease of 300 to 500 kcal per day provides a weight loss of 0.5 to 1 lb per week with a 6-month 10% weight reduction for BMI 25 to 30. A decrease of 500 to 1000 kcal per day provides weight loss of 1 to 2 lb per week with a 6-month 10% weight reduction for BMI 30 to 35.

■ To calculate a 500 kcal per day deficit:
Calculate the **resting energy expenditure (REE):**

$(10 \times$ weight [kg]$) + (6.25 \times$ height [cm]$) - (5 \times$ age [years]$)^* =$ REE*
$= +5$ for men and -161 for women

■ Estimate **total caloric need** to maintain weight.

total caloric need $=$ REE $\times$ activity factor
(activity factor $= 1.6$ for men and 1.5 for women)

■ Calculate **adjusted caloric intake:**

total caloric need $- 500$ kcal $=$ caloric energy deficit[7]

Caloric balance should first be undertaken through a diet to decrease energy intake and exercise to increase energy expenditure.

■ The Mediterranean Diet is high in fruits, vegetables, nuts, whole grains, and olive oil. Adopting this diet has been demonstrated to lower weight and blood pressure, improve lipid profiles and insulin resistance, and lower markers of inflammation and endothelial function.[8]

■ The DASH diet limits daily sodium intake to 2,400 mg and is rich in fruits, vegetables, low or nonfat dairy, and also includes whole grains; lean meats, fish and poultry; nuts and beans. The DASH diet has been shown to improve triglycerides, diastolic blood pressure, and fasting glucose in addition to leading to weight loss.[9]

■ Low glycemic index diets replace refined grains with whole grains, fruits, and vegetables and eliminate high-glycemic beverages. In addition to weight-loss benefits, choosing low glycemic index foods in place of conventional or high glycemic index foods has a clinically useful effect on medium-term glycemic control in patients with diabetes. The incremental benefit is similar to that offered by pharmacologic agents that also target postprandial hyperglycemia.[10]

Pharmacotherapy

In selected patients who have failed to achieve weight loss goals through diet and exercise alone, medication is an appropriate adjunct to a low-calorie diet, physical activity, and behavior modification. Weight loss medications create an energy deficit through reduced food consumption or reduced absorption.

- Sympathomimetic drugs reduce food intake by causing early satiety through a centrally acting anorectic mechanism:
  - Phentermine stimulates the release of norepinephrine. Dosed at 8 mg tid with meals or 15 to 37.5 mg in the morning, phentermine is chemically an amphetamine and a schedule IV narcotic. It is recommended that use be limited to 12 weeks or less. Contraindications to the use of phentermine include obesity comorbitities, cardiovascular disease, and hypertension.
  - Sibutramine acts by increasing serotonin and norepinephrine levels in the brain through reuptake inhibition. The serotonergic action, in particular, is thought to influence appetite, but has not been shown to affect depression. Dosed at 5 to 15 mg per day, sibutramine is chemically related to amphetamine and is a schedule IV narcotic, but is approved for long-term use. It has been demonstrated to increase both systolic and diastolic blood pressure, and should be avoided in patients with heart disease. Use of sibutramine with weight loss has been associated with a graded decrease in serum triglyceride and low-density lipoprotein (LDL) cholesterol concentrations.[11]
- Reduced absorption in gastrointestinal (GI) tract
  - Orlistat is the only available medication that influences fat absorption. Through the inhibition of pancreatic lipases ingested fats are not hydrolyzed to fatty acids and glycerol; thus it is not absorbed and is excreted as fecal fat. Dosed at 50 to 200 mg with meals, orlistat provides a dose-dependent reduction of fat absorption by approximately 30%. Orlistat use by patients with diabetes has been demonstrated to reduce weight and decrease hemoglobin A1c over placebo.[12]
  - There is no evidence to support the use of combination therapy for improved weight loss outcomes.[13,14]

Surgical Intervention

For patients with a BMI greater than 40, or BMI greater than 35 with serious medical comorbidities, who have not been successful with diet, exercise, and medical management, consultation to a bariatric surgeon should be considered. Appropriate candidates should be well informed and motivated for both the surgical process and the subsequent weight loss. The three surgical procedures currently in use are:

- The Roux-en-Y gastric bypass creates a small stomach pouch and allows food to bypass some of the small intestine.
- Gastroplasty decreases the overall size of the stomach to create a feeling of fullness after eating a small amount of food leading to decreased caloric intake and weight loss.
- Lap-banding gastroplasty places a plastic band around the stomach that is connected to a subcutaneous pouch. This pouch is inflated with saline to apply a variable level of constriction to the stomach.

Postoperative complications of bariatric surgery include infection, anemia, vitamin B deficiencies, inadequate weight loss, and gallstone formation due to rapid weight loss. The family physician should ensure that dietary changes, physical activity, and behavior modification are a part of the overall strategy for weight reduction to ensure maintenance of weight loss over time.

Patient Education

Follow-up, in the form of office visits, telephone contact, and written communication, is an important component of a successful weight loss program. Encourage social support through family and friends, newsletters, the Internet, weight loss groups, and exercise partnerships.

Contraindications to Weight Loss

Absolute contraindications to weight loss are terminal illness and anorexia nervosa. Temporary contraindications include pregnancy and lactation; unstable psychiatric, medical, or surgical status; and bulimia nervosa. Patients with osteopenia or osteoporosis should undergo discussion of risk and undertake medical management to maintain bone mineral density.

OBESITY MANAGEMENT ACROSS THE LIFE SPAN

BMI is not an accurate measure of body fat in children who have not achieved full height. Increasing numbers of children are overweight and will continue this trend into their adult years, placing them at higher risk to develop comorbid conditions early in life. Emphasis on healthy eating habits and physical activity can help children maintain normal weight while supplying adequate nutrition for growth and development.

Elderly persons are at increased risk of becoming overweight with loss of physical activity and decreased energy expenditure. Regular, moderate exercise and a diet low in fat and high in fiber can control weight while providing for nutritional needs. Issues of polypharmacy, drug interactions, and age-related physiologic factors should be considered before medication is prescribed for obese elderly patients.

References

1. Mokdad AH, Serdula MK, Dietz WH, et al. The spread of the obesity epidemic in the United States, 1991–1998. *JAMA* 1999;282:1519–1522.
2. Baskin ML, Ard J, Franklin F, et al. National prevalence of obesity: prevalence of obesity in the United States. *Obesity Rev* 2005;6(1):5.
3. Calle EE, Thun MJ, Petrelli JM, et al. Body mass index and mortality in a prospective cohort of U.S. adults. *N Engl J Med* 1999;341:1097–1105.
4. http://www.surgeongeneral.gov/topics/obesity/calltoaction/1_2.htm#table1.
5. Grundy SM, Hansen B, Smith SC, et al. Clinical management of metabolic syndrome: report of the American Heart Association/National Heart, Lung, and Blood Institute/American Diabetes Association conference on scientific issues related to management. *Circulation* 2004;109:551.
6. U.S. Preventive Services Task Force. *Guide to clinical preventive services.* 2nd ed. Washington, DC: Office of Disease Prevention and Health Promotion; 1996.
7. Willett WC, Dietz WH, Colditz GA. Guidelines for healthy weight. *N Engl J Med* 1999;341:427–434.
8. Esposito K, Marfella R, Ciotola M, et al. Effect of a Mediterranean-style diet on endothelial dysfunction and markers of vascular inflammation in the metabolic syndrome: a randomized trial. *JAMA* 2004;292:1440.
9. Seim HC, Pi-Sunyer FX. Management of obesity. *Am Fam Physician Monogr* 1999; 2:11.
10. Azadbakht L, Mirmiran P, Esmaillzadeh A, et al. Beneficial effects of a dietary approaches to stop hypertension eating plan on features of the metabolic syndrome. *Diabetes Care* 2005;28:2823.
11. Brand-Miller J, Hayne S, Petocz P, et al. Low-glycemic index diets in the management of diabetes: a meta-analysis of randomized controlled trials. *Diabetes Care* 2003;26: 2261–2267.
12. Bray GA, Blackburn GL, Ferguson JM, et al. Sibutramine produces dose-related weight loss. *Obesity Res* 1999;7:189.
13. Kelley DE, Bray GA, Pi-Sunyear FX, et al. Clinical efficacy of orlistat therapy in overweight and obese patients with insulin-treated type 2 diabetes: A 1-year randomized controlled trial. *Diabetes Care* 2002;25:1033.
14. Wadden RA, Berkowitz RI, Wombie LG, et al. Effects of sibutramine plus orlistat in obese women following 1 year of treatment by sibutramine alone: a placebo-controlled trial. *Obesity Res* 2000;8:431.

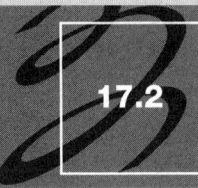

DIABETES MELLITUS

17.2

John P. Sheehan, Margaret M. Ulchaker,
Charles Kent Smith

CLASSIFICATION

- **Type 1 (insulin-dependent) diabetes mellitus** (DM) is characterized by insulin deficiency due to autoimmune pancreatic β-cell destruction.
- **Type 2 (non–insulin-dependent) DM** is characterized by insulin resistance and variable insulin secretory defects. Obesity (specifically abdominal), hypertension, and dyslipidemia often coexist (metabolic syndrome, previously known as Reaven syndrome X).
- **Gestational DM** (see Chapter 14.6)
- **Secondary DM** (not covered in this chapter)

INITIAL APPROACH TO THE PATIENT

- **Clinical history** yields important clues to the presence and correct classification of DM.
  - Type 1 DM
    - Recent onset of polydipsia, polyuria, significant weight loss, fatigue, and ketonuria occurs in a patient generally younger than 30 years.
    - Clinical duration of symptoms is relatively short despite a long prodrome of autoimmune pancreatic islet destruction.

  - Type 2 DM
    - Patient may present with polydipsia, polyuria, history of weight gain or loss, fatigue, glycosuria, obesity (especially abdominal), hypertension, dyslipidemia, positive family history of DM, or previous gestational DM in a patient generally older than 40.
    - Clinical duration of mild hyperglycemia with minimal symptoms may be prolonged in such a way that patients may present with DM complications (peripheral neuropathy, retinopathy, nephropathy).

  - Gestational DM (see Chapter 14.6)
  - Secondary DM. Consider DM in the context of the primary condition.

- **Physical examination**
  - The presence of DM complications noted on a careful initial physical examination at time of diagnosis strongly favors a diagnosis of type 2 DM. Unfortunately, DM complications at diagnosis remain common, confirming long-standing undiagnosed DM.

- **Laboratory diagnosis**
  - Fasting serum glucose ≥126 mg per dL on two occasions in ambulatory setting.
  - Casual serum glucose ≥200 mg per dL on two occasions in ambulatory setting.
  - A 2-hour postload plasma glucose (glucose tolerance test no longer routinely needed to diagnose DM).
  - Indications
    - Equivocal serum glucose levels, especially in the presence of other stigmata of metabolic syndrome.
    - Presence of complications suggestive of DM when casual serum glucose and fasting serum glucose are nondiagnostic.
    - Diagnostic when 2-hour postload glucose ≥200 mg per dL
    - Patient status and preparation
      - Usual state of health (no exogenous glucocorticoid therapy or total parenteral nutrition)
      - Dietary carbohydrate intake of 300 g daily for the 3 days prior

- Overnight fast of 8 hours
- Ingestion of 75 g of anhydrous glucose with 300 mL water to prevent nausea or emesis. Phlebotomy for serum glucose in sodium fluoride tube 2 hours after glucose ingestion.

- The hemoglobin A_{1c} is not a diagnostic criterion for DM. Therefore, a normal hemoglobin A_{1c} does not rule out a diagnosis of DM.
- Other abnormalities of glucose tolerance
  - Impaired glucose tolerance
    - Fasting plasma glucose <126 mg per dL
    - 2-hour postload (75 g anhydrous glucose) plasma glucose of ≥140 mg per dL and ≤199 mg per dL

  - Impaired fasting glucose
    - Fasting plasma glucose ≥100 mg per dL and <126 mg per dL

- **Laboratory classification.** Clinical history, physical examination, ambient glucose levels, and degree of ketosis usually suffice for appropriate diagnostic classification. In equivocal settings, C-peptide or insulin levels (low in type 1 patients) coupled with glutamic acid decarboxylase antibodies and pancreatic islet cell antibodies (positive in 90% of new-onset type 1 DM patients) allows correct classification.
- **Treatment goals.** Since publication of the Diabetes Control and Complications Trial (DCCT), the Epidemiology of Diabetic Complications Trial (EDIC) (the extension of the DCCT), the United Kingdom Prospective Diabetes Study (UKPDS) and numerous position statements from the American Diabetes Association, the ultimate goal for all patients, with few exceptions, is normalization or near-normalization of blood glucose levels within the constraints of hypoglycemia. Exceptions may include extremes of age, limited life expectancy, and advanced diabetic complications, including cardiac and cerebrovascular disease. Intensive patient training by a skilled team is vital to the safety and efficacy of the treatment plan.
  - Short-term goals are (a) correction of hyperglycemia and ketosis, (b) elimination of hypoglycemia, and (c) reintegration of patient into society.
  - Long-term goals include preservation of residual insulin production in type 1 patients through early physiologic insulin replacement, facilitating long-term optimal glycemic control and forestalling "brittleness." Key is attainment and maintenance of normal or near-normal body weight to optimize insulin sensitivity, minimize insulin requirements, and minimize cardiovascular risk. It is helpful to obtain optimization of physical fitness through individualized realistic exercise schedules for optimal weight maintenance, insulin sensitivity, and cardiovascular risk. Prevention of microvascular complications occurs through optimal glycemic control, normotension, and avoidance of excess sodium and protein intake. Prevention of macrovascular disease is achieved via aggressive conventional risk factor reduction. Early detection and prompt intervention once complications occur.

- **Patient counseling, education, and motivation.** Patient training programs in the following areas are vital for short- and long-term goal achievement: pathophysiology of DM and the prevention of complications; therapeutic options for optimal control and lifestyle flexibility; dietary instruction/counseling; exercise integration; foot care; and sick-day and minor-illness management. Patients must be well versed in integration of these principles into their daily lives.

MANAGEMENT OF TYPE 1 DIABETES MELLITUS: INSULIN CONSIDERATIONS

- **Indications for outpatient initiation of insulin** include the following: patient is not vomiting, has no evidence of clinical dehydration, has no evidence of diabetic ketoacidosis (DKA), and the necessary support staff are readily available. It is impossible to accurately predict insulin sensitivity based on weight alone. Conservative initial starting doses in an otherwise well patient are in the range of 0.25 to 0.5 unit per kg of body weight.

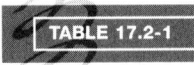

Activity	Classification	Name	Onset (h)	Peak (min)	Duration (h)
Short-acting	Insulin	Regular	0.5–1.0	150–210	6
Rapid-acting	Insulin analogue	Aspart	0–0.25	60–90	3–5
		Glulisine	0–0.25	60–90	3–4
		Lispro	0–0.25	60–90	3–5
Intermediate-acting	Insulin	NPH	1–3	6–8[a]	10–19
Long-acting	Insulin	Detemir	2–4	None	up to 24
	Insulin analogue	Glargine	2–4	None	24–36

[a] Considerable fluctuations in day-to-day kinetics depending on absorption.

- **Choice of insulin.** Human insulin is the only insulin available in the United States. Some patients report being less aware of their hypoglycemia with human (as opposed to animal) insulin, although the issue remains controversial. See Table 17.2-1 for insulin types and kinetics. The table reflects the kinetics seen in actual clinical practice rather than those reported by the manufacturers in nondiabetic individuals.
- **Injection site** principles are important for insulin absorption rate.
  - Site selection
    - Buttocks are the preferred site for bedtime injections of intermediate-acting insulin to minimize the risk of nocturnal hypoglycemia via (a) slow absorption, (b) avoidance of the 2 A.M. counterregulatory nadir, and (c) optimization of control of dawn surge in hepatic glucose output (dawn phenomenon).
    - Upper abdomen is preferred for the other injections because of (a) its more rapid insulin absorption and (b) better control of the early postprandial glucose level. Upper arms can be used as an alternative.
    - Avoid injecting into legs and buttocks before meals due to slower absorption from these sites.
  - Site consistency. Patients must be instructed regarding the consistent use of anatomical regions for premeal and bedtime injections with adequate site rotation within these regions to prevent lipohypertrophy. Injection site selection is less of an issue with newer analogues—the rapid-acting analogue (RAA) glulisine and the long-acting analogues glargine and detemir.

- **Insulin injection timing issues**
  - Use of the subcutaneous site versus physiologic portal insulin results in delay in insulin absorption and an unavoidable mismatch between onset and peak of the insulin action and the onset and peak of blood glucose rise after carbohydrate ingestion.
  - Injection interval
    - RAA insulin (aspart, glulisine, lispro) 0 to 10 minutes premeal, due to their rapid onset of action. Glulisine insulin injected up to 20 minutes after the start of a meal has similar kinetics to regular insulin injected 30 minutes premeal.
    - Regular insulin 30 to 40 minutes premeal helps to improve postprandial glycemic control.
  - A small snack (15 g carbohydrate) at the peak of the insulin action—3 hours for regular insulin and 6 to 8 hours for Neutral Protamine Hagedorn [NPH]—prevents hypoglycemia at this high-risk time.

- **Intensive insulin therapy programs**
  - Multiple daily insulin injections

- Principles
  - The use of multiple injections results in (a) smaller individual insulin doses, (b) more physiologic matching of carbohydrate and insulin, and (c) reduced risk of hypoglycemia. Evidence continues to accrue suggesting that early physiologic insulin replacement "rests" the pancreas, decreases insulitis, and preserves any residual β-cell function. The better postprandial control that can be achieved with intensive insulin therapy (as compared to conventional therapy) may reduce microvascular and macrovascular risk even with comparable hemoglobin A_{1c} levels.

- Program options
  - The tid program with NPH
  - Two thirds of total daily dose is given in the morning. One third of dose is RAA/regular insulin. Two thirds of dose is NPH insulin (isophane insulin suspension) insulin.
  - One third of total daily dose is given in the evening with half of the dose as RAA/regular insulin before supper and half of the dose as NPH given between 10 P.M. and 1 A.M.
  - Ratios must be modified pending patient's preferred mealtime carbohydrate distribution.

- The qid program: (a) Premeal dose (tid) of regular insulin titrated to carbohydrate intake and (b) bedtime NPH (20% of total daily dose)
- The qid program: (a) Premeal dose (tid) of RAA insulin titrated to carbohydrate intake and (b) bedtime insulin glargine/detemir (40% total daily dose)

■ Continuous subcutaneous insulin infusion (CSII) or insulin pump therapy
- Indications
  - Failure of multiple daily insulin injection regimens
  - Exuberant dawn phenomenon
  - Need for convenience and flexibility
  - Pregnancy
  - Preconception

- Setup
  - RAA insulin is programmed at set hourly basal rates to control hepatic glucose output in the fasting state and attain control of hepatic glucose production liver (approximately 40% to 60% total daily dose).
  - Remainder of dose is premeal/snack RAA insulin titrated to carbohydrate intake.
  - RAA insulin used nearly exclusively due to superior kinetics.

■ **Insulin adjustment**
  ■ Baseline dose
  - Doses of RAA, regular, NPH, glargine, or detemir insulin can be readily adjusted based on premeal, postprandial, and bedtime home blood glucose test results. Assuming a total daily dose of 0.5 unit per kg body weight, supplementing the baseline dose by 1 unit of insulin will drop an elevated blood glucose by approximately 50 mg per dL.
  - Algorithm
    - Home adjustment algorithm for the patient using supplemental RAA/regular insulin:
      - Use before meals and at bedtime. Example: In a patient taking 0.5 unit insulin per kg body weight, the following calculations apply:
        - Premeal dosing. Add 1 unit of RAA/regular insulin for every 50 mg per dL elevation in blood glucose above 120 mg per dL; that is, at 170 mg per dL, add 1 unit RAA/regular; at 220 mg per dL, add 2 units RAA/regular.
        - At bedtime. Add 1 unit of RAA/regular insulin for every 50 mg per dL elevation in blood glucose above 150 mg per dL; that is, at 200 mg per dL, add 1 unit RAA/regular; at 250 mg per dL, add 2 units RAA/regular.

- In the context of frequent follow-up, optimal control can be achieved with gradual insulin titration. Once achieved in the newly diagnosed patient, insulin requirements may gradually decline ("honeymoon phase"). Although insulin therapy can be discontinued for weeks to (occasionally) months, it may not be prudent to do so entirely. Maintaining a dose as low as 0.2 unit per kg body weight in divided doses may prevent progressive insulitis and delay complete loss of β-cell function.

MANAGEMENT OF TYPE 1 DIABETES MELLITUS: DIETARY CONSIDERATIONS

- **Basic principles.** Dietary recommendations continue to change somewhat, with the current emphasis on individualization and carbohydrate counting while maintaining low fat (<35% of total daily calories), high fiber, and moderate protein intake. Better matching of insulin to intake of total carbohydrate through gram counting of carbohydrate allows the incorporation of modest amounts of sucrose in the diet.
- **Ideal body weight (IBW).** Several formulas exist for estimation of IBW. A simple nomogram is as follows:
  - Female IBW
    - Assume 100 lb for first 5 feet of height.
    - Add 5 lb for every inch in height above 5 feet.
    - A 5 ft 5 in. tall woman should weigh 125 lb.
  - Male IBW
    - Assume 106 lb for first 5 feet of height.
    - Add 6 lb for every inch in height above 5 feet.
    - A 5 ft 8 in. tall man should weigh 154 lb.
  - Add 10% for a large-framed individual; subtract 10% for a small-framed individual.
- **Caloric requirements**
  - Caloric requirements vary with age, sex, IBW, level of physical activity, and concurrent illness.
  - Formulas for calculation. The Harris–Benedict equation approximates well, but a simpler formula follows:
    - IBW (lb) × 10 = resting energy expenditure (REE) calories.
    - Activity factor: Add 10% for inactivity, 30% for moderate activity, and 50% for significant activity (e.g., manual labor, intense exercise).
    - Total caloric requirements = REE + activity factor − 500 kcal per day for a 1 lb per week weight loss
- **Nutrient distribution.** Carbohydrate should be 45% to 65% of total daily calories, whereas fat should account for less than 35% and protein for 10% to 35% of total daily calories.
- **Priorities of patient training**
  - Emphasize carbohydrate counting and consistency with three meals. Add 15-g carbohydrate snacks to cover insulin peaks (regular/NPH), in the context of an appropriate total caloric intake.
  - Other priorities include fat gram counting and maintenance of low fat intake (goal is less than 35% of total intake). Sodium intake goal is less than 2000 mg per day. Optimizing fiber intake and limiting excess protein intake are also important.

MANAGEMENT OF TYPE 1 DIABETES MELLITUS

Home blood glucose monitoring (HBGM) considerations:

- **Basic principles**
  - Accuracy in HBGM is critical to safety and success of intensive therapy.
  - Frequency
    - Minimum of four tests per day should be done before meals and at bedtime.
    - Testing 1 hour after a meal is necessary to accurately determine the adequacy of the premeal Lispro insulin doses.
    - Additional testing is done when hypoglycemia or hyperglycemia is suspected.

- Periodic 2 A.M. and 4 A.M. tests
- Prior to driving

■ Meters are easy to use and have "no blot" technology, thus eliminating timing by the patient. The blood volume required has progressively decreased, with some meters requiring as little as 0.3 μL. Test time can be as little as 5 seconds. Many meters have memories that can store a large volume of results and can download data to personal computers. Patients must follow manufacturer's instructions carefully to achieve accurate results.

■ Sources of error in HBGM: Improper cleansing of finger; failure to wipe away first drop of blood when alcohol is used to cleanse finger; volume of blood applied to strip is too much or too little; meter is not calibrated to strip lot number; damaged strips resulting from exposure to heat, light, humidity, or cold; out-of-date strips; meter not properly cleaned; and failure to use glucose control solutions to verify strip accuracy.

■ Patient precision is vital to successful use of the insulin algorithm and sick-day management.

MANAGEMENT OF TYPE 1 DIABETES MELLITUS: EXERCISE CONSIDERATIONS

■ **Physical fitness** is a goal for all individuals with DM. Benefits of exercise include improvement of insulin sensitivity, aid in weight control, and reduction of cardiovascular risk and stress. Safe exercise plans must be individualized based on age, cardiovascular status, foot problems, neuropathy, and retinopathy. Even increased activity, such as grocery shopping, results in a lowering of blood glucose levels. Uncompensated physical activity is a very common cause of hypoglycemia.

■ **Insulin adjustment for exercise or activity.** Use for planned physical activity.
- Reduce insulin dose that is active during the exercise by 1 to 2 units for every 20 to 30 minutes of exercise.
- Occasionally, individuals have a delayed or sustained response to physical activity such that their bedtime insulin dose may need to be reduced by 1 to 2 units following, for example, evening physical activity.
- Insulin pump patients have the option to program a temporary reduction in their basal insulin infusion rates. Temporary basal rates must be programmed 45 to 60 minutes prior to the planned activity.

■ **Carbohydrate adjustment for exercise or activity**
- Use for either planned or spontaneous activity.
- Augment carbohydrate intake as follows: Add another 15-g carbohydrate snack (over and above the planned snacks) for every 20 to 30 minutes of physical activity, depending on the intensity of activity.

STANDARD OF CARE FOR FOLLOW-UP

Once glycemic control has been established, maintenance of glycemic control depends on the frequency of follow-up.

■ Minimum visit frequency is once every 3 months.

■ Review history; perform an interim physical examination; identify patient errors and omissions; adjust the patient's insulin dosage, diet, and exercise program; and do ongoing patient counseling. Laboratory evaluations should include hemoglobin A_{1c} every 3 months and annual assessments of urine microalbumin/creatinine ratio, thyroid-stimulating hormone, blood chemistries, and lipids (full panel). In addition, an electrocardiogram (ECG) and ankle–brachial indices (see following section) should be obtained annually.

DAWN PHENOMENON

■ **The dawn phenomenon** is a markedly elevated fasting blood glucose secondary to an exuberant rise in hepatic glucose output. This hyperglycemia results from a surge in counterregulatory hormone concentrations (catecholamines, growth hormone, and cortisol) in the absence of nocturnal hypoglycemia.

- **Treatment**
  - Delaying the timing of bedtime insulin dose until closer to midnight and titrating up the bedtime NPH, glargine, or detemir insulin usually suffices. In some instances, however, the dose increase results in hypoglycemia prior to the dawn surge. Continuous subcutaneous insulin infusion is ideal, so that basal rates can be pre-programmed to coincide with the patient's individual dawn surge.

SOMOGYI PHENOMENON

- **The Somogyi phenomenon** is posthypoglycemia hyperglycemia due to a surge in counterregulatory hormones, rather than insulin "run-out" or overtreatment with excess carbohydrate.
- **Strategy.** Perform HBGM at 2 A.M. and 4 A.M. in addition to premeal and bedtime HBGM. If the Somogyi phenomenon is identified, a dose reduction of the bedtime injection is indicated, coupled perhaps with a shift in the timing of the injection as late as possible (midnight or thereafter), with emphasis on the lower buttocks as the injection site of choice if NPH insulin is being used.

HYPOGLYCEMIA

Recurrent. In a well-designed, physiologic, individualized treatment program, most episodes are related to patient error.

- **Patient-related errors** include insulin–carbohydrate mismatch, delayed or missed meals, missed snacks, uncompensated exercise, erratic insulin injection site rotation, and lack of adequate HBGM (inaccurate tests or low frequency of HBGM).
- **Nonpatient-related problems** include unpredictable absorption or kinetics of NPH or lente insulin or possibly insulin autoantibodies. This is best treated by utilizing a quid program with insulin glargine or detemir.
- **Hypoglycemia unawareness**
  - Hypoglycemia can be a major problem in intensive therapy. In most cases, it is reversible to varying degrees through program revisions designed to eliminate hypoglycemia.
  - Once hypoglycemia has been eliminated for a reasonable period, the patient's subjective awareness and counterregulatory response improve, with the exception of the glucagon response. Improvement in hypoglycemia awareness facilitates safe lowering of ambient glucose levels and hemoglobin A_{1c}.

DIABETIC KETOACIDOSIS (DKA)

Prevention and management. DKA is a syndrome of hyperglycemia, ketonemia, and ketonuria of varying intensity that results in death in 10% of cases.

- Causes. Minor illnesses are the most common cause, such as upper respiratory and urinary tract infections. Major illnesses (e.g., myocardial infarction) are a less common cause. Most cases of severe DKA can be averted through aggressive attention to the sick-day management guidelines (refer to Special Issues, below).
- Treatment
  - If intractable emesis occurs, take the following measures:
    - Administer early intravenous hydration with 1 to 2 L of normal saline fluid (in emergency room or office).
    - Administer SC insulin bolus, not IV insulin bolus, as the half-life of an IV bolus of regular insulin is only 5 minutes.
    - Administer parenteral or rectal antiemetics.
    - Do not delay. Delay in seeking therapy is the major factor in severe DKA episodes, which result in costly hospitalizations in intensive care units and even death.
- Identify and address the underlying illness. Rule out silent myocardial infarction or occult sepsis as cause of DKA.
  - Correct the volume depletion.
    - Give 1 to 2 L of normal saline in the first 1 to 2 hours to correct hypotension and establish good urine output. In children and adolescents, give 500 mL of normal saline per hour for the first 1 to 2 hours.

- Total volume deficit is frequently 5 to 6 L. In most individuals, volume can be replaced over 12 to 24 hours, depending on the underlying cardiac and renal status.
- Failure to adequately rehydrate and correct ketosis completely is a common cause of rapid DKA relapse.

■ Insulin treatment. Start a low-dose IV infusion at the rate of 0.1 unit/kg/hour to result in a 100 mg/dL/hour fall in blood glucose. Adequately dilute the insulin to allow fine titration (50 units human regular insulin in 500 mL normal saline). This dosage overcomes the common clinical problem of having 1 unit per hour be the lowest infusion rate possible. To maintain a sufficiently high insulin dose to correct ketosis without hypoglycemia, the intravenous fluids must be changed to dextrose 5% or 10% when blood glucose level falls below 250 mg per dL.

■ Electrolyte replacement
- Potassium replacement may be initiated once urine output is documented. Use 20 to 40 mEq per L IV fluids and monitor serum values q2h.
- Bicarbonate therapy is indicated only for severe acidosis (pH < 7.2) or a bicarbonate concentration of less than 5 mEq per L. The goal is to raise pH above 7.2, not to achieve total correction; 40 to 80 mEq per m^2 of bicarbonate may be infused over 2 hours and the levels reassessed. Bicarbonate should not be given by IV push because that could result in cerebral edema, which is often fatal.
- Phosphate repletion has more theoretical than proven practical benefits unless severe depletion is present (serum phosphorus < 0.5 mg/dL).
- Magnesium repletion. If deficiency is severe (serum magnesium level < 1.0 mEq/L) or the patient is symptomatic (seizures, tetany, cardiac arrhythmias), then replace with magnesium chloride at a dose of 1 mEq/kg/24 hours, assuming normal renal function.

■ Monitor DKA progress. Clinical and laboratory monitoring of the patient should be documented on a flow sheet. Laboratory parameters should be followed at least every 2 hours until stability emerges.

HYPERGLYCEMIC HYPEROSMOLAR NONKETOTIC COMA

■ **Characteristics.** This development occurs in type 2 DM patients, most commonly with underlying renal insufficiency or cerebrovascular disease (cerebrovascular accident or subdural hematoma). The degree of dehydration is more severe than that of DKA. Blood glucose levels range from 600 to 2,000 mg per dL, and ketosis is absent.

■ **Treatment** is similar to that for DKA in terms of IV fluids, insulin, and electrolytes, but hydration rates must be lower.
- The initial infusion rate of normal saline should not exceed 1 L per hour to expand the extracellular space, with the IV fluid being switched to half normal saline once blood pressure is stable and good urine output is established. Fluid should be replaced over a 24-hour period.
- Often insulin therapy is not needed on an ongoing basis once the acute metabolic derangement has been corrected and any underlying precipitating illness treated or resolved.

RECURRENT DIABETIC KETOACIDOSIS OR BRITTLE DIABETES MELLITUS

Nonadherence to a well-designed treatment program or lack of same is the cause. If, after comprehensive repeat patient counseling, the problem persists, then occult psychologic issues, such as marital disharmony or dysfunctional family, should be explored. The assistance of a psychologist or psychiatrist experienced in diabetes management is essential.

INITIAL MANAGEMENT OF TYPE 2 DIABETES MELLITUS

■ **Minimally decompensated presentation**
- Clinical picture includes obesity and mild to moderate hyperglycemia with or without symptoms. Treatment strategies include patient education, training, and motivation; an individualized hypocaloric diet with diet training; and an exercise plan tailored to the individual. Emphasize permanent lifestyle modification.

- **Moderately decompensated presentation**
  - Clinical picture. Obesity, severe symptomatic hyperglycemia (fasting blood glucose >300 mg/dL), and mild dehydration or decompensation calls for more urgent lowering of blood glucose levels, largely for symptomatic relief and reversal of the glucotoxic effect of the prior sustained hyperglycemia on pancreatic islet insulin secretion and periphera; insulin action.
  - Treatment strategies
    - Temporary insulin therapy with daily glargine/detemir or prebreakfast and bedtime dosing of NPH insulin at a starting daily dose of 0.5 unit per kilogram of weight and an algorithm for hyperglycemia similar to that for type 1 DM patients will rapidly yield symptomatic relief and reversal of islet and peripheral/target organ glucotoxicity. Prescribe an individualized hypocaloric diet with diet training and an exercise plan. The long-term goal is tapering and withdrawal of insulin, assuming that glycemic control can be maintained with diet and oral agent therapy.
- **Severely decompensated presentation**
  - Clinical picture shows a severely symptomatic patient with blood glucose levels exceeding 500 mg per dL, marked dyslipidemia (serum triglycerides >1,000 mg/dL), and hyperosmolality with absence of ketosis.
  - Treatment strategies
    - Intravenous fluids and insulin (similar to DKA) in the hospital setting are necessary for acute reversal of the metabolic derangement, followed later by a switch to daily insulin glargine/detemir or prebreakfast and bedtime dosing of NPH insulin.
    - Start patient training and education with an individualized hypocaloric diet and exercise plan. The long-term goal is tapering and withdrawal of insulin, assuming that glycemic control can be maintained with diet and oral agent therapy.
- **Consider pharmacotherapy for obesity** (sibutramine or orlistat) in patients who are not losing weight.
- **Special situation: The nonobese type 2 diabetic patient.** Patients who are at less than 120% IBW may benefit from modest weight loss toward IBW, with a hypocaloric diet and exercise training program. Exercise may be especially beneficial to these patients, many of whom are relatively insulinopenic and poor responders to oral agents. Frequently these patients will require basal insulin therapy with glargine/detemir insulin, and many will need to progress to full insulin replacement akin to an individual with type 1 DM.

DIETARY MANAGEMENT OF TYPE 2 DIABETES MELLITUS

- **The IBW and caloric requirements** are the same as those for type 1 DM patients. Reduction in daily caloric intake by 500 calories will facilitate a 1 lb per week weight loss.
- **Goals in obese patients**
  - Reduction in body weight
    - Strategies. Reduce fat intake through fat gram counting, high fiber intake, reduced sodium intake, and the use of artificial sweeteners and low-fat products.
    - A reduction of even 5% to 10% in weight can have a major impact on the clinical course of a type 2 patient. Patients need not reduce to IBW to achieve euglycemia, but the closer they are, the better all the other markers of the metabolic syndrome will be (e.g., dyslipidemia, hypertension).
  - Manage concurrent dyslipidemia and hypertension.
- **Very low-calorie diets** are occasionally used in specialty centers for the more difficult or noncompliant patients. Recidivism remains common.

EXERCISE THERAPY FOR TYPE 2 DIABETES MELLITUS

All of the benefits of exercise for the type 1 patient apply even more to the type 2 patient, with the added benefit of raising the frequently depressed high-density lipoprotein (HDL) cholesterol. Adherence to an ongoing exercise routine is one of the most powerful predictors of maintenance of weight loss. The importance of exercise capacity and survival must be stressed.

PHARMACOTHERAPY OF TYPE 2 DIABETES MELLITUS (TABLE 17.2-2)

■ **Insulin sensitizers**
  ▒ Metformin
    • Indication. Metformin therapy is indicated for obese (>120% IBW), diet-failure patients with type 2 DM who are free from liver disease, have good renal function (normal serum creatinine, normal estimated glomerular filtration rate, and normal measured creatinine clearance), and have no underlying chronic hypoxic condition (e.g., chronic obstructive pulmonary disease, asthma, or advanced congestive heart failure). Lactic acidosis is a risk if any of these underlying conditions exist; hence, the contraindication. Metformin should be discontinued on

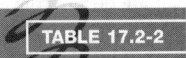 **TABLE 17.2-2   Oral Agents Used to Treat Diabetes Mellitus**

Medication	Usual recommended starting dose	Usual maintenance dose	Maximum daily dose	Dose frequency
Biguanide				
Metformin	500 mg bid	1,000 mg bid	2,550 mg	bid or tid
Metformin xr	500 mg qd	1,000–2,000 mg qd	2,000 mg qd	qd
Thiazolidinediones (glitazones)				
Rosiglitazone	2 mg bid	2–4 mg bid	8 mg	bid preferred; can be qd
Pioglitazone	15 mg qd	30–45 mg qd	45 mg	qd
α-Glucosidase inhibitors				
Acarbose	25 mg tid	50–100 mg tid	300 mg	tid
Miglitol	25 mg tid	50–100 mg tid	300 mg	tid
Repaglinide	0.5 mg tid 0–15 min premeal	2–4 mg tid 0–15 min premeal	16 mg	bid-qid pending meal/snack frequency
Nateglinide	120 mg tid premeal	120 mg tid premeal	360 mg	tid with meals
Sulfonylureas				
Glimepiride	1 mg qd	4–8 mg qd	8 mg	qd or bid
Glipizide GITS	2.5 mg qd	10–20 mg qd	20 mg	qd or bid
Glipizide	5 mg bid	10–20 mg bid	40 mg	bid
Micronized glyburide	1.5 mg bid	3–6 mg bid	12 mg	bid
Glyburide	2.5 mg qd	5–10 mg bid	20 mg	bid
Tolbutamide	500–1,000 mg	500–3,000 mg	3,000 mg	bid or tid
Tolazamide	100–250 mg	100–1,000 mg	1,000 mg	qd or bid
Acetohexamide	250–500 mg	250–1,500 mg	1,500 mg	qd or bid
Chlorpropamide	100–250 mg	100–500 mg	750 mg	qd

the day of any iodinated dye-load procedure or surgery and should be withheld for 48 hours after the procedure. Metformin should not be restarted until a normal posttest/surgery serum creatinine is confirmed. Metformin should also be withheld during treatment for pneumonia or acute myocardial infarction. Metformin is contraindicated in individuals with known hypersensitivity to the drug or any of its components.

- Mode of action. Metformin is an insulin sensitizer with a primary mode of action of controlling hepatic glucose output. It is an antihyperglycemic agent. It is not a hypoglycemic agent; therefore, it cannot cause hypoglycemia when used as monotherapy.
- Dosing
  - Use as monotherapy or in combination with sulfonylureas or insulin. Combination therapy results, on average, in an additional 50 mg per dL lowering of blood glucose and an additional 1.0% to 1.5% lowering of hemoglobin A_{1c}.
  - Initial dose (500 mg bid with food) can be titrated to a maximum of 2550 mg in an 850 mg tid dosing schedule. Maximum effective dose is seen at 1000 mg bid.
  - An extended-release preparation is now available to facilitate dosing convenience and reduce frequency of diarrhea.
- Other effects. Metformin facilitates weight loss and an improvement in the lipid profile.
- Adverse effects. Gastrointestinal (GI) side effects of nausea, flatus, and diarrhea can occur but are usually self-limited (1 to 2 weeks). Side effects can be minimized by taking the agent with food or using an extended-release preparation. Long-term discontinuation rate due to GI side effects is only 3% to 4%.

▨ Thiazolidinediones (glitazones)
- Indications. Therapy with rosiglitazone or pioglitazone therapy is indicated for obese (>120% IBW) diet-failure patients with type 2 DM who are free of liver disease, hepatic transaminases ≤1.5 times the upper limit of normal, and who have good left ventricular function. Therapy is contraindicated in patients who have New York Heart Association class III or IV congestive heart failure. Glitazones are contraindicated in individuals with known hypersensitivity to the drug(s) or any of their components. They can be used safely in patients with end-stage renal disease.
- Mode of action. Glitazones are insulin sensitizers that activate peroxisome proliferator–activated receptors (PPARs). Clinical effect from this activation is delayed, and the maximal effect of a given dose level may not be seen for 8 to 12 weeks. The primary mode of action of glitazones is to enhance skeletal muscle glucose uptake both directly and also indirectly via reduction in free fatty acids. At higher doses they also reduce hepatic glucose output. They are antihyperglycemic and as such when used as monotherapy or in combination with metformin cannot cause hypoglycemia.
- Dosing
  - Rosiglitazone
    - Initial dose of 2 mg bid can be titrated to 4 mg bid. Can be given qd but better glucose lowering effect noted with bid dosing in clinical trials.
    - Dosing independent of food intake.
    - Can be used as monotherapy or in combination with metformin, sulfonylureas, or insulin.
  - Pioglitazone
    - Initial dose of 15 mg qd can be titrated to 45 mg qd.
    - Dosing independent of food intake.
    - Can be used as monotherapy or in combination with metformin, sulfonylureas, or insulin.
- Adverse effects
  - Idiosyncratic hepatic dysfunction. The first glitazone troglitazone was voluntarily removed from the U.S. market by its manufacturer in March 2000, secondary

to the occurrence, among a small number of treated patients, of fulminant hepatic failure resulting in transplantation and/or death. The incidence of elevations in hepatic transaminases in treated patients was 2%. Rosiglitazone and pioglitazone have a lower risk of elevations in hepatic transaminases (0.35% and 0.26%). Current recommendations are for monitoring of hepatic transaminases at baseline and then periodically thereafter.

- Pedal edema. Edema, varying from trace to 4+, can develop as a consequence of glitazone therapy. No predisposing factors appear to exist. Patients who experience edema with one glitazone may occasionally tolerate another. Frequently, starting at a low dose with slow titration can help. This edema can potentially precipitate congestive heart failure in susceptible patients. The risk of edema is increased with concurrent use of calcium-channel blockers and NSAIDs.
- Dilutional anemia
- Weight gain. The weight gain seen with glitazone therapy in some patients appears to be in excess of that expected from reduction/elimination in glycosuria.

■ α-Glucosidase inhibitors

- Indications. Acarbose and miglitol are generally indicated as second-line pharmacologic treatment for individuals with type 2 DM who have previously failed diet therapy. Contraindications include cirrhosis, inflammatory bowel disease, other bowel disease, and malabsorption and known hypersensitivity to the drugs or any of their components.
- Mode of action. α-Glucosidase inhibitors interfere with digestion and absorption of dietary carbohydrate. Therefore, their primary effect is on postprandial blood glucose levels. They are antihyperglycemic agents and as such when used as monotherapy or in combination with metformin (acarbose only) cannot cause hypoglycemia. However, hypoglycemia can occur when acarbose is used in combination with a sulfonylurea or insulin. When hypoglycemia occurs, it must be managed with pure glucose because the digestion and absorption of alternative carbohydrates will be blocked.
- Dosing
  - Starting dose of 25 mg tid to be taken with the first bite of each meal.
  - Titration to 50 mg tid, up to a maximum dose of 100 mg tid.
  - May be used as monotherapy or in combination with sulfonylureas. Acarbose may also be used in combination with metformin or insulin.
- Adverse effects include flatus and nausea, which lessen over time. Small numbers of patients experience an elevation in transaminases (usually in individuals with a body weight of less than 60 kg).

■ Secretagogues

- Sulfonylureas
  - Indications. Although in the past sulfonylureas were considered to be first-line pharmacotherapeutic agents for type 2 DM, new treatment patterns generally utilize these drugs as second-line agents in the setting of mild to moderate hyperglycemia. Their use is contraindicated in patients with elevations in hepatic transaminases. A relative contraindication is sulfa allergy. Caution must be used in the setting of end-stage renal disease. Sulfonylureas are contraindicated in individuals with known hypersensitivity to these medications.
  - Mode of action is augmentation of pancreatic insulin secretion.
  - Dosing. See Table 17.2-2.
  - Adverse effects are weight gain and hypoglycemia. Hypoglycemia frequency is reduced with glimepiride. The first-generation agents (chlorpropamide, tolazamide, tolbutamide, and acetohexamide) are now rarely used because they carry a poor side-effect profile, including protein binding issues, syndrome of inappropriate secretion of antidiuretic hormone, and the chlorpropamide flush.
- Fixed combinations of glyburide/metformin and glimiperide/rosiglitazone are available.
- Repaglinide

- Indications. Patients with type 2 DM who have failed dietary therapy. Contraindicated in individuals with known hypersensitivity to the drug or any of its components. No sulfa moiety. Can be used in patients with sulfa allergy/sulfonylurea allergy.
- Mode of action. Binding to a specific islet cell receptor results in more rapid secretion of insulin in response to food eaten as compared with sulfonylureas. Effect is seen especially on postprandial and to a lesser extent on fasting glucose levels
- Dosing
  - Initial dose of 0.5 mg taken 0 to 15 minutes before a meal can be titrated to a maximum dose of 4 mg taken 1 to 15 minutes before a meal or snack for a maximal daily dose of 16 mg.
  - Must be dosed in conjunction with food to have optimum glucose-lowering effect.
  - Can be used as monotherapy or in combination with metformin or glitazones.
  - Adverse effects. Hypoglycemia can occur, but does so less frequently than with sulfonylureas due to the rapid onset and shorter duration of action. This is especially pertinent when patients delay or miss meals. In addition, the lack of an increase in basal insulin secretion lowers the risk of hypoglycemia.

- Nateglinide
  - Indications. Type 2 DM inadequately controlled by diet. Contraindication is hypersensitivity to nateglinide or any of its components. No sulfa moiety. Can be used in patients with sulfa allergy/sulfonylurea allergy. Can be used as monotherapy or in combination with metformin or glitazones.
  - Mode of action. The phenylalanine derivative nateglinide binds to the potassium channel in the islet, resulting in more rapid insulin secretion from the pancreatic islets. It uniquely restores early insulin secretion, which is lost early in the course of type 2 DM. Early insulin secretion is very important in the regulation of hepatic glucose production postprandially.
  - Dosing
    - 120 mg tid prior to meals. 60 mg tid prior to meals may be used in patients who are near goal hemoglobin A_{1c} when initiating treatment.
  - Adverse effects
    - Hypoglycemia is the most common side effect and is seen at a much lower rate than that with any other secretagogue.

- **Insulin**
  - Insulin source. All insulin should be human insulin.
  - Long-term insulin therapy indications.
    - Insulinopenic nonobese type 2 DM patients who have failed optimum diet, exercise, and oral agent therapy are best managed on insulin programs described for type 1 DM patients.
    - Insulin is indicated in secretagogue-failure patients in whom metformin and/or glitazones are contraindicated, are not tolerated, or have failed.
  - Dosing schedules. Several dosing schedules have been advocated, and all have a tendency to progressive weight gain and attendant increasing insulin requirements to try to maintain glycemic control. Administration of NPH, glargine, or detemir insulin at bedtime facilitates the best control of dawn hepatic glucose output, thereby minimizing islet glucotoxicity and maximizing islet insulin secretory response to daytime sulfonylureas. Should this regimen fail to give adequate control, any of the regimens outlined for type 1 DM patients may be used, with the exception of CSII (see above). A rare indication for the use of CSII in type 2 DM is the lean insulinopenic patient.

- **New agents**
  - Exenatide. Exenatide is a 39 amino acid glucagons-like peptide 1 analogue that enhances glucose-dependent insulin secretion, suppresses glucagon secretion, delays gastric emptying, and promotes satiety. Exenatide improves both first-phase and second-phase insulin secretion resulting in improved postprandial and overall glycemic control. Exenatide is indicated for type 2 DM patients who are using metformin or

a sulfonyluea or a combination of both who have not achieved adequate glycemic control. Exenatide is administered as a subcutaneous injection at a dose of 5 μg within 60 minutes of the morning and evening meals. The dose can be increased after 1 month to 10 μg bid. GI side effects include nausea, vomiting, and diarrhea. Exenatide is not recommended for patients with severe renal impairment (30 mL/min) due to severe GI side effects.

■ Pramlintide. Pramlintide is an analogue of the neuroendocrine hormone amylin that is cosecreted by the pancreatic β-cells in response to food intake. Pramlinitide delays gastric emptying, suppresses glucagon secretion, and reduces food intake via central modulation of appetite. Pramlintide improves postprandial glucose and overall glycemic control and is indicated for individuals with type 1 DM or type 2 DM as an adjunct to insulin therapy. In type 2 DM patients, it may be used with a sulfonylurea or metformin therapy. In type 1 DM patients, pramlintide should be initiated at a dose of 15 μg SC immediately prior to major meals with titration in 15 μg increments to a maintenance dose of 30 to 60 μg premeal as tolerated. In patients with type 2 DM, pramlintide should be initiated at a dose of 60 μg SC immediately prior to major meals and increased to 120 μg premeal as tolerated. Concurrent insulin therapy increases the risk of insulin-induced hypoglycemia, especially in patients with type 1 DM. Reduction in premeal insulin by 50% is recommended to minimize the risk of hypoglycemia. Frequent HBGM is needed to ensure safety and efficacy. Nausea is the most common treatment-emergent adverse event that limits dose titration or ongoing use of pramlintide. No dose adjustments are needed for patients with moderate to severe renal impairment (creatine clearance 20 to 50 mL/min).

■ Inhaled human regular insulin (Exubera). This is indicated for the treatment of adult patients with type 1 and type 2 DM. In type 1 DM patients, inhaled insulin must be used in a regimen that includes a longer-acting basal insulin. In type 2 DM patients, inhaled insulin can be used as monotherapy with meals or in combination therapy with oral agents or longer-acting insulins. Initial meal-time dosing is based on the patient's body weight and ranges from 1 to 6 mg per meal; 1 mg of inhaled insulin is approximately equivalent to 3 units of subcutaneous regular insulin. Inhaled insulin should be dosed within 10 minutes of each meal. Pulmonary function should be assessed at baseline, with patients having a forced expiratory volume in 1 second (FEV_1) or lung defusing capacity of carbon monoxide (DL_{CO}) <70% predicted contraindicated for therapy with inhaled insulin. Inhaled insulin is contraindicated in patients who smoke or who have discontinued smoking within the past 6 months. Pulmonary function should be rechecked at 6 months and annually thereafter. A decline of ≥20% in FEV_1 from baseline should prompt the discontinuation of inhaled insulin. Patients must be trained on the proper handling and care of the inhalation powder and inhalation device.

SPECIAL TESTING IN DIABETES

■ **Ankle–brachial indices** are part of the standard of care because of their predictive value, not only for peripheral vascular disease (PVD) but also for coronary artery disease and cardiovascular death risk. Blood pressures are measured with a mercury sphygmomanometer and hand-held Doppler at both the dorsalis pedis and posterior tibial arteries and compared with that obtained at the brachial artery. Any reduction in the ankle–brachial index (ankle pressure divided by brachial pressure) below 0.9 is significant and warrants intensive risk factor modification.

■ **Stress testing**
  ■ Stress testing will only detect severe flow-limiting disease, which is responsible for less than 30% of all acute infarcts. The majority of acute myocardial infarctions result from plaque rupture in individuals with nonhemodynamically significant degrees of stenosis.
  ■ Despite the above limitations, stress testing is warranted under certain circumstances as per the American Diabetes Association Consensus Development Conference on the Diagnosis of Coronary Heart Disease in People with Diabetes.

- Routine stress testing is not indicated in the asymptomatic diabetic patient with one or no risk factors (as listed below) and a normal resting ECG and 0 to 1 risk factors (as listed below).
- Stress testing is warranted under the following situations:
  - Typical or atypical (dyspnea or exertional fatigue) symptoms.
  - Resting ECG suggestive of ischemia or prior infarction.
  - Peripheral or carotid occlusive disease.
  - Sedentary lifestyle, age ≥35, and planning to begin a vigorous exercise program.
- Conventional cardiac risk factors do not help identify asymptomatic patients with abnormal perfusion imaging on stress testing. Additionally, there is currently no evidence to suggest that stress-testing asymptomatic patients improves outcomes or leads to better utilization of available therapies. Accordingly, intensive risk factor modification for both asymptomatic and symptomatic patients is appropriate to include angiotensin-converting enzyme (ACE) inhibitor therapy for patients >55 years of age without hypertension and other cardiovascular risk factors to reduce the risk of cardiovascular events.

SPECIAL ISSUES

■ Foot care
- The critical interplay of three pathophysiologic processes—neuropathy, ischemia, and sepsis—results in injury predisposition and potential amputation.
- Patient should be instructed to inspect and wash feet daily; to use lotion on plantar and dorsal surfaces but not on intertriginous areas; to keep nails trimmed; and to seek podiatric care if needed.
- Patient should be instructed not to soak feet, walk barefoot, or do "bathroom surgery."

■ Sick-day guidelines
- Perform HBGM at a minimum qid; ideally q4h.
- Monitor urine ketones with voiding or monitor serum ketones with the Precision Xtra meter.
- Maintain aggressive oral fluid intake to prevent onset of hyperglycemia or ketosis: 1 cup salted broth every hour to replace fluids and electrolytes; 2 cups hourly is needed if urine ketones are moderate or higher.
- Always take full baseline insulin dose.
- Add more insulin per algorithm; increase algorithm (i.e., take 2 units of RAA/regular insulin per 50 mg per dL elevation in blood glucose) if making no or slow progress.
- Replace solid carbohydrates with clear liquid carbohydrates (such as regular ginger ale, regular soda, regular gelatin) if necessary.
- Obtain early medical evaluation for underlying illness.
- Obtain early emergency intervention with intravenous fluids if emesis reoccurs (more than three episodes) or diarrhea is intractable.
- The goal is prevention of DKA, which has up to a 10% mortality per episode.

COMPLICATIONS OF DIABETES MELLITUS

■ Hypertension in DM (see Chapter 9.1)
- In type 1 DM patients, hypertension implies the presence of microalbuminuria or nephropathy until proven otherwise.
- Treatment
  - ACE inhibitors have a special role in preserving renal function in type 1 DM patients based on an excellent study with captopril.
  - Calcium-channel blockers are warranted in cases of intolerance of or contraindications to ACE inhibitors or inadequate blood pressure control with these agents. They may have renal protective effects.
  - Angiotensin II receptor blockers (ARBs) are useful when ACE inhibitors are not tolerated, the most common reason being cough.

- β-Blockers have generally been avoided by endocrinologists unless there are specific indications (e.g., following myocardial infarction) because of symptom masking and delay in recovery of hypoglycemia in type 1 DM patients and worsening dyslipidemia and PVD in type 2 DM patients. However, the combination blocker carvedilol has unique properties that almost negate the potential negatives.
- Diuretics can be used in low dose without increasing insulin resistance.
- α-Blockers may be useful add-on therapy (not monotherapy) for patients not achieving goal with first-line agents.

■ Dyslipidemia (see Chapter 17.4)

- In type 1 DM, in the absence of nephropathy, dyslipidemia is generally only associated with poor glycemic control. If dyslipidemia is present, it usually indicates a concurrent familial dyslipidemia, which must be aggressively treated along conventional lines.
- Type 2 DM treatment priorities per current guidelines revolve around the following:
  - Low density lipoprotein cholesterol (LDL-C) lowering with therapeutic lifestyle changes with statins as the preferred initial intervention to achieve at least a 30% reduction in LDL-C regardless of baseline LDL-C. Cholesterol absorption inhibitors may be added or substituted in the case of statin intolerance. Alternative agents include niacin and fenofibrate.
  - High density lipoprotein cholesterol (HDL-C) elevating with therapeutic lifestyle changes, with the addition of niacin or fibrates.
  - Triglyceride lowering with therapeutic lifestyle changes, optimization of glycemic control, the addition of fibrates, niacin, or high-dose statins, especially for patients with LDL-C elevations.
  - In the past, niacin has been contraindicated in diabetes due to its adverse effect on glucose control. However, the long-acting formulation of niacin extended-release tablets appears to have good clinical effect in terms of lowering triglycerides and raising HDL-C with minimal adverse effects on glucose control.

■ Proteinuria

- Type 1 DM
  - The presence of proteinuria greater than 500 mg per 24 hours, regardless of presence of hypertension, is a Food and Drug Administration (FDA)-approved indication for the use of captopril 25 mg tid. Other ACE inhibitors probably have similar benefits, although definitive long-term data are lacking.
  - Reduction of dietary protein intake toward 0.8 g per kilogram of body weight is prudent.
- Type 2 DM. Management strategies are similar to those of type 1, with additional data present on the use of ARBs regarding renal protection.

■ Microalbuminuria

- As an elevated urine microalbumin/creatinine ratio is a strong predictor of the progression to clinical proteinuria, its presence is an indication for ACE inhibitor treatment. Clinical trial data support their use in patients with type 1 or type 2 diabetes.

■ Retinopathy

- An annual dilated ophthalmologic examination is indicated for all, with laser therapy being well established in the preservation of vision. In the UKPDS, improved blood pressure control was positively associated with reduced microvascular complication risk. Although not FDA-approved, the benefits of ACE inhibitor treatment in slowing the progression of retinopathy was noted in the EUCLID trial.

■ Neuropathy (see Chapter 6.9). Symptomatic pain may be controlled with:

- FDA-approved for diabetic peripheral neuropathic pain
  - Pregabalin, an anticonvulsant structurally related to gabapentin has been found in clinical studies to benefit diabetic peripheral neuropathy pain as well as postherpetic neuralgia. Pregabalin should be dosed at 50 mg tid and may be increased to 100 mg tid based on tolerability and efficacy. A lower starting dose and gradual increase to a lower maximum dose should be considered in patients

with renal impairment. It is a Schedule V controlled substance due to a very small percentage of patients in clinical trials experiencing euphoria.

- Duloxetine, a selective serotonin and norephinephrine reuptake inhibitor with antidepressant properties, has been found in clinical trials to benefit diabetic peripheral neuropathic pain. Duloxetine should be dose at 60 mg qd irrespective of meals. A lower starting dose and gradual titration should be considered in patients with renal impairment.

■ Not FDA-approved for neuropathic pain but commonly prescribed:

- Venlafaxine XR a selective serotonin and norephinephrine reuptake inhibitor can be used starting at a dose of 37.5 mg qd and titrating to an effective dose of 150 to 225 mg daily.
- Gabapentin, an anticonvulsant, can be used starting at a dose of 100 to 300 mg hs and titrating to a maximum dose of 800 mg tid. Doses must be significantly reduced in the setting of reduced creatinine clearance.
- Tricyclic antidepressants (e.g., amitriptyline), starting at low doses of 10 to 25 mg at bedtime and titrating up, pending patient tolerance.
- Additional daytime pain relief can be obtained with topical capsaicin cream or dextropropoxyphene–acetaminophen (Darvocet N-100), or both.

PREGNANCY PLANNING (SEE CHAPTER 14.6)

The congenital abnormality rate and risks of macrosomia can be reduced almost to nondiabetic levels through euglycemia at the time of conception and throughout pregnancy. This is best achieved through an intensive program of (a) RAA premeal and bedtime NPH insulin, or (b) CSII. Individuals with type 2 DM should discontinue all oral agents and initiate intensive insulin therapy prior to conception. Additionally, ACE inhibitors and other antihypertensives should be discontinued preconception. Methyldopa and labetolol are agents frequently used preconception and throughout pregnancy.

INDICATIONS FOR SPECIALTY REFERRAL

These include inadequate support staff (diabetes team) to provide comprehensive diabetes care, failure to achieve glycemic control goals, recurrent hypoglycemia or DKA, or hyperglycemic hyperosmolar nonketotic coma, and diabetic complications (e.g., nephropathy, retinopathy, refractory dyslipidemia, refractory hypertension, unusual neuropathies, peripheral vascular disease, coronary artery disease).

NETWORKING TO OPTIMIZE DIABETES CARE

Physicians alone cannot provide all the care and counseling needed by patients with DM. Physicians need to identify community resources to assist in the modern multidisciplinary team-care approach: nurse educators (certified diabetes educators) who are hospital based or private practice based, dietitians (certified diabetes educators), psychologists, social workers, podiatrists, and endocrinologists.

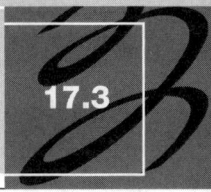

THYROID DISORDERS
Carrie Riah, Lois Starr

17.3

GENERAL PRINCIPLES

Definition
Disorders of the thyroid gland include states of hyperthyroidism, hypothyroidism, and euthyroidism. The thyroid is a common site of disease making it imperative for the family physician to be capable of identifying systemic symptoms. The thyroid itself may be enlarged (goiter), have nodules, or have benign or malignant tumors.

Anatomy
Embryologically, the thyroid gland is derived from an evagination of the floor of the pharynx descending along the midline. The median isthmus connects the two lateral lobes. In most people there is also a pyramidal lobe that extends superiorly from the isthmus. Oxygenated blood is supplied by the superior and inferior thyroid arteries. Venous drainage is then completed by the superior, middle, and inferior thyroid veins.

Epidemiology
Hyperthyroidism occurs 10 times more often in females than males with an annual incidence of 1:1,000 females. Hypothyroidism occurs in approximately 20:1,000 females and 2:1,000 males annually. The incidence of hypothyroidism increases with age, while hyperthyroidism occurs most commonly between 20–50 years of age.

HYPERTHYROIDISM

Diagnosis
Etiology
- **Graves disease** is the most common cause of hyperthyroidism in iodine-sufficient areas usually affecting women of reproductive age. It is a diffuse toxic goiter and is caused by abnormal thyroid-stimulating immunoglobulin binding to thyroid-stimulating hormone (TSH) receptors on the follicular cells, resulting in diffuse excessive stimulation of thyroid hormone production as well as enlargement of the gland itself. Graves disease consists of the following: hyperthyroidism, ophthalmopathy (puffiness of the lids, chemosis, proptosis, extraocular muscle weakness), and dermopathy.
- **Toxic multinodular goiter** is usually a mild hyperthyroidism in which there is a large, asymmetric, nodular goiter.
- **Toxic thyroid adenoma** is a hyperfunctioning follicular adenoma. It is usually a firm, large, solitary nodule.
- **Painless lymphocytic thyroiditis** is most common in the postpartum period and has a high recurrence rate with subsequent pregnancies. It usually presents with an initial hyperthyroid phase, a subsequent hypothyroid phase, and eventually a recovery of normal thyroid function.
- **Subacute thyroiditis** (de Quervain) is often accompanied by fever, myalgia, and a history of an upper respiratory tract infection. The thyroid gland itself is painful and tender.
- **Exogenous hyperthyroidism** should be suspected when there are symptoms present, yet absence of a goiter and absence of a suppressed radioactive iodine uptake (RAIU) test.
- **Pituitary tumors, ovarian teratomas (struma ovarii), iatrogenic (lithium therapy), and excessive ingestion of iodine–induced hyperthyroidism** are rare causes, but should be considered when more common causes are ruled out.

659

Clinical Presentation

An increase in thyroid hormone concentration causes an increase in tissue oxygen consumption that raises heat production and also increases metabolism. This can cause excessive diaphoresis, palpitations, fatigue and weakness, heat intolerance, oligomenorrhea, frequent bowel movements, anxiety, insomnia, and irritability. Eyelid retraction, hyperreflexia, a fine tremor, and proximal muscle weakness may also be present.

Apathetic thyrotoxicosis is an atypical presentation of hyperthyroidism, usually seen in elderly patients. Patients exhibit apathy, muscle rigidity, depression, dementia, anorexia, marked weight loss, and constipation. Thyrotoxic crisis, though rare, may be life-threatening. This condition is often accompanied by fever, seizures, vomiting, diarrhea, jaundice, and even coma.

Physical Examination

Hyperthyroidism can cause numerous systemic effects. The cardiovascular effects often include sinus tachycardia, a widened pulse pressure (due to increased systolic blood pressure and decreased diastolic pressure), as well as arrhythmias (most commonly atrial fibrillation or premature ventricular contractions) due to increased myocardial excitability. On exam, it is also important to look for onycholysis, pretibial myxedema, tremor, lid lag, proptosis, goiter, thyroid tenderness, hyperreflexia, warm or moist skin, and gynecomastia. Thyrotoxicosis for an extended period of time may also cause osteopenia. Also, it is important to listen for a bruit over the arteries of the thyroid, as they are commonly present in Graves disease.

Laboratory Evaluation

To diagnose hyperthyroidism biochemically, most commonly there is a suppressed or undetectable TSH level and an increased serum level of free T_4 (thyroxine). If there are normal free T_4 levels, the serum free T_3 (triiodothyronine) levels should be obtained. Occasionally, a patient may have hyperthyroid symptomatology, a suppressed TSH, normal free T_4 index, but elevated T_3—this is T_3 toxicosis. A low TSH level alone is not diagnostic for hyperthyroidism as it can be found to be decreased in dopamine or glucocorticoid therapy or secondary hypothyroidism.

Serum thyroglobulin is usually used as a tumor marker to follow up on thyroid carcinomas (see below), but it is also useful if the TSH is suppressed and the RAIU is low. The thyroglobulin level is high in lymphocytic thyroiditis and is low in exogenous hyperthyroidism.

TSH receptor autoantibody tests—TSI (thyroid-stimulating immunoglobulin) or TRab (thyroid receptor antibody)—are positive in 80% of patients with Graves disease and are diagnostic of this disorder. TSI levels can also be measured in infants born to women with Graves disease. The antibody tests are of special importance in pregnant women in whom one cannot perform an RAIU study.

When subacute thyroiditis is in the differential diagnosis, an erythrocyte sedimentation rate (ESR) level may be helpful as this is usually markedly elevated in that condition.

Imaging

Ultrasonography may be used to evaluate thyroid nodules and goiters. Graves disease may demonstrate an altered blood flow that can also be demonstrated via ultrasound.

Diagnostic Procedures

Radioactive iodine I 131 uptake (RAIU) study is done after thyroid function tests have been done, the thyrotropin levels are suppressed, and the diagnosis is not clear. This test evaluates hyperthyroidism by separating the high RAIU uptake disorders from the low RAIU uptake disorders. The RAIU is elevated in Graves disease, toxic adenomas, toxic multinodular goiters, TSH-secreting pituitary adenomas, metastatic follicular thyroid carcinomas, and trophoblastic tumors. The RAIU is low in subacute thyroiditis, lymphocytic thryoiditis, exogenous hyperthyroidism, recent iodine load (contrast dye, diet), and struma ovarii. Low RAIU disorders are the cause of hyperthyroidism only 5% of the time.

Thyroid scanning shows a diffuse, homogeneous distribution in Graves disease (diffuse toxic goiter), multiple areas of increased uptake in toxic multinodular goiter, and a single area of increased uptake in toxic adenoma. It can also be used to evaluate ectopic thyroid tissue (struma ovarii) or to follow up on thyroid cancer. It can be done with either pertechnetate or radioactive iodine.

Treatment

Medications

Thionamides (propylthiouracil and methimazole) are used to treat hyperthyroidism and work by blocking thyroid hormone synthesis and may also decrease the production of TSI. Propylthiouracil at high doses also decreases the peripheral conversion of T_4 to T_3. Thionamides are used to lower thyroid hormone levels in anticipation of radioactive iodine therapy or surgery or as long-term therapy in Graves disease with the goal of inducing a remission of the hyperthyroid condition. Because the drugs only work temporarily and spontaneous remission is a possibility, treatment is given for 12 to 18 months and then a trial discontinuation is initiated. More than half of patients relapse in the first 6 months.

Monitor patients for relapse every 4 to 6 weeks for the first 3 to 6 months, and then every 3 months for the first year following cessation of the antithyroid drugs (ATD). If the patient remains euthyroid, annual monitoring is continued indefinitely. If relapse of hyperthyroidism occurs, alternative therapy is recommended.

Adverse side effects include rash, urticaria, nausea, transient leukopenia (not a harbinger of agranulocytosis), and, less commonly, arthralgias, hepatic necrosis, or cholestatic jaundice. Agranulocytosis is idiosyncratic, occurs in 0.4% of patients, and is usually seen within the first 3 months of therapy. Routine monitoring of white blood cells during the initial 3 months is recommended. If agranulocytosis is detected, it is usually reversible upon discontinuation of the drug but may recur with use of the alternative ATD. Agranulocytosis can develop in hours and a severe sore throat is often the first symptom. Methimazole is often preferred because of its longer half-life and at doses of less than 30 mg per day may have a lower risk of agranulocytosis. It is important to perform pregnancy tests on women of reproductive potential because thionamides are contraindicated. These medications cross the placenta and may disrupt thyroid hormone synthesis in the fetal thyroid.

β-**Adrenergic antagonists**, or β-blockers, provide rapid control of sympathetic-mediated hyperthyroid symptoms and are administered to those with severe symptoms and those awaiting more definitive treatment. Propranolol (nonselective) given in doses of 20 to 40 mg PO q6h is very effective and is prescribed most commonly. Propanolol should not be used alone in the patient with hyperthyroidism as it does not prevent a potentially life-threatening thyrotoxic crisis.

Iodides are not routinely used to treat hyperthyroidism because they may cause a paradoxic increase in thyroid hormone levels. The organic iodide radiographic contrasts agents iopanoic acid and ipodate sodium are used more often than the inorganic potassium iodide. All of the iodides block the peripheral conversion of T_4 to T_3 and suppress hormone. Usually they are used as adjunctive therapy before emergent surgical procedures or to decrease thyroid vascularity prior to surgery for Graves disease.

Nonoperative Treatment

Radioactive iodine (I-131) is effective thyroid gland ablating treatment. It is commonly used as initial therapy for Graves disease, toxic adenoma, or toxic multinodular goiter, or as an alternative therapy for the patient with Graves disease who fails to obtain or maintain a remission with thionamides. Using radioactive iodine effectively will leave the patient hypothyroid. Adverse effects include a painful thyroiditis that may develop within days after treatment, as well as a transient worsening of hyperthyroid symptoms. Radioactive iodine is contraindicated in women who are pregnant, plan to become pregnant within 6 months, and those who breastfeed.

Surgery

Surgical excision is recommended in patients with contraindications to radioactive iodine therapy, those with very large goiters, and also for those who cannot tolerate or are not responsive to thionamides. Thionamides are the first-line treatment of thyrotoxicosis in pregnancy; however, the lowest dose should be employed. Surgery is often considered in the second and third trimester of pregnancy if reasonable doses of antithyroid drug therapy are not working. The goal of the surgery is to reduce the amount of thyroid gland so that euthyroid levels of thyroid hormone are secreted by the tissue left behind. A "necklace" incision extends to the sternocleidomastoid muscles bilaterally to access the gland. Although there is a very low surgical risk, the rare complications are serious. If the recurrent laryngeal nerve is injured, there can be vocal cord paralysis. Permanent hypothyroidism and hypoparathyroidism can also occur.

Follow-Up

After hyperthyroidism is treated by one of the above modalities, it is critical to follow up with thyroid function tests to ensure that the patient is euthyroid. This is very important because postablation and postoperative hypo- or hyperthyroidism is common and should be treated appropriately.

HYPOTHYROIDISM

General Principles

Definition

Clinical hypothyroidism is present when characteristic physical findings are evident and laboratory analysis supports the diagnosis. Hypothyroidism can have a primary, secondary, or tertiary etiology. Subclinical hypothyroidism lacks physical characteristics, but is detected by laboratory analysis.

Epidemiology

Clinical hypothyroidism is evident in up to 2% of women and 0.2% of men. Subclinical hypothyroidism has an approximate prevalence of 4% to 8.5%. The prevalence of both clinical and subclinical hypothyroidism is higher in women. In addition, prevalence increases with age.

Etiology

Hypothyroidism can have a primary, secondary, or tertiary etiology. Primary hypothyroidism results from a defect in the thyroid gland itself. The most common cause of primary hypothyroidism is Hashimoto thyroiditis. Other causes of primary hypothyroidism include radiation exposure, radioactive ablation therapy, iodine deficiency or excess, subacute thyroiditis, and medications. Secondary hypothyroidism results from a defect in the pituitary gland causing a deficiency in TSH production. Some causes of secondary hypothyroidism include Sheehan syndrome, a pituitary neoplasm, radiation exposure, and tuberculosis. Tertiary hypothyroidism results from a defect in the hypothalamus causing a deficiency in thyrotropin-releasing hormone (TRH) production. Tertiary hypothyroidism can be caused from a neoplasm, radiation exposure, or a granuloma.

Diagnosis

Clinical Presentation

Historic findings that are suggestive of hypothyroidism include fatigue, weakness, cold intolerance, weight gain, dry skin, coarse hair, decreased sweating, constipation, muscle cramps, arthralgias, menorrhagia, and impaired cognition.

Physical Examination

Physical exam findings consistent with hypothyroidism include bradycardia, cool skin, brittle nails, periorbital edema, carpal tunnel syndrome, slow speech, loss of the outer third of eyebrows, depression, and delayed relaxation of deep tendon reflexes.

Laboratory Studies

As initial diagnostic tests, a TSH level and free T_4 level should be obtained. Primary hypothyroidism can be diagnosed based on an elevation in TSH greater than twice the normal level. Subsequently, a decrease in free T_4 will also be observed. Secondary hypothyroidism presents with a decreased or normal TSH level and a decreased free T_4 level. Tertiary hypothyroidism will also present with a normal or decreased TSH level and a decreased free T_4 level; however, if the TRH level is measured, it will be normal or decreased. A TRH stimulation test may be used to differentiate secondary from tertiary hypothyroidism. Subclinical hypothyroidism presents with a normal free T_4 level, but an elevation in TSH.

Other laboratory studies may be affected by a hypothyroidism state. Cholesterol and triglyceride levels are often elevated. Anemia and hyponatremia can be observed. Creatinine phosphokinase (CPK) may be elevated in addition to lactate dehydrogenase (LDH), aspartate aminotransferase (AST), and alanine aminotransferase (ALT) levels. If the hypothyroidism is due to Hashimoto thyroiditis, antithyroid peroxidase antibodies are present in the serum.

Treatment
Medications
Therapy for clinical hypothyroidism is best accomplished with levothyroxine. Levothyroxine is a synthetic isomer of T_4. The use of levothyroxine precludes the need for T_3 because T_3 is produced via peripheral deiodination of T_4. Dosage requirements for levothyroxine vary according to the patient's age and weight. Elderly individuals usually require a lower dosage. If a patient has known or suspected cardiovascular disease, a low dose should initially be used to prevent angina pectoris. In general, therapy should begin at a low dose. The dosage can be increased if necessary after analyzing thyroid levels 6 to 8 weeks after the initial dose.

Subclinical hypothyroidism treatment with levothyroxine is recommended if the TSH levels are greater than 10 μ per L. If TSH levels are between 4.5 and 10 μ per L, no firm guidelines direct treatment. Patients can follow thyroid hormone levels every 6 to 12 months for an elevation in TSH levels. If patients have elevated lipid levels, symptoms of hypothyroidism, or positive antithyroid peroxidase antibodies, treatment with levothyroxine should be considered.

Follow-Up
Adequate replacement therapy is assured by remeasuring TSH levels 6 to 8 weeks after a specific dose has been started. If the TSH level remains elevated, the dose is increased. If the TSH level is suppressed, the dose is decreased. The goal of levothyroxine replacement therapy is normalization of TSH. Suppression of TSH is avoided due to the increased risk of accelerated osteoporosis, induction of cardiac arrhythmias, and increase in left ventricular mass.

Complications
Myxedema coma is severe hypothyroidism complicated by marked hypothermia, hypotension, bradycardia, hypoventilation, and unresponsiveness. Even if treated early, mortality rates are approximately 20% to 50%. Supportive measures should be started immediately and include assisted ventilation, warming devices, volume repletion for hypotension, and glucocorticoids if adrenal insufficiency is suspected. Intravenous levothyroxine should be started immediately.

THYROIDITIS

- **Subacute thyroiditis,** also known as de Quervain thyroiditis, is the result of a viral infection of the thyroid gland. Women are four times more affected than men. The average age of diagnosis is 40 to 50 years. A prodromal phase characterized by pharyngitis, myalgias, fatigue, and low-grade fever precedes the development of a tender goiter with neck pain often radiating to the ear. Due to cytotoxic damage of the follicular cells, about half of individuals initially exhibit hyperthyroidism due to the release of preformed T_3 and T_4. When preformed T_3 and T_4 are depleted, transient hypothyroidism may follow. In the majority of cases, full recovery results. Laboratory studies illustrate an elevated sedimentation rate and C-reactive protein level in addition to a mild anemia and leukocytosis. Treatment consists of providing nonsteroidal anti-inflammatory drugs (NSAIDs) for pain. If no resolution of pain occurs within 1 week, prednisone can be utilized. β-adrenergic antagonists are used for symptomatic treatment.
- **Acute suppurative thyroiditis** is the result of a bacterial, fungal, mycobacterial, or parasitic infection of the thyroid gland. Patients present with a warm, erythematous, tender thyroid gland as well as systemic signs of infection. Laboratory studies illustrate an elevated sedimentation rate and elevated white blood cell count with a left shift. Treatment includes appropriate antimicrobial therapy with possible surgical drainage.
- **Radiation-induced thyroiditis and trauma-induced thyroiditis** are the result of the destruction of thyroid parenchyma with subsequent release of preformed T_3 and T_4. Radiation-induced thyroiditis can occur following radioactive iodine therapy or following radiation to the head and neck area for cancer treatment. Trauma-induced thyroiditis results from physical force. Treatment includes NSAIDs or prednisone for pain and β-adrenergic antagonists for symptomatic relief.
- **Hashimoto thyroiditis,** also known as chronic lymphocytic thyroiditis, is an autoimmune condition characterized by infiltration of the thyroid by lymphocytes. Women are seven times more affected than men. The average age of diagnosis is 40 to 60 years.

Patients present with painless enlargement of the thyroid gland. Hypothyroidism or euthyroidism may be clinically evident at presentation. Laboratory studies illustrate the presence of antithyroid peroxidase antibodies in 90% to 95% and antithyroglobulin antibodies in 20% to 50% of affected individuals. Treatment with levothyroxine is indicated for patients with clinical hypothyroidism, subclinical hypothyroidism with a TSH greater than 10 μ per L, and progressive goiter enlargement.

- **Postpartum thyroiditis and silent sporadic thyroiditis** are probably the result of an autoimmune condition. About 5% to 7% of women develop postpartum thyroiditis. A firm, painless goiter is usually present 2 to 6 months after delivery. Women may experience hypothyroidism (43%), hyperthyroidism (32%), or hyperthyroidism followed by hypothyroidism (25%). The hyperthyroid variant occurs most frequently 3 months postpartum whereas the hypothyroid variant occurs most frequently at 6 months postpartum. About 80% of patients have normal thyroid function at 1 year postpartum. Laboratory studies illustrate a normal sedimentation rate while 80% have positive antithyroid peroxidase antibodies. Treatment includes beta-blockers for hyperthyroid symptom management and levothyroxine for clinical hypothyroidism. Caution should be used when prescribing beta-blockers to breastfeeding mothers as it is secreted into the breast milk. Silent sporadic thyroiditis is similar to postpartum thyroiditis; however, it does not occur during pregnancy.

- **Drug-induced thyroiditis** results from the use of amiodarone, interferon-alpha, interleukin-2, and lithium. This destructive thyroiditis may result in hyperthyroidism or hypothyroidism and usually resolves with discontinuation of the offending agent.

- **Riedel thyroiditis** results in extensive fibrosis of the thyroid gland and adjacent structures. The etiology is unknown. Women are four times more affected than men. The average age of diagnosis is 30 to 60 years. Clinically, the patient exhibits a fixed, rock-hard painless goiter with signs of esophageal and tracheal compression. Approximately two thirds of patients illustrate positive antithyroid peroxidase antibodies. An open biopsy is often needed for diagnosis. Surgical intervention may be necessary to relieve compression of the esophagus and trachea.

THYROID NODULE

General Principles

Epidemiology
Clinically evident thyroid nodules can be found in 5% of the adult population. Solitary thyroid nodules are malignant in approximately 10% of these cases. In children younger than 13, thyroid nodules are rare, but the incidence of cancer in these children reaches approximately 20%.

Diagnosis

Clinical Presentation
Historic findings that are suggestive, but not diagnostic, of malignancy include a family history of thyroid cancer, history of irradiation to the head and neck region, patient age younger than 20 or older than 60 years, rapid nodule growth, or presence of distant metastases.

Physical Examination
Physical findings suspicious for malignancy include a very firm irregular nodule, fixation to adjacent structures, vocal cord paralysis, or enlarged regional lymph nodes.

Laboratory Studies
A fine-needle aspiration biopsy (FNAB) and TSH levels are recommended as initial diagnostic tests in most adults presenting with a thyroid nodule. Unless the patient has signs and symptoms of thyrotoxicosis, a TSH level and FNAB should both be obtained. In the case of suspected thyrotoxicosis, a TSH level should be measured to confirm the diagnosis followed by a RAIU study. A calcitonin level should be obtained if there is a family history of medullary carcinoma. An ultrasound can be obtained to determine the presence of other nodules, nodule consistency (cystic vs. solid), and thyroid anatomic structure. In children younger than 13, the use of FNAB remains controversial. An ultrasound is recommended in this age group to further examine thyroid anatomy as well as nodule consistency and number. Due to the high incidence of malignancy in these children, further preoperative studies are not recommended, as surgical excision is currently the mainstay of treatment.

The first step in diagnosis is analyzing the TSH level. If the TSH level is elevated, the thyroid nodule is hypofunctioning. Because hypofunctioning thyroid nodules represent malignancies in 10% to 20% of cases, FNAB results should be reviewed for further diagnostic information. Similarly, if the TSH level is normal, the patient's FNAB results should be reviewed. If the TSH level is decreased, the thyroid nodule is hyperfunctioning. Of hyperfunctioning thyroid nodules, 1% are malignant. A RAIU study is recommended in this case to determine whether the nodule is "hot" or "cold." Individuals with "cold" nodules should have a FNAB completed.

In analyzing the FNAB results, the pathologic structure of the tissue can determine whether the nodule is benign or malignant. If the FNAB results illustrate a cellular pathology, follicular adenoma and follicular carcinoma are both diagnostic possibilities. In this case, a hypofunctioning nodule as determined by TSH levels favors malignancy and surgical excision. A hyperfunctioning nodule as determined by TSH levels necessitates further studies including a RAIU study. If FNAB results are nondiagnostic, repeat FNAB testing is necessary with possible ultrasound-guided aid.

Treatment

If the thyroid nodule represents a malignancy, surgical excision is necessary. Postoperative therapy is often malignancy dependent. Levothyroxine suppression therapy is recommended to decrease TSH levels and subsequent thyroid gland stimulation. Imaging studies as well as calcitonin and thyroglobulin levels, if applicable, are important for surveillance of metastasis or recurrence. If the thyroid nodule is benign, levothyroxine suppression therapy and clinical observation with or without ultrasound monitoring should be considered.

SPECIAL CONSIDERATIONS

- Occasionally abnormal thyroid function tests can be found in patients who have a number of nonthyroidal illnesses or conditions, including caloric restriction, recent surgery, chronic liver disease, chronic renal disease, diabetes mellitus, infections, malignancy, psychiatric disorders, and with certain drugs (β-adrenergic blockers, amiodarone, phenytoin, glucocorticoids, dopamine, cholecystographic dyes, and heroin). These patients are not generally pharmacologically treated and the laboratory abnormalities typically resolve with improvement of the underlying cause.
- Whenever a patient has acute behavioral changes consider thyrotoxicosis as a potential cause.
- If a patient presents with signs and symptoms of dementia or depression, rule out hypothyroidism as a potential etiology.
- Thyrotoxicosis symptoms may be overlooked in pregnancy as they may be mistaken for normal changes.

References

1. American Association of Clinical Endocrinologists and the American College of Endocrinology. AACE clinical practice guidelines for the evaluation and treatment of hyperthyroidism and hypothyroidism. *Endocr Pract* 1994;9:1137–1141.
2. Bartalena L, et al. Relation between therapy for hyperthyroidism and the course of Graves ophthalmopathy. *N Engl J Med* 1998;338:73–78.
3. Bindra A, Braunstein GD. Thyroiditis. *Am Fam Physician* 2006;73:1769–1776.
4. Bunevicius R, et al. Effects of thyroxine as compared with thyroxine plus triiodothyronine in patients with hypothyroidism. *N Engl J Med* 1999;340:424–429.
5. Cooper DS. Subclinical thyroid disease: a clinician's perspective. *Ann Intern Med* 1998;129:135–138.
6. Merce J. Cardiovascular abnormalities in hyperthyroidism. *Am J Med* 2006;119:e25.
7. Sakiyama R. Thyroiditis. In: Conn RB, Borer WZ, Synder JW, eds. *Current diagnosis.* 9th ed. Philadelphia: WB Saunders; 1997:756–760.
8. Ladenson PW, et al. Comparison of administration of recombinant human thyrotropin with withdrawal of thyroid hormone for radioactive iodine scanning in patients with thyroid carcinoma. *N Engl J Med* 1997;337:888–896.
9. Wilson GR, Curry RW. Subclinical thyroid disease. *Am Fam Physician* 2005;72:1517–1524.
10. Wu SY, Weiss RE. Radioiodine imaging in the primary care of thyroid disease. *Postgrad Med* 2006;119:80–87.

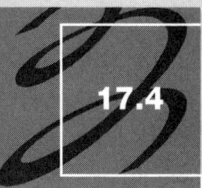

17.4

DYSLIPIDEMIAS
Marvin Moe Bell

GENERAL PRINCIPLES

Hypercholesterolemia is a major risk factor for coronary heart disease (CHD). High levels of low-density lipoprotein (LDL) cholesterol are the main target for cholesterol-lowering therapy. Low levels of high-density lipoprotein (HDL) cholesterol and high levels of triglycerides (TGs) are additional risk factors for CHD. The benefit of treating people with dyslipidemias has been demonstrated in both primary prevention (people without CHD) and secondary prevention (people with known CHD) trials. Guidelines for detection, evaluation, and management of high blood cholesterol have been published by the National Cholesterol Education Program and are generally followed in this chapter.[1]

- Recommended for all adults older than 20 years, every 5 years.
- Obtain fasting lipid profile (total cholesterol, LDL cholesterol, HDL cholesterol, and TGs)
- LDL is calculated as follows (valid if TGs less than 400 mg/dL): LDL = total cholesterol−HDL—(TGs/5).
- If screening opportunity is nonfasting, measure total cholesterol and HDL.
- People with total cholesterol (≥200 mg per dL or HDL <40 mg per dL require a follow-up fasting lipid profile.

DIAGNOSIS

- **Document CHD risk factors:**
  - Established CHD or diabetes (considered equivalent risk as established CHD)
  - Nonmodifiable risks: Age (men older than 45, women older than 55), family history of premature CHD (first degree relative, male < age 55, female < age 65)
  - Modifiable risks: Cigarette smoking, hypertension, low HDL (less than 40 mg/dL).
  - Protective factor: HDL more than 60 mg per dL.
  - Categorize for treatment based on LDL and risk factors:
  - Mbl2 > LDL less than 100 mg per dL is the goal for people with established CHD or diabetes. (LDL less than 70 mg/dL is an optional goal for very high-risk people.)
  - LDL less than 130 mg per dL is the goal for people without CHD but with two or more risk factors.
  - LDL less than 160 mg per dL is the goal for people without CHD and with fewer than two risk factors.
  - A useful, computer-based tool to assess risk and guide treatment decisions can be found on the National Heart, Lung, and Blood Institute web site.[2]

MANAGEMENT PRINCIPLES

Rule out and treat secondary causes of hyperlipidemia (especially with marked hypertriglyceridemia):

- Endocrine: type 2 diabetes, hypothyroidism (see Chapters 17.2 and 17.3)
- Renal: nephrotic syndrome, chronic renal failure (see Chapter 12.7)
- Lifestyle: alcoholism, anabolic steroids (see Chapters 5.3 and 5.7)
- Statins are first-line therapy for virtually all people with established CHD to rapidly reduce LDL levels below the goal of 100 mg per dL.
- Therapeutic lifestyle changes (TLC) are important and should be tried for several months before considering drug therapy for primary prevention. Dietary modification, weight loss, and increased physical activity are key components of TLC.

- Delay drug therapy in premenopausal women and young adult men with high LDL who are otherwise at low risk for CHD.
- Consider drug therapy in high-risk postmenopausal women and elderly people with high LDL who are otherwise in good health.

DIETARY THERAPY

- Healthy diet recommendations for the general public are the same as those of a step I diet, which includes the following:
  - Reduce total fats to less than 30% of calories and saturated fats to less than 10% of calories (limit meat to 6 oz/day, use lean cuts of beef and pork with fat trimmed, remove skin from poultry, avoid fried foods and highly saturated oils such as palm or coconut, and use low-fat dairy products).
  - Reduce cholesterol to less than 300 mg per day (limit egg yolks to four per week, and avoid organ meats).
  - Substitute monounsaturated fats in the diet (olive and canola oils are good sources).
  - Increase complex carbohydrates to 55% to 60% of calories (fresh fruit, vegetables, and whole-grain products).
- Water-soluble fiber in the diet or as a supplement can help to lower LDL. Sources include oat bran, beans, fruit, and psyllium (Metamucil).
- A more restricted step II diet may be tried with the assistance of a dietician, if cholesterol control is inadequate and the patient is willing. Saturated fats are limited to 7% of calories and cholesterol to 200 mg per day.

DRUG THERAPY FOR ELEVATED LOW-DENSITY LIPOPROTEIN LEVEL

- Statins are well proven to reduce both cardiac and overall mortality rates.[3] Bile acid sequestrants (resins) and nicotinic acid (niacin) have been shown to reduce major coronary events. Ezetimibe is an alternative that has not been shown to reduce morbidity or mortality.
- For primary prevention, consider addition of a drug if TLCs (diet and exercise) fail to lower LDL to goal levels within 3 to 6 months. Encourage their use when LDL remains greater than 190 mg per dL (4.9 mmol/L) or greater than 160 mg per dL in people with two other CHD risk factors.
- If response to the first drug is inadequate, a drug from another class or a combination of drugs from different classes may be tried. Resins used with statins or nicotinic acid have been very safe and effective. Combination of statins with nicotinic acid or fibrates increases the risk of myopathy.

HYPERTRIGLYCERIDEMIA

- TG levels are defined as follows:
  - Normal: less than 150 mg per dL (1.7 mmol/L)
  - Borderline high: 150 to 199 mg per dL (1.7 to 2.2 mmol/L)
  - High: 200 to 499 mg per dL (1.7 to 5.6 mmol/L)
  - Very high: greater than 500 mg per dL (5.6 mmol/L)
- Very high TGs warrants therapy to reduce the risk of pancreatitis. Treatment of borderline or high TGs to reduce CHD risk remains controversial but is often recommended.
- Therapy includes exercise, weight reduction, alcohol restriction, and treatment of contributing causes. Omega-3 fatty acids or niacin are preferred in resistant cases.

ISOLATED LOW HIGH-DENSITY LIPOPROTEIN (<40 MG/DL)

- Recommend smoking cessation, exercise, weight loss if obese, and avoidance of androgens and progestins.
- A low-fat, high-carbohydrate diet can lower HDL. Replacing carbohydrates with healthy fats may increase HDL.
- Medications are generally not effective at increasing HDL when the TG level is normal.

FORMULARY OF LIPID-LOWERING DRUGS

- Statins (HMG-CoA reductase inhibitors)
  - Advantages. These agents are extremely effective in lowering LDL and may prevent atherosclerotic plaque rupture. They are well tolerated and reduce overall mortality in primary and secondary prevention.
  - Problems. Statins are expensive. Elevation of liver function tests (LFTs) to three times normal occurs in 1% to 2% of patients (monitor LFTs and use caution with liver disease). Myositis or myopathy with high serum creatinine phosphokinase (CPK) develops in 0.5% of patients, more often when statins are used with niacin or fibrates. Warn patients and check CPK if muscle soreness occurs.
  - Dosing (Table 17.4-1)
- Bile acid sequestrants (resins)
  - Advantages. Bile acid sequestrants lower LDL, are very safe, and can be used in combination with any other class of lipid-lowering drug.
  - Problems. These agents may raise TGs; often cause constipation, bloating, nausea, or heartburn; may reduce absorption of other medications (thiazides, digoxin, thyroxine, and warfarin should be taken 1 hour before or 4 hours after a resin).
  - Dosages. Take cholestyramine 4 g or colestipol (Colestid) 5 g (one scoop or packet) orally bid with liquids and a meal to start; gradually increase to a maximum of 8 to 16 g bid for cholestyramine or 15 g bid for colestipol. Colestipol also comes as 1-g tablets dosed 2 to 16 g per d. Colesevelam (WelChol) requires four to seven 625-mg tablets daily.
- Nicotinic acid (niacin)
  - Advantages. Niacin does it all: lowers LDL, lowers TGs, raises HDL, is inexpensive, and is available over the counter.
  - Problems include flushing (often resolves over time, aspirin 325 mg 30 minutes before dose may prevent flush), dyspepsia (avoid in patients with peptic ulcer disease), hyperglycemia (use caution in diabetics), hyperuricemia (use caution with gout), and liver function abnormalities (may be worse with sustained-release niacin, monitor LFTs).
  - Dosage. Take 250 mg orally bid with meals to start, gradually increase to 500 to 1000 mg orally tid. Extended-release niacin (Slo-Niacin, Niaspan) taken at bedtime may reduce flushing but is more costly.
  - Niacinamide is ineffective for cholesterol reduction.
- Ezetimibe
  - Advantages. Lowers LDL by inhibiting cholesterol absorption. Generally well tolerated. Safe to combine with statins.
  - Problems. Fairly expensive. Effect on cardiac and overall mortality is unknown.
  - Dosage of ezetimibe (Zetia) is 10 mg daily.

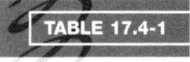 **TABLE 17.4-1**   Statins (HMG-CoA Reductase Inhibitors) Dosing (mg)

	Usual starting dose	Dosing range
Atorvastatin (Lipitor)	10 or 20	10–80
Fluvastatin (Lescol)	20 or 40	20–80
Lovastatin (Mevacor)	20 in evening	10–80
Pravastatin (Pravachol)	40	10–80
Rosuvastatin (Crestor)	10	5–40
Simvastatin (Zocor)	20 to 40	5–80
HMG-CoA, 3-hydroxy-3-methylglutaryl coenzyme A.		

- Omega-3 fatty acids—include eicosapentaenoic acid (EPA) and docosahexaenoic acid (DHA)
  - Advantages. Omega-3 fatty acids effectively lower TGs and have been shown to reduce both cardiac and overall mortality.[3]
  - Problems. New formulation is expensive. May cause eructation, may increase risk of bleeding for patients on aspirin or other blood thinners.
  - Dosage of omega-3-acid ethyl esters (Omacor) is 4 g daily, either divided or taken all at once.
- Fibric acid derivatives (fibrates)
  - Advantage. Fibrates effectively lower TGs, fenofibrate lowers LDL.
  - Problems. Noncardiac mortality is increased by fibrates. Gemfibrozil may raise LDL. Use with caution in liver or renal disease; may cause cholelithiasis.
  - Dosage of fenofibrate is 43 to 201 mg once daily with a meal, and gemfibrozil (Lopid) is 600 mg bid 30 minutes before a meal.

References

1. Expert Panel on Detection, Evaluation, and Treatment of High Blood Cholesterol in Adults. Executive summary of the third report of the National Cholesterol Education Program (NCEP) Expert Panel on the Detection, Evaluation, and Treatment of High Blood Cholesterol in Adults (Adult Treatment Panel III). *JAMA* 2001;285:2486–2497.
2. http://www.nhlbi.nih.gov/guidelines/cholesterol/profmats.htm.
3. Studer M, Briel M, Leimenstoll B, et al. Effect of different antilipidemic agents and diet on mortality. *Arch Intern Med* 2005;165:725–730.

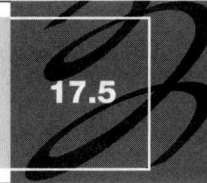

HYPERCALCEMIA
J. Steven Cramer
17.5

GENERAL PRINCIPLES

Definition

Hypercalcemia is considered by most laboratories to be a **calcium concentration greater than 10.5 mg per dL.**

Epidemiology

In a population of hospitalized patients hypercalcemia was related to **malignancy** (46%), **primary hyperparathyroidism** (35%), **thiazide diuretics** (8%), **elevated levels of 25-hydroxy-vitamin D$_3$ levels** (6%), **immobilization** (2%), and **other/unknown** causes (4%).[1]

Etiology

Hypercalcemia occurs when bone resorption exceeds the kidneys' ability to excrete the excessive calcium load, with decreased renal excretion of calcium, or with increased absorption of calcium from the gut.

Classification

- High bone turnover. Immobilization, hyperthyroidism, thiazides, vitamin A intoxication
- Malignancy. Solid tumors (breast, lung, kidney), hematologic (myeloma, lymphoma, leukemia)
- Parathyroid. Adenoma/neoplasia, lithium, familial
- Renal failure. Aluminum intoxication, milk-alkali syndrome, secondary hyperparathyroidism
- Vitamin D. Granulomatous diseases (sarcoidosis, tuberculosis), excess intake of vitamin D

DIAGNOSIS

Clinical Presentation

Symptoms and signs often reflect the underlying disease but vary with the serum level of **ionized calcium** (the physiologically active form) and with the rate of development of hypercalcemia.

History

Hypercalcemia may present as an acute or chronic illness with **lethargy, nausea, vomiting, polydypsia, and polyuria.**

Physical Examination

Impaired renal function, nephrocalcinosis, muscle atrophy, bradycardia, electrocardiographic changes (e.g., short QT), or subtle psychological symptoms (e.g., anxiety, indecisiveness, loss of energy, excessive worry, irritability) may be seen. Other symptoms (e.g., anorexia, weight loss, bone pain) may be due to hypercalcemia but often are directly due to the underlying disease.

Laboratory Studies

Obtain **ionized calcium levels** (4.6 to 5.1 mg/dL). Almost half of serum calcium is protein bound and a 1 g per dL rise in serum protein will result in a 0.8 mg per dL rise in serum calcium level, but mathematical corrections are notoriously inaccurate.[2] Be aware that **prolonged tourniquet** application can result in hemoconcentration and a **spurious hypercalcemia.** Parathyroid hormone **(PTH) immunoassay** will identify hypercalcemia secondary to hyperparathyroidism (>60 ng/L).

Differential Diagnosis

Diabetes mellitus.

Treatment

The cornerstone of treatment is **management of the underlying cause.** If the patient has limited symptoms and signs, management of the underlying disease is often all that is required. **Hospitalization** is indicated if the patient has **serious signs** (e.g., confusion, psychosis, dehydration, azotemia).[3] Patients with hyperparathyroidism should be treated by physicians who are experienced in the medical and surgical treatment of that disorder.

Medications

Acute hypercalcemia usually reflects increased osteoclastic activity such as malignancy and suggested treatment includes:

- Hydration with normal saline (NS) at 300 to 500 mL per hour is an appropriate initial therapy, if the patient's cardiac status permits.
- This can be **followed by a saline diuresis** with NS or half NS (as indicated by serum electrolytes) and furosemide (20 to 40 mg q2–4h). Fluid intake and output must be carefully monitored.
- **Corticosteroids** can be effective for hypercalcemia associated with malignancies and sarcoidosis, but the onset of action may be delayed for several days. They are ineffective for primary hyperparathyroidism; 40 to 100 mg per day of prednisone or equivalent is given in four divided doses.
- **Intravenous bisphosphonates** are the drugs of choice for decreasing osteoclastic activity and include:
  - **Pamidronate disodium,** 60 to 90 mg IV over 24 hours, monitor creatinine prior to each dose, and wait 7 days between treatments.
  - **Zoledronic acid,** 4 mg IV over >15 minutes; may repeat in 7 days.
  - **Salmon calcitonin,** 4 IU/kg IM or SQ q12h, if you are looking for a quicker onset of action than pamidronate. Administration follows a 5 IU test dose and therapeutic utility can be limited by anaphylaxis, bronchospasm, and hypersensitivity reactions.
- **Other possible medications:**
  - **Plicamycin,** 15 to 25 µg/kg/day IV qd over 4 to 6 hours for 3 to 4 days
  - **Gallium nitrate,** 200 mg/m^2/day IV for 5 days

Surgery

The vast majority of surgically correctable cases of hypercalcemia will result from **primary hyperparathyroidism.** An NIH-sponsored consensus development panel has proposed guidelines for surgery in asymptomatic primary hyperparathyroidism.

- A serum calcium 1.0 mg per dL greater than the upper limit of normal
- A 24-hour urinary calcium >400 mg, a creatinine clearance reduced by 30%
- A bone mineral t-score ≤2.5 at any site and age <50.[4]

Operative

Surgery is rapidly moving away from the standard full neck exploration under general anesthesia for identification of all four parathyroid glands to **minimally invasive parathyroidectomy** (MIP). This utilizes a combination of high resolution ultrasound and [99] Tc-labeled Sestamibi-SPECT (single-photon emission computed tomography) imaging to precisely localize the affected gland. This allows for a small incision, local anesthesia with unilateral neck exploration in an ambulatory setting. Successful removal of the suspect gland can be ascertained using pre- and post-PTH levels with rapid PTH assays.[5]

Special Therapy

Hemodialysis against a low-calcium bath may be required in severe or refractory cases of hypercalcemia.

Risk Management

In **asymptomatic patients** with hyperparathyroidism who do not meet the criteria for surgery a **conservative approach is supported** by a longitudinal study. Approximately one quarter of initially asymptomatic patients will develop symptomatic disease over the subsequent 5 to 10 years. The remainder will have stable asymptomatic disease with no significant increase in serum calcium levels, urinary calcium excretion, or decrease in renal function or bone density.[6]

Follow-Up

Patients followed conservatively with **asymptomatic hypercalcemia** secondary to primary hyperparathyroidism should be **followed annually** using the consensus panel evaluations to determine whether surgery is required.

Results

Surgery usually results in a prompt return of the calcium level to normal. The rate of recurrent kidney stones is decreased significantly and bone density with increase 12% to 14% over the subsequent 3 to 4 years.[7]

Complications

Results of surgery by expert parathyroid surgeons are generally excellent. **Injury to the recurrent laryngeal nerve** can occur as can postsurgical hypoparathyroidism. Postoperative **symptomatic hypocalcemia** can occur in those with severe primary hyperparathyroidism but is rare in mild disease.

References

1. Blind E, Raue F, Zisterer A, et al. [Epidemiology of hypercalcemia. Significance of the determination of intact parathyroid hormone for differential diagnosis]. *Dtsch Med Wochenschr* 1990;115(46):1739–1745 [in German].
2. Slomp J, van der Voort PH, Gerritsen RT, et al. Albumin-adjusted calcium is not suitable for diagnosis of hyper and hypocalcemia in the critically ill. *Crit Care Med* 2003;31:1389–1393.
3. Bilezikian JP. Management of acute hypercalcemia. *N Engl J Med* 1992;326:1196.
4. Bilezikian JP, Potts Jr JT, Fuleihan GE, et al. Summary statement from a Workshop on Asymptomatic Primary Hyperparathyroidism: a perspective for the 21st century. *J CLin Endocrinol Metab* 2002;87(12):5353–5361.
5. Ariyan CE, Sosa JA. Assessment and management of patients with abnormal calcium. *Crit Care Med* 2004;32[suppl]:S146–S154.
6. Silverberg SJ, Shane E, Jacombs TP, et al. A 10-year prospective study of primary hyperparathyroidism with or without parathyroid surgery. *N Engl J Med* 1999;341:1249–1255.
7. Bilezikian JP. Asymptomatic primary hyperparathyroidism [clinical practice]. *N Engl J Med* 2004;350(17):1746–1751.

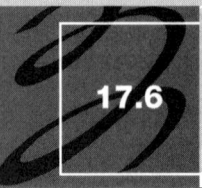

17.6

OSTEOPOROSIS
Fred E. Heidrich, Susan M. Ott

GENERAL PRINCIPLES

Definition
Osteoporosis (OP) is a syndrome in which bone strength is decreased and fractures may occur after minimal trauma.

Anatomy
Hip fractures and vertebral compression fractures are the most serious consequences. Also common fracture sites include the distal forearm and proximal humerus.

Epidemiology
At age 50, one third of women have osteopenia (see below). At age 65 years, 40% are normal, 40% have osteopenia, and 20% have osteoporosis. Only 10% of 80-year-old women have a "normal" bone density. The lifetime risk of hip fracture for an average 50-year-old person is 15% for White women and 6% for men; risks are lower for those of African descent.

Fractures
The fractures due to osteoporosis occur mostly in the latter half of life, but bone loss begins in the third decade. **Maximizing bone gained in childhood and adolescence and minimizing losses in the middle years** of life are key to bone health in old age.

Classification
Bone density is best assessed by **dual energy x-ray absorptiometry (DEXA)** at the hip. Other techniques include peripheral or spinal DEXA and quantitative ultrasound. Results: T-scores (number of standard deviations, sd, from a young woman's mean value) and Z-scores (sd from an age-matched mean). WHO definitions of osteoporosis for menopausal White women:

- **Osteopenia:** Decreased bone density more than 1 sd below mean for young women (T-score < –1)
- **Osteoporosis:** Bone density more than 2.5 sd below mean (T-score < –2.5)
- **Established OP:** Fracture in addition to low bone density

Pathophysiology
Bone is a metabolically active tissue, in which **osteoclasts resorb bone** and **osteoblasts lay down new bone.** This lets bone **remodel after injury** or in response to stressors, and **serve as a reservoir** of calcium. When bone resorption exceeds formation over a period of time, the bone loses density and strength.

Etiology
- **Aging** is the most common cause of osteoporosis.
- Other risk factors:
    - Gonadal hormone deficiency (gonadal failure, surgical or natural menopause, oligomenorrhea (<4 periods per year, including extreme athleticism, anorexia or use of depot-medroxyprogesterone)
    - Bone-thinning drugs (glucocorticoids, anticonvulsants, antineoplastics, heparin, and medications that decrease gonadal hormones)
    - Low weight
    - Heredity and race (parent with hip fracture; White or Asian race)
    - Female gender
    - Inactive lifestyle

- Tobacco use
- Low calcium intake
- OP may be secondary to many disease states (see differential diagnosis).

Mechanisms of Injury

Hallmark is **fracture from a degree of injury not usually expected to result in fracture,** for example, a fall from standing height.

DIAGNOSIS

Diagnosis of OP sometimes can be made based on a history of low impact fracture and no other obvious cause (see Differential Diagnosis). DEXA can also define. Although bone density is currently the standard way to quantify OP, other bone properties such as microstructural integrity also play a role in OP.

Clinical Presentation

OP is usually detected by a **screening bone density,** or after a person has a **typical fracture with minimal trauma.** Efforts to intervene early, however, depend on recognition of risks for bone loss before fractures occur.

History

Look for **risk factors and secondary causes** (see Etiology and Differential Diagnosis). A history of an osteoporotic fracture is a strong predictor of future fracture. A woman with a vertebral compression fracture is four times more likely to have a new vertebral fracture as a woman of the same age and bone density with no pre-existing fracture. Such compression fractures are often asymptomatic; two thirds of such patients do not note any increase in pain associated with the fracture, but it is nonetheless an important indicator of risk.

Physical Examination

Look for:

- Kyphosis
- Height loss >2 to 3 inches
- Protruding abdomen
- About 60% of women with spinal compression fractures are unaware of their occurrence. Height loss of up to 2 to 3 inches may be seen with disc thinning of aging, but greater loss can indicate osteoporosis.

Laboratory Studies

- **Basic evaluation.** Complete blood count (CBC), electrolytes serum 25-OH-vitamin D, thyroid-stimulating hormone, phosphate, and calcium are normal, but alkaline phosphatase may be temporarily elevated following a fracture. Check testosterone in men.
- **Other tests.** Occasionally useful in OP evaluation are urinary calcium (normally 50 to 250 mg/day), parathyroid hormone (PTH), and serum and urinary protein electrophoresis (for myeloma). Tests of bone resorption rate (such as pyridinolines or collagen telopeptides) and formation rate (osteocalcin or bone specific alkaline phosphatase) may occasionally guide therapy but cannot be used for screening individual patients.

Imaging

The U.S. Preventive Services Task Force USPSTF recommends **routine bone density screening** for all women starting at age 65, and for those a higher risk at age 60. Consensus still pending for men.

Monitoring

DEXA scanning can be used in observation of those at risk or to monitor progress in treatment. A person must change more than 5% to be sure a change is not merely machine imprecision; therefore, testing is usually done at intervals of 2 or more years. If a woman at age 65 has normal bone density, further monitoring is unnecessary unless her risk profile changes.

Surgical Diagnostic Procedures

Bone biopsy is occasionally used where the diagnosis is in doubt.

Differential Diagnosis

Many causes of secondary osteoporosis or other bone weakening states can present as low impact fractures. Consider metastatic lesions, multiple myeloma, immobilization, weight loss, renal or hepatic failure, intestinal malabsorption, renal calcium loss, gonadal deficiency, and excesses of cortisol, parathormone, or thyroxine. Alcoholism should always be considered, particularly when OP occurs in young people or middle-aged men. Many of these conditions can be excluded by history and physical examination.

TREATMENT

Behavioral

Calcium is not sufficient to prevent OP, but is an important adjuvant. Recommended daily intake is 500 mg for children aged 1 to 3; 800 to 1,300 mg for ages 4 to 18; 1,000 mg for ages 19 to 50; and 1,200 mg thereafter. Quick assessment of dietary calcium intake: 300 mg for each serving of dairy product and 200 mg for the rest of the diet. Calcium carbonate in the most cost-effective supplement, and is best absorbed with food. Vitamin D is important in calcium absorption and neurologic function. Persons lacking sun exposure and those older than age 70 are at risk for vitamin D deficiency and should take 400 to 800 IU vitamin D daily, administered as part of most multiple-vitamin preparations. Avoid vitamin A intake greater than the recommended daily allowance (RDA).

People at risk for **falls** should be counseled regarding footwear (laced, low heel, traction sole), vision aids, and environmental hazards (poor lighting, floor-level obstructions, slippery surfaces, lack of handrails, cool temperature). Medicines that affect alertness or cause postural syncope must be minimized in elderly people. Elderly people are more prone to postural hypotension after a large meal. Protective hip padding can reduce hip fractures.

Lifestyle

- **Weight-bearing exercise** (walking, running, dancing, aerobic exercise, sports, weight lifting, Tai Chi—as appropriate) has skeletal, cardiovascular, muscular, and emotional benefits for all age groups. Reasonable goal: 30 to 60 minutes, 4 to 6 times per week. Discourage smoking and overconsumption of alcohol. Discourage unnecessary weight loss despite cultural fashions, as women who lose weight also lose bone density. The kyphosis of established osteoporosis results in a protruding abdomen, which patients may misinterpret as excess fat.

Medications

- **Bisphosphonates** are the most commonly used therapy for OP. A halving of fracture rates is seen in men and women with osteoporosis. They decrease fracture rates for at least 5 years of use. They do, however, decrease both bone formation and resorption, with a very long half-life (over 10 years) in bone and longer-term effects remain uncertain. Alendronate (35 or 70 mg weekly), risedronate (35 mg weekly), and ibandronate (150 mg monthly) are the oral bisphosphonates currently approved for treating OP and are quite similar. They should be taken with a full glass of water on an empty stomach, and 30 minutes should pass before any other oral intake. The patient should avoid reclining for at least 30 minutes after the dose to prevent esophagitis. Avoid using in pregnancy, renal failure, or hypocalcemic states, and ensure adequate intake of both calcium and vitamin D. Duration of treatment is controversial but many advocate a "drug holiday" after 5 years.
- **Hormonal replacement therapy (HRT)** results in about a 50% reduction in fractures, but adverse effects may limit their use. HRT is mainly indicated early in menopause in women who also want relief from hot flushes, but after age 60 the initiation of estrogen carries a risk of myocardial infarction so this is not recommended. A dose of 0.625 mg conjugated estrogens daily or equivalent can promote increases in bone density, and smaller doses (0.3 mg) can be helpful in stabilizing density. Bone loss similar to that at natural menopause occurs on cessation of HRT, so other management is indicated when HRT is stopped in women using it for OP.

- **Raloxifene,** 60 mg daily, is effective at decreasing vertebral fracture rates in post-menopausal women, although hip fracture rates are not reduced. It does not stimulate breast or uterine neoplasia, but does have prothrombotic characteristics similar to estrogen, and can worsen hot flushes. Raloxifene halves the incidence of breast cancer in studies lasting up to 8 years.
- **Calcitonin** has been found helpful in reducing vertebral fractures. Bone density gains are not as great as those for other agents. It is given intranasally, 200 units daily.
- **Testosterone** in men can result in increased bone density but may have adverse effects on serum lipids and hematocrit, and should be avoided in men with a history of prostate cancer. Men with demonstrated low testosterone may be treated with intramuscular or transdermal testosterone.
- **Teriparatide** is a potent stimulator of bone formation. It may be considered in men or women failing standard therapy. It is given by daily subQ injection, for up to 24 months. It should be avoided in pregnancy, hypercalcemia, Paget disease, active gout, and in persons with a history of bone cancer or bone irradiation. At the conclusion of therapy with teriparatide it is important to then administer an osteoclast inhibitor (such as a bisphosphonate) for several years to avoid a rapid loss state.

Surgery

Percutaneous infusions of cement (vertebroplasty or kyphoplasty) have been advocated to treat acute vertebral compression fractures. These procedures carry a risk of spinal cord damage, and possibly higher risk of compression of adjacent vertebra. Long-term benefits have not been shown to be better than standard therapy, and further studies are needed.

Special Therapy

- Thiazide diuretics decrease renal calcium excretion. Effects on bone density are beneficial but modest. If an antihypertensive is indicated, possible bone benefits may enter into the choice of agents. These drugs can improve bone density in patients with high urine calcium.
- **Hip pads** prevent hip fractures in elderly people if they wear the padding.

Referrals

Consider specialty referrals for patients with **secondary osteoporosis** where assistance is needed with the underlying cause and for cases where **fractures or density losses continue despite therapy.**

Physical Therapy

Gait and balance training may prevent falls and thus fractures. **Spinal extension exercises** and instruction in **lifting technique** may prevent vertebral crush fractures. Brief bed rest and local heat complement analgesics in managing compression fractures. In cases of severe kyphosis, back bracing may provide comfort.

Patient Education

- Calcium/vitamin D
- Exercise for bones, strength, flexibility, and balance
- Understanding DEXA
- How to take bisphosphonates

SPECIAL CONSIDERATIONS

- **Chronic steroid users:** Bone losses greatest during first 6 months of therapy with doses of prednisone of 5 mg per day or greater. Management includes **minimizing the dose** of steroid given, maintaining **physical activity,** and aggressive implementation of **preventive and therapeutic strategies** above. Patients may suffer fractures even with normal bone density.
- **Hypercalciuria** may be aggravated by high-dose vitamin D and helped by thiazides. In worrisome cases, measurements of vertebral or hip bone density may guide use of bisphosphonate or hormonal therapy.

References

1. Ott SM. Osteoporosis and bone physiology. http://courses.washington.edu/bonephys/.
2. Osteoporosis prevention, diagnosis, and therapy. NIH Consensus Statement 2000 March 27–29;17(1):1–36.
3. U.S. Department of Health and Human Services. Bone health and osteoporosis: a report of the Surgeon General. Rockville, MD: U.S. Department of Health and Human Services, Office of the Surgeon General, 2004. Available online at http://www.surgeongeneral.gov/library/bonehealth/content.html.
4. Boonen S, Laan RF, Barton IP, et al. Effect of osteoporosis treatments on risk of non-vertebral fractures: review and meta-analysis of intention-to-treat studies. *Osteoporos Int* 2005;16:1291–1298.
5. U.S. Preventive Services Task Force. Screening for osteoporosis in postmenopausal women: recommendations and rationale. September 2002. Agency for Healthcare Research and Quality, Rockville, MD. Available at http://www.ahrq.gov/clinic/3rduspstf/osteoporosis/osteorr.htm.
6. Writing Group for the Women's Health Initiative Investigators. Risks and benefits of estrogen plus progestin in healthy postmenopausal women: principal results from the Women's Health Initiative randomized controlled trial. *JAMA* 2002;288:321–333. See also: Effects of conjugated equine estrogen in postmenopausal women with hysterectomy: the Women's Health Initiative randomized controlled trial. *JAMA* 2004;291(14):1701–7012.

Disorders of the Blood 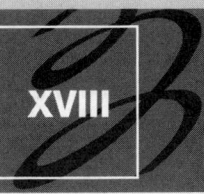 **XVIII**

IRON DEFICIENCY ANEMIA
S. Shekar Chakravarthi
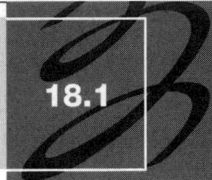 **18.1**

GENERAL PRINCIPLES[1,2]

Definition

Anemia is a condition where the number of red blood cells, amount of hemoglobin, or volume of red blood cells is less than normal. In iron deficiency anemia the cause is inadequate iron. The acceptable hemoglobin cutoffs defining the condition are age and gender dependent.

- Adult male: 14 g per dL (declines slightly with age)
- Adult female: 12 g per dL
- Pregnant female: 11 g per dL
- Age 6 months to 2 years: 10.5 g per dL
- Age 2 years to 12 years: 11.5 g per dL

Epidemiology

Worldwide, iron deficiency is the most common cause of anemia. Anemia of chronic disease is more prevalent in the Western world and has to be differentiated from iron deficiency anemia. These two types of anemia may coexist.

Pathophysiology

Iron deficiency results in a defective synthesis of hemoglobin and smaller red cells (microcytic) with less hemoglobin within the cell (hypochromic).

Etiology

Increased requirements, inadequate dietary iron, malnutrition, low iron stores, eating disorders, pica, and lead poisoning are common causes in infants and children. In adults, common causes of gastrointestinal (GI) blood loss are the use of nonsteroidal anti-inflammatory drugs, peptic ulcer disease, angiodysplasia, diverticulosis, malignancy, and, rarely, parasites such as hookworms. Frequent blood donations and phlebotomies, surgical procedures, and, in females, menstrual disorders, pregnancy, and lactation can lead to iron deficiency. The daily loss of iron in an adult is about 1 mg, and menstrual loss can be an additional 20 mg per month. Normally less than 10% of the daily dietary intake of iron is absorbed.

DIAGNOSIS

Clinical Presentation

With an insidious onset and gradual progression of symptoms the body can compensate and tolerate low hemoglobin (less than 7 gm/dL). In elderly individuals,[3] some of these signs and symptoms may be subtle or dismissed as age related. A detailed *history and physical* examination is essential. *Symptoms* may include weakness, leg cramping, malaise, fatigue, dyspnea on exertion, palpitations, dizziness, chest pain, headaches, pago-phagia (ice eating), and pica. *Signs*: Tachycardia, systolic murmur, and even high-output failure may be the cardiac signs. Epithelial changes include pallor of the conjunctiva, lips, nail beds, and palmar skin creases. Dry skin, and nail changes such as brittle and spoon-shaped nails (koilonychia) are also found. Angular stomatitis, glossitis, and, rarely, dysphagia from pharyngeal and esophageal webs may also be present.

Laboratory

- The test result would depend on the stage of development of iron deficiency. The classic hypochromic microcytic picture develops when iron stores are exhausted. Anisocytosis, poikilocytosis, and target cells may be present on the peripheral smear. Increased red cell distribution width with a low mean corpuscular volume is suggestive of iron deficiency anemia.
- Serum ferritin level is decreased to less than 12 μg per L (normal: 18 to 300 μg/L). A low serum ferritin indicates iron deficiency; however, ferritin, which is an acute phase reactant, may be elevated in the presence of inflammation and malignancy.
- Iron binding capacity (IBC) is increased, usually to more than 375 μg per dL (normal: up to 300 μg/dL).
- Serum iron is decreased, often to less than 60 μg per dL (normal: 100 μg/dL).
- Transferrin saturation is decreased to less than 16%.
- Reticulocyte count, which is indicative of red blood cell replacement and bone marrow function, is decreased when iron stores are exhausted.
- Erythropoietin level is normal or high.
- Transferrin receptor level is increased.
- Erythrocyte protoporphyrin is increased.
- Local laboratory values for normal range may differ.
- Bone marrow biopsy is not usually necessary but would demonstrate absence of iron stores. In anemia of chronic disease, serum iron may be low but the IBC is not elevated. Hemoglobin electrophoresis will detect thalassemias, and lead testing will help rule out lead poisoning.

Differential Diagnosis

Thalassemia, anemia of chronic disease, and sideroblastic anemia.

TREATMENT

In the adult, iron deficiency could represent GI blood loss; therefore, appropriate workup should be initiated and the cause addressed. With the initiation of iron replacement therapy, reticulocyte count should rise within a week and a 2 g per dL hemoglobin increase should be seen in 3 weeks. To replenish the stores, continue replacement for 6 months. Treatment failures are due to noncompliance, malabsorption, inadequate dosing, ongoing blood loss, or incorrect diagnosis. Occult GI blood loss should be further evaluated to exclude malignancies. A poor response to exogenous erythropoetin could be due to underlying iron deficiency. Iron, vitamin B_{12}, and folate must be supplemented when treating anemia of chronic disease with erythropoetic agents.

Iron Replacement

Oral

This is the preferred method of replacing the iron stores gradually. Ferrous sulfate, which is inexpensive and commonly used, is better tolerated when given with meals. GI side effects are dose related and include nausea and constipation. Ferrous sulfate 325 mg (65 mg of elemental iron) started once daily may be titrated up weekly to three times a day. Target dose is 150 to 200 mg of elemental iron per day. Foods, milk, coffee, and tea reduce absorption and vitamin C enhances absorption. Ferrous fumarate 300 mg (100 mg of elemental iron) or ferrous gluconate 300 mg (37 mg of elemental iron) may be better tolerated than ferrous sulfate. Drugs such as histamine-2 blockers, proton pump inhibitors, antacids, and methyldopa reduce absorption.

For children, iron supplements in the form of drops, elixir, and syrup are available. The regimen for management of iron deficiency in children is 3 to 6 mg/kg/day of elemental iron in divided doses. Liquid preparations are given by dropper or straw to prevent staining of teeth.

Parenteral[1,4]
In the presence of severe side effects, GI intolerance, or poor absorption due to inflammatory bowel disease, iron may be given parenterally. Iron gluconate (125 mg) or iron sucrose (100 mg) can be given intravenously over 5 to 10 minutes and be repeated one to three times a week until 1,000 mg is given. These formulations are preferred over iron dextran. Iron dextran may also be given intramuscularly using the Z technique, or as a total calculated dose, diluted in saline solution, and infused over a few hours.

The formula for the total dose of iron required is as follows:

$$\text{Dose (mg)} = [15 - \text{patient's Hgb (g/dL)}] \times \text{body wt (kg)} \times 3$$

A test dose of 25 mg is given (required for iron dextran). If no allergic reaction is noted, a 100 to 125 mg dose may be given daily. Although most reactions are mild, life-threatening anaphylactic reactions may occur, more commonly with iron dextran. Arthralgias, myalgias, and phlebitis may occur as a delayed reaction. Severe reactions have been noted in patients with collagen vascular disease.

Prevention
Breast milk or formula should be encouraged during the first year of life, as cow's milk is a poor source of iron. Along with a diet rich in iron, supplemental iron should be provided when the requirement is high, such as during infancy and growth spurts, in people who donate blood on a frequent basis, in menstruating girls and women, and in pregnant and lactating women.

References
1. Cook JD. Diagnosis and management of iron-deficiency anemia. *Best Practice Res Clin Hematol* 2005;189(2):319–332.
2. Umbreit J. Iron deficiency—a concise review. *Am J Hematol* 2005;78:225–231.
3. Brit Ger Soc. Commentary, Iron def anemia in older people—inv, mgt and treatment. *Age Aging* 2002;31:87–91.
4. Silverstein SB, Rodgers GM. Parenteral iron therapy options. *Am J Hematol* 2004; 76:74–78.

MEGALOBLASTIC ANEMIA
Nicole N. Paulman, Roger A. Paulman

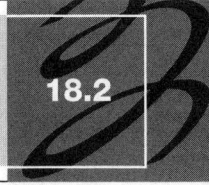

18.2

GENERAL OVERVIEW

Megaloblastic anemia is a disorder caused by impaired DNA synthesis. Macrocytic anemia is a general term for anemia with mean corpuscular volume (MCV) of greater than 100 fL. There are many causes of macrocytosis, one of which is megaloblastic anemia. Other causes include liver disease, alcoholism, hypothyroidism, hemolysis, and aplastic anemia. Megaloblastic anemias typically have an MCV >110 fL and hypersegmented neutrophils can be seen on the peripheral smear. Vitamin B_{12} (cobalamin) and folic acid (pteroylmonoglutamic acid) are both crucial in the synthesis of DNA. Deficiencies in either are the two most common causes of megaloblastic anemia.

VITAMIN B$_{12}$ DEFICIENCY

General Principles

Vitamin B$_{12}$ is a substance that is widely used by the body in DNA synthesis and nerve cell processes. It cannot, however, be produced by the body and therefore must be present in the diet. The only source of cobalamin is animal products, such as meat and dairy. The minimum daily intake is 2.5 μg, the average diet provides 5 to 15 μg per day. Parietal cells in the stomach produce intrinsic factor that binds with cobalamin and together they travel to the terminal ileum where absorption occurs. This vitamin is stored predominantly in the liver and is utilized by bone marrow and nervous tissue among others. The body stores approximately 4 to 5 mg of cobalamin, so it generally takes years of deficiency to result in clinically significant disease.

Causes of Vitamin B$_{12}$ Deficiency

The most common cause is **pernicious anemia.** Pernicious anemia is a specific disease disorder caused by deficient or absent intrinsic factor, due to atrophy of gastric mucosa or antiparietal cell or anti-2-intrinsic factor antibodies. It is most common in those of African American and Northern European descent. It most commonly presents in those age >60 and very rarely <30. Other causes of B$_{12}$ deficiency include:

- Inadequate dietary content (alcoholics, strict vegans)
- Gastrectomy (removal of intrinsic factor producing parietal cells)
- Malabsorption (ileal resection, Crohn disease, sprue—especially tropical sprue in those living nearer the equator)
- Cobalamin degradation (bacterial overgrowth, fish tapeworm infection—*Dyphyllobothrium latum,* especially in Scandinavians)
- Food-bound malabsorption (increased gastric pH prevents B$_{12}$ cleavage from food particles leading to decreased absorption, i.e., patients on proton pump inhibitors, H$_2$ blockers, elderly with achlorhydria is actually quite common)

Manifestations of Cobalamin Deficiency

B$_{12}$ deficiency may affect up to 15% of the adult population older than age 65. Vitamin B$_{12}$ deficiency is likely to take as many as 5 years to present given the large body stores.

- **Hematologic.** Anemia leading to weakness, dizziness, heart failure, fatigue, palpitations, pallor, etc. Macrocytosis that may not occur if concurrent iron deficiency or thalassemia. Hypersegmented (>5 lobes) neutrophils.
- **Gastrointestinal.** Red beefy, sore tongue, anorexia, diarrhea.
- **Neurologic.** Paresthesias, peripheral neuropathy, and if affecting spinal cord, ataxia and signs of posterior and lateral column involvement. Neurologic symptoms can be the most worrisome as they may not resolve despite appropriate therapy. Anemia need not be present to have neurologic sequelae of B$_{12}$ deficiency.

Laboratory Findings

- Anemia (hemoglobin <12g/dL in women, <14 g/dL in men)
- Macrocytosis (MCV >100)
- Decreased vitamin B$_{12}$ levels (<200 pg/mL with symptoms)
- Elevated homocysteine and methylmalonic acid levels are often more sensitive than absolute B$_{12}$ levels. (B$_{12}$ is critical in the conversion of homocysteine to methionine, used in folate metabolism.)
- Schilling test of historical significance but is of little clinical benefit.
- Anti-intrinsic factor antibody in patient serum is 100% specific for pernicious anemia.

Treatment

- Treat the underlying disorder if appropriate.
- B$_{12}$ replacement has traditionally been accomplished through intramuscular injections: 1 mg daily for 1 to 2 weeks, followed biweekly for 1 month, followed by monthly for life. New studies have shown oral B$_{12}$ to be as effective as IM injections, absorbed through

a yet unknown pathway. Oral B_{12} can be accomplished through daily administration of 1 to 2 mg.

Follow-Up

Annual complete blood count (CBC) and vitamin B_{12} serum levels should be checked. Patients with true pernicious anemia should have endoscopic follow-up due to an increased incidence of gastric cancer.

FOLIC ACID DEFICIENCY

General Principles

Folic acid is a vitamin used in the synthesis of DNA. It is widely used throughout the body, but especially in places of high turnover such as bone marrow. Required daily intake of folate is 50 µg; however, needs may increase severalfold during times of increased metabolic demand such as pregnancy. Total body stores are 5 to 20 mg with half of the body's supply stored in the liver. This means that when malnourished, the body will be depleted in a few months. Folate can be found predominantly in fruits and vegetables, and since 1998 in all enriched grain products by order of the Food and Drug Administration (FDA).

Causes of Folate Deficiency

- Inadequate intake (alcoholics, elderly "tea and toast," teenagers "junk food")
- Increased requirements (pregnancy, infancy, malignancy)
- Malabsorption (sprue, small bowel disease such as Crohn disease)
- Impaired folate metabolism (alcohol, methotrexate, trimethaprim, triamterene, pentamidine, rare enzyme deficiencies)

Manifestations of Folate Deficiency

Symptoms are identical to those of cobalamin deficiency as the end result is megaloblastic anemia. The one important distinction is the lack of neurologic deficits in folate deficiency.

Laboratory Findings

- Anemia
- Macrocytosis
- Hypersegmented neutrophils
- Low folate levels (normal serum values 6 to 20 ng/mL). Levels less than 4 ng per mL are considered diagnostic.
- Red blood cell folate level is often a more accurate indicator of long-term stores as serum levels often fluctuate.

Treatment

Evaluate and treat causes of folate deficiency when appropriate. Oral replacement is the mainstay of treatment although parenteral folate may be given as an IM injection in certain cases. Therapy is initiated and maintained at 1 to 5 mg per day. If vitamin B_{12} deficiency is also present, replacement of this should occur concomitantly to prevent neurologic complications.

Follow-Up

- Recommend adequate dietary intake
- CBC after 1 to 2 months to allow correction of anemia

Other Causes of Megaloblastic Anemia

- Medications inhibiting DNA synthesis (antineoplastic and antiviral agents)
- Myelodysplastic syndrome
- Metabolic disorders (Lesch-Nyham syndrome, etc.)

References

1. Babior BM, Bann HF. *Harrison's principles of internal medicine.* 16th ed. 2005: New York: McGraw-Hill.
2. Oh RC, Brown DL. Vitamin B_{12} deficiency. *Am Fam Physician* 2003;67:979–986.
3. Smith DL. Anemia in the elderly. *Am Fam Physician* 2000;62.

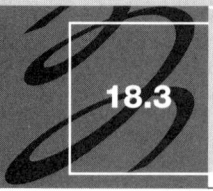

18.3 BLEEDING DISORDERS
Angela W. Tang, Daniel T. Lee

GENERAL PRINCIPLES

Bleeding disorders are caused by abnormalities in coagulation factors, platelets, or blood vessels and result in bleeding anywhere in the body. Such disorders may be inherited or acquired. Occasionally, an asymptomatic patient is found to have an abnormal platelet or coagulation study that generates concern.

DIAGNOSIS

History

- **Bleeding episodes** should be characterized.
- Not all easy bruising is abnormal. **Spontaneous bruising** on the trunk or bruising of areas greater than 3 cm in diameter on the extremities is more likely pathologic.
- **Childhood onset** of symptoms and a **family history** of bleeding problems suggest an inherited disorder. When an inherited disorder is mild, it may not be evident until adulthood or until significant trauma or surgery occurs.
- **Other important aspects of history** are prior transfusion need and bleeding responses to surgery, dental procedures, childbirth, and menstruation.
- **Underlying diseases** such as infection and liver dysfunction can lead to acquired bleeding problems.
- A thorough **review of medications,** including antiplatelet agents—aspirin, non-steroidal anti-inflammatory drugs (NSAIDs), clopidogrel, and ticlopidine—and anticoagulant drugs is essential.
- **Symptoms of significant blood loss,** such as lightheadedness, dyspnea, and chest pain, may trigger more urgent inpatient evaluation.

Physical Examination

- The **central nervous system (CNS), gastrointestinal (GI) tract, joints, deep tissue, skin, and mucous membranes** should be evaluated for bleeding.
- **Petechiae, mucocutaneous bleeding, or slow oozing after trauma** suggests deficient platelet number or function.
- On the other hand, **deep or visceral bleeding** (hemarthroses, deep hematomas) is indicative of a problem with coagulation factors.
- There may be evidence of **accompanying medical problems,** such as infections, malignancy, and liver and renal disease.

Laboratory Studies

- **Prothrombin time (PT)** and **activated partial thromboplastin time (aPTT)** evaluate coagulation factors.
- A **complete blood count (CBC)** assesses platelet number.
- **Bleeding time** will be prolonged (more than 7 minutes) in qualitative platelet dysfunction, thrombocytopenia, and von Willebrand disease.
- The **peripheral smear** confirms CBC abnormalities and may provide additional diagnostic clues (schistocytes in disseminated intravascular coagulation, large platelets in idiopathic thrombocytopenic purpura).

TREATMENT

- The choice of **outpatient versus inpatient** management depends on the severity and location of bleeding.

- **Hemodynamic compromise** or **marked anemia** requires supportive therapy.
- **Management of underlying etiologies** or concurrent medical problems is often imperative in improving the bleeding disorder.
- Patients should **avoid aspirin-containing products and NSAIDs** in bleeding disorders unless otherwise indicated.
- **Contact sports** should be avoided in significant bleeding disorders.
- Patients requiring frequent blood product transfusions should have their **HIV and hepatitis B and C status** checked, and if nonimmune, hepatitis B vaccination can be performed.
- A **hematology consult** should be considered for severe, chronic, or familial bleeding problems.

COAGULATION DISORDERS

Hemophilia A

Definition

Hemophilia A is an X-linked disease due to **deficiency of coagulation factor VIII.** As a rule, only men and boys are affected, but occasionally female carriers are clinically affected.

Clinical Presentation

The **bleeding tendency varies** with factor VIII levels. Patients with mild hemophilia (5% to 50% of normal concentrations) bleed only in response to major trauma or surgery. Patients with moderate hemophilia (1% to 5%) bleed in response to mild trauma or surgery, and those with severe hemophilia (less than 1%) bleed spontaneously.

Laboratory Studies

Laboratory findings are **prolonged aPTT** and **decreased factor VIII assay.**

Treatment

Selection and dosing of therapy depend on severity of bleeding and levels of factor VIII and factor VIII inhibitor. Hematology consultation can guide treatment. For patients with severe hemophilia, chronic prophylactic treatment may be desired.

- **Cryoprecipitate** 1 to 2 bags per 10 kg q8 to 12h for 1 to 3 days or longer can raise factor VIII levels.
- **Desmopressin acetate (DDAVP)** 0.3 μg per kg IV may raise factor VIII levels prior to minor surgery in mild hemophiliacs and can be readministered in 8 hours.
- Purified IV human and porcine **factor VIII concentrates** may be given, although effectiveness may be limited when significant factor VIII inhibitors are present. Recombinant DNA-derived clotting factors are available, eliminating the risks of viral transmission.
- For patients with significant inhibitor levels, **recombinant activated factor VIIa (rFVIIa)** or activated **prothrombin complex concentrates (APCCs)** may be used to bypass the inhibitor. Plasmapheresis or immunoadsorption can temporarily lower inhibitor levels.
- **ε-Aminocaproic acid** is an inhibitor of fibrinolysis that can be used as an adjunct to factor VIII concentrate or DDAVP.

Hemophilia B

Definition

Hemophilia B is an X-linked bleeding disorder due to **deficiency of coagulation factor IX.** It is clinically identical to hemophilia A but less common. Acquired factor IX deficiency may occur concomitantly with deficiencies of factors II, VII, and X and in patients with vitamin K deficiency.

Laboratory Studies

Laboratory findings are **prolonged aPTT** and **decreased factor IX assay.**

Treatment

- **Factor IX concentrates,** available as recombinant preparations to eliminate risks of viral transmission, are administered.

- **Fresh frozen plasma (FFP)** contains low levels of factor IX activity and may be used in patients with mild disease.
- DDAVP is ineffective in management of hemophilia.

Factor XI Deficiency

Definition
Factor XI deficiency is an autosomal recessive bleeding disorder common in Ashkenazi Jews. The correlation between bleeding propensity and factor levels is less consistent than for hemophilia A and B. Spontaneous hemorrhage and hemarthrosis are rare.

Laboratory Studies
The **aPTT** is prolonged. **Factor XI assay** is usually decreased to less than 10% in homozygotes and to 20% to 60% in heterozygotes.

Treatment
Give **FFP** 10 to 20 mL per kilogram body weight initially, and 5 to 10 mL/kg/day maintenance. Factor XI activity level of 30% is usually sufficient for hemostasis.

Prothrombin (Factor II) and Factors V, VII, X, and XIII and Fibrinogen Deficiencies
These are exceedingly rare coagulation disorders that may sometimes present with spontaneous hemorrhage. The treatment mainstay is FFP, although factor concentrates are available for deficiencies of factors II, VII, and X.

Circulating Anticoagulants
Antibodies may inhibit specific coagulation factors, prolonging the aPTT or PT. **Factor VIII inhibitor** is the most common inhibitor that causes bleeding. Lupus anticoagulant prolongs aPTT but causes excessive thrombosis rather than bleeding. Inhibitors may be detected when adding normal plasma to patient plasma fails to correct prolonged coagulation times (1:1 dilution test). Management of bleeding may involve massive plasma or concentrate infusion, use of activated prothrombin complex concentrates, plasmapheresis, and immunosuppression.

Vitamin K Deficiency
Vitamin K has an important role in hemostasis as a cofactor in the γ-carboxylation of glutamic acid residues for coagulation factors II, VII, IX, X, protein C, and protein S. Vitamin K deficiency may develop within a week if both intake and endogenous production of vitamin K are eliminated. Vitamin K deficiencies may occur with warfarin use, postsurgical states, antibiotic therapy, biliary obstruction, liver disease, nutritional deficiencies, and malabsorption syndromes, such as inflammatory bowel diseases and ingestion of nonabsorbed fat substitutes in diet foods.

Laboratory Studies
The PT is prolonged. The aPTT may be prolonged if the deficiency is severe. Assays for factors II, VII, IX, and X are typically low if measured.

Treatment
- Mild deficiencies may be corrected with **vitamin K,** 10 to 20 mg PO.
- Severe bleeding should be managed by transfusion of **FFP,** 15 mL per kg IV initially, followed by 5 to 8 mL per kg q8-12h as needed, along with vitamin K administration.
- Vitamin K may be given PO, SC, IM, or IV. If given IV, administer slowly, 1 mg every 2 to 5 minutes, to decrease the risk of anaphylaxis.
- Hospitalized patients at risk for vitamin K deficiency should receive prophylactic vitamin K 10 mg PO or SC weekly.

Liver Disease
Many patients with acute or chronic liver disease develop hemostatic abnormalities. The bleeding disorder may range from asymptomatic to significant hemorrhage.

Laboratory Studies
The PT and aPTT are prolonged from decreased clotting factor synthesis. Thrombo cytopenia, decreased fibrinogen concentration, and prolonged bleeding time may be seen. Platelet dysfunction may also occur.

Treatment

- **Vitamin K** 10 to 20 mg SC can be tried, although it may be ineffective.
- **FFP** may transiently improve hemostatic function for the actively bleeding patient.
- **Platelet transfusions** may be required if the patient is thrombocytopenic, actively bleeding, or about to undergo surgery.
- The value of DDAVP, fibrinolytic inhibitors, and conjugated estrogens remains uncertain.
- Certain causes of bleeding may require **targeted therapy,** such as sclerotherapy for esophageal varices.

Disseminated Intravascular Coagulation (DIC)

DIC is the consequence of activation of both the coagulation and fibrinolytic systems and may be a life-threatening condition. Usually a predominance of bleeding or thrombosis exists. DIC occurs secondarily to an initiating event, such as malignant neoplasm, infection, leukemia, obstetric complications, liver disease, shock, connective tissue diseases, massive trauma, snake bite, or extensive tissue damage, such as burns or frostbite.

Laboratory Studies

Laboratory findings include decreased **fibrinogen** (often the cardinal manifestation of DIC that correlates closely with bleeding), elevated **fibrin degradation products (FDPs)** including **D-dimer, thrombocytopenia,** prolonged **PT** and **aPTT,** and **schistocytes** (fragmented red blood cells) on blood smear.

Treatment

Treatment of the underlying condition is paramount. Use of cryoprecipitate, FFP, and platelet transfusions is considered in the event of major bleeding. Heparin is indicated if there are thrombotic complications.

Von Willebrand Disease (VWD)

VWD is a family of predominantly autosomal dominant disorders characterized by **deficient or defective von Willebrand factor (vWF).** vWF facilitates platelet adhesion by linking platelet membrane receptors to vascular subendothelium, and it serves as the plasma carrier for factor VIII. The severity of bleeding is highly variable even within an individual patient over time.

Laboratory Studies

Bleeding time may be prolonged but correlates poorly with bleeding risk. Prolonged **aPTT** may occur. Reduced **ristocetin cofactor activity (vWF activity)** is the most sensitive and specific test. Measurements of **vWF antigen, vWF multimers,** and **ristocetin-induced platelet agglutination** are useful for the subclassification of vWD.

Treatment

- **Oral contraceptives** may be given to women. They mimic the hormonal changes of pregnancy, increasing vWF and factor VIII levels.
- **DDAVP,** 0.3 μg per kg IV or SC, increases vWF concentrations two- to fivefold. A nasal spray is now available, making administration easier. DDAVP is contraindicated in patients with type IIB or severe type III vWD because of the potential for exacerbating thrombocytopenia.
- **Certain factor VIII concentrates** that contain vWF in high-molecular-weight form have been used successfully.
- **Cryoprecipitate** 1 to 3 bags per 10 kg per day replaces vWF.
- Cryoprecipitate or factor VIII concentrate may need to be continued for 5 to 10 days following major surgery or trauma.
- **ε-Aminocaproic acid** may help stabilize clots once they have formed.

PLATELET DISORDERS

Thrombocytopenia is defined as a platelet count less than 150,000 per μL. In general, platelet counts greater than 50,000 per μL are not associated with significant bleeding. Severe spontaneous bleeding usually does not occur with platelet counts exceeding 20,000 per μL in the absence of other hemostatic abnormalities. Bleeding may also occur despite normal platelet counts if there is a qualitative defect in platelet function.

Drug-Induced Thrombocytopenia

Thrombocytopenia has been associated with the use of heparin, quinidine, thiazide diuretics, alcohol, H_2 antagonists, estrogens, trimethoprim–sulfamethoxazole, quinine, gold salts, phenytoin, rifampin, ticlopidine, sulfonamides, and chemotherapeutic agents. Many other drugs have been implicated on rare occasions.[1] Thrombocytopenia usually resolves within days of discontinuation of drug unless there is slow excretion of the drug. Prednisone, 1 mg per kg PO qd, may decrease the duration of thrombocytopenia in some cases. Plasma exchange or platelet transfusions may be considered if hemorrhage is severe.

Autoimmune ("Idiopathic") Thrombocytopenia (ITP)

ITP is a disorder of antibody-mediated platelet destruction. This syndrome occurs primarily in otherwise healthy patients. Less commonly, autoimmune platelet destruction occurs with other diseases, including thyroid disease, pregnancy, HIV infection, malignancies, granulomatous disorders, systemic lupus erythematosus, and other rheumatologic disorders. The presence of lymphadenopathy or splenomegaly should trigger a search for secondary causes of thrombocytopenia.

Acute ITP

- **Acute ITP** usually occurs in **children** and often follows a viral infection of the preceding 3 weeks.
- Most cases **resolve spontaneously** within 6 months.
- **Platelet count is often less than 20,000 per μL.** Peripheral smear shows large platelets.
- **Treat** with prednisone 1 to 3 mg/kg/day and γ-globulin 0.4 to 1.0 g/kg/day IV. Platelet transfusions are usually reserved for severe hemorrhage.

Chronic ITP

- **Chronic ITP** is usually seen in adults, and spontaneous remissions are rare.
- **Platelet count usually is greater than 20,000 per μL** but may drop lower.
- **Initial treatment** is traditionally **prednisone** 1 to 2 mg/kg/day PO. A 4-day course of **dexamethasone** 40 mg PO qd achieves sustained improvements in platelets for some adults and avoids the side effects of chronic steroids.[2] Immunoglobulin, splenectomy, danazol 200 mg PO tid, immunosuppressive therapy, and anti-Rh(D) antibodies may be considered, depending on the severity of the disease.

Thrombotic Thrombocytopenic Purpura (TTP)

TTP is a life-threatening disorder characterized by thrombocytopenia, microangiopathic hemolytic anemia, neurologic abnormalities, fever, and renal dysfunction. Most patients have only part of this classic pentad of abnormalities. Peripheral smear shows fragmentation of red blood cells (RBCs). High lactate dehydrogenase (LDH) and reticulocyte count result from hemolysis.

Treatment

- Initial therapy **must** include **plasmapheresis** if available or **FFP infusion** until plasmapheresis is available.
- Treat renal failure, seizures, and hypertension with **supportive measures.**
- Platelet transfusions are avoided and severe anemia is treated with platelet depleted RBCs.
- Glucocorticoids are sometimes used.

Hemolytic Uremic Syndrome (HUS)

HUS is closely related to thrombotic thrombocytopenic purpura, but renal failure is the predominant manifestation and there are no neurologic disturbances. It is usually preceded by diarrhea. Dialysis for renal failure may be required.

Other Causes of Thrombocytopenia

Other causes of thrombocytopenia include hypersplenism, transfusions, DIC, nutritional deficiencies of folic acid or vitamin B_{12}, bone marrow infiltration due to myelophthisic disease (e.g., tuberculosis, metastatic carcinoma, myelofibrosis), primary hematopoietic disorders (e.g., leukemia, aplastic anemia, myelodysplasia, multiple myeloma), radiotherapy, and various viral, bacterial, and rickettsial infections. Therapy is directed at the underlying disorder.

Qualitative Platelet Disorders

Abnormal platelet function with normal platelet counts may occur with uremia, liver disease, cardiopulmonary bypass surgery, paraproteinemia, and myeloproliferative disorders. It may also occur with the use of drugs such as NSAIDs, aspirin, ticlopidine, clopidogrel, β-lactam antibiotics, alcohol, antihistamines, calcium-channel blockers, dipyridamole, and quinidine. Therapy is directed at the underlying disease or at removing the offending agent. Treatments that have been of use in some of the above conditions include DDAVP, corticosteroids, conjugated estrogen, cryoprecipitate, and platelet transfusions, if indicated.

ABNORMALITIES OF VASCULAR STRENGTH OR STRUCTURE

Bleeding in the absence of a hematologic defect may occur when vascular strength or structure is abnormal. For example, **senile purpura** presents with dark purple, irregularly shaped areas of skin bleeding on sun-exposed areas in elderly people. **Purpura simplex** presents with ecchymoses of the legs in healthy females, especially during menses. Management of these conditions consists of reassurance and possibly avoidance of antiplatelet medications. **Cushing syndrome** and **scurvy** also may present with abnormal skin bleeding, and treatment is directed at the underlying condition. **Osler–Weber–Rendu disease** (hereditary hemorrhagic telangiectasia) is an autosomal dominant disorder associated with bleeding from abnormal capillaries in the GI tract and nasal mucosa. Patients with **Marfan and Ehlers–Danlos syndromes** have fragile skin vessels, easy bruisability, and a tendency to form aneurysms of large arteries with potential rupture.

References

1. George JN, El-Haruke MA, Aster RH. Thrombocytopenia due to enhanced platelet destruction by immunologic mechanisms. In: Beutler E, ed. *Williams hematology.* 5th ed. New York: McGraw-Hill; 1995:1332.
2. Cheng Y, Wong RSM, Soo YOY, et al. Initial treatment of immune thrombocytopenia purpura with high dose dexamethasone. *N Engl J Med* 2003;349:831–836.

THE LEUKEMIAS

Joseph T. Cheatle, Christopher Smith

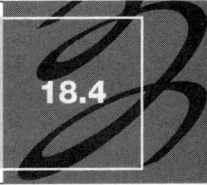

18.4

$\mathscr{T}$he leukemias are a group of illnesses characterized by the malignant infiltration of bone marrow by abnormal cell lines that produce high numbers of leukocytes, which are often nonfunctional. These disorders are categorized according to the type of cells produced, and the chronic or acute clinical course of the disease. Any cell line can be affected. The following is an overview of the most common leukemias found in children and adults.

ACUTE LEUKEMIAS IN CHILDHOOD

Acute Lymphoblastic Leukemia (ALL)

ALL is characterized by replacement of bone marrow with neoplastic lymphoid cells. ALL is the most common childhood malignancy with a peak incidence at age 2 to 5 years. Up to 80% of children achieve 5-year event-free survival.

- **Presentation:** Pallor, fatigue, bleeding, fever, bone pain, adenopathy, arthralgias, and hepatosplenomegaly.
- **Diagnosis:** Characteristic appearance of the bone marrow aspirate with >20% lymphoblasts.

- **Management:** Risk-based stratification; usually includes high-dose induction chemotherapy with vincristine, prednisone or dexamethasone, and l-asparaginase, with central nervous system (CNS) prophylaxis with intrathecal methotrexate or radiation.
- **Prognosis:** Indicators include age at diagnosis (children aged 1 to 9 years fare better than infants or children older than 10 years), sex (girls fare better than boys), race (whites fare better than blacks), and white blood cell count at the time of diagnosis (best if under 50,000/μL). A good indicator of lasting remission is rapid response of cell counts to chemotherapy.
- **Complications:** Opportunistic infections, cytomegalovirus, dehydration, and thrombocytopenia during treatment; long-term survivors may show cognitive impairment from intrathecal irradiation.

Acute Myelogenous Leukemia (AML)

AML is a heterogeneous group of disorders characterized by replacement of bone marrow with neoplastic hematopoietic cells. Approximately 15% to 20% of childhood leukemias are classified as AML.

- **Presentation:** Similar to that of ALL.
- **Diagnosis:** Characteristic appearance of bone marrow aspirate with >20% myeloblasts.
- **Management:** High-dose induction chemotherapy, often with cytarabine and anthracycline, and CNS prophylaxis with intrathecal chemotherapy or radiation.
- **Prognosis:** Increased incidence with chromosomal abnormalities (e.g., Down syndrome, Klienfelter syndrome), chromatin fragility disorders (e.g., ataxia telangiectasia), and exposure to alkylating agents (average 4 to 6 years after exposure).
- **Complications:** Myelosuppression, leukostasis with initially high white blood cell (WBC) counts, and infection. Long-term monitoring of cardiac, renal, and auditory function may be required.

ACUTE LEUKEMIAS IN ADULTS

Acute Lymphoblastic Leukemia (ALL)

ALL is characterized by replacement of bone marrow with neoplastic lymphoid cells. Any patient older than 10 is considered high risk with a poorer prognosis. Definitive diagnosis is crucial, as this disease is often confused with AML, hairy cell leukemia, and lymphoma, all of which have very different treatments and prognoses. B-cell subtypes are more common than T-cell subtypes.

- **Presentation:** Fatigue, poor wound healing, anemia, neutropenia, and thrombocytopenia.
- **Diagnosis:** Characteristic appearance of the bone marrow aspirate with >20% lymphoblasts. Recurrences can be outside the bone marrow.
- **Management:** Induction chemotherapy that may include vincristine, prednisone, anthracycline, and/or L-asparaginase. CNS prophylaxis is usually performed. If remission is achieved, an allogenic bone marrow transplant (BMT) may be considered. For recurrence, induction is repeated.
- **Prognosis:** Based on cytogenetics, age, WBC count, and time to remission.
- **Complications:** Anemia, thrombocytopenia, disseminated intravascular coagulation, infection (pay careful attention to dental hygiene), neutropenic fever (use broad-spectrum antibiotics), and tumor lysis syndrome. BMT recipients are susceptible to graft-versus-host disease. Long-term survivor: relapse, secondary malignancy, infertility, psychologic and intellectual problems, and neuropathy and cardiomyopathy due to chemotherapy.

Acute Myelogenous Leukemia (AML)

AML is a heterogeneous group of disorders characterized by replacement of bone marrow with neoplastic hematopoietic cells. If untreated, AML will result in death. The incidence increases with age; the most common age of diagnosis is 60. About 60% to 70% of patients achieve remission with treatment, with 15% 5-year survival. Subtypes include myeloblastic, promyelocytic (APL), monocytic, myelomonocytic, megakaryoblastic, and erythroleukemia.

- **Presentation:** Fatigue, anorexia, weight loss, fever, recurrent infections, abnormal hemostatic signs, elevated WBC count.
- **Diagnosis:** Characteristic appearance of bone marrow aspirate with >20% myeloblasts.
- **Management:** Chemotherapeutic regimens commonly include daunorubicin and/or cytarabine; APL is treated with all-trans retinoic acid (ATRA).
- **Prognosis:** Advancing age is associated with poorer prognosis; increased incidence with chromosomal abnormalities (e.g., Down syndrome, Klienfelter syndrome), chromatin fragility disorders (e.g., ataxia telangiectasia), and exposure to alkylating agents (average 4 to 6 years after exposure).
- **Complications:** Hemorrhagic complications including disseminated intravascular coagulation and thrombocytopenia, tumor lysis syndrome, careful attention to hygiene and dental care is needed with prophylactic antibiotics for dental work, prolonged decreased WBC count may be treated with granulocyte colony-stimulating factor.

CHRONIC LEUKEMIAS IN ADULTS

Chronic Myelogenous Leukemia (CML)

CML may be an indolent disease that progresses to acute phase and blast crisis (blasts >20%) over a period of weeks to years. About 90% to 95% of patients test positive for Philadelphia chromosome, a reciprocal translocation between the long arms of chromosomes 9 and 22. Median age at diagnosis is 67 years.

- **Presentation:** Clinical symptoms may be absent; increased WBC count may be found incidentally. Some patients present with fatigue, weight loss, night sweats, or splenomegaly.
- **Diagnosis:** Bone marrow aspirate, identifying clonal expansion of hematopoietic stem cells with the characteristic translocation between chromosomes 9 and 22.
- **Management:** Treatment is based on the age of the patient and stage of disease.
  - If patient is asymptomatic, no treatment may be given.
  - Allogenic BMT is the only curative treatment, and is considered in patients <65 years of age.
  - When BMT is not feasible, therapy options include imatinib mesylate and α-interferon. Imatinib mesylate targets cells with the Philadelphia chromosome, inducing apoptosis. Early trials have shown remarkable remission rates, and imatinib is now the preferred therapy for the chronic phase of CML. Long-term studies of imatinib are pending. Patients in acute phase or blast crisis are less sensitive to imatinib therapy.
  - Combination chemotherapy, including hydroxyurea, is used in patients who do not tolerate imatinib or to rapidly reduce WBC counts and symptoms.
  - Treatment of blast crisis is generally ineffective (median survival 6.6 months). Imatinib treatment and intensive combination chemotherapy are indicated, with consideration of BMT if remission is achieved.
- **Prognosis:** Indicators of poorer prognosis include certain genetic abnormalities, splenomegaly, increased number of blasts (circulating or in bone marrow), older age, male gender, and elevated lactate dehydrogenase (LDH).
- **Complications:** Splenomegaly, anemia, thrombocytopenia, infection, pulmonary fibrosis, hyperuricemia, and evolution to acute phase and blast crisis. Disease progression is associated with worsening symptoms.

Chronic Lymphocytic Leukemia (CLL)

CLL is the most common leukemia in the Western world. About 95% of cases arise from B cells. Various forms of lymphoma may present as chronic leukemia, and the distinction between these classifications may be tenuous. The median age at diagnosis is 64 to 70 years old, and CLL rarely occurs in patients under 25 years of age.

- **Presentation:** Clinical symptoms may be absent, with an increased WBC count found incidentally. Lymphadenopathy, hepatomegaly, and splenomegaly are common at diagnosis.
- **Diagnosis:** Sustained monoclonal lymphoctyosis (absolute lymphocyte count usually >10,000/µL). Bone marrow aspirate can be used to confirm the diagnosis.

- **Management:** Treatment is based on the patient's age and symptoms.
  - No treatment may be given if the patient is asymptomatic.
  - In symptomatic patients, combination chemotherapy is used. Regimens may include chlorambucil and fludarabine (alone or in combination), steroids, cyclophosphamide, and monoclonal antibodies. Allogenic BMT may be used in young patients, or those with poorer prognoses.
- **Prognosis:** Indicators of poorer prognosis include certain genetic abnormalities, lymphadenopathy, organomegaly, and bone marrow failure.
- **Complications:** Hematologic autoimmune disorders, pancytopenia, anemia, thrombocytopenia, generalized lymphadenopathy, opportunistic infections, and secondary malignancies, including treatment-induced leukemias.

Hairy Cell Leukemia

This chronic disease originates in B cells and affects primarily middle-aged men.

- **Presentation:** May include fatigue, anemia, bleeding, splenomegaly, pancytopenia, or, occasionally, leukocytosis.
- **Diagnosis:** Based on bone marrow aspirate with cells demonstrating prominent cytoplasmic projections (hairy cells).
- **Management:** Not required in some cases. If treatment is indicated, the usual agents are α-interferon, 2-chlorodeoxyadenosine, and pentostatin. Indications for treatment include anemia, thrombocytopenia, neutropenia, infection, tissue infiltration, massive splenomegaly, and symptoms of autoimmune disease.
- **Prognosis:** Generally good, with about 85% 5-year survival.
- **Complications:** Infection, including fungal and opportunistic infections, especially during and immediately following treatment.

ADDITIONAL RESOURCES

The National Cancer Institute web site at http://cancernet.nci.nih.gov is an excellent source of treatment information for leukemias and is updated monthly. The PDQ Cancer Treatment Statements are especially helpful in providing useful information in an office setting.

Infectious Diseases 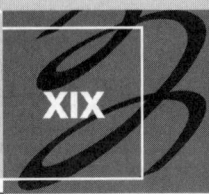 XIX

VIRAL UPPER RESPIRATORY INFECTIONS, INFLUENZA, AND FLU  19.1
George L. Kirkpatrick

INFLUENZA VIRUS
General Principles
Epidemiology
- RNA virus of predominantly two subtypes, A and B, but type C has been identified
- *Morbidity & Mortality Weekly Report* **gives physicians advance warning of the pattern of spread around the world**
- In United States occurs from December to February
- Overwhelming number of new similar cases with typical symptoms over a brief period of time

Diagnosis
Clinical Presentation
The Flu
- Influenza has characteristic set of clinical findings
- Onset is sudden
- Shivering, sweating, headache, aching in orbits, and general malaise and misery
- Fever to 102°F and higher in children
- Most consistent signs are polymyalgias, weakness, and malaise
- Cough from tracheobronchitis often quite severe

Bronchiolitis
- Age below 2 years
- Begins as mild cough and tachypnea
- Respirations become rapid and shallow with a prolonged expiratory phase
- Infants cannot suck or drink well because of the effort to breathe and may become dehydrated
- Findings include intercostal retractions, nasal flaring, and rales on auscultation
- Chest x-ray shows only hyperinflation

Pneumonia
- **Pneumonia can be a frequent and severe presentation.**
- More people die of heart disease than pneumonia during an influenza epidemic.

Laboratory Studies
- Viral cultures of respiratory secretions require 5 to 10 days and are 60% sensitive.
- Rapid enzyme immunoassay tests are available everywhere, are 75% sensitive, and provide results in less than and hour.
- Reverse-transcriptase polymerase chain reaction (RT-PCR) tests available in larger labs, are 80% to 90% sensitive, and report-out next day.

Treatment
- Management of flu requires both antiviral agents and symptomatic **medications.**
  - Decongestants, analgesics, and antitussives
  - Narcotics for severe myalgias and cough
  - Bronchiolitis may require ventilator support

Antiviral Agents
- Based on local testing or reports in *Morbidity & Mortality Weekly Reports*
  - For type A influenza use amantadine (Symmetrel) or rimantadine (Flumadine) 100 mg twice a day; elderly and renal compromised patients require half that dose; children up to age 10 require 3 mg/lb/day.
  - For type A or B use zanamivir (Relenza) applied intranasally two puffs q12h, or oseltamivir (Tamiflu) orally 75 mg bid for 5 days; for renal impairment use 75 mg daily for 5 days.
  - Oseltamivir may be used down to age 1 year; weight-related dosing.
  - Zanamivir down to age 5 years.

Prevention
- Transmission by hand contact
  - Virus survives on countertops for 4 to 6 hours
  - Hand washing reduces viral spread
  - Masks are not useful

- Immunization by new specific vaccine annually
  - Worldwide active subtypes chosen for vaccine
  - High-risk groups:
    - Elderly individuals and children with chronic disease.
    - Control by immunizing all school children or military personnel and employees of large companies.
    - Immunologic senescence in frail elderly prevents immune response to vaccine.
    - Prophylactic medications are more effective.

- **Prophylaxis**
  - Amantadine and rimantadine 100 mg twice a day can be used prophylactically when influenza type A is known to be predominant in the area.
  - Oseltamivir may be more practical for prophylaxis to prevent both types A and B.

RESPIRATORY SYNCYTIAL VIRUS (RSV)
General Principles
Epidemiology
- Single-stranded RNA paramyxovirus
- Two antigenically distinct groups (types A and B)
- Group A viruses are more severe in infants
- Winter and spring incidence, peak in January
- Pattern of outbreaks is a steady trickle of cases over several weeks to several months

Diagnosis
Clinical Presentation
Bronchiolitis
- RSV is responsible for the great majority of cases of acute bronchiolitis.
- Rhinorrhea and nasal congestion follow an incubation period of 4 to 5 days.

- After 2 to 3 days of mild symptoms youngsters experience acute respiratory distress with wheezing, cough, and inspiratory stridor, associated with tachypnea and hyperinflation of the lungs.

Bronchitis

- After age 2, Bronchitis becomes the most common clinical presentation, and RSV is second only to influenza as the most common cause.

Fever and Respiratory Distress

- In elderly patients, the symptoms become severe with higher fever, respiratory distress, more severe cough, and occasionally respiratory failure requiring intubation and respiratory support.
- Death from either cardiovascular collapse or overwhelming pneumonia is seen in elderly patients, particularly those with heart or lung diseases.

Asthma

- RSV and to a lesser extent rhinoviruses, coronaviruses, and parainfluenza viruses play a causative role in the origination of asthma in young children.
- Trigger exacerbations in later life.

Laboratory Studies

- Nasopharyngeal washings may be cultured
  - RSV detected in 7 to 10 days

- Rapid enzyme-linked immunoassay
  - RSV identified in a few hours
  - Nasal swab or nasopharyngeal washings
  - Abbott test pack RSV or directigen RSV by Becton-Dickinson

- RT-PCR is a very sensitive technique that requires about 24 hours for reporting and may be picked-up from a nasal or throat swab.

Treatment

- Supportive. Mild cases should be treated with outpatient hydration and rest and cough medication.
- Hospitalize if respiratory distress develops or the patient becomes dehydrated.
- Oxygen is the cornerstone of treatment for hospitalized patients.
- Antibiotics have no place in therapy.
- Ribavirin (Virazole) as a continuous aerosol using 6 g in 300 mL of water in a croup tent 6 to 20 hours per day up to 6 days or delivered by ventilator to intubated patients is a controversial treatment.
  - Conflicting reports of efficacy
  - Not cost-effective

- **Steroids are also controversial**
  - Frequently used, but no evidence of effectiveness
  - Wide range of dosages used

Prevention

- Transmission by large droplet inoculation of nose or eyes, or contact with contaminated surfaces or fomites.
- Virus recovered from countertops up to 6 hours.
- Hand washing prevents transmission.
- Virus shedding lasts on average 7 days from symptom onset.
- RSV is inactivated by many detergents, soaps, weak bleach solutions, and 70% alcohol.

PARAINFLUENZA VIRUS

General Principles

Epidemiology

- Single-stranded RNA paramyxoviruses
- Group of four subtypes; type 3 is endemic, types 1 and 2 cause a seasonal pattern in the summer and fall, type 4 is uncommon and hard to identify.
- By age 3 most children have experienced infection with types 1, 2, and 3.
- Brief incubation period after inoculation

- Virus remains in upper respiratory epithelial cells, uncommon to spread systemically
- Unlikely to produce a febrile response

Diagnosis
Clinical Presentation
- Croup (laryngotracheobronchitis) is most common presentation, and is most likely caused by a parainfluenza virus type 1.
  - Primarily children 6 months to 3 years old
  - Mostly fall and spring
  - Children present with 1- to 3- day history of rhinorrhea and congestion, associated with a barking cough and hoarseness
  - Fever is low
  - May be tachypnic
  - Severe stridor suggests bronchiolitis

- Asthma may be initiated by parainfluenza viruses in early childhood
  - Expiratory tight sounds
  - Wheezing and breathlessness
  - Persistent cough

- **Episodic croup has an explosive onset in an otherwise healthy young child.**
  - Barking cough and inspiratory difficulty
  - Usually late evening
  - No fever or other symptoms
  - Responds quickly to warm mist in a steamed-up bathroom or being carried around out in the cool night air.
  - Rare to require medication
  - Symptoms do not redevelop until the next episode months or years later.
  - Frightening family experience
  - Look for coexisting underlying illnesses

- Bronchiolitis, laryngitis, pharyngitis, and parotitis are occasionally caused by parainfluenza viruses.

Laboratory Studies
- Viral cultures of nasopharyngeal washings may be positive in 4 to 14 days.
- Immunofluorescent testing may be available in larger medical centers.
- RT-PCR testing is very sensitive, but not widely available as yet.

Imaging
- Lateral neck radiographs demonstrate hypopharyngeal overdistension and subglottic narrowing.
- Frontal neck views demonstrate the classic "pencil-tip" sign in the subglottic area. Also called "steeple sign."

Treatment
- Episodic croup responds to warm mist or cool night air.
- More severe episodes may require racemic epinephrine 0.25 to 0.5 mL of a 2.25% solution in 3 mL of normal saline as an aerosol.
  - Watch for rebound airway constriction.

- Dexamethasone 0.6 mg per kg IM one time is frequently given, although somewhat controversial.
- Oxygen by mask at low flow rates is useful in the more severe cases.
- Antibiotics, antivirals, and antihistamines are contraindicated.
- Reassurance for frightened young parents is very helpful.

Prevention
- Parainfluenza viruses are stable in small-particle aerosols that can contaminate humidifiers, and be inhaled from a cough. They are also stable on environmental surfaces for 4 to 6 hours.
- Good hand washing is essential.

- Masks can be helpful.
- A vaccine for type 3 viruses is being developed.

RHINOVIRUSES AND CORONAVIRUSES

General Principles

Epidemiology

- Rhinoviruses are nonenveloped RNA picornaviruses with more than 100 subtypes.
- Coronaviruses are single-stranded RNA viruses that have just a few subtypes.
- Neither has much of a pattern of spread, both are found worldwide with peak incidence in September and a lesser peak in April.

Diagnosis

Clinical Presentation

- **Common cold.** This includes symptoms of sneezing, tearing, nasal stuffiness, postnasal drainage, sore throat, hoarseness, and cough.
- **Laryngitis.** May be the only manifestation of the infection.
- **Malaise,** headache, and sore throat. Suggest infection by a coronavirus.
- **Severe acute respiratory syndrome (SARS).** Caused by a novel coronavirus and produces a highly fatal pneumonia with high fever and respiratory distress.
- **Exacerbation.** Of asthma by either virus.

Laboratory Studies

- Viral cultures are difficult and of limited usefulness.
- Early in an infection reverse transcriptase polymerase chain reaction (RT-PCR) has excellent sensitivity, but as the viral load decreases later in the illness enzyme-linked immunoassays (ELISA) become sensitive enough and offer excellent specificity to confirm the type of infection encountered.

Treatment

- Antibiotics are of no benefit.
- Steroids reduce airway inflammation and give symptomatic relief.
  - Pleconaril, a novel antipicornavirus agent may become available as it has potent antiviral activity.

ADENOVIRUSES

General Principles

Epidemiology

- Adenoviruses are double-stranded DNA viruses.
- 41 serotypes and more than 100 subtypes.
- Year-round occurrence, but spring and winter prevalence.
- Certain types, especially type 3, 4, 7, 11, and 21, cause epidemics of specific respiratory illnesses.
- More than half of all school-aged children have antibodies to the common respiratory types.
- Also causes gastrointestinal (GI), cardiovascular, and genitourinary (GU) illnesses.

Diagnosis

Clinical Presentation

- Acute respiratory disease that includes fever, coryza, sore throat, and cough, usually fairly mild symptoms.
- Includes a significant incidence of diarrhea.
- Bronchiolitis due to types 7 and 21 may lead to permanent bronchiolar damage.
- Pharyngoconjunctival fever due to types 3 and 7 is a syndrome of pharyngitis, cough, fever, headache, myalgias , malaise, and conjunctivitis.
- Conjunctivitis is always present, but other symptoms vary in their expression and intensity.
- Virus types 3 and 7 are found in lakes and poorly chlorinated swimming pools.
- Symptoms last about 7 days.
- Epidemic keratoconjunctivitis caused by types 8, 19, and 37 can be the typical "pink-eye" seen coming from daycare centers and schools.

Laboratory Studies
- Culture requires 21 days for results.
- Monoclonal antibodies in the Bartels Viral Respiratory Screening and Identification Kit detect RSV, influenza A and B, parainfluenza 1, 2, and 3, and adenoviruses in a few hours from a throat swab.
- A similar rapid direct immunofluorescence assay is available from Diagnostic Products Corp. (PATHO DX RVP).
- RT-PCR is the most sensitive test, but is not widely available.

Treatment
- For the most part is symptomatic.
- Antibiotics are of no use.
- Soothing eye drops can be helpful.
- Cidofovir a toxic antiviral (Vistide) is available for IV use in very ill patients.

Prevention
- Aerosolized droplets, surface contact, and fecal–oral transmission are common in children and virus can be isolated from respiratory secretions for up to several weeks.
  - Prevention involves blocking all three routes.
  - Prevention has not been very successful.
  - Military personnel have access to vaccine for types 4 and 7 but civilians do not as yet.
- Good swimming pool chlorination.

HUMAN META PNEUMOVIRUS (hMPV)

General Principles
Epidemiology
- hMPV is a nonsegmented RNA virus in the paramyxovirus family.
- First identified in 2001 from respiratory samples submitted from young children sick with mild respiratory symptoms.
- It is attracted to and remains with respiratory epithelial cells.
- By age 5 all children show evidence of past infection.

Diagnosis
Clinical Presentation
- Mild common colds to bronchiolitis to pneumonia.
- Does induce asthma and croup exacerbations.

Laboratory
- Not found by viral culture very effectively.
- RT-PCR is rapid and specific, but only available at few centers.

Treatment
- Symptomatic except, severe pneumonia, which may require ribavirin.

Prevention
- By good hand washing especially during winter months.

References
1. Louie JK, Hacker JK, Gonzales R. Characterization of viral agents causing acute respiratory infection in a San Francisco University Medical Center Clinic during the influenza season. *Clin Infect Dis* 2005;41(6):812–818.
2. Hu JJ, Kao CL, Lee, PI. Clinical features of influenza A and B in children and association with myositis. *J Microbiol Immunol Infect* 2004;37(2):95–98.
3. Yang TY, Lu CY, Kao CL. Clinical manifestation of parainfluenza infection in children. *J Microbiol Immunol Infect* 2003;36(4):270–274.
4. Pratter MR. Cough and the common cold. Accp evidence-based clinical practice guidelines. *Chest* 2006;129(1 Suppl):72s–74s.
5. Paes BA. Current strategies in the prevention of RSV disease. *Pediatr Respir Rev* 2003;4(1):21–27.

6. Gentile DA, Villalobos E. Cytokine levels during symptomatic viral upper respiratory tract infection. *Ann Allergy Asthma Immunol* 2003;91(4):362–367.
7. Azevedo AM, Durigon EL. Detection of influenza, parainfluenza, adenovirus, and RSV during asthma attacks in children older than two years old. *Allergol Immunopathol* (Madr.) 2003;31(6):311–317.
8. Billaud G, Peny S, Legay V. Detection of rhinovirus and enterovirus in upper respiratory tract samples using a multiplex nested PCR. *J Virol Methods* 2003;108(2): 223–228.
9. Anzueto A, Niederman MS. Diagnosis and treatment of rhinovirus respiratory infections. *Chest* 2003;123(5):1664–1672.
10. Wedzicha J, Donaldson GC. Exacerbations of chronic obtrusive pulmonary disease. *Respir Care* 2003;48(12):1204–1213.
11. Kahn JS, McIntosh K. History and recent advances in coronavirus discovery. *Pedatr Infect Dis J* 2005;24(11 Suppl):5223–5227.
12. Savolainen C, Blomquist S, Hovi T. Human rhinoviruses. *Paediatr Respir Rev* 2003;4(2): 91–98.
13. Alto WA. Human metapneumovirus: a newly described respiratory tract pathogen. *J Am Board Fam Pract* 2004;17(6):466–469.
14. Lau SK, To WK, Tse PW. Human parainfluenza virus 4 outbreak and the role of diagnostic tests. *J Clin Microbiol* 2005;43(9):4515–4521.
15. Principi N, Bosis S, Espositos. Human metapneumovirus in paedeatric patients. *Clin Microbiol Infect* 2006;25(4):354–359.
16. Foulongne V, Guyon G, Rodiere M, Segondy M. Human metapneumovirus infection in young children hospitalized with respiratory tract disease. *Pediatr Infect Dis J* 2006;25(4): 354–359.
17. Arroll B. Non-antibiotic treatment for upper-respiratory tract infections (common cold). *Respir Med* 2005;99(12):1477–1484.
18. Lindquist SW, Demmler EJ. Parainfluenza virus and the chameleon of medicine. *Infect Med* 1998;15(11):778–786.
19. Hashem M, Hall CB. Respiratory syncytial virus in healthy adults: the cost of a cold. *J Clin Virol* 2003;27(1):14–21.
20. Respiratory consequences of rhinovirus infection. Greenberg SB. *Arch Intern Med* 2003; 163(3):278–284.
21. Ogra PL. Respiratory syncytial virus: the virus, the disease and the immune response. *Paediatr Respir Rev* 2004;(5 Suppl A):119–126.
22. Papadopoulos NG, Psarras S. Rhinovirus in the pathogenesis of asthma. *Curr Allergy Asthma Rep* 2003;3(2):137–145.
23. Black CP. Systematic review of the biology and medical management of RSV infection. *Respir Care* 2003;48(3):209–231.
24. Williams JV, Wang CK, Yang CF. The role of human metapneumovirus in upper respiratory tract infections in children: a 20-year experience. *J Infect Dis* 2006;193(3): 387–395.
25. Melbye H, Hvidsten D, Holm A. The course of C-reactive protein response in untreated upper respiratory tract infection. *Br J Gen Pract* 2004;54(506):653–658.
26. Delmar C, Glasziou P. Upper respiratory tract infection. *Clin Evid* 2003;6:1747–1756.
27. Lemanske RF Jr. Viruses and asthma: inception, exacerbation, and possible prevention. *J Pediatr* 2003;142(2 Suppl):53–57.

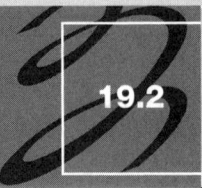

19.2 GASTROENTERITIS
Charles E. Henley

GENERAL PRINCIPLES

Diarrhea due to gastroenteritis is one of the leading causes of infant mortality worldwide and results in the hospitalization of more than 200,000 children each year in the United States.[1]

Causative agents of gastroenteritis include rotavirus, which causes sporadic viral gastroenteritis; Norwalk virus, which causes epidemic viral gastroenteritis; and enteric adenovirus, the second most common cause of viral gastroenteritis in young children. Rotavirus is the most common cause of gastroenteritis and affects mainly infants and young children. It can be severe enough to require hospitalization, whereas Norwalk virus causes a self-limiting, mild illness that can affect both adults and children and tends to occur in family, school, or community outbreaks.

DIAGNOSIS

Clinical Presentation

Viral gastroenteritis usually presents with symptoms of nausea, vomiting, and crampy abdominal pain of varying intensity due to excessive fluid in the upper gastrointestinal tract and increased peristalsis. Blood and fecal leukocytes are usually not present in the stool.[2] In this way it can be differentiated from most of the bacterial pathogens that are inflammatory and invade the mucosa of the colon, producing a bloody diarrhea. Other physical signs besides the voluminous nonbloody stools are those associated with dehydration, such as decreased urination, mental status changes, dry mucosal membranes, and lethargy. A history of daycare exposure, foods eaten, and recent exposure to antibiotic use is also important. Patients with bloody diarrhea, abdominal tenderness, and fever or severe dehydration should be hospitalized.

Diagnostic testing should be focused rather than all-inclusive. If the history and examination of the stool for blood and leukocytes lead to the conclusion that the diarrhea is noninflammatory, then routine stool cultures may be an expensive waste of time.

- **Laboratory tests** are not helpful in differentiating between inflammatory and noninflammatory diarrhea, but the plasma glucose, creatinine, and electrolytes of sodium, potassium, and HCO_3 are useful in assessing volume and acid–base status.
- **Viral detection** is expensive and may be unnecessary, but the best test for rotavirus is the enzyme-linked immunosorbent assay, which detects viral antigens.

TREATMENT

Because the course of viral gastroenteritis is self-limiting, the goals of therapy are to replace fluids and electrolytes lost secondary to the diarrhea. Most patients can be treated at home with oral rehydration therapy (ORT).

- **Mild to moderate dehydration** can be managed with ORT, even in the face of continued vomiting. It is rapid, safe, and inexpensive and can be used no matter what the patient's serum sodium is at the onset of therapy. Several ORT solutions, such as Pedialyte and Rice-Lyte, are commercially available, with 45 and 50 mEq per L of sodium, respectively. ORT has also been used successfully in more severe dehydration, but if there are signs of shock, uremia, ileus, or fluid loss greater than 10 mL/kg/hour, then treatment with intravenous fluids (normal saline or half normal with dextrose) is indicated. The World Health Organization (WHO) has recommended a recipe for ORT using easily obtained materials: 3 to 4 teaspoons salt, 4 tablespoons sugar, 1 teaspoon baking powder, 1 cup orange juice, 1 L clean water. This solution is relatively high in sodium (90 mmol/L) and should be reduced in salt if there is concern about retention of sodium and water.

■ **Refeeding.** The question of when and how to initiate feedings again can be simplified by following certain guidelines. ORT can be continued during the diarrhea, even if there is nausea and vomiting. Breastfeeding should continue uninterrupted, in addition to ORT. Formula-fed infants should have a lactose-free, full-strength formula reintroduced after 6 to 24 hours of ORT. The American Academy of Pediatrics recommends starting with a 1:1 dilution and gradually progressing to full strength. If the diarrhea worsens, return to ORT and gradually refeed with dilute formula, up to full strength over 6 to 72 hours. In weaned children, foods such as rice, wheat noodles, and bananas are good initially, but lactose-containing foods, caffeine, and raw fruits should be avoided for 24 to 48 hours.[3]

■ **Antidiarrheal agents** should be used with caution. Anticholinergic agents are generally ineffective and are contraindicated in children. Absorbents, such as kaolin and pectin (Kaopectate), may create more formed stools but may not actually cause a reduction in fluid loss or duration of the diarrhea. Antisecretory agents, such as bismuth subsalicylate (Pepto-Bismol), can increase intestinal sodium and water reabsorption and block the effects of enterotoxins. Antimotility agents, such as loperamide (Imodium) and diphenoxylate plus atropine (Lomotil), work by decreasing intestinal motility and reducing the distention that causes cramping and pain associated with gastroenteritis. Side effects include drowsiness, tachycardia, and paralytic ileus. Antimotility agents should be avoided in infants and used cautiously, if at all, in older children or adults because they can increase the morbidity associated with certain bacterial diseases, such as shigellosis.

■ **Vaccines.** In 1998, the U.S. Food and Drug Administration approved a vaccine for rotavirus (Rotoshield), which was subsequently withdrawn due to its association with intussusception. Since then two new vaccines have been developed and tested in one of the largest vaccine trials ever completed.[4] Rotateq, a pentavalent vaccine from Merck & Co., is dosed orally at 2, 4, and 6 months of age. A monovalent vaccine from GlaxoSmithKline, Rotarix, is also given orally in two doses 1 to 2 months apart. The incidence of intussusception during the safety trials for both vaccines has been insignificant compared to placebo.[5,6]

SPECIAL CONSIDERATIONS

■ **Food-borne gastroenteritis.** The etiology of food-borne gastroenteritis includes such viruses and bacteria as *Staphylococcus aureus, Salmonella typhi, Clostridium difficile,* and their enterotoxins, as well as some parasites, such as *Giardia lamblia.* These illnesses are usually associated with ingestion of undercooked meats, contaminated seafood or water, or foods left unrefrigerated. Because most cases of food-borne gastroenteritis resolve with supportive care alone, an extensive workup may be unnecessary except for public health concerns; or if one suspects botulism, which requires therapy with a specific antibody to the neurotoxin; or for patients who exhibit signs of extreme toxicity.

■ **Patients with AIDS** commonly have gastrointestinal symptoms that may be caused by an array of agents such as *Salmonella, Mycobacterium avium, Cytomegalovirus, Cryptosporidium, Isospora belli,* and *Campylobacter jejuni.* They are also at risk for *Clostridium* infection as a result of frequent antibiotic use. Therapy should be focused on the treatable causes of the diarrhea and the therapeutic measures that alleviate morbidity, such as the previously discussed antidiarrheal agents. Attention should also be paid to prevention of the spread of gastrointestinal infection, especially in hospitalized patients where there is potential for fecal–oral transmission of enteric pathogens.[7]

References

1. Taterka JA, Cuff CF, Rubin DH. Viral gastrointestinal infections. *Gastroenterol Clin North Am* 1992;21:303.
2. Park SI, Giannella RA. Approach to the adult patient with acute diarrhea. *Gastroenterol Clin North Am* 1993;22:483.

3. Laney DW Jr. Approach to the pediatric patient with diarrhea. *Gastroenterol Clin North Am* 1993;22:508.
4. Glass R, Parashar UD. The promise of new rotovirus vaccines. *N Engl J Med* 2006:354(1): 75–77.
5. New rotovirus vaccines close to roll out. *Am Med News*, Feb. 27, 2006:33,35.
6. RotaTeq's adoption by FPs uncertain. *Fam Pract News* 2006;36(6):1,8.
7. Smith PD. Infectious diarrheas in patients with AIDS. *Gastroenterol Clin North Am* 1993;22:535.

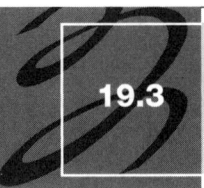

19.3 INFECTIOUS MONONUCLEOSIS
Jeffrey G. Jones

DEFINITION

Infectious mononucleosis (IM) is the symptomatic infection caused by Epstein–Barr virus (EBV). EBV is usually asymptomatic in infants and children, but commonly causes symptoms in young adults.[1] Like other human herpes viruses, EBV causes both acute and latent infections. EBV is associated with the pathogenesis of several lymphomas and nasopharyngeal cancer, and can manifest in a variety of ways in the immunosuppressed.[1,2]

DIAGNOSIS

The diagnosis of infectious mononucleosis is made via clinical, hematologic, and serologic means.

Clinical Manifestations

- The classic triad is fever, sore throat or pharyngitis, and lymphadenopathy.
- Other manifestations can include malaise (43% to 67%), splenomegaly (50% to 63%), headache (37% to 55%), anorexia (10% to 27%), myalgias (12% to 22%), hepatomegaly (6% to 14%), palatal enanthem (5% to 13%), nausea (2% to 17%), and rash (0% to 15%).[3] Rash is very common if ampicillin or amoxicillin is given.[4]

Hematologic Manifestations

- White blood cell (WBC) count is usually elevated 2 to 3 weeks after infection and is often 12,000 to 18,000 cells per µL. It is composed largely of monocytes and lymphocytes.
- Atypical lymphocytosis is a hallmark of IM, and occurs in most cases. Atypical lymphocytes may also be associated with acute HIV-1 infection, cytomegalovirus infection, toxoplasmosis, viral hepatitis, mumps, rubella, and drug reactions.
- Mild thrombocytopenia is seen in about 50% of patients.

Serologic Manifestations

- **Monospot test.** The Monospot test is a latex agglutination test that measures production of heterophile antibodies during acute and recent EBV infection. The use of this test can be limited because of false-negative readings (due to slow or no production of heterophile antibody) and a false-positive readings (due to cross-reactivity with other illnesses, such as lymphoma or hepatitis). Commercially available kits have fairly good operational characteristics.
- **EBV-specific antibodies.** Antibodies are formed to the structural proteins of EBV and can be useful in diagnosis, especially if the heterophile is negative. These tests are more expensive and require referral to laboratories.
- **Viral capsid antigens (VCA).** Antibodies to VCAs (VCA-IgM and, later, VCA-IgG) are elevated during acute infection with EBV. IgM is undetectable after 3 months and peaks

generally in 3 to 4 weeks. Therefore, VCA-IgM titer is the most predictive tool for early diagnosis of acute primary infection.

- **Early antigens—diffuse (D) and restricted (R).** Early anti-D correlates with severe disease. Anti-R is usually not present. These antibodies can be markers for atypical EBV infections or malignancies.
- **Nuclear antigen (NA or EBNA).** The antibody is undetectable during acute illness. Nuclear antigen develops after 3 to 4 weeks and persists for life.

TREATMENT

- **Therapy** for infectious mononucleosis is largely supportive because the disease is usually self-limited. Bed rest is recommended during the febrile stage, and strenuous exercise should be avoided for at least 3 to 4 weeks, especially if splenomegaly is present.
- **Medications,** in general, are of little benefit, with the exception of acetaminophen or ibuprofen to control pain symptoms and fever. Aspirin should be avoided to avert the rare and potentially fatal Reye syndrome.
- **Antibiotics** are of no value in mononucleosis, except in patients with secondary bacterial infection. As referenced above, amoxicillin is strongly associated with a rash, which does not appear to represent an allergic reaction.
- **Corticosteroids,** although advocated by some physicians, should be avoided unless severe complications develop, such as airway obstruction, hemolytic anemia, severe thrombocytopenia, and aplastic anemia. It is not yet clear how corticosteroids alter immune response and eventual risk of malignancy.
- **Intravenous γ-globulin** for immune thrombocytopenia refractory to corticosteroids is effective.[5]

Complications

Although infectious mononucleosis is usually self-limited, several complications may develop during the course of the illness.

- **Upper airway obstruction** from tonsillar enlargement and generalized inflammation, severe thrombocytopenia, and severe hemolytic anemia can be life-threatening complications. Prednisone is generally given in these situations at dosages of 60 to 80 mg per day for 5 to 7 days, then tapering over 14 days. Any potential benefit derived from the use of corticosteroids in the management of these complications should be balanced against any side effects.[6]
- **Insertion of an artificial airway** appears to be replacing emergency tonsillectomy as a first-line treatment in patients with complete airway obstruction.
- **Spontaneous or traumatic rupture of the spleen** is rare, occurring in 0.1% to 0.5% of patients with confirmed IM. Because of the risk of hemorrhage, splenectomy is the treatment of choice for rupture.[7] Sports, especially contact sports, and physically demanding tasks should be avoided during the acute infection and for as long as splenomegaly persists, given the risk of traumatic rupture. An ultrasound of the abdomen is more sensitive than physical examination in detecting splenomegaly, and can be useful in determining return to work or sports.[8]
- **Hepatitis** resulting from EBV infection is not usually severe, and transaminase levels are generally less than 10 times the upper limit of normal. Supportive measures should be taken and other possible causes ruled out in patients who present with jaundice or abnormal liver function tests.

References

1. Cohen JI. Epstein-Barr virus infection. *New Engl J Med* 2000;343:481.
2. Macsween KF, Crawford DH. Epstein-Barr virus—recent advances. *Lancet Infect Dis* 2003;3:131.
3. Johannsen EC, Schooley RT, Kaye KKM. Epstein-Barr virus (infectious mononucleosis). In: Mandell GL, Bennett JE, Dolin R. *Bennett's principles and practice of infectious diseases.* 6th ed. Philadelphia: Elsevier; 2005:1801–1820.
4. Patel BM. Skin rash with infectious mononucleosis and ampicillin. *Pediatrics* 1967; 40:910.

5. Cyran EM, Rowe JM, Boom RE. Intravenous gamma globulin treatment for immune thrombocytopenia associated with infectious mononucleosis. *Am J Hematol* 1991; 38:124.
6. Maddern BR, et al. Infectious mononucleosis with airway obstruction and multiple cranial nerve paresis. *Otolaryngol Head Neck Surg* 1991;104:529.
7. Rutkow IM. Rupture of the spleen in infectious mononucleosis. *Arch Surg* 1978;113:718.
8. Haines JD. When to resume sports after infectious mononucleosis. How soon is safe? *Postgrad Med* 1987;81:331.

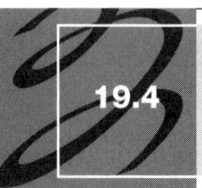

HUMAN IMMUNODEFICIENCY VIRUS INFECTIONS AND THE ACQUIRED IMMUNODEFICIENCY SYNDROME

19.4

Paul Lyons

GENERAL PRINCIPLES

Human immunodeficiency virus (HIV) is a retrovirus that infects human lymphocytes and other cells, causing progressive immune dysfunction resulting in acquired immunodeficiency syndrome (AIDS). AIDS is characterized by opportunistic infections, malignancies, and other clinical manifestations. Without treatment, the latency period from initial HIV infection to the development of AIDS may be as long as a decade.

Epidemiology

All patients should be assessed for risk factors for HIV including intravenous drug use, unprotected/at-risk sexual activity, occupational exposures, and maternal HIV status (for newborns). Physician-initiated discussion of safe sex and drug use are appropriate at well-adolescent and health care maintenance visits, and may influence patient behavior. About 40% of patients diagnosed with HIV meet criteria for AIDS at the time of initial diagnosis. All pregnant patients (and those considering pregnancy) should be encouraged to undergo screening as a routine part of preconception/prenatal care.

DIAGNOSIS

HIV Testing

HIV testing should be offered to all patients, especially those with a history of injection drug use or at-risk sexual activity. A positive screening test result (enzyme-linked immunosorbent assay) is confirmed by Western blot or other specific test. Patients almost always test positive within 6 to 12 weeks of exposure (median time to seroconversion approximately 9 weeks), although there are reports of delayed seroconversion. Greater than 95% will seroconvert within 6 months. HIV infection is generally considered to have been ruled out with a final negative test at 6 months. Viral load testing via RT-PCR may be indicated in some circumstances especially in patients with suspected acute HIV infection.

■ **Initial history** should be comprehensive, highlighting concomitant infections—sexually transmitted diseases, tuberculosis (TB), hepatitis, and opportunistic infections—travel, drug allergies, illicit drug use, and psychiatric illness, and, for women, Pap smears and past pregnancies. Social history should assess impact of infection on support systems, work history, etc. Review of systems for fever, night sweats, recurrent oral or vaginal candidiasis, diarrhea, lymphadenopathy, and dermatitis may help in disease staging, as may physical examination of the mouth, skin, lymph nodes, and abdomen. Particular attention should be paid to history of AIDS-related conditions including recurrent/diffuse zoster, esophageal candidiasis, invasive cervical cancer, Kaposi sarcoma, or chronic herpes simplex.

- **Laboratory screening.** Confirmatory HIV serology should be considered. A complete blood cell count and platelet count, renal and liver chemistries, fasting glucose and lipid panel, albumin, as well as syphilis and hepatitis B and C serologies should be obtained. Baseline CD4 lymphocyte count and viral load (VL) should be determined with two measurements. Genotypic resistance testing should be considered prior to the initiation of antiretroviral therapy. Skin testing for TB should be performed annually. Cervical Pap smears should be performed every 6 months for the first year, then annually if normal.

MANAGEMENT

Management of HIV-infected patients. With the advent of potent combination antiretroviral therapy, HIV is becoming a chronic disease necessitating long-term care for many patients. Expert consultation is encouraged for clinicians with little experience in managing HIV disease. Advice regarding the treatment of HIV-infected patients is also available from the National HIV Telephone Consultation Service ("Warmline") at (800) 933-3413.

Antiretroviral Therapy

Antiretroviral agents comprising four distinct drug classes that interfere with viral replication and slow HIV disease are available. Potent regimens have been shown to suppress viral replication, elevate CD4 cells, and reconstitute the immune system. Treatment initiation is dependent on three factors: HIV-related symptoms, CD4 count, and VL levels. Current guidelines suggest combination antiretroviral therapy for symptomatic patients and for asymptomatic patients with CD4 counts less than 200 regardless of VL level. For asymptomatic patients with CD4 between 200 and 350 providers should discuss the risks and potential benefits of treatment. For patients with CD4 count above 350 treatment may be considered if the VL > 100,000. Current guidelines suggest deferring treatment for patients with CD4 > 350 and VL < 100,000.[1] Therapy can be considered for patients with acute or early (<1 year) infection as well. Thus, if and when to initiate antiretroviral therapy is a complex decision that should be individualized. Combination therapy with three agents from two classes of drugs is the standard of care for initial therapy. Second- and third-line regimens, chosen when viral resistance develops, are increasingly difficult to tolerate. The optimal regimen balances potency with tolerability to promote maximum adherence. Complex drug interactions with and among antiretroviral agents must also be addressed. Genotypic and phenotypic resistance testing may also be helpful in designing an optimal antiretroviral regimen.[1,2] Rapid development of new agents requires frequent revision of treatment guidelines, available on standard web sites (Table 19.4-1).

- **Nucleoside reverse transcriptase inhibitors (NRTIs).** These drugs inhibit reverse transcriptase by competing with host nucleotides. The agents in this class are zidovudine (azidothymidine, AZT; 300 mg bid), lamivudine (3TC; 150 mg bid), stavudine (d4T; 20 to 40 mg bid), didanosine (ddI; 400 mg qd), abacavir (ABC; 300 mg bid), emtricitabine (FTC), and tenofovir (TDF). Zalcitabine (ddC) is infrequently used due to its relative inefficacy. Lactic acidosis has been identified as a rare but potentially fatal side effect of all drugs in this class. All drugs in this class have also been associated with lipodystrophy. Common side effects include gastrointestinal (GI) intolerance with AZT

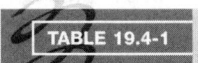

TABLE 19.4-1   **Useful Internet Resources**

www.cdc.gov

www.hivatis.org

www.hivinsite.ucsf.edu

www.hopkins-aids.edu

www.medscape.com

www.ucsf.edu/hivcntr

www.aidsinfo.nih.gov

and ddI; peripheral neuropathy with ddI, ddC, and d4T; pancreatitis with ddI; and bone marrow suppression with AZT. ABC can cause a potentially fatal hypersensitivity reaction characterized by fever, rash, nausea, and malaise. Patients who have discontinued ABC should not be rechallenged with this agent.

- **Nonnucleoside reverse transcriptase inhibitors (NNRTIs).** These drugs inhibit reverse transcriptase by binding to it and changing its shape. The agents in this class are nevirapine (Viramune, NVP; 200 mg bid), efavirenz (Sustiva, EFV; 600 mg qd), and delavirdine (Rescriptor, DLV; 400 mg tid). DLV is rarely used because of relative inefficacy and frequent dosing. Rash (including occasional Stevens–Johnson syndrome) and increased transaminase levels are common class side effects. EFV can cause central nervous system (CNS) side effects. These drugs all affect the P450 system, so drug interactions must be considered.
- **Protease inhibitors (PIs).** These drugs inhibit protease, thereby preventing formation of new virus. The agents in this class are saquinavir (Fortovase or Invirase, not recommended as a single protease inhibitor), indinavir (Crixivan 800 mg q8h), ritonavir (Norvir, 600 mg bid), nelfinavir (1,250 mg bid), and amprenavir (Agenerase; 1600 mg bid). Lopinavir (Norvir) is a second-generation protease inhibitor formulated as Kaletra in combination with ritonavir and dosed at 400/100 mg bid. Additional agents in this class include tipranavir (Aptivus, 500 mg bid with ritonavir 200 mg bid) and fosamprenavir (Lexiva, 700 to 1,400 mg bid), Class side effects include GI intolerance, hyperglycemia/diabetes mellitus, fat redistribution, hyperlipidemia, and liver function test (LFT) abnormalities. Drug-specific side effects include diarrhea with nelfinavir and lopinavir, paresthesias with ritonavir and amprenavir, rash with amprenavir, and nephrolithiasis with indinavir. These drugs, especially ritonavir, can inhibit enzymes in the P450 system, so drug interactions need to be carefully considered. Such drug interactions can be employed to therapeutic advantage when a combination of protease inhibitors is used.
- **Fusion inhibitors.** These drugs are the newest addition to antiretroviral therapy but are not currently considered first-line therapy for HIV.

Immunizations

Influenza and pneumococcal vaccines are recommended. Hepatitis B vaccine is indicated for hepatitis B seronegative patients. Live virus vaccines are generally contraindicated in patients with AIDS but should not be withheld when indicated in less immunocompromised patients. Measles–mumps–rubella (MMR) vaccine use is not contraindicated.

Prophylaxis against Opportunistic Infections

Prophylaxis against *Pneumocystis carinii* pneumonia (PCP) is indicated when the CD4 count falls to less than 200 cells per μL, or following an episode of PCP.[3] Trimethoprim-sulfamethoxazole (TMP-SMX), one double-strength (DS) tablet daily, is the drug of choice; alternatives include single-strength (SS) TMP-SMX, TMP-SMX DS three times weekly, dapsone—check for glucose-6-phosphate dehydrogenase (G6PD) deficiency before administering—with or without pyrimethamine, or inhaled pentamidine if no other options are available. Toxoplasmosis prophylaxis is indicated for patients with positive *Toxoplasma* titers who have a CD4 count less than 100. TMP-SMX is an effective prophylactic agent against *Toxoplasma gondii*; alternative prophylaxis is usually with dapsone plus pyrimethamine and folinic acid. Prophylaxis against *Mycobacterium avium complex* (MAC) disease is indicated for a CD4 count less than 50; clarithromycin and azithromycin are the preferred agents. Increasing evidence suggests that prophylaxis against these illnesses can be safely discontinued in individuals who respond to combination antiretroviral therapy with a sustained rise in their CD4 count greater than the CD4 thresholds noted above.

COMPLICATIONS OF HIV DISEASE

Systemic

- **Fungal infections** with *Cryptococcus neoformans, Histoplasma capsulatum, Blastomyces dermatitidis,* and *Coccidioides immitis,* often with disseminated disease in blood, bone marrow, liver, spleen, and CNS, require management with amphotericin B and/or oral azole drugs (itraconazole, fluconazole).

- **MAC disseminated infection** typically presents with progressively worsening constitutional symptoms such as fevers, night sweats, and weight loss in patients with a CD4 count less than 50. Bone marrow involvement is common. MAC is generally managed with ethambutol plus either clarithromycin or azithromycin; rifabutin, ciprofloxacin, or amikacin can be added for severe infections.

- *Mycobacterium tuberculosis* **infection** (TB) can occur early or late in the course of HIV disease. With advanced HIV disease, disseminated TB is more common than the localized pulmonary form. TB involving the bone marrow, GI tract, pericardium, CNS, or lungs is most common. Initial treatment with a four-drug regimen, including isoniazid, pyrazinamide, ethambutol, and rifampin or rifabutin for the first 2 months, is generally recommended, followed by an additional 7 months of therapy based on sensitivity results.[4] Directly observed therapy should be considered if compliance is a concern. Potentially dangerous drug interactions between rifampin and some antiretroviral agents often require substitution of rifabutin for rifampin. Guidelines regarding the treatment of tuberculosis, especially HIV-related tuberculosis, change frequently; updated CDC guidelines on the management of comorbid tuberculosis and HIV disease can be found at http://www.cdc.gov (also see Chapter 10.4).

- **Weight loss and wasting** are almost universal in AIDS. Opportunistic infections and malignancies, inadequate oral intake, chronic diarrhea, and depression can accelerate the wasting process. Consultation with a nutritionist can be helpful. Megestrol and tetrahydrocannabinol can promote increase in weight by improving appetite; resistance exercise training has shown more benefit in increasing lean body mass. Growth hormone can also increase lean body mass, but it is expensive and the safety of its long-term use unclear.[5]

- **Kaposi sarcoma (KS),** while typically confined to the dermis, can involve the viscera as well (see below).

- **Hematologic** complications of HIV infection commonly include leukopenia, anemia, and, less commonly, thrombocytopenia. Destruction of CD4 cells, HIV-mediated disruption of the hematopoietic system, low erythropoietin levels, anemia of chronic disease, and bone marrow suppression by HIV-related medications, opportunistic infections (such as MAC or B19 parvovirus), or malignancies should all be considered in the differential diagnosis of hematologic abnormalities. Treatment is generally directed at the underlying cause; granulocyte colony-stimulating factor can be used for significant neutropenia (absolute neutrophil count less than 500).

- **Skin disease.** KS typically presents as raised or flat violaceous lesions on the skin and/or hard palate (see below). Sometimes a biopsy is needed to distinguish KS from bacillary angiomatosis, which results from *Bartonella henselae* infection. Perioral and anogenital recurrent herpes simplex virus (HSV) infections are treated with oral acyclovir; intravenous acyclovir or foscarnet can be used for refractory or resistant infections. Herpes zoster infection confined to one or two dermatomes is treated with oral acyclovir, but disseminated infections or those involving the eye should be treated with IV acyclovir. Staphylococcal folliculitis and seborrheic dermatitis are more common in HIV infection. Cutaneous reactions to medications are common, including maculopapular or urticarial rashes, erythema multiforme, fixed drug eruptions, or more severe reactions such as the Stevens–Johnson syndrome or toxic epidermal necrolysis.

- **Oral cavity diseases** include candidiasis (thrush), KS, hairy leukoplakia, aphthous ulcers, and periodontal disease. Thrush can appear as erythematous patches or white plaques. Treatment with topical clotrimazole is usually effective, but systemic treatment with ketoconazole or fluconazole is sometimes required. Oral and esophageal aphthous ulcers often respond to prednisone; thalidomide has shown benefit for these conditions as well.

- **Eye disease.** Cytomegalovirus (CMV) retinitis occurs in persons with advanced HIV disease (CD4 < 50). Patients may note floaters, visual defects, or frank peripheral or central vision loss. Induction therapy with IV ganciclovir or foscarnet, followed by maintenance therapy with IV or oral ganciclovir or IV foscarnet can be effective in halting or slowing disease progression. Ganciclovir intraocular implants are convenient and similarly effective, and early data suggest that valganciclovir is an effective oral alternative to IV ganciclovir for induction therapy. *Treponema pallidum, Toxoplasma gondii,* and fungi are also associated with symptomatic disease and ophthalmologic findings.

- **Pulmonary disease**
  - **Pneumocystis carinii pneumonia (PCP)** most commonly occurs in patients with a CD4 count less than 200. Patients usually present with nonproductive cough, fever, and progressive dyspnea. Chest radiograph shows infiltrates or diffuse interstitial involvement but can be normal. Diagnosis is confirmed with induced sputum, bronchoalveolar lavage, or biopsy specimens. The treatment of choice is TMP-SMX; adjuvant prednisone therapy improves survival in patients with PaO_2 less than 70 mmHg. Second-line therapies for PCP include intravenous pentamidine, dapsone and trimethoprim, dapsone and trimetrexate, or clindamycin and primaquine.
  - **Bacterial pneumonia.** *Mycobacterium tuberculosis* (TB) can occur early or late in the course of HIV disease. Pulmonary infiltrates should be carefully evaluated for TB because of the severity of its course in HIV-infected persons, as well as the public health implications. Typical bacterial pneumonias, especially those caused by *Streptococcus pneumoniae, Haemophilus influenzae,* and *Staphylococcus aureus,* are common in HIV disease. Standard antibiotic therapy is usually effective.
  - **Fungal infections.** Pulmonary involvement with *Cryptococcus, Histoplasmosis, Aspergillus, Blastomyces,* or *Coccidioides,* while not as common as PCP or bacterial pneumonias, should be considered in patients with low CD4 counts.
  - **KS** can cause pulmonary disease, occasionally without dermal lesions. Radiographs characteristically show reticulonodular interstitial disease with pleural effusions.

GI Disease

- **Candidal esophagitis** causes dysphagia, odynophagia, and retrosternal pain. Response to empirical therapy with fluconazole or ketoconazole establishes the diagnosis and avoids endoscopic evaluation. Treatable HSV and CMV infections, which can cause painful ulcerations, are identified by endoscopic biopsy. Aphthous ulcers have a similar presentation and can be treated with prednisone and/or thalidomide.
- **Diarrhea,** often with severe weight loss, occurs in more than half of AIDS patients. Bacterial stool cultures can identify *Salmonella, Campylobacter,* and *Shigella* species. In patients with fever, blood cultures should also be obtained. *Clostridium difficile* enteritis, identified by *C. difficile* antigen in stool, is managed with oral metronidazole. Stool tests for ova and parasites can reveal *Entamoeba histolytica, Giardia lamblia,* and other infectious agents that respond to usual therapies. *Cryptosporidium* infection produces watery diarrhea, abdominal pain, nausea, and vomiting; treatment with paromomycin or azithromycin might help, but the most effective intervention appears to be potent antiretroviral therapy. Symptomatic control of diarrhea with diphenoxylate hydrochloride with atropine, loperamide, tincture of opium, or octreotide can be helpful. Sigmoidoscopy with biopsy and culture is indicated when results of initial stool studies are negative. CMV enterocolitis is often accompanied by diarrhea, weight loss, abdominal pain, fever, and anorexia, and can lead to severe complications such as perforation. Ganciclovir and foscarnet provide limited benefit.

Neurologic Disease

- **Cryptococcus neoformans** causes meningoencephalitis in 6% to 10% of AIDS patients, usually in patients with a CD4 count less than 100. The most common symptoms are fever, headache, and altered mental status. Meningeal signs and symptoms are uncommon. Serum and cerebrospinal fluid cryptococcal antigen is positive in 95% and 90% of patients, respectively. Acute treatment with amphotericin B for 2 weeks (minimum), usually with flucytosine, followed by fluconazole for 8 to 10 weeks is recommended. Patients with mild disease, low cerebrospinal fluid titers, and normal mental status can be treated initially with fluconazole alone. Lifetime maintenance therapy with fluconazole is currently recommended to prevent reoccurrence of disease; the safety of discontinuing lifelong suppressive therapy against cryptococcosis in patients who enjoy a sustained immunologic response to combination antiretroviral therapy is under investigation.
- **Toxoplasma gondii** encephalitis usually presents in patients with a CD4 count less than 100. Symptoms and signs include altered sensorium, seizures, focal motor or sensory abnormalities, cerebellar dysfunction, or neuropsychiatric manifestations. Empirical therapy is recommended for patients with multiple ring-enhancing lesions on computed

tomography (CT) scans or magnetic resonance images; CNS lymphoma presents similarly and should be considered if empirical antitoxoplasmosis therapy is not effective. Treatment with pyrimethamine and folinic acid plus either clindamycin or sulfadiazine is continued for 6 to 8 weeks. Clinical or radiographic improvement can be expected within 2 to 3 weeks. Failure to respond usually generates an evaluation for lymphoma. Maintenance therapy with pyrimethamine and clindamycin or sulfadiazine is required to prevent relapse.

- **AIDS dementia complex (ADC)** is a common condition in advanced AIDS. It is characterized by cognitive, motor, and behavioral dysfunction. Early manifestations include difficulties with concentration and memory. Eventually, performance of complex tasks becomes more difficult; slowing of thought processes and verbal response is typical. As the disease progresses, motor impairment and behavioral disturbances can become severe. The condition may respond to potent combination antiretroviral therapy, ideally including at least two antiretroviral agents that cross the blood–brain barrier.
- **Distal symmetric polyneuropathy (DSPN)** presents as painful or burning paresthesias in a stocking-glove distribution on the extremities. It usually begins in the lower extremities but can include the upper extremities as well. DSPN is a common adverse effect of combination antiretroviral therapy, especially to regimens including d4T and ddI, but can also be caused by HIV itself. The most effective therapeutic options include tricyclic antidepressants and gabapentin.
- **Progressive multifocal leukoencephalopathy (PML),** caused by infection by JC virus, occurs late in the course of HIV disease. PML usually develops insidiously with a single focus (e.g., limb weakness, ataxia, visual defects) but can progress to multiple foci, delirium, seizures, and death. Prolonged survival and remission has been reported with effective combination antiretroviral therapy.

Gynecologic Disease

Chronic vaginal candidiasis, recurrent HSV infection, and condyloma acuminatum are common. Cervical dysplasia can progress rapidly in HIV-infected women, resulting in cervical neoplasia. Pelvic inflammatory disease can be difficult to diagnose because leukocytosis is uncommon (see also Chapters 13.1 and 13.5).

Malignancies

KS is the most common AIDS-associated malignancy. Treatment modalities include radiation therapy, cryotherapy, intralesional chemotherapeutic drug injections, systemic chemotherapy, and α-interferon therapy. Non-Hodgkin lymphoma often presents at an advanced stage, behaves aggressively, and responds poorly to treatment. Primary CNS lymphoma is usually managed with radiation but can be difficult to distinguish from *T. gondii* encephalitis.

SPECIAL CONSIDERATIONS

Pregnancy and HIV

Women with advanced HIV disease are at risk for having low-birth-weight infants, prematurity, chorioamnionitis, and fetal demise. Perinatal transmission occurs in about 25% of births unless antiretroviral therapy is given. Zidovudine therapy during pregnancy, labor, and delivery and for the newborn during the first 6 weeks of life can decrease the risk of perinatal transmission to approximately 8%. Combination antiretroviral therapy may further decrease transmission and may be indicated to promote maternal health.[6] An appropriate regimen can be chosen with the help of an expert consultant. Invasive procedures that might promote transmission, such as fetal scalp monitoring, scalp sampling, and episiotomy, should be utilized only when clearly indicated. Caesarean section should be offered to all HIV-infected women with a viral load greater than 1000 but has increased morbidity in HIV-positive women. Breastfeeding is contraindicated because it promotes transmission of HIV.

HIV in Children

Polymerase chain reaction, repeated at designated intervals, can be used to diagnose HIV in most infants by 4 months of age.[7] Common early manifestations of HIV infection in children include oral candidiasis, lymphadenopathy, hepatosplenomegaly, fever, diarrhea, recurrent bacterial infections, failure to thrive, and developmental delay.

References
1. Guidelines for the use of antiretroviral agents in HIV-1. May 4, 2006. Available at: http://aidsinfo.nih.gov.
2. Hirsch MS, Brun-Vezinet F, D'Aquila RT, et al. Antiretroviral drug resistance testing in adult HIV-1 infection. *JAMA* 2000;283:2417–2444.
3. U.S. Centers for Disease Control and Prevention. 2002 USPHS/IDSA guidelines for the prevention of opportunistic infections in persons infected with human immunodeficiency virus: U.S. Public Health Service and Infectious Diseases Society of America. *MMWR* 2002;51(No.RR-8).
4. U.S. Centers for Disease Control and Prevention. Prevention and treatment of tuberculosis among patients infected with human immunodeficiency virus: principles of therapy and revised recommendations. *MMWR* 1998;47(No. RR-20).
5. Goldschmidt RH, Dong BJ. Treatment of AIDS and HIV-related conditions: 2000. *J Am Board Fam Pract* 2000;13:274–298.
6. Public Health Service Task Force recommendations for the use of antiretroviral drugs in pregnant HIV-1 infected women for maternal health and interventions to reduce perinatal HIV-1 transmission in the United States. November 17, 2005. Available at http://aidsinfo.nih.gov.
7. Guidelines for the use of antiretroviral agents in pediatric HIV infection. November 3, 2005. Available at http://aidsinfo.nih.gov.

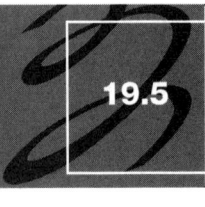

19.5   SYPHILIS
Megan R. Mahoney

GENERAL PRINCIPLES

Definition

Syphilis is a complex systemic illness caused by the spirochete *Treponema pallidum*. Because of its variable clinical presentations, it has earned the name "the great imitator" or "the great impostor."

Epidemiology

The Centers for Disease Control and Prevention (CDC) have reported a steady increase in the incidence of syphilis since 2000, largely among men with HIV coinfection and high-risk sexual behavior. During 2003–2004, the rate of primary and secondary syphilis increased almost 12% among men, and has remained stable among women. The rate of early syphilis was 5.6 times higher among African Americans than among whites in 2004. The highest rate of early syphilis occurred in southern states, accounting for 47.5% of total primary and secondary syphilis cases reported in 2004.[1]

Classification

- **Primary syphilis:** An incubation period of 3 weeks is followed by the appearance of a painless skin lesion known as a *chancre* (papules that ulcerate), which lasts 3 to 90 days at the site of inoculation (usually in the genital area). It is usually accompanied by regional lymphadenopathy. The patient is contagious and bacteremic during this period. Transmission occurs in about one third of those exposed.[2,3]
- **Secondary syphilis:** A secondary bacteremia develops 2 weeks to 2 months after the appearance of the chancre. It is usually associated with systemic signs, such as generalized

skin rash, mucocutaneous lesions, and lymphadenopathy. Relapses of secondary syphilis in untreated patients are not uncommon.[3,4]

- **Latent syphilis:** Without treatment, the infection becomes subclinical, detectable only by reactive serologic tests, for a period of 10 to 40 years. The latent stage is further subdivided into early latent (<1 year after exposure) and late latent syphilis (of unknown duration or >1 year after exposure). Treatment recommendations differ according to stage.[5]
- **Tertiary syphilis:** Approximately one fourth of untreated infected persons will develop tertiary syphilis, characterized by cardiovascular and gummatous disease, involving virtually any organ system except the nervous system.[5]
- **Neurosyphilis:** Neurosyphilis is syphilis infection of the nervous system and can arise at any stage of disease.
- **Congenital syphilis:** The incidence of mother-to-child transmission of syphilis in the United States and other developed countries is now relatively low since testing for syphilis is part of routine prenatal care. Additional serologic testing and sexual history at 28-week gestation and at delivery might be warranted in populations at high risk for congenital infection.

Etiology

Treponema pallidum is a thin, motile spirochete that has poor survivability outside of the host. The organism is transmitted from mucocutaneous lesions, and enters the body through epithelial surfaces of genital, anorectal, oropharyngeal and other cutaneous sites. Syphilis is rarely transmitted percutaneously.[6]

DIAGNOSIS

Clinical Presentation, History, and Physical Examination

Patients are symptomatic during primary, secondary, tertiary, and congenital infection. Patients with latent syphilis, by definition, are asymptomatic and diagnosed only by serologic tests.

- **Primary syphilis:** The syphilitic chancre is a painless, indurated, clean-based ulcer. The chancre appears at the site of inoculation. The chancre can be several millimeters to 2 cm in diameter. Although regional lymphadenopathy is common in primary syphilis, it is not an essential for the diagnosis. Without treatment, the chancre usually resolves in 3 to 6 weeks.[2,5]
- **Secondary syphilis:** Its manifestations include lymphadenopathy, mucocutaneous lesions (ulcers and flattened eroded lesions known as "mucous patches") in mouth or throat, and a maculopapular rash on the palms and soles is highly suggestive of syphilis, although the rash can be of any kind except vesicular. It may start on the trunk and spread to the extremities in a pityriasis rosea-like pattern. Systemic symptoms, such as malaise, low-grade fever, sore throat, headache, generalized lymphadenopathy, and arthalgia, occur in most patients. Other manifestations can occur, such as hepatosplenomegaly, cardiac arrhythmia, nephritis, cystitis, iritis, uveitis, prostatitis, and gastritis.[2,6]
- **Tertiary syphilis:** Cardiovascular manifestations of tertiary syphilis are uncommon. They include aortitis, aortic dilatation and regurgitation, and nonatherosclerotic coronary ostial stenosis. Gummas, also uncommon, are granulomatous lesions of the skin, skeletal, hepatic and respiratory systems that represent a delayed sensitivity reaction with local destruction.[2,6]
- **Neurosyphilis:** Neurologic involvement can occur at any stage of syphilis. Examples of neurologic presentations are cranial nerve palsies, including Argyll Robertson pupils (small irregular pupils that are nonreactive to light but reactive to accommodation) and auditory symptoms; signs or symptoms of meningitis; tabes dorsalis, which is well-characterized as a wide-based "steppage" gait and signifies destruction of the dorsal roots of the spinal column; bladder or bowel incontinence; optic abnormalities, such as neuroretinitis, optic neuritis, or uveitis; peripheral neuropathy; shooting pains; personality change; speech disturbances; facial tremor; hyperactive reflexes; meningovascular stroke syndromes; and seizures.[2,6]

- **Congenital syphilis:** *In utero* sequelae of congenital syphilis include hydrops fetalis (usually diagnosed by ultrasound before 18 weeks), stillbirth, and prematurity. However, most infants with congenital syphilis are usually not symptomatic until the first months of life. Congenital syphilis during early infancy can manifest as rhinitis, skin, oral and visceral lesions, bone abnormities, chorioretinitis, hepatosplenomegaly, and nephritic syndrome. If left untreated, late manifestations develop after 2 years of age, which include mental retardation, dental abnormalities, hydrocephalus, and bony deformities such as frontal bossing.[2,6]

Laboratory Studies

Direct visualization of *Treponema pallidum* by darkfield examination or direct fluorescent antibody tests of biopsied lesions is the gold standard of diagnosis. However, interpretation requires considerable expertise, and most often indirect methods of diagnosis, such as serologic tests, are employed.

- Presumptive diagnosis is possible with the following two types of serologic tests.
  - VDRL and RPR tests are nontreponemal tests (i.e., the interaction of the spirochete with host tissue yields an antibody against a lipoidal antigen). VDRL and RPR tests have sensitivities of 78% and 86%, respectively, and are used for screening. They become positive 4 to 6 weeks after infection and 1 to 3 weeks after the appearance of the primary lesion. The titers correlate well with the disease activity but can be falsely negative at the very early or late stage, initially due to developing antibody response and later due to waning antibody response. Common causes of false positives are viral infectious, pregnancy, malignancy, immunizations, connective tissue disorders, and intravenous drug use.[3]
  - FTA-ABS and microhemagglutination: *Treponema pallidum* (MHA-TP) tests are used to confirm a positive VDRL or RPR. MHA-TP is positive in 76% of patients with primary syphilis, and the FTA-ABS is positive in 84%. Compared with nontreponemal tests, treponemal tests may become positive earlier in the course of the infection. These tests do not correlate well with disease activity and should not be used to monitor treatment response. The FTA-ABS remains positive for life in most people despite treatment. Consider other sexually transmitted diseases, including HIV infection, in all patients diagnosed with syphilis.[3]

- For the diagnosis of **neurosyphilis**, cerebrospinal fluid (CSF) evaluation is required.
  - CSF examination is indicated for any patients with neurologic or ophthalmic symptoms or signs potentially attributable to syphilis. Other indications for CSF evaluation include tertiary syphilis without neurologic symptoms, treatment failure, and HIV coinfection, according to some experts. All children with syphilis should have a CSF examination to exclude neurosyphilis, with a review of birth and maternal medical records to determine if syphilis was acquired perinatally.[5,6]
  - When CSF evaluation is performed, it should include determination of protein and glucose levels, cell count, and VDRL. The VDRL is associated with a high false-negative rate, and can be used to should not be used to exclude neurosyphilis.[5]
  - An elevated CSF leukocyte count (more than five white blood cells per mm²), a CSF protein measurement greater than 40 mg per dL (40 mg/L) and low CSF glucose levels are consistent with neurosyphilis. The CSF should not be tested routinely for RPR nor treponemal-specific antibodies (MHA-TP or FTA-ABS), because false-positive tests occur frequently.[5,6]

- All **sexual contacts** occurring within 3 months for primary syphilis, within 6 months for secondary syphilis, and within 1 year for early latent disease should be tested for possible treatment.[7]
- The workup for **congenital syphilis** should include a complete CBC with differential, CSF analysis for VDRL, cell count and protein, and other tests as indicated, such as long bone radiography, chest radiography, liver function testing, cranial ultrasonography, ophthalmologic examination, and auditory brainstem response.[6]
  - A diagnosis can be confirmed when *T. pallidum* has been identified from darkfield microscopy or fluorescent antibody test of lesions, placenta, umbilical cord, or any other tissue from the infant.[6]

■ A presumptive diagnosis can be made in any infant whose mother had untreated or inadequately treated syphilis at delivery, regardless of symptoms or signs in the infant, or in any infant or child who has a reactive specific treponemal test for syphilis *and* any of the following: evidence of congenital syphilis on physical examination; evidence of congenital syphilis on long bone radiographs; reactive CSF VDRL; elevated CSF cell count or protein (without other cause); or reactive test for FTA-ABS-IgM using fractional serum.[6]

Differential Diagnosis

For **primary syphilis,** the differential diagnosis for a genital ulcer includes genital herpes (usually painful with a red base), chancroid (typically painful with sharp undermined borders), and lymphogranuloma venerum (usually painless and shallow). The presentation of **secondary** and **tertiary syphilis** can be similar to a wide array of inflammatory and infectious syndromes. **Neurosyphilis** must be considered in the workup of any neurologic condition.

TREATMENT

Medications

Parenteral penicillin G (Bicillin L-A) is the drug of choice for management of all stages of syphilis. The **Jarisch-Herxheimer** reaction (fever, hypotension, headache, and myalgias) can occur within 24 hours after appropriate therapy, particularly in patients with early syphilis. This reaction is thought to be the result of an inflammatory response to the destruction of treponemes. It can be treated symptomatically with antipyretics, but there is no known preventive treatment. Patients should be advised that this is not a manifestation of penicillin allergy.[5]

■ For **primary, secondary,** and **early latent syphilis,** the treatment regimen is as follows:
  ■ For adults, benzathine penicillin G, 2.4 million units IM in a single dose.
  ■ Children are given benzathine penicillin G, 50,000 units per kilogram (up to the adult dose) IM in a singe dose.[3]

■ For **late latent syphilis** or latent syphilis of unknown duration, the treatment regimen is as follows:
  ■ For adults, benzathine penicillin G, 2.4 million units IM every week for 3 weeks.
  ■ For penicillin-allergic nonpregnant adults, doxycycline 100 mg twice daily for 2 weeks or tetracycline 500 mg four times day for 4 weeks.
  ■ Children are given benzathine penicillin G, 50,000 units per kilogram (up to the adult dose) IM every week for 3 weeks.[3]

■ For **tertiary syphilis,** the treatment regimen is as follows;
  ■ For adults, benzathine penicillin G, 2.4 million units IM every week for 3 weeks.
  ■ For penicillin-allergic nonpregnant adults, doxycycline 100 mg twice daily for 2 weeks or tetracycline 500 mg four times day for 2 weeks.[3]

■ For **neurosyphilis,** the treatment regimen is as follows:
  ■ Aqueous crystalline penicillin G, 18 to 24 million units daily (2 to 4 million units every 4 hours) for 10 to 14 days, followed by benzathine penicillin G, 2.4 million U IM weekly for 3 weeks.[3]

■ For **congenital syphilis,** the treatment regimen is as follows:
  ■ Aqueous crystalline penicillin G, 50,000 units/kg/dose IV every 8 to 12 hours for 10 to 14 days; *or* procaine penicillin G 50,000 units/kg/dose IM per day in a single dose for 10 days.
  ■ Treatment for congenital syphilis is recommended in the absence of confirmatory serologic testing when the mother has untreated syphilis; when the mother has a fourfold or greater increase in nontreponemal titer; when she was treated with erythromycin or other nonpenicillin regimen during pregnancy; or if the mother was treated for syphilis within the month prior to delivery.[3,5]

■ For **penicillin-allergic patients,** the treatment regimen is as follows:
  ■ For penicillin-allergic nonpregnant adults, doxycycline 100 mg twice daily for 2 weeks or tetracycline 500 mg four times day for 2 weeks for primary, secondary, and early latent syphilis. Extend treatment to 4 weeks total if treating tertiary syphilis.

■ Penicillin-allergic pregnant women, patients with neurosyphilis, HIV-infected patients and children, should undergo penicillin desensitization orally or intravenously, and be treated with penicillin. The procedure should be treated as a medical emergency, taking place in a medical setting.[3]

Patient Education and Counseling

Comprehensive health education and prevention services are imperative to combat the spread of syphilis. Patients should be advised that the highest risk of syphilis transmission is unprotected sex with one who has multiple partners. Other risk factors include sexual activity that occurs in exchange for drugs, high-risk sexual activity among adolescents and men who have sex with men, and sexual behavior in correctional facilities.[1]

Follow-Up and Monitoring

No studies have established the absolute laboratory criteria for successful therapy. However, evidence from large epidemiologic studies suggests obtaining serum VDRL or RPR titers at 6, 12, and 24 months after treatment. The titers are both qualitative and quantitative and can be ensued to monitor response to treatment. The tests are not interchangeable. The test that is used initially must be used for subsequent testing. It is expected that patients will become nonreactive following treatment; however, some patients demonstrate a **serofast** reaction, maintaining persistently low titers for life (usually 1:8 or less). Other causes of reactive tests posttreatment include reinfection, HIV coinfection, and undiagnosed neurosyphilis.[6]

■ In patients treated for **primary** and **secondary syphilis,** a fourfold decrease in antibody titers should be seen by 6 months, and those with **early latent syphilis** should have a fourfold decrease by 1 year posttreatment. In the absence of a fourfold change in titers, which is equivalent to a change of two dilutions (from 1:16 to 1:4), retreatment should be considered.[2,3]

■ Successful treatment of **late latent** and **tertiary syphilis** should lead to a decrease fourfold by 12 to 24 months. If titers increase fourfold, fail to drop at least fourfold within 12 to 24 months, or syphilitic signs and symptoms develop, treatment should be considered a failure and retreatment should be considered.[3]

■ For **neurosyphilis,** predicting the response to treatment is somewhat more complicated. The purpose of treatment is to arrest further disease progression, and attempt to reverse the ongoing symptoms. Patients should be monitored with CSF examination every 6 months for decreasing cell count if CSF pleocytosis was initially present. If there is no decrease in 6 months or failure to return to normal in 2 years, retreatment should be considered.[3]

SPECIAL CONSIDERATIONS

For **HIV-infected** persons, the clinical and laboratory presentations of syphilis in HIV-infected persons are generally similar to those in persons who are not infected with HIV. There are reports of HIV-infected patients who have persistent or recurrent syphilis despite appropriate antisyphilitic therapy.[5]

References

1. Centers for Disease Control and Prevention. *Sexually transmitted disease surveillance 2004 supplement, syphilis surveillance report*. Atlanta, GA: U.S. Department of Health and Human Services, Centers for Disease Control and Prevention; December 2005.
2. Mandell GL, Bennett JE, Dolin R. *Bennett's principles and practice of infectious disease*. 6th ed. Philadelphia: Elsevier; 2005:2773–2781.
3. Krigger KW. *Manual of family medicine*. Philadelphia: Lippincott Williams & Wilkins; 2002.
4. Myint M, Bashiri H, Harrington RD, et al. Relapse of secondary syphilis after benzathine penicillin G: molecular analysis. *Sex Transm Dis* 2004;31(3):196–199.
5. Birnbaum NR, Goldschmidt RH, Buffett WO. Resolving the common dilemmas of syphilis. *Am Fam Physician* 1999;59:2233–2240.
6. Cohen J, Powderly WC. *Infectious diseases*. 2nd ed. London: Mosby; 2004:720.
7. Brown DL, Frank JE. Diagnosis and management of syphilis. *Am Fam Physician* 2003;286.

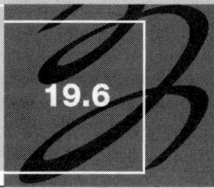

GENERAL PRINCIPLES

Gonorrhea continues to be a very prevalent sexually transmitted disease in the United States and the rest of the world. Despite efforts to control this disease, the trend toward lower incidence reversed itself in 1998. The rate had been decreasing for the previous 13 years. In the United States, for the year 1998, the incidence of gonorrhea increased by 9% as reported by the Centers for Disease Control (CDC) in June 2000.[1] The incidence rate was not consistent across states but was up overall. Highest rates are found in urban areas, age less than 24, with multiple sexual partners having unprotected intercourse. Rates for women are highest between ages 15 and 29. Rates for men are highest between ages 20 and 24. There is approximately a 20% resistance to penicillin or tetracycline. Resistance to quinolones is greater than 40% in some Asian countries. There has been an increase in resistance to azithromycin since 1992.[2] There is a high association with coinfection with *Chlamydia,* which should also be treated.

Etiology

Gonorrhea is caused by *Neisseria gonorrhoeae.* This is a Gram-negative coccus (gonococcus), which usually occurs in pairs. There is an association with polymorphonuclear cells (PMNs). The culture is performed on enriched media, such as Mueller–Hinton or Modified Thayer–Martin. The organism is strictly aerobic. Unlike the meningococcus, there is no polysaccharide capsule. It may be cultured from many areas, including urethra, cervix, throat, rectum, and conjunctiva. In addition to culture diagnosis, there is also a rapid antigen test available. Serologic testing is available, but it takes longer than other tests to return a result and may delay treatment.

DIAGNOSIS

History at Presentation

Symptoms may be related to location of infection. This is usually associated with a mucopurulent discharge, but such discharge may not always be present. Some individuals may not have any symptoms.

- Urethritis often presents with a purulent or mucopurulent discharge; however, some patients, especially male patients, may be asymptomatic.
- Cervicitis usually is associated with a purulent or mucopurulent discharge, but patients may be asymptomatic. This is often associated with symptoms of urethritis as well. May also be associated with pelvic inflammatory disease (PID) (see Chapter 13.5).
- Pharyngitis presents with enlarged tonsils, pain, and purulent exudates, usually associated with oral–genital contact. Frequently involves enlarged cervical lymph nodes.
- Conjunctivitis is often the result of transmission from mother to infant at the time of delivery. There is significant swelling and erythema of the conjunctiva and lids, with copious purulent discharge. If not managed, may lead to corneal ulceration.
- Monoarthropathy results from hematogenous spread of the disease. This occurs in approximately 1% to 2% of infections. These patients appear septic and often have positive blood cultures. The arthropathy is frequently wandering but tends to remain with a single joint. There may also be associated systemic involvement. Rarely, it progresses to endocarditis or meningitis.
- Diagnosis is usually begins with confirmation of the presence of urethritis,[1] and the presence of purulent or mucopurulent discharge.
- Gram stain of urethral secretions demonstrates five or more white blood cells (WBCs) per oil immersion field. Documentation of the presence of WBCs containing intracellular

Gram-negative diplococci is classic. Patients may have positive leukocyte esterase on voided urine or microscopic exam with at least 10 WBCs per high-power field. If these criteria are absent, diagnosis can be deferred pending culture or rapid antigen testing. Treatment is based on results.

- Treatment for patients whose diagnosis does not include urethritis should be recommended only for high-risk individuals with poor likelihood of follow-up. These individuals should be treated for both gonorrhea and chlamydial infection. Partners should also be empirically treated.

TREATMENT

The CDC[2] recommends that all patients being treated for gonorrhea should also be treated for chlamydial infection because of the high incidence of coinfection. This can be done without testing for *Chlamydia*. Chlamydial coinfection is associated with 10% to 30% of gonococcal infections. Consideration should be given to looking for other sexually transmitted diseases, such as syphilis and HIV infection, as well as hepatitis B.

- Uncomplicated infections are usually managed with ceftriaxone (Rocephin) 125 mg IM as a single dose and doxycycline 100 mg orally twice a day for 7 days. A single dose of azithromycin (Zithromax) 1.0 g orally may be substituted for the doxycycline for improved compliance. Options for the ceftriaxone include cefixime 400 mg orally as one dose, ciprofloxacin (Cipro) 500 mg orally as one dose, ofloxacin (Floxin) 400 mg orally as a single dose, or levofloxacin (Levaquin) 250 mg orally as a single dose. Test of cure is not required. Patients with persistent symptoms should be evaluated for resistant organisms. Treatment failure is often a result of reinfection or coinfection with other organisms, such as *Chlamydia*. Sexual partners will require treatment, and intercourse should be avoided until completion of therapy.
- Uncomplicated pharyngeal infections should be treated with ceftriaxone (Rocephin) 125 mg IM as a single dose or with ciprofloxacin (Cipro) 500 mg orally as a single dose.
- Pregnant patients should not be treated with quinolones or tetracyclines. Ceftriaxone is safe in pregnancy, as are erythromycin and azithromycin (see also Chapter 22.2).
- Patients who are HIV-positive should receive the same treatment as HIV-negative individuals.
- Conjunctivitis in adults may be managed with ceftriaxone 1 g IM as a single dose. The eyes should then be irrigated with saline solution once.
- Patients with disseminated gonococcal infection (DCI) should be hospitalized and treated for presumptive chlamydial infection as well. Treatment should be ceftriaxone 1 g IM or IV daily until 12 to 24 hours after the patient improves, at which time oral therapy may be begun. Alternatives include cefotaxime 1 g IV q8h, ceftizoxime (Cefizox) 1 g IV q8h, ciprofloxacin 400 mg IV q12h, ofloxacin 400 mg IV q12h or levofloxacin 250 mg IV daily. Oral therapy may be cefixime 400 mg twice a day, ciprofloxacin 500 mg twice a day, ofloxacin 400 mg twice a day, or ofloxacin 500 mg orally daily.
- Meningitis or endocarditis should be treated with IV medications. Treatment of choice is ceftriaxone 1 to 2 g IV q12h.
- Ophthalmia neonatorum is frequently caused by chlamydial infection, but gonorrhea should be considered. Topical therapy alone is not adequate. Recommended treatment is ceftriaxone 25 to 50 mg/kg IV or IM as a single dose (maximum dose 125 mg). Prophylaxis may be silver nitrate 1%, erythromycin 0.05%, or tetracycline 1% as a single treatment.
- Prophylaxis for infants born to infected mothers is recommended. A single dose of ceftriaxone 25 to 50 mg per kg IV or IM up to a maximum of 125 mg is used. Mother and infant should be evaluated for concurrent chlamydial infection.
- Children may be treated with ceftriaxone 125 mg IM as a single dose if weight is less than 45 kg. If the child weighs more than 45 kg, the adult dose of 250 mg ceftriaxone is used.

References

1. CDC fact sheet on antimicrobial resistance and *Neisseria gonorrhoeae*. Available online at www.cdc.gov/std/Gonorrhea.
2. U.S. Centers for Disease Control and Prevention. 2002 guidelines for treatment of sexually transmitted diseases. *MMWR* 2002;51(No. RR-6).

CHLAMYDIA INFECTION

Sally Weaver

19.7

GENERAL PRINCIPLES

Chlamydia species are obligate intracellular **bacteria** that cause several diseases. *Chlamydia trachomatis, Chlamydia pneumoniae,* and *Chlamydophila psittaci* (formerly known as *Chlamydia psittaci*) are species that cause infections in humans. **Many persons** with urogenital chlamydial infections are **asymptomatic** or experience mild symptoms but can still suffer significant sequelae. **Sequelae** include pelvic inflammatory disease (PID), chronic pelvic pain, infertility, or ectopic pregnancy **in women** and epididymitis or Reiter syndrome (reactive arthritis, conjunctivitis, and urethritis) **in men.**

Epidemiology

- **C. trachomatis** genital infection is the **most frequently reported infectious disease** in the United States. *It is a reportable disease in every state.*
  - Nearly **1 million cases** were reported in 2004. The actual annual prevalence is around 3 million due to underreporting and underdiagnosis. The **highest prevalence** is among 15- to 24-year-old women (approximately 6% infected). Approximately **70%** of genital *Chlamydia* infections are **asymptomatic.** *C. trachomatis* infections make an individual five times **more likely to contract HIV** if the individual is exposed. Up to 40% of untreated women will develop **PID.**
  - *Chlamydia* **screening and treatment may reduce PID** incidence by 50%. Posttreatment **repeat infections usually result from reinfection** and are associated with an elevated risk of PID and other complications. Men most commonly have urethral infections. **Nongonoccocal urethritis** (NGU) in men is often (15% to 55%) caused by *Chlamydia.* There is a decreasing prevalence with increasing age. Women and men can develop acute or chronic **conjunctivitis** when exposed to infectious genital secretions during oral–genital sexual contact or autoinoculation. Women and men who practice receptive **anal intercourse** can develop **proctitis** or proctocolitis. *Chlamydia* serovars L1, L2, and L3 cause **lymphogranuloma venereum** (LGV), which is rare in the United States. **Infected infants** develop **conjunctivitis** 5 to 12 days after exposure and chlamydial **pneumonia** presents as early as 2 weeks or as late as 4 months after delivery. Although perinatally transmitted *Chlamydia* infections may persist for >1 year, **sexual abuse** must also be **considered in preadolescent children** infected with *C. trachomatis.*

- **C. pneumoniae** causes **lower respiratory tract infection** most commonly in school-age children and adults.
- **Psittacosis** is caused by *Chlamydophila psittaci,* a **zoonotic infection** acquired from infected birds.

DIAGNOSIS

Clinical Presentation

- Exposure to *C. trachomatis* usually occurs through sexual intercourse. The cervix, urethra, and rectum are initial sites of infection in women.
  - **History: Women** are symptomatic or can have dysuria, vaginal discharge, abdominal pain, or vaginal bleeding after intercourse. **Men** are asymptomatic or can have mild to severe symptoms of **dysuria** and penile discharge. Symptoms of **proctitis** or proctocolitis include rectal pain, discharge, and tenesmus.
  - Physical examination in women is normal or can show cervical friability, green or yellow endocervical mucopus (from **mucopurulent cervicitis**), abdominal

tenderness, or cervical motion and adnexal tenderness consistent with PID. Testicular and/or epididymal pain, which is typically unilateral, is present with **epididymitis.** Physical examination may be normal or can show white, gray, or clear urethral discharge. Tenderness and swelling of the epididymis are present with epididymitis.

■ *Chlamydia* **conjunctivitis** shows unilateral or bilateral conjunctival erythema, mucopurulent discharge, and preauricular adenopathy on physical examination.

■ In proctitis, tenderness on rectal examination is often present.

■ **LGV** causes a self-limited **genital ulcer** followed by tender inguinal adenopathy located above and below the inguinal ligament. The adenopathy frequently becomes suppurative.

■ Infected **infants** who present with *Chlamydia* **conjunctivitis** may have tearing, erythematous conjunctiva, purulent discharge, and eyelid swelling. Infants with chlamydial **pneumonia** present with paroxysmal cough and tachypnea without fever. Physical findings include rales and sometimes wheezing. Approximately 50% of infants with chlamydial pneumonia also have conjunctivitis.

■ **C. pneumoniae** symptoms include pharyngitis, hoarseness, and headache. Cough is prominent and can persist for weeks to months if the infection is not managed effectively. Pneumonia and bronchitis can also be present.

■ **Psittacosis** symptoms include fever, chills, headache, nonproductive cough, malaise, and myalgias. complications include confusion, abdominal pain, hepatitis, endocarditis, and Stevens–Johnson syndrome.

Laboratory Studies

■ **All sexually active women under age 26,** and those older but with risk factors (new or multiple sex partners) should be **screened annually** for *Chlamydia* infection (and gonorrhea). Women who are **pregnant** should be tested at their first prenatal visit. The **endocervix** is the preferred site of specimen **collection in women,** and the **urethra** the preferred site **in men.**

■ Sexually active **adolescent boys** can be screened with the leukocyte esterase test on urine. A positive test result necessitates further testing for chlamydial and gonorrheal infection to determine the cause of the infection.[2]

■ **C. trachomatis is diagnosed by** enzyme immunoassay (EIA), direct fluorescent antibody (DFA) tests, nucleic acid hybridization tests (DNA probe), polymerase chain reaction (PCR), ligase chain reaction (LCR), transcription-mediated assay (TMA), and cell culture.

■ PCR and LCR tests detect *C. trachomatis* in first-catch urine (the first 10 to 30 mL of the urine stream) with a sensitivity comparable to that for a specimen obtained by urogenital swab.

■ Cell culture is recommended for diagnosis of infections of the rectum and in cases of sexual assault or abuse.

■ **Microimmunofluorescence IgM antibody serology** specific to *Chlamydia* is also available, with a titer of 1:32 or greater suggestive of infection. A fourfold rise of acute and convalescent antibody titer is diagnostic.

■ During the **female physical examination,** collect specimens for Pap smear, Gram stain, or *Neisseria gonorrhea* first.

■ Clean the cervix with a sponge or large swab. Insert the appropriate swab 1 to 2 cm into the endocervical canal and rotate against the canal wall for 10 to 30 seconds. Do not touch vaginal surfaces while withdrawing the swab.

■ Collect **specimens from the urethra** by gently inserting the appropriate swab 1 to 2 cm into the female urethra or 2 to 4 cm into the male urethra and rotate the swab in one direction for 5 seconds.

■ Collect **specimens for** the diagnosis of chlamydial **conjunctivitis** from the **everted eyelid.** Do not collect exudate alone.

■ Giemsa-stained scraping from the conjunctiva assists with the **diagnosis of chlamydial conjunctivitis** but is less sensitive than culture, DFA, or EIA.

■ **LGV** is diagnosed by isolating the LGV strain from the urethra, cervix, ulcer, or node and by serology.

- **C. pneumoniae** infection is **diagnosed by cell culture** preferably from the nasopharynx.
- **C. psittaci** infection is **diagnosed by serology or cell culture.**

TREATMENT

Behavioral—Prevention

- **Abstinence** from sexual intercourse (oral, vaginal, or anal sex) is the most reliable way to avoid transmission of sexually transmitted diseases such as *Chlamydia*. Other **behavioral changes to prevent STDs** include delaying the age of first intercourse, decreasing the number of sexual partners, selecting partners carefully, being knowledgeable about HIV infection and other sexually transmitted diseases, and using condoms.
- **Male condoms**, when used consistently and correctly, are effective for reducing the transmission of *Chlamydia*.
- **Vaginal contraceptive sponges** may help protect against cervical *Chlamydia*.
- Because chlamydial infections may be asymptomatic and sequelae significant, identification and treatment of infected individuals before they infect their sexual partners or before pregnant women infect their babies is important. Instruct **patients treated** for chlamydial infection to **abstain from intercourse for 7 days** after single-dose treatment or until completion of their treatment with other regimens and until all of their sex partners have been treated.
- **Treat all sexual partners of the previous 60 days** preceding onset of symptoms in the infected patient or treat the latest sexual partner even if last sexual contact occurred more than 60 days previously.

Medications

Table 19.7-1 presents medications.

TABLE 19.7-1	Medications	
Infection	**Primary antibiotic treatment**	**Alternative regimens**
C. trachomatis urethral, endocervical, rectal infections	Azithromycin (Zithromax), 1 g PO single dose, or doxycycline (Vibramycin), 100 mg PO bid for 7 days (These have equal efficacy, but azithromycin should always be available to give patients when there is a question of compliance.)	Erythromycin[a] base (E-Mycin, Eryc) 500 mg PO qid for 7 days, or erythromycin[a] ethylsuccinate (EES) 800 mg PO qid for 7 days, or ofloxacin[b] (Floxin) 300 mg PO bid for 7 days, or levofloxacin[b] (Levaquin) 500 mg a day for 7 days
C. trachomatis during pregnancy[c]	Erythromycin base 500 mg PO qid for 7 days or amoxicillin (Amoxil) 500 mg PO tid for 7 days	Erythromycin base 250 mg PO qid for 14 days, or erythromycin ethylsuccinate 800 mg PO qid for 7 days (or 400 mg qid for 14 days), or azithromycin, 1 g PO single dose
LGV	Doxycycline, 100 mg PO bid for 21 days	Erythromycin base 500 mg PO qid for 21 days
Chlamydia conjunctivitis[d] or pneumonia in infants/children	Erythromycin suspension (EES, EryPed) 50 mg/kg/day PO in 4 divided doses for 10–14 days[1]	

(continued)

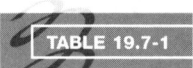

TABLE 19.7-1	Medications *(Continued)*	
Infection	**Primary antibiotic treatment**	**Alternative regimens**
C. pneumoniae	Doxycycline 100 mg PO bid for 7 days or erythromycin base 500 mg PO qid for 7 days, or erythromycin ethylsuccinate 800 mg PO qid for 7 days	Fluoroquinolones taken for 7–14 days have also been shown to be effective
C. psittaci[e]	Doxycycline 100 mg PO bid	Tetracycline 500 mg qid

[a]Consider retesting 3 weeks after completion of treatment with erythromycin because side effects can lead to decreased patient compliance. False positives on retesting can occur if tests are conducted <3 weeks after completion of therapy due to excretion of dead organisms.
[b]Ofloxacin and levofloxacin are not recommended for adolescents ≤18 years or in pregnant or lactating women.
[c]CDC recommends retesting 3 weeks after completion of treatment.
[d]Ocular prophylaxis does not prevent transmission of *Chlamydia* from and infected mother to her infant.
[e]Erythromycin is the best alternative for patients in whom tetracyclines are contraindicated, although its *in vivo* efficacy has not been determined. Continue treatment for 10–14 days after defervescence.

References

1. Centers for Disease Control and Prevention. Sexually transmitted diseases treatment guidelines—2002. *MMWR Recomm Rep* 200;51(RR-6):1–78.
2. Centers for Disease Control and Prevention. Sexually transmitted disease surveillance 2004 supplement, chlamydia prevalence monitoring project. Atlanta, GA: U.S. Department of Health and Human Services, Centers for Disease Control and Prevention; December 2005.
3. File TM Jr, Tan JS, Plouffe JF. The role of atypical pathogens: *Mycoplasma pneumoniae*, *Chlamydia pneumoniae*, and *Legionella pneumophila* in respiratory infection. *Infect Dis Clin North Am* 1998;12:569.
4. Latham-Sadler BA, Morell VW. Community-acquired respiratory infections in children. *Primary Care Clin Office Pract* 1996;23:837.
5. Smith KA, Bradley KK, Stobierski MG, et al. Compendium of measures to control Chlamydophila psittaci (formerly *Chlamydia psittaci*) infection among humans (psittacosis) and pet birds. *J Am Vet Med Assoc* 2005 Feb 15;226(4):532–539.

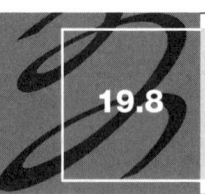

19.8 HERPESVIRUS INFECTIONS
Peggy R. Cyr, Ann K. Skelton

GENERAL PRINCIPLES

Definition

Herpes simplex virus (HSV) affects more than one third of the world population and is responsible for a wide array of disease, with effects ranging from discomfort to death. Primary infection causes local viral replication with painful itchy vesicles, seeding of regional neural ganglia, and possible viremia. A unique property of all HSV is the ability to establish lifelong latency in neural ganglia and periodically reactivate.

Classification

The three most common types are HSV-1 (affinity for oral sites), HSV-2 (affinity for genital sites), and varicella zoster virus (VZV). Several specific clinical syndromes associated with herpes viruses are listed below.

HERPES SIMPLEX

Epidemiology

HSV infects through direct contact of mucous membranes and secretions and has an incubation period of 2 to 14 days. It can be excreted asymptomatically at the time of primary or recurrent infection.

Diagnosis

Clinical Presentation

- **Gingivostomatitis** is usually caused by HSV-1. Primary infection is manifested by fever, cervical adenopathy, and oral, facial, labial, and buccal vesicular lesions, which heal by crusting in 1 to 2 weeks. Intraoral lesions are ulcerative. Most cases occur at age 1 to 5 years, but HSV-1 should be considered in a young adult with ulcerative pharyngitis.
- **Herpes labialis** (cold sores, fever blisters) is usually due to recurrent HSV-1. A prodrome of tingling and itching precedes the appearance of vesicles on the lip. Lesions may be brought on by stress, fever, ultraviolet light, trauma, and immunosuppression.
- **Genital infection** is typically caused by HSV-2 and is sexually transmitted. If seen in a preadolescent, one must think of possible sexual abuse. Primary infection causes systemic symptoms of fever, malaise, and lymphadenopathy. Lesions develop on male and female genitalia. Primary perianal HSV-2 infections and proctitis are more common in male homosexuals. Primary infection lasts 2 to 3 weeks. Recurrent infection is less intense, has rare systemic manifestations, and lasts 1 to 2 weeks.
- **Herpetic whitlow,** a viral paronychia characterized by vesicles, occurs by autoinoculation or by direct contact with infected persons.
- **Herpes gladiatorum** is transmitted by close physical contact in sports such as wrestling and may be seen in almost any skin site, but particularly head, neck, thorax, and upper extremities.
- **Ocular HSV** presents as a unilateral keratoconjunctivitis with pain, photophobia, chemosis, blurred vision, and tearing (see also Chapter 7.1). HSV is the most common cause of corneal blindness in the United States.
- **HSV encephalitis,** the most serious and feared type of HSV infection, starts with a nonspecific febrile illness and headache that progresses to seizures and focal neurologic signs.
- **Neonatal herpes infections** are the result of intrapartum contact with genital HSV or postpartum contact with hospital staff or others shedding HSV. With a primary genital infection, 30% to 60% of neonates are infected, compared with only 1% to 3% if the infection is recurrent. Consider HSV in an infant showing signs of sepsis; only one third of neonates with HSV have typical skin lesions.
- **In the immunocompromised host,** prolonged and destructive lesions are found in typical locations and contiguous structures (e.g., esophagus and lungs).

History

Check for history of close contact with an affected person. Also check for history of HSV in the past for recurrent lesions.

Physical Examination

The physical findings depend on the syndrome, but oral ulcers in stomatitis and gouped vesicles on an erythematous base in other presentations are common.

Laboratory Studies

Tzanck smear is obtained by scraping cells from the base of a vesicle. Look for viral inclusions or multinucleated giant cells. Results are rapid but the test is only 60% sensitive. **Viral culture** of lesions and other areas of the body, such as mouth, eyes, urine, cerebrospinal fluid (CSF), and cervix, is the gold standard for diagnosis, although sensitivity is only 70%

to 80%. Isolation of HSV in tissue culture is the gold standard. Results are available in 2 to 7 days. **The enzyme-linked immunosorbent assay (ELISA)** shows a rise from acute to convalescent titers. Limitations include inability to detect early infection and to distinguish HSV-1 from HSV-2. **Polymerase chain reaction of CSF** is the diagnostic method of choice for central nervous system (CNS) infections, with a specificity of 100% and a sensitivity greater than 95% at the time of clinical presentation.[1]

Differential Diagnosis
Contact dermatitis and cellulitis are two conditions to consider.

Treatment
Prevention
Infection control measures include careful hand washing to prevent transmission, contact isolation for neonates who have been exposed or who are infected, and use of condoms to prevent spread of HSV-2. **Caesarean section** prevents vertical transmission for women with an active herpetic lesion during labor. The use of **continuous acyclovir** during the last month of pregnancy in women with recurrent HSV decreases the risk of outbreaks and decreases the need for Caesarean section delivery.[2] **Excluding athletes** from play with active herpes outbreaks decreases transmission. **Vaccine** development is under way.

Medications
Table 19.8-1 presents medications for treatment.

Special Therapy
Oral suppressive antiviral therapy controls symptomatic disease in the source partner and reduces the likelihood of disease in the susceptible partner by between 48% and 75%.[4]

Referrals
An ophthalmologist referral should be done for eye involvement.

Counseling
Discuss the possibility of recurrences and potential triggers. Provide information on sexual transmission and on congenital transmission risks.

VARICELLA (CHICKENPOX)

Epidemiology
Transmission occurs by inhalation of infected respiratory secretions or direct contact with lesions of varicella or zoster. Incubation occurs over an average of 14 to 16 days, ending with development of rash. Patients are infectious from 5 days before onset of rash until lesions have crusted. Varicella affects 90% of household contacts. Generally, immunity is lifelong after infection.

Diagnosis
Clinical Presentation
Chickenpox presents with a prodrome of low-grade fever, malaise, and headache that may precede rash by a few days. Skin lesions develop first on the face and trunk. Skin complications include scarring and bacterial superinfection. CNS complications, including Reye syndrome, occur in 1 in 1,000 cases. Pneumonia occurs in 1 in 400 adults. The mortality rate is 10% and in immunocompromised patients 30%. **Congenital varicella syndrome** occurs in 2% of affected pregnancies, with limb hypoplasia, ocular atrophy, and psychomotor retardation. **Neonatal varicella** occurs when the mother develops varicella around the time of delivery; it has a mortality up to 30%.

History
Recent exposure to others with history of the disease, presence of fever and rash, and absence of vaccination against varicella support the diagnosis.

Physical Examination
Lesions in all stages, from vesicles to crusting lesions are found on the face, trunk, and extremities. The vesicles are on an erythematous base.

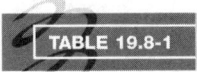

TABLE 19.8-1	Treatment for Herpesvirus Infections[3]		

Viral infection	Drug of choice	Dosage	Duration (d)
Herpes simplex virus (HSV)			
Orolabial herpes in immunocompetent recurrence	Penciclovir (Denavir) Docosanol (Abreva)	1% cream applied q2h w/a apply 5 times a day until healed	4
Genital			
First episode	Acyclovir (Zovirax)	400 mg PO tid or 200 mg PO 5×/d[a]	7–10
	or Famciclovir[b] (Famvir)	250 mg PO tid	7–10
	or Valacyclovir (Valtrex)	1 g PO bid	7–10
Recurrence	Acyclovir	400 mg PO tid or 200 mg 5 times per day or 800 mg bid	5
	or Famciclovir	125 mg PO bid	5
	or Valacyclovir	500 mg PO bid or 1 gm per day	5
Chronic suppression	Acyclovir	400 mg PO bid	—
	or Famciclovir	250 mg PO bid	—
	or Valacyclovir	500 mg–1 g PO daily	—
Mucocutaneous disease in immuno-compromised	Acyclovir	5 mg/kg IV q8hb	7–14
		or 400 mg PO 5×/d	7–14
Encephalitis	Acyclovir	20 mg/kg IV q8h	14–21
Neonatal	Acyclovir[b]	20 mg/kg IV q8h	10–21
Acyclovir resistant	Foscarnet (Foscavir)	40 mg/kg IV q8h	14–21
		5 mg/kg IV once weekly	14
Acyclovir and foscar-net-resistant HSV	Cidofovir (Vistide)		
Keratoconjunctivitis	Trifluridine (Viroptic)	1 drop of 1% solution topically q2h, up to 9 drops/d	10
	Vidarabine	1/2 in. q3h with a maximum of 5 times per day until healed	
Varicella-zoster virus (VSV)			
Varicella	Acyclovir	20 mg/kg (800 mg max. qid)	5
Herpes zoster	Valacyclovir	1 g PO tid	7
	or Famciclovir	750 mg once daily or 500 mg PO bid, or 250 mg TID	7
	or Acyclovir	800 mg PO 5×/d	7–10
Varicella or zoster in immunocompromised	Acyclovir	10 g/kg IV q8h[c]	7
Acyclovir resistant	Foscarnet	40 mg/kg IV q8h	10

[a]For severe initial genital herpes, intravenous acyclovir (5 mg/kg q8h for 5–7 d) can be used. Dosage reduction is recommended for creatinine clearance less than 50 mL/min.
[b]For children <12. 10mg/kg IV every 8 hours × 7 days.
[c]Pediatric dosage is 500 mg/m^2 q8h for 7–10 days.

Laboratory Studies
See above.

Differential Diagnosis
The differential diagnosis includes contact dermatitis, cellulites, and other viral exanthems.

Treatment
Prevention
- Avoidance of VZV during the host's contagious period and vaccinating within 72 to 120 hours of exposure reduce infection.
- Active immunization with a live virus vaccine (Varivax 0.5 mL SC for children 12 months to 12 years of age; 0.5 mL, twice, 4 to 8 weeks apart for those older) results in 94% immunity; duration of immunity is not known.
- Passive immunization with varicella-zoster immune globulin (VZIG, 1 vial = 125 units = 1.25 mL, 125 units/10 kg up to 625 units, with minimum of 1 vial, IM), administered within 96 hours of a significant exposure, is indicated for neonates, pregnant women, and immunocompromised patients.

Medications
See Table 19.8-1.

Counseling
Patients should be counseled about avoiding transmission to others, and about prevention of superinfection. Aspirin should be avoided because of risk of Reye syndrome.

HERPES ZOSTER (SHINGLES)
Epidemiology
Reactivation of VZV resulting in zoster is associated inversely with immunocompetence and proportionately with age. Factors that decrease immune function are chemotherapy, chronic steroid use, HIV infection, and malignancies. Recurrent shingles occurs in 5% of immunocompetent patients.

Diagnosis
Clinical Presentation
- Severe pain, tingling, or itching precedes the development of clustered vesicles on an erythematous base in one to three adjacent dermatomes. Lesions evolve and crust over 10 to 14 days.
- Zoster *sine herpete,* or characteristic pain without rash, occurs infrequently. Infection can be confirmed by serologic testing. Disseminated zoster, with more than 20 lesions in dermatomes removed from the primary dermatome, occurs in up to 40% of immunocompromised hosts.
- Cranial nerve involvement produces symptoms referable to the nerve involved.
- Involvement of the ophthalmic branch of cranial nerve V may cause visual impairment or blindness.
- The presence of the Hutchinson sign (vesicles on the side and tip of the nose) is an indication that ocular involvement is likely, and slit-lamp examination is mandatory.
- Ramsay Hunt syndrome, involvement of cranial nerves VII and VIII, produces vesicles on the pinna, ear canal, and tongue. This can result in facial palsy, tinnitus, vertigo, and impairment of taste and hearing.
- Postherpetic neuralgia (PHN) is characterized by pain persisting 4 to 6 weeks beyond crusting of lesions. It is more common in older patients, occurring in more than 50% of persons older than 60 years.
- Unusual complications include CNS and visceral involvement. Pregnancy-related shingles usually has a benign course, with low risk of VZV infection in the fetus.

History
Prior history of chickenpox and absence of varicella immunization support the diagnosis.

Physical Examination

Grouped vesicles on an erythematous base are found in a dermatomal distribution in various stages.

Laboratory Studies

See above.

Treatment

- **Prevention** is achieved by primary prevention of varicella infections. In elderly individuals with a history of varicella, reactivation as zoster may be reduced by boosting immunity with varicella vaccine. A vaccine has now been approved to reduce the risk of zoster in patients over 60.
- **Medications.** Table 19.8-1 lists medications for treatment of zoster. Analgesics help reduce acute pain. Systemic steroids have demonstrated no additional benefit in reduction of PHN. Studies examining amitriptyline, narcotics, capsaicin, anticonvulsants, and percutaneous nerve stimulation for PHN were of fair to poor quality and no conclusions could be drawn from these studies.[5]
- **Special therapies.** Local treatment with wet compresses of water or 5% Burlow solution is helpful.
- **Referral.** Patients with eye involvement should be referred to an ophthalmologist.
- **Counseling** should include a description of postherpetic neuralgia.

References

1. Whitley RJ, Kimberlin DW, Ruizman B. Herpes simplex viruses. *Clin Infect Dis* 1998;26: 541–555.
2. Wenner C, Nashelsky J. FPIN's clinical inquiries: antiviral agents for pregnant women with genital herpes. *Am Fam Physician* 2005;72:1807.
3. Brady RC, Bernstein DI. Treatment of herpes simplex virus infections. *Antiviral Res* 61:73–81.
4. Patel R. Antiviral agents for the prevention of the sexual transmission of herpes simplex in discordant couples. *Curr Opin Infect Dis* 2004;17:45–48.
5. Holten KB, Britigan DH. FPIN's clinical inquiries: treatment of herpes zoster. *Am Fam Physician* 2006;73:882.

LYME DISEASE

Robert Sheeler

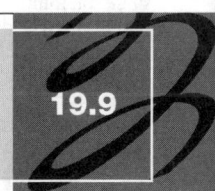

19.9

GENERAL PRINCIPLES

Lyme disease is a multisystem spirochetal illness caused by the organism *Borrelia burgdorferi*. Primary manifestations are systemic and cutaneous. Delayed rheumatologic, neurologic, cardiac, and other complications may follow, especially if the primary illness is unrecognized or untreated. Lyme disease is a tick-borne illness with *Ixodes* genus ticks believed to be the primary or sole agent of transmission.

Definition

The spectrum of Lyme disease can range from asymptomatic seroconversion to chronic central nervous system disease with dementia. Any infection with *B. burgdorferi* can be considered to be Lyme disease. Rash occurring less than 3 days from the initial tick bite is usually reaction to tick salivary proteins not Lyme disease.

Pathophysiology (Epidemiology)

Lyme disease in North America is believed to be caused by *B. burgdorferi*. Different *Borrelia* subspecies may play a role in Lyme disease in Europe. In the United States Lyme disease is most likely to occur in endemic areas in New England, the upper Midwest, and the Northern California/Pacific Northwest regions. Coinfection with other organisms such as *Babesia, Anaplasma, Ehrlichia,* and *Bartonella* may complicate the treatment and response to therapy for Lyme disease. Chronic disease may occur either from untreated or incompletely treated sequestered infection or possibly from triggering destructive autoimmune processes.

DIAGNOSIS

Clinical manifestations. Joint involvement occurs in up to 70% of untreated patients, usually 2 to 24 months from exposure. The arthritis is oligoarticular and migratory, with symptoms in the involved joints lasting days to months. Large joints, especially the knees, are most frequently involved. About 10% of patients with Lyme arthritis progress to a more chronic erosive rheumatoid picture. Acute and chronic neurologic involvement may occur, usually 4 weeks or more after exposure. Lyme neuroborreliosis most commonly manifests as cranial or peripheral neuropathy. Bell palsy is the most frequently observed sequelae and may be bilateral. Lyme meningitis, encephalitis, vasculitis, chronic encephalopathy, and other sequelae have been reported as have acute psychosis and chronic neuropsychiatric manifestations. Cardiac involvement generally presents with various degrees of heart block from first to third degree. Typical onset is 4 weeks after exposure. The heart block is usually self-limited. Some patients may require temporary pacemaker support. Myocarditis develops in a minority of patients. Various ophthalmologic syndromes are also possible.

History

The diagnosis of Lyme disease remains contingent on potential exposure to an endemic area and appropriately timed clinical manifestations. History should include the presence or absence of an early systemic illness, cutaneous, cardiac, neurologic, psychiatric, and joint complaints.

Physical Examination

The skin should be examined for erythema multiforme (EM) lesions, which can be either single or multiple, 3 to 70 cm in diameter, often originating at the site of the initial bite within 3 to 30 days. EM lesions are pathognomonic and usually precede seroconversion. Unfortunately, EM lesions are likely present in 50% or less of cases. Various atypical rashes and late stage rashes such as acrodermatitis chornicum atrophicum are also known to occur. Cardiac exam can show bradycardia in cases of heart block. Neurologic exam should include cranial and peripheral nerves as well as assessment of neuropsychiatric status in chronic cases. Joints may be painful but normal to exam early in the illness or hot, red, and swollen later on.

Laboratory Studies

Currently available testing for Lyme disease is less than ideal. Two-stage testing involving screening with enzyme-linked immunosorbent assay (ELISA) followed by confirmation with Western blot testing may increase specificity, but has sensitivity as low as 50%, especially early in the disease. Serial testing using Western blot with the demonstration of the presence of increasing bands is suggestive of ongoing exposure to *Borrelia* antigens and chronic infection, but antibiotic treatment can blunt serologic response and sequestered infections such as those in the central nervous system may have negative peripheral serology despite ongoing active infection. Polymerase chain reaction (PCR) testing of cerebrospinal fluid (CSF) and joint fluid can be useful if positive but also has relatively low sensitivity.

Genetics

There is literature that argues both for and against the role of certain HLA types being predisposed to increased long-term sequelae, especially chronic joint problems.

Differential Diagnosis

In systemically ill patients, the differential diagnosis includes Rocky Mountain spotted fever, syphilis, babesiosis, tularemia, relapsing fever, Colorado tick fever, and ehrlichiosis. Concomitant infections with *Borellia* and *Babesia, Anaplasma, Ehrlichia,* and *Bartonella* have been reported and can complicate both diagnosis and treatment outcomes. Southern tick-associated rash illness (STARI) is similar to Lyme disease in apparently being tick transmitted and having a similar EM type rash. But longer-term sequelae of the type reported in Lyme disease do not seem to be present. It is thought to represent infection with a different *Borrelia* species—*B. lonestari*—and to be transmitted by the Lone Star tick (*Amblyomma americanum*) although this has yet to be fully proven.

More chronic presentations of Lyme disease when joint involvement is predominant should raise the possibility of rheumatologic diseases, especially rheumatoid arthritis and systemic lupus erythematosus.

TREATMENT

Medication

Prophylactic treatment of tick bites is controversial, one study recommended a single dose of doxycycline. For practitioners who choose to treat preventively 10 to 14 days of doxycycline or amoxicillin are likely to be more effective in avoiding late sequelae. For early Lyme disease (adults and children of adult weight over 9 years): Give doxycycline 100 mg bid, amoxicillin 500 mg tid, or cefuoxime axetil 500 mg bid for 21 to 30 days. (Avoid doxycycline in pregnant and lactating women and children under 9 years of age.) For more serious, advanced, or persistent disease give ceftriaxone 2 g per day for 14 to 28 days. Response to treatment of more complex disease may not occur for several weeks after treatment. Treatment of persistent disease with longer courses of oral and parenteral antibiotics and with combinations of antibiotics has been tried. The advisability of this is highly controversial with strong advocates both for and against such practices. Treatment in children 8 years or younger: early or mild disease can be treated with amoxicillin 50 mg/kg/day divided tid for 21 to 30 days or cefuoxime axetil 30 mg/kg/day divided bid for 21 to 30 days (not to exceed 1 g/day). For advanced and persistent disease give ceftriaxone 75 to 100 mg/kg/day for 14 to 28 days (max 2 g/day).

Complications

Long-lasting rheumatologic syndromes resembling rheumatoid arthritis and chronic neuropsychiatric syndromes are the most feared complications. Substantial persisting fatigue is also seen in a certain percentage of patients.

Patient Education

Patients should be educated to recognize the early and late onset symptoms of Lyme disease and to seek treatment for them promptly. Protective clothing, various repellents, and frequent tick checks can all decrease the likelihood of acquiring Lyme disease. The sole marketed vaccine for Lyme disease, LYMErix, has been removed from the market. Second-generation vaccines are under development.

References

1. DePietropaolo D, Powers J, Gill J, et al. Diagnosis of Lyme disease. *Del Med J* 2006;78: 11–18.
2. Halperin J. Central nervous system Lyme disease. *Curr Neurol Neurosci Rep* 2005;5: 446–452.
3. Hu L. Lyme arthritis. *Infect Dis Clin North Am* 2005;19:947–961.
4. Stricker RB Lautin A, Burrascano J. Lyme disease: point/counterpoint. *Expert Rev Anti-infect Ther* 2005;3:155–165.

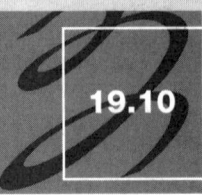

ROCKY MOUNTAIN SPOTTED FEVER
Ashley J. Falk, Nathan P. Falk

GENERAL PRINCIPLES

Definition
Rocky Mountain spotted fever (RMSF) is a potentially fatal, tick-borne illness caused by *Rickettsia rickettsii*.

Epidemiology
- Most prevalent in the southeastern and south central states
- 1454 cases of RMSF reported to the Centers for Disease Control and Prevention in 2004[1]
- Incidence is highest in children ages 5 to 9 years[2]
- Most common between the months of April and September
- Two principal vectors for bacterial transmission within the United States
  - The wood tick (*Dermacentor andersoni*) in the western United States
  - The dog tick (*Dermacentor variabilis*) in the eastern and southern United States

Etiology
- Caused by the Gram-negative obligate intracellular bacterium *R. rickettsii*

DIAGNOSIS

Clinical Presentation
- Based on clinical signs and symptoms after an incubation period of 4 to 12 days (mean 7 days).
- Classic presentation is rapid onset of headache and fever followed in 2 to 3 days by rash.
- Other symptoms are nonspecific and may include myalgias, nausea, vomiting, malaise, sore throat, nonproductive cough, and pleuritic chest pain.
- Classic triad of fever, headache, and rash present in less than 50% of cases at initial presentation.[3]

History
- A tick bite is recalled by 50% to 70% of patients.[2]

Physical Examination
- Rash initially appears on the distal extremities (palms, soles, wrists, ankles, and forearms) and consists of small, pink, blanchable macules.
- Rash later spreads centripetally to the trunk, neck, and face.
- Lesions become maculopapular and petechial and may then coalesce and form large ecchymotic areas and ulcerations.
- From 5% to 15% of patients may never develop a rash.[4]

Laboratory Studies
- Primarily a clinical diagnosis as there are no completely reliable tests in the early phase of illness when therapy should be initiated.
- Skin biopsy
  - May be used if rash is present, however, very few laboratories have the ability to perform, so often of little or no use in initial patient management
  - 100% specific, 60% sensitive (very low sensitivity once treatment has been initiated)[5]
- Serologic testing
  - Confirmation may be done using indirect fluorescent antibody testing.[6]
  - Overall sensitivity is 95% and is available through most state health departments.

- False negatives may occur during the first 5 days of symptoms as antibody response not yet detectable or if treatment is initiated within 48 hours of symptom onset as these patients may never develop an antibody response.

- General laboratory testing is nonspecific but may reveal thrombocytopenia, hyponatremia, elevated liver transaminases, azotemia, and an increased, decreased, or normal white blood cell count.

Differential Diagnosis

Measles, meningococcemia, streptococcal infection, parvovirus infection (Fifth disease), roseola, enteroviral infection, viral meningitis, ehrlichiosis, drug reaction, infectious mononucleosis, leptospirosis, immune thrombocytopenic purpura, immune complex vasculitis, or bacterial sepsis

TREATMENT

Medications

- Antibiotics should be initiated immediately when there is suspicion of RMSF rather than waiting for confirmatory testing, especially in patients from endemic areas with fever and rash during the summer months.[4]
- Delay in initiating therapy may increase mortality, especially in children.[7]
- **Adults** (and children weighing >45 kg): Doxycycline 100 mg bid or tetracycline 500 mg qid or chloramphenicol 500 mg qid for at least 7 days or 2 days after fever is gone.[8]
  - Fluoroquinolones may be effective, but should not be used first line because of a lack of evidence.[4]
- **Children.** Doxycycline 2.2 mg per kg IV/PO bid or tetracycline 10 mg per kg qid

Complications

Multisystem illness may occur including renal failure, pneumonitis, adult respiratory distress syndrome, myocarditis, hepatitis, gastrointestinal bleeding, diarrhea, skin necrosis, coagulopathy, hemolysis, encephaliltis, and seizure.

SPECIAL CONSIDERATIONS

- **Prevention.** No vaccine exists and routine prophylaxis following tick exposure is not recommended as less than 1% of ticks in endemic areas are infected with *Rickettsia*.
- Patients reporting tick bites should inform their physician if they develop fever, headache, or rash within 14 days of exposure.

References

1. CDC. Summary of provisional cases of selected notifiable disease, cumulative, week ending December 18, 2004. *MMWR Morb Wkly Rep* 2004;53:1185.
2. Walker DH. Tick-transmitted infectious diseases in the United States. *Annu Rev Public Health* 1998;19:237.
3. Abramson JS, Givner LB. Rocky Mountain spotted fever. *Pediatr Infect Dis J* 1999; 18:539.
4. Thorner AR, Walker DH, Petri WA. Rocky Mountain spotted fever: state of the art clinical review. *Clin Infect Dis* 1998;27:1353.
5. Bratton RL, Corey GR. Tick-borne disease. *Am Fam Physician* 2005;71:2323.
6. Kirkland KB, Wilkinson WE, Sexton DJ. Therapeutic delay and mortality in cases of Rocky Mountain spotted fever. *Clin Infect Dis* 1995;20:1118.
7. Consequences of delayed diagnosis of Rocky Mountain spotted fever in children—West Virginia, Michigan, Tennessee, and Oklahoma, May–June 2000. *MMWR Morb Wkly Rep* 2000;49:885.
8. Gilbert DN, Moellering RC, Eliopoulos GM, et al. *The Sanford guide to antimicrobial therapy.* Sperryville, MD: Antimicrobial Therapy Inc.; 2006.

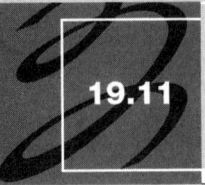

19.11

PARASITIC DISEASES
Matthew R. Anderson, Manel Silva

GENERAL PRINCIPLES

Definition
A parasite is an organism that lives on or in another living organism (the host) while doing that host some harm. Medically important parasites include the single-celled protozoans, arthropods, and helminths (roundworms or flatworms). Although commonly thought of as intestinal pathogens, parasites produce clinical syndromes as diverse as seizures and heart failure.

Anatomy
Parasitic infections can involve multiple organs depending on the life cycle of the organism. Parasitic infection and symptomatology by organ system:

- **Skin.** Dermatitis *(Ascaris, Capillaria hepatica,* hookworms, *Strongyloides,* chigoe flea, cutaneous and visceral larva migrans, *Dracunculus,* lice, *Mansonella,* scabies, mites), migratory pruritic swellings *(Loa loa),* subcutaneous nodules, skin ulcers and scars (cutaneous leishmaniasis, *Dracunculus, Dirofilaria, Onchocerca,* sparganum, *Taenia, Trypanosoma brucei gambiense),* swimmer's itch (schistosomiasis), pruritus and skin depigmentation (onchoceriasis), temporal and periorbital swelling with conjunctivitis (acute *Trypanosoma cruzi* infection), facial and periorbital edema during acute infection *(Trichinella),* and ulcers (cutaneous and mucocutaneous leishmaniasis, *T. gambiense, Dracunculus, Tungiasis)*
- **Central nervous system.** Meningoencephalitis (African trypanosomiasis, *Acanthamoeba, Angiostrongylus, Naegleria,* cerebral malaria, schistosomiasis), new-onset seizures or focal neurologic signs consistent with a space-occupying lesion (cysticercosis, malaria, toxoplasmosis, trichinosis, hydatid and coenurus cysts, *Sparganosis)*
- **Eyes.** Vitreous infestation (onchocercosis, ascariasis, ocular toxocariasis), conjunctivitis *(Loa loa),* keratoconjunctivitis and corneal ulcers (caused by free-living amebas), uveitis, choroiditis and choroidoretinitis (toxoplasmosis), anterior uveitis *(Wuchereria bancrofti)* periorbital swelling, and conjunctivitis *(Trypanosoma cruzi)*
- **Hematologic.** Microcytic anemia (malaria, babesia, hookworm, *Trichuris,* trypanosomes), macrocytic anemia (fish tapeworms), leukopenia (malaria, visceral leishmaniasis), eosinophilia (invasive helminths especially schistosomasis and *Trichinella, Dientamoeba fragilis,* and *Isospora belli)*
- **Lymphatic.** Elephantiasis (lymphatic filariasis), lymphadenopathy (African trypanosomiasis, *Mansonella ozzardi,* toxoplasmosis, visceral leshmaniasis)
- **Respiratory.** Loeffler syndrome *(Ascaris lumbricoides, Strongyloides),* pneumonitis (hookworms, *Pneumocystis, Strongyloides),* chest pain and hemoptysis (paragonimiasis), pulmonary mass lesion *(Dirofilaria,* echinococcosis, paragonimiasis), tropical pulmonary eosinophilia (filariasis)
- **Cardiovascular.** Heart block, congestive heart failure *(Trypanosoma cruzi)*
- **Intestinal.** Appendicitis *(Ascaris, Trichuris,* pinworms); colic, diarrhea, and vomiting *(Capillaria philippinensis, Cryptosporidium,* intestinal flukes, *Isospora belli, Strongyloides, Cyclospora, Giardia);* mucoid and bloody diarrhea (amebiasis), bloody stool (schistosomiasis), obstruction *(Ascaris, Hymenolepis nana, Taenia saginata);* colitis *(Trichuris);* pruritus ani *(Enterobius)*
- **Hepatobiliary.** Liver abscess or cyst (Entamoeba *histolytica,* cysticercosis, hydatid disease), biliary obstruction *(Ascaris lumbricoides),* portal hypertension (schistosomes), hepatosplenomegaly (malaria, babesiosis, *Capillaria hepatica,* visceral leishmania, visceral larva migrans, Katayama fever in acute schistosomiasis)

- **Genitourinary.** *Chyluria* (lymphatic filariasis), hematuria (schistosomes), prostatitis, urethritis, and vaginitis (trichomonads)
- **Musculoskeletal.** Myositis (trichinosis, toxoplasmosis, Chagas disease), cysts (*Echinococcus, cysticercosis*)

Transmission

Transmission of parasites may occur via the fecal–oral route, through the skin, by blood transfusions or organ transplants, or by a suitable local vector such as a mosquito.

Epidemiology

- **Populations at risk.** International travelers (especially those traveling outside of industrialized countries and major cities), missionaries, and immigrants are at particular risk. Backpackers who drink untreated groundwater are at risk for acquiring *Giardia,* amebiasis, guinea worm, and *Cryptosporidium* as well as bacterial pathogens.
- Residents of institutions, including daycare centers, group homes, and nursing homes, are at risk for acquiring *Giardia,* amebiasis as well as bacterial pathogens spread by fecal contamination. People who engage in oral–anal sex are at risk for acquiring *Entamoeba. histolytica* and *Giardia lamblia* as well as viral pathogens such as hepatitis A, and bacteria such as *Shigella.*
- **Risk by geographic area.** For information about specific risks in various geographic regions, consult the U.S. Centers for Disease Control and Prevention (CDC) web page (http://www.cdc.gov/travel/) or the World Health Organization (WHO) web page (http://www.who.int/ith/en/).
- **Immunosuppressed patients** show increased susceptibility to some parasites. This group includes malnourished individuals, patients with cancer, patients on steroids, and patients with AIDS (discussed later in the chapter).

Screening and Prevention

- Routine testing for asymptomatic parasite carriage in travelers or food handlers is not recommended because of the low yield.
- Individuals with a high likelihood of exposure to parasites (missionaries, refugees, and immigrants arriving from endemic regions) can be treated empirically for intestinal helminths. Although not Food and Drug Administration (FDA)-approved for this indication, a single dose of albendazole (400 mg taken orally) may be superior to treating only those with positive ova and parasite examinations; testing is more expensive and results in fewer carriers receiving treatment.[1]
- Individuals with suspected exposure to *Giardia,* amebiasis, or platyhelminths may need repeated stool exam for ova and parasites or testing for *Giardia* antigen.

Prevention Advice

- Travelers should avoid inhaling water while swimming, or swimming with open cuts or abrasions. They should not to swim in freshwater areas where schistosomiasis is endemic.
- In areas where chlorinated or filtered tap water is not available, and hygiene and sanitation are poor, people should drink canned or bottled beverages, or beverages made with boiled water such as tea or coffee. Decontamination options include processing water with a micropore filter, boiling, or treating water with chorine or iodine.
- To prevent fecal–oral transmission of diseases, strict hand washing should be practiced.
- For mosquito-borne diseases, the best strategy is to avoid getting bitten. Travelers should use clothing that covers extremities and sleep under bed nets; ideally these items should be pretreated with Permethrin. DEET-containing repellants are probably the best agents for use on the skin. Mosquito activity is highest at dawn and dusk.
- Travelers should avoid foods that may harbor parasites, especially raw or undercooked foods. Salads and cut fruits are potentially a source of infections. Travelers should avoid consuming foods from street vendors, as well as unconventional foods or animal products.
- Infants under 6 months benefit from exclusive breastfeeding to prevent parasitic infections.
- Travelers should obtain prophylactic vaccines and medicines if traveling to endemic areas and consult with a travel clinic if they have any predisposing illnesses that increases their risks.

DIAGNOSIS

History

The most important step in assessing risk is to obtain a careful history about the patient's social and physical environment (including exposure to immigrants from endemic areas), travel history including duration of potential exposure, and personal habits. It is unnecessary to rule out parasitic infection for asymptomatic individuals who were never in environments where they might have been infected. Personal medical history and potential increased risks are also important in risk assessment. Because parasitic infections can affect diverse systems, a thorough review of systems may be necessary to obtain the appropriate differential (see Clinical Presentations below). If this history suggests a risk for parasitic disease, the clinician must then determine which parasites are potential pathogens.

- **Parasites seen in stool.** Roundworms or flatworm segments can be passed in stool. Specimens brought in by patients should be preserved in 70% alcohol and sent to a diagno-stic laboratory. Objects such as earthworms or mucus plugs can be mistaken for parasites.
- **HIV infection.** HIV infection with certain parasites has been associated either with increased susceptibility or more severe disease. The major parasitic infections include *Toxoplasma gondii, Cryptosporidium* spp., *Cyclospora* spp., *Isospora belli,* visceral leishamaniasis, *Trypanosoma cruzi, Microsporum* spp., *Strongyloides stercoralis, Plasmodium* species.

Laboratory Studies

Diagnosis of Symptomatic Infection

- The CDC Division of Parasitic Diseases maintains an excellent web site on the diagnostic evaluation of parasites (http://www.dpd.cdc.gov/dpdx/).
- Appropriate lab work should be obtained for symptomatic patients with risk factors for parasitic disease. In U.S. laboratories, only about 1% of ova and parasite tests indicate the presence of some form of parasite; most of these are nonpathogenic protozoans.
- Clinically useful diagnoses come almost exclusively from outpatients or hospitalized patients within 3 days of their admission. Testing asymptomatic patients is not recommended.

Office Examination

- **Stool examination (ova and parasites).** Three separate stool samples taken every other day increase the likelihood of finding pathogens. Examination of a fresh stool specimen permits visualization of short-lived motile forms that cannot be found in preserved or refrigerated specimens. Purged stools that are examined immediately are superior to preserved specimens, especially when one is looking for ameba; magnesium citrate can be used as a purgative. Ideally a thin, fresh slide of feces should be examined within an hour of collection looking for trophozoites and amebas. Then a drop of Gram iodine or Lugol solution is added to provide better visualization of cysts. Part of the sample should be placed in separate preservative containing vials according to supplied directions and sent to a reference laboratory. Care should be taken to avoid contamination with urine or water. Testing for *Cryptosporidium* and *Cyclospora* cysts requires special staining.
- **The cellophane tape test** is used to detect *Enterobius* (pinworm) and *Taenia saginata* eggs. Clear cellophane (Scotch) tape is placed with the sticky side down on the unwashed perianal area, preferably in the early morning before bathing or after defecation. The tape is placed (again sticky side down) on a microscope slide, which is examined for eggs. Adult pinworms can be seen with this technique. Sensitivity is improved by repeating the examination on subsequent days.

Clinical Laboratory Examination

- **Stool examination (ova and parasites).** Various techniques exist for concentrating and staining stool specimens. When looking for helminth eggs, one or two concentrated preserved specimens is usually sufficient. Table 19.11-1 provides a guide to the interpretation of findings in the ova and parasite examination.
- **Antigen tests** for amebiasis, cryptosporidiosis, giardiasis, and trichomoniasis are now available in many clinical laboratories. Antigen tests often have better sensitivity than microscopy and are considered the test of choice for giardiasis.
- **Blood smear.** Blood smear is indicated for malaria (thick and thin film done at time of fever), filariasis (blood drawn during hours of periodic release, usually midnight),

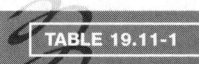

| **TABLE 19.11-1** | Interpreting Stool Ova and Parasite Results |

Definite pathogens	Pathogens primarily in immunosuppressed hosts	Pathogenicity disputed	Nonpathogens
Cryptosporidium parvum	*Balantidium coli*	*Blastocystis hominis*	*Chilomastix mesnili*
Cyclospora spp.	*Microsporidia* spp.		*Endolimax nana*[a]
Dientamoeba fragilis			*Entamoeba coli*
Entamoeba histolytica			*Entamoeba dispar*
Enterobius vermicularis			*Entamoeba hartmanni*
Giardia lamblia			*Iodamoeba buetschlii*
Isospora belli			

Note: The presence of a "nonpathogenic" organism implies fecal contamination of the food or water supply and therefore may be clinically significant.
[a]Morphologically similar to *Entamoeba histolytica* by light microscopy.

trypanomiasis and babesiosis. For periodic fevers, blood drawing must be timed appropriately for the clinical syndrome.

- **Directed biopsy** is often necessary for diagnosis of parasites that do not colonize the intestinal tract. Leishmaniasis can be diagnosed by microscopic evaluation of sections from lesions (spleen or bone marrow or skin biopsy) stained with Giemsa and methanol, or by culture of biopsied lesions. *Trypanosoma brucei* (sleeping sickness) can be diagnosed from biopsies of lymph nodes, bone marrow, or spleen. *Entamoeba histolytica* can be diagnosed by biopsy of the liver, lung, or colon. When examination of stools is negative, an endoscopic aspirate may demonstrate *Giardia* or *Strongyloides*.
- **Skin test.** Cutaneous infection with leishmaniasis can be detected by the Montenegro skin test (similar to the PPD). It stays positive for lifetime and is negative in visceral leishmaniasis.
- **Sputum samples** can be useful in identifying PCP, *Paragonimus westermani* eggs, *Stronglyoides* larvae, hookworm larvae, and rarely Entamoeba histolytica. Bronchoscopic samples obtained early in the morning have a higher yield.
- **Urine specimens** can be examined to look for *Schistosoma haematobium* eggs (collected near noontime) or *Trichomonas vaginalis*.
- **Vaginal swab** is indicated in female patients to assess for *Trichomonas vaginalis* infections; antigen tests are also available.
- **Endoscopy** may reveal *Giardia* and *Strongyloides* in patients where the ova and parasite exam is negative.
- **Other testing modalities.** Antibody, antigen, as well as molecular diagnostic techniques are available for a variety of parasitic infections. For details consult the CDC Division of Parasitic Diseases (http://www.dpd.cdc.gov/dpdx/HTML/DiagnosticProcedures.htm).
- **Eosinophilia.** Helminths that invade tissue can produce eosinophilia. Among these are *Dientamoeba fragilis, Isospora, Trichinella, Schistosomisis,* and *Filariasis.*

Imaging

Imaging can be useful for diagnosis and for localization for biopsies. A chest radiograph or computed tomography (CT) scan of the chest may suggest parasites that cause respiratory and cardiovascular findings. Abdominal ultrasound or CT of abdomen may be useful for those parasites causing hepatobiliary and spleen findings. A head CT may suggest parasites causing central nervous system pathologies.

TREATMENT

Parasitic infections are reviewed periodically by the *Medical Letter on Drugs and Therapeutics.* Its recommendations are available free online at www.medletter.com in the "Public Reading Room."

SPECIAL CONSIDERATIONS
Common Parasitoses
Giardia Lamblia
In about 60% of patients, *Giardia* produces no symptoms (asymptomatic cyst passer) and infection resolves spontaneously. Acute giardiasis (1 to 3 weeks after infection) presents with watery diarrhea and other abdominal symptoms. These symptoms may last for months. Chronic giardiasis presents with symptoms of malabsorption and lactose intolerance.

Diagnosis. Fecal examination may reveal trophozoites or cysts and should be done in all patients. Examination of three stool samples is only 85% sensitive in chronic giardiasis so that enzyme immunoassay (EIA) testing for *Giardia* antigen is now considered the test of choice. If stool tests are negative, but clinical suspicion is high, more invasive testing may be necessary and referral to a gastroenterologist should be considered.

Treatment. Metronidazole (Flagyl), 250 mg tid for 5 days (pediatric dose is 15 mg/kg/day in three doses for 5 days), or Nitazoxanide 500 mg bid for 3 days (pediatric dose varies by age).

Enterobius Vermicularis
Pinworms cause intense anal pruritus, usually at night. They can occasionally be visualized as threadlike worms that migrate outside the anus at night. Diagnosis is generally via visualization of pinworm eggs using the cellophane tape test (see above). Treat both adults and children with mebendazole (Vermox), 100 mg PO, repeated in 2 weeks or albendazole 400 mg once, repeated in 2 weeks. It is recommended to treat the entire family if one individual is infected.

Ascaris Lumbricoides
Ascaris is the world's most common intestinal worm. Infections are usually asymptomatic, but large infestations can cause intestinal obstruction. Worms occasionally migrate into the biliary tree, causing cholangitis. Diagnosis is by stool ova and parasite examination. Treat with albendazole 400 mg once or mebendazole (Vermox), 100 mg PO bid for 3 days. Pediatric and adult doses are the same.

Entamoeba Histolytica
Amebiasis usually results in asymptomatic colonic infection. When *E. histolytica* invades the intestinal wall, it produces colitis with clinical presentations ranging from dysentery to perforation. Amebas can spread hematogenously to any organ in the body; liver abscesses are the most common extraintestinal manifestation.

Diagnosis. Performed by ova and parasite examination of stool or of aspirates obtained during colonoscopy. The mucus portion is more likely to contain amebas than the other parts of the stool. For abscesses, ultrasound-directed needle aspiration or serology, or both, may be necessary. *E. dispar,* which is morphologically indistinguishable from *E. histolytica,* is nonpathogenic.

Treatment. Asymptomatic intraluminal infection is usually treated with iodoquinol (Yodoxin) 650 mg tid × 20 days or paromomycin (Humatin) 25 to 35 mg/kg/day divided tid and given over 7 days. Symptomatic disease is treated with metronidazole (Flagyl), 750 mg tid for 7 to 10 days (pediatric dose 35 to 50 mg/kg/day in three doses for 10 days). Alternative treatment for severe intestinal disease or hepatic abscess is tinidazole, 600 mg bid or 800 mg tid for 5 days (pediatric dose, 50 to 60 mg/kg, maximum, 2 g, daily for 3 days).

Isospora Belli, Cyclospora Cayetanensis, and Blastocystis Hominis
These are protozoans that can cause diarrhea and intestinal cramping. Whether *Blastocystis* is truly a pathogen remains in dispute.

Diagnosis. Made by ova and parasite stool examination.

Treatment. Both *Isospora* and *Cyclospora* are treated with co-trimoxazole (Bactrim, Septra), 160/800 mg PO qid for 10 days. *B. coli* is treated with tetracycline, 500 mg qid for 10 days.

Delusional Parasitosis
A psychiatric condition in which patients insist that there are bugs or insects crawling on their bodies or into body openings. Patients may bring samples of these (nonexistent) insects inside match-boxes or envelopes (the "match box" sign). Treatment is difficult; antipsychotics are generally recommended.

Reference
1. Muennig P. The cost effectiveness of strategies for the treatment of intestinal parasites in immigrants. *N Engl J Med* 1999;340:773–779.

Injuries and Violence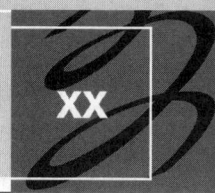

BITES OF HUMANS AND ANIMALS
Richard W. Pretorius, Amber M. Tyler, Thomas Paul Forks

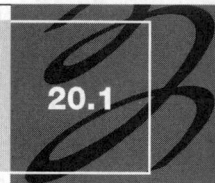

*T*here are approximately 3 million animal bites per year in the United States, and approximately half of all Americans will be bitten by an animal at some time during their lives. The vast majority (80% to 90%) of these bites are from dogs, usually the family pet or an animal known to the victim.[1] Dog and cat bites are responsible for 1% of all emergency room visits, and approximately 1% of dog bites and 6% of cat bites will require hospitalization. The remainder of animal bites suffered by human beings are inflicted by various wild and domestic animals, including farm animals, foxes, coyotes, skunks, rodents, and reptiles. Snakes account for approximately 45,000 bites annually in the United States, but less than 20% of these bites are inflicted by poisonous snakes.

Prophylactic antibiotics for cat or dog bites have not been shown to be effective in controlled trials.[2] Antibiotics may prevent hand infection, particularly if there is a delay in obtaining medical attention. Human bites, other than the hand, do not appear to have any higher risk of infection than animal bites.[2] Deeper wounds can carry increased risk of infection,[3] which is usually polymicrobial involving several genera of bacteria, fungi, viruses, spirochetes, and rickettsia. Other potential complications include tenosynovitis, cellulitis, sepsis, arthritis, osteomyelitis, and fractures of underlying bony structures. Peritonitis and meningitis have also occurred in patients as a result of bites that have penetrated the abdominal cavity or the thin cranial bone of children.

HUMAN BITES

Epidemiology

The majority (80%) of human bites result from closed-fist injuries sustained during fist fights. The resulting lacerations are typically 3 to 8 mm in length, overlie the third metacarpophalangeal joint of the dominant hand, and are frequently infected by the time the patient seeks medical care. Bacteria are often introduced into the joint when the joint capsule is broken and may spread into the deeper spaces of the hand when the digits are extended. Swelling and edema may decrease mobility of the involved digit. These injuries often have a poor prognosis as patients typically present for medical care after infection has occurred. The majority of the remaining bites (15%) are "love nips." These accidental, occlusional bites are commonly seen on the genitalia, breasts, shoulders, arms, and hands. Occlusional bites found on children are usually inflicted by other children. The intercanine distance of occlusional bites on children should be measured. An intercanine distance of 3 cm or greater suggests a bite from an adult, and the child should be evaluated for abuse.

Treatment

The mainstay of treatment is cleansing with povidone–iodine and thorough irrigation with a large volume of sterile saline, 500 mL for small wounds and a liter or more for larger wounds. With all bites, infected wounds should be cultured prior to irrigation, but the routine culture of uninfected wounds is not recommended.[4] Human bites may be left open to close by secondary intention. Although this method has the least incidence of infection, it is accompanied by the greatest scar formation and longest healing time (i.e., several weeks for complete healing). Delayed primary closure has a slightly higher risk of infection. Primary closure has a significant risk of infection and is not advised in the treatment of hand bites, although it may be used in areas with excellent blood supply, such as the face. After dressing the wound, the hand should be splinted in a position of function to maximize the length of the involved tendon and muscle. It is advisable to elevate all hand bites, especially when swelling is present. The lack of elevation when the bitten area is swollen frequently leads to treatment failures. Patients should be re-evaluated within 24 hours. Radiographs of the bite site should be obtained to rule out underlying fractures and the presence of foreign bodies, joint space air, and osteomyelitis. In contrast to hand injuries, studies have indicated that human bites to the face can be closed immediately after appropriate irrigation and cleansing, even when presenting late.[5]

α-Hemolytic streptococci are the most common organisms cultured from infected hand injuries. Other bacteria commonly cultured from these injuries include *Staphylococcus aureus, Eikenella corrodens, Haemophilus influenzae,* and β-lactamase-producing oral, anaerobic bacteria.

Outpatient Antibiotic Therapy

All patients with closed-fist injuries and occlusional bites to the hand or fingers, even when presenting within 8 hours of the injury and before overt signs of infection occur, should be considered for antibiotic prophylaxis for 5 to 7 days. This is best accomplished with amoxicillin–clavulanate potassium (Augmentin, 875/125 mg) 1 pill orally twice daily for 10 days for adults and (600/42.9 mg/5 ml) 45 mg/kg orally bid for children. Alternatively, a second-generation cephalosporin, such as cefuroxime axetil (Ceftin), may be used at a dosage of 250 to 500 mg every 12 hours in adults and 20 to 30 mg/kg/day in divided doses in children.

Hospitalization

Intravenous antibiotics are necessary for all patients with clinically infected hand wounds. A surgeon should be consulted for bites over joints, especially the metacarpophalangeal joint, due to the frequent need for early surgical intervention with intrasynovial irrigation and drain placement. Aerobic and anaerobic cultures must be obtained before starting antibiotics. Intravenous antibiotic options include ampicillin sodium/sulbactam sodium (Unasyn) 1.5 to 3.0 g every 6 hours, cefoxitin (Mefoxin) 1 to 2 g every 6 to 8 hours, cefotetan disodium (Cefotan) 1 to 2 g every 6 to 12 hours, and imipenem–cilastatin (Primaxin) 500 mg every 6 hours.[6] Patients with diabetes who do not respond to initial treatment with oral antibiotics should be considered for coverage with gentamicin (Garamycin) 2 g per kg load, then 1.7 mg per kg every 8 hours, or similar aminoglycoside antibiotic, because these patients frequently have Gram-negative infections.

DOG BITES

Epidemiology

Dogs are responsible for 80% to 90% of animal bites to humans. Annually, 10 to 20 deaths from dog bites occur.[7] The majority of these deaths result from the exsanguination associated with head and neck bites in children younger than 4 years. Elderly patients are also at increased risk. Tears, avulsions, punctures, scratches, and crush injuries may also be present. The overall risk of infection is about 5%,[2] with a greater risk in patients older than 50 years who delay seeking treatment for bites of the upper extremity[8] and in patients whose wounds require surgical repair.[9]

Treatment

All wounds should be thoroughly cleaned and irrigated. Devitalized tissue should be debrided and the wound thoroughly examined for foreign bodies. Dog bites to the hand, wrist, and foot should be left open to close by secondary intention. Bites to the face and other areas with excellent blood supply that appear clinically uninfected may undergo primary closure. Children with severe facial or neck injuries from dog bites should be considered for primary closure under general anesthesia. In children with dog bites to the head by a moderate- to large-sized dog, evaluation with radiographs or computed tomography (CT) scan should be considered to evaluate for a potential open skull fracture. Positive cultures have been obtained in 90% of clinically infected wounds.[9] One study found that *Pasteurella multocida* was isolated in 53% of cases, whereas *Streptococcus* was cultured in 29%, and *Staphylococcus* in about 24%.[9] Another study[10] found that α-hemolytic streptococci were the most frequently isolated organisms. Patients with poorly functioning immune systems are at risk for the development of *Capnocytophagia canimorsus* sepsis (examine peripheral smear for bacilli) and disseminated intravascular coagulation and should be immediately hospitalized at their initial presentation for treatment of the bite. Anaerobic bacteria, including *Bacteroides, Fusobacterium, Peptostreptococcus,* and *Eubacterium,* have also been cultured from infected dog bite wounds.

Outpatient Antibiotic Therapy

Antibiotic therapy should be administered to patients with moderate to severe bites; bites on the hands, neck, or face; bites that appear clinically infected; and immunocompromised patients. The routine culturing of uninfected wounds is not recommended as they often grow multiple organisms and will not assist in guiding the treatment of an infection if one occurs. Facial bites have a relatively low risk of infection (7%); consequently, some authors feel that these wounds should be managed with reconstructive surgery without prophylactic antibiotics.[11] Amoxicillin–clavulanate potassium (Augmentin), 250 to 500 mg every 8 hours, is the drug of choice for outpatient therapy. Children are dosed at 20 mg/kg/day in divided doses. Penicillin V potassium (Pen-Vee K), 250 to 500 mg for every 6 hours, and ampicillin (Omnipen), 250 to 500 mg every 8 hours (in children, 50 to 100 mg/kg/day), are other possible choices. In the absence of overt infection, a 3- to 5-day prophylaxis regimen is prudent for crush injuries or injuries that involve the hand or a joint.

Hospitalization

Hospitalization is indicated for patients with systemic manifestations of infection and in patients with severe cellulitis or in whom the infection has spread rapidly and has not responded to outpatient therapy. Intravenous antibiotic therapy can be accomplished with ampicillin sodium/sulbactam sodium, 1.5 to 3.0 g every 6 hours. Alternative intravenous antibiotics include ceftriaxone sodium (Rocephin), given 1 to 2 g once daily or administered in divided doses. Children may be administered 50 to 75 mg per kg once daily or in divided doses.

CAT BITES

Epidemiology

Cats are involved in approximately 400,000 bites to humans annually. The majority of cat bites occur on the arms, forearms, and hands. Feline canine teeth are sharp and pointed, which facilitates the penetration of bones and joints. The resulting puncture wounds are difficult to clean and irrigate adequately, and 50% of these bites become infected. Patients may develop septic arthritis and osteomyelitis following a cat bite.[12] Other patients have developed *Pasteurella* meningitis, pneumonia, and prosthetic joint infections after a cat bite.

Treatment

Puncture wounds should be carefully irrigated, although care must be taken to prevent extravasation of fluid and bacteria into surrounding tissues. Puncture wounds should be left open to heal by secondary intention. *Pasteurella multocida* is the most common bacterium isolated from the oral cavity and teeth of cats.[13] This organism can cause an intense inflammation with a rapidly expanding cellulitis. A purulent drainage is noted in approximately 40% of patients. Cultures frequently show growth of *Pasteurella* within 24 hours of the bite.[2] Wounds that become infected 24 hours postbite usually culture *Staphylococcus* or *Streptococcus*.[14] Other isolates cultured from cat bite wounds include *Eikenella* and various Gram-negative enteric bacteria and anaerobic bacteria, including *Bacteroides* and *Actinomyces*. *Bartonella henselae*, the etiologic agent of cat-scratch disease, may be inoculated in both cat scratches and bites.[15] Infection with this agent may also result in a reactive arthritis with polyarthralgia of the knees and elbows.[16]

Outpatient Antibiotic Therapy

The drug of choice for the outpatient treatment of cat bites is amoxicillin–clavulanate potassium, 250 to 500 mg every 8 hours. Children are dosed at 20 mg/kg/day in divided doses based on the amoxicillin component.

Hospitalization

Severely infected bites requiring hospitalization may be treated with ceftriaxone sodium (Rocephin), 1 to 2 g in adults and 50 to 75 mg/kg/day in children. Tularemia has also been shown to be transmitted by cat bites and scratches[17] and should be considered where bites have failed to improve with appropriate treatment. This kind of infection is most appropriately managed with streptomycin, 1 g per kg every 12 hours IM or IV for 7 to 14 days. Children should be dosed at 15 mg/kg/day IM in two divided doses for 10 days. In adults, *Bartonella henselae* infections should be managed with erythromycin 500 mg qid or doxycycline 100 mg bid. Children may be treated with erythromycin 30 to 50 mg/kg/day in divided doses.

EXOTIC PETS

Epidemiology

The ownership of exotic pets in the United States is rapidly increasing. Approximately 3% of U.S. homes keep exotic pets.[18] The most common exotic pets are reptiles such as iguanas, monitor lizards, anoles, and chameleons. Some unusual mammals are kept as pets as well, including rats, chinchillas, hedgehogs, and simians.

Treatment

As with all other bites, the mainstay of treatment is copious irrigation with sterile saline and debridement if necessary. Because exotic pets are far less common than cats and dogs, their bites are not seen very often, and the treatment of these bites has not been well studied. It is generally recommended that the bites of simians be treated the same as a human bite because their oral flora is very similar. Lizards, on the other hand, harbor unusual subtypes of salmonella. Routine prophylaxis of these bites is not necessary. If a lizard bite does become infected, the antibiotic treatment should provide coverage for salmonella.[18] Clindamycin 450 mg four times a day for adults or 20 to 30 mg per kg in divided doses four times a day is one option.

SNAKE BITES

Epidemiology

Poisonous snakes, found in every state except for Maine, Alaska, and Hawaii, inflict approximately 7,000 to 8,000 bites yearly in the United States resulting in 9 to 15 deaths. Up to 50% of poisonous snake bites are "dry bites" and do not result in envenomation. Snake venoms are complex mixtures of enzymes that result in the disruption of cell membranes, precipitation of free hemoglobin, muscle and local tissue necrosis, thrombocytopenia, abnormal clotting times, and—in severe cases—death. Patients may experience breathing difficulties, perioral tingling, weakness, diplopia, nausea, vomiting, and muscle fasciculations of the tongue, face, and upper chest and arms after pit viper envenomation. Patients may also experience a metallic taste in the mouth. Patients will commonly experience severe pain and marked swelling at the bite site.

Treatment

A poisonous snake bite is a medical emergency. Field treatment includes having the victim stop physical exertion and resting, calmly reassuring, splinting of the bitten extremity below heart level, considering loose application of a wide lymphatic constriction band (that easily allows two fingers between the skin and the band) and transporting to the nearest emergency facility. Cryotherapy, restricting arterial or venous blood flow, and incision and suction are contraindicated.

- Emergency treatment includes an assessment of envenomation, cleansing of the wound, and administration of antivenom where indicated. Bites from pit vipers (rattlesnakes, cottonmouths, copperheads) are primarily hemotoxic in nature. Hallmark findings of pit viper envenomation are pain and swelling. If pain and swelling are not present within 30 minutes of a pit viper bite, the patient was probably not envenomated. Patients thought to have received a dry bite can be observed for an additional 2 to 4 hours and can be treated as outpatients if no signs of envenomation occur with 8 hours of the bite.[19] Patients remaining asymptomatic may be safely discharged home after routine wound care has been accomplished. However, coral snake bites are primarily neurotoxic. Patients envenomated by coral snakes may show minimal signs and symptoms for several hours. Hospitalization (24-hour observation) is indicated for patients of coral snake bites even when it is suspected that the patient received a dry bite. Serial measurements of the bitten extremity should be made and recorded at 15- to 30-minute intervals. Envenomation may be graded as follows: grade 1, no envenomation; grade 2, mild envenomation with pain and edema extending up to 6 inches from the bite site during the first 12 hours; grade 3, moderate envenomation with edema extending up to 12 inches from the bite site accompanied by nausea, vomiting, prolonged bleeding times, and decreases in platelet counts and hematocrit; and grade 4, severe envenomation with marked swelling and extensive systemic involvement.
- **Antivenom administration.** Not all venomous bites require the administration of antivenom. The major indications would be rapid progression of swelling, coagulation defect, neuromuscular paralysis, and cardiovascular collapse. A new Fab affinity-purified, mixed crotalid antivenom has recently become available (CroFab) and has shown promise in the management of moderate crotalid envenomation.[19] This antivenom has been shown to quickly reverse the local effects of the venom and has the unique capacity to completely reverse the neurotoxicity associated with bites of the Mojave rattlesnake. When a decision to administer polyvalent Crotalidae antivenom has been made, the patient must first be given a skin test with 0.1 mL of a 1:10 saline solution of horse serum intradermally. It is preferable to perform skin testing in the emergency room or intensive care unit because of the risk of anaphylaxis. A syringe of 0.3 to 0.5 mL of a 1:1,000 solution of epinephrine must be available for management of anaphylaxis. Prior to starting the antivenom, a complete blood count, prothrombin time, partial thromboplastin time, electrolytes, blood urea nitrogen, urinalysis, and arterial blood gases should be done. Blood should also be typed and cross-matched. Two large-bore intravenous lines of normal saline or lactated Ringer solution are typically started, and a Foley catheter should be inserted for accurate urine measurements. Grade 2 envenomations may require up to 6 vials of antivenom, whereas grade 3 and 4 envenomations may require up to 15 and 30 vials, respectively. Antivenom is only effective when administered intravenously and should not be injected intramuscularly, subcutaneously, or directly into the bite site. There is no maximal dose of antivenom. The patient's condition must be continuously re-evaluated after each antivenom dosing. A small vial of venous blood (5 to 10 mL) may be collected after each dose of antivenom dosing. If this blood clots after 20 minutes, no additional antivenom is needed.[20] In cases where the patient develops an allergy to the antivenom and has sustained a severe poisoning, the antivenom can be temporarily stopped while the patient is treated with intravenous diphenhydramine (Benadryl), 10 to 50 mg in adults and 5 mg/kg/day in children. The antivenom may then be restarted at a lower rate.
- **Antibiotic prophylaxis.** Antibiotic prophylaxis may be accomplished with intramuscular ceftriaxone sodium, 1 to 2 g per day in adults and 50 to 75 mg/kg/day in children.

VACCINATION PROPHYLAXIS

Tetanus

It is important to determine the patient's tetanus vaccination status.[21] Patients who have completed the primary three-shot regimen will need a booster shot if it has been 10 or more years since their last shot. A wound that is large and dirty needs a booster if it has been longer then 5 years since their last one. If the patient has not completed the primary three-shot series, that series should be started when the patient presents for treatment. If the wound is small and clean, beginning the vaccination series is adequate. If the wound is large and/or dirty the patient should be given be given human tetanus immune globulin (250 units for adults and children). The vaccine and immune globulin should be administered at separate sites that are distant from the other so that they do not interfere with each other.

Rabies

Rabies prophylaxis includes both vaccination and human rabies immune globulin (RIG).[22,23] There are three commercially available vaccines in the United States: RabAvert, Rabies vaccine absorbed, and Imovax Rabies. All are effective but it is recommended that the brand of vaccine is not switched in the middle of the vaccination series. There are two commercially available brands of RIG: BayRab and Imogam Rabies-HT. If a patient has been previously immunized against rabies, a single booster injection is adequate. If there is no history of vaccination and the patient has a high-risk bite, then the patient is given the vaccine on days 0, 3,7,14, and 28. Additionally the patient should be given RIG as a single dose of 20 IU per kg. As much of the RIG as possible is infiltrated around the wound, and the rest injected IM at a site distant from the vaccine. The difficult part is determining which bites need rabies prophylaxis. The best source for an answer to this is the local public health department. Some basic guidelines include bites from any dog, wild animal, or bat that is not available for observation. If the animal is available, prophylaxis can be held for up to 10 days to allow for observation and examination to determine if the animal was carrying rabies. One absolute indication is for people who have been in a room with a bat and it cannot be determined if a bite, scratch, or mucous membrane exposure has occurred (Advisory Committee on Immunization Practices recommendation). This includes small children, the disabled, intoxicated persons, and anyone who awakens to find a bat in the room. Bats have very small sharp teeth and it can be very difficult to determine if a bite occurred.

References

1. Gandhi RR, Liebman MA, Stafford BL, et al. Dog bite injuries in children: a preliminary survey. *Am Surg* 1999;65:9.
2. Medeiros I, Saconato H. Antibiotic prophylaxis for mammalian bites. *Cochrane Database Syst Rev* 2001;(2):CD001738.
3. Dire DJ. Emergency management of dog and cat bite wounds. *Emerg Med Clin* 1992;10:719.
4. Hagen M, Goldstein E, Sanford JP. Bites from pet animals. *Hosp Pract* 1993;28:79.
5. Donkor P, Bankas DO. A study of primary closure of human bite injuries to the face. *J Oral Maxillofac Surg* 1997;55:5.
6. Kahn RM, Goldstein EJ. Common bacterial skin infections: diagnostic clues and therapeutic options. *Postgrad Med* 1993;93:175.
7. Weiss HB, Friedman DI, Coben JH. Incidence of dog bite injuries treated in emergency departments. *JAMA* 1988;279:1.
8. Callaham ML. Treatment of common dog bites: infection risk factors. *JACEP* 1978;7:83.
9. Dire DJ, Hogan DE, Riggs MW. A prospective evaluation of risk factors from dog-bite infections. *Acad Emerg Med* 1994;1:3.
10. Goldstein EJ. Bite wounds and infection. *Clin Infect Dis* 1992;14:633.
11. Wolff KD. Management of animal bite injuries of the face: experience with 94 patients. *J Oral Maxillofac Surg* 1998;56:7.
12. Choda Kewitz J, Bia FJ. Septic arthritis and osteomyelitis from a cat bite. *Yale J Biol Med* 1988;61:6.
13. Galloway RE. Mammalian bites. *J Emerg Med* 1988;6:325.

14. Aghababian RV, Conte JE. Mammalian bite wounds. *Ann Emerg Med* 1980;9:79.
15. Piemont Y, Heller R. Bartonellosis: I. Bartonella henselae. *Ann Biol Clin Paris* 1998;56:6.
16. Jendro MC, Weber G, Brabant T, et al. Reactive arthritis after cat bite: a rare manifestation of cat scratch disease-case report and overview. *Z Rheumatol* 1998;57:3.
17. Capellan J, Fong IW. Tularemia from a cat bite: case report and review of feline associated tularemia. *Clin Infect Dis* 1993;16:472.
18. Kelsey J, Ehrlich M, Henderson SO. Exotic reptile bites. *Am J Emer Med* 1997; 15:536.
19. Singletary EM, Rochman AS, Bodmer JCA, Holstege CP. Envenomations. *Med Clin North Am* 2005;89:1195.
20. Warrell DA, Fenner PJ. Venomous bites and stings. *Br Med Bull* 1993;29:423.
21. www.cdc.gov/ncidod/dvrd/rabies. Accessed July 4, 2006.
22. Rupprecht CE, Gibbons RV. Prophylaxis against rabies. *N Engl J Med* 2004; 351:2626.
23. www.cdc.gov/nip/vaccine/tetanus. Accessed July 4, 2006.

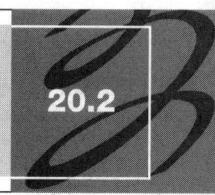

BURNS
Eric D. Morgan
20.2

GENERAL PRINCIPLES
Epidemiology
Each year in the United States 2.5 million people seek medical care for burns. Although 95% of burn victims do not require hospitalization, burns can be devastating. They are the third leading cause of accidental death and can cause life-long scarring and disfigurement. Major risks of death consist of smoke inhalation injuries, shock due to inadequate fluid resuscitation, and infection.

Severity Classification
The severity of the burn should be categorized as minor, major, or severe. This is based on the subcategorizations of burn depth and size, as well as special considerations (burn location, other medical problems, special burn situations).

- **Minor burns** can be treated as outpatients:
  - <10% total body surface area (TBSA) partial-thickness burn in a child
  - <15% TBSA partial-thickness burn in an adult
  - <2% full-thickness burn in a child or adult, not involving eyes, ears, face, or genitalia
- **Moderate burns** should be admitted to the hospital:
  - 10% to 20% TBSA partial-thickness burn in a child
  - 15% to 25% TBSA partial-thickness burn in an adult
  - 2% to 10% TBSA full-thickness burn in a child or adult
  - Suspected inhalation injury
  - High-voltage electrical injury
  - Circumferential partial or full-thickness burn
  - Medical problem predisposing to infection (e.g., diabetes, sickle cell disease)
- **Major burns** should be referred to a burn center:
  - >20% TBSA partial-thickness burn in a child
  - >25% TBSA partial-thickness burn in an adult
  - >10% full-thickness burn in a child or adult
  - Full-thickness burn involving eyes, ears, face, or genitalia
  - Known inhalation injury
  - High-voltage electrical burns
  - Significant associated injuries (fracture or other trauma)

Pathophysiology

The depth of the burn determines the need for medical interventions as well as the risk for complications. Burn depth can be viewed as **superficial** (epidermal involvement only), **Superficial** and **deep partial-thickness** (involving the superficial or deep dermal layers), and **full-thickness** (destroys the entire dermis). Burn depth estimation revisions are often necessary in the first 24 to 72 hours, especially if involving thin-skinned areas.

Burns to **thin-skinned areas** should always be treated initially as at least partial-thickness. Thin-skin areas include volar forearm surfaces, medial thighs, perineum, ears, and burns in children less than age of 5 and adults over the age of 55.

Mechanisms of Injury

Most burns are due to thermal injuries, such as scalding water or fires. Electrical burns due to high voltage can cause significant damage to muscles, including the heart. **High-voltage burns** are characterized by entry and exit burn sites; if none is present, then the patient would have a high-voltage injury that still places the patient at risk for occult muscle damage.

DIAGNOSIS

Clinical Presentation

Remove any hot or burned clothing. Immediately begin cooling using cool water-soaked gauzes; avoid ice and freezing to prevent frostbite.

History

Burn victims from closed spaces are at greater risk for smoke inhalation. The time of injury is important for determining fluid resuscitation during the first 8 hours following injury.

Physical Examination

Minor, moderate, or major burns should be categorized by classifying injuries as superficial, superficial partial-thickness, deep partial-thickness, and full-thickness (see "classification," below). It is important to estimate the burn size of all partial-thickness and full-thickness burns. Examination is necessary for signs of smoke inhalation (persistent coughing, wheezing, dyspnea, hoarseness, facial burns, sooty mucus, and laryngeal edema).

Burn size is expressed as a percentage of TBSA. Ignore superficial burns. The **rule of nines** method is an appropriate way to estimate TBSA in adults; each leg represent 18% TBSA, each arm 9%, the anterior and posterior trunk each 18%, and the head 9%. For small burns, the surface of the patient's palm represents 0.4% of the TBSA. With electrical burns, all tissue in between the entry and exit wounds should be considered and treated as full-thickness burns.

Laboratory Studies

In an electrical injury, evaluate for occult rhabdomyalosis by checking blood creatinine kinase (CK) levels. Arterial blood gas (ABG) can access for carbon monoxide poisoning and pulmonary status should be evaluated in suspected smoke inhalation.

Imaging

Electrocardiogram (ECG) should be done if an electrical injury has occurred.

Monitoring

- A total of 12 to 24 hours of cardiac monitoring is warranted after an electrical injury if the ECG has any abnormalities.
- Observe patients with suspected inhalation injury for 12 to 24 hours if unable to directly visualize the airway (see below).

Surgical Diagnostic Procedures

Fiberoptic laryngoscopy and bronchoscopy can assess the extent of airway injury and assist with intubation with suspected smoke inhalation victims. If unavailable, monitor for declining pulmonary function using serial peak expiratory flow rates and repeat ABGs.

Depth Classification

Burns are classified according to the depth of the burn. Hallmarks distinguishing burn depth are as follows:

- **Superficial burns** are painful, dry, red, and blanch with pressure. They usually take 3 to 6 days to heal without scarring.
- **Superficial partial-thickness burns** are painful to temperature and air. They usually blister and are moist, red, weeping, and blanch with pressure. They heal in 7 to 21 days; scarring is unusual although pigment changes may occur.
- **Deep partial-thickness burns** are painful to pressure only. They almost always blister (easily unroofed), are wet or waxy dry, and have variable color from patchy cheesy white to red. They do not blanch with pressure. They take more than 21 days to heal, and scarring may be severe.
- **Full-thickness burns** are usually painless. The skin is waxy white to leathery gray to charred and black, is dry and inelastic, and does not blanch with pressure. Healing is very slow, if at all, and may require skin grafting if more than 2% of the total body surface is involved. Scarring is very severe with contractures.

TREATMENT

Initial treatment of minor burns consists of cooling, cleansing, appropriate dressing, and pain management. Moderate and severe burns require intravenous (IV) fluid resuscitation. All patients should be assessed for smoke inhalation with aggressive management of airway.

Medications

Superficial burns do not require infection prophylaxis. All other burns benefit from applying a topical antibiotic.

- **1% silver sulfadiazine** (SSD) is a good first-line agent, but avoid using near eyes or mouth; in persons with sulfonamide hypersensitivity; and in pregnant women, newborns, and nursing mothers.
- **Bacitracin** is an effective alternative topical antibiotic in these individuals.

Administer a **tetanus booster** to all burn victims who are not current with tetanus immunization.

Pain control should focus on both an around-the-clock regimen, as well as a rescue medication before dressing changes and during increased physical activity.

Surgery

Full-thickness burns greater than 2 cm usually requires skin grafting. Timing of the procedure is crucial: Skin grafting begun within 72 hours is beneficial for nonscald burns in children and adults younger than 30 years old. Observe all other nonscald full-thickness burns for 8 to 10 days. Wait 2 weeks before performing surgery in children with hot water scald burns; earlier interventions in this group have resulted in worse outcomes.

Nonoperative

Airway management is critical in patients with major burns. Intubation should not be delayed if severe inhalation injury or respiratory distress is present or anticipated.

Prevention of shock using aggressive **fluid resuscitation** is crucial in those with moderate to major burns.

- In the first 24 hours, give IV crystalloid solution (e.g., Ringer lactate). An estimate of the amount of fluid required is 4 mL per kg of body weight for each percentage point of TBSA burned. Give half of the total calculated fluid in the first 8 hours.
- In the second 24 hours, give IV fluids to maintain baseline fluid needs and urinary output. The crystalloid solution can be changed to 5% dextrose in water 0.45% normal saline with 20 mEq of potassium chloride per liter.
- Maintain hourly urine output at 0.5 mL per kg in adults and 1.0 mL per kg in children weighing less than 25 kg; those with electrical injuries should have an hourly urine output of 1.0 to 1.5 mL per kg.

- The use of colloids (e.g., albumin) appears to offer no advantage over the use of crystalloids.

    All burn wounds should be cleaned. Washing using mild soap and tap water is preferred. Skin disinfectants (Hibiclens, Betadine) can actually inhibit the healing process and are discouraged.

    Remove ruptured blisters. Intact blisters should be left undisturbed unless there are signs of infection. If blisters persist without resorption past 2 weeks, refer to a surgeon as there could be an underlying deep partial burn warranting grafting. Avoid needle aspiration of blisters.

Special Therapy

Dressings. Superficial burns do not require wound dressings. Simple skin lubricants (e.g., aloe vera cream) are sufficient. All partial and full-thickness burns should have dressings.

- Apply a fine-mesh gauze (e.g., Telfa) after the burn has been cleansed and a thin layer of topical antibiotic applied. Hold the dressing in place using either a tubular net bandage or gauze wraps lightly applied.
- Change dressings whenever they become soaked with excessive exudates or other fluids. Topical antibiotics should be removed gently with dressing changes.
- Deep wounds may require biologic dressings or skin graftings.

    After epithelialization occurs, use a nonperfumed moisturizing cream until natural lubricating mechanisms return. Avoid the use of preparations high in lanolin.

Referrals

Refer minor burn patients to a surgeon with burn care expertise if a full-thickness burn greater than 2 cm is discovered or at 2 weeks if wound epithelialization has not begun. Wound complications can also be the grounds for referral. Full-thickness burns less than 2 cm diameter can be allowed to heal by contracture when it is in a nonfunctional, noncosmetic area and the skin is not thin.

Follow-Up

See patients the day after injury to adjust pain medications and assess dressing change competence. Visits can then be weekly until wound epithelialization occurs. More frequent follow-up is required if there is insufficient pain control, any concern about the patient or family's ability to provide care, or if synthetic or biologic dressings have been used.

Complications

- All suspected **burn infections** warrant aggressive management to include admission and parenteral antibiotics. Burn infections are prone to sepsis and will extend the depth and extent of the burn. Diagnosing infection in burn patients is challenging. It should be suspected whenever increasing erythema, edema, pain, or tenderness is associated with lymphangitis, fever, malaise, or anorexia.
- **Necrotic tissue** in deep burn wounds may cause progressive tissue injury as well as increasing the risk for infection. Wound excision and grafting is usually beneficial.
- **Hypertrophic scarring** is usually inevitable whenever epithelialization takes longer than 2 weeks in black and young children, and 3 weeks in all others. Early application of pressure is recommended. Refer patients promptly if the wound misses its epithelialization milestone or if hypertrophic scarring appears.

References

1. Alderson P, Schierhout G, Roberts I, et al. Colloids versus crystalloids for fluid resuscitation in critically ill patients. *Cochrane Database Syst Rev* 2000;2:CD000567.
2. Baxter CR. Managment of burn wounds. *Dermatol Clin* 1993;11:709–714.
3. Deitch EA. The management of burns. *N Engl J Med* 1990;323:1249–1253.
4. Deitch EA, Wheelahan TM, Rose MP, et al. Hypertrophic burn scars: analysis of variables. *J Trauma* 1983;23:895–898.
5. Desai MH, Rutan RL, Herndon DN. Conservative treatment of scald burns is superior to early excision. *J Burn Care Rehabil* 1991;12:482–484.

6. Hartford CE. Care of outpatient burns. In: Herndon D, ed., *Total burn care.* Philadelphia: WB Saunders; 1996:71–80.
7. Mertens DM, Jenkins ME, Warden GD. Outpatient burn management. *Nurs Clin North Am* 1997;32:343.
8. Miller K, Chang A. Acute inhalation injury. *Emerg Med Clin North Am* 2003;21: 533–537.
9. Monafo WW. Current concepts: initial management of burns. *N Engl J Med* 1996; 335:1581–1586.
10. Muller MJ, Herndon DN. The challenge of burns. *Lancet* 1994; 343:216–220.
11. Pushkar NS, Sandorminsky BP. Cold treatment of burns. *Burns Incl Therm Inj* 1982; 9:101–110.
12. Rockwell WB, Ehrlich HP. Should burn blister fluid be evacuated? *J Burn Care Rehabil* 1990;11:93–95.
13. Ulmer JF. Burn pain management: a guideline-based approach. *J Burn Care Rehabil* 1998;19:151–159.
14. Waitzman AA, Neligan PC. How to manage burns in primary care. *Can Fam Physician* 1993;39:2394–2400.

SMOKE INHALATION AND CARBON MONOXIDE POISONING   20.3

Richard W. Pretorius, Jefferey D. Harrison

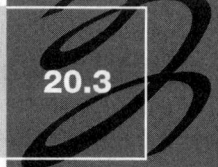

SMOKE INHALATION

General Principles

The inhalation of heated gas and the products of combustion can cause serious respiratory injury and are responsible for the majority of fire deaths, more so than surface burns and their complications. Any patient with carbon deposits in the mouth, singeing of nasal hair or other findings suspicious for significant smoke inhalation should be admitted to the hospital for observation, treatment, and possible intubation. Approximately one third of patients admitted to burn units have smoke inhalation as a compounding complication. Injuries to the lung parenchyma can be caused by hypoxia, heat, and chemicals.

Pathophysiolocy/Etiology

- **Impaired tissue oxygenation** results from the carbon monoxide and—with increased frequency—cyanide found in smoke. It can be immediately life-threatening.
  - Carbon monoxide (CO) accounts for over half of the fatalities in smoke inhalation (see "Carbon Monoxide Poisoning").
  - Suspect cyanide, which impairs cellular oxidative metabolism, when plastics or organic chemicals are fuels,[1] especially with high temperature and low oxygen settings.
- **Thermal injury** results from the inhalation of heated gases.
- The supraglottic mucosa has little protection from heated gases that often results in edema and airway obstruction within 18 to 24 hours after exposure.
- Because smoke is dry with a low specific heat and the upper airway has excellent heat exchange properties, the subglottic tissues are generally protected from thermal injury, although steam inhalation can result in tracheobronchial burns.
- Elective intubation needs to be considered early in all patients with suspected thermal injury.
- **Chemical injury primarily** is caused by insoluble irritant gases that affect the lower airways.

- Insoluble irritant gases include aldehydes, amines, chlorine, hydrochloric acid, and sulfur dioxide.
- There may be a delay between exposure and clinical manifestation.

Diagnosis of Smoke Inhalation

History
- Positive predictive factors for significant smoke inhalation include unconsciousness, entrapment or being in an enclosed space, and exposure to known toxins.[2]

Physical Examination
- Facial burns, singeing of eyebrows and nasal vibrissae, carbonaceous sputum, and oropharyngeal carbon deposits are suggestive of inhalation injury.
- Cyanosis, tachypnea, stridor, wheezing, and crackles are suggestive of the need for aggressive treatment; however, these signs are infrequently found despite the presence of significant injury.

Laboratory Studies
- Carboxyhemoglobin testing should be carried out on all patients. Elevated levels ($>2\%$) should raise suspicion regarding the presence of other toxins (e.g., CO and cyanide).
- Arterial blood gases. Hypoxemia and elevated alveolar–arterial ($P_AO_2–P_aO_2 > 15$ mm) gradient are frequently seen in inhalation injury, although they are insensitive indicators of injury and do not predict clinical outcome.
- Pulse oximetry can also be used as a noninvasive measure of oxygenation,[1] but may be normal despite the presence of carboxyhemoglobin as CO displaces oxygen from hemoglobin but does not change the concentration of oxygen dissolved in the blood.

Imaging
- Chest radiography generally is an insensitive initial test and should be reserved for hospitalized patients and those with suspected thoracic injury.

Diagnostic Procedures
- Bronchoscopy with direct fiberoptic visualization of the upper and lower airway provides an assessment of the extent of injury. Since the appearance of the subglottic tissues is an unreliable predictor of the need for ventilation, laryngoscopy may suffice for management decisions.[3]

Treatment

Protocol
- **Immediate.** Early mortality occurs from asphyxiation due to CO and cyanide.
- Remove patient from offending environment.
  - Provide 100% oxygen until carboxyhemoglobin level is in the normal range. Maintain a partial pressure of oxygen (PO_2) greater than 75.
  - If cyanide poisoning is present, induce methemoglobinemia. This can be expedited by contacting the local poison control center.

- **Early.** Upper airway obstruction causing fatal injury occurs in the first 8 to 48 hours after exposure.
  - Direct laryngoscopy provides the most accurate assessment of upper airway injury.
  - Endotracheal intubation should be performed if laryngoscopy reveals even minimal early swelling or obstruction because swelling will continue for the first 24 hours. If direct laryngoscopy is unavailable, endotracheal intubation should be strongly considered if findings are suggestive of inhalation injury.[2]
  - Humidified oxygen or air should be given to thin the viscous bronchorrhea that is produced by injured airways.
  - Bronchodilators (albuterol 5% solution, 0.5 mL) may have variable effects, depending on whether obstruction is due to edema or bronchospasm. There is no contraindication to its use in smoke inhalation.
  - Steroids and prophylactic antibiotics are contraindicated.
  - Antibiotics are indicated for proven infection, which tends to occur with the onset of bronchorrhea 2 to 3 days after the injury.

- **Late.** Adult respiratory distress syndrome is a late complication.

CARBON MONOXIDE POISONING

General Principles

CO, which causes up to 80% of fatalities from smoke inhalation, is a colorless, odorless, tasteless, nonirritating gas produced by incomplete combustion of carbonaceous materials. It is responsible for 500 accidental and 5000 suicidal deaths in the United States every year. The CO molecule has 210 times the affinity of oxygen for hemoglobin. Toxic effects are due to tissue hypoxia as carboxyhemoglobin is incapable of carrying oxygen and interferes with oxygen release.

Diagnosis

Clinical Presentation

Although exposure levels do not consistently correlate with carboxyhemoglobin levels and symptoms, the following associations are commonly seen:

- Mild exposure (1% to 15% carboxyhemoglobin) causes headache, dizziness, and nausea.
- Moderate exposure (16% to 40% carboxyhemoglobin) causes severe headache, nausea, vomiting, loss of coordination, and unconsciousness.
- Severe exposure (40% to 60% or greater carboxyhemoglobin) causes seizures, coma, and death.[3]

History

History may include suicidal or accidental exposure to auto exhaust, smoke inhalation, or exposure to a poorly vented heater or appliance.

Laboratory Findings

- Increased carboxyhemoglobin level. Normal levels are 1% to 3%; levels in smokers are 5% to 6%.
- Patients may have a normal arterial partial pressure of oxygen (PaO_2).
- Pulse oximetry should be considered unreliable; it cannot differentiate oxyhemoglobin from carboxyhemoglobin.

Management

Medications

- Remove the patient from exposure, maintain vital functions, and support ventilation artificially if necessary. Patient should remain quiet so as to decrease oxygen consumption.
- Administer 100% oxygen until carboxyhemoglobin is less than 5%; 40% to 50% of the body's CO can be eliminated in 1 hour with high-dose oxygen.

Special Therapy

- Hyperbaric oxygen can reduce the half-life of CO to 22 minutes, although it cannot be routinely recommended due to equivocal trials.[5] Despite unproven benefit, it can be considered for severe cases including CO > 40%, loss of consciousness, severe metabolic acidosis (pH < 7.1), and end-organ ischemia. Due to the increased binding of CO to fetal hemoglobin, consider hyperbaric oxygen for CO >20% in the pregnant patient.
- Consider transfusion of blood or packed cells to increase the oxygen-carrying capacity of the blood.
- Cerebral edema should be managed with diuretics and steroids.

Follow-Up

Monitor the patient after severe exposure for the following neurologic symptoms: tremors, mental deterioration, and psychotic behavior.

References

1. Haponik EF. Smoke inhalation. *Am Rev Respir Dis* 1988;138:1060.
2. Committee on Trauma. Injuries due to burns and cold. In: *ATLS manual,* 7th ed. Chicago: American College of Surgeons; 2003.
3. Inhalation injury: diagnosis. *J Am Coll Surg* 2003;196:307.
4. Harrington JT. *Consultation in internal medicine.* Boston: BC Decker, 1990:437.
5. Juurlink DN, Buckley NA, et al. Hyperbaric oxygen for carbon monoxide poisoning. *Cochrane Database Syst Rev* 2006:2.

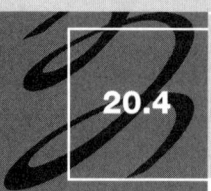

20.4 DOMESTIC VIOLENCE
Jennifer M. Joyce

GENERAL PRINCIPLES

Domestic violence is defined as "a pattern of behavior used to establish power and control over another person through fear and intimidation, often including the threat or use of violence."[1] It is the most common cause of nonfatal injury to women in the United States. A woman's lifetime risk for abuse is 22%.[2] Nearly 5.3 million incidents occur each year among women 18 years of age and older and 3.2 million occur among men.[3] Between 17% and 31% of women and up to 30% of men experience violence in same-sex partnerships.[4]

Domestic violence is not a disease present in the body; rather it is a health-related risk factor.[5] A public health approach seeks to identify a combination of individual, relational, community, and societal factors that contribute to the risk of being a victim or perpetrator of domestic violence.[3] Abuse is a common and complex public health issue. Awareness of the prevalence of violence in all sectors and of its effects will assist family physicians and others to address this important health issue effectively.

DIAGNOSIS

Risk factors for domestic violence are outlined in Table 20.4-1.

TREATMENT

- **Physicians should be aware of risk factors and associated symptoms.** The U.S. Preventive Services Task Force (USPSTF) found insufficient evidence to recommend for or against routine screening of women for intimate partner violence. However, the American Academy of Family Physicians notes that it is imperative that family physicians be aware of the prevalence of violence in all sectors of society, be alert for its effects in their encounters with virtually every patient, and be capable of providing an appropriate response when these issues are identified. With this awareness, physicians are able to work to prevent violence for patients who are at risk within their practices and commu-nities.[6]
- **In the case of an injury.** Suspect domestic abuse if unexplained injuries are present or if the patient's explanation seems implausible. Ask directly, "Did someone hurt you?" Talk with the patient privately and provide enough space to answer your questions. If a patient discloses abuse, be explicit that physical and sexual violence are never acceptable. Offer assurance and unconditional positive regard. Skill in establishing rapport and communication are critical to help a woman feel comfortable and safe. Accept her answers; reaffirming your desire to understand and help when you can. Remember, abuse and violence are **never** easy to talk about.
- **Look for domestic abuse "red flags."** Abused persons may avoid eye contact or seem overly agitated or wary in their encounters with physicians. They may also not show up for appointments or have an appointment canceled by a partner. An abuser may attempt to stay close at hand or be overly vigilant during an examination to monitor what is said to the physician.
- **Complete documentation.** A physician's notation in the medical record should include an objective report of the abuse history as reported by the patient, detailed drawings of physical findings, laboratory and radiologic findings, and any photographs of abuse injuries. Document in the chart that the symptoms or injuries treated are abuse related and request a follow-up appointment.

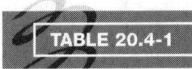

TABLE 20.4-1	Domestic Violence Risk Factors	

Risk type	Victimization	Perpetration

Individual	Prior history
	Being female
	Young age
	Heavy alcohol/drug use
	High-risk sexual behavior
	Being less educated
	Unemployment
	For men: different ethnicity
	  from partners
	For women: greater education
	  than their partners
	Being Native American/Alaskan
	  or African American
	Verbally abusive, jealous, or
	  possessive partner
		Low self-esteem
		Low income
		Low academic achievement
		Involvement in aggressive
		  behavior
		Heavy alcohol/drug use
		Depression
		Anger/hostility
		Personality disorders
		Few friends/social isolation
		Economic stress
		Belief in strict gender roles
		Desire for power/control
		Victim of physical/psychologic
		  abuse (strongest predictor)

Relational	Couples with income,
	  educational, or job status
	  disparities
	Dominance and control of
	  the relationship by the male
		Marital conflict
		Marital instability
		Dominance and control of
		  the relationship by the male
		Economic stress
		Unhealthy family relationships
		  and interactions

Community	Poverty
	Low social capital
	Weak community sanctions
	  against domestic violence
		Poverty
		Low social capital
		Weak community sanctions
		  against domestic violence

Societal	Traditional gender norms	Traditional gender norms

Associated signs and symptoms with intimate partner violence

Acute injuries	Psychologic	Nonspecific

Multiple bruises/
  anatomical sites
  involved
Firearm wounds
Knife wounds
Fractures
	Acute/chronic anxiety
	Depression
	Posttraumatic stress disorder
	Suicidal ideation
	Sleep disturbance
	Substance abuse
		Abdominal/chest/pelvic pain
		Headaches
		Insomnia/fatigue
		Choking sensation

SPECIAL CONSIDERATIONS

- **Know your state's legal requirements.** Every state has legislation designed to protect victims of domestic violence, because spouse and partner abuse has been defined as a criminal act. Physicians must be aware of the specific laws and support services for abused persons available in their practice community. Remember to obtain informed consent from an abused person before disclosing the abuse diagnosis to a third party or the police.
- **Assess the safety of children in the home.** It is also imperative to assess the risk to children who are in the home. "Children who witness violence are at risk for developmental delay, school failure, violent behavior and a variety of psychiatric disorders."[7] Ask directly whether or not children are safe in the home. If the children have been mistreated or are at risk for abuse, refer them to an emergency shelter or child protection services.

■ **Assess psychologic needs.** Determine whether an abused person is using drugs or alcohol or is suicidal. Each requires urgent and appropriate intervention.

■ **Knowledge of community service providers.** In caring for an abused patient, the physician's primary role is to provide that person with good medical care and safe, reliable information about support services. These community service providers have been specifically trained to help survivors of domestic violence. Respect an abused person's ability to make appropriate choices. It is up to a victim to decide if and when he or she will leave a violent partner.

■ **Work to make the office a safe place to discuss domestic abuse.** Work with local service providers to obtain sensitive posters and educational materials. Provide patients with educational materials about family violence and community resources. Ensure that these materials are offered in ways that allow patients privacy to access them. Placing them in bathrooms as well as waiting rooms is important. Local agencies may help you with this educational outreach. There are excellent on line resources such as "The Family Violence Prevention Fund" (www.endabuse.org) or "The National Coalition Against Domestic Violence" (www.ncadv.org). These can be useful tools for working with women and men who experience interpersonal violence in their intimate relationships.

■ Domestic violence is a common problem and a complex public health issue that must be recognized and treated with sensitivity. In addition to recognizing abuse-related injuries and symptoms, family physicians can provide patients with life-saving information on community resources available to address domestic violence.

References

1. National Coalition against Domestic Violence. Available online at www.ncadv.org.
2. Kyriacou DN, et al. Risk factors for injury to women from domestic violence. *N Engl J Med* 1999;341:25.
3. National Center for Injury Prevention and Control. Intimate partner violence; fact sheet. Available online at www.cdc.gov/ncipc/factsheets/ipvfacts.htm.
4. Burke LK, Follingstad DR. Violence in lesbian and gay relationships: theory, prevalence, and correlational factors. *Clin Psychol Rev* 1999;19:5.
5. Tacket A, Wathen CN, MacMillan H. Should health professionals screen all women for domestic violence? *Plos Med* 2004;1:1–4.
6. AAFP policy statement: family and intimate partner violence and abuse (2002) (2004). Available online at http://www.aafp.org/online/en/home/policy/policies/f/familyandintimatepartner-violenceandabuse.html.
7. U.S. Preventative Service Task Force. Recommendations: screening for family and intimate partner violence 2006. Available online at www.ahcpr.gov/clinic/3rduspstf/famviolence/famviolrs.htm.

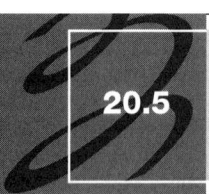

20.5 CHILD ABUSE
Pamela Dull, Maria R. Conroy

GENERAL PRINCIPLES

Child abuse is a common problem encountered in the family physician's office. Because it cuts across all racial, economic, educational, and religious backgrounds and because the presentation of abuse varies widely, providers should include child abuse in the differential diagnosis of many presenting problems.

Definition and Classification

As defined by federal law, child abuse is "any recent act or failure to act on the part of the parent or caretaker which results in death, serious physical or emotional harm, sexual abuse or exploitation; or an act or failure to act which presents an imminent risk of serious harm." **Neglect** is failure to provide for a child's basic needs, be it **physical, medical, emotional,** or **educational.** Abuse can be **physical,** such as punching, beating, kicking, biting, burning, shaking, or otherwise physically harming a child. **Emotional** abuse is an act or omission by the parents or other caregivers that have caused, or could cause, serious behavioral, cognitive, emotional, or mental disorder. **Sexual** abuse includes fondling a child's genitals, intercourse, incest, rape, sodomy, exhibitionism, and commercial exploitation through prostitution or the production of pornographic materials.[1]

Prevalence

In 2004, it is estimated that approximately 3 million reports of child abuse or neglect were filed and about 872,000 children were confirmed victims. That same year, 1490 children died due to the abuse or neglect![2] That's a rate of 2.03 deaths per 100,000 children. This is comparable to the rate of 2.00 deaths from any cause per 100,000 children in the national population for 2003.[3] About 79% of the perpetrators were parents. Those highest at risk are children between birth and 3 years old.[2]

According to Nation Committee for the Prevention of Child Abuse (NCPCA) 1996 Annual Fifty State Survey, neglect is the most common type of reported and substantiated form of abuse.[4]

The Third National Incidence Study (NIS 3) of Child Abuse and Neglect showed that a child's risk of experiencing harm causing abuse or neglect in 1993 was one and a half times the risk in 1986 (NIS 2). Physical abuse more than doubled, emotional abuse, physical and emotional neglect increased more than two and one half times from 1986 to 1993. The total number of children seriously injured and the total number endangered both quadrupled during this time. The number of undisclosed incidents of sexual abuse is believed to be large owing to the stigma and criminal behavior involved.[5]

Risk factors for abuse include children with complex medical problems or development delays. Unwanted or difficult to control children are also more likely to be abused. Caregivers with stress such as single parent or teen parents are more likely to abuse.[6]

Girls are sexually abused three times more than boys. As regards emotional neglect and serious injury, boys are at a higher risk than girls. Children are consistently vulnerable to sexual abuse from age 3 on. There were no significant race differences in the incidence of maltreatment or maltreatment-related injuries uncovered in either the NIS 2 or the NIS 3.[5]

Children in the largest families were physically neglected three times more than single child families. Children from families with annual incomes less than $15,000 per year versus $30,000 per year were over 22 times more likely to experience some form of maltreatment. Children from low-income families are 18 times more likely to be sexually abused, 56 times more likely to be educationally neglected, and 22 times more likely to be seriously injured from maltreatment.[5]

DIAGNOSIS

Clinical Presentation

Presentations are variable with head trauma, abdominal trauma, or fractures. Nonspecific symptoms such as sleep disturbance, abdominal pain, enuresis, encopresis, and phobias should also be kept in mind. It's important to interview child and caregiver separately if possible and in a nonjudgmental manner. Documentation verbatim is important.[7]

History

History can be highly variable and may not be obvious. A history that is inconsistent with the injury(ies) is the hallmark of physical abuse. However, some key questions can help point to those at risk for abuse. If there has been a delay between an injury and seeking help without a reasonable explanation, look for abuse. If the history between caregivers or health personnel is inconsistent, consider further evaluation. Last, check if the child's behavior and interactions are age-appropriate and check for the presence of any unexplained injuries. If any of these four areas reveal suspect answers, then probe further for possible abuse or neglect. Having a questionnaire sticker on emergency room charts with these questions on it increased compliance with documentation of screening.[8] Document history as much as possible in quotes.

Physical Examination

"First do no harm," a rule that should be applied when examining any patient especially abused/neglected patients. Make sure the evaluation will not result in additional trauma. Explaining to the child beforehand helps alleviate apprehensions. Interview the caregiver first to give the child a chance to relieve or decrease the child's anxiety. Do not interview children younger than 3 years old.[9]

The skin is the most commonly injured system. Careful examination of clothed areas may reveal trauma. Bruises that are on uncommonly injured areas or in the shape of a handprint or cord loop are suspicious. Circumferential immersion or "glove" distribution burns or burns from a blunt instrument frequently are indicative of abuse. Careful documentation of location, size, shape, and color should be noted. Photographs need to be clearly labeled. Retinal hemorrhages also are suspicious for abuse known as "shaken-baby syndrome."[6]

If sexual abuse is suspected within the previous 72 hours, then forensic evidence should be collected. If more than 72 hours have passed without any acute injuries, an emergency physical exam is not necessary. Forensic exams beyond 72 hours are unlikely to yield anything useful.[6] Magnification and illumination are key for the genitalia exam. An otoscope or colposcope can provide both. A Wood lamp may be useful to detect semen. Prepubertal girls are better examined in the "frog-leg, while sitting on caregiver's lap or prone knee–chest position. Many sexually abused children will have a normal exam.[7]

Laboratory Studies

Patients with a history of easy bruising should have a bleeding disorder workup with a complete blood count (CBC), prothrombin time, partial thromboplastin time, and bleeding time.[6] Rapid tests are not appropriate in the context of a child sexual abuse (CSA) evaluation because of their higher potential for false-positive results.[10] Cultures remain the criterion standard and are valuable from a forensic evidence standpoint. Depending on the contact suspected and the clinical situation, recommended testing to consider includes the following:

- Gram stain of vaginal and/or anal discharge
- Genital, anal, and pharyngeal culture for gonorrhea
- Genital and anal culture for *Chlamydia*
- Serology for syphilis
- Wet prep of vaginal discharge for *Trichomonas vaginalis*
- Culture of lesions for herpes virus
- Serology for HIV (based on suspected risk)
- Pregnancy[10]

Imaging

The most basic imaging in suspected child abuse is the skeletal survey, which includes frontal and lateral views of the skull and single frontal views of the long bones, lateral spine, frontal chest, and abdomen. Any symptomatic or visually abnormal area would also be imaged. Surveys are for children without symptoms, but suspicion of abuse. If the survey is negative and the suspicion is high for abuse, then a bone scan may be helpful, especially for rib, spine, pelvic, or acromion fractures. If there is a history of head trauma but no neurologic findings, magnetic resonance imaging (MRI) is the recommended choice of imaging. If there are neurologic symptoms or findings, then an immediate noncontrast brain computed tomography (CT) scan is needed. MR imaging may needed if the CT is negative. For visceral injuries, a contrast abdominal CT is recommended.[11]

Monitoring

The victim's physical and emotional well-being needs to be evaluated at follow-up. Let the child know that the abuse is *not* his or her own fault.

Differential Diagnosis

Differential diagnosis of excessive bruising includes hemophilia, ITP, von Willebrand disease, and Henoch–Schonlein purpura. Metabolic congenital disorders such as osteogenesis imperfecta, Ehlers–Danlos syndrome, and rickets my cause fractures similar to abuse. Dermatologic considerations include photodermatitits, Mongolian spots, vascular malformations, and subcutaneous fat necrosis. Other mimics of child abuse include bullous impetigo, staphylococcal scalded skin syndrome, and petechia or purpura from systemic bacterial or viral infections.[6]

TREATMENT

Treatment should be directed toward the injury(ies). If the child is in immediate danger, acute hospitalization and/or removal from the home (to relatives, neighbors, or foster care) may be necessary. With children sexually abused, wait for results of sexually transmitted disease (STD) testing before treating. Adolescents may be prophylactically treated for gonorrhea and *Chlamydia*. Consider emergency postcoital contraception if appropriate.

Reporting

All 50 states have some type of mandatory reporting law; however, specifics of which law enforcement or child protective agency needs to be notified vary among them. Web references can help physicians take proper steps in notifying their proper authorities as needed. There is also a Childhelp USA National Child Abuse Hotline that will help one find out where and how to report at 800-4-A-CHILD. Note that failure to report can result in criminal and civil liability. Inform parents or caregivers of the need to report. Most states have "good faith" immunity for those who report. False reports can lead to prosecution.[1,12] Note: it's the role of the child protecting agency to determine if there's been abuse, not the physician's!

Referrals

Community resources are useful and may include community centers, shelters, foster care, or parenting hotlines. Besides phone books and social service centers, national web sites have helped pool resource listings by state. Primary care providers can help coordinate care.[1]

References

1. http://nccanch.acf.hhs.gov/topics/reporting/index.cfm. Accessed May 3, 2006.
2. U.S. Department of Health and Human Services, Administration on Children, Youth and Families. Child maltreatment 2004. Washington, DC: U.S. Government Printing Office; 2006.
3. http://www.childwelfare.gov/can/prevalence.cfm. Accessed June 20, 2006.
4. http://www.yesican.org/stats.html. Accessed June 20, 2006.
5. http://www.childwelfare.gov/pubs/statsinfo/nis3.cfm. Accessed June 20, 2006.
6. Pressel DM. Evaluation of physical abuse in children. *Am Fam Physician* 2000;61: 3057–3064.
7. Lahoti SL, McClain N, Girardet R, et al. Evaluating the child for sexual abuse. *Am Fam Physician* 2001;63:883–892.
8. Benger JR, Pearce AV. Simple intervention to improve detection of child abuse in emergency departments. *BMJ* 2002;324:780–782.
9. http://www.guideline.gov/summary/summary.aspx?doc_id=7583&nbr=004453&string=child+AND+abuse. Accessed June 20, 2006.
10. http://www.emedicine.com/ped/topic2649.htm#section~clinical. Accessed June 20, 2006.
11. ACR practice guideline for skeletal surveys in children. Available online at http://www.acr.org. Accessed May 15, 2006.
12. http://www.smith-lawfirm.com/mandatory-reporting.htm. Accessed May 31, 2006.

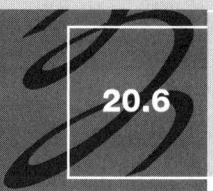

EVALUATION AND MANAGEMENT SEXUAL ASSAULT VICTIM
Sandra Christina Ogata

GENERAL PRINCIPLES

Definition

According to the U.S. Department of Health and Human Services, sexual assault is defined as any sexual act performed by rape and child molestation. Sexual assault is the most underreported violent crime.[1]

Many misconceptions are perpetuated about sexual assault. The most common is the assumption that rape is motivated by sexual desire. Rape is a violent crime, motivated by the need for power and control or by anger.[2]

Epidemiology

The vast majority of information and statistics relate to female rape victims. Prevalence studies suggest that at least 20% of all adult women and 23% of adolescent women have experienced some form of sexual abuse or assault during their lifetimes.[3] One in three women will be a victim of sexual assault sometime in her life.[4] One in four women will experience rape or attempted rape during her college years.[5]

The estimated incidence of assault on males is 7% to 10% of reported rapes. About 50% of rape victims have some acquaintance with their attackers.[3]

Tintinalli and Hoelzer's study of 372 rape victims reported that only 7% of all injuries were gynecologic injuries. Genital injuries are not an inevitable consequence of rape, and lack of genital injuries does not imply consensual intercourse.[3] Only 1% to 2% require hospitalization.[2,3,6]

DIAGNOSIS

History

Evidence beyond 48 to 72 hours after an assault often is difficult to recover or may be invalid. It is imperative to document the time frame (from time of assault to medical examination) and to encourage victims to proceed with evidence collection as soon as possible.[7] Multidisciplinary sexual assault team may be available in some medical centers.[1,8,9]

Informed consent or refusal should be obtained for each of the following components of the sexual assault evaluation.[1]

- Medical evaluation and treatment
- Reporting the crime
- Performing a physical examination
- Photo documentation
- Evidence collection: The patient has the right to decline the collection of any and all specimens. However, to give the patient the ability to make an informed decision, it is important to explain to the patient that this is the only time to gather certain forensic evidence.
- Transferal of evidence to law enforcement personnel
- The history should focus on explicit details of the sexual assault for forensic purposes. Avoid legal terms such as "rape" or "abuse."
- Provide a quiet, secure, and private environment. Allow 30 to 60 minutes for the history and the physical examination.[10]
- The following details of the history should be obtained[5]
  - Circumstances of the assault: date, time, location, use of weapons, force, restraints or threats

- Whether or not the victim experienced loss of consciousness or memory loss
- Specifics regarding oral, vaginal, or anorectal contact or penetration along with the presence or absence of ejaculation and or condom use
- If the patient has had recent intercourse (less than 3 days) prior to the attack, it may confuse laboratory analysis of sperm, acid phosphatase, and genetic typing
- Victims should be asked if they have showered or bathed, changed clothing, eaten, used toothpaste or mouthwash, used enemas, changed or removed a tampon, sanitary pad, or barrier contraceptive device since the assault.
- Last menstrual period, contraceptive use, and gynecologic history are necessary for the investigation.

Physical Examination

Most hospitals have a standard rape kit with instructions to help guide the clinician through the collection and preservation of evidence for forensic evaluation.[3] Once the kit is opened, the "chain of evidence" must be maintained; evidence cannot be left unattended.[11]

Note that history of sexual assault with no physical findings may still be consistent with the sexual assault. Accurately document the assessment of the patient, remembering that the lack of obvious injuries does not preclude the possibility that sexual assault took place.[2]

The physical examination should be performed thoroughly and compassionately. A female chaperone should be present for a male physician. The patient should undress for the examination with a sheet beneath her to capture any failing debris for medical evidence. Only the victim should handle her or his clothes. Clothing can be collected up to 1 month after the assault, provided the items have not been laundered. Clothing should be placed in paper bags to avoid bacterial growth on blood or semen stains.[11]

The physical examination should describe the patient's emotional state. The examiner should document any evidence of trauma; a body map may be helpful. If possible, photographs of injuries should be taken with the patient's consent. As many of 29% of rape survivors will have nongenital injuries.[2,12–14]

Always begin in a nonthreatening location such as ears, eyes, nose, and throat. Swab oral cavity if oral penetration took place, swab the oropharynx for semen retrieval and gonorrhea testing. Even if the teeth were brushed or mouthwash used sperm may be recovered up to 6 hours later.[1,7,15]

The breasts, external genitalia, vagina, anus, and rectum should be carefully examined. Genital trauma occurs more commonly in postmenopausal women.[14] The most common sites of vaginal injury include the posterior vagina, anus, and the labia minora. Engorgement of the clitoris and or labia may last for 1 to 2 hours after injury. Colposcopic examination can enhance detection of areas of milder genital trauma. Toluidine blue can be used to detect small vulvar lacerations. Lacerations expose the deeper dermis containing nuclei that absorb this stain. Prior to insertion of the speculum (this should be lubricated with saline only because the jelly may be spermicidal) the dye is applied to the posterior fourchette with gauze. A linear blue stain will highlight the vulvar lacerations.[16]

A wet mount should be done to check for the presence of bacterial vaginosis, trichomonads, yeast, and sperm. Motile sperm may be seen up to 8 hours postcoitus and nonmotile sperm can be detected beyond 72 hours. The absence of sperm may indicate that the assailant had undergone a vasectomy. Vaginal swabbing should be collected during pelvic examination for *Chlamydia* and *Neisseria gonorrhoeae*. If blood is present, anoscopy or sigmoidoscopy and rectal digital examination should be performed based on patient's history.[3,16]

In a male victim obtain rectal aspiration in case of anal assault, injection of sterile saline into the rectum and then aspiration. Swabs from the victim's penis should be collected and may be examined for saliva if there is a history of oral copulation.[3]

If available, use a Wood lamp to examine the patient's thighs for fluorescing semen and urine stains. Swab any highlighted areas.

With a comb provided in the rape kit, the patient should comb the pubic area to collect any foreign hair. In addition, the patient should pluck approximately 15 to 20 pubic hairs to serve as samples for reference.[16]

Blood samples are drawn for DNA testing, blood typing, and pregnancy testing.[1]

In summary, collected samples should include[5]:

- The victim's clothing
- Swabs and smears from the buccal mucosa, vagina, and rectum and from other areas highlighted by ultraviolet light
- Combed specimens from the scalp and pubic hair
- Fingernail scrapings and clippings
- Control samples of the victim's scalp and pubic hair
- Whole blood sample
- Saliva sample

Laboratory Studies[1,2,11,15]

- Pregnancy test is recommended to all women of childbearing age and to rule out an established pregnancy; 1% to 5% of sexual assaults result in pregnancy.
- VDRL or RPR test should be obtained at the time of the initial visit and repeated 6 weeks, 3, and 6 months later.
- Hepatitis serology.
- HIV at the initial visit and repeated at 3, 6, and 12 months form the date of exposure. There is a risk of less than 1% of infection at one-time sexual encounter.
- Acid phosphatase detection in vaginal washing is helpful in cases of azoospermic ejaculations.
- Glycoprotein 30 is unique to the male and is produced in large quantities by the prostate. Its presence indicates that coitus occurred within the past 48 hours.
- Genetic typing from ABO blood group, DNA.
- Gamma-hydroxybutyrate (GHB), flunitrazepam ("date rape drug") serum, and/or urine level. GHB it is a central nervous system depressant approved as an anesthetic in some countries; however, with the exception of investigational research, it is not approved for any use in the United States.
- Drugs of abuse and alcohol level in serum, urine, and toxicology.

TREATMENT

Behavioral

The patient may have nonspecific symptoms, such as sleep disturbance, nightmares, emotional lability, fatigue, self-blame, shame, fear, or sexual dysfunction.[4] Children who are sexually assaulted or abused may display variable nonspecific symptoms and/or physical findings.[17]

Medications

- Pregnancy prophylaxis: Most postcoital pregnancy interventions are ineffective after 72 hours. One recommended treatment is to administer 100 μ of ethinyl estradiol and 0.5 mg of levonorgestrel, which is then repeated 12 hours later. Plan B is a regimen of 0.75 mg of levonorgestrel then repeated 12 hours later; this is more effective with fewer side effects than the first.[3]
- Sexually transmitted disease prophylaxis for gonorrhea, chlamydial, and syphilis infection. Empiric therapy, per Centers for Disease Control (CDC) guidelines, includes ceftriaxone 125 mg IM for gonorrhea and either azithromycin 1 g PO (single dose) or doxycycline 100 mg PO twice daily for 7 days for *Chlamydia*. Trichomoniasis therapy if present on wet mount: metronidazole 2 g PO (single dose).[1,6,9]
- Hepatitis B vaccine (if patient was not previously vaccinated) at the time of visit, then repeated at 1 and 6 months; hepatitis B immunoglobulin should be reserved for patients who have been exposed within 14 days and or high-risk exposure.[9]
- HIV prophylaxis is controversial because of presumed low risk of transmission and the lack of evidence proving the efficacy of antiretroviral drugs after sexual assault.[3] Postexposure prophylaxis (PEP) may consist of zidovudine and lamivudine; each medication should be given simultaneously for 4 weeks and not commence beyond 72 hours from the time of exposure. The CDC recommends that patients be given an initial prescription for PEP for only 3 to 7 days with short-term follow-up for further counseling.[1,6,9]

Referral

Provide patients with oral and written medical discharge instructions. Include a summary of the exam (e.g., evidence collected, tests conducted, medication prescribed or provided, information provided, and treatment received), medication doses to be taken, follow-up appointments needed or scheduled, and referrals. The discharge form could also include contact information and hours of operation for local advocacy programs.[4,18]

Follow-Up

An optimal time for a first medical follow-up contact is 24 to 48 hours following discharge.[4,18]A medical visit should occur within 2 weeks of the acute evaluation; ongoing psychologic and counseling support should be provided. A male victim should be referred to an urologist or proctologist. A child should be referred to a pediatrician.

Follow-up appointment should include[10,18]

- Pregnancy testing
- STD testing for patients who develop interim symptoms or who declined initial evaluation

Complications

Many victims can experience rape trauma syndrome. In the first phase, days to weeks, symptoms may include anger, fear, anxiety, physical pain, sleep disturbance, anorexia, shame, guilt, and intrusive thoughts. The second phase, "reorganization," which may last for months, includes physical and emotional symptoms. Patients may experience muscu-loskeletal, genital, pelvic and or abdominal pain, anorexia, and insomnia. Dreams and nightmares are common and phobias may develop. Patients may develop posttraumatic stress disorder, depression (50% of victims), or anxiety symptoms. Sexual dysfunction has been reported in 24% to 40% of victims up to 6 years after the assault.[4,7]

References

1. U.S. Department of Justice, Office on Violence against Women. A national protocol for sexual assault medical forensic examinations adult/adolescents. September 2004, NCJ 206554.
2. Geist RF. Sexually related trauma. *Emerg Med Clin North Am* 1988;6:439.
3. Fled Haus KM. Female and male sexual assault. In: *Emergency medicine—a comprehensive study guide*. 5th ed. McGraw-Hill, New York; 2000:1952–1955.
4. Burgess AW, Holmstrom LL. Rape: crisis and recovery. Bowie, 1979; Robert J Brady.
5. Up to date. Evaluation and management of rape victims. www.Update.com.
6. U.S. Department of Health and Human Services/Public Health Service. *MMWR* April 4, 1997;46(13).
7. Evaluation and management of sexually assaulted or sexually abused patient. American College of Emergency Physicians. Available online at www.acep.org.
8. National Sexual Violence Resource Center. Available online at www.nsvrc.org.
9. CDC. Gamma Hydroxy Butyrate Use-New York and Texas, 1995–1996." April 14, 1997/46 (13);281–283. Accessible at: http://www.cdc.gov/mmwr/preview/mmrhtm/00047106.htm
10. Enos WF, Beyer JC. Management of the rape victim. *Am Fam Physician* 1978;18:97–102.
11. Hochbaum SR. The evaluation and treatment of the sexually assaulted patient. *Emerg Med Clin North Am* 1987;5:601.
12. Council on Scientific Affairs, American Medical Association. Violence against women: relevance for medical practitioners. *JAMA* 1992;267:3184.
13. Rambow SM, Atkison D, Frost TH, et al. Female sexual assault: medical and legal implications. *Ann Emerg Med* 1992;21:727.
14. Ramim SM, Stain Stone IC, et al. Sexual assault in postmenopausal women. *Obstet Gynecol* 1992;80:860.
15. The California medical protocol for examination of sexual assault and child sexual abuse victims; 2001:98.
16. Dupre AR, Hampton HL, Morrison H, et al. Sexual assault. *Obstet Gynecol Surv* 1993;48:640–648.
17. Berkowitz CD. Abuse and neglect of children. In: *Emergency medicine—a comprehensive study guide*. 5th ed. McGraw-Hill, 2000;115–117.
18. Support services: the Rape Abuse and Incest National Network (RAINN at 1-800-656-HOPE) and the National Coalition Against Sexual Assault (NCASA at 717-728-9764).

Occupational and Environmental Problems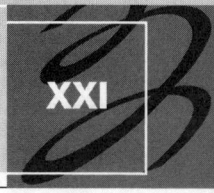

XXI

DISABILITY DETERMINATION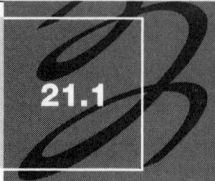
Joanne Williams

21.1

GENERAL PRINCIPLES

Definition

The definition of disability is multifactorial. It is generally accepted as the inability or altered ability to perform a given task successfully; the gap between what a person can do and what he or she needs or wants to do.

Disability determination is an important medical function that not only affects the patient, but also has greater economic ramifications on the patient, the employer, and the economy, in general. Determination of disability is a specialized activity often requiring the use of medical specialists who provide detailed information to a team of workers who evaluate and assign a disability or impairment rating.

The other definitions required to fully appreciate this topic are listed below.

The goal of disability determination is the normalization and equalization of the more than 6 million people, worldwide, with disabilities. It is felt that all persons should have the same rights, obligations, and equal opportunities as other members of society. Efforts to accomplish this equity are due to different socioeconomic circumstances and, in the United States, are due to different provisions regarding disability as determined by the various states.

- **Normal.** The range or zone of function representing healthy functioning; varies with age, gender, environmental conditions. It can be defined based on an individual or population perspective.[1] The preinjury or preillness state is considered the baseline.
- **Impairment.** "A loss, loss of use, or derangement of any body part, organ system or organ function." Impairment is considered permanent when it has reached maximal medical improvement (MMI). The assessment can be objective, such as a fracture, or subjective, such as fatigue or pain.[1] The physician ascribing the percent work disability must be familiar with the specific job duties of the patient as well as the specific activities that the patient can or cannot do, in light of the impairment.
- **Disability.** A broad definition given to persons with various limitations in their ability to meet social or occupational demands. It is the end of the continuum from normal to impairment, to functional limitation, to disability.

■ **Handicap.** A function of the relationship between persons with disabilities and their environments[2]; a legal and policy term describing people living with disabilities.

Evaluating impairment is an exact and tedious task. An expert may be required to best evaluate the patient and accurately assess the degree of disability or rating or percentage of impairment.

The **activities of daily living (ADL) and the instrumental ADL** scales are used to assess patients and their functional limitations. Self-care, communication, physical activity, sensory function, nonspecialized hand activities, travel, sexual function, and sleep. Impairment percentages or ratings are issued based on these activities.

History

After a more than 20-year debate, Social Security exempted disabled persons from making Social Security contribution but allowed them to remain eligible to receive old-age pensions at age 65. Thus, disability was defined at the "inability to engage in any substantial gainful activity because of any medically determinable physical or mental impairment that can be expected to be of long, continued, and indefinite duration"[3] (Social Security Amendments. P.L. 761, Title 1, Section 215(i), Par.3, Washington, DC, 1954).

In 1972, benefits were substantially increased and Medicare benefits were made available to those who had received disability benefits for more than 2 years. Currently, the administration of worker compensation programs varies by state, but is generally administered by a special state agency. Contested claims may employ referees or hearing officers who are highly skilled in worker compensation law and medicine.

Americans with Disabilities Act (ADA) is a civil rights law that was passed in 1990. It protects persons with disabilities, temporary or permanent, from discrimination and mandates accommodations for disabled employees, customers, clients, and patients. This comprehensive act uses a functional approach to disability and encompasses provisions for adequate communication, architectural design of buildings including entrances and exits, and streets and curbs.

Organizations such as the Centers for Disease Control have partnered with the World Health Organization to determine and develop values, goals, and definitions, as well as goals and principles of treatment.

Communication and understanding of one's role in the process of disability determination are crucial to the process. The physician or other health care provider is the person who provides medical information regarding the patient's claim of impairment or disability to the adjudicator who is expected to make the final decision about a patient's disability. The adjudicator also relies on a team of individuals to help provide the information necessary to make that ultimate determination. Often it is necessary to refer the patient to a specialist to make the appropriate assessment. These include, but are not limited to radiologist, physical therapist, occupational nurse or safety specialist, human resource personnel, social workers, psychologists, and vocational rehabilitationists.

Anatomy

Depends on problem or organ system involved (Table 21.1-1).

Epidemiology

The lack of a definite, consistent agreed-upon definition of disability makes it difficult to gather accurate statistics about the number of disabled persons in the country. The Current Population Survey (CPS) defines disability in terms of one's ability to work. It found that disabilities were more prevalent in persons with less education, in minorities, and slightly higher among women. Back disabilities are the leading cause of work disability.

The National Health Interview Survey (NHIS) has carried out self-reporting survey continuously since 1957. In 1995, these data suggested that 14.7% of the population had some had some kind of limitation in activity due to a chronic condition. Additionally, about 2 million disabled persons resided in institutional facilities, This study also found that rates were higher for males, blacks, low-income, and older individuals.

At the high end, the Survey of Income and Programs Participation (SIPP) panel study estimated that 20.6% of the 1995 population had a disability; 9.9% of them a severe disability.

Using the prevalence approach, the aggregate costs of disability in 1980 was estimated at $177 billion, about 6.5% of the gross domestic product. Pain and suffering are difficult to evaluate.[3]

Classification

Where possible, this information has been put into the chart shown in Table 21.1-1. The information is not expected to be exhaustive or complete, by any means, but aims more to provide an appreciation of the vastness of nature of the problems and a way to approach a comprehensive handling of the issues.

Mechanisms of Injury

The causes and consequences of disability vary. Disability may be due to the following:

- Congenital abnormality
- Chronic medical condition
- Psychiatric illness
- Falls, violence, or other trauma
- Overuse
- Exposure (environmental, chemical, including medication)
- Sports injury
- Iatrogenic
- Consequence of aging

TREATMENT

Behavioral

The goal of behavioral treatment is always to help the patient obtain and maintain the highest level of functioning without the least amount of discomfort. This may include lifestyle changes, improving diet, exercising, maintaining health weight, participating in group therapy.

Medications

Coordinated prescribing is important. It is desirable to avoid using narcotics and medications with a high addiction potential.

Surgery

The nature of the surgical procedure would depend on the specific disability.

Nonoperative

These would include behavioral changes such as weight loss, diet modification, physical therapy, and exercise.

Referrals

Depending on the nature of the patient's impairment, referrals may be necessary or desirable. Some of the more common referrals are with physical therapy, pain clinics, help groups, one or more specialists dealing with the patient's particular diagnosis. Ideally, there will be ongoing communication between the referring and primary physician, and follow-up with both physicians.

Counseling

Counseling plays a large and important role in the ongoing management of chronic health issues. It is useful in managing or helping to alleviate problems associated with the depression that so often accompanies chronic illness or disability. Counseling also helps to treat posttraumatic stress disorder, and may be helpful in sorting out cases of suspected malingering.

Patient Education

For all patients, a clear assessment of the problem, reasonable expectations of improvement or of the expected course of the illness, and the complete treatment plan should be given and explained. This should be reviewed and updated at the follow-up visits.

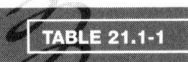 **TABLE 21.1-1**   **Disability Determination**

	Sx/CC	History	Physical exam	Lab	Imaging	Monitoring	Surgical diagnosis procedure
Cardiovascular system	SOB, fatigue, pain, edema	Long-standing hypertension; arrhythmia; family history	Heart murmur, S3 or S4 gallops, JVD	Chemistries, CBC, cardiac enzymes, troponin, TSH, BNP	ECG, cardiac echo, stress test	Follow-up with cardiology and PCP; labs, chest x-ray, ECG, echos	Cath
Respiratory system	SOB, fatigue, pain	Environmental or occupational exposure		ABG, O_2 saturation	ECG, cardiac echo, stress test	PFT; O_2 sat; chest x-ray; peak flow	
Digestive system	Pain, nausea, vomiting	Family history, ingestion of alcohol, or exposure to toxins	Abdominal pain, hemoccult pos. stool guiaic	Chemistries, CBC	EGD, colonoscopy, barium studies	Gastrointestinal follow-up; possible repeat studies; tumor markers	
Genitourinary system	Pain, blood in urine or feces, urinary frequency or nocturia; pelvic or rectal pain	Family history; abnormalities noted on self-exam or exam by health practitioner; risky sexual practices	Erythema or foreign body in urethra; abnormal prostate exam or pelvic exam	U/A, urine C&S	Pelvic or scrotal U/S	Cancer tumor markers, follow-up exams	Cystoscopy
Skin	Itch, pain, rash or some skin perturbation	Exposure to toxins; medical history	Rash, excoriation, skin lesion	RPR, heavy metal screening, skin scraping	Photographs of lesions	Regular exams by dermatologist	Biospy and pathology report
Hematopoietic system	Weakness, bruising, fevers		Conjunctival pallor, ecchymoses, lymphadenopathy	CBC with diff; B_{12}, iron studies; coagulation studies	Chest x-ray	CBC; hematologist visits	Bone marrow
Endocrine system	Diabetes, thyroid, morbid obesity	Medical history		Chemistries, TFTs		Regular monitoring of thyroid functioning; HGBA1C	Aspiration, tissue biopsy
ENT	Pain, decreased or loss of hearing, chronic or recurrent infections	Self-awareness of abnormalities or noted on screening exam		CBC, cultures	CT scan, MRI		Nasolaryngoscopy
Visual system	Low vision, glaucoma; diabetic retinopathy; blindness	Screening exams or self-awareness of abnormalities	Complete ophthalmologic exam	± Blood glucose	CT scan, MRI	Follow-up eye exams	
Neurologic systems—Central nervous system and movement disorders	Pain, headache, dizziness; loss of sense of smell, taste, balance	Complaints of decreased function or symptoms		CBC, RPR, HIV, chemistries, B_{12}, folate	CT scan, MRI; EEG	Alleviation of pain/Sx, ability to function	

Pathophysiologic findings	Differential diagnosis	Treatment: behavioral	Medications	Referrals	Patient education and counseling	Complications
Infection, tumors, valvular heart disease, abnormal ECG, echo, cardiac cath	Congestive heart failure, valvular heart disease	Lifestyle modification: low sodium/ low cholesterol diet, weight control, exercise	Control blood pressure, diuretics, ACE inhibitor or ARB, ASA, antilipid meds	Cardiologist, cardiothoracic surgeon	Diet, exercise, info on lifestyle modification changes, cardiac rehab	Severe disease, refractory to medical treatment
				Pulmonologist	Tobacco cessation, pulmonary rehab	
			PPIs; H2 blockers	GI	Diet, modify angle of bed and activities around meals	
Calculi, inflammation or infection, tumors				GU		
Abnormal pathology report from excised lesions				Derm		
	Anemia, leukemia, lymphoma; thrombotic disorder; HIV; acquired immunno-deficiency			Heme/Onc		
	Diabetes; thyroid or parathyroid disease; obesity; pheochromo-cytoma			Endocrine, surgeon as needed		
				ENT		
				Ophthalmologist		
				Neurology, neurosurgery		

(continued)

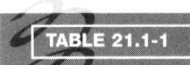

TABLE 21.1-1 **Disability Determination** *(Continued)*

	Sx/CC	History	Physical exam	Lab	Imaging	Monitoring	Surgical diagnosis procedure
Neurologic systems— Peripheral	Pain or tingling in an extremity	Patient complaint	Focal neurologic findings; may be normal	CBC, RPR, HIV, chemistries, B_{12}, folate	CT scan, MRI, EMG/NCS; EEG	Alleviation of pain/Sx, ability to function	
Mental and behavioral psychiatric diagnosis	DSM IV diagnosis	Past medical history; family report or family history	Abnormal mental status exam and psychiatric assessment; psychologic testing	CBC, RPR, HIV, chemistries, B_{12}, folate	CT scan, MRI, EEG	Regain/maintain stable mental functioning	
Addictions— Drugs, prescribed medications	Impaired function	Overusage of prescribed pain meds	Abnormal mental status exam and psychiatric assessment; psychologic testing	Drug screen		Pain clinic	
Drugs— Illegal use	Impaired function	Possible involvement with the law or patient's job	Abnormal mental and psychiatric evaluation	Drug screen		Drug testing, group therapy and/or individual counseling	
Addictions— Alcohol	Impaired function	Possible involvement with the law or patient's job	Abnormal mental and psychiatric evaluation	Drug screen; blood alcohol			
Musculoskeletal system— Spine	Pain, deformity, limited range of motion	May have history of trauma or decreased ability to perform job duties or activities of daily living	Decreased range of motion	Tuberculosis skin test; arthritis profile	Radiographs, CT scan, MRI	Healing of fractures, regaining function, alleviating pain	
Musculoskeletal system— Upper extremity	Pain, deformity, limited range of motion	May have history of trauma or decreased ability to perform job duties or activities of daily living	Decreased range of motion	Arthritis profile	Radiographs, CT scan, MRI	Healing of fractures, regaining function, alleviating pain	
Musculoskeletal system— Lower extremity	Pain, deformity, limited range of motion	May have history of trauma or decreased ability to perform job duties or activities of daily living	Decreased range of motion	Arthritis profile	Radiographs, CT scan, MRI	Healing of fractures, regaining function, alleviating pain	
Chronic fatigue	Fatigue, inability to function	History of prior infection	Complete physical exam, generally normal	CBC, chemistries, TSH, HIV, hepatitis profile; viral cultures	Chest x-ray, CT scan	Maintaining or regaining function; ability to do activities of daily living	

Pathophysiologic findings	Differential diagnosis	Treatment: behavioral	Medications	Referrals	Patient education and counseling	Complications
				Neurology, neurosurgery		
				Psychiatry/ psychology		
		Group therapy, psych assessment, counseling	Antidepressants, pain meds, as needed	Pain clinic; psychiatry	Exercise	
		Group therapy, psych assessment, counseling		Psychiatry/ psychology		
		Group therapy, psych assessment, counseling		Psychiatry/ psychology		
				Ortho, neurosurgery		
				Ortho, PT, pain clinic		
				Ortho, PT, pain clinic		
	Infection, depression, presentation of other disease		Pain meds, muscle relaxants	PT, counseling		

Follow-Up

Follow-up with the primary physician and consultants, as needed, is an important part of the patient's improvement. This should be coordinated between all involved parties, especially regarding pain medication, and there should be ongoing, bidirectional communication about the patient and his or her condition and treatment expectations. One of the goals of follow-up is to ensure that the patient is not lost to appropriate care. There may be insurance issues or other problems that can develop during periods of prolonged care. New problems may develop that would need to be addressed. These would be identified, evaluated, and treated by the team of physicians.

Complications

Again, the nature of the possible complication depends on the nature of the problem, impairment, or disability. Some of the more common, more general complications are as follows:

- Chronic pain
- Lack of improvement
- Patient becomes psychologically disabled or impaired or loses the will to get better
- Patients desire not to return to work; may not match functional abilities
- Question of malingering or patient's apparent impairment does not match the objective physical findings or the mechanism/nature of injury

SPECIAL CONSIDERATIONS

Older patients have special needs and situations; there are two groups: elderly individuals who become disabled and the disabled who age and become elderly. Some of the health challenges that are affected by or that are of particular concern to an older population include: stroke, traumatic brain injury, spinal cord injuries, amputation, posthip fracture, and postjoint replacement. Added to their problems are the location of and provisions needed for rehabilitation of the older patient.[4]

References

1. AMA. *Guides to the evaluation of permanent impairment.* 5th ed. Cocchiarella L, Andersson G, eds. American Medical Association; Philadelphia: 2002.
2. World Health Organization. International classification of functioning, disability and health; includes information on rehabilitation and care of the disabled person. Available online at http://www.who.int/classifications/icf/en/.
3. Demeter S, Andersson G, eds. *Disability evaluation.* 2nd ed. St. Louis, MO: Mosby; 2003.
4. Cruise C, Sasson N, Lee M. Rehabilitation outcomes in the older adult. *Clin Geriatr Med.*
5. Anfang S, Wall B. Psychiatric fitness-for-duty evaluations. *Psychiatr Clin North Am* 2006;4(9):675–693.
6. Pain in patient groups frequently treated by physiatrists. *Phys Med Rehab Clin North Am* 2006;17(2):275–285.
7. Sattinger A, Sinclair LB, Lollar DJ, eds. Healthy people 2010 disability and secondary conditions focus area 6: reports and proceedings, Sept. 20–21, 2002 and Dec. 4–5, 2000. Atlanta GA: National Center on Birth Defects and Developmental Disabilities, Centers for Disease Control; 2003.
8. Sinclair LB. Disability and ethnic minorities: Analysis of the literature, 1990–2000. *Neurorehab Neural Repair* 2005;19(1):64S–65S.
9. The standard rules on the equalization of opportunities for persons with disabilities. Adopted by the United Nations General Assembly, 48th session, resolution 48/96, annex, of 20 December 1993.

HELPFUL INTERNET SITES

www.geriatric.theclinics.com
www.dir.ca.gov/CHSWC/AMAGuides_WorkersCompBrochure.pdf
www.occupationalmedicine.com
www.acoem.org
www.who.int/classifications/icf/en/

PESTICIDE AND RELATED POISONING
Jason L. Musser

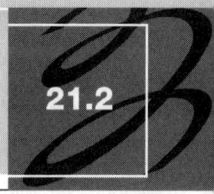

GENERAL PRINCIPLES

Pesticides represent hundreds of chemicals mixed into thousands of formulations targeted at a specific pest, crop, or structure. They are used throughout the world in home, office, industrial, agricultural, and military applications. These chemicals are used in gaseous, liquid, and in solid forms. The range of chemicals includes organophosphates, elements, organochlorides, carbamates, dipyridyls, chlorophenoxy compounds, anticoagulants, hydrocarbons, and more.

Epidemiology

A person's presence in an area where pesticides are used does not necessarily mean that there will be exposure. Exposure does not necessarily mean there will be adequate contact to produce the physiologic changes of poisoning. Poisoning may not automatically lead to impairment or disability.

Pathophysiology

As in all poisonings, time and amount of exposure will influence the effects on the patient's systems. Organophosphates and carbamates are acetylcholinesterase inhibitors used in insecticides and nerve agents. Organophosphates immediately penetrate the central nervous system (CNS) and permanently inactivate acetylcholinesterase, producing acute cholinergic symptoms from the accumulation of acetylcholine in the body. Whereas organophosphates enter the CNS immediately, carbamates do not and their action on the enzyme is reversible leading to limited toxicity.

Symptoms

The effects of the increased acetylcholine are felt by the muscarinic and nicotinic receptors producing miosis and mydriasis, bradycardia or tachycardia, salivation, lacrimation, urination, nausea, vomiting, bronchorrhea, bronchospasm, weakness, hypertension, and diaphragmatic failure.[1] The most life-threatening concerns are the bronchorrhea, bronchospasm, and respiratory insufficiency. Effects on the CNS include headache, confusion, delirium, seizures, and coma. Many pesticides and nerve agents are formulated to resist degradation and thus stay around in the area and on persons who have come in contact with the chemical. Decontamination, both at the site and again upon arriving at a medical facility, should be considered a highest priority in order to protect others from harm.

DIAGNOSIS

Mild poisonings are associated with few symptoms and normal vital signs. Moderate poisonings are associated with more severe symptoms, objective signs, and normal vital signs. Severe poisonings are associated with multiple complaints, objective signs, and unstable vital signs. Exercise caution as some pesticides may exhibit delayed onset of symptoms and signs. Signs and symptoms are detailed in the pathophysiology section above for organophosphates. The signs and symptoms of other pesticide and related poisonings vary and the diagnosis is many times made upon history alone. In suspected poisonings where the substance is not known and the clinical picture is confusing, consulting the poison control center and local toxicologists is highly recommended. In any poisoning, early communication with the poison control center is advisable as it will have the latest information on diagnosis and treatment.

- **Initial care** involves evacuation, decontamination, and treatment.
  - **Remove from exposure.** Persons who are exposed must leave immediately and stay away until the area is safe.

- ▓ **Decontamination.** Each exposed person should bathe thoroughly, with careful attention to the hair. Clothing should be removed and be treated as hazardous waste. If exposed, the eyes need to be aggressively irrigated.
- ▓ **Emergency care** should be instituted as soon as practicable. Responders must be careful not to expose themselves.

History

- Contact the employer or applicator for the name of the formulation and the material safety data sheet (MSDS).
- Question how the exposure occurred, with emphasis on the exact mechanism of exposure, cause and effect relationship of exposure and symptoms, previous exposures and poisonings, and drug- or alcohol-related problems.
- Symptoms (and signs) may vary by the type of formulation to which the person was exposed, the length and concentration of exposure, and decontamination. Nausea, vomiting, fatigue, and vertigo are common to most poisonings but may also represent other diseases as well as psychogenic illness. The classic symptoms of salivation, lacrimation, urination, and diarrhea—the SLUD syndrome seen in organophosphate poisoning—may not be seen in low-concentration poisoning of short duration, although the person may have fatigue and vertigo.

Physical Examination

- **Skin.** Rashes should be carefully described and secondary changes caused by scratching and treatment documented. Halogenated hydrocarbons can produce chloracne, often confused with acne vulgaris.
- **Respiratory.** Inhalation of dusts, mists, and gases may cause instantaneous or delayed bronchospasm.
- **Gastrointestinal (GI).** Nausea, vomiting, diarrhea, and abdominal pain occur as a result of eating contaminated food or by direct ingestion of poison in attempted suicides and homicides.
- **Neurologic.** Acute or delayed polyneuropathy and chronic lapses in concentration and memory can result from exposure to organophosphates and halogenated hydrocarbons.
- **Ocular.** Sprays or mists to the eyes can cause problems ranging from simple conjunctivitis to corneal opacities.

Laboratory Tests

Laboratory tests are of limited usefulness and care should not be delayed waiting for them. Urine and blood pesticide levels are costly, must be collected as soon after exposure as possible, may take weeks to produce results, and may be negative even in well-documented exposures. Blood, liver, and kidney test results may be clouded by the presence of other diseases and may be abnormal in only the most severe poisonings. Cholinesterase (ChE) activity tests are useful only in organophosphate and carbamate poisoning and are most effective when used in a monitoring program for applicators where baselines have been established. A person can have a 60% drop in ChE activity levels and still stay in "normal" ranges. A postexposure series of tests demonstrating a dip with recovery may be the only laboratory response elicited. ChE activity levels can also be affected by cocaine use and the taking of medications.

Research

Whenever possible, physicians should learn the name of the chemical and its properties before embarking on nonemergency treatment. Sources include the MSDS, reference texts, poison control centers, telephone numbers on the pesticide container, TOXLINE, and MEDLINE.

TREATMENT

As previously stated, the cornerstone of pesticide treatment is decontamination, stabilization, and supportive care. In more severe cases this may include airway and circulation support. Decontamination should not be ignored in the hospital setting. Gastric elimination of the substance, if ingested, should be performed. See Chapter 3.3 for specific elimination options. Mild poisonings may be able to be evaluated and followed on an outpatient basis, depending on the poison. Individuals may require only decontamination, reassurance, antiemetics for nausea and vomiting, and steroids for rash. Observe for a minimum of 2 hours. Contact with the poison control centers will help determine if this is an option, as many pesticides have delayed action and an initially stable patient may not stay that way for long.[2] Moderate symptoms (to include eye irritation without intense blepharospasms, minor skin erythema, and small blisters less than 2 cm in size) should be observed for 24 hours for any deterioration in clinical condition.

Severe poisonings (from early eye irritation worsening to severe blepharospasm, obvious skin blister, weakness, neurologic involvement, and respiratory difficulty) require hospitalization and intensive physiologic support.[2] Elimination enhancement, forced diuresis, exchange transfusion, and chelation are replete with complications and should be considered only when the patient's condition is severe, on an inpatient basis, when the specific agent has been identified, and after consulting toxicology experts. Atropine is the hallmark of initial treatment in organophosphate and carbamate poisoning. It does not reverse the nicotinic effects but does help control secretions in cases of respiratory distress from bronchorrhea, bronchospasm, and respiratory insufficiency. The initial dosage is 2 to 4 mg IV every 2 to 5 minutes as needed for control of airway secretions. Glycopyrrolate can be considered instead of atropine in cases of no CNS involvement. Nerve agent poisonings generally require less atropine. More lipid soluble poisons may require large doses of atropine (up to a total of 40 to 100 mg/day). Continuous IV infusion of atropine, starting at 0.05 mg/kg/hour and titrated, can also be used in severe cases.[1]

Pralidoxime (2-PAM) is required in patients with significant muscle weakness in organophosphate poisoning and allows for the reactivation of cholinesterases if it is given before irreversible binding of the toxin occurs (24 to 48 hours depending on the specific agent). Initial dosing is 1 to 2 g IV over 10 to 20 minutes followed by 200 to 500 mg per hour infusion.[1]

Complications

Respiratory paralysis, weakness, and depressed reflexes can occur 24 to 96 hours after resolution of the severe crisis and general support is all that is required with resolution of this within 1 to 3 weeks. Delayed neurotoxicity and polyneuropathy can occur up to 1 to 3 weeks later with variable recovery.[1]

Follow-Up

Serial examinations to follow chronic problems may be necessary, especially with neurologic and respiratory involvement. Work impairments and disability status must be documented. The possibility of fraud must be considered and documented if discovered.

SPECIAL CONSIDERATION

In jurisdictions where required, reports must be made to the appropriate agencies in accidental poisonings. Intentional poisoning and any suspected terrorist or malicious poisoning should be immediately reported to the appropriate authorities.

References

1. Zimmerman JL. Poisonings and overdoses in the intensive care unit: general and specific management issues. *Crit Care Med* 2003;31(12).
2. Baker DJ. Critical care requirements after mass toxic agent release. *Crit Care Med* 2005;33(1 Suppl):S66–74.
3. Barthold CL, Schier JG. Organic phosphorus compounds—nerve agents. *Crit Care Clin* 2005;21(4):673–689.
4. Fry DE. Chemical threats. *Surg Clin North Am* 2006;86(3).
5. Lessenger JE. Pesticide and related poisoning. In: *Manual of family practice*. 2nd ed. Philadelphia: Lippincott Williams & Wilkins; 2001.

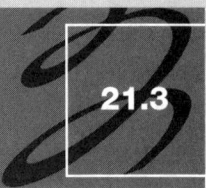

OCCUPATIONAL LUNG DISEASES
Trang H. Nguyen, David C. Randolph

*T*he most common occupational lung diseases are asthma, hypersensitivity pneumonitis, toxic pneumonitis, pneumoconiosis (asbestosis, coal worker's pneumoconiosis, and silicosis), work-related pulmonary infections, and lung cancer.[1] Because these patients may present with nonspecific or undifferentiated pulmonary symptoms, documentation of the nature and duration of exposure is essential. As these illnesses may present years after the occupational exposure, a detailed past medical and occupational history is required.[2-4]

OCCUPATIONAL ASTHMA
General Principles
Definition
Occupational asthma is characterized by variable airflow limitation and bronchial hyper-responsiveness caused by conditions attributable to a particular work environment. The variable airflow obstruction is reverse spontaneously or with treatment.
There are generally two different subtypes of occupational asthma.

- Allergic (long latency)
  - Large-molecular-weight sensitizers (examples: plant allergens, insect, animal)
  - Low-molecular-weight sensitizers (examples: di-isocyanates and acid anhydrides)
- Irritant-induced asthma (no latency)
  - Reactive airways dysfunction syndrome (RADS)
  - Not-so-sudden irritant-induced asthma

Note: Pre-existing asthma made worse by the workplace exposure is NOT considered occupational asthma.

Mechanism
- **Early phase.** Allergen–immunoglobulin E (IgE) mast cell interaction causes cytokines production. This cause an increase in vascular permeability and bronchoconstriction. As a result, macrophages and T lymphocytes are recruited.
- **Late phase.** CD4 lymphocyte cytokines will lead to increase in IgE, mast cell, and eosinophils production. TH1 and TH2 lymphocytes will recruit more leukocytes to the site to cause chronic inflammation.

Epidemiology
This condition accounts for approximately 25% to 50% of all occupational lung disease and is responsible for approximately 5% to 15% of all asthma cases.

Etiology
More than 250 plausible causes have been associated with occupational asthma. The most common of these are isocyanates, wood dust, dyes, irritant gases and fumes (e.g., chlorine and ammonia), flour, animal dander, and latex. Isocyanates (di-isocyanates) are responsible for more cases of occupational asthma than any other single substance; approximately 5% of workers exposed to volatile isocyanates develop asthma.[5]

Diagnosis
Clinical Presentation
Most common symptoms of asthma are cough (also nocturnal cough), wheezing, chest tightness, and shortness of breath. Respiratory symptoms that occur within 1 hour after

work begins or 6 to 8 hours later are consistent with but not diagnostic of occupational asthma. Symptoms that worsen during the workweek but improve during weekends or vacations are suggestive of occupationally induced asthma.

History
History includes the exposure to substances known to cause occupational asthma, as well as the duration and intensity of exposure. Because many products contain multiple chemicals, the Material Safety Data Sheet (MSDS) should be obtained from the company's safety officer and reviewed for known causative agents. Timing is important, as there may be a latency versus no latency period. When did the symptoms begin? What makes symptoms worse or better? Also important are a personal history of asthma, atopy, hay fever, other pulmonary disorders, family history of asthma, medications, environment at home, and personal habits.

Physical Examination
Expiratory wheezing, shortness of breath, atopic dermatitis, nasal polyps, sinusitis.

Diagnostic Testing
Lung Function Tests
- Changes to demonstrate *reversible airway obstruction*
- 12% increase in forced expiratory volume in 1 second (FEV_1) with absolute value ≥ 200 mL postbronchodilations
- Positive nonspecific bronchoprovocation tests ($PC_{20} \leq 8$ mg/mL)
- Improvement in $FEV_1 \geq 20\%$ after a trial of steroids
- 20% change in peak expiratory flow measured while at work for 2 weeks and while off work for 2 weeks

Immunologic Studies
- Skin prick test. Best when the workplace allergen extracts are well characterized. Sensitivity specificity (SN) 74%, SP 89% for large-molecular-weight allergens.
- Radioallergosorbent test (RAST). SN 57%, SP 86% for large-molecular-weight allergens.
- Basophil histamine release test. SN 78%, SP 93% for large-molecular-weight allergens.

Inhalation Provocation Tests. Specific inhalation challenge is the gold standard to confirm occupational asthma. A decrease of FEV_1 of 20% is considered a positive test.

Nonspecific Inhalation Challenge. Patient breathing a sequence of nebulized mists containing progressively increased concentrations of bronchoconstricting agents such as methacholine or histamine.

Imaging
The chest radiograph is useful to exclude other pulmonary conditions or complications of asthma.

Differential Diagnoses
Includes pre-existing asthma, allergy to indoor allergens, hypersensitivity pneumonitis, bronchiolitis obliterans, byssinosis, organic toxic dust syndrome, and metal fume fever.

Treatment
Medications
Include inhaled agents such as β-agonists, corticosteroids, and mast cell membrane stabilizers. Noninhaled agents include leukotriene antagonists, theophylline, and systemic corticosteroids.

Prevention of occupational asthma is preferable to management of bronchospasm. Early detection of reversible airway disease may facilitate a plan to prevent chronic symptoms. Complete avoidance of the offending substance is the primary means of preventing recurrence of symptoms. This may be accomplished by transferring the worker from the specific area of causation. Alternatively, the work area may be changed, such as by making an open system into a closed system or by improving or redirecting the ventilation. Personal protective equipment and high-efficiency particulate air (HEPA) filters may be used in certain circumstances.

HYPERSENSITIVITY PNEUMONITIS (EXTRINSIC ALLERGIC ALVEOLITIS)

General Principles

Definition

Hypersensitivity pneumonitis encompasses a group of occupational lung diseases that include farmers' lung, bird fanciers' disease, Japanese summer-type hypersensitivity pneumonitis, humidifier lung, bagassosis, and mushroom workers' lung. Agricultural workers are at particularly increased risk for these disorders.

Mechanism

The hypersensitivity pneumonitis is caused by hyperimmune reactions of the lung tissues to inhaled antigens. It is an interstitial granulomatous lung disease caused by repeated inhalation of antigens in organic dusts. These antigens are typically of fungal or animal protein origin.

Epidemiology

Difficult to estimate, and the tendency is probably to underestimate the incidence.

Etiology

Usually due to contamination of vegetable produce with microbes when stored in damp, humid, and moldy climate.

Diagnosis

Clinical Presentation

Hypersensitivity pneumonitis can be categorized as acute, subacute, and chronic. Acute hypersensitivity pneumonitis consists of flulike signs and symptoms including cough, fever, chills, myalgias, malaise, dyspnea, and tachycardia within 3 to 8 hours after exposure to an environmental antigen. Subacute and chronic hypersensitivity pneumonitis can include progressive shortness of breath and chronic cough.

Physical Examination

- **Acute.** Auscultation usually reveals bilateral inspiratory crackles with fever.
- **Subacute and chronic.** Weight loss, clubbing of nails, inspiratory crackles, rhonchi, squawks with auscultation, and signs of corpulmonale in advanced situation.

Diagnostic Testing

Chest radiograph may reveal diffuse infiltrates mostly in the lower lung fields. Spirometry reveals decreased lung volumes with a decrease in vital capacity revealing a restrictive defect. In chronic state, obstructive, restrictive, or mixed pattern may be seen. High-resolution computed tomography (HRCT) is important in the diagnosis of hypersensitivity pneumonitis. HRCT indicates ground-glass patchy infiltrates along with a mosaic pattern in the lower zones of the lung. Bronchoscopy with brochoalveolar lavage is now the standard in the diagnosis of hypersensitivity pneumonitis. In hypersensitivity pneumonitis, the ratio of T-suppressor subtype lymphocytes CD4+/CD8+ is usually less than 1.

Differential Diagnosis

Includes organic dust toxic syndrome, sarcoidosis, miliary tuberculosis (TB), *Pneumocystis carinii* pneumonia, bronchiolitis obliterans with organizing pneumonitis, and berylliosis.

Treatment

Includes corticosteroids, oxygen, and bronchodilators. Workers who have severe symptoms or hypoxemia require hospitalization for more aggressive treatment.

Prevention

Avoidance of exposure to the precipitating antigen is best. In some circumstances use of respirators will reduce exposure to relatively safe levels.

TOXIC PNEUMONITIS

Organic Agents

Other conditions in this category include Mill fever, Monday morning fever, grain fever, swine confinement, farmers fever, humidifier fever, and mycotoxicosis. Organic dust toxic syndrome (ODTS) is also known as toxin fever and toxic pneumonitis.[1]

General Principles

Etiology. Usually very high exposure to organic dust such as bacteria, fungi, and toxins. Workers in textile, grain, livestock, and horticulture industries are at risk.

Diagnosis

History. Symptoms normally occur on the first day of returning to work from some period of time off (therefore, sometimes it is called Monday morning fever) and very high moldy dust seen by workers.

Clinical Presentation. Usually a flulike reaction, fever, myalgias, chest tightness, cough, headache, nausea normally 4 to 12 hours after the initial exposure.

Physical Examination. The patient may have fever (38.5 to 40.0°C), increased respiratory rate, and bibasilar crackles, while wheezing is often not present.

Diagnostic Testing. Spirometry. Mild restrictive pattern, mild decreased in total lung capacity and diffusion capacity. Chest radiographs can be normal or patchy infiltrates. Broncho alveolar lavage (BAL) may be helpful.

Differential Diagnosis. Includes viral syndrome, pneumonia, and allergic alveolitis.

Treatment

Acutely, paracetamol or nonsteroidal anti-inflammatory drugs (NSAIDs) as needed. Corticosteroids are *not* recommended.

Prevention. Causal agent should be identified to prevent recurrences. Consider modifying job tasks and using respiratory protection.

Prognosis. The course is usually benign with no long-term sequelae.

Chemical Agents

Also known as chemical-induced lung injury. There are three subtypes:

- Inhalation fevers
- Acute chemical pneumonitis
- Subacute toxic pneumonitis

Inhalation Fevers (Metal Fume Fever and Polymer Fume Fever)
General Principles

- **Etiology.** Metal fume fever is due to direct inhalation of heated zinc (zinc oxide) or exposure to fumes of heated Teflon, plastics, polymers, and polyurethane. Welders and metal trade workers are at increased risk.

Diagnosis

- **Clinical presentation.** Flulike symptoms occur, and may include ocular or respiratory irritant symptoms, fever, chills, headaches, malaise, nausea, cough, sore throat, and muscle aches occurring 4 to 8 hours after exposure.
- **Physical examination.** Ascultation of the lung is often normal. Crackles may be heard in severe cases.
- **Diagnostic testing.** Chest radiographs may show transient infiltrates. Spirometry test can be normal.
- **Differential diagnosis.** Includes asthma and hypersensitivity pneumonitis.

Treatment

Anti-inflammatory medication as needed.

- **Prevention.** Discourage smoking in the workplace. Metal fumes should be kept below the occupational threshold limit value.
- **Prognosis.** Usually self-limiting, benign course.

Acute Chemical Pneumonitis

Etiology. Acute chemical pneumonitis can be caused by irritant gases (NH_3, SO_2, HCl, Cl_2, H_2S, O_3, NO_2), organic chemicals (acetic acids, aldehydes, isocyanates, amines, tear gas, organic solvents, and agrichemicals), metallic compounds (mercury, metallic oxides, halides, hydrides), and complex mixtures (fire smoke, pyrolysis products, solvent mixtures).

Diagnosis

- **Clinical presentation.** Includes irritation of eyes, nose, throat, cough, hoarseness, wheezing, and chest pain.
- **Physical examination.** Ascultation of the lung can be normal or wheezing, rhonchi can be heard.
- **Diagnostic testing.** Chest radiographs can be normal. Spirometry test is consistent with obstructive or mixed patterns.

Treatment

Steroids are used for severe conditions.

Subacute Toxic Pneumonitis

Other conditions in this category: acute silicosis, Ardystil syndrome, and nylon flock worker's lung.[1]

Pneumoconiosis. Describes the group of pulmonary diseases caused by the deposition of dust in the lungs. The dusts that cause pneumoconiosis are asbestos, coal dust, silica, beryllium, graphite, aluminum, and others. Asbestos, coal dust, and silica have affected the largest number of workers. The ILO has standardized procedures for radiologic evaluation of pneumoconiosis, and the NIOSH National Coal Workers' Health Surveillance Program has adopted these standards along with specific certification requirements for radiologists.[1]

Asbestosis. Asbestosis is a diffuse fibrotic condition of the lung caused by naturally occurring fibrous mineral silicate. The prevalence of asbestosis is variable and depends on the type of asbestos fiber, the type of industry, dose of exposure, and age. The highest prevalence was found among insulation workers. The main occupational exposures have been asbestos mining, asbestos removal, building demolition, textile and tile manufacturing, shipbuilding, pipefitting, and application of asbestos fireproofing and insulation. The latency period for the disease is generally 15 to 20 years. Other diseases associated with asbestos are carcinoma of the lung, malignant mesothelioma, and benign pleural lung disease (pleural plaques, pleural thickening, and pleural effusion).[1]

- **Diagnosis.** Based on the following criteria from the American Thoracic Society:
  - A reliable history of asbestos exposure
  - Appropriate duration from time of exposure to time of disease detection
  - Chest radiographys with type s, t, u, small irregular opacities of a profusion of I/I or greater
  - Restrictive pattern on lung function test with forced vital capacity (FVC) less than normal limit
  - DL_{CO} less than normal limit
  - Bilateral inspiratory crackles audible in posterior lower lung fields

The usual duration of exposure before changes are visualize on chest x-rays is at least 15 years. The greater and longer duration of exposure, the more severe the disease and the greater the number of workers who will develop the disease.

- **Clinical presentation.** Patients present with cough, shortness of breath, thoracic pain, or hemoptysis.
- **Physical examination.** Findings include inspiratory crackles in the lower lung fields. Clubbing of the fingers may be seen occasionally.
- **Diagnostic testing.**
  - **Chest x-rays.** Small, irregular opacities can be visualized in lower lung fields. Honeycombing may be seen in severe stage. However, posteroanterior (PA) chest x-rays have poor sensitivity and specificity. HRCT with 1-mm sections is more accurate at detecting asbestosis in asymptomatic subjects.
  - **Spirometry test.** Restrictive pattern with decreased in total lung capacity (TLC), FVC, and DL_{CO}.
- **Differential diagnosis.** Hypersensitivity pneumonitis, connective tissue disorders, and idiopathic pulmonary fibrosis.

- **Treatment.** Only supportive care, as there is no effective treatment. Smoking should be avoided.
  - **Prevention** of asbestosis is accomplished by controlling asbestos dust and preventing workers from coming into direct contact with asbestos particles. This usually requires workers to wear protective suits and respirators when performing tasks such as removal of insulation. The 1995 Occupational Safety and Health Administration asbestos standard requires employers to provide medical surveillance for employees who work with or around asbestos for more than 30 days in a year.
  - **Prognosis.** Progression of disease is dependent on the total dose of exposure, fiber type, and susceptibility of the individual. The severity on chest x-rays has been shown to correlate positively with probability disease progression.

Coal Worker's Pneumoconiosis (CWP). Is an interstitial lung disease due to chronic exposure to coal dusts. Black lung is the term used in the Federal Coal Mine Health and Safety Act, which defines the coal miners' benefits program. Coal dust can result in a spectrum of conditions, including simple or complicated pneumoconiosis, progressive massive fibrosis (PMF), chronic bronchitis, and emphysema. Occupations including underground mining, face working, roof bolting, and tunnel drilling are at increased risk of exposure.[1]

- **General principles**
  - **Epidemiology.** The prevalence in the United States is approximately 10%.
  - **Mechanisms.** Coal dust targets macrophages and epithelial cells, which become activated, releasing reactive oxygen species, cytokines, and proteases that damage lung tissue.
- **Diagnosis.** Based on occupational exposure to coal dust, symptoms, and radiologic findings.
  - **Clinical presentation.** Patients present with productive cough and shortness of breath with exertion.
  - **Physical examination.** No specific findings may be noted. In advance stage of complicated CWP, findings of emphysematous changes can be present.
  - **Diagnostic testing.** Chest radiograph may show round, small densities in the upper zones initially with middle and lower zones involvement at later stages. PMF is associated with increased radiologic nodularity, sometimes coupled with bullous emphysematous changes. Computed tomography (CT) of the chest has higher sensitivity than chest radiography in simple CWP. Advanced disease is associated with both obstructive and restrictive impairment of lung function with decreases in FEV_1 and FVC, and decreased diffusion capacity.
- **Treatment.** Treatment of persons with CWP, PMF, and emphysema caused by coal dust is largely unsatisfactory, although standard bronchodilator therapy may be useful.
  - **Prevention.** Prevention is done by dust control primarily by ventilation and respiratory protection. Periodic medical examinations are now required of all coal mine workers. Workers who have early radiologic evidence of CWP (e.g., simple CWP) should be removed from the exposure, which effectively halts development of disease.
  - **Prognosis.** Simple CWP categories 1, 2, and 3 and complicated CWP category A can be expected to have the same life expectancy as the general population.
- **Related disorders.** CWP have been associated with rheumatoid disease (Caplan syndrome), tuberculosis, bronchitis, and emphysema.

Silicosis. Silicosis is a chronic fibrotic disease of the lungs caused by exposure to free crystalline silica. Compounds that contain silica are sand, quartz, and certain mining products. The disease is usually seen after 10 to 30 years of exposure. It may be seen in an accelerated pattern if exposure has been intense. Industrial sources of free silica include mining, stonework, sandblasting, foundry work, and glass manufacturing.[1]

- **Diagnosis**
  - **Clinical presentation.** Due to prolonged exposure, most workers are older than 40 years at presentation. Productive cough.

- **Physical examination.** Physical findings include crackles and wheezes. In advanced stages, emphysematous changes may develop.
- **Diagnostic testing.** Spirometry is usually normal in early disease. In more advanced stages, restrictive pattern can be expected. Chest radiographs show small, round opacities in upper zone with hilar enlargement. Eggshell calcification of the hilar nodes is characteristic of silicosis. End-stage silicosis is characterized by progressive decline in pulmonary capacity with the development of fibrotic masses in the upper lung fields.
- **Differential diagnosis.** Includes sarcoidosis, histoplasmosis, tuberculosis, other pneumoconiosis, and chronic fungal diseases.

- **Treatment.** Treatment of silicosis is supportive. Workers with any degree of silicosis should be prevented from working in areas of silica dust, although the disease may progress despite this measure.
  - **Prevention.** Controlling exposure to silica dust through the use of strict environmental control techniques is important.
  - **Prognosis.** Disease progression is dependent on the type of silica, intensity and duration of exposure, and susceptibility of the host.

Occupational Nontuberculous Lung Infections

- **General principles.** Etiologic agent can come from different sources.
  - Human (influenza, *Streptococcus*, and *Chlamydia* pneumonia)
  - Animal (anthrax, *Coxiella burnettii,* brucellosis, psittacosis, tularemia, and plague)
  - Environment (sporotrichosis, coccidiodonycosis, legionellosis)
  - **Clinical presentation.** Usual presentation includes fever, chills, malaise, weight loss, cough, chest pain, and shortness of breath.

- **Diagnosis.** Diagnosis of occupational lung infections involves a detailed history of exposure, physical examination, chest radiograph, appropriate cultures, and serologic testing.
- **Treatment.** Treatment of these infections requires precise diagnosis based on cultures and is usually amenable to standard treatment.
  - **Prevention.** Prevention of occupational lung infections may require respiratory protection in the presence of potential exposure. Consider vaccine availability and safety. Monitor and control potential for pathogen transmission.

References

1. Hendrick DJ, Sherwood B, eds. *Occupational disorders of the lung, recognition, management, and prevention.* Philadelphia: WB Saunders; 2002.
2. U.S. Centers for Disease Control and Prevention. Work related lung disease surveillance report. Washington, DC: U.S. Department of Health and Human Services; 1999.
3. Levin SM, Kahn PE, Lax MB. Medical examination for asbestos-related disease. *Am J Ind Med* 2000;37:6.
4. Beckett WS, Bascom R. Occupational lung disease. *Occup Med State Art Rev* 1992;7:2.
5. Bernstein DI, Jolly A. Current diagnostic methods for diisocyanate induced occupational asthma. *Am J Ind Med* 1999;36:459.

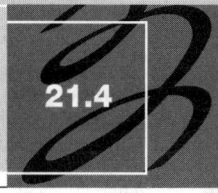

HEAT-RELATED SYNDROMES
Quinn Saigh

21.4

GENERAL PRINCIPLES

Heat-related syndromes occur when the effects of environmental and metabolic heat result in illness. When the ambient temperature rises above 95°F, the evaporation of sweat is the body's only effective mechanism of heat dissipation. High humidity limits the evaporation of sweat.

Dehydration, medications that limit sweating (antihistamines, anticholinergics, phenothiazines), poor conditioning, obesity, sleep deprivation, alcoholism, chronic disease, and extremes of age all compromise the ability to tolerate heat load.

MINOR SYNDROMES

- **Heat cramps.** Patients complain of brief, intense cramps that last approximately 1 to 3 minutes in severely stressed muscles. In addition, patients may experience muscle twitches and tenderness. Workers and athletes are typically affected after profuse sweating from vigorous physical activity/exercise, which causes fluid and electrolyte depletion. Physical exam may reveal cool and moist skin, but body temperature will be within the normal range. Laboratory data may show hyponatremia, hemoconcentration, and an elevated blood urea nitrogen (BUN) and creatinine. Heat cramps respond well to rest and an oral fluid and electrolyte replacement. Gradual heat acclimation, increased dietary salt, and ongoing fluid replacement are preventive measures.

- **Heat edema** refers to swelling of the feet and ankles that occurs with heat stress in addition to prolonged sitting or standing. This condition is most commonly seen in elderly and nonacclimatized individuals. Heat edema is a benign condition that responds well to rest in a cool environment, elevation of the lower extremities, and support stockings. Diuretics should be avoided in patients with edema secondary to heat exposure. Diagnostic workup for more serious conditions (congestive heart failure, liver failure, kidney failure, etc.) is warranted if additional physical signs and symptoms are present that support these diagnoses.

- **Heat syncope** occurs at high temperatures with vigorous physical activity/exercise, which causes volume depletion and cutaneous vasodilation. Ultimately, dilation of the vascular space leads to compromised venous return and, subsequently, loss of consciousness. Advanced age and dehydration are common precipitating factors. In addition, medications like anticholinergics and diuretics are often contributory to heat syncope and should be adjusted accordingly. On physical exam, patients may present with a weak pulse, hypotension, and cool skin secondary to volume depletion, but body temperature will not be elevated. Management consists of putting the patient in a cool environment in the recumbent position. In addition, the patient should receive oral and/or intravenous fluid replacement and close observation. In extreme heat, maintaining adequate hydration, rising gradually from lying or sitting positions, and wearing support hose may all help to prevent recurrences of syncope.

MAJOR SYNDROMES

Heat Exhaustion

Clinical Presentation

Heat exhaustion symptoms include profuse sweating, cutaneous flushing, nausea, vomiting, headache, muscle weakness, dizziness, and visual disturbances.

775

Diagnosis

A patient with heat exhaustion will present with a clear sensorium without neurologic findings. In this case, core body temperature is often elevated. Tachycardia, hyperventilation, and hypotension occur in serious cases of heat exhaustion.

Management

The patient must be immediately taken to a cool environment with excess clothing removed and sponged with tepid water. Oral rehydration should be initiated at a rate of 1 L per hour for several hours. Serious cases are best managed by transporting the patient to an emergency medical facility more equipped to manage these patients. Hemoconcentration, azotemia, and oliguria are corrected by initiation of intravenous rehydration with either dextrose in normal saline or dextrose in half-normal saline. Caution should be taken in elderly individuals to avoid complications associated with fluid overload.

Exercise-Associated Hyponatremia

Clinical Presentation

Endurance athletes and sportspeople are usually aware of the dangers associated with heat-related illnesses. In an attempt to compensate for dehydration, these people may inadvertently consume excessive fluid during periods of exertion, and exercise-associated hyponatremia may ensue. Early symptoms include nausea, vomiting, headache, dizziness, lack of coordination, and confusion. Serious progressive symptoms include combative behavior, lethargy, seizures, and coma. Deterioration commonly occurs after physical exertion during the treatment phase.[1]

Diagnosis

Exercise-associated hyponatremia should be a consideration when a patient presents with mental status changes after exposure to extreme heat. Examination of these patients is relatively benign with a low to normal body temperature, stable blood pressure and pulse, moist mucous membranes, and normal blood pressures. Low serum sodium is diagnostic for this condition, with symptoms typically occurring when the serum sodium concentration falls below 130 mmol per L. Severe symptoms are associated with a serum sodium concentration of less than 125 mmol per L.

Management

Fluid administration should be withheld until clinical hyponatremia is proven. If heat exhaustion is also on the differential diagnosis, a 250-cc bolus of normal saline is a reasonable treatment measure. This bolus of fluid will help to manage heat exhaustion without worsening hyponatremia. Mild hyponatremia can be treated with fluid restriction and, in some cases, administration of normal saline. Severe symptomatic hyponatremia requires 3% NaCl at approximately 1 mL/kg/hour. Frequent serum sodium monitoring is indicated to achieve a gradual rise in serum sodium. Sodium levels should not exceed 10 mmol per L for the first 24 hours.

Complications

Obtundation, seizures, and coma commonly occur with acute and severe hyponatremia. Intensive care support may be necessary to properly monitor these patients. Rapid correction of hyponatremia may result in central pontine myelinolysis (CPM), a condition characterized by quadriparesis, swallowing dysfunction, and mutism.

Heatstroke

Clinical Presentation

- Classic heatstroke victims are those with chronic diseases, patients with limited mobility, obese patients, and elderly patients. Other people affected include alcoholics, patients taking certain medications (e.g., sedatives, diuretics, anticholinergics, antipsychotics), and drug abusers. During periods of extreme heat, these individuals become progressively dehydrated until their body's cooling mechanisms fail. Physical exam will often reveal skin that is hot and dry without sweating, and these patients will also have a core body temperature of greater than 40.5°C (105°F). In addition, patients are often tachypnic, tachycardic, and hypotensive.

- Exertional heatstroke victims are unacclimitized individuals who overexert themselves in conditions of extreme heat. In this case, sweating may be profuse or absent, and core body temperature may be lower than 40.5°C (105°F). Similar to classic heatstroke victims, these patients may also be tachypnic, tachycardic, and hypotensive.

Diagnosis

Heatstroke victims have a core body temperature of greater than 40.5°C (105°F) with accompanying acute neurologic findings ranging from irritability and confusion to a deep coma. In these patients, seizures are very common.

Management

- **Prehospital treatment.** Heatstroke victims must be immediately cooled to a core body temperature of 39°C (102°F).[2] Treatment consists of removing unnecessary clothing, spraying the body with tepid (20 to 25°C) water, and enhancing airflow across the patient during transport to an emergency facility.
- **Airway, breathing, and circulation.** Respiratory assistance with intubation is often required for critically ill patients. Continuous cardiac monitoring and oxygen therapy should be initiated. Fluid resuscitation is started with dextrose in normal saline or dextrose in half-normal saline. Core temperature is continuously measured with a flexible rectal probe. A Foley catheter is inserted to monitor urine output.
- **Immediate cooling.** Core temperature should be lowered at least 0.1°C per minute to the target temperature of 39°C (102°F). Cooling can be accomplished by one of two methods.
  - Evaporative cooling involves spraying the uncovered patient with lukewarm water and using fans to blow air across the body.[3]
  - Ice-water baths consist of placing the patient in a tank of ice water, relying on the rapid conduction of heat into water. Shivering and agitation, more common in iced baths, is effectively controlled with intravenous diazepam (Valium), 5 to 10 mg IV every 5 minutes.

- Baseline laboratory tests should include a complete blood count, complete metabolic profile, arterial blood gases, chest radiography, electrocardiography, cardiac isoenzymes, prothrombin time, partial thromboplastin time, fibrin degradation products, creatine kinase, urinalysis, and urine myoglobin.

Complications

- Cardiovascular instability requires continuous monitoring with a Swan–Ganz catheter and a central line. For persistent hypotension with low cardiac index, low-dose isoproterenol infusion is appropriate.[4]
- Low or absent urine output, hematuria, and proteinuria are signs of renal damage.
- Rhabdomyolysis, a common complication of exertional heatstroke, results in dark urine, intense muscle pain, myoglobinuria, and high serum creatine kinase. Renal damage should be treated with fluid administration in an attempt to maintain a high urine output (more than 50 mL/hour). With myoglobinuria, urine alkalinization with sodium bicarbonate and mannitol 12.5 to 25.0 g should be initiated.
- Hepatic injury is a common complication. Resulting jaundice usually occurs within 1 to 3 days following heatstroke.
- Computed tomographic scanning of the head and possibly lumbar puncture are recommended for patients with persistent coma, seizures, or a focal neurologic deficit.
- Serial clotting studies are indicated for patients with petechiae, purpura, hematemesis, or epistaxis. Early coagulopathies are treated with fresh frozen plasma and platelet transfusions.
- Disseminated intravascular coagulation is a relatively common complication of patients with exertional heatstroke. In this instance, heparin has been shown to be effective in some cases.
- Increasing airway resistance, pulmonary infiltration, and decreased oxygen saturation characterize adult respiratory distress syndrome, another complication of heatstroke. These patients should be started on mechanical ventilation with positive end-expiratory pressure.

Prevention

A National Weather Service heat index of over 90°F should be considered hazardous. Exposure to direct sunlight can raise the temperature an additional 15°F. Patients with any physical impairment or limitation and those taking medications that decrease their ability to sweat should avoid heat and drink plenty of liquids. More active individuals can minimize their risk of heat-related illness by gradually acclimating themselves to the heat over a period of 10 to 14 days, drink plenty of water before and during exposure to the heat, and wear vapor-permeable, light clothing. Endurance athletes and sportspeople should replenish fluid losses with frequent and small quantities of fluid, but should not exceed 0.5 to 1 L per hour. A commercially available carbohydrate electrolyte beverage may be beneficial in the case of prolonged physical exertion.[5]

References
1. Backer HD, Shopes E, Collins SL, et al. Exertional heat illness and hyponatremia in hikers. *Am J Emerg Med* 1999;17:532.
2. Vicario SJ, Okabajue R, Haltom T. Rapid cooling in classic heatstroke: effect on mortality rates. *Am J Emerg Med* 1986;4:394.
3. Khogali M, Weiner JS. Heat stroke: report on 18 cases. *Lancet* 1980;2:276.
4. Khosla R, Guntupalli KK. Heat-related illnesses. *Crit Care Clin* 1999;15:251.
5. Vrijens DM, Rehrer NJ. Sodium-free fluid ingestion decreases plasma sodium during exercise in the heat. *J Appl Physiol* 1999;86:1847.

Therapeutic Choices XXII

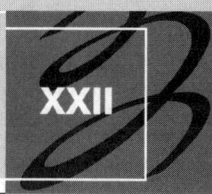

BACTERIAL ENDOCARDITIS PROPHYLAXIS
Bruce M. Bushwick

22.1

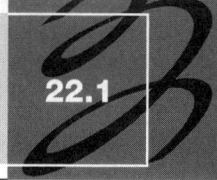

GENERAL PRINCIPLES

Definition

Bacterial endocarditis is an infection of the endocardium. The infection can develop on heart valves, septal defects, or on mural endocardium. There are no definitive controlled clinical trials of prevention strategies in humans, but animal models, *in vitro* studies, and clinical experience suggest that risk for infection can be reduced by the use of prophylactic antibiotics in at-risk individuals. Optimal prevention strategies remain a subject of controversy in academic medicine.[1,2]

Etiology

Bacterial endocarditis is believed to result from transient bacteremia from organisms such as enterococci, viridans streptococci, *Staphylococcus aureus, Staphylococcus epidermidis,* or *Pseudomonas aerugenosa.* Individuals at risk for the infection have a damaged or altered endothelial surface that is colonized and infected by bacteria. The subsequent inflammation causes vegetations to develop on the endocardial surface that are composed of platelets, fibrin, and bacteria. The vegetations cause structural damage and can embolize throughout the body resulting in systemic disease.[3] Risk of developing endocarditis is inferred based on the probability of a procedure causing transient bacteremia that seeds an at-risk cardiac lesion and whether the procedure is anecdotally associated with endocarditis.[4]

Epidemiology

The exact incidence is not known. Between 10,000 and 20,000 patients develop endocarditis each year in the United States.[3]

DIAGNOSIS

History

- Administer prophylactic antibiotics to patients who have conditions associated with an increased risk of endocarditis and who undergo bacteremia-associated procedures. Transesophageal echocardiography can facilitate risk stratification.

779

- Administer prophylactic antibiotics optionally to patients with high-risk conditions who undergo procedures not usually associated with endocarditis that involve the lower respiratory (including flexible fiberoptic bronchoscopy), genitourinary (including vaginal hysterectomy and vaginal delivery), or gastrointestinal tract (including transesophageal echocardiography and endoscopy).
- Administer prophylactic antibiotics in additional circumstances if clinical judgment warrants.
- When performing a bacteremia-associated procedure in the presence of infected tissue, antibiotic choice should cover the most likely pathogen causing the infection.
- Consider parenteral route of administration for lower gastrointestinal or genitourinary procedures in high-risk patients.

Classification

- High-risk patients are those with:
  - A previous infection with endocarditis
  - A history of cardiac valve replacement surgery
  - A history of surgically constructed systemic-pulmonary shunts or conduits
  - Complex cyanotic congenital heart disease such as single ventricle conditions, transposition of the great arteries, or tetralogy of Fallot

- Moderate-risk patients are those with:
  - Acquired cardiac valve disease
  - Hypertrophic cardiomyopathies
  - Other congenital abnormalities not mentioned under high-risk patients, above
  - Mitral valve prolapse with valvular regurgitation and/or thickened leaflets

- Bacteremia-producing procedures that predispose patients with high- or moderate-risk conditions to developing endocarditis
  - Dental procedures involving dentogingival manipulation or endodonics
  - Respiratory tract procedures
  - Tonsillectomy and/or adenoidectomy
  - Operations involving the respiratory mucosa
  - Nasal packing
  - Cosmetic piercing of tongue or oral mucosa in high-risk patients
  - Gastrointestinal tract procedures
  - Sclerotherapy for esophageal varices
  - Esophageal dilatation of stricture
  - Endoscopic retrograde cholangiography with biliary obstruction
  - Biliary tract surgery
  - Operations involving the intestinal mucosa
  - Gallstone lithotripsy
  - Genitourinary tract procedures
  - Cystoscopy
  - Urethral dilatation
  - Urethral catheterization or surgery if urinary infection is present
  - Prostate surgery or biopsy

- Other procedures
  - Incision and drainage of infected tissue
  - Vaginal delivery in the presence of infection

TREATMENT (ADAPTED FROM THE AMERICAN HEART ASSOCIATION WEB SITE[5])

Dental, Oral, Upper Respiratory Tract, or Esophageal Procedures (Adults)

- The standard regimen is amoxicillin, 2.0 g PO 1 hour before procedure. If unable to take oral medications, use ampicillin, 2.0 g IV or IM within 30 minutes before procedure.

- If amoxicillin/penicillin allergic, use azithromycin or clarithromycin, 500 mg PO 1 hour before procedure or clindamycin, 600 mg PO 1 hour before procedure. If unable to take oral medications, use clindamycin, 600 mg IV within 30 min of starting procedure.

Genitourinary or Gastrointestinal Procedures (Adults)

- For high-risk patients: Ampicillin, 2.0 g IV or IM, plus gentamicin, 1.5 mg per kg IV (not to exceed 120 mg) within 30 minutes of starting procedure, then ampicillin, 1.0 g IV or IM 6 hours later (or amoxicillin, 1 g PO).
- For high-risk patients who are ampicillin allergic: Vancomycin, 1.0 g IV (over 1 to 2 hours) completed within 30 minutes of starting procedure plus gentamicin, 1.5 mg per kg IV or IM (not to exceed 120 mg) within 30 minutes of starting procedure.
- For moderate-risk patients (treatment for these patients is optional for gastrointestinal tract procedures), use amoxicillin, 2.0 g PO 1 hour before procedure, or ampicillin, 2.0 g IV or IM within 30 minutes of starting procedure.
- For moderate-risk patients who are allergic to ampicillin use vancomycin, 1.0 g IV (over 1 to 2 hours) completed within 30 minutes of starting procedure.

Complications

There are patient-dependent risks of adverse reactions to the antibiotics administered prior to the procedure. No prevention strategy is perfect. Patient education should include a discussion of emerging symptoms of endocarditis should prophylactic efforts fail.

Patient Education

- In patients who are at risk, an effective oral health program should be promoted to minimize bacterial seeding from chronically inflamed tissues.
- Charts of at-risk patients should be clearly identified. For convenience, keep an outline of prophylactic antibiotic choices on the chart to facilitate prescribing.
- When endocarditis prophylaxis is given, the rationale for treatment, including risks and benefits, should be explained to the patient. Early signs and symptoms of endocarditis should be reviewed, such as unexpected fevers, night sweats, chills, weakness, myalgias, arthralgias, or malaise, so that emergent infections can be rapidly identified and treated.

SPECIAL CONSIDERATIONS

Modification of initial dose in pediatric patients (total dose not to exceed adult dose; second dose in pediatric patients should be one half the initial dose).

- Amoxicillin or ampicillin, 50 mg per kg
- Azithromycin or clarithromycin, 15 mg per kg
- Clindamycin, 20 mg per kg
- Gentamicin, 1.5 mg per kg
- Vancomycin, 20 mg per kg

References

1. Durack DT. Antibiotics for prevention of endocarditis during dentistry: time to scale back? *Ann Inter Med* 1998;129:829–831.
2. Morris AM, Webb GD. Antibiotics before dental procedures for endocarditis prophylaxis: back to the future. *Heart* 2001;86:3–4.
3. Fowler VG Jr, Scheld WM, Bayer AS. Endocarditis and intravascular infections. In: Mandell G, Bennett J, Dolin R, eds. 2004; Oxford publisher: Churchill-Livingstone, Oxford: *Principles and practice of infectious diseases.* 6th ed. chap 74.
4. Gould FK, et al. Guidelines for the prevention of endocarditis: report of the Working Party of the British Society for Antimicrobial Chemotherapy. *J Antimicrob Chemother* 2006;57:1035–1042.
5. www.americanheart.org (American Heart Association web site).
6. Dajani AS, et al. Prevention of bacterial endocarditis. Recommendations by the American Heart Association. *JAMA* 1997;277:1794–1801.

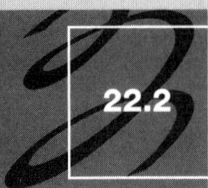

MEDICATION USE DURING PREGNANCY
Marilyn S. Darr, Jacintha S. Cauffield

*I*n general, common sense suggests that medication use during pregnancy should be limited. Nevertheless, pregnant women sometimes present with clinical syndromes that may warrant drug therapy.

The U.S. Food and Drug Administration (FDA) has established five categories for drugs based on their potential for causing birth defects in infants born to women who use the drugs during pregnancy. The categories are as follows[1]:

- **A** Controlled studies in women fail to demonstrate a risk to the fetus in the first trimester, and fetal harm appears remote (e.g., folic acid, levothyroxine).
- **B** Animal studies have not demonstrated a fetal risk, but there are no human studies in pregnant women, or animal studies have shown an adverse effect that was not confirmed in human studies (e.g., amoxicillin, ceftriaxone, cetirizine, and loratidine).
- **C** Animal studies show adverse effects, and there are no controlled studies in women. Drugs should be given only if benefit outweighs the potential risk to the fetus (e.g., budesonide, propranolol, and pseudoephedrine).
- **D** Positive evidence of human fetal risk exists, but benefits may outweigh risks in certain situations (e.g., carbamazepine, lithium, phenytoin, propylthiouracil, and valproic acid).
- **X** Studies or experience have shown fetal risk that clearly outweighs any possible benefits (e.g., ACE inhibitors, isotretinoin, methotrexate, misoprostol, thalidomide, and warfarin).

Drugs used in pregnancy and others that should be avoided are discussed here by system category. Commonly used herbal agents considered safe and those to avoid are listed at the end of the chapter. Most medications are followed by the FDA category in parentheses if available. Clinicians who prescribe medications during pregnancy should observe the following guidelines: Try to avoid any medication during the first trimester. Use single, noncombination agents. Choose topical treatments (if available) over oral. Use the lowest effective dose. Remember, use medication only if the benefit appears to outweigh the risk.

INFECTIOUS DISEASE

- **Colds (upper respiratory tract infection).** The best treatment is symptomatic management with fluids, humidity, and rest. If absolutely necessary, first-generation antihistamines, particularly chlorpheniramine (B) appear safest, but cetirizine (B) (Zyrtec) and loratidine (B) (Claritin) are reasonable alternatives. If a decongestant is indicated, use a topical agent first. If an oral decongestant is necessary, pseudoephedrine (C), 30 to 60 mg PO every 6 to 8 hours, has the best safety record. Preparations containing guaifenesin (C) or dextromethorphan (C) may be used for the management of cough.[2,3] *Avoid* iodine-containing expectorants (e.g., potassium iodide) (D) because of the potential for thyroid toxicity in the newborn, and also *avoid* alcohol-containing products.
- **Pneumonia (community acquired).** *Streptococcus pneumoniae, Mycoplasma pneumoniae,* and *Chlamydia pneumoniae* are the most common bacterial organisms. *Haemophilus influenzae* is commonly found in patients who smoke. For empirical outpatient treatment, use azithromycin (B) (Zithromax), 500 mg followed by 250 mg

per day PO for 4 days. Alternative treatment includes cefuroxime (B) (Ceftin), 500 mg PO bid, amoxicillin/clavulanic acid (Augmentin), 875/125 mg PO bid. These alternative antibiotics are *not* active against *Mycoplasma pneumoniae* or *Chlamydia pneumoniae*. *Avoid* clarithromycin (C), tetracycline (D), and quinolones (C) (see also Chapter 10.2).

- **Sexually transmitted diseases[4]**
    - **Chlamydial infection.** Manage with amoxicillin (B), 500 mg PO tid for 7 days, or erythromycin base (B) (Eryc, E-Mycin), 500 mg PO qid for 7 days. Alternative regimen is azithromycin (B) (Zithromax), 1 g orally. Repeat culture 3 weeks after completion of antibiotic course. *Avoid* erythromycin estolate (Ilosone), doxycycline (D), and quinolones (C).
    - **Genital warts, external (*Condyloma acuminata*).** Safe treatments during pregnancy include topical bi- or trichloracetic acid weekly, cryotherapy, or liquid nitrogen. *Avoid* podophyllin (C), podofilox (C) (Condylox), and imiquimod (C) (Aldara).
    - **Gonorrhea (GC) (uncomplicated).** Treat for both GC and *Chlamydia* with ceftriaxone (Rocephin) (B), 125 mg IM or cefixime (Suprax) (B), 400 mg PO single dose plus azithromycin (B), 1 g orally. Women who cannot tolerate a cephalosporin should be administered a single 2-g dose of spectinomycin (B) IM. Reculture after treatment. *Avoid* quinolones and tetracyclines.
    - **Herpes genitalis.** For severe first episode, late-onset disease in the second or third trimester, or disseminated herpes simplex virus infections, use of acyclovir (B) (Zovirax) appears justified. Famciclovir (B) (Famvir) and valacyclovir (B) (Valtrex) are newer agents with better absorption. Doses vary with indication. If daily suppressive therapy at 36 weeks appears justified, use acyclovir, 400 mg PO bid.
    - **Pediculosis (*Phythirus humanus capitis* or "head lice" and *P. pubis* or "crabs").** Treat with topical, poorly absorbed permethrin (B) 5% (Elimite) cream or pyrethrins with piperonyl butoxide (C) (Nix) 1% liquid. Wash hair, apply lotion for 10 minutes, then rinse off. *Avoid* lindane (B) (Kwell) due to the potential for neurotoxicity and aplastic anemia.
    - **Scabies (*Sarcoptes scabei*).** Treat with topical permethrin (B) (Elimite) 5% cream. Apply to entire skin from chin to toes. Leave on for 8 to 10 hours. Avoid crotamiton (C) (Eurax) and lindane (Kwell).
    - **Syphilis.** Manage primary, secondary, and latent infection of less than 1-year duration with benzathine penicillin (B) (Bicillin LA), 2.4 million U IM. Higher doses are used in late latent or when the duration of disease is unknown. There is no alternative to penicillin in pregnancy. If there is a penicillin allergy, skin test and desensitize if necessary. Follow patient with monthly venereal disease research laboratory (VDRL), and if there is a fourfold increase in titer, retreat (see also Chapter 19.5).

- **Urinary tract infection (uncomplicated).** Empirical treatment includes oral cephalexin (B) (Keflex), 500 mg tid, amoxicillin/clavulanate (B) (Augmentin), 250 mg tid, or nitrofurantoin (B) (Macrodantin), 50 to 100 mg qid.[4] Treat for 7 to 10 days. Trimethoprim–sulfamethoxazole (C) (Bactrim, Septra) can also be used, but *avoid* near-term due to risk of kernicterus. Obtain a repeat urine culture after treatment. *Avoid* quinolones (C), which are associated with fetal cartilage damage, and doxycycline (D) due to offspring teeth staining and maternal hepatotoxicity (see also Chapters 12.1 and 12.2).[5]

- **Vaginitis** (see also Chapter 13.1)
    - **Bacterial vaginosis.** Manage with metronidazole (C) (Flagyl), 250 mg PO bid for 7 days or clindamycin (B) (Cleocin), 300 mg PO bid for 7 days. *Avoid* metronidazole in the first trimester. Use oral metronidazole and clindamycin, *not* topical in pregnancy.
    - **Candidiasis.** Treat with topical agents, such as clotrimazole (B) (Mycelex, Gyne-Lotrimin), miconazole (Monistat) (C), and terconazole (Terazol) (C) vaginal cream. Use vaginally every night for 7 days. Avoid oral fluconazole (Diflucan) (C) until more data are available.
    - ***Trichomonas vaginalis*.** Metronidazole (C), as a single 2-g dose or 500 mg PO bid for 7 days, is the treatment of choice. Avoid this agent in the first trimester. For symptomatic relief in the first trimester, try clotrimazole (B) suppositories.

RESPIRATORY DISORDERS

■ **Allergic rhinitis.** Allergic rhinitis can affect up to one third of women of childbearing age. First-line therapy includes intranasal cromolyn (B) (Nasalcrom) or beclomethasone (C) (Vancenase AQ, Beconase AQ). If symptoms are not controlled, then antihistamines, such as chlorpheniramine (B), loratadine (B), and cetirizine (B) can be used. Pseudoephedrine (C) (Sudafed), 30 to 60 mg PO qid has the best safety record if an oral decongestant is required.[3]

■ **Asthma.** It is safer for pregnant women with asthma to be treated than to have symptoms. Like nonpregnant patients, management is stepwise. Whenever possible, treatment should be by inhalation rather than oral. Preferred agents include short-acting beta-agonist albuterol (C) (Ventolin, Proventil), and inhaled corticosteroids, particularly budesonide (C) (Pulmicort). For add-on, but not preferred therapy, use cromolyn (B) (Intal), long-acting beta-agonist salmeterol (C) or formoterol (C), leukotriene D4 antagonist zafirlukast (Accolate) (B) or montelukast (Singulair) (B), or theophylline (C). During exacerbations, IV and oral glucocorticoids may be used in the usual manner. Zileuton (C) (Zyflo) should be *avoided* during pregnancy (see also Chapter 10.1).[6]

GASTROINTESTINAL DISORDERS

■ **Nausea and vomiting.** Attempt conservative measures, including small frequent meals, a bland diet, and acupressure wristbands or acupressure on the volar surface of the forearm. Ginger tea up to 1 g per day (about 4 cups) may help. Initial medications include pyridoxine (A), 25 mg PO q8h, and phosphorated carbohydrate solution (Emetrol), 1 to 2 tablespoons PO every 15 minutes to five doses. Safe antiemetics include doxylamine (A) 10 mg PO q6h prn, meclizine (B) (Antivert), 25 mg Po q6h prn, promethazine (C) (Phenergan), 25 mg PO/IM/PR every 4 to 6 hours prn, or metoclopramide (B) (Reglan), 10 mg PO qid. Ondansetron (B) (Zofran) has been used in patients whose symptoms are refractory to other therapy.[7]

■ **Gastroesophageal reflux (GERD).** GERD can affect 50% to 80% of pregnant women. Treatment includes routine antireflux measures. Antacids and alginic acid (Gaviscon) are first-line agents. Antacids may interfere with iron absorption. H_2 receptor antagonists cimetidine (B) (Tagamet), 400 mg PO at bedtime, and ranitidine (B) (Zantac) 150 mg PO bid, have the most published data in terms of human experience. In refractory cases, the proton pump inhibitors lansoprazole (B) (Prevacid), pantoprazole (B) (Protonix), esomeprazole (B) (Nexium), and omeprazole (C) (Prilosec) can be used (see also Chapter 11.2).

■ **Constipation.** Nonpharmacologic management, including physical activity, increased fiber and fluid intake, and education are preferred. A supplemental fiber, preferably calcium polycarbophil, and docusate (C) are the preferred first-line agents. For refractory symptoms, lactulose (B), sorbitol, bisacodyl, and senna (C) may be used.

■ **Diarrhea.**[2] Attempt conservative measures, such as fluid replacement and bland diet, first. If medication is need, kaolin/pectin (B) (Kaopectate) is the preferred agent. For refractory symptoms, loperamide (B) (Imodium) can be used. *Avoid* bismuth salicylate (C) (Pepto Bismol) and atropine/diphenoxylate (C) (Lomotil).

■ **Inflammatory bowel disease.** Active Crohn disease and ulcerative colitis can have an adverse impact on pregnancy. First-line treatment in active disease is sulfasalazine (B) (Azulfidine), 500 mg PO qid, or mesalamine (B) (Asacol), 800 mg PO tid, and rectal or systemic glucocorticoids.[5] Like other sulfonamides, sulfasalazine is considered category D near term because of the theoretical risk of kernicterus. Folic acid 1 mg PO bid is advised in women receiving sulfasalazine. Adverse fetal effects have been documented with the use of 6-mercaptopurine, azathioprine, and cyclosporine. Methotrexate (D) is *contraindicated*. Consultation with a gastroenterologist is warranted in active disease (see also Chapter 11.9).[8]

ENDOCRINE DISORDERS

■ **Diabetes.** Diet is the cornerstone of management. If medication is needed, insulin (B) is the drug of choice. Avoid or limit oral agents (see also Chapter 17.2).

- **Thyroid disorders** (see also Chapter 17.3)
    - **Hypothyroidism.** Oral levothyroxine (A), 0.1 to 0.20 mg per day, is the thyroid preparation of choice. Other preparations are associated with increased side effects.
    - **Hyperthyroidism.** Propylthiouracil (PTU) (D) is preferred over methimazole (Tapazole) (D), due to a possible lower incidence of major malformations and slower placental transfer. Adjust PTU to the lowest dose effective to maintain a free T4 in the upper one third of normal to slightly elevated range. *Avoid* beta-blockers, such as propranolol (C) (Inderal), during the first trimester. Monitor for intrauterine growth retardation. The use of radioactive iodine (X) is *contraindicated*. Endocrinology consultation for management issues is recommended.[9]

NEUROLOGIC AND PSYCHIATRIC DISORDERS

- **Headaches, migraine.** Nondrug therapies, such as relaxation, sleep, massage, ice packs, and biofeedback, should be tried first. If drug therapy is needed, the most acceptable analgesic is acetaminophen (B) (Tylenol), 1000 mg at first sign of headache. An antiemetic may also be required, such as promethazine (C) (Phenergan) or metoclopramide (B) (Reglan). *Avoid* aspirin (C) and nonsteroidal anti-inflammatory drugs, especially in the last trimester (category D) due to risk of premature closure of ductus arteriosus. In severe cases, hydrocodone (C) and meperidine (C) may be given for short-term use only. Prophylactic treatment is rarely indicated. Ergotamine (D) and serotonin 5-HT$_1$ receptor agonists such as sumatriptan (C) are *contraindicated* in pregnancy[10] (see also Chapter 6.1).
- **Depression.** Psychotherapy is considered first-line treatment for depression during pregnancy. Fluoxetine (Prozac) (C), 20 mg per day PO, appears to be relatively safe and should be the agent of first choice. The selective serotonin-reuptake inhibitors (SSRIs) sertraline (C) (Zoloft) and citalopram (C) (Celexa) also appear safe, but data on humans are limited. Controlled trial data on bupropion (C) and venlafaxine (C) are also limited. Tricyclic antidepressants (TCAs), including nortriptyline (C), desipramine (C), amitriptyline (D) and imipramine (D) should be used *very* judiciously, due to unsubstantiated teratogenic activity. *Avoid* paroxetine (D) due to an FDA advisory of possible fetal ventricular septal defect and monoamine oxidase (MAO) inhibitors[11] (see also Chapter 5.2).

HERBAL AGENTS (SEE ALSO CHAPTER 22.3)

- Herbal agents generally recognized as safe (GRAS) for use as a food supplement by the FDA include chamomile, garlic, ginger, and mints.
- Herbal agents to avoid in pregnancy include but are not limited to bitter orange, black and blue cohosh, cascara, chondroitin, dong quai, ginseng, dihydroepiandrosterone, feverfew, ginkgo, goldenseal, guarana, horse chestnut, kava kava, passionflower, St. John's wort, soy isoflavones, and valerian.[12]

References
1. Briggs GG, Freeman RK, Yaffe SJ. *Drugs in pregnancy and lactation*, 7th ed. Baltimore: Lippincott Williams & Wilkins; 2005.
2. Black RA, Hill DA. Over-the-counter medications in pregnancy. *Am Fam Physician* 2003;67:2517.
3. Gilbert C, Mazzotta P, Loebstein R, et al. Fetal safety of drugs used in the treatment of allergic rhinitis. A critical review. *Drug Saf* 2005;28:707.
4. U.S. Centers for Disease Control and Prevention. Sexually transmitted diseases treatment guidelines 2002. *MMWR* 2002;51(RR-6).
5. Delzell JE, Lefevre ML. Urinary tract infections during pregnancy. *Am Fam Physician* 2000;61:713–721.
6. National Asthma Education and Prevention Program. Managing asthma during pregnancy: recommendations for pharmacologic treatment—update 2004 (NIH Publication No. 05-3279). Accessed at http://www.nhlbi.nih.gov/health/prof/lung/asthma/astpreg.htm.

7. Mazzotta P, Magee LA. A risk-benefit assessment of pharmacological and non-pharmacological treatments for nausea and vomiting of pregnancy. *Drugs* 2000; 59:781.

8. Steinlauf AF, Present DH. Medical management of the pregnant patient with inflammatory bowel disease. *Gastroenterol Clin North Am* 2004;33:361.

9. LeBeau SO, Mandel SJ. Thyroid disorders during pregnancy. *Endocrinol Metab Clin North Am* 2006;35:117.

10. Fox AW, Diamond ML, Spierings ELH. Migraine during pregnancy. Options for therapy. *CNS Drugs* 2005;19:465.

11. Ryan D, Milis L, Misri N. Depression during pregnancy. *Can Fam Physician* 2005; 51:1087.

12. The Pharmacist's Letter/Physician's Letter Natural Medicines Comprehensive Database. Available online at http://www.naturaldatabase.com. Accessed June 28, 2006.

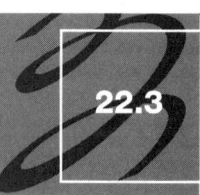

22.3 HERBAL MEDICINE
Mari A. Ricker, Wendy Kohatsu

GENERAL PRINCIPLES

- **Variety.** Herbs come in many different forms: whole fresh, whole dried, encapsulated powder, extract tablets, teas, tinctures, juice, essential oils, decoctions, lyophilized herb, standardized extract, cold and hot infusions, and topical preparations.
- **Standardization.** In an attempt to ensure consistency of herbal dosing, herbs are standardized to a constituent marker within the herb. For example, St. John's wort is often standardized to an active component known as hypercin. Standardized products will reflect that they contain 0.3% hypercin in their St. John's wort.

INDICATIONS/CONTRAINDICATIONS: DOSING AND ADMINISTRATION (TABLE 22.3-1)

- **Normal dosage.** Unless noted differently on the packaging, a dosage is given for oral intake for an adult weighing approximately 150 pounds (70 kg).
- **Dosing for children/elderly.** There are several rules that can be used for determining the appropriate dose:
  - **Young's rule.** *Children*: The fraction of the adult dose is the child's age divided by the child's age plus 12. For example, 500 mg tid is the adult dose. For a 7-year-old child the fraction is 7/(7 + 12) = 7/19. So the appropriate dose would be approximately 180 mg tid for a 7-year-old child.
  - **Cowling's rule:** *Children 12 to 18*: Take the age of the child at the child's next birthday and divide by 24 to determine the fraction. For example, 500 mg tid for a 14-year-old (at next birthday) child would be 14/24 or 300 mg tid approximately.
  - **Clark's rule:** *Elderly or weight adjustment:* Using the patient's weight in pounds, you can divide the weight by 150 to calculate the fraction. For example, 500 mg tid, a 94-pound woman would have a fraction of 94/150 and a dose of approximately 300 mg tid.

SIDE EFFECTS

See Table 22.3-1.

TABLE 22.3-1

Some Commonly Used Herbal Products: Uses and Precautions$^{\alpha}$

Herb	Most common uses	Dose	Interactions/precautions/contraindications
Black cohosh *Cimicifuga racemosa*	Used to manage the symptoms of menopause, best studies in Germany for up to 6 mo. Used for premenstrual symptoms and dysmenorrhea, less well studied. Used to induce menses, poor studies.	Clinical studies have used a commercially prepared standardized extract from Germany, Remifemin, 20-mg tablet BID.	Maximum effect achieved in 4–8 wk. Limit use to 6 mo (German Commission E). Evidence of estrogenic activity is conflicting. German *in vitro* studies show that Remifemin amplifies tamoxifen's induced proliferation inhibition on the estrogen receptors of breast cancer cells. However, the following are uncertain: (a) if black cohosh has estrogen-like protection for osteoporosis or cardiovascular diseases; (b) if black cohosh can be combined with hormone replacement therapy; (c) if patients with a uterus need progesterone protection for endometrial cancer prevention. Contraindicated in pregnancy and breastfeeding. Side effects: mild GI. Black cohosh is not blue or white cohosh.
Echinacea *Echinacea angustifolia* or *E. pallida* or *E. purpurea*	Used orally to prevent or treat URIs. Limited studies suggest nonspecific immune stimulant activity. Used topically for wound healing in burns and abscesses.	Dosing depends on *Echinacea* species, plant part, and extraction process. Echinacea root extract of 1:5 tincture with 50% ethanol is indicated in Germany for the supportive treatment of flu-like infections at a dose equivalent to 900 mg of crude drug daily. Echinacea juices are indicated for the supportive treatment of recurrent upper and lower respiratory infections at a dose of 6–9 mg/d.	German Commission E recommendations: (a) limit use to 8 consecutive weeks; (b) discourage use in individuals with immune or autoimmune illnesses, such AIDS, HIV infection, multiple sclerosis, and tuberculosis. (Controversial because no studies demonstrate or confirm this.) Avoid in patients allergic to Asteraceae/Compositae family (ragweed, chrysanthemums, marigolds, daisies, etc.). Anaphylactic reactions have occurred. In Germany, intravenous formulations may compromise diabetes control. Not demonstrated in oral echinacea formulations. May inhibit oocyte fertilization and alter sperm DNA and should be avoided in couples attempting to conceive. Side effects: some GI.

(continued)

TABLE 22.3-1 Some Commonly Used Herbal Products: Uses and Precautions$^\alpha$ *(Continued)*

Herb	Most common uses	Dose	Interactions/precautions/contraindications
Garlic *Allium sativum*	Used for lowering mild hypertension and cholesterol.	One raw clove per day. Prolonged cooking will inactivate the ingredients thought to be beneficial. Benefits in studies from garlic in pill form have been conflicting because different processes have been used to prepare garlic pills, resulting in pills with different pharmacologic actions.	Safe in amounts consumed in food. Some products may have antithrombotic activity, so avoid use in patients taking anticoagulants. Can lower blood glucose in patients with diabetes. Undesirable garlic taste and smell can occur even with so-called "odorless" products.
Ginkgo *Ginkgo biloba*	Used to improve memory in mild to moderate dementia (good studies). Less evidence, but possibly effective for use in peripheral vascular disease, reversing SSRI-induced sexual dysfunction (men and women), and treatment for depression in elderly patients. Claims to improve mental alertness and overall brain function are unsubstantiated.	120–240 mg/d of concentrated standardized extract.	Side effects include mild GI complaints, headache, dizziness, palpitations, and allergic skin reactions. Large doses might cause restlessness, diarrhea, nausea, vomiting, lack of muscle tone, and weakness. Bleeding is often mentioned as a side effect of ginkgo, but very few cases have been reported. Until further studies are performed, patients on NSAIDs, aspirin, or anticoagulants should avoid ginkgo. To avoid transient headache and dizziness, start with low dose and increase over 8 wk.
Ginger *Zingiber officinale*	Used for motion sickness and joint pain, studies show possible effectiveness. Used to reduce postoperative nausea and vomiting, conflicting evidence. Prevention and treatment of chemotherapy-induced nausea, no conclusive data.	For motion sickness: 1-g tablet or capsule 30 min prior to travel, then 1/2 g every 4 h. Maximum dose 4 g/d.	Caution in patients with gallstones, ginger increases flow of bile. Large doses can cause heartburn. Inhibits platelet aggregation: clinical significance and/or potential interaction with anticoagulants, unknown.

Herb			
	Use for nausea in pregnancy is controversial, no conclusive evidence of safety.		
Ginseng Several species, e.g., *Panax ginseng*	Used to improve the body's response to stress. Called an "adaptogen." Many studies of poor quality.	Preparations vary widely.	When considering reports of adverse reactions, keep in mind that ginseng has been the most commonly adulterated herbal product in the United States. Reports of adverse reactions include breast tenderness in women; nervousness, excitation, heart palpitations, insomnia, and increased blood pressure; postmenopausal bleeding. Germany recommends limiting duration of use to 3 mo because of the possibility of hormone-like or hormone-inducing effects. Antiplatelet effects, be careful with blood-thinning drugs. May have hypoglycemic effects.
Kava *Piper methysticum*	Used for anxiety, restlessness, stress and muscle relaxant, poor studies.	Extracts standardized to 30% or 70% kava lactones. Doses vary, usually 100–300 mg/d.	May reduce reaction time while driving. Alcohol should not be consumed concomitantly. May have additive CNS depressant effects with prescription tranquilizers, muscle relaxants, valerian, St. John's wort. No evidence for physical dependence. Heavy, prolonged use can result in dermatitis. High doses can result in a drunken-like state. Avoid in pregnancy, lactation, and depression.
Ma huang *Ephedra sinica*	Commonly used today in the United States as an appetite suppressant. Primary active ingredient is the alkaloid ephedrine. Ephedrine produces amphetamine-like actions: stimulates CNS, produces mydriasis, enhances myocardial contraction and heart rate, causes bronchodilation, decreases GI	The FDA recommends using ephedra-containing products for a maximum of 7 d and in amounts not exceeding 8 mg of ephedrine every 6 h or 24 mg/d. (Much more is consumed if patients follow the instructions for Metabolife.)	Not recommended for weight loss. The FDA issued warnings against the use of ephedra as an appetite suppressant and advises that intake over the recommended amount may result in heart attack, stroke, seizure, or death. The FDA prohibits the marketing of ephedrine with other CNS stimulants, such as caffeine and yohimbine. However, herbal weight loss products package ma huang with guarana, a caffeine-containing herb.

(continued)

Herb	Most common uses	Dose	Interactions/precautions/contraindications
	motility, and stimulates peripheral vasoconstriction with an associated rise in blood pressure.		
Milk thistle *Silybum marianum*	Fruit and seed promoted for treatment of acute and chronic liver conditions by the German Commission E. Studies show likely effective when used orally for dyspeptic complaints, bile duct inflammation, and treating toxic, inflammatory, or chronic liver conditions (cirrhosis due to hepatitis, alcohol, or drugs, etc.).	Daily dose of 200–400 mg standardized by the amount of silymarin extract (70%–80%).	No serious adverse effects have been seen with milk thistle. Can cause an allergic reaction in individuals sensitive to the Asteraceae/Compositae family (ragweed, chrysanthemums, marigolds, daisies, etc.). Silymarin decreases elevated serum transaminase laboratory values.
Saw palmetto *Serenoa repens*	Used for the symptoms of BPH. Clinical studies provide evidence of moderate scientific quality that commercial extracts of saw palmetto are more effective than placebo in relieving lower urinary tract symptoms of BPH, frequency, urgency, dysuria, nocturia, and impaired urinary flow. Improvement of symptoms can take up to 2 months of treatment.	Daily dose 320 mg or 160 mg bid of a commercial liposterolic extract standardized to 70%–95% free fatty acids.	No reported side effects or drug interactions. Contrary to earlier warnings, saw palmetto has no significant effect on serum prostate-specific antigen levels. It does not affect overall prostate size, but shrinks the inner prostatic epithelium and may have anti-inflammatory and antiandrogen properties. Studies show no side effects or drug interactions, but be aware of potential α-adrenergic or endocrine blocking effects. Simultaneous use with prescription medications to treat BPH like finasteride is not recommended.
St. John's wort *Hypericum perforatum*	Orally for mild to moderate depression. Topically, oil preparations used for bruises, burns, and neuralgia.	Adults: Up to 1000 mg daily, standardized to 0.3%. Commercial products available in whole-herb form; also standardized to hypericin and hyperforin.	Superior to placebo and as effective as low-dose TCAs and possibly as effective as SSRIs. Associated with fewer side effects than synthetic antidepressants. Do not use in pregnancy: historical records include St. John's wort in herbal formulas for inducing abortion. Animal studies show slight uterine effects.

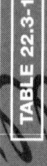

		Pediatric: 200–400 mg/d. German Commission E does not recommend use in children younger than 12 yr.	Possibly increases photosensitivity in patients with fair complexions. Reports suggest that St. John's wort extracts are potent inducers of hepatic enzymes. St. John's wort can decrease plasma cyclosporine levels (reports of transplant rejections); reduce serum digoxin, theophylline, and amitriptyline levels; decrease protease inhibitors (indinavir); and decrease the effectiveness of warfarin. Breakthrough bleeding in women on oral contraceptive pills; unknown if this results in contraceptive failure.

Dietary supplements

Creatine	Used to increase physical muscle performance during brief, high-intensity exercise or work.	Dose: 20–30 g/d for 1 wk max., then 3 g/d maintenance.	Creatine is present in red meat and is synthesized in the body from arginine, glycine, and methionine. It is metabolized to creatinine. Vegetarians, those without a large dietary intake of creatine, and untrained athletes gain the most advantage. Side effects include mild GI and muscle cramping. Dehydration is a risk because creatine causes muscles to retain water. Therefore, hydration is important when using creatine. The effects of chronic creatine administration have not been adequately studied.
Chromium	May benefit patients with type 2 diabetes mellitus who are chromium deficient but use limited because currently no reliable diagnostic test exists to determine chromium deficiency. Potentiates insulin action, increasing insulin receptor sensitivity. American Diabetes Association says, "The only known circumstance in which chromium replacement has a beneficial effect on glycemic control	Currently do not know the content of chromium in the U.S. diet or how to monitor chromium levels or status. Studies have looked at doses of 175–1000 µg/d. The recommended daily allowance is 50–200 µg. Chromium picolinate is the most easily absorbed form.	Studies show benefit in gestational and type 2 diabetes mellitus. In 19 randomized controlled trials in which individuals received between 175 and 1000 µg/d chromium for duration of 6–64 wk, there was no evidence of any toxic effects. Lowers the hyperglycemia caused by steroids. No adverse reactions reported.

(continued)

Herb	Most common uses	Dose	Interactions/precautions/contraindications
	is for people who are chromium deficient as a result of long-term parenteral nutrition. However, it appears that most people with diabetes are not chromium deficient and therefore chromium supplementation has no known benefit." (1998)		
Glucosamine sulfate	Used to manage pain, inflammation and to retard or reverse degenerative joint changes in osteoarthritis.	500 mg tid. Takes at least 1 mo to see results. Although chondroitin sulfate and glucosamine sulfate are frequently marketed together, there is no evidence that the combination has greater benefit than either product alone.	Compared head to head with NSAIDs and shown to be as effective, with fewer side effects. Takes longer to achieve benefit with glucosamine, but benefits persist longer. Few side effects; possible constipation. Animal studies show increased insulin resistance: clinical significance unknown. Many of the "joint mixtures" also contain potassium.
Omega-3 fatty acids	Used for a variety of inflammatory-related conditions.	Fish oil: Doses vary, 1–4 g/d; capsules typically contain EPA and DHA fish oil.	Adverse effects: Some of the supplements have other vitamins and minerals added. When used with anticoagulants, NSAIDs, and aspirin, can increase bleeding risk. Lowers blood sugar.
Flax seed oil Fish oil	Insufficient evidence. Likely effective for modest antihypertensive effect and decreased mortality after myocardial infarction (29%–42%). Has been shown with one fish meal a day or fish meal as well as fish oil capsules. American Heart Association recommends use with triglycerides > 1000.	Flax seed oil: 1 tbs of oil or capsule bid-tid. Oil must be refrigerated and cannot be used in cooking. Polyunsaturated fatty acid—precursor.	Potential side effects: fishy odor, GI upset. May increase bleeding time. Increase in calories and weight gain. May increase LDL cholesterol in some individuals (meta-analysis and summary of trials showed an average of 4 g/day increased LDL by 5%–10%). May decrease immune response. Unrefined fish oil preparations may contain pesticides.

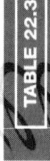

Possible effectiveness:

Rheumatoid arthritis: modest but significant improvements in joint symptoms and decreases the amount of NSAIDs needed.

GI: lowers relapse rate of Crohns disease.

GU: treat painful menses, to prevent recurrent miscarriage associated with antiphospholipid antibodies.

To treat symptoms of chronic fatigue syndrome; to reduce albuminuria in individuals with diabetic nephropathy; when taken orally with other therapy for bipolar disorder.

Pulmonary: lowers smokers' risk of chronic obstructive pulmonary disease. It has been suggested that depletion of omega-3 fatty acids may be of etiologic importance in depression, aggression, schizophrenia, and other mental and neurologic disorders. Studies are ongoing.

Ineffective for asthma, lupus, atopic dermatitis, psoriasis.

References

1. German Commission E Monographs. Austin, TX: American Botanical Council; 1998.
2. Natural medicines comprehensive database. Stockton, CA: Prescriber's letter, 2000. Available online at http://www.naturaldatabase.com. Access through www.prescriber-sletter.com can subscribe to print, web, or both.
3. DerMarderosian A. *The review of natural products by facts and comparisons.* St. Louis: Wolters Kluwer; 1999.
4. Rotblatt M, Ziment I. *Evidence-based herbal medicine.* Philadelphia: Hanley and Belfus; 2002.
5. Krinsky DL, LaValle JB, et al. *Natural therapeutics pocket guide.* 2nd ed. Hudson, OH: Lexi-Comp; 2003.
6. Donald Brown ND. *Herbal prescriptions for health and healing.* Prima Health; Roseville: 2003.

WEB ADDRESSES

American Botanical Council: http://www.herbs.org/
U.S. Pharmacopeia: http://www.usp.org
Food and Drug Administration (FDA): http://vm.cfsan.fda.gov

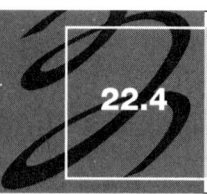

22.4 MANAGEMENT OF ACUTE AND CHRONIC NONMALIGNANT PAIN
Janey M. Purvis

GENERAL PRINCIPLES

Definition

Pain is defined as an "unpleasant sensory and emotional experience which we primarily associate with tissue damage or describe in terms of such damage, or both." Pain can be classified by duration (acute or chronic) or by mechanism (nociceptive or neuropathic). Pain is one of the most common reasons to seek medical care, and primary care physicians manage most of the acute and chronic pain in the United States. More than 85 million Americans have chronic pain, at a cost to the U.S. economy of more than $100 billion per year in direct costs and lost productivity. Despite the frequency and cost, most patients are still treated suboptimally.

ACUTE PAIN

Acute pain is the **"normal, predicted physiological response to a noxious chemical, thermal or mechanical stimulus** and typically is associated with invasive procedures, trauma and disease. It is generally time-limited." It is caused by tissue injury from trauma, disease process, or surgical procedures. Injured peripheral sensory nerves transmit signals to the dorsal horn, which course up the spinal cord through the medulla, thalamus, and finally to the cerebral cortex **where pain is perceived or experienced.** Multiple mechanisms and neurochemicals are involved (see chronic pain), providing potential locations for therapeutic interventions.

Evaluation of acute pain determines the source/etiology of pain and enables the diagnosis of the underlying condition. This includes:

- A **complete history and physical examination** focused on pain location (onset, duration, character, location, relieving and stimulating factors)
- **Investigations** appropriate to history (radiologic, laboratory)
- Initial **pain assessment** (Figure 22.4-1), which guides acute pain management

Acute pain treatment goal is to **relieve patient discomfort, while facilitating recovery/healing,** and depends on the etiology of the pain.

A. 0–10 Numeric Pain Intensity Scale

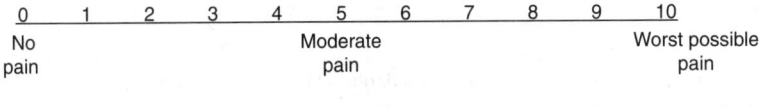

| 0 | 1 | 2 | 3 | 4 | 5 | 6 | 7 | 8 | 9 | 10 |

No
pain

Moderate
pain

Worst possible
pain

B. Visual Analog Scale

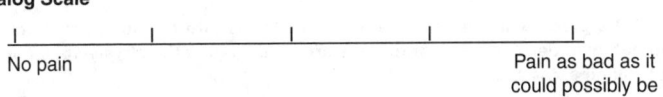

No pain

Pain as bad as it
could possibly be

Figure 22.4-1. Pain assessment scales. Simple, valid for measuring most accurate and reliable if patient reported. Useful for monitoring treatment effects. Wong-Baker Faces Pain Scale may be used for children, elderly individuals, or semiconscious patients who may give less reliable responses.

- **Short-term treatment** is the norm, using a flexible, practical treatment plan discussed with the patient and family. Consultation with a specialist is required if spinal analgesia, complex neural blockade, or continuous analgesic infusion will be utilized.
- **Pre-emptive pain treatment** for surgery is known to reduce postoperative pain. Postoperative-controlled analgesia **(PCA)** by self-administered intravenous opioids is effective, and commonly used. Initial **pain assessment** (see Figure 22.4-1), repeated at frequent intervals directs treatment. Early, adequate treatment may reduce the development of chronic pain syndromes. Current evidence suggests that neuronal damage may occur with acute injury and chronic neuropathic effects may be averted by acute use of drugs for neuropathic pain, that is, tricyclics or antiseizure. Pharmacologic plus nonpharmacologic treatment combination is considered to be most effective.

   Pharmacologic treatments are the mainstay of treatment, guided by pain level (see Figure 22.4-1) and the World Health Organization (WHO) Analgesic Ladder (Table 22.4-1).

- Anti-inflammatories are frequently used as most acute pain is accompanied by inflammation
- Opioid analgesics are used for moderate to severe acute pain
- Topical modalities (Lidocaine patch, Capsaicin cream) and muscle relaxants may be effective
- Regularly scheduled doses initially, then taper dose or use weaker analgesics as pain decreases
- Document responses and treatments

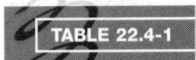

TABLE 22.4-1	WHO Analgesic Ladder

Step 1: Mild pain (0–3 on Pain Assessment Scale)
  Nonopioid
  ± adjuvant

Step 2: Moderate pain (4–6 on Pain Assessment Scale)
  Weak-opioid + nonopioid
  ± adjuvant

Step 3: Severe pain (7–10 on Pain Assessment Scale)
  Strong opioid + nonopioid
  ± adjuvant

World Health Organization Analgesic Ladder provides basis for treatment by pain intensity. Used appropriately, 80% to 90% of pain is controllable.

Nonpharmacologic treatments are useful adjuncts to pharmacotherapy:

- RICE (rest/immobilization, ice, compression, elevation)
- Heat
- Massage and relaxation
- Transcutaneous electrical nerve stimulation (TENS)/stimulation
- Range of motion exercises
- Early mobilization and exercise program

"The process whereby acute pain transforms into chronic pain is complex and not completely understood. The process is affected by genetic, physiologic, neurological and psychological factors."

CHRONIC PAIN

Chronic pain is "a state in which **pain persists beyond the usual course** of an acute disease or healing of an injury, or that may or may not be associated with an acute or chronic pathologic process that causes continuous or intermittent pain over months or years." **Chronic noncancer pain (CNCP)** is unrelated to a cancerous or terminal pain process. CNCP may be classified by mechanism (nociceptive, neuropathic but is often a combination). CNCP affects 15% to 30% of the U.S. population, is 1.5 times more common in women, and is usually localized to the lower back, neck, joints, head, abdomen, or pelvis. Chronic pain syndromes such a fibromyalgia, and peripheral nerve pain syndromes such as post herpetic neuropathy (PNH), trigeminal neuralgia, diabetic neuropathy, and poststroke pain are commonly seen in primary care. CNCP increases with age (osteoarthritis) and more than two thirds of patients have two or more pain sites. The loss of physical, personal, social, and occupational function is devastating to the patient and society in general.

Pathophysiology of CNCP is characterized **by pain signals that persist despite objective healing, or absence of tissue pathology.** Abnormal pain signals develop in peripheral tissue, the spinal dorsal horn, sensory thalamus, and/or the cerebral cortex. **"Sensitization"** of peripheral and central neurons causes altered detection, sensitivity, activation, excitation and inhibition of pain signals. Emotional and psychologic aspects have a **neurobiologic** basis and modulate the perception of pain. Mechanisms, neurochemicals, and receptors provide potential treatment targets: (glutamate, aspartate, norepinephrine, bradykinin, prostaglandins, histamine, N-methyl-D-asparate, serotonin, mu, kappa, and sigma opioid receptors, gamma-aminobutyric acid, endorphins, kephalins, endocannabinioids, calcium and sodium channels).

Nociceptive pain utilizes opioid receptors. **Neuropathic pain** is due to damaged peripheral or central nerves; described as "burning, shooting, lancinating, crawling, icy, shock-like, numbness and tingling, pins and needles."

Evaluation of the Patient with Chronic Pain

Comprehensive medical history (history of pain condition—onset, duration, character, location, relieving and stimulating factors; investigations, treatments, responses, consultations), including:

- Past medical history (comorbid conditions)
- Psychosocial history (drugs and alcohol, history of psychologic diagnoses, family support, work)
- Family history (pain/substance use/medical and psychiatric disorders)
- Pain intensity (see Figure 22.4-1)
- Impact of pain on sleep, mood, physical abilities, activities of daily living (ADL), relationships, and occupation
- **Complete physical examination** (focus on area of pain, range of motion)
- **Review and verify** past medical records
- Establish pain condition **diagnosis**
- Develop and **document a treatment plan**

Treatment of Chronic Pain

Chronic pain treatment goal is to **improve function and quality of life by reducing pain intensity.** A **multifactorial,** individualized plan is most effective. Patient education and participation is essential; discuss and document *realistic* treatment goals. A 50% reduction in pain and improvement in function is considered attainable.

- **Physical treatments.** Physical therapy, manipulation, **exercise,** and TENS/stimulation, stretching. Surgical therapies include nerve blocks, trigger point injections, and spinal infusions.
- **Psychologic treatments.** Cognitive–behavioral therapy, goal setting, relaxation techniques, biofeedback, yoga, meditation, and hypnosis
- **Alternative therapies.** Acupuncture, reflexology, and chiropractic
- **Occupational** therapies or work conditioning programs
- **Medication** is based on pain assessment scales and the WHO Analgesic Ladder (see Figure 22.4-1 and Table 22.4-1).
  - Combinations of drugs with different mechanisms **"rational polypharmacy"** is most effective
  - **Adjuvant medications play key role** (analgesia, potentiation of other analgesic effects, effective for sleep disorders, depression, and neuropathic pain)
  - **Neuropathic pain** responds well to antidepressants (not selective serotonin-reuptake inhibitors, SSRIs) and anticonvulsants, opioids are partially effective and nonsteroidal anti-inflammatory drugs (NSAIDs) usually ineffective
  - **Treat depression and anxiety** (>60% chronic pain patients), and **sleep** disorders (common)
  - If nonpharmacologic treatments and nonopioids ineffective, **opioid use is indicated**

Opioid use issues commonly affect provider practice. The increased use of opioids in pain management parallels the noted increase in **opioid abuse** in the United States. Both undertreatment and overtreatment are considered below standard of care. The decision to use opioids must be carefully thought out. The **benefits of opioid use must outweigh risks,** and there must be a **"legitimate medical purpose."** Providers must be able to recognize **addictive disorders, medication misuse, and diversion.**

Treatment Approach for Opioid Use in CNCP
Follow **"Model Guidelines for Opioid Use in Chronic Pain"** (or state board guidelines).

- **Complete evaluation,** chronic opioid indications, and justification
- **Treatment plan.** Nonpharmacologic and medications
- **Informed consent and agreement.** Opioid agreement (see below)
- Periodic review. Responses, changes in function, side effects, **aberrant behaviors**
- **Behaviors suggestive of abuse**
  - Decreased function
  - Unsanctioned dose escalations
  - Angry confrontations with staff
  - Early refills
  - Missed appointments
  - Lost or stolen prescription
  - Stealing/borrowing medications
  - Tampering with prescriptions
  - Multiple providers or emergency visits
  - Abnormal urine drug test
  - Noncompliance with nondrug therapies
- **Consultation** if necessary
- **Records (documentation).** Accurate, complete, accessible, and available for review
- **Comply with Drug Enforcement Agency (DEA)**
- Ensure patient is **appropriate candidate** for opioids (currently studying screening tools)
- **Risk factors** most predictive for abuse/ addiction:
  - Past/present history of substance abuse
  - Family history of substance abuse
  - Tobacco abuse and need for cigarette within 1 hour of waking
  - Others: Psychiatric illness, history of legal problems, motor vehicle accidents

- In **high-risk patients,** tailor approach (strict conditions, frequent visits, and prudent drug choice)
- Most experts agree that **patients with substance abuse issues still require pain management.**

Opioid Agreement/Informed Consent
- Document and sign discussion of risks and benefits of opioid use
- Understand and discuss addiction/dependence/tolerance/pseudoaddiction and abuse
- Document **conditions of opioid prescriptions** (one prescriber, office attendance, rules for telephone refills, early refills, lost or stolen meds, use of illicit substances, random urine drug testing, consequences of agreement violation)
- **Understand the meaning of urine drug testing.** Many patients who abuse medications and violate opioid agreements do *not* show aberrant behaviors.

Medication Selection
- Determine appropriate total dose with **short-acting opioids** (consult conversion tables)
- **Convert to long-acting** for consistent pain control
- Use short acting opioids for **breakthrough pain**
- Augment with adjuvants and NSAIDs **"rational polypharmacy"**
- If suboptimal effect, **"opioid rotation"** may be effective
- **Anticipate and treat side effects**
  - **Addiction.** Primary, chronic, neurobiologic disease, with genetic, psychosocial, and environmental factors influencing its development and manifestations. It is characterized by behaviors that include the following: impaired control over drug use, craving, compulsive use, and continued use despite harm. Physical dependence and tolerance are normal physiologic consequences of extended opioid therapy for pain and are not the same as addiction.
  - **Physical dependence.** State of adaptation that is manifested by drug class-specific signs and symptoms that can be produced by abrupt cessation, rapid dose reduction, decreasing blood level of the drug, and/or administration of an antagonist. Physical dependence, by itself, does not equate with addiction.
  - **Pseudoaddiction.** The iatrogenic syndrome resulting from the misinterpretation of relief-seeking behaviors as though they are drug-seeking behaviors that are commonly seen with addiction. The relief-seeking behaviors resolve upon institution of effective analgesic therapy.
  - **Substance abuse.** Substance abuse is the use of any substance(s) for nontherapeutic purposes or use of medication for purposes other than those for which it is prescribed.
  - **Tolerance.** Tolerance is a physiologic state resulting from regular use of a drug in which an increased dosage is needed to produce a specific effect, or a reduced effect is observed with a constant dose over time. Tolerance may or may not be evident during opioid treatment and does not equate with addiction.
- **Reassessment. Record** responses, changes in function, side effects, effect on **quality of life factors** (sleep, mood, activity, relationships, work), that is, Brief Pain Inventory (Short Form); see Web Sites.
- **Assess for aberrant behaviors,** address issues if present
- **Review and revise treatment plan and goals regularly**
- **Referral** to specialist if management issues, or for consultation. Pain clinics use multidisciplinary approach; studies suggest increased return-to-work rates. Refer for management difficulties, ineffective treatments, or consultation. Managed care programs may not cover.
- Maintain up to date medical knowledge in this rapidly evolving field.

PHARMACOLOGIC THERAPY
Nonopioids
- **NSAIDs.** Nonselective/selective (Cox-2) are effective for **mild to moderate pain** (lowest dose, shortest time possible). They act synergistically with opioids, allowing a decreased required opioid dose (Table 22.4-2).

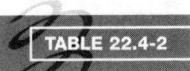

TABLE 22.4-2	Commonly Prescribed NSAIDs and Dosages		
Common NSAIDs	**Usual dose**	**Max. dose/day**	**Comments**
Acetylsalicylic acid (aspirin, Empirin)	325–650 mg q4h	4,000 mg	R, G
Celocoxib (Celebrex)	100 mg bid	400 mg	CI sulfa allergy
Choline magnesium trisalicylate (Trilisate)	1,000–1500 mg bid	3,000 mg	S
Diclofenac and misoprostol (Arthrotec)	50/200 mg tid- 75/ 200 qid 225 mg diclofenac	CI in pregnant	
Ibuprofen (Motrin, Advil, Nuprin)	400–800 mg tid-qid	2,400 mg	S
Indomethacin (Indocin, Indocin SR)	25–50 mg tid SR75 mg bid	200 mg	R, S, G
Ketorolac (Toradol) (IM/IV)	10 mg q4-6h 15–30 mg q6h	40 mg 120 mg	G, up to 5 days G, up to 5 days
Nabumetone (Relafen)	1 g qd-bid	2 g	
Naproxen (Naprosyn, Aleve, Anaprox)	250–500 mg bid	1,500 mg	S, G
Salsalate (Disalcid, Salflex)	1,000 mg bid-tid	3,000 mg	G
Acetaminophen (Tylenol)	325–650 mg q4h	4,000 mg	R, S, G Liver toxicity in healthy adults >10 g, caution if heavy alcohol safe use in pregnancy and in stable mild liver disease, monitor liver and renal function

Abbreviations: R, rectal dosing available; G, generic available; S, suspension available; IV, intravenous; IM, intramuscular; SC, subcutaneous; q, every; h, hours; d, day; bid, twice a day; tid, three times a day; qid, four times a day; CI, contraindicated; qhs, at bedtime.

- **Serious adverse effects:** Nephrotoxicity, gastrointestinal (GI) bleeding and ulcers, congestive heart failure, allergic reactions, hepatotoxicity, bronchospasm, and anti-coagulation– not choline magnesium trisalicylate (Trilisate) or Cox-2.
- **Increased risk** in patients with congestive heart failure, renal or liver disease, and in elderly patients.
- **GI complications** are higher in elderly individuals, or if there is a history of peptic ulcer disease and chronic steroid use. Consider cytoprotection (misoprostil, proton pump inhibitor or H2 blocker). GI effects *may* be lower with Cox-2 inhibitors (Celebrex).
- Recent concerns of **increased risk of cardiovascular events** (all NSAIDS). There is no risk in short-term use for acute pain and no cardiovascular risk factors. Ibuprofen **may** be the safest.

Weak Opioid Plus Nonopioid

Combination drug use is limited by the maximum dose of nonopioid (NSAID or acetaminophen). They must be **titrated to effect and side effects. Side effects** include **constipation, respiratory depression, nausea, and sedation** (see Opioids). Multiple preparations and doses are available (see Physicians Drug Reference/ePocrates). Common examples are as follows:

- **Codeine** (DEA III):
    - + acetylsalicylic acid (ASA): Empirin #3, Empirin #4
    - + Acetaminophen: Tylenol #2, Tylenol #3, Tylenol #4
- **Hydrocodone** (DEA III):
    - + ASA: Lortab ASA
    - + Acetaminophen: Hyco-pap, Lorcet, Lortab, Vicodin
    - + Ibuprofen: Vicoprofen
- **Oxycodone** (DEA II):
    - + ASA: Percodan, Percodan-Demi
    - + Acetaminophen: Percocet, Roxicet, Tylox
- **Tramadol**
    - + Acetaminophen: Ultracet
    - **Tramadol** (Ultram). Weak opioid, potentiates serotonin and norepinephrine (no DEA schedule). Caution in elderly patients, renal and liver dysfunction; avoid in opiate dependent; seizures may occur with antidepressants.
- **Propoxyphene** (DEA IV)
    - + Acetaminophen: Darvocet-N50, Darvocet-N100 (abuse potential and questionable analgesic advantage over non-opioids, possible NMDA activity)

Opioids

Opioids are the **"cornerstone of therapy for moderate to severe pain"** (Table 22.4-3). Use caution in renal dysfunction and in the elderly patients. **Constipation is inevitable.** Treat pre-emptively with bowel regimen—stool softener + stimulant (i.e., senna), plus high fluid intake. **Respiratory depression** is short-lived, antagonized by pain and occurs in opioid-naïve patients. **Nausea and sedation** resolve over time but recur if dose increases. **Hypogonadism** occurs but is rare; check testosterone levels if needed.

- Regularly dosed **long-acting** opioids are preferred, with short acting for breakthrough, acute, or episodic pain.
- Oral and transdermal **routes** are preferred.
- **Appropriate dose relieves pain, with minimal side effects.**
- **Methadone** is noneuphoric, has less abuse potential, and some effects on neuropathic pain. **Titrate slowly and start with low doses.**
- Meperidine (Demerol) use is not advised (short action, toxic metabolite, and poor oral effect.)
- **Starting doses** are lower than equianalgesic doses below.
- **Observe for addiction, tolerance, dependence, and abuse, all are DEA Schedule II.**

Agonist-Antagonists

Pentazocine (Talwin) and Butorphanol (Stadol). Use is limited due to low effectiveness, short action, dysphoria, and abuse potential.

Adjuvant Medications

Enhance analgesia, control side effects, and treat other symptoms often associated with chronic pain. They are effective for neuropathic pain.

- **Antidepressants**
    - Use to treat depression, anxiety, sleep disturbance, and neuropathic pain. May have some analgesic properties. Role of SSRIs unclear; treat depression.
    - Tricyclics: Amitriptyline (Elavil) (avoid in elderly patients), desipramine (Norpramin), nortriptyline, doxepin. Start at 25 to 50 mg qhs, up to 300 mg qd. Caution in elderly patients, cardiac conduction problems, narrow angle glaucoma (electrocardiogram useful). Side effects: dry mouth, blurred vision, constipation, urinary retention, arrhythmias.
    - Others: Duloxetine (Cymbalta) and venlafaxine (Effexor) effective for neuropathic pain and fibromyalgia.

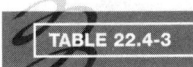

| TABLE 22.4-3 | Equianalgesic Doses (DEA II) |

Equianalgesic doses	Oral	Parenteral	Comments
Morphine	30 mg q3–4h	10 mg SC/IM/IV q4h	R 10–20 mg q4h, S, G
Morphine, long acting (MS Contin, Oramorph)	15–30 mg q8–12h	N/A	Do not cut/chew/crush
Codeine	30 mg q3–4h	10 mg SC/IM q3–4h	
Oxycodone (Roxicodone)	30 mg q3–4h	N/A	S, G
Oxycodone, long acting (OxyContin)	10 mg q12h	N/A	Increase dose q1–2d
Hydrocodone (Vicodin, Lortab)	30 mg q3–4h	N/A	
Hydromorphone (Dilaudid)	7.5 mg q3–4h	1.5 mg IV/SC/IM q3–4h R, G	
Levorphanol (Levo-Dromoran)	4 mg q6–8h	2 mg SC q6–8h	G, half-life 6 h
Methadone (Dolophine, Methadose)	20 mg q6–8h	10 mg SC/IM q6–8h	G, potent, inexpensive
Fentanyl (Duragesic) transdermal	25–100 μg q72h, start at 25, increase q3–6d, rotate sites, takes 12 h		
Fentanyl (Actiq) transmucosal lozenges	600 μg lozenge, max. 4 qd		

Dose ratio of 1:4 (1 mg oral methadone = 4 mg oral morphine) if oral morphine dose <90 mg/d; 1:8 if oral morphine dose is 90–300 mg/d; 1:12 if oral morphine dose is >300 mg/d. See Table 24.4-2 for abbreviations.

- ■ **Anticonvulsants**
  - ■ Effective for neuropathic pain, doses vary
  - ■ Gabapentin (Neurontin). Effective for postherpetic neuralgia, pregabalin (Lyrica)
  - ■ Lamotrigine (Lamictal), topiramate (Topmax), phenytoin (Dilantin), valproic acid (Depakote)
  - ■ Carbamazepine (Tegretol; monitor complete blood count): Side effects: dizziness, sedation, cognitive difficulties
- ■ **Topical Agents**
  - ■ Capsaicin (Zostrix) 0.75% topical: Apply tid-qid. May cause burning, erythema, or hyperalgesia, full effectiveness takes 6 weeks
  - ■ Lidocaine patches 5% applied 12 hours per day useful for postherpetic neuralgia, promising in acute conditions
- ■ **Muscle Relaxants**
  - ■ May reduce muscle pain and spasm; short term and acute use, doses vary.
  - ■ Cyclobenzaprine, baclofen (Lioresal) may be useful in lancinating, paroxysmal neuropathic pain. Tizanidine (Zanaflex) may be effective in fibromyalgia.

WEB SITES

www.painmed.org
www.aapainmanage.org
www.medsch.wisc.edu/painpolicy
www.fsmb.org/pain.htm
www.ampainsoc.org
www.painandhealth.org
www.painedu.com

References

1. Ballantyne JC, Mao J. Opioid therapy for chronic pain. *N Engl J Med* 2003;349; 1943–1953.
2. Cancer Pain Guideline Panel. Management of cancer pain: adults. *AHCPR Clin Pract Guidelines* 1994;9.
3 Katz NP, et al. Behavioral monitoring and urine toxicology testing in patients receiving long-term opioid therapy. *Anesth Analg* 2003;97(4):1097–1002.
4. Federation of State Medical Boards of the United States, Inc. Model guidelines for the use of controlled substances for the treatment of pain. 2004. Available online at www.fsmb.org/pain/htm. Accessed June 12, 2006.
5. Gourlay D, Caplan YH, Heit HA. Urine drug testing in primary care. Monograph. California Academy of Family Practice. 2003. Available online at www.alaskaafp.org. Accessed June 13, 2006.
6. Wisconsin Medical Society Task Force on Pain Management. Guidelines for the assessment and management of chronic pain. *Wisc Med J* 2004;103:13–42.

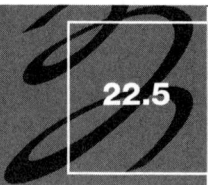

22.5 END-OF-LIFE CARE
Marc Tunzi, James J. Helmer

GENERAL PRINCIPLES

Everybody dies. The aim of end-of-life care is to make life's last transition as easy and meaningful as possible for dying patients and their families. Physical, psychologic, and social problems should be prevented, when possible, and managed actively, when not. Death is not failure; not properly caring for dying patients is failure. End-of-life care generally refers to the medical care of patients with a life expectancy of 6 to 12 months or less. Many aspects of end-of-life care planning apply to everyone but especially to geriatric patients and to patients with chronic diseases. Similarly, certain aspects of end-of-life care symptom and problem management apply to patients who are severely ill but are not yet considered terminally ill.

COMMUNICATION AND PLANNING ISSUES

- **Break bad news in a quiet, unhurried, comfortable setting.** Find out what patients know, and how much they want to know, before delivering information in a sensitive but straightforward manner, using clear language. Check for patients' understanding and emotional response. Schedule follow-up.[1]
- **The goals of care** for end-of-life patients and their families are to maximize comfort and function and to minimize pain and suffering. Achieving these goals relies on effective communication and planning.
  - Discuss expectations and the goals of care directly with patients who have decision-making capacity (see below). When possible, patients should be empowered to control their own treatment and to resolve conflicts among competing goals of care (see below).

- Discuss expectations and treatment goals with families and friends after discussing them with patients first. Exceptions to this are when it is not possible to communicate directly with patients (see below) and when patients explicitly want family present for the discussion.
- Be sensitive to cultural differences in end-of-life care values and practices. In addition to encouraging patients and families to consider community resources and pastoral care, clinicians must be sensitive to how their own social, moral, and religious values influence life-and-death decision making with their patients.
- "Be there." All patients and families experience a wide range of emotions during the dying process. Anger, denial, depression, and bargaining are typical reactions.[2] In addition, personal psychosocial problems, interpersonal family relationships, and the timeline of the death (whether chronic or acute) all influence how patients and families react. The family physician's continued presence and validation of these reactions—even when other medical specialists are involved in patient management—may be therapeutic for everyone.

- **Ethical planning issues.** Addressing patients' desires about end-of-life care and life-sustaining treatment should be part of health care maintenance performed during regular office visits. These issues may be introduced as a sort of "informed consent" for the future by making such statements as, "I discuss life-sustaining treatments and advance directives, such as the living will and the power of attorney for health care, with all my patients; do you have any questions about them?" or "I discuss medical values with all my patients; have you ever discussed them with your family?"
  - Personal values ultimately guide patient decision making. Patients must be asked whether they want to live at all costs or whether they might compromise some life expectancy for a better quality of life. Patients must also be asked about a variety of other potentially competing values, such as maintaining mobility and physical independence, maintaining the ability to think clearly and communicate with others, being treated in accordance with their cultural and religious/spiritual beliefs, not becoming a burden on family, and avoiding unnecessary pain and suffering.
  - Advance directives are written or oral instructions that enable patients to guide their future health care decisions in the event that they cannot do so themselves.
    - Living wills are documents that allow patients to choose one of two or three scenarios for their end-of-life care (choices vary by state): Do everything medically possible to maintain life; do no extraordinary intervention but maintain comfort and allow death to occur "naturally"; or do no extraordinary intervention but continue nutrition and hydration in addition to other comfort care. In most states, laws require a patient to be diagnosed as terminal (prognosis less than 6 to 12 months) by two physicians for a living will to be legally binding.
    - Durable powers of attorney for health care (DPAHC) are legal documents that enable patients to appoint another specific individual (known as a proxy, agent, or surrogate) to make decisions for them, should they be unable to do so for themselves. These documents are most effective when patients and their surrogates have thoroughly discussed treatment options so that the standard of substituted judgment may be applied (see above). Many DPAHC documents include a "living will" section within them. Patients do not need a lawyer to complete a DPAHC.
    - Oral directives are the most common kind of advance directives and are often sufficient in guiding terminal care decisions. Unfortunately, the legal benefits of oral directives to family and friends vary by state and may not be upheld in cases of a family dispute or family-physician disagreement. Oral directives to physicians, on the other hand, *when clearly documented in the medical record,* are usually honored by the courts. This documentation should include a description of the patient's medical condition and clear evidence of the patient's decision-making capacity (see above).[3]
  - Medical decision-making capacity refers to the ability to make a rational decision about medical treatment options. Capacity should be viewed on a sliding scale: a patient may have the ability to understand and make decisions about some treatment options but not others, and this ability should be re-evaluated for each

pending decision. Determining capacity requires assessment of a patient's ability to accept responsibility for making the treatment decision; to understand the medical situation and prognosis; to understand the alternatives for care; to communicate a clear decision from those alternatives; and to discuss how the decision fits his or her general goals and values. Appropriate questions include, "What can you tell me about your condition?" "What is your understanding of this treatment and why do you think it is right for you?" "What can you tell me about the alternatives we've discussed?" Medical decision-making capacity should not be confused with *competency*, which is a legal status determined by a court of law.

■ Surrogacy. When an individual does not have medical decision-making capacity, surrogate decisions must be made. When possible, a legal surrogate, appointed by the patient in a DPAHC, should make decisions. A living will or other clearly documented advance directive may also guide care. When these are not available, surrogate decision makers should generally follow the traditional family hierarchy: spouse, parents or children, siblings, other relatives, and friends. The two standards most often used for making surrogate decisions are substituted judgment ("If the patient were still able to make decisions for herself, what would she want in this situation?") and best interests ("What do you think is the best thing to do for the patient, all things considered?"). Of the two, substituted judgment is usually thought to be superior, although it requires intimate knowledge of the patient to be accurate. It also produces less guilt because it focuses the decision-making process back on the patient and away from the family.

MEDICAL CARE ISSUES

■ **Symptom and problem management** should focus on comfort and function, not on achieving a particular physiologic effect. Information about symptoms must be solicited; patients may be too afraid, proud, weak, or tired to divulge symptoms on their own but will usually discuss them if asked. A formal palliative care consult should be considered when clinically significant symptoms and problems persist.[4]

■ **Pain** should be prevented when possible (e.g., pain due to bedsores or futile treatments), and treated promptly when not (also see Chapter 22.4). Visual or numeric pain intensity scales may help assess pain severity. Before treating, however, other symptoms should be assessed as well; sometimes "pain" is really anxiety, fatigue, loneliness, dyspnea, nausea, constipation, or another condition. When prescribing pain medications, low-potency agents should be used first and advanced quickly as needed. Side effects (epigastric burning, nausea, constipation, unwanted sedation) should be monitored closely. Both duration of action and the best delivery system (liquid, pill, tablet, rectal suppository, transdermal) should be carefully considered. The routine use of pain medication in end-of-life patients is much more effective than "as needed" (prn) use and is preferred. Drug dependency is not an issue. As-needed pain medication should be reserved for "breakthrough" pain above a patient's baseline. The goal of complete pain relief must be weighed against the competing goals of function and alertness. See Chapter 22.4 for pain medication choices and dosages.

■ **Anxiety and agitation** may be due to hypoxemia, pain, or a specific patient fear (see Chapter 5.1). Treatment, when needed, will depend in part on the patient's other symptoms: some pain and nausea medications, for example, may also be anxiolytic. Treatment may also depend on how much sedation is wanted. Severe agitation should be re-evaluated every 24 hours. Medication choices for treating anxiety and agitation include short-acting benzodiazepines, such as lorazepam, 1 to 2 mg PO bid-qid, or alprazolam, 0.25 to 0.5 mg PO bid-qid—orally disintegrating tablet (ODT) available; sedating antidepressants, such as amitriptyline, 10 to 100 mg PO at bedtime (watch for anticholinergic side effects) or trazodone, 50 to 100 mg PO bid-tid; and neuroleptics, such as haloperidol, 1 to 5 mg PO bid-tid, risperidone (Risperdal), 0.5 to 4 mg PO bid (ODT available), quetiapine (Seroquel) 25 to 50 mg PO bid, or olanzapine (Zyprexa), 2.5 to 10 mg PO qd (ODT available).

- **Nausea and vomiting** may be due to constipation or gastritis, diets of excessive volume, diets that may have become intolerable (e.g., dairy products), or opiate pain medications. Choices for antinausea medication include prochlorperazine (Compazine), 5 to 10 mg PO qid or 25 mg per rectum (PR) bid-tid; metoclopramide (Reglan), 5 to 10 mg PO qid; or ondansetron (Zofran), 4 to 8 mg PO, via tablets or solution, q12h. Ondansetron 4 mg IV or droperidol (Inapsine), 0.5 to 2.0 mg IV or IM (watch QT interval on electrocardiogram, ECG) over 2 to 5 minutes may be used for refractory vomiting.
- **Constipation** may be due to bowel obstruction, lack of stool water or fiber content, or slowed bowel transit time caused by inactivity or opiate pain medications. Increasing dietary fiber, either naturally or with supplements such as psyllium, may help—but it may also worsen constipation in patients with poor gut motility, causing a "soft" impaction. Significant impactions, hard or soft, should be manually removed. Magnesium laxatives (Milk of Magnesia, magnesium citrate) should not be used on a long-term basis. The osmotic agents lactulose or sorbitol 70% solution, 15 to 30 mL PO qd-bid may be used intermittently. Other medications include stool softeners, such as docusate sodium (Colace), 100 mg PO qd-bid; motility agents, such as metoclopramide (see above), bisacodyl (Dulcolax, Correctol, Feen-a-mint), 10 mg PO or PR qd-bid, or senna preparations 15 to 30 mg qd-bid, either alone as tablets, syrup, liquid, or granules (Senokot, Ex-lax) or in combination with docusate (Peri-colace, Senokot-S); and enemas.
- **Bladder problems.** Urinary retention may be treated with intermittent catheterizations, a chronic indwelling catheter changed every month, cholinergic agents such as bethanecol (Urecholine), 10 to 50 mg PO tid-qid, or alpha-adrenergic antagonists such as terazosin (Hytrin), 1 to 10 mg PO qhs, doxazosin (Cardura) 1 to 8 mg PO qhs, or tamsulosin (Flomax) 0.4 to 0.8 mg PO qhs. Xylocaine jelly should be considered for catheter changes. Condom catheters are not recommended. Assessment of urinary spasm or overactive bladder and urge incontinence should begin with evaluation for overdistention with an ultrasound measurement of postvoid residual. Fecal impaction may also lead to urinary obstruction and should be assessed. Symptoms may be managed behaviorally, with bladder training or biofeedback, or pharmacologically, with anticholinergic agents such as oxybutynin (Ditropan), 5 mg PO bid-tid, tolterodine (Detrol, Detrol-LA), 1 to 4 mg PO qd-bid, trospium (Sanctura) 20 mg PO qhs-bid, or solifenacin (VESIcare) 5 to 10 mg PO qd.
- **Dyspnea** is best treated with supplemental oxygen. Patients with worsening dyspnea should be assessed for the patency of their oxygen delivery system, fluid overload, pneumothorax, pleural effusion, or other medical problem. Morphine sulfate (see Chapter 22.4) is the drug of choice to decrease the sensation of air hunger; low doses of liquid morphine to the buccal mucosa may be enough for some patients. Respiratory secretions, sometimes known as the "death rattle" in patients shortly before death, may be diminished by decreasing hydration or by administration of atropine or scopolamine, 0.2 to 1.0 mg sublingual or subcutaneous q 4 to 6 hours, or scopolamine transdermal patch, 1.5 mg q 1 to 3 days.
- **Nutrition.** Few activities and treatments provoke as many emotions as those associated with nutrition. Food is often seen as a sign of life and hope, and not eating or withholding nutrition is seen as a sign of despair or abandonment. End-of-life patients often have decreased hunger and thirst, however, and should control their own dietary intake. Studies have not shown that forced feeding prolongs life; in fact, for some cancers, increased feeding may speed the rate of cancer growth. Decisions on the use of tube feedings or hyperalimentation in patients who are unable to eat should be guided by the concept of benefits versus burdens (see below). Potential benefits of nutrition in terminal patients include maintaining and increasing strength and function. Potential burdens include increasing patient anxiety by forcing food and the risks of gastric distention and aspiration. Alert patients who are anorectic should be evaluated for pain control, oral candidiasis, depression, and constipation. Symptoms of dry mouth may be managed with glycerine swabs or mouthwash or cautious use of viscous lidocaine (Xylocaine). Thirst may be relieved with ice chips or sips of water.

- **Ethical treatment issues**
  - **Do not resuscitate (DNR) order** refers to the withholding of cardiopulmonary resuscitation (CPR) in the event of a cardiac or pulmonary arrest. Before writing a DNR order, the patient's clinical condition and prognosis, a description of what CPR entails, and an estimate of the patient's likely chance for survival should be discussed with the patient and family and documented in the medical record. Studies suggest that when CPR is attempted, approximately 14% of patients survive to discharge and 86% die acutely. Survival rates for elderly patients and for patients with metastatic cancer, sepsis, or elevated creatinine are much lower.[3] Patients who choose not to be resuscitated should be reassured that other treatments will not be affected by this decision. If not already completed, advance directives should be addressed. Although some communities have out-of-hospital "DNR bracelet" programs, patients who are still at home should be advised that if an ambulance is called and emergency medical services personnel respond, CPR may be automatically initiated; depending on the clinical situation, these patients and families should be instructed to call their physician or hospice or home health nurse first.
  - **Withholding versus withdrawing care.** There is no ethical difference between withholding and withdrawing care that cannot or has not achieved its desired effect. Psychologically, however, it usually *feels* different to withdraw care. Clear communication about expectations is critical. The judicious use of treatment time trials may also be helpful. If a particular treatment is tried over a predetermined, fixed period of time and if at the end of that time the desired outcomes are not achieved, the treatment may be discontinued without guilt. In general, the concept of "benefits versus burdens" should guide decisions on the appropriateness of care. This involves engaging the patient, family, and health care team in listing the pluses and minuses of an intervention and weighing them against each other to determine use.
  - **Determination of futility** depends on who decides what is futile: the patient, the family, or the physician. A treatment may be physiologically futile but may be extremely important to a patient's sense of hope or may give a family enough time to gather together. On the other hand, a patient or a family who strongly values life at all costs might insist on an intervention that clearly has no benefit but does have great burdens (e.g., administering chemotherapy to a patient with metastatic cancer who is now failing medical therapy for sepsis). If clear communication with the patient and family does not resolve disagreements regarding futile care, an ethics consultation should be obtained (see below). Alternatively, care may be transferred to another physician who feels able to meet the patient's or family's treatment requests.
  - **Ethics consultation** should be considered whenever there are persistent disagreements or conflicts in patient care. In some hospitals, consultation is performed by an ethics committee, whereas in others, it is performed by a professional clinical ethicist. Decisions about DNR status and withholding or withdrawing care are the most common reasons for requesting an ethics consultation.
  - **Euthanasia and physician-assisted suicide** are beyond the scope of this manual. However, if a patient inquires about them, the opportunity should be used to explore the reasons behind the request. Often, these patients have great fears about pain, isolation, or becoming a physical or financial burden to their families. Some may have treatable depression. Others may simply need a clarification of their medical problems and a discussion of their medical care plans.

- **Home and hospice care**
  - Family members are the primary caregivers for most end-of-life patients. Family physicians may enlist caregiver resource centers and other community agencies to support families in this role.
  - Home health services may include nursing assessment of the patient's clinical status and home environment; teaching about medications, other treatments, diagnosis, and prognosis; social service evaluation of financial issues and individual or family counseling needs; and occupational and physical therapy evaluation and treatment.
  - Hospice programs are a Medicare-covered benefit that provides full-spectrum, interdisciplinary, team-based services for dying patients and their families. In addition

to usual home care services, hospice emphasizes the dying process itself, particularly addressing pain control, pastoral care, and bereavement support for the family. Hospice is appropriate for a patient who has progressively lost weight, suffered a significant reduction in function, been repeatedly hospitalized for symptom management, or whose disease has progressed to a point where the family is experiencing great stress in providing the necessary care. To be eligible for hospice, patients must have a survival prognosis of less than 6 months, and patients and families must decline further aggressive treatment. Very often, however, hospice referrals are made "too late"—shortly before death—to have maximum benefit for patients and families. Although most hospice care is home based, reasons to consider short-term inpatient hospice care include providing a respite for the family, intervening in a home or family crisis situation, or providing intensive symptom management for pain, nausea, vomiting, and other acute problems.

- **Determination of death**
    - Traditionally, death has been clinically defined as the absence of spontaneous pulse and blood pressure (no circulatory function) and the absence of spontaneous breathing (no respiratory function). Often, the absence of pupillary responses (no brain function) is added.
    - Brain death criteria have been established in most states because intensive care life support systems may physiologically sustain certain organs even after a patient's cerebral functions have been permanently lost. These clinical criteria generally include coma that is documented to be irreversible (i.e., not due to drugs or hypothermia), absence of motor function and reflexes (though spinal cord reflexes may still be intact), and absence of brainstem function, established by apnea and the lack of pupillary and oculovestibular reflexes.[5]
        - Electroencephalograms and other studies may be confirmatory but are not usually required. However, some hospitals do require formal neurologic consultation before allowing a patient to be declared brain dead. Organ donation is sometimes an issue with brain-dead patients whose other organs remain viable. In these cases, death should first be declared by a physician clearly unassociated with the transplant team, and the discussion of organ donation should follow.
    - Persistent vegetative state (PVS) refers to the condition wherein patients have no obvious cortical function but do have residual brainstem activity that allows them to maintain circulatory and respiratory functions and many neurologic reflexes. Clinically, these patients still have a heart beat, can still breathe, can still constrict their pupils, and may posture with pain or loud noise; however, they are unable to think, actually feel pain, or have any awareness or purposeful activity. The diagnosis requires repeated examinations and neurologic consultation. Recovery from PVS rarely occurs after 6 months following anoxic brain injury (e.g., after a cardiac arrest) or after 12 months following traumatic brain injury. *Very* rare recoveries have been reported, however.[6] The treatment provided to patients in PVS should be based on advance directives, if present, and clear and honest family discussions if not. Although it may be completely appropriate to withhold or withdraw medical interventions from patients in PVS, unilateral withholding and withdrawal by the medical team involves the complex issue of futility and is not universally accepted.

BEREAVEMENT AND FOLLOW-UP ISSUES

- **Autopsy** should be considered when the physician or the patient's family wants certainty about the cause of death to confirm the clinical diagnosis, to evaluate the level of response to a particular treatment, or to be reassured that care was appropriate and death unavoidable. Legally, the local coroner's office must be notified when an individual dies without medical attendance, when the attending physician is unable to state the cause of death, or when death follows an accident or injury, including suicide or homicide. Asking about autopsies should be simple and direct, emphasizing the considerations outlined previously. The discussion should follow family notification of the death and preferably occur in person (though, in most states, consent for autopsy may be obtained over the phone). If an autopsy is performed, a family conference should be arranged afterward to discuss the findings. The costs of an autopsy are usually not covered by health insurance plans. However, many hospitals provide autopsies as a quality control measure at no charge.

■ **Family follow-up issues** focus on promoting the tasks of bereavement, which include feeling sadness and pain, accepting the reality of the loss, and redirecting time and energy from caring for the deceased to other activities. Reassuring family members that they will not be abandoned, normalizing their reactions, and encouraging open communication are all helpful. Appropriate comments include "It's OK to feel both sad and angry" and "Death is hard to understand; have you talked with your family or minister about how you're handling things?"

■ **Physician follow-up issues.** The death of a patient who has had a very complicated course of disease or with whom the physician has developed a close relationship is often a great personal loss. Complicating this loss may be a sense of guilt or personal failure. Just as family and friends must grieve to recover, physicians too should be allowed to grieve by discussing a patient's death with staff, colleagues, or their own families, if appropriate. Attending a patient's funeral service should be considered a means of both assisting the physician's own grief work and showing support for the patient's family.

References

1. Buckman R. *How to break bad news: a guide for health care professionals.* Baltimore: Johns Hopkins University Press; 1992.
2. Kubler-Ross E. *On death and dying.* New York: Macmillan; 1969.
3. Lo B. *Resolving ethical dilemmas.* 3rd ed. Baltimore: Williams & Wilkins; 2005.
4. Doyle D, Hanks G, Cherny N, et al. *Oxford textbook of palliative medicine.* 3rd ed. New York: Oxford University Press; 2003.
5. Wijdicks EFM. The diagnosis of brain death. *N Engl J Med* 2001;344:1215–1221.
6. Wade DT, Johnston C. The permanent vegetative state: practical guidance on diagnosis and managment. *BMJ* 1999;319:841–844.

INTERNET RESOURCES

www.eperc.mcw.edu. Medical College of Wisconsin End of Life/Palliative Care Education Resource Center

www.aahpm.org. American Academy of Hospice and Palliative Medicine

Note: Page numbers followed by "f" refer to illustrations; page numbers followed by "t" refer to tables.